Functional BOLD MRI

Scott H. Faro • Feroze B. Mohamed
Editors

Functional BOLD MRI

Principles and Applications

Springer

Editors
Scott H. Faro, MD
Department of Radiology
Functional Brain Imaging Center
Temple University School of Medicine
Philadelphia, PA, USA

Feroze B. Mohamed, PhD
Department of Radiology
Functional Brain Imaging Center
Temple University School of Medicine
Philadelphia, PA, USA

ISBN 978-1-4939-1994-9 ISBN 978-1-4939-1995-6 (eBook)
DOI 10.1007/978-1-4939-1995-6
Springer New York Heidelberg Dordrecht London

Library of Congress Control Number: 2014951837

Printed on acid-free paper

Springer is part of Springer Science+Business Media (www.springer.com)

Preface

In the past two decades there have been numerous technological developments and the establishment of fundamental clinical and cognitive magnetic resonance imaging protocols to understand brain functions. The next decade, the beginning of the twenty-first century, will continue the great momentum of brain research. This is currently one of the most exciting and progressive times of scientific advancement in the field of brain function,in which the development and application of Blood Oxygen Level-Dependent (BOLD) fMRI are the driving forces.

The field of BOLD fMRI has two major areas of research interest and applications. The first is within the field of cognitive neuroscience, which focuses on understanding all aspects of mental processes involved in awareness, reasoning, and acquisition of knowledge and behavior. The second is the use of BOLD fMRI in the medical sciences to localize eloquent regions in the brain for a large variety of clinical applications. This book focuses primarily on describing the basic principles of BOLD fMRI imaging and the new and developing clinical applications of fMRI.

This book contains 21 chapters and is separated into 4 main sections. The first section provides an introduction to the physical principles of BOLD fMRI imaging as well as a review of scanning methodologies, data analysis, challenges and limitations of BOLD, neurovascular uncoupling, functional connectivity, and clinical challenges. The second section presents a pictorial neuroanatomical atlas of the basic motor, sensory, and cognitive activation sites within the brain. This section gives a new clinical scientist a familiarity with some of the more clinically relevant brain activation sites that are discussed in subsequent chapters. The third section reviews all the current and future clinical applications of BOLD fMRI. These chapters include the clinical fields of language, memory, fMRI WADA, visual pathway, brain mapping of eloquent cortex, pediatric applications, auditory pathways, epilepsy, psychiatric disorders, neurodegenerative disorders, pharmacological applications, and cognitive neuroscience applications. The fourth section reviews many BOLD fMRI paradigms that can be used for clinical and cognitive BOLD fMRI experiments.

There has never previously been a noninvasive technique with high spatial and temporal resolution to define brain activation. One of the current primary indications for BOLD fMRI is to localize language centers in the frontal lobe and temporal lobes and the sensory-motor cortex in the frontal-parietal lobe region. This is becoming a commonplace procedure for pre-surgical evaluation in temporal lobe epilepsy and regional masses. Please note that most of the BOLD fMRI images are presented in radiological coordinates (the left side of the image represents the right side of the subject). Images presented in neurologic coordinates (the left side of the image represents the left side of the subject) are indicated.

The field of BOLD fMRI is relatively young, and it has grown to be a vital tool for clinical and cognitive neuroscience research. It is our hope that this book will give a thorough introduction to this exciting field and will be a reference, to all physicians and cognitive neuroscientists, for the emerging clinical applications of BOLD fMRI.

Philadelphia, PA

Scott H.Faro, MD
Feroze B. Mohamed, PhD

Acknowledgements

I am grateful to my dear wife Paula for her remarkable patience and continued support for my projects.

I would like to thank my dear friend and first scientific mentor, Dr. Anita Pruzan-Hotchkiss, who taught me that any question or scientific inquiry, no matter how far-fetched it may seem, has merit. I would also like to thank my mentors from my molecular biology graduate program, diagnostic radiology residency, and adult and pediatric neuroradiology fellowship training programs for their encouragement in my academic pursuits. These individuals lead by example and fostered my great interest in teaching and research.

I would also like to thank all of the contributors of this book, for their participation is truly a labor of love, and a special thanks to Feroze Mohamed, my longtime friend and colleague who has supported me and our work during the past 20+ years of trials and tribulations.

Lastly, I would like to thank all our friends at Springer, especially Janet Foltin, who share our goal to produce this book on an important and fascinating topic of the physical principles and clinical applications of BOLD fMRI.

Scott H. Faro, MD

I am extremely grateful to Shaila for playing the roles of spouse, friend, and counselor over the years. She was a great sounding board during the years it took to compile this book. Another person I owe my deepest gratitude is Professor Simon Vinitski, who not only generously guided me in the research project for my doctoral work but also inspired me to pursue academia with undeterred zeal. I also cannot but mention my parents, Mohamed and Subaidha Ali, without whose encouragement I would not be here writing and compiling work for this book.

More specifically, I would like to thank the authors of the various chapters of this book. They should know that this book is essentially a reflection of their work, which, in many instances, is the result of years of research.

I would be remiss if I did not mention Scott Faro, whose friendship and assistance have influenced a good deal of my academic work.

Finally, I wish to express my appreciation to Janet Foltin at Springer Publishing for her coordination to make this book a reality.

Feroze B. Mohamed, PhD

Contents

Contributors

Geoffrey K. Aguirre, MD, PhD Department of Neurology, Hospital of the University of Pennsylvania, Philadelphia, PA, USA
aguirreg@mail.med.upenn.edu

Nolan R. Altman, MD Department of Radiology, Miami Children's Hospital, Miami, FL, USA
nolan.altman@mch.com

Peter A. Bandettini, PhD Section on Functional Imaging Methods, Laboratory of Brain and Cognition, National Institutes of Health, Bethesda, MD, USA
Bandettini@nih.gov

Byron Bernal, MD, CCTI Department of Radiology, Miami Children's Hospital, Miami, FL, USA
byron.bernal@mch.com

Jeffrey R. Binder, MD Department of Neurology, Medical College of Wisconsin, Milwaukee, WI, USA
jbinder@mcw.edu

Susan Y. Bookheimer, PhD Department of Psychiatry and Biobehavioral Sciences, David Geffen School of Medicine at UCLA, Los Angeles, CA, USA
Sbook@ucla.edu

Anthony J.W. Chen, MA, MD Department of Neurology, VA Medical Center – San Francisco, Helen Wills Neuroscience Institute, University of California, San Francisco, Berkeley, CA, USA
Anthony.chen@va.gov

R. Todd Constable, PhD Diagnostic Radiology, Biomedical Engineering, and Neurosurgery, The Anlyan Center, Yale University School of Medicine, New Haven, CT, USA
todd.constable@yale.edu

Mark D'Esposito, MD Brain Imaging Center, Helen Wills Neuroscience Institute, University of California, Berkeley, Berkeley, CA, USA
despo@berkley.edu; http://bic.berkeley.edu/despolab/

Edgar A. DeYoe, PhD Department of Radiology, Medical College of Wisconsin, Milwaukee, WI, USA
deyoe@mcw.edu

Scott H. Faro, MD Department of Radiology, Functional Brain Imaging Center, Temple University School of Medicine, Philadelphia, PA, USA
faros@tuhs.temple.edu

Jorn Fierstra, PhD Candidate Rudolf Magnus Institute of Neuroscience, University Medical Center Utrecht, Utrecht, The Netherlands
jornfierstra@gmail.com

Division of Neuroradiology, Division of Neurosurgery, Toronto Western Hospital, University Health Network, Toronto, ON, Canada

Lotfi Hacein-Bey, MD Radiological Associates of Sacramento Medical Group Inc., Sacramento, CA, USA

Deborah A. Hall, BSc, PhD National Biomedical Research Unit in Hearing, Ropewalk House, Nottingham, UK
deb.hall@nottingham.ac.uk

Division of Psychology, School of Social Sciences, Nottingham Trent University, Nottingham, UK

Michelle Hampson, PhD Department of Diagnostic Radiology, Yale University, New Haven, CT, USA
michelle.hampson@yale.edu

Joy Hirsch, PhD Departments of Radiology, Neuroscience, and Psychology, Columbia University Medical Center, New York, NY, USA
joyhirsch@yahoo.com

Stephen E. Jones, MD, PhD Department of Neuroradiology, Cleveland Clinic, Cleveland, OH, USA
Joness19@ccf.org

Andrew S. Kayser, MD, PhD Department of Neurology, Ernest Gallo Clinic & Research Center, University of California at San Francisco, Emeryville, CA, USA
akayser@gallo.ucsf.edu

Jacob Kean, PhD Department of Physical Medicine and Rehabilitation, Indiana University Center for Neuroimaging, Rehabilitation Hospital of Indiana, Indiana University School of Medicine, Indianapolis, IN, USA
jakean@indiana.edu

Seong-Gi Kim, PhD Department of Radiology, University of Pittsburgh, Pittsburgh, PA, USA
kimsg@pitt.edu

Karsten Krakow, MD, PhD Asklepios Neurologische Klinik Falkenstein, Königstein, Germany
k.krakow@asklepios.com

Melissa Lopez-Larson, MD Department of Psychiatry, The Brain Institute, University of Utah, Salt Lake City, UT, USA
melissa.lopez-larson@hsc.utah.edu

Mary Jo Maciejewski, PhD Center for Brain Health, University of Texas at Dallas, Dallas, TX, USA
mjm091000@utdallas.edu

Shamseldeen Y. Mahmoud, MD Department of Radiology, Cleveland Clinic, Cleveland, OH, USA
mahmous@ccf.org

Assiut University, Asyut, Egypt

Muhammed Malik, BS Department of Radiology, Temple University School of Medicine, Philadelphia, PA, USA
muhammed.malik@gmail.com

Jedediah Mathis Department of Radiology (Neuro Lab), Medical College of Wisconsin, Milwaukee, WI, USA

Brenna C. McDonald, PsyD, MBA Department of Radiology and Imaging Sciences, Indiana University School of Medicine, Indianapolis, IN, USA
mcdonalb@iupui.edu

Karen Medler Neurolab, Department of Biophysics, Medical College of Wisconsin, Milwaukee, WI, USA
kmedler@mcw.edu

David John Mikulis, MD Division of Neuroradiology, University Health Network: Toronto Western Hospital, University of Toronto, Toronto, ON, Canada
mikulis@uhnres.utoronto.ca

Toronto Western Hospital, University of Toronto, Toronto, ON, Canada

Feroze B. Mohamed, PhD Department of Radiology, Functional Brain Imaging Center, Temple University School of Medicine, Philadelphia, PA, USA
feroze@temple.edu

Wade Mueller, MD Department of Neurosurgery, Medical College of Wisconsin, Milwaukee, WI, USA

Michael D. Phillips, MD Research and Academic Affairs, Imaging Institute, Department of Radiology, Cleveland Clinic, Cleveland, OH, USA
phillim@ccf.org

Alexander B. Pine, PhD Cleveland Clinic Lerner College of Medicine, Cleveland, OH, USA

Nader Pouratian, MD, PhD Department of Neurosurgery, University of California, Los Angeles, CA, USA
npouratian@mednet.ucla.edu

Danielle Reitsma Department of Radiology, Medical College of Wisconsin, Milwaukee, WI, USA
dreitsma@mcw.edu

Shannon L. Risacher, BS Department of Radiology and Imaging Sciences, Indiana University School of Medicine, IU Center for Neuroimaging, Indianapolis, IN, USA
srisache@iupui.edu

Betty Jo Salmeron, MD Neuroimaging Research Branch, National Institute on Drug Abuse, Baltimore, MD, USA
bsalmeron@mail.nih.gov

Andrew J. Saykin, PsyD, ABPP/CN Center for Neuroimaging, Department of Radiology and Imaging Sciences, Indiana University School of Medicine, Indianapolis, IN, USA
asaykin@iupui.edu

Xilin Shen, PhD Associate Research Scientist, Department of Diagnostic Radiology, Yale University, New Haven, CT, USA
xilin.shen@yale.edu

Dan J. Stein, MD, PhD Department of Psychiatry and Mental Health, University of Cape Town, Groote Schuur Hospital (J-2), Cape Town, South Africa
dan.stein@uct.ac.za

Viktor Szeder, MD, PhD Division of Stroke, Department of Neurology, Columbia University Medical Center, New York, NY, USA

John L. Ulmer, MD Medical College of Wisconsin, Milwaukee, WI, USA
julmer@mcw.edu

Heather A. Wishart, PhD Brain Imaging Laboratory, Department of Psychiatry, Dartmouth Medical School, Lebanon, NH, USA
Heather.A.Wishart@dartmouth.edu

Yihong Yang, PhD FMRI Section, Neuroimaging Research Branch, National Institute on Drug Abuse, NIH, Baltimore, MD, USA
yihongyang@mail.nih.gov

Michael Yannes, BS Department of Radiology, Temple University School of Medicine, Philadelphia, PA, USA
michael.yannes@gmail.com

Deborah A. Yurgelun-Todd, PhD Department of Psychiatry, The Brain Institute, University of Utah, Salt Lake City, UT, USA
deborah.yurgelun-todd@hsc.utah.edu

Part I

BOLD Functional MRI: Physical Principles

Principles of BOLD Functional MRI

1

Seong-Gi Kim and Peter A. Bandettini

Introduction

The idea that regional cerebral blood flow (CBF) could reflect neuronal activity began with experiments of Roy and Sherrington in 1890 [1]. This concept is the basis for all hemodynamic-based brain imaging techniques being used today. The focal increase in CBF can be considered to directly relate to neuronal activity because the glucose metabolism and CBF changes are closely coupled [2]. Thus, the measurement of CBF change induced by stimulation has been used for mapping brain functions. Although it often assumed that cerebral metabolic rate of oxygen utilization ($CMRO_2$) and CBF changes are coupled, Fox and colleagues unexpectedly found that an increase in CBF surpassed an increase in $CMRO_2$ in humans during somatosensory and visual stimulation [3, 4]. Consequently, a mismatch between CBF and $CMRO_2$ changes results in an *increase* in the capillary and venous oxygenation level, which can be used for brain mapping. In 1990, based on rat brain studies during stimulation at 7 T, Ogawa and colleagues at AT&T Bell Laboratories reported that functional brain mapping is possible with the venous blood oxygenation level-dependent (BOLD) magnetic resonance imaging (MRI) contrast [5, 6]. The BOLD contrast relies on changes in deoxyhemoglobin (dHb) contents, which act as an endogenous paramagnetic contrast agent [7–9]. Therefore, changes of the local dHb contents in the brain lead to alterations in the MRI signal intensity.

Application of the BOLD contrast to human functional brain mapping followed shortly [10–12]. Since then, functional magnetic resonance imaging (fMRI) has been the tool of choice for visualizing neural activity in the human brain due to its high sensitivity and easy implementation. However, the BOLD signal is dependent on various anatomical, physiological, and imaging parameters [13], thus its interpretation with respect to physiological parameters is not straightforward. To utilize fMRI techniques efficiently and interpret fMRI data accurately, it is important to examine underlying physiology and physics. In this chapter, we discuss the source of the fMRI signal and improvement of BOLD techniques.

Physiological Changes

Since fMRI measures the hemodynamic response induced by increased neural activity, it is important to understand a chain of events from task to fMRI.

S.-G. Kim, PhD (✉)
Department of Radiology, University of Pittsburgh, 3025 East Carson Street, Pittsburgh, PA 15203, USA
e-mail: kimsg@pitt.edu

P.A. Bandettini, PhD
Section on Functional Imaging Methods, Laboratory of Brain and Cognition, National Institutes of Health, 10 Center Drive, Building 10, Room 1D80, Bethesda, MD, 20892, USA
e-mail: Bandettini@nih.gov

S.H. Faro and F.B. Mohamed (eds.), *Functional BOLD MRI: Principles and Applications*,
DOI 10.1007/978-1-4939-1995-6_1, © Springer Science+Business Media New York 2015

Task and/or stimulation induce synaptic and electric activities at localized regions, which will trigger an increase in CBF, cerebral blood volume (CBV), $CMRO_2$, and cerebral metabolic rate of glucose (CMR_{glu}). Although the exact relationship between neural activity and vascular/metabolic change is not known, it is well-accepted that the change in CMR_{glu} is a good indicator of neural activity. Since the CMR_{glu} change is linearly correlated with the CBF response [2], a change in CBF is a good indicator of neural activity.

CBF is defined as an amount of blood moving into capillaries within 100 g tissue per minute (unit: ml blood/[100 g tissue·min]). During increased neural activity, arterial blood vessels dilate and blood velocity also increases. CBF can be measured with various imaging methods with the use of exogenous blood tracers. CBV is defined as an amount of blood within 100 g tissue (unit: ml blood/100 g tissue) and comprises arterial, capillary, and venous blood volumes. Although CBV differs for different brain regions, it ranges 3–5%. As the capillary blood volume cannot be measured easily, it can be divided into arterial and venous CBV. Since venous blood volume constitutes of ~75% of the total blood volume [14], it is often assumed that the venous blood volume change is dominant during stimulation [15]. However, recent MRI and microscopic studies during neural stimulation [16, 17] show that arterial CBV change is dominant. Change in total blood volume can be measured using exogenous contrast agents. The relationship between CBV and CBF changes can be described as

$$\left[\frac{\Delta \mathrm{CBV}}{\mathrm{CBV}} = \left(\frac{\Delta \mathrm{CBF}}{\mathrm{CBF}} + 1\right)^{b} - 1,\right]$$

where ΔCBV/CBV and ΔCBF/CBF are relative CBV and CBF changes [18]. Constant β differs for different brain regions, but has been used to be 0.38, which was determined from the entire brain of anesthetized monkeys [18]. Thus, CBV and CBF changes can be calculated from each other.

Oxygen is transported mostly with binding with hemoglobin and it is delivered to tissue at the capillary level by diffusion. Arterial oxygen saturation level is close to 1.0. The venous oxygenation level (Y) is dependent on a difference between oxygen supply by CBF and oxygen utilization in tissue. During stimulation, the change of venous oxygenation level can be determined from changes of both CBF and $CMRO_2$ in the following manner [19]:

$$\frac{\Delta Y}{1-Y} = \frac{\Delta CBF/\mathrm{CBF} - \Delta \mathrm{CMRO_2}/\mathrm{CMRO_2}}{\left(\Delta \mathrm{CBF}/\mathrm{CBF}+1\right)}. \quad (1.1)$$

When the relative CBF is much larger than $CMRO_2$ change, ΔY is highly correlated with CBF change. If relative changes in CBF and $CMRO_2$ are similar, then an oxygenation level change is close to zero. Since the BOLD signal change is related to ΔY (see later), $\Delta CMRO_2/CMRO_2$ may be determined from BOLD and CBF changes.

Functional Imaging Contrasts

MRI signal intensity in a given voxel (S) can be described as a sum of signals from different compartments weighted by functions of relaxation times,

$$S = \sum_i \mathrm{V}_i \rho_i \mathrm{fn}(T_{1i}^*) \mathrm{fn}(T_{2i}^*), \quad (1.2)$$

where subscript i is the extravascular tissue, intravascular arterial blood, intravascular venous blood, and cerebrospinal fluid (CSF) compartment, V is the partial volume fraction, ρ is the spin density, and T_1* and T_2* are apparent longitudinal and transverse relaxation times, respectively. Thus, the signal change can be induced by a change in partial volume fraction, T_1*, and/or T_2*. Changes in partial volume fractions may be observed when water spins redistribute between compartments with vastly different signal intensities and have been used for some CBV-weighted fMRI studies (see section on "CBV-weighted fMRI"). Changes in T_1* can be induced by CBF changes, while T_2* can be changed by modulation in paramagnetic dHb contents (see Table 1.1). Both intravascular (IV) and extravascular (EV) signals will contribute to fMRI signals, and its relative contributions are

Table 1.1 Physiological changes and its corresponding MR responses

Physiology	MR-related effects	MR parameters
Increase in CBF	Increase in inflow effects Increase in venous oxygenation	Decrease in blood and tissue apparent T_1 Increase in blood and tissue $T_2/T_2{}^*$
Increase in $CMRO_2$	Decrease in venous oxygenation	Decrease in blood and tissue $T_2/T_2{}^*$
Increase in CBV	Increase in partial blood volume fraction Increase in deoxyhemoglobin content	Decrease in tissue partial volume fraction Decrease in tissue $T_2/T_2{}^*$

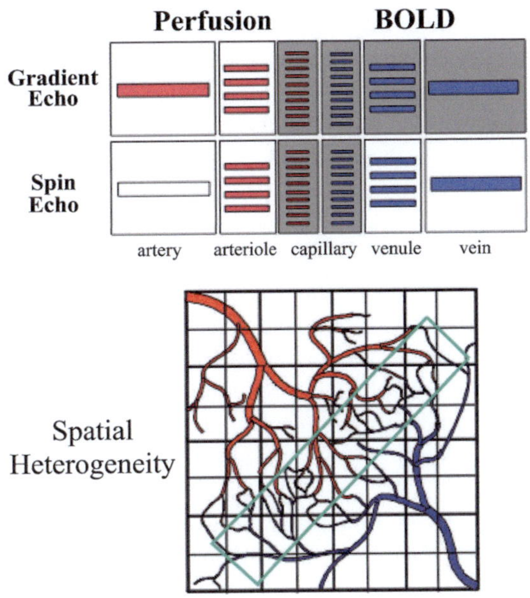

Fig. 1.1 Intravascular (IV) and extravascular (EV) signal contributions to perfusion (CBF) and BOLD signals [59] and hypothetical vascular structures across imaging pixels. In perfusion-weighted images, the IV component of all arterial vessels (*red*) and EV component (*gray*) of capillaries will constitute. When spin-echo data collection is used, spins in large vessels will not be refocused, removing signal contribution from very large arteries. Further removal can be achieved by using bipolar flow-crushing gradients. In BOLD images, IV (*blue*) and EV (*gray*) components of all-sized venous vessels will contribute when gradient-echo data collection is used. When spin-echo data collection is utilized, the EV effect of large vessels can be minimized. Spatial heterogeneity of vascular distributions exists (*bottom figure*); in some pixels (*see black grids*), large vessels are dominant, while some pixels contain mostly capillaries. When neural activity occurs at tissue level, demarked by a *green rectangle*, only capillary-level signal change will locate the actual neural activity area. Containing large vessels may shift activation to nonspecific vessel area. Reprinted with permission from Bandettini PA. The temporal resolution of Functional MRI. In: Moonen CTW, Bandettini PA, eds. Functional MRI. New York: Springer, 1999; 205–220

dependent on imaging techniques and parameters (see Fig. 1.1). The goal of fMRI studies is to detect changes in capillary and tissue signals, since large vessels can be far away from the site of elevated neuronal activity. Dilution by blood draining from "inactive" areas should reduce nonspecific draining-vein effects and thus limit its spatial extent [20]. Therefore, it is important to minimize intravascular and extravascular contribution of large vessel signals to high-resolution fMRI. However, in low-resolution studies, containing small-sized vessel signals enhances functional sensitivity, which is often preferable.

T_1-Weighted Perfusion fMRI

Inflow-based fMRI approach will be discussed in this section. An inflow effect into the region of interest will shorten apparent T_1. Using this property, time-of-flight angiographic images can be obtained. When the inflow time is relatively long such as 1 s, labeled spins by RF pulse(s) move into capillaries in the imaging slice and exchange with tissue water spins. Thus, CBF can be measured noninvasively using arterial water as a perfusion tracer [21–25]. Perfusion MRI techniques include continuous arterial spin tagging [21], flow-sensitive alternating inversion recovery (FAIR) [23, 24], and various other techniques [22, 25]. The general principle behind all arterial spin-labeling (ASL) techniques is to differentiate the net magnetization of endogenous arterial water inflowing to the region of interest from the stationary magnetization of tissue. For this, two images are acquired, one with arterial spin labeling and the other without labeling. In the most widely utilized FAIR technique, because of its simple implementation, two T_1-weighted inversion recovery (IR) images are acquired; one with a nonselective (global) inversion pulse and the other with a slice-selective inversion pulse. The longitudinal magnetization following a nonselective inversion pulse and a slice-selective inversion pulse recovers by R_1 ($=1/T_1$) and R_1^* ($=1/T_1^*$), respectively, where R_1^* is equal to R_1 + CBF/λ, where λ is the tissue–blood partition coefficient (typically 0.9–0.95 ml blood/g tissue). In functional activation studies, labeled and control images are alternately and repeatedly acquired during both control and task periods. The intensity difference between labeled and control images, which is directly related to CBF, is determined during control (DS_{cont}) and stimulation periods (DS_{st}). Stimulation-induced relative CBF changes can be described as ΔCBF/CBF = (DS_{st} $S_{cont}-1$) [23].

Relative CBF changes measured by FAIR (see Fig. 1.2 for finger movements) agree extremely with those measured by $H_2{}^{15}O$ positron emission tomography (PET) in the same region and subject during the identical stimulation task [26]. Thus, the perfusion-weighted MRI technique is an excellent approach to detect relative CBF changes induced by neural activity or other external perturbations. Further, since small arterioles and capillaries are very close to neuronally active tissue, it is expected that tissue-specific CBF signal improves spatial specificity of functional images [27]. Additionally, slow baseline intensity changes not related to neural activity can be removed by subtracting subsequently acquired images [23].

Although perfusion-based approaches can be utilized for fMRI studies, there are many shortcomings. First, large vascular contribution exists because labeled blood fills up arterial vasculature before it travels into capillaries (see also Fig. 1.1) [28]. This arterial vascular contribution can be reduced by using spin-echo data collection or eliminated using bipolar gradients or post-labeling delay, but the suppression of arterial vascular signals will decrease the sensitivity of perfusion-weighted images. However, labeled blood will fill up large vasculature during control and stimulation; thus, no functional signal changes are expected in large arterial vessels (see Fig. 1.2). Second, the proper perfusion contrast is only achieved when enough time is allowed for the labeled arterial spins to travel into the region of interest and exchange with tissue spins. This makes it difficult to detect changes in CBF with a temporal resolution greater than T_1 of arterial

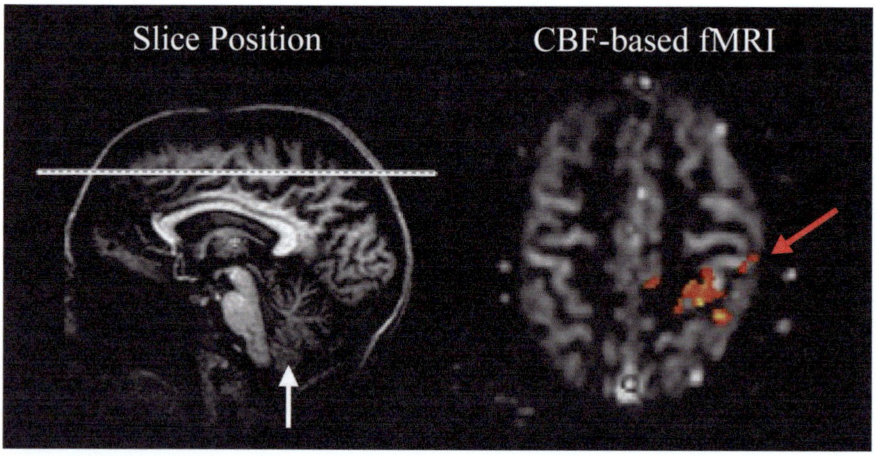

Fig. 1.2 CBF-weighted functional image during finger movements [60]. To obtain the perfusion contrast, flow direction (indicated by a *white upward arrow*) has to be considered. Five mm-thick transverse planes were selected for CBF-based fMRI studies. The background image (*in the right panel*) is weighted by CBF; higher signal areas have higher inflow rates. Functional activity areas were located at gray matter in the contralateral primary motor cortex indicated by a *red arrow*. Interestingly, no large signal changes were observed at the edge of the brain, which was often seen in conventional BOLD functional maps. Reprinted with permission from Kim S-G, Tsekos NV, Ashe J: Multi-slice perfusion-based functional MRI using the FAIR technique: Comparison of CBF and BOLD effects. NMR in Biomedicine 1997;10:191–196

blood, resulting in poor temporal resolution and consequently ineffective signal averaging. Third, in multi-slice application, transit times to different slices are different, which may cause errors in the quantification of CBF [29], which can be overcome using a post-labeling delay [25, 30]. However, relative CBF changes measured by multi-slice FAIR (without post-labeling delay) agree extremely with those measured by PET, suggesting that the change in transit time is not a significant confound [26]. Despite shortcomings, perfusion-weighted fMRI is an attractive method for mapping relative CBF changes.

CBV-Weighted fMRI

CBV-weighted fMRI can be obtained using blood contrast agents. The first human fMRI data were obtained by CBV-weighted fMRI with the intravascular injection of Gd-DTPA [31]. In animal studies, iron oxide nanoparticles have been used as a long half-life intravascular contrast agent [32, 33]. Unlike in the BOLD case, iron oxide concentration in blood does not change with alterations in blood flow and oxygen consumption induced by neuronal activity. Thus, only when the blood volume changes, the content of these particles in an imaging voxel is perturbed. During steady-state condition, established following the infusion of an intravascular contrast agent, an increase in CBV during stimulation will induce an increase in the content of contrast agents, and consequently a *decrease* in MRI signal. Although the use of contrast agents is not preferable for human fMRI studies, CBV-weighted fMRI shows high specificity for active neuronal sites. The highest CBV response is localized at cortical layer IV, where microvessel density, metabolic response, and synaptic inputs are greatest [34], and at "active" orientation-selective columns, where activation-induced neural activity is greatest [35, 36]. These findings indicate that CBV may be an attractive approach for high-resolution fMRI studies in humans.

The vascular space occupancy-dependent (VASO) technique was recently proposed for obtaining endogenous CBV-weighted contrast [37]. VASO images are acquired by an IR sequence at the blood nulling point, leaving only tissue magnetization. When CBV increases during stimulation, a partial fraction of tissue (extravascular space) concomitantly decreases, resulting in a decrease in MRI signals during stimulation. Thus, a relative change in CBV can be obtained with the VASO technique.

This technique has some shortcomings [38]. At higher magnetic fields, T_1 values of blood and tissue water are longer and relatively similar. When blood magnetization is nulled, only small tissue magnetization remains at high fields, leading to poor SNR. An additional difficulty with higher magnetic fields is the increased BOLD signal, which counteracts the negative VASO signal changes and further reduces its sensitivity. In the case that CSF contains in voxels, a change in CSF volume fraction will contribute to errors in CBV quantification. Although the quantification of CBV responses is difficult at high fields, its dynamic properties can be obtained.

T_2* and T_2-Weighted BOLD fMRI

It is well known that, with typical fMRI acquisition parameters, the BOLD response is particularly sensitive in and around large draining veins because the BOLD effect is sensitive to a change in paramagnetic dHb contents [19]. To understand the spatial resolution and magnitude of BOLD-based fMRI, it is important to examine the anatomical source of the BOLD signal. The BOLD contrast induced by dHb arises from both intravascular (IV) and extravascular (EV) components (see Fig. 1.1). Since the exchange of water between these two compartments (typical lifetime of water in capillaries > 500 ms) is relatively slower than the imaging time (echo time < 100 ms), MRI signals from these are treated as separate pools.

Intravascular BOLD Component

During fMRI measurements, water rapidly exchanges between red blood cells (RBC) with paramagnetic dHb and plasma (average water residence time in RBCs = ~5 ms) and travels along space with different fields by diffusion, e.g., diffusion distance – i.e., 6 × diffusion constant × diffusion time$^{1/2}$ – during ~50 ms measurement time = ~17 μm with diffusion constant of ~1 μm^2/ms. This process is referred to as "dynamic" (time irreversible) averaging. All water molecules inside the vessel will experience the similar "dynamic averaging," resulting in the reduction of T_2 of blood water in the venous pool. T_2 of blood water for $Y = 0.6$ is ~127 ms at 1.5 T [39], ~31 ms at 3 T [40], ~12–15 ms at 7 T [41], and ~5 ms at 9.4 T [42], while T_2 value of gray matter water is 90 ms at 1.5 T [43], 71 ms at 3 T [44], 55 ms at 7 T [45], and 40 ms at 9.4 T [42]. When spin-echo time is set to T_2 of gray matter, it is evident that the blood contribution to MRI signals decreases dramatically with an increase in magnetic field.

In addition to the T_2 change induced by dHb, the frequency change is observed. When a blood vessel is considered as an infinite cylinder, frequency shift $\Delta\omega$ induced by dHb within and around the vessel is depicted in Fig. 1.3. It should be noted that frequency (ω) and magnetic field (B) are interchangeable because $\omega = \gamma B$, where γ is the gyromagnetic ratio. Inside the blood vessel, the frequency shift will be expressed by

$$\left[\Delta w_{in} = 2\pi\,\Delta\,\chi_o(1-Y)w_o\left(cos^2 q - \frac{1}{3}\right),\right] \quad (1.3)$$

where $\Delta\chi$o is the maximum susceptibility difference between fully oxygenated and fully deoxygenated blood, Y is the fraction of oxygenation in venous blood, ω_o is the applied magnetic field of the scanner in frequency units ($\omega_o = \gamma B_o$), and θ is the angle between the applied magnetic field (B_o) and vessel orientation. Assuming a hematocrit level of 0.38 and the susceptibility difference between 100% oxyhemoglobin and 100% dHb of 0.27 ppm [9], $\Delta\chi$o in whole blood is 0.1 ppm. In a given voxel, many vessels with different orientations exist. These random orientations cause phase dispersion (rather than a net phase shift), therefore causing a reduction in T_2*. However, a very large vessel will have its own phase shift depending on oxygenation level and orientation. Using this property, Haacke and his colleagues determined an oxygenation level from a large vein perpendicular to B_0 [46].

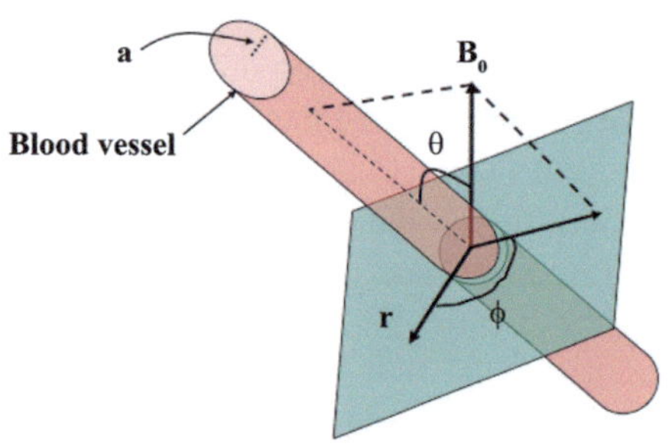

$\Delta\omega_{in} = 2\pi\Delta\chi_0\,(1\text{-}Y)\omega_0(\cos^2\theta - 1/3)$

$\Delta\omega_{out} = 2\pi\Delta\chi_0\,(1\text{-}Y)\omega_0(a/r)^2(\sin^2\theta)(\cos 2\phi)$

Fig. 1.3 Diagram of a blood vessel and the parameters that determine the susceptibility effect induced by deoxyhemoglobin irons in red blood cells at a distance r from the center of a vessel. The vessel with a radius of a is oriented at angle θ from the main magnetic field B_0. φ is the angle between r and plane defined by B_0 and the vessel axis. Intravascular and extravascular frequency shifts are shown in equations. $\Delta\chi_0$: susceptibility difference between 100% oxygenated and 100% deoxygenated blood (ppm); ω_0: frequency of B_0; and Y: venous oxygenation level

Extravascular BOLD Component

At any location outside the blood vessel, the frequency shift is described by

$$\Delta w_{out} = 2p\Delta c_0(1-Y)w_o\left(\frac{a}{r}\right)^2 (\sin^2 q)(\cos 2f), \quad (1.4)$$

where a is the radius of blood vessel, r is the distance from the point of interest to the center of the blood vessel, and φ is the angle between r and the plane defined by B_o and the vessel axis. The dephasing effect is dependent on the orientation of vessel; vessels running parallel to B_0 ($\theta = 0°$) do not have the EV effect, while those orthogonal to B_0 will have the maximal frequency shift (see Fig. 1.4). At the lumen of vessels ($r = a$), $\Delta\omega_{out}$ is identical and independent of vessel sizes. At $r = 5a$, the susceptibility effect is 4% of the maximally available $\Delta\omega_{out}$; the same frequency shift will be observed at 15 μm away

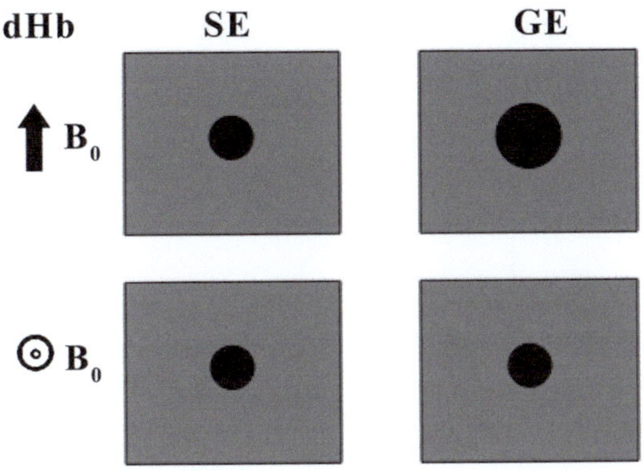

Fig. 1.4 Spin-echo (SE) and gradient-echo (GE) images of a 1-mm diameter capillary filled with blood with 100% deoxyhemoglobin (dHb). These images are not actual MRI data, but produced based on Ogawa et al. data [7]. Deoxyhemoglobin induces susceptibility effects within and outside the capillary. In all spin-echo and gradient-echo images, signal intensity within the capillary is low due to dynamic averaging. The signal intensity outside the capillary is not affected by dHb in spin-echo images because static dephasing effect is refocused. However, the signal outside the capillary is dependent on capillary orientation in gradient-echo images (see Fig. 1.3). When the capillary is oriented parallel to B_0, no signal change outside the capillary is observed in gradient-echo image, while the capillary is oriented orthogonal to B_0, the effect of dHb to MR signals outside the capillary is the largest

from a 3-μm radius capillary and 150 μm around a 30-μm radius venule (see Fig. 1.5). This shows why the dephasing effect around a larger vessel is more spatially extensive. The EV contribution from large vessels to conventional BOLD signal is highly significant, regardless of magnetic field strength. During echo time for fMRI studies (e.g., ~50 ms), water molecules diffuse tens micrometers (e.g. ~17 μm), which are shorter than the entire range of susceptibility gradients around the 3-μpm radius capillary. Thus, tissue water around *capillaries* will be "dynamically" averaged over the many different fields (i.e., no net phase change as the IV component). However, tissue water around *large vessels* will be locally averaged during an echo time, because the diffusion distance covers only a small range of susceptibility gradients around the 30-μm radius venule (see small circles with dephasing information in Fig. 1.5). Within a voxel, many different dephasing effects are averaged; this process is often referred to as time-reversible static averaging. The static dephasing effect can be removed at an echo time by refocusing with the 180° RF pulse. The EV

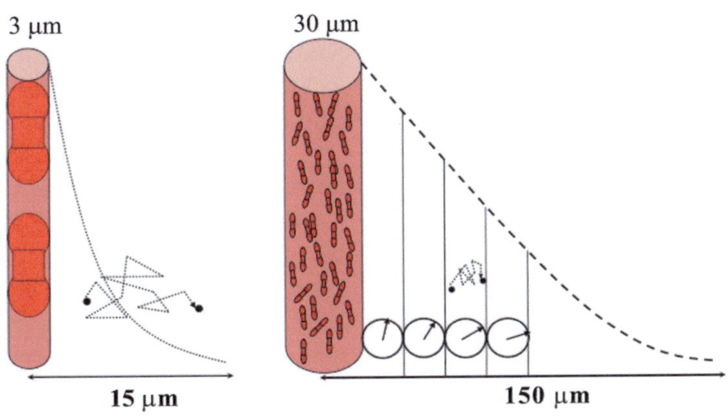

Fig. 1.5 Extravascular dephasing effects from a 3-μm radius capillary versus a 30-μm radius venule [33]. Magnitude of susceptibility effect (decay lines from vessels) is shown as a function of distance. Water spins inside and outside vessels are diffused during TE; hypothetical Brownian-motion-like displacement of a water molecule is shown. No net phase shift is observed around the capillary. However, phase shift around large vessels is dependent on distance from the venule (shown in averaged phases in *circles*); the dephasing effect is larger at closer to a vessel. This static dephasing effect can be removed by a refocusing RF pulse in the spin-echo sequence. Extravascular diffusion-dominant susceptibility effect around small vessels is observed in both gradient-echo and spin-echo images, while the static dephasing effect around large vessels is only detectable in gradient-echo images. Reproduced with permission from Kim S-G, Ugurbil K: High-resolution functional magnetic resonance imaging of the animal brain. Methods 2003;30:28–41

contribution of large vessels can be reduced by using the spin-echo technique (see Fig. 1.4).

In a given voxel, MRI signals with different dephasing effects (i.e., frequency shifts) induced by numerous vessels will be summed, resulting in a decrease in T_2*. Signal in the voxel at echo time (TE) can be described as

$$S(\mathrm{TE}) = \sum_i S_{0_i} \mathrm{e}^{-\mathrm{TE}/T_2} \mathrm{e}^{-iw_i\mathrm{TE}} \approx S_0 \mathrm{e}^{-\mathrm{TE}/T_2^*} \quad (1.5)$$

where i is the subvoxel index and ωTE indicates the phase shift at TE. The summation of MRI signals is performed over numerous subvoxel i, which designates the small volume element within the voxel (e.g., hypothetically a volume with a small circle with phase shift in Fig. 1.5). If the variation of ω within the voxel is relatively large, the MR signal will be decayed approximately with a single exponential time constant T_2*. Measured R_2* (=1/T_2*) is a sum of R_2 (=1/T_2) and susceptibility-induced R_2' (=1/T_2'). Based on Monte Carlo simulation [19, 47], the dephasing effect within a voxel can be simplified into R_2' change as

$$\left[R_2' = \frac{1}{T_2'} = a \times \mathrm{CBV}\left\{\Delta c_0 w_0 (1-Y)\right\}^g,\right] \quad (1.6)$$

where α and γ are constants. The power term γ is 1.0 for time-reversible "static" averaging domain and 2.0 for time-irreversible "dynamic" averaging domain [19, 47]. All venous vessels will have a power term of 1.0–2.0 [19, 47]. When water molecules sufficiently diffuse through different frequency areas during TE, γ will be close to 2.0. A larger change in R_2' induces a larger BOLD fMRI signal change; a larger increase in Y during stimulation, a higher magnetic field, and a higher baseline CBV will induce a higher BOLD response.

Spin-echo (SE) and gradient-echo (GE) BOLD signal changes in a function of vessel size can be seen in Fig. 1.6 [48]. At capillaries, R_2 (=1/T_2) is similar to R_2* (=1/T_2*). However, when vessel size increases above 5–8 μm diameter (which is related to diffusion time and susceptibility gradient), R_2 is reduced, while R_2* remains high [19]. Thus, extravascular SE BOLD signals predominantly originate from small-size vessels including capillaries, while extravascular GE BOLD signals dominate from large veins.

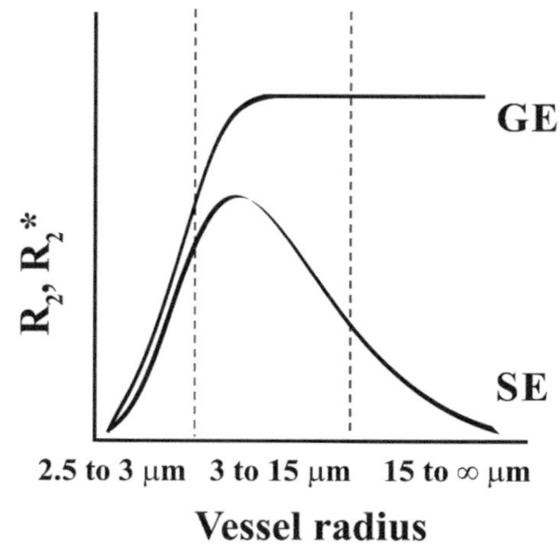

Fig. 1.6 Spin-echo (SE) and gradient-echo (GE) BOLD signal changes as a function of vessel size [48]. GE BOLD fMRI (R_2*) is sensitive to all sizes of vessels containing dHb. Peak response in SE BOLD (R_2) is dependent on susceptibility gradient and diffusion distance; peak shifts to a smaller vessel size at a higher susceptibility gradient, while it shifts to a larger vessel size at a longer echo time. Reprinted with permission from Bandettini PA, Wong EC: Effects of biophysical and physiologic parameters on brain activation-induced R2* and R2 changes: Simulations using determistic diffusion model. Int J Imaging Systems Technology 1995;6:133–152

Spin-Echo Versus Gradient-Echo BOLD

As we discussed already, GE BOLD signals consist of EV and IV components of venous vessels, regardless of the vessel size. A 180° RF pulse refocuses the dephasing effect around large vessels, and thus the SE BOLD image contains the EV signals of small-size vessels with diffusion-related time-irreversible averaging and the IV signals of all-size vessels (see Fig. 1.1). The IV component can be reduced by setting an echo time of >3T_2* or 3T_2 of blood. Thus, at ultrahigh fields, the IV component can be significantly reduced because venous blood T_2* and T_2 decrease faster than corresponding tissue T_2* and T_2 when magnetic field increases. The IV contribution to the BOLD responses can be examined using bipolar gradients [49]. These gradients induce velocity-dependent phase shifts in the presence of flow and consequently reduce signals from blood because of inhomogeneous velocities within a vessel and the presence of blood vessels of different orientations within a voxel. Based on fMRI studies with bipolar gradients, the BOLD fMRI signals at 1.5 T originate predominantly from the IV component (70–90%) [47, 49, 50], while those at 7 and 9.4 T come mostly from the EV component [42, 51]. With relatively high sensitivity of SE BOLD at high fields, high-resolution functional maps can be obtained from human and animal brains at 7 and 9.4 T [52, 53].

After removing the IV component in the BOLD signal, the EV component remains. In GE BOLD fMRI, the EV effect around large vessels is linearly dependent on B_0, while the EV effect around small vessels is supralinearly dependent on B_0. Thus, at a higher B_0, the extravascular contribution of small-vessel-related signals increases. However, even at 9.4 T, the EV effect around large vessels is still significant in GE BOLD fMRI [54]. In SE BOLD fMRI, the EV effect around small vessels is supralinearly dependent on B_0, while that around large vessels is minimized. Thus, the SE technique is more specific to parenchyma than GE BOLD fMRI [54]. When high-spatial specificity is required for mapping sub-millimeter functional structures, the SE BOLD technique at high fields is preferable [34]. As the dephasing effect around vessels is refocused, the sensitivity of SE BOLD signal is significantly reduced. Even if respective optimized echo times are used for GE and SE BOLD fMRI, the GE BOLD technique provides the higher signal change even at ultrahigh magnetic fields such as 9.4 T [34]. For supramillimeter resolution studies, the GE BOLD technique is the choice of tools because of high sensitivity, even if its spatial specificity may compromise.

BOLD Versus CBF Versus CBV fMRI

In most fMRI studies, BOLD is the most appropriate tool because of its high sensitivity and easy implementation. However, the BOLD method has some shortcomings. As seen in (16.6), the BOLD signal change is sensitive to baseline physiological parameters such as oxygenation level and blood volume (Y and CBV), anatomical parameters such as vessel size and orientation, and MR-related parameters and techniques such as magnetic field and echo time. Thus, BOLD fMRI signal changes may not be compared across different cortical regions and subjects (especially normal subjects versus patients). Thus, the most prevalent approach is to compare BOLD responses across different tasks in the same brain regions. Owing to large variations of BOLD signal changes, it is difficult to perform longitudinal fMRI studies. Similar concerns are raised in CBV-based fMRI, as the BOLD contribution to CBV-based VASO measurements is significant. Also, the quantification of CBV changes is highly sensitive to blood T_1 value and CSF contamination. Thus, CBV-based VASO technique is not likely to be viable for longitudinal functional imaging studies. These problems can be overcome using CBF-based fMRI techniques, albeit low sensitivity. Since a single physiological parameter is measured, it is independent of imaging parameters and methods as well as magnetic field. Thus, CBF-based fMRI is more suitable for longitudinal studies than BOLD and CBV fMRI. CBF-based fMRI is often used to complement BOLD fMRI. CBF-based fMRI measures ΔCBF/CBF, and BOLD fMRI can measure $\Delta Y/(1-Y)$, if other parameters (see 16.6) are known. Combining CBF and BOLD fMRI, oxygen consumption changes can be determined (see 16.1). Thus, both hemodynamic and metabolic responses may be determined from fMRI data.

Contrast-to-Noise Ratio

Important consideration of fMRI is contrast-to-noise ratio (neural activity-induced signal change relative to temporal signal fluctuation). To increase the detectability of fMRI, an increase of neural activity-induced change and decrease of noise are crucial. Neural activity-induced signal is dependent on both image contrast and imaging techniques used for fMRI. In the T_2*-based BOLD measurements, the signal change induced by neural activity (ΔS) can be described by

$$[\Delta S = S_{cont} \times \left(-TE \times \Delta R_2^*\right),] \quad (1.7)$$

where S_{cont} is the signal intensity during the control period and can be described as $S_0\exp(-\text{TE}/T_2^*)$, TE is the echo time and ΔR_2^* is the change in the apparent transverse relaxation rate. Signal change is maximal when a gradient echo time is set to T_2^* of tissue at resting conditions. When spin echo imaging techniques are used, ΔR_2^* is replaced by ΔR_2. ΔS for spin-echo BOLD fMRI will be maximal by setting TE of tissue T_2. In CBF-based techniques, $\text{TE}\Delta R_2^*$ should be substituted by $\text{TI}\Delta R_1^*$, where TI is the spin-labeling time (i.e., the inversion time for pulsed labeling methods), and ΔR_1^* is the change in the apparent longitudinal relaxation rate. ΔS is maximized by setting TI of tissue T_1. In all fMRI techniques, the contribution of large vessels increases ΔS. Depending on the constraint of spatial resolution, the MR technique with the highest ΔS should be chosen. Since the contribution of small intracortical veins is likely localized within 1.5 mm to the site of activation [55], contribution of small veins can improve SNR for supramillimeter spatial resolution. In typical fMRI studies with supramillimeter spatial resolution, the removal of only large surface arteries and veins may be necessary.

Sources of temporal noises include random white noise, physiological fluctuations, bulk head motion, and system instability, if it exists. Random noise is independent between voxels, while other noise sources may be coherent among voxels, resulting in spatial and temporal correlation. In fMRI, coherent noises are the major source of signal fluctuation. Bulk head motion can be reduced by head constraint and corrected using post-processing approaches. Physiological noise, which is mainly due to respiration and cardiac pulsation, can be reduced by post-processing. Minimal head motions during scanning are important for successful fMRI studies.

Spatial and Temporal Resolution of fMRI

Spatial Resolution

Spatial resolution of fMRI is dependent on SNR and intrinsic hemodynamic response. The intrinsic limit of spatial specificity of hemodynamic-based fMRI can be dependent on how finely CBF is regulated. Recent studies suggest that intrinsic CBF changes are specific to sub-millimeter functional domains [27]. Especially, the highest CBF change was observed in the middle of the cortex, cortical layer IV, not at the surface of the cortex during various stimulations [56, 57]. Among the available hemodynamic fMRI approaches, the CBF-based signal is likely to be the most specific to neuronal active sites because most of signals originate from tissue and capillaries. Both CBV response and SE BOLD signal without large vessel contribution will have similar spatial specificity to the CBF-weighted signal [57, 58]. It should be noted that large vessel contribution is closely dependent on the volume of activation region. If the activation region is large, then dHb from the active region can travel far away without dilution, while if the activation region is small, then the draining issue will not be serious, allowing high-resolution functional mapping with GE BOLD fMRI.

Temporal Resolution

Since hemodynamic responses are sluggish, it is difficult to obtain very high temporal resolution even if images can be obtained rapidly. Typically, hemodynamic signal changes are observed at 1–2 s after onset of stimulation and reaches maximum at 4–8 s (see Fig. 1.7). The exact time of neural activity cannot be easily obtained from hemodynamic responses because hemodynamic response varies depending on vascular structures

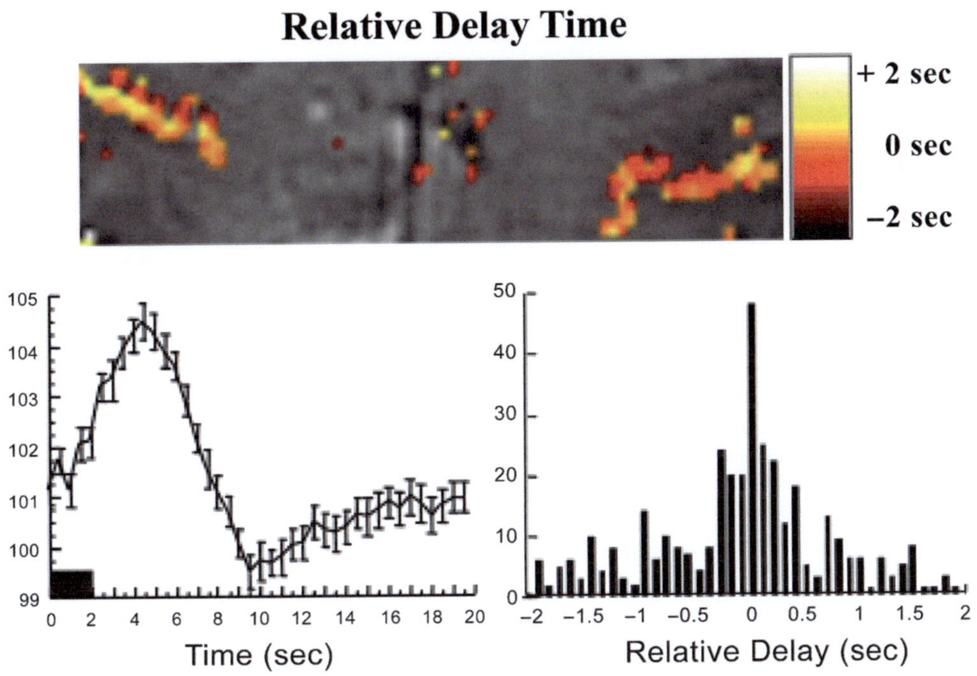

Fig. 1.7 Heterogeneity of hemodynamic dynamics [59]. Two-second bilateral finger movements were performed at 3 T. Delay time of GE BOLD fMRI signal changes was obtained in the motor cortical areas. Although an average delay time is ~1 s, there is a large variation in delay times shown in delay map as well as histogram. In histogram and the delay map, relative hemodynamic delay time (not actual delay time) was calculated, which means average of all relative delay times = 0 s. Large variations in delay times are due to different vascular responses and draining effects. Reprinted with permission from Bandettini PA. The temporal resolution of Functional MRI. In: Moonen CTW, Bandettini PA, eds. Functional MRI. New York: Springer, 1999;205–220

and reactivity (see Fig. 1.7). The important question is to determine sequential neural activities of different cortical regions. If the hemodynamic response times in all regions and in all subjects were the same, neuronal activities could be directly inferred from fMRI time courses. However, this may not be true in all regions and in all subjects (see Fig. 1.7), and thus differences in fMRI time courses may be simply related to intrinsic hemodynamic response time differences, hampering temporal studies. Typical temporal resolution of hemodynamic-based fMRI is on the order of a second.

Conclusion

Advancement of imaging technologies allows detections of various vascular physiological parameters induced by neural activity (see Table 1.2 for a summary of key studies on the advancement of fMRI techniques). Fortunately, tissue-based hemodynamic response is relatively specific to neuronal active sites. Thus, sub-millimeter spatial resolution can be achieved. Since hemodynamic response is slow, its temporal resolution cannot be reached at a level of neural activity time scale, but can be on the order of a second.

Table 1.2 Summary of key literature

Authors	Article title	Significance
Belliveau et al. [31]	Functional mapping of the human visual cortex by magnetic resonance imaging. Science 1991;254:716–9.	This is the first human fMRI paper with the use of contrast agent, and is a historically important paper.
Detre et al. [21]	Perfusion imaging. Magn Reson Med 1992;23:37–45.	This is the first arterial spin-labeling paper. Principle of arterial spin labeling is described, and quantitative CBF in rats was measured.
Ogawa et al. [10]	Intrinsic signal changes accompanying sensory stimulation: functional brain mapping with magnetic resonance imaging. Proc Natl Acad Sci USA 1992;89(13):5951–5.	One of the first human BOLD fMRI papers. This paper demonstrates that functional activation maps can be obtained with MRI noninvasively.
Kwong et al. [11]	Dynamic magnetic resonance imaging of human brain activity during primary sensory stimulation. Proc Natl Acad Sci USA 1992;89(12):5675–9.	One of the first human fMRI papers. This paper shows that BOLD and inflow contrasts can be used for functional mapping in humans.
Boxerman et al. [47]	The intravascular contribution to fMRI signal change: Monte Carlo modeling and diffusion-weighted studies in vivo. Magn Reson Med 1995;34:4–10.	Shows computer simulations of SE vs. GE BOLD fMRI, and experimental data.
Kim [23]	Quantification of relative cerebral blood flow change by flow-sensitive alternating inversion recovery (FAIR) technique: application to functional mapping. Magn Reson Med 1995;34:293–301.	This paper reported quantitative CBF changes during stimulation. Advantages of ASL approach over BOLD fMRI are described.
Ogawa et al. [13]	On the characteristics of functional magnetic resonance imaging of the brain. Annu Rev Biophys Biomol Struct 1998;27:447–74.	Review article. Detailed biophysical source of the BOLD contrast is described.
Duong et al., [56]	Functional MRI of calcium-dependent synaptic activity: Cross correlation with CBF and BOLD measurements. Magn Reson Med 2000;43:383–92.	CBF fMRI is specific to neural active sites determined by calcium-sensitive manganese-enhanced MRI.
Lu et al. [37]	Functional magnetic resonance imaging based on changes in vascular space occupancy. Mag Reson Med 2003;50:263–74.	Describes a CBV-based fMRI technique without the use of contrast agent.

Acknowledgements Supported by the National Institutes of Health.

References

1 Roy CS, Sherrington CS. On the regulation of blood supply of the brain. J Physiol. 1890;1:85–108.

2 Raichle ME. Circulatory and metabolic correlates of brain function in normal humans. In: Handbook of physiology, The nervous system, vol. V. Bethesda: American Physiological Society; 1987. p. 643–74.

3 Fox PT, Raichle ME. Focal physiological uncoupling of cerebral blood flow and oxidative metabolism during somatosensory stimulation in human subjects. Proc Natl Acad Sci USA. 1986;83:1140–4.

4 Fox PT, Raichle ME, Mintun MA, Dence C. Nonoxidative glucose consumption during focal physiologic neural activity. Science. 1988;241:462–4.

5 Ogawa S, Lee T-M, Kay AR, Tank DW. Brain Magnetic Resonance Imaging with Contrast Dependent on Blood Oxygenation. Proc Natl Acad Sci USA. 1990;87:9868–72.

6 Ogawa S, Lee T-M, Nayak AS, Glynn P. Oxygenation-sensitive contrast in magnetic resonance image of rodent brain at high magnetic fields. Magn Reson Med. 1990;14:68–78.

7 Ogawa S, Lee TM. Magnetic resonance imaging of blood vessels at high fields: in vivo and in vitro measurements and image simulation. Magn Reson Med. 1990;16(1):9–18.

8 Thulborn KR, Waterton JC, Mattews PM, Radda GK. Oxygenation dependence of the transverse relaxation time of water protons in whole blood at high field. Biochem Biophys Acta. 1982;714:265–70.

9 Pauling L, Coryell CD. The magnetic properties and structure of hemoglobin, oxyhemoglobin and carbonmonoxyhemoglobin. Proc Natl Acad Sci USA. 1936; 22:210–6.

10 Ogawa S, Tank DW, Menon R, et al. Intrinsic signal changes accompanying sensory stimulation: functional brain mapping with magnetic resonance imaging. Proc Natl Acad Sci USA. 1992;89(13):5951–5.
11 Kwong KK, Belliveau JW, Chesler DA, et al. Dynamic magnetic resonance imaging of human brain activity during primary sensory stimulation. Proc Natl Acad Sci USA. 1992;89(12):5675–9.
12 Bandettini PA, Wang EC, Hinks RS, Rikofsky RS, Hyde JS. Time course EPI of human brain function during task activation. Magn Reson Med. 1992;25: 390–7.
13 Ogawa S, Menon RS, Kim S-G, Ugurbil K. On the characteristics of functional magnetic resonance imaging of the brain. Annu Rev Biophys Biomol Struct. 1998;27:447–74.
14 Lee S-P, Duong T, Yang G, Iadecola C, Kim S-G. Relative changes of cerebral arterial and venous blood volumes during increased cerebral blood flow: Implications for BOLD fMRI. Magn Reson Med. 2001;45:791–800.
15 Buxton RB, Wong EC, Frank LR. Dynamics of blood flow and oxygenation changes during brain activation: The balloon model. Magn Reson Med. 1998;39: 855–64.
16 Kim T, Masamoto K, Hendrich K, Kim S-G. Arterial versus total blood volume changes during neural activity-induced cerebral blood flow change: implication for BOLD fMRI. J Cereb Blood Flow Metab. 2007;27:1235–47.
17 Hillman EM, Devor A, Bouchard MB, et al. Depth-resolved optical imaging and microscopy of vascular compartment dynamics during somatosensory stimulation. Neuroimage. 2007;35(1):89–104.
18 Grubb RL, Raichle ME, Eichling JO, Ter-Pogossian MM. The effects of changes in PaCO2 on cerebral blood volume, blood flow, and vascular mean transit time. Stroke. 1974;5:630–9.
19 Ogawa S, Menon RS, Tank DW, et al. Functional brain mapping by blood oxygenation level-dependent contrast magnetic resonance imaging. A comparison of signal characteristics with a biophysical model. Biophys J. 1993;64(3):803–12.
20 Turner R. How much cortex can a vein drain? Downstream dilution of activation-related cerebral blood oxygenation changes. Neuroimag. 2002;16:1062–7.
21 Detre JA, Leigh JS, Williams DS, Koretsky AP. Perfusion imaging. Magn Reson Med. 1992;23:37–45.
22 Edelman RR, Siewert B, Darby DG, et al. Qualitative mapping of cerebral blood flow and functional localization with echo-planar MR imaging and signal targeting with alternating radio frequency. Radiology. 1994;192:513–20.
23 Kim S-G. Quantification of relative cerebral blood flow change by flow-sensitive alternating inversion recovery (FAIR) technique: application to functional mapping. Magn Reson Med. 1995;34:293–301.
24 Kwong KK, Chesler DA, Weisskoff RM, et al. MR perfusion studies with T1-weighted echo planar imaging. Magn Reson Med. 1995;34:878–87.
25 Wong E, Buxton R, Frank L. Quantitative imaging of perfusion using a single subtraction (QUIPSS and QUIPSS II). Magn Reson Med. 1998;39:702–8.
26 Zaini MR, Strother SC, Andersen JR, et al. Comparison of matched BOLD and FAIR 4.0 T-fMRI with [^{15}O]water PET brain volumes. Med Phys. 1999;26:1559–67.
27 Duong TQ, Kim D-S, Ugurbil K, Kim S-G. Localized cerebral blood flow response at submillimeter columnar resolution. Proc Natl Acad Sci USA. 2001;98: 10904–9.
28 Ye FQ, Mattay VS, Jezzard P, Frank JA, Weinberger DR, McLaughlin AC. Correction for vascular artifacts in cerebral blood flow values by using arterial spin tagging techniques. Magn Reson Med. 1997;37:226–35.
29 Buxton R, Frank L, Wong E, Siewert B, Warach S, Edelman R. A general kinetic model for quantitative perfusion imaging with arterial spin labeling. Magn Reson Med. 1998;40:383–96.
30 Alsop D, Detre J. Reduced transit-time sensitivity in noninvasive magnetic resonance imaging of human cerebral blood flow. J Cereb Blood Flow Metab. 1996;16:1236–49.
31 Belliveau JW, Kennedy DN, McKinstry RC, et al. Functional mapping of the human visual cortex by magnetic resonance imaging. Science. 1991;254:716–9.
32 Mandeville JB, Marota JJ, Kosofsky BE, et al. Dynamic functional imaging of relative cerebral blood volume during rat forepaw stimulation. Magn Reson Med. 1998;39(4):615–24.
33 Kim S-G, Ugurbil K. High-resolution functional magnetic resonance imaging of the animal brain. Methods. 2003;30:28–41.
34 Zhao F, Wang P, Hendrich K, Ugurbil K, Kim S-G. Cortical layer-dependent BOLD and CBV responses measured by spin-echo and gradient-echo fMRI: insights into hemodynamic regulation. Neuroimage. 2006;30:1149–60.
35 Zhao F, Wang P, Hendrich K, Kim S-G. Spatial specificity of cerebral blood volume-weighted fMRI responses at columnar resolution. Neuroimag. 2005; 27:416–24.
36 Fukuda M, Moon C-H, Wang P, Kim S-G. Mapping iso-orientation columns by contrast agent-enhanced functional MRI: reproducibility, specificity and evaluation by optical imaging of intrinsic signal. J Neurosci. 2006;26:11821–32.
37 Lu H, Golay X, Pekar J, Van Zijl P. Functional magnetic resonance imaging based on changes in vascular space occupancy. Mag Reson Med. 2003;50:263–74.
38 Jin T, Kim SG. Improved cortical-layer specificity of vascular space occupancy fMRI with slab inversion relative to spin-echo BOLD at 9.4 T. Neuroimag. 2008;40:59–67.
39 Wright GA, Hu BS, Macovski A. Estimating oxygen saturation of blood in vivo with MR imaging at 1.5 T. J Magn Reson Imag. 1991;1:275–83.
40 Zhao J, Clingman C, Närväinen M, Kauppinen R, van Zijl P. Oxygenation and hemotocrit dependence

of transverse relaxation rates of blood at 3 T. Magn Reson Med. 2007;58:592–7.
41 Ogawa S, Lee TM, Barrere B. Sensitivity of magnetic resonance image signals of a rat brain to changes in the cerebral venous blood oxygenation. Magn Reson Med. 1993;29:205–10.
42 Lee S-P, Silva AC, Ugurbil K, Kim S-G. Diffusion-weighted spin-echo fMRI at 9.4 T: microvascular/tissue contribution to BOLD signal change. Magn Reson Med. 1999;42:919–28.
43 Breger RK, Rimm AA, Fischer ME, Papke RA, Haughten VM. T_1 and T_2 Measurements on a 1.5 Tesla Commercial Imager. Radiology. 1989;171:273–6.
44 Gelman N, Gorell J, Barker P, et al. MR imaging of human brain at 3.0 T: preliminary report on transverse relaxation rates and relation to estimated iron content. Radiology. 1999;210:759–67.
45 Yacoub E, Shmuel A, Pfeuffer J, et al. Imaging brain function in humans at 7 Tesla. Magn Reson Med. 2001;45:588–94.
46 Haacke EM, Lai S, Reichenbach JR, et al. In vivo measurement of blood oxygen saturation using magnetic resonance imaging: a direct validation of the blood oxygen level-dependent concept in functional brain mapping. Hum Brain Mapp. 1997;5:341–7.
47 Boxerman JL, Bandettini PA, Kwong KK, et al. The intravascular contribution to fMRI signal change: Monte Carlo modeling and diffusion-weighted studies in vivo. Magn Reson Med. 1995;34:4–10.
48 Bandettini PA, Wong EC. Effects of biophysical and physiologic parameters on brain activation-induced R2* and R2 changes: Simulations using determistic diffusion model. Int J Imaging Syst Technol. 1995; 6:133–52.
49 Song AW, Wong EC, Tan SG, Hyde JS. Diffusion weighted fMRI at 1.5 T. Magn Reson Med. 1996; 35(2):155–8.
50 Zhong J, Kennan RP, Fulbright RK, Gore JC. Quantification of intravascular and extravascular contributions to BOLD effects induced by alteration in oxygenation or intravascular contrast agents. Magn Reson Med. 1998;40(4):526–36.
51 Duong TQ, Yacoub E, Adriany G, Hu X, Ugurbil K, Kim S-G. Microvascular BOLD contribution at 4 and 7 T in the human brain: Gradient-echo and spin-echo fMRI with suppression of blood effects. Mag Reson Med. 2003;49(6):1019–27.
52 Yacoub E, Harel N, Ugurbil K. High-field fMRI unveils orientation columns in humans. Proc Natl Acad Sci USA. 2008;105:10607–12.
53 Moon CH, Fukuda M, Park SH, Kim SG. Neural interpretation of blood oxygenation level-dependent fMRI maps at submillimeter columnar resolution. J Neurosci. 2007;27(26):6892–902.
54 Zhao F, Wang P, Kim SG. Cortical depth-dependent gradient-echo and spin-echo BOLD fMRI at 9.4 T. Magn Reson Med. 2004;51(3):518–24.
55 Duvernoy HM, Delon S, Vannson JL. Cortical blood vessels of the human brain. Brain Res Bull. 1981; 7(5):519–79.
56 Duong TQ, Silva AC, Lee S-P, Kim S-G. Functional MRI of calcium-dependent synaptic activity: Cross correlation with CBF and BOLD measurements. Magn Reson Med. 2000;43:383–92.
57 Jin T, Kim SG. Cortical layer-dependent dynamic blood oxygenation, cerebral blood flow and cerebral blood volume responses during visual stimulation. Neuroimag. 2008;43:1–9.
58 Lee S-P, Silva AC, Kim S-G. Comparison of diffusion-weighted high-resolution CBF and spin-echo BOLD fMRI at 9.4 T. Magn Reson Med. 2002;47:736–41.
59 Bandettini PA. The temporal resolution of functional MRI. In: Moonen CTW, Bandettini PA, editors. Functional MRI. New York: Springer; 1999. p. 205–20.
60 Kim S-G, Tsekos NV, Ashe J. Multi-slice perfusion-based functional MRI using the FAIR technique: Comparison of CBF and BOLD effects. NMR Biomed. 1997;10:191–6.

fMRI Scanning Methods

2

Alexander B. Pine and Feroze B. Mohamed

Introduction

The constant challenge in the field of neuroscience is to advance the understanding of working mechanisms of the human brain and of what enacts such complex functions as perception, emotions, and behavior. In areas of clinical psychology, neurophysiology, and neurosciences, the ultimate interest is to describe neuronal functions qualitatively and quantitatively in normal conditions and various disorders, and subsequently apply such knowledge for diagnostic and therapeutic purposes.

A number of imaging techniques have been developed to investigate these complex functions and characterize neuronal activity of the human brain. In recent years, technical advances have tremendously enhanced capabilities of magnetic resonance imaging (MRI) equipment in regard to detection of minute physiological features, unprecedentedly widening the application spectrum of this modality. MRI and nuclear magnetic resonance (NMR) systems with superconducting magnets operating at field strengths of 7 T [1] and 9 T [2] for human and up to 21 T [3] for animal studies are becoming available, allowing extremely fine spatial resolution and considerably improved signal-to-noise ratios (SNRs). Multichannel low-noise detection electronics coupled with ultrafast signal collection algorithms are paving the way for new sensitive imaging techniques toward observations of highly detailed static morphological features and dynamic markers of physiological events and brain activity.

Various achievements have led to the development of functional MRI (fMRI) methods. The basis of fMRI methods lies in susceptibility of magnetic resonance signal to physiological surrogates of neuronal activity. The most explored, developed, and utilized fMRI method detects tiny changes in magnetic properties of hemoglobin as it transitions between oxygenated to deoxygenated states. This method is aptly called blood-oxygenation-level-dependency (BOLD) fMRI.

Brain activity as represented by synaptic firings is associated with increased energy demands, which under normal conditions are satisfied by way of oxidative glucose metabolism. At the onset of brain activity in a particular region, local feeding arterioles dilate increasing blood flow in downstream capillaries. Although at the no-stimulus baseline all capillaries are already perfused, regional brain activity increases blood flow through the capillaries in an immediate vicinity of active neurons. The amount of oxygen brought by this influx is in excess of what is consumed through oxidative

A.B. Pine, PhD
Cleveland Clinic Lerner College of Medicine, 9500 Euclid Avenue, Cleveland, OH 44195, USA

F.B. Mohamed, PhD (✉)
Department of Radiology, Functional Brain Imaging Center, Temple University School of Medicine, 3401 North Broad Street, Philadelphia, PA 19140–5103, USA
e-mail: feroze@temple.edu

S.H. Faro and F.B. Mohamed (eds.), *Functional BOLD MRI: Principles and Applications*, DOI 10.1007/978-1-4939-1995-6_2, © Springer Science+Business Media New York 2015

glucose metabolism. As a result, overall fraction of oxygenated hemoglobin is increased. In the configuration with bound oxygen, ferrous iron of a heme molecule changes its conformation and becomes progressively more diamagnetic (less paramagnetic) as more oxygen molecules bind. Under the influence of the magnetic field of an MR scanner, diamagnetism of oxygenated hemoglobin (oxyhemoglobin) leads to reduced magnetic susceptibility. The magnetic susceptibility introduces tiny variations to the local magnetic field and affects MR signal relaxation times, most notably T_2 and T_2*. Such dependence may be taken advantage of in fMRI experiments using imaging methods purposefully producing T_2* and T_2 contrasts. Depending on application objectives, relaxation and magnetic resonance-related properties of a target, the gradient-echo formation mechanisms can be used to achieve T_2* contrast, while the spin-echo formation algorithms are employed to produce the T_2-weighted contrast.

Quality and observational value of an fMRI study depend on assortment of parameters and factors prescribed in a form of MR imaging pulse sequences. Such a sequence is a piece of software program that directs the MR scanner's data acquisition system to collect MR signal, which is sensitized to a particular property of a target by a set of instructions within the sequence. These instructions specify appropriate manipulations with magnitude and phase of the sample's bulk magnetization.

It is of particular importance in an MR experiment to achieve a high signal-to-noise (SNR) ratio and tissue, or functional, contrast. Higher SNR is achieved by adjusting pulse sequence parameters to either increase the amount of detected signal or reduce that of concurrent noise. Higher contrast is achieved by sensitizing MR signal to a specific target and, in some cases, by suppressing that of the target's surroundings. Similarly, to gain functional information, for instance in a typical BOLD experiment, type, structure, and timing of a pulse sequence's manipulations are optimized to collect most data when the MR signal related to a studied set of functions is the strongest.

Generation of MR Signal

In a typical imaging experiment, a sample is placed into a strong constant magnetic field, also known as B_0. Interacting with this field, intrinsic magnetic fields of hydrogen nuclei assume precessional motion around the direction of B_0. Precessing nuclei are also called spins. When a sample is placed in such a field, it is *magnetized*. Spins inside the sample become oriented either "parallel" or "antiparallel" in respect with the direction of B_0 (Fig. 2.1a). Those nuclei aligned with B_0 are said to be in the lower energy state, while those oriented in the opposite direction are in the higher energy state. Subjected to Brownian collisions with surroundings and among themselves, spins constantly switch between lower and higher energy states and, thus, along- or against-B_0 orientations. Despite such random interactions, when magnetic fields of individual nuclei are summed together taking their direction into account, there is a small but essential excess of spins aligned with B_0 (in the order of 10^{18} nuclei in 9 g of water). This excess is called *bulk* or *net magnetization* M_0 (Fig. 2.1b) and is essential for the generation of MR signal.

MR signal is generated through cycles of concerted nuclear energy transitions, which occur via absorption/emission of electromagnetic photons. While sufficient to magnetize a sample and build the bulk magnetization, static field B_0 alone is unable to impart synchronized energy transitions or influence the orientation of the bulk magnetization, which remains aligned with B_0 as long as it is the only magnetic field present. To induce energy transitions, a transient *oscillating* magnetic field is applied. The frequency of this field is equal to ("resonates" with) the frequency of spin precession around B_0. This transient oscillating magnetic field is also often referred as radio-frequency (RF) pulse.

When RF pulse interacts with lower energy-state spins, some of them absorb a portion of energy and transition to the higher energy state. A spin that assumed a higher energy state is said to be "excited," and such an RF pulse referred to as an *excitation pulse*. Importantly, excited nuclei

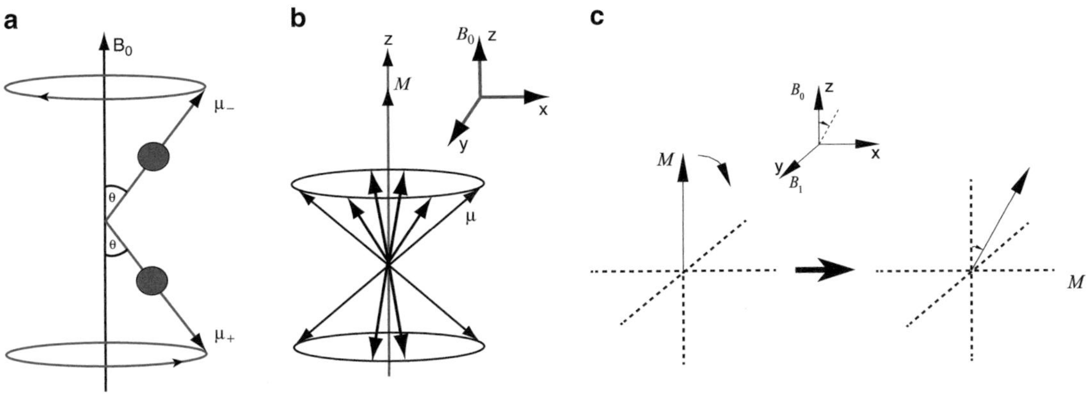

Fig. 2.1 Graphical representation of (**a**) nuclear precession, (**b**) bulk magnetization, (**c**) tipping of bulk magnetization

change their orientation to the "antiparallel" relative to B_0. When a large number of individual spins assume the higher energy state and change their orientation, the orientation of bulk magnetization also changes, since it is the directional sum of orientations of individual nuclei. The strength, duration, and the frequency spectrum of an excitation pulse determine the number of spins entering the higher energy state and assuming the anti-B_0 orientation. This number in turn determines how far the bulk magnetization is rotated away from its longitudinal alignment with B_0 to create the transverse component of the bulk magnetization. Such rotation of bulk magnetization can also be seen as *precessional motion* around the axis of the RF pulse's magnetic field. For example, an RF pulse applied "along *y* axis" rotates the bulk magnetization's vector in the *XZ* plane. The degree of deflection of the bulk magnetization away from B_0 is conventionally expressed as a "flip angle." When the flip angle is 90°, the bulk magnetization immediately after the RF pulse makes the right angle with B_0 and, thus, is fully converted from the *longitudinal* to the *transverse* plane (Fig. 2.1c).

The RF pulse is turned on only for a very brief period of time. When it is turned off, two independent *relaxation* processes act to restore the sample's nuclear equilibrium: the *longitudinal regrowth* and *transverse decay*. The longitudinal component of the magnetization grows back and returns to its B_0-aligned equilibrium state via nuclear interactions among themselves and with surrounding structures. During these interactions spins give up energy and return to the low-energy state. The transverse component of magnetization decays as precessing spins gradually lose coherence by getting out-of-phase with each other and becoming uniformly distributed in the transverse plane leading to no net transverse magnetization. Such loss of coherence occurs due to variations in precessional frequencies of individual spins. Precessional frequency may be affected by interactions between nuclei and impurities encapsulated in the lattice structure. However, interactions among neighboring spins remain the most perturbing factor. All these types of disturbances cause microscopic magnetic field variations from the location occupied by one spin to that with another. Because the rate at which spins precess about B_0 is determined by local magnetic fields, spatial magnetic field variations affect precessional rates of spins. They precess somewhat faster in regions with stronger local fields, while those seeing weaker fields precess slower. As a result, spin coherence breaks down and spins scramble and spread out in the transverse plane in a process called "dephasing." Since the total transverse magnetization is the vector sum of transverse components of all nuclear magnetic fields, the transverse component of the bulk magnetization gradually decreases to zero when individual spins go out of phase with each other and become uniformly distributed in the transverse plane.

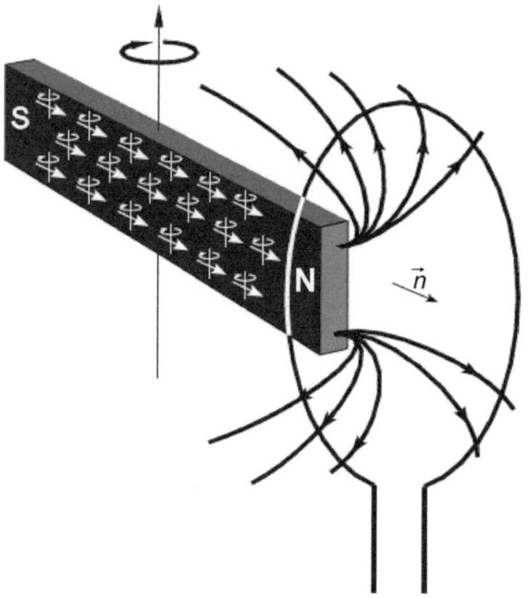

Fig. 2.2 Flux in the coil

Coherently precessing nuclei can be seen as a large magnet (Fig. 2.2). If a wire loop is placed near a sample, a current is induced in the wire every time the magnetization sweeps through the loop's wire. This current is the principal source of the MR signal. The induced current contains a spectrum of frequencies, since it is produced by nuclei precessing at various precessional frequencies.

Beyond the process of excitation/reemission and detection of MR signal, the principle purpose of MR imaging is to build an image of a three-dimensional sample. An image is essentially a spatial representation of a sample's properties, for example water content. The basic principle of spatial localization of MR signal is based on the dependence of the precessional frequency on the strength of magnetic fields that act on individual spins. If a sample is placed into a magnetic field that varies in a known fashion along a single direction, precessional frequencies of spins are changed proportionally at every point of space along that direction, representing a spectrum of precessional frequencies. Spatial distribution of frequencies can be modulated by three *linearly* varying magnetic fields called *gradients*, which are oriented at the right angle to each other. Combined, these fields establish unique three-dimensional spatial dependence of precessional frequencies on position in space. Consequently, MR signal produced by spins subjected to a spatially varying magnetic field contains a spectrum of frequencies. Analyzed for frequency content, the amplitude of MR signal produced by spins at a certain position can be determined. This process known as *spatial-frequency encoding* was first described by Paul Lauterbur, for which he shared the 2003 Nobel Prize in Physiology and Medicine with Sir Peter Mansfield.

The gradients are used to define a three-dimensional *k-space*, in which raw MR signal is *frequency-encoded.* The *k*-space, just as its conventional Euclidean spatial counterpart, is used to localize MR signal. In contrast to the Euclidian space, where the location of each MR signal source is given in terms of its spatial *xyz* coordinates, coordinates of raw frequency-encoded MR signal samples are determined by precessional frequencies, which are in turn are established using gradient fields. These coordinates are known as *k indices*, and together they represent a matrix with MR samples as its elements as shown in Fig. 2.3b, where MR signal samples are represented by solid circles. The *k*-space is filled with MR signal samples acquired in the presences of various combinations of gradients, and therefore, *k*-space indices. After a particular MR signal sample is acquired and recorded into the raw signal matrix, one or more *k*-indices is incremented, and the next MR signal sample is acquired and stored in the successive element of the matrix. The *k*-indices are advanced by changing amplitudes and timing of the gradient fields, and the process continues until the entire *k*-space matrix is filled with MR signal samples. The process of MR signal acquisition and construction of the raw signal matrix is often called the *k-space coverage*. The *k*-space can be covered in a variety of ways. The most typical coverage path utilized in the majority of conventional pulse sequences is the *sequential line-by-line traversal*. This pattern describes the *k*-space coverage, in which the order MR signal samples are placed in the *k*-space diagram appears as a line, as shown by the *green* arrow on the right of Fig. 2.3b.

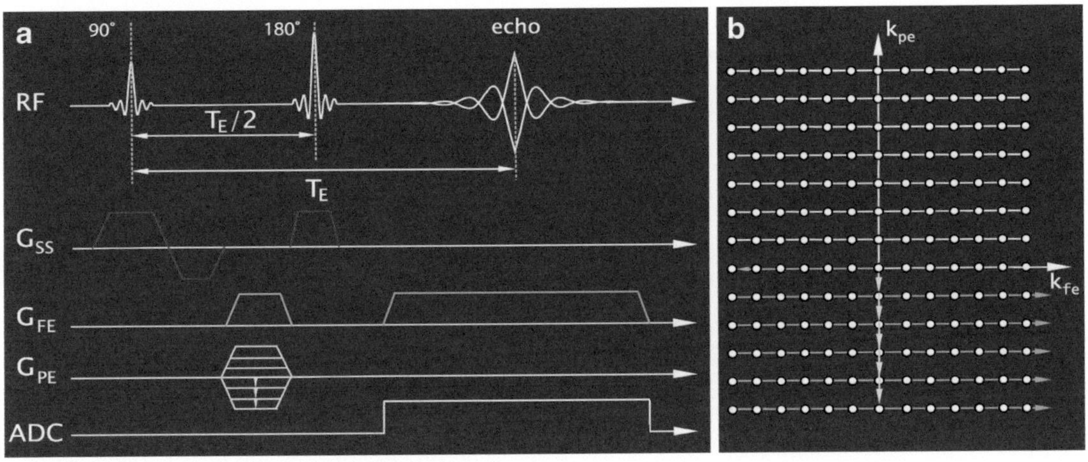

Fig. 2.3 Spin-echo pulse sequence: (**a**) time diagram, (**b**) *k*-space

In order to implement this type of the coverage, one of the gradients (usually phase-encoding, G_{pe}) is turned on for a period of time and with amplitude needed to get the value of the corresponding k_{pe} index advanced to the location of the necessary *k*-space line. Such a move is shown by yellow gradient lobes on the pulse sequence graphics and corresponding arrows in the k-space diagram in Fig. 2.3. At the same time, frequency-encoding gradient is applied to "move" the index k_{fe} along just selected *k*-space line to the location of the matrix element that corresponds to a first-to-be-acquired MR signal sample. This advancement is shown in *light blue color*. In order to conserve imaging time, these two gradients, called *y*- and *x-offset* gradient pulses, are applied simultaneously and immediately after the slice-selective excitation, respectively.

During the signal acquisition period, the detection circuitry and the analog-to-digital converter (ADC) are turned on to receive and digitize the RF signal from the precessing spins. Simultaneously, the frequency encoding gradient is turned on to encode precessional frequencies. The signal is sampled and recorded into elements of the raw MR signal matrix according to the *k*-space indices, which are in turn established by the gradient's amplitude-time product.

Because the signal sampling takes finite time, longitudinal and transverse relaxations may have an effect on MR signal during acquisition and have to be taken into account. In particular, if the time it takes to complete the acquisition of all samples necessary for image reconstruction is comparable with that of T_2, the transverse component of MR signal deteriorates during sampling, rendering MR signal in later-acquired samples negligible. To prevent significant deterioration of MR signal during signal sampling, the coverage of the *k*-space is performed in several iterations, or *segments*. In a typical and the most simple *k*-space coverage, each segment corresponds to a single *k*-space line. MR signal acquisition is completed "along" such a line within a single repetition period. During the acquisition, only one of the *k*-space indices, k_{fe}, is incremented, while the other in-plane index, k_{pe}, is kept constant. When all necessary MR signal samples along the line are acquired, the process moves onto the next iteration that begins with the next excitation RF pulse. This time, the amplitude of the phase encoding gradient is incremented so that the corresponding index k_{pe} is advanced to the next *k*-space line. Further on, the detection circuitry is turned on in the presence of the frequency-encoding gradient, and MR signal is sampled along another *k*-space line.

The conversion of frequency-encoded raw MR signal to its spatially encoded format is performed by a three-dimensional Fourier transformation. Such a process is known as *image reconstruction*.

Spin-Echo and Gradient Echo Imaging Methods

Conventional spin-echo and gradient-echo signal formation algorithms are versatile in producing a number of contrasts for various tissue targets. Spin-echo imaging pulse sequences are used in anatomical studies to produce T_1, T_2, and proton density (PD)-weighted images; gradient-echo imaging pulse sequences are employed in formation of T_2* and T_2 image contrasts, although it is used to render T_1 image contrast as well, especially in higher field strength systems.

Both mechanisms of MR signal formation, spin- and gradient-echo, are sensitive to BOLD-associated microscopic field variations in magnetic susceptibility due to changing blood oxygen content.

Spin-Echo Formation Mechanism

The spin-echo (SE) formation mechanism requires at least two RF pulses. The first pulse is used to deflect the bulk magnetization from its longitudinal orientation into the transverse plane. Without further manipulations following the withdrawal of an RF pulse, nuclei begin to lose their precessional coherence in the transverse plane, and dephase relative to each other, bringing the transverse component of the bulk magnetization and consequently MR signal to naught. Disappearance of coherence following an excitation RF pulse in the absence of any further manipulations with spins is called *free induction decay (FID)*, and it can be recorded as MR signal. In typical SE sequences, however, spin coherence is partly recreated using another RF pulse, and MR signal is recorded as a signal *echo*. MR signal is recorded during echo rather than free induction decay to allow precessing spins become affected by T_1 and T_2 relaxation processes, which are the basis of tissue contrast.

Consider the evolution of transverse magnetization and phases of individual spins as illustrated in Fig. 2.4. At $t = 0$ a 90° RF pulse (magnetic field B_1^y) is applied to the sample along the y axis. As pointed out earlier, this field, like B_0, imparts the precessional motion around itself forcing the bulk magnetization to rotate around the y axis in the XZ plane. At the end of the rotation, the transverse component of the bulk magnetization (M_1) is oriented along the x axis. Upon conclusion of the RF pulse, spins with different precessional frequencies start to progressively deflect from their original orientation along the x axis. If this process continues uninterrupted, the transverse coherence is lost as described earlier. However, a 180° RF pulse applied along the x axis (B_1^x) can partially restore the lost coherence.

The process of how the phase coherence and transverse magnetization are lost and restored to form an echo is illustrated in Fig. 2.4. The two spins, s and f, experience slightly different magnetic fields and, therefore, precess at different frequencies. If the magnetic field in the location occupied by the spin s is weaker than that seen by the spin f, the precessional frequency of the spin s is lower than that of the spin f, and the spin f precesses faster, getting ahead of the spin s. These two spins can be realigned again if the faster-recessing spin f is repositioned behind the spin s, and given a period of time to "catch up" with the slower-precessing spin s. This action is accomplished by applying an RF pulse along the x axis that "flips" the spins on the other half of the transverse plane. This flipping motion is essentially a precession around the x axis in the YZ plane, and can be exerted by a 180° pulse applied along the x axis (Fig. 2.4, *top row*, *center box*). Immediately following such a pulse, the spin that was ahead (f) is now lagging behind the slower one (s) by the same phase angle it has just prior the 180° RF pulse. Following the pulse, the two spins continue to move in the same direction under the influence of B_0, clockwise in the figure, and at the same rates if the magnetic field seen by both spins remains unchanged. The faster spin is eventually going to catch up with the slower one in exactly the same amount of time that elapsed between the two pulses. As the spins get closer to each other, their coherence grows back, and the overall magnetization starts to build up again. Spins become fully aligned, or *refocused* at the moment of time known as *echo time*, which in

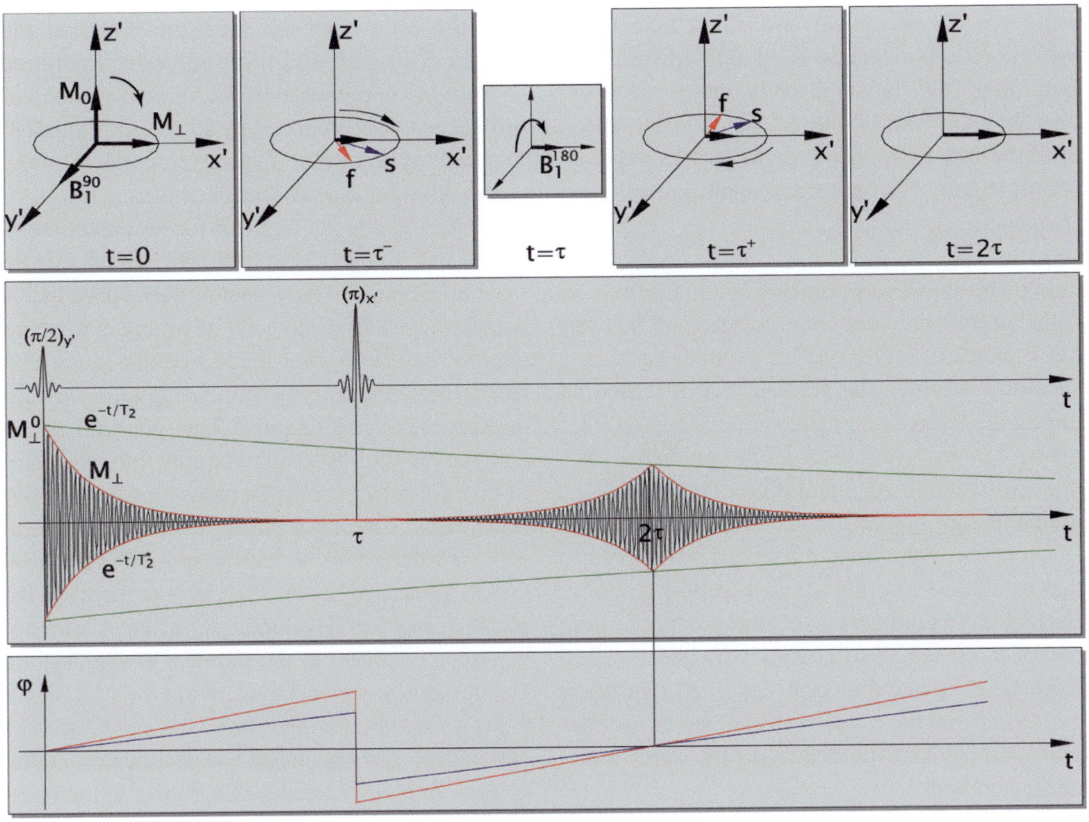

Fig. 2.4 Spin echo: evolution, MR signal, spin phase dynamics

this particular scenario type of the spin echo happens at $T_E = 2\tau$.

As shown in the middle row of Fig. 2.4, the refocusing RF pulse is applied after individual spins have been "scrambled," and most of the transverse magnetization has vanished. The refocusing pulse can be applied even before the transverse magnetization is fully destroyed. In either case, after the refocusing RF pulse, the magnetization grows back gradually.

MR signal recovered at the echo time is only partially restored relative to the amplitude of MR signal immediately following the first RF pulse, as shown in Fig. 2.4. Indeed, complete refocusing of spins is only possible when magnetic fields seen by the two spins, *f* and *s*, do not change over time. In reality, however, magnetic fields in locations of each spin vary slightly over time between the first RF pulse and the echo. Because of random field fluctuations, complete realignment of spins at the echo time is not possible, and the degree of coherence at the echo time is always less than 100%.

A pulse sequence that implements spin-echo signal formation mechanism is shown in Fig. 2.3a. Typically, a 90° excitation RF pulse is applied. There are two excitation regimes, *selective* and *nonselective*, with selectivity referring to the spatial preference of the excitation. The nonselective regime is invoked when no special arrangements are made to associate precessional frequencies of spins with their positions, and applied RF pulse affects all nuclei within the sample. Such a nonselective pulse is called *hard pulse*.

In order to spatially differentiate and act on a subpopulation of nuclei, their precessional frequencies are made position-dependent using gradient fields that vary from one location in space to another in a pattern predetermined by a pulse sequence. Because there is a direct association between local magnetic field and precessional frequency, the latter also becomes position-dependent. If one of the gradients is turned on concurrently with the excitation RF pulse as shown in Fig. 2.4, only nuclei with precessional frequencies matching those in the frequency spectrum of the applied RF pulse "sense" the pulse. The *selective excitation*, as this process is called, is applied when only a portion of the sample's nuclei is needed to be excited, such as a slice or a volume. The gradient that is turned on during the RF pulse is called *slice selection* (G_{ss}) gradient. Two similar *in-plane* gradients, *frequency encoding* (G_{fe}) and *phase encoding* (G_{pe}) gradients, are applied to modulate precessional frequencies in other two directions orthogonal to that established by the slice selection gradient. Each of these gradients associates positions along one of three spatial directions with precessional frequencies in that direction. Such an association permits spatial localization of MR signal sources via assessment of the detected MR signal's frequency content.

In the description of the spin-echo formation mechanism and the corresponding pulse sequence, it was presumed that the center of the acquisition window coincides with the center of the *k*-space line. The center of the *k*-space line corresponds to an MR signal sample that has only been partially encoded with spatial information, as one of indices, namely k_{fe}, is zero. The center of the acquisition window is taken as a point of time when the phase dispersion created by offset gradients is fully compensated by the rephasing lobe of the readout gradient. Only in this case does it become possible to fully eliminate the phase dispersion accrued due to fixed local field inhomogeneities. Indeed, if the first half of the read-out (frequency-encoding) gradient lasts exactly as long as the *x*-offset gradient and has the same amplitude, the phase imparted by the gradients is zero in the center of the acquisition window. On the contrary, the phase dispersion developed due to fixed local field inhomogeneities between the excitation and refocusing pulses is nullified by the rephasing pulse to form what was described as the spin echo. Therefore, when the echo time coincides with the center of the *k*-space line, with all other sources of the phase aberrations compensated, the overall phase disturbance is only imposed by irreversible random fluctuations due to the T_2 relaxation that is solely responsible for overall image contrast.

However, it is not required for the echo time to match the moment when the MR signal sample that corresponds to the center of the *k*-space line is acquired. The spin echo can be arranged to occur slightly before or after that particular sample by respectively moving the refocusing pulse toward or away the excitation pulse. The spin echo is then also moved with it, as it invariably trails the refocusing pulse by exactly the same time as the latter follows the excitation pulse. Such an offset spin echo is referred to as the *asymmetric spin echo* (ASE). No longer in an ASE pulse sequence is the phase dispersion developed out of local inhomogeneities balanced at the moment of passing the *k*-space line's center, thus leaving the MR signal slightly dephased at that time. Since it is the very MR signal sample located in the center of the *k*-space line that contributes the most to the overall image contrast, the magnetic susceptibility effects will be reflected in the final image. Therefore, besides T_2 contrast, an additional T_2* weighting is introduced into MR signal, thus making the ASE pulse sequence more sensitive to the BOLD effect.

It is possible, regardless of the echo position in the acquisition window, to cover several lines in a single iteration. The corresponding pulse sequence diagram is shown in Fig. 2.5. This sequence collects MR signal in a train of echoes by having a manifold of refocusing pulses applied to redirect spin dynamics multiple times after a single excitation pulse. Each echo is formed for different *k*-space line. The first echo is generated the same way a single spin echo is formed. At the end of the acquisition period, a *rewinder* gradient is applied in the phase-encoding direction that cancels the effect of the preceding phase-encoding gradient. This operation essentially resets the k_{pe} index back to zero. Following the first echo, spins are allowed to continue to dephase. At some point into the dephasing process another 180° refocusing pulse is transmitted.

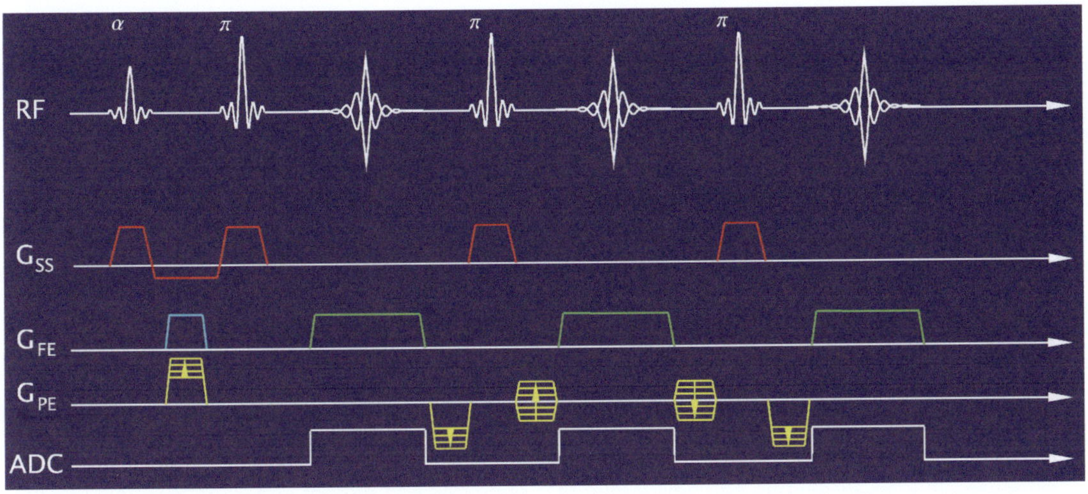

Fig. 2.5 Fast spin-echo timing diagram

The effect of this pulse on spins is exactly the same as that of the original refocusing pulse: it swaps around faster and slower precessing spins. Immediately after the refocusing pulse another phase-encoding gradient is applied. This time its amplitude is set to advance the k_{pe} to a different k-space line. The number of formed echoes and, thus, the number of covered k-space lines is given as *echo train length* (ETL). Several echoes can be generated following a single RF excitation pulse before T_2 relaxation introduces a significant effect. Although there are multiple variations of a multiecho acquisition scheme, such an arrangement is generally referred as *turbo* spin-echo pulse sequence because it greatly reduces the acquisition time.

When the entire raw signal matrix is completed for the selected slice, the process is started anew either to acquire and average more signal for the same slice or to proceed on to another slice.

Contrast Characteristics of Spin-Echo Sequences

Vascular Effects

As mentioned earlier, spin echo is formed by restoring spin coherence and bulk magnetization using a "refocusing" pulse that brings out-of-phase spins back in phase with each other. If the precessional frequency of a particular spin is fixed throughout the acquisition, the phase angle acquired by this spin before a refocusing pulse can be entirely balanced out by the phase displacement accumulated after the refocusing pulse. Spin coherence and bulk magnetization can only be fully restored if precessional frequencies of all spins remain constant throughout the repetition period. In reality, however, the precessional frequency of spins constantly experiences tiny variations that are largely imparted by diffusion. A diffusing water molecule drifts randomly through spatially varying magnetic field modulated by several physical factors, including magnetic susceptibility caused by the BOLD effect.

The degree to which diffusion influences spin-echo MR signal depends on the spatial range of inhomogeneities compared to the distance traveled by a water molecule during acquisition period. If a magnetic field varies significantly only over distances that are far larger than the distance traveled by a water molecule, it is likely that nuclear spins of this molecule would experience similar magnetic field before and following the refocusing pulse. In this case, the spin echo is fully or nearly fully refocused, and MR signal carries little or only a negligible imprint of field inhomogeneities. Conversely, a spin is bound to experience varying magnetic field if a distance it travels during acquisition is larger than the spatial scale of inhomogeneities. In this case, its precessional frequency is unlikely to remain constant, thus contributing to incomplete refocusing and attenuated MR signal.

A water molecule diffuses about 20 μm in 100 ms, which is the typical acquisition time. In the vicinity of vessels larger than 20 μ(mu)m in diameter, a water molecule spends a relatively longer period of time in the same field than in the vicinity of smaller vessels and capillaries measuring 10 to 20 μ(mu)m in diameter, where a spin experiences a varying field. Consequently, spin echo from spins located near smaller vessels and capillaries is refocused to a lesser degree, and MR signal is relatively weaker. For capillaries with a lumen diameter below 10 μ(mu)m, phase dispersion is even stronger as water molecules diffuse through larger field variations. However, in this case the *average* phase dispersion encountered by spins is very similar, as it is more likely that they experience the same field variations and, therefore, accumulate similar, if not the same, phase angle over the acquisition period. That the phase angle remains the same or nearly the same means that within-acquisition spin coherence is maintained. Therefore, spin-echo MR signal coming from areas of very small vessels, namely less than 5 μ(mu)m in diameter, is comparable to that acquired near the largest vessels, and dips to its minimum around vessels that measure about 20 μ(mu)m in diameter. Owing to such a bell-shaped dependence of spin-echo MR signal on the vessel size, spin-echo sequences are desirable to use in BOLD experiments, as spin-echo MR signal is sensitized to BOLD-related oxy/deoxygenation exchanges that occur in capillaries.

Flow Effects

MR signal formed in spin-echo sequences is sensitive to inflow effects. Inflow effects refer to variations in MR signal secondary to blood flow rather than BOLD effect. Inflow can affect MR signal when blood flowing from regions not exposed to an excitation pulse brings undisturbed spins into the volume with exited spins. Undisturbed spins that enter the imaging volume between excitation and refocusing RF pulses are exposed only to the latter RF pulse. This RF pulse acts as intended for excited spins restoring transverse coherence. However, this is the first pulse seen by fresh washed-in spins, and as such, it acts to excite them. Excited washed-in spins are not likely to substantially contribute to MR signal during the current excitation–reemission cycle because they do not get refocused. The MR signal contribution from a portion of spins excited within the imaging volume, but washed out by incoming blood before the refocusing pulse was applied, is also insignificant, since it remained dephased and did not undergo the refocusing outside the selected volume.

The actual number of spins leaving and entering the imaging volume depends on timing characteristics of the sequence, size, and position of the selected imaging volume and blood flow velocity. If the time between the excitation and refocusing pulses is relatively short, a smaller number of excited spins is replaced by fresh ones, and the MR signal is suppressed to a lesser degree. From another perspective, the time between the two pulses is equal to half of the echo time. Therefore, it is optimal to keep the echo time short enough to reduce inflow-induced MR signal loss but long enough to collect a sufficient amount of the MR signal with BOLD contrast. It was shown that such an optimal echo time is on the order of the T_2 relaxation time of a tissue under examination [4].

Since the echo time is usually much shorter than the repetition time for the spin-echo sequences, the inflow-induced MR signal suppression would become significant only for relatively high flow velocities, which do not typically occur in the capillaries and small venulae, which are the primary source of the BOLD contrast.

Gradient Echo Formation Mechanism

A refocusing RF pulse is essential for the spin-echo formation, as it restores phase coherence and leads to the reappearance of transverse magnetization and MR signal. However, the rephasing action and refocusing effect of an RF pulse can also be achieved using gradient fields to modulate spin phase. The MR signal is then recovered in the form of a *gradient echo* generated only through gradient reversals.

In a system with four spins, as shown in Fig. 2.6, a gradient field makes spins in the north half precess slower than those in the south half.

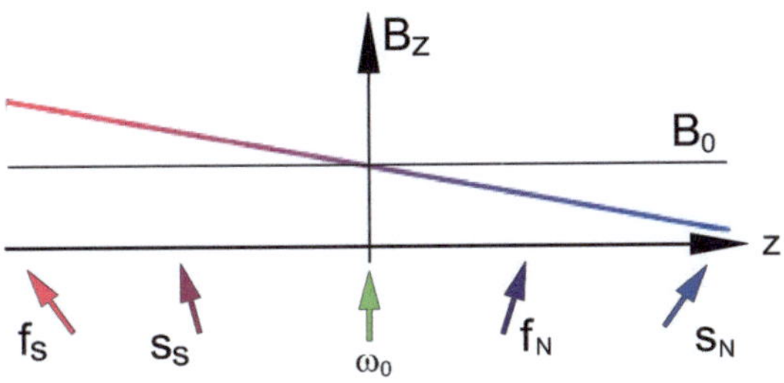

Fig. 2.6 The gradient field and its effect on precessional frequencies

Indeed, when an additional gradient field is superimposed on the static B_0, the two south spins experience higher than B_0 field, and they precess slightly faster in regard to a spin unaffected by the gradient field (shown in the center). Of these two south spins, the one closer to the center of the field, s_s, precesses at a rate slower than f_s because the field deviation at the location of the former spin is smaller, and its precessing frequency is closer to that of the unaffected spin. Similarly, for the north half, where the magnetic field is weaker than B_0, spins precess generally slower than in the south half, with the one further from the center of the field, s_N, precessing slower than the f_N spin. With such a dependence on the gradient field, the concept of gradient echo can be explained phenomenologically and graphically as illustrated in Fig. 2.7.

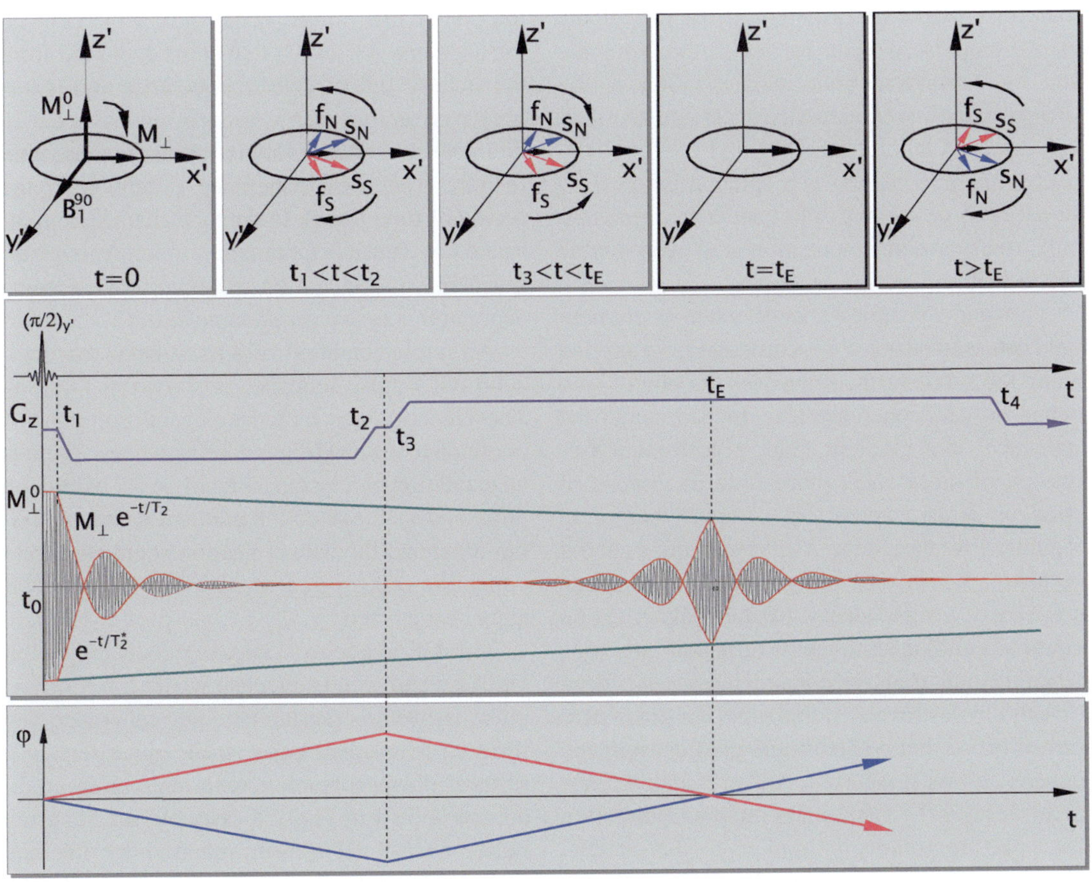

Fig. 2.7 Gradient echo: evolution, MR signal, spin phase dynamics

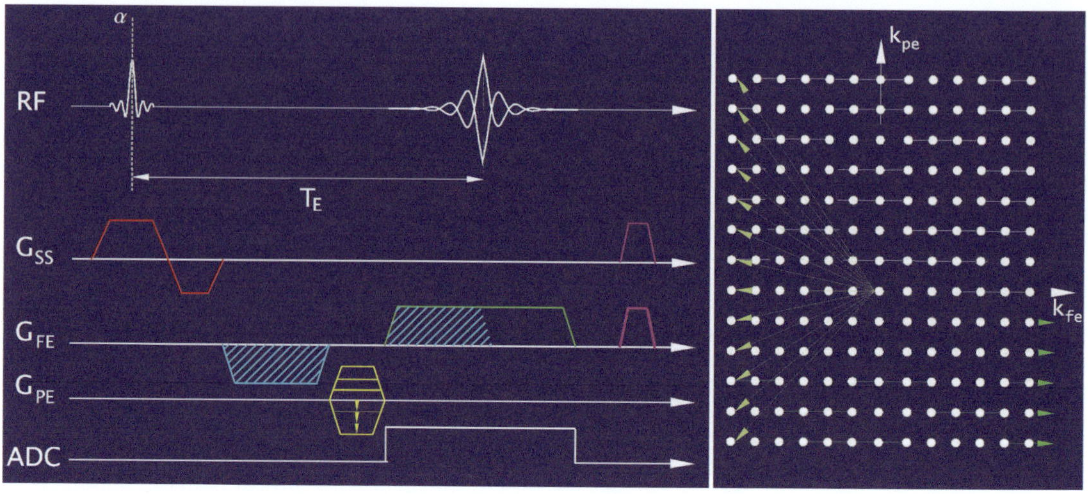

Fig. 2.8 Gradient echo timing diagram

An excitation RF pulse applied at $t = 0$ converts the longitudinal magnetization into the transverse plane. Immediately at the end of the excitation pulse all spins precess at the same rate and the transverse bulk magnetization is the strongest. However, naturally occurring spatially varying field inhomogeneities and energy dissipating interactions between spins affect precessional rates destroying spin coherence, reducing bulk transverse magnetization and recoverable MR signal.

The spin dynamics change when a gradient field is turned on at $t = t_1$. A gradient field applied along the z axis further increases the rate of spin dephasing and coherence loss. Indeed, under the influence of a gradient field, precessional frequency of those spins that reside in regions of stronger fields exceeds that of spins located in regions of weaker fields. As a result, spins get out of phase. Because of the general loss of phase coherence, a rapid decay of the magnetization continues until the gradient is turned off at $t = t_2$, when the bulk transverse magnetization has been essentially destroyed. At this time, the gradient is turned off so that no additional gradient-induced coherence loss is incurred. At $t = t_3$ another gradient field of the same magnitude and direction but opposite polarity is applied to the sample. This gradient field forces previously fast-moving spins to slow down and assume precessional frequency of the spins that were earlier trailing during the dephasing period. In a similar manner, the previously slow-moving spins are now "chasing" those that moved faster during the dephasing segment. Assuming that spins dephased from the state of full transverse coherence and ignoring irrecoverable energy-dissipating losses due to interactions between spins, spins rephase and recreate transverse coherence exactly after the period of time it took to dephase them. The reinstated coherence is tantamount to a restored bulk transverse magnetization and, thus, newly formed echo, in this case a *gradient echo*.

An implementation of a most basic gradient-echo (GE) pulse sequence is shown in Fig. 2.8. The GE sequence includes several components common to all imaging pulse sequences. There is an excitation block consisting of an RF excitation pulse and a slice selection gradient with a rephasing lobe, and the data collection segment during which the echo is generated and associated MR signal is detected.

The GE sequence lacks a refocusing pulse. Unlike a spin-echo sequence where a refocusing pulse is used to reestablish spin coherence and form an MR signal echo, a GE pulse sequence restores phase coherence with alternating gradients as shown in Fig. 2.8. Without a refocusing pulse, overall RF power released by the coil and absorbed by tissues during gradient-echo sequence execution is reduced, making gradient-echo sequence safer. Reduced energy deposition in GE sequences is especially salient when performed in higher field strength scanners (3 Tesla and up), where substantial amounts of RF energy are required to perturb longitudinal equilibrium magnetization. Reduction of RF energy emission allows one to pack more RF pulses closer together and, therefore, speed up signal acquisition without exceeding established *specific absorption rate* (SAR) limits.

The absence of a refocusing pulse affects sensitivity of gradient-echo sequences to magnetic field inhomogeneities. The main effect of a refocusing RF pulse is cancellation of phase angles accumulated by dephasing spins. Therefore, a spin-echo sequence is inherently insensitive to MR signal contributions from *fixed* inhomogeneities. On the contrary, because it lacks a refocusing pulse, a GE sequence is sensitive to field inhomogeneities and magnetic susceptibilities. Overall phase change introduced by gradients themselves by the echo time is zero, since a phase change during the dephasing segment is offset by the opposite phase change during the rephasing segment. However, any amount of spin phase advanced or retarded due to factors other than gradients fields, such as effects of sample-related magnetic susceptibilities, remain uncompensated at the echo time. This is because neither refocused nor compensated, phase angles continue to develop through the entire echo formation period and, thus, are nonzero at the echo time, effectively reducing the MR signal.

GE sequences are generally shorter than SE sequences. Timing parameters of a pulse sequence are determined by the duration of individual components of the sequence such as RF pulses, signal detection periods, and gradients. The amount of phase angle imparted by a gradient is determined by its amplitude-time product: stronger gradients need less time to impart a given phase angle. Since spin coherence in GE sequence is achieved by nullifying spin phase changes with gradient reversals, the repetition time T_R can be made shorter by using stronger but shorter gradients. While shorter gradients help reduce the overall sequence run time, transverse spin coherence is given less time to die down at the end of the signal detection period and before an excitation pulse of the next repetition period is applied. Such lingering transverse magnetization may persist through and contribute to signal echoes formed in subsequent repetition periods. However, such contributions may not be desired because persisting transverse magnetizations with imprints of relaxation processes and gradient-induced phase accumulated over several repetition periods may lead to unwanted mixing of signal echoes with various relaxation and gradient weightings, and ultimately result in imaging artifacts and reduction of MR signal.

There are two ways to mitigate unwanted effects of lingering transverse magnetization on MR signal echoes. One approach uses either additional gradient fields ("spoilers") alone or coupled with quasi-random flip angle RF pulses to *irreversibly* scramble remaining bulk transverse magnetization components at the end of the repetition period [5]. In this case, only the longitudinal component contributes to fresh bulk transverse magnetization during the next repetition period. Alternatively, the net phase change imparted by gradient fields can be eliminated if transverse components of the bulk magnetization at the end of the repetition period are brought back to the orientation they occupied immediately after the excitation pulse. In this case, there is no gradient-induced phase dispersion, and MR signal only carries imprints of tissue-specific relaxation properties. The most trivial pulse sequence, in which gradient-induced phase changes are compensated in one of three gradient directions using a gradient with an opposite polarity is shown in Fig. 2.9. The new gradient has the same magnitude as the initial phase encoding gradient field but applied in the opposite direction, and acts to compensate the phase change introduced by the initial phase-encoding gradient step. Full refocused transverse magnetization is attained by rendering zero the net phase change along all three directions. This approach is implemented in the pulse sequence shown in Fig. 2.10. Such a sequence contains a train of equally spaced RF pulses and gradient structures balancing phase in all three directions. Having phase of the transverse magnetization at the end of the repetition period restored to its prepulse value improves overall transverse coherence and preserves signal-to-noise ratio while maintaining

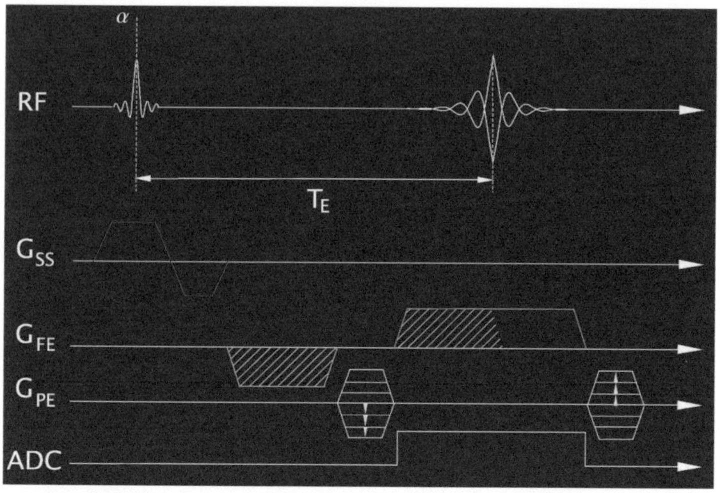

Fig. 2.9 FISP pulse sequence timing diagram

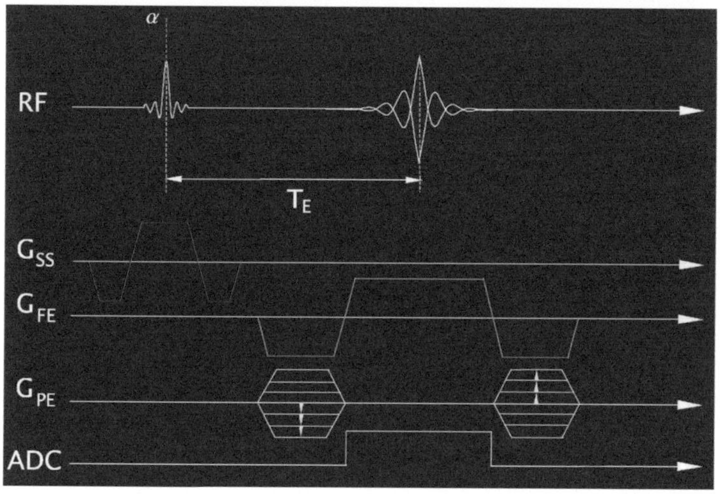

Fig. 2.10 trueFISP pulse sequence timing diagram

the repetition time in the order of few milliseconds. It has been showed that such balanced sequences are capable of recovering strong BOLD signal [6].

Contrast Characteristics of Gradient Echo Sequences

Vascular Effects

As in the case with SE pulse sequences, microscopic phase variation experienced by diffusing water molecules as they randomly move through magnetic field inhomogeneities established by nearby vessels affect GE MR signal. If the spatial extent of field variations created by venules span distances larger than a diffusing molecule travels on average, it experiences very similar fields at any point of its trajectory. Without a refocusing pulse to balance out the accumulated phase, the average phase displacement acquired by molecules due to offset fields linearly increases as a function of time, and is not compensated at the end of the acquisition period leading to weakened MR signal. When water molecules traverse fields with spatial extent comparable to average length of their trajectory, phase offsets gained by water molecules are very similar, and therefore, the range of phase offsets is minimal. In this case, a majority of spins accumulate similar phase angles and their average phase dispersion is minimal, keeping relatively strong spin coherence and, therefore, MR signal in the vicinity of small vessels. Relative insensitivity of GE MR signal to field variation around small vessels contrasts with that of SE echo MR signal, which is sensitive to diffusion effects occurring around small capillaries.

Inflow Effects

As in the case of SE pulse sequences, MR signal recovered as GE echo is sensitive to blood flow effects, which can confound BOLD contributions to MR signal. GE MR signal from vessels generally appears higher than that from stationary surrounding tissues. This is caused by the condition called *signal saturation.*

A rapid succession of excitation RF pulses can reduce the amount of recoverable MR signal from stationary tissues. Each RF excitation pulse brings a portion of longitudinal magnetization into the transverse plane. If the time between RF pulses is shorter than that needed for the full recovery of the longitudinal magnetization, each subsequent RF pulse acts on smaller longitudinal magnetization than the previous one. On the contrary, since the flip angle is kept constant, each RF pulse brings the same portion of the longitudinal magnetization into the transverse plane. After a series of RF pulses the amount of longitudinal magnetization available for the transfer into the transverse plane is significantly reduced. This portion is determined by the duration between two RF pulses, the flip angle of RF pulses, and relaxation characteristics of tissues. Reduced prepulse longitudinal magnetization translates into smaller postpulse transverse magnetization, which in turn leads to reduced amount of available MR signal from stationary tissues. The signal is said to be saturated. On the contrary, fresh blood spins entering an imaging slice are not saturated at all because they did not experience all previous excitations. Upon entering the imaging volume, spins within flowing blood become slightly saturated as they pass through it. Since less saturated spins are capable of returning higher MR signal than more saturated, MR signal coming from blood appears hyperintense compared with that from more saturated stationary tissues.

The degree of saturation sustained by blood spins depends on blood flow velocity, the repetition interval (T_R), and the flip angle of RF pulses. MR signal increases when a sufficient number of unsaturated spins enter an imaging slice over several T_R periods. In the case of the relatively short T_R or fast blood flow, MR signal from blood increases due to partial desaturation with fresh spins. However, the longer the T_R period, the greater number of saturated spins recover and contribute to the prepulse longitudinal magnetization decreasing the degree of saturation. Increased prepulse longitudinal magnetization leads to higher MR signal from stationary tissues and diminished contrast between stationary tissues and blood. In the case of relatively slower blood flow such as capillary flux, the transit time is reduced and blood spins that entered the imaging slice experience a relatively larger number of RF pulses, also becoming more saturated. In this case, the contrast between stationary tissues and blood is also reduced.

Echo Planar Imaging Methods

Generic gradient echo sequence displayed in Fig. 2.8 acquires n MR signal samples per an excitation period. In order to create an $n \times n$-pixel image, the acquisition has to be repeated n times [7]. Even though gradient-echo sequences discussed so far can be used to detect gross BOLD-related MR signal, originated from areas capable of producing a relatively robust signal, such as visual or motor cortices, they are proved to be unfittingly sluggish to adequately resolve rather fine BOLD effects elicited by swift subtle cognitive and behavioral processes.

A pulse sequence tailored for imaging of physiological markers of transient events and processes would acquire MR signal needed to reconstruct the entire image in the shortest time possible, while lasting sufficiently long to

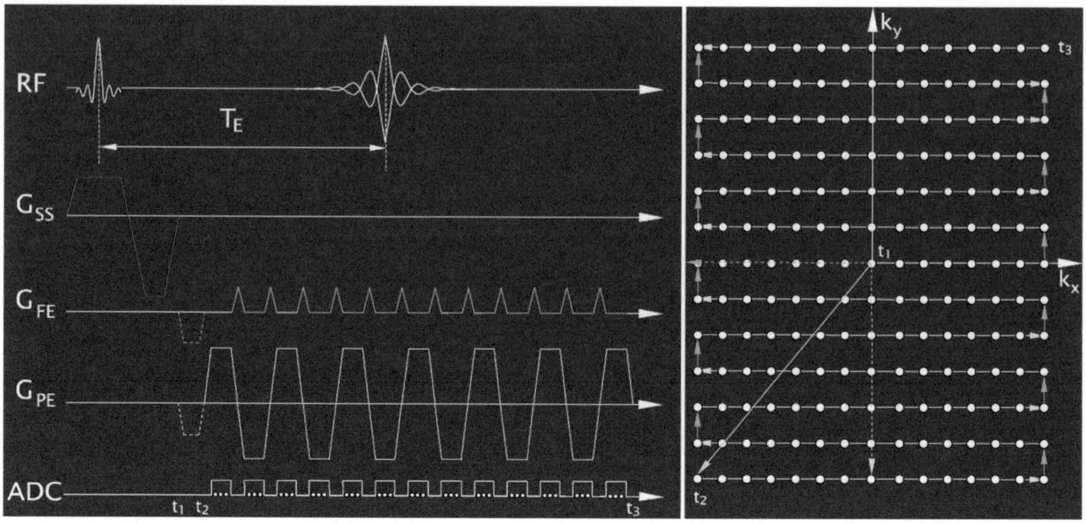

Fig. 2.11 EPI pulse sequence timing diagram

capture an imprint of BOLD-inducing factors in MR signal. The demand for higher temporal resolution necessitates very rapid MR signal sampling. The shortest acquisition time is attained when all MR signal samples needed to reconstruct an entire image are acquired following a single excitation pulse. The group of imaging methods that acquire all required MR signal samples and fill the entire *k*-space in a single passing make up a class of *echo planar imaging* (EPI) techniques.

It is noteworthy to mention that even though EPI methods belong to a distinct class of imaging techniques, they are neither based on nor establish entirely new acquisition principles. EPI pulse sequences use the same echo-formation mechanisms as spin- or gradient-echo methods to collect all MR signal samples following a single RF pulse, thus offering a drastic improvement in acquisition time.

EPI Imaging Pulse Sequences

A generic EPI pulse sequence follows the design shown in Fig. 2.11. Initially a pair of gradients is applied in both the phase and frequency-encoding directions to advance to the first sample point of the first *k*-space line. Then an oscillatory gradient is applied along the frequency-encoding direction so that the train of echoes is generated, each for every gradient lobe, positive or negative. Such a waveform of the read-out gradient establishes alternating directions of traversing read-out lines, while brief phase-encoding gradient pulses move from one *k*-space line to another in the phase-encoding direction. Such waveforms of the phase- and frequency-encoding gradients draw the *zigzag k*-space trajectory shown in the right of Fig. 2.11. Each echo is produced in the same fashion as the gradient echo using a bipolar dephasing-rephasing gradient structure. Even though an echo is formed during each gradient lobe, only the central or *primary* echo, where the net gradient encoding is zero in both phase and frequency-encoding directions, is taken to calculate the echo time. This is because MR signal gained during this echo is the largest and determines the image contrast.

The greatest challenge in the design of EPI sequences is imposed by the effect of the intrinsic decay owing to the T_2* relaxation that accounts for MR signal dropout across the entire image. Indeed, every MR signal echo is attenuated by the signal decay during the acquisition, including that acquired during the central echo. Since this echo determined the image contrast, the overall signal dropout is determined by the amount of the MR signal lost to the T_2* relaxation at this echo. Thus, the effective T_E assigned to the time of the primary echo defines the overall loss of the MR signal.

The extent of MR signal dropout depends on the T_2*-relaxation decay profile. The amount of T_2*-induced spin dephasing during the acquisition is determined by the position of the primary echo relative to the RF pulse. The further in time the primary echo is, the stronger is BOLD-induced spin phase offset. On the contrary, if the primary echo is timed too far away from the RF pulse, MR signal is destroyed by inhomogeneities.

In EPI sequences, all MR signal samples are obtained within a single acquisition window that may last up to 200 ms. The length of the acquisition window determines the amount of the image blurring caused by T_2* relaxation. In the beginning of the acquisition window, the loss of coherence due to T_2* relaxation is minimal since little time elapsed after the RF pulse. During the acquisition spins progressively dephase acquiring the imprint of the T_2* relaxation, some of which is induced by the BOLD effect. Therefore, during the acquisition MR signal is modulated by T_2* decay, which can be large enough to cause significant differences between magnitude of MR signal samples acquired in the beginning and the end of the acquisition window. This variation causes image blurring. In order to mitigate blurring, the length of the acquisition window is shortened. It may be accomplished by faster sampling of MR signal. The contrariety of the faster sampling is reduced image signal-to-noise ratio. Alternatively, the length of the acquisition window can be abridged by lowering the image resolution. In this case, the number of MR samples acquired during each echo is reduced, and the acquisition window is shortened. For the same field-of-view coverage with lower resolution, in-plane voxel size has to be increased, which leads to a larger number of spins in each voxel. With more spins in each voxel, per-voxel MR signal and SNR is higher. On the contrary, degree of intravoxel inhomogeneity within a larger voxel is also higher since leading to a wider spectrum of precessional frequencies and, therefore, faster T_2* relaxation. Faster T_2* allows for shorter T_E to maintain the SNR. On the contrary, T_E has to be long enough to let MR signal accumulate sufficient imprint of the BOLD effect.

There are several EPI pulse sequence designs. The sequence shown in Fig. 2.11 is *gradient echo-recalled* EPI since it employs gradient-echo formation mechanism to produce MR signal. This is the most commonly used imaging method in functional neuroimaging applications and research due to several reasons. MR signal generated by this type of EPI sequence design carries robust T_2* contrast even though some amount of the T_2 weighting is inevitably present due to overall irreversible transverse decay. Prevailing T_2*-weighted contrast component is due to sensitivity of the GE echo-formation mechanism to local field inhomogeneities. Gradient-recalled EPI sequences are very appropriate for collection of BOLD-related MR signal changes sought in the functional imaging because the nature of the BOLD contrast is rooted in tiny field inhomogeneities imparted by variations in oxy/deoxyhemoglobin-induced blood susceptibility.

Similar to generic gradient-echo sequences, flip angles smaller than 90° can be used in gradient-recalled EPI designs without suffering large MR signal losses. The smaller flip angle makes it possible to shorten the T_R period, as less time is needed to restore the original longitudinal relaxation. Alternatively, a larger number of slices can be covered over the same T_R period. The optimal flip angle at which the gradient-echo generated MR signal reaches its maximum, the *Ernst angle*, can be calculated to provide the best contrast possible [7].

The EPI spatial encoding mechanism can be used to form spin echoes by placing all necessary gradient structures following an excitation and refocusing RF pulses as shown in Fig. 2.12. The contrast-defining properties of a spin-echo recalled EPI sequence are similar to those of a regular spin-echo pulse sequence. In particular, even though spin-echo pulse sequences appear to be most susceptible to inhomogeneities imparted by small capillaries, overall image contrast generated by this pulse sequence shows relatively little sensitivity to field inhomogeneities.

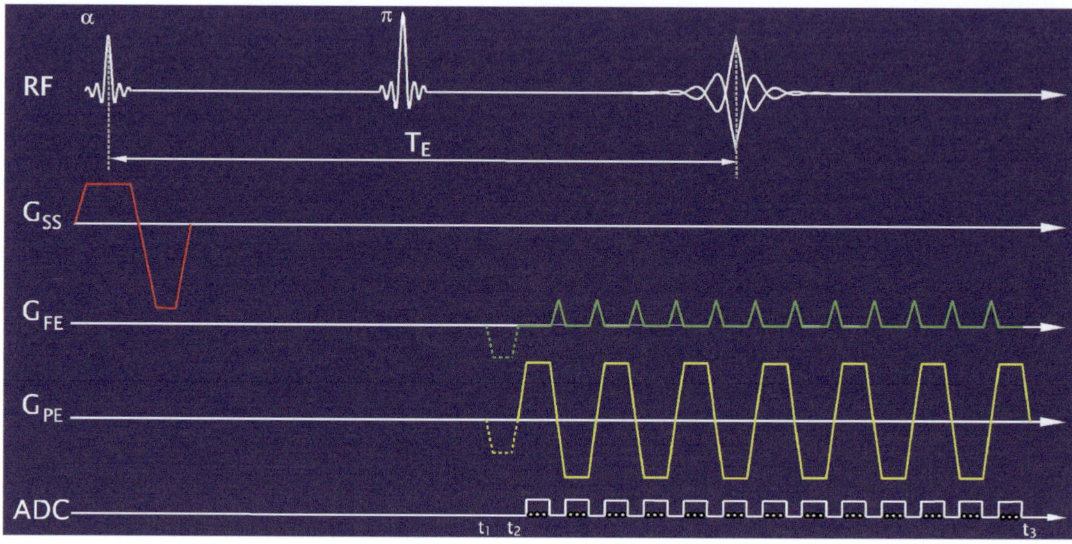

Fig. 2.12 Spin-echo EPI pulse sequence timing diagram

Somewhat more sensitive to BOLD-related changes is an *asymmetric spin-echo* sequence. A key feature that differentiates such a sequence from a typical spin-echo pulse sequence is the temporal misalignment between the *k*-space center and the central echo. Such a mismatch is usually achieved by advancing the refocusing pulse and EPI MR signal collection structures towards the excitation pulse. In this case, there is a certain amount of T_2* dephasing present at the moment of the contrast-defining central echo of the EPI readout echo train, thus imprinting BOLD-related inhomogeneities into MR signal contrast.

Spiral Echo Planar Imaging Methods

EPI sequences are used to collect all necessary MR signal samples needed to reconstruct an image following a single excitation pulse. Specific designs of EPI sequences depend on what trajectory is chosen to cover the *k*-space [8]. One of the trajectories proven effective in the implementation of fast imaging technique and producing relatively high BOLD-related SNR resembles a *spiral,* as shown in Fig. 2.13. A pulse sequence that utilizes such a trajectory is, thus, called *spiral* EPI pulse sequence. These sequences have been found effective in cardiovascular, renal [9, 10] and multiple functional brain imaging studies [11, 12]. Imaging with spiral algorithms excels in these applications because of its

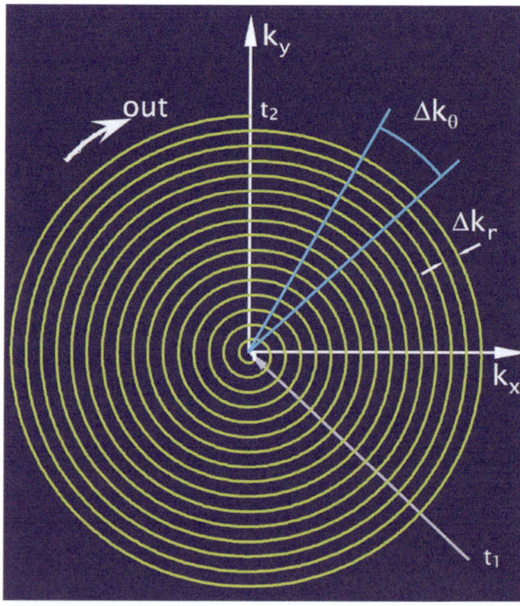

Fig. 2.13 *k*-Space diagram of spiral EPI sequence

relatively low sensitivity to motion and flow, and efficient use of gradient power [13]. The spiral sequences do not constitute a whole new class of imaging methods. Rather, they should be considered as a subset of EPI techniques because of many similarities between their designs, including collection of the MR signal corresponding to a large portion of the *k*-space with time-varying gradients following a single excitation pulse.

The simplest type of the spiral trajectory is so-called *Archimedean spiral*, although many other shapes of spiral trajectories exist. For instance, to reduce physiologic noise effects, the vicinity of the *k*-space center is often oversampled by implementing a larger number of windings around the *k*-space's center, thus increasing the coverage density and fidelity of MR signal. To achieve an optimal density throughout the *k*-space, and keep acquisition time from growing long, varying sampling density spiral trajectories were proposed [14].

There are two ways to follow the spiral, from the center to the periphery of the *k*-space (spiral-out) and in the opposite direction (spiral-in). The spiral-out pulse sequence traverses the *k*-space center in the beginning of the acquisition period and, therefore, obtains the contrast-defining echo immediately following the excitation pulse. In such a design, there is very short time to develop an appreciable imprint of the T_2* relaxation; the FID signal is strong and any motion did not have enough time to have an impact on the spatial encoding. On the contrary, following the spiral in the opposite direction, from the periphery to the *k*-space center, leads to accumulation of the T_2* relation imprint that sensitizes the image contrast to the field inhomogeneities.

Each of these traversals has benefits and limitations that should be considered in the context of a specific application. In cardiac imaging, for example, where motion and flow artifacts could be severe, a pulse sequence capable to limit contributions thereof to MR signal is advantageous. Therefore, the spiral-out design is more desirable in cardiac and abdominal studies. On the contrary, if the contrast-defining primary echo comes too soon after the excitation pulse, BOLD-induced phase offsets are negligible, thus limiting their effect on the MR signal. Therefore, in BOLD studies, the *spiral-in* pulse sequences are preferred.

There is, however, a significant drawback associated with such a design. Namely, if the entire *k*-space is sampled over a single trajectory, overall MR signal may experience considerable T_2* decay leading to decreased SNR. The solution to this particular predicament is to split the acquisition into several parts, covering the *k*-space in segments, so that the last echo appears earlier but still at the end of the acquisition period. This approach reduces nonuniformity effects and increases the SNR. However, cardiac motion and respiration give rise to undesirable image-to-image variations.

Several pulse-sequence designs were proposed to accommodate the better of two traversals. For instance, one of the designs is a two-segment acquisition that includes the spiral-in segment followed by the spiral-out portion. In this case both echoes, at the end of the spiral-in segment and at the beginning of the spiral-out portion occur one after the other. MR signal collected during the leading spiral-in section is not severely decayed but still reflects T_2* relaxation. MR signal recovered in the consecutive spiral-out segment does not experience any substantial inhomogeneity effects and returns strong SNR. The two *k*-space segments covered in both segments are later combined and transformed into the image. Such an image can reflect BOLD imprint while sustaining sufficient MR signal magnitude without substantial degradation due to the T_2* relaxation.

Conclusion

In summary, this chapter gives an overview of the various pulse sequences that currently are used today in fMRI BOLD imaging, as well as their characteristics (see Table 2.1 for summary of important scanning method articles). The appropriate choice of the pulse sequence and its optimal parameters are key factors in maximizing the BOLD signal for every fMRI experiment performed.

Table 2.1 Key articles of scanning methods

Authors	Article title	Significance
Oppelt et al. 1986 [5]	FISP: a new fast MRI sequence. Electromedica 1986;54:15–18.	First paper to demonstrate FISP sequence.
Bandettini et al. 1994 [4]	Spin-echo and gradient-echo epi of human brain activation using bold contrast: a comparative study at 1.5 T. NMR Biomed. 1994;7:12–20.	The paper compared the flow effects on SE and GRE BOLD signal.
Noll et al. 1995 [11]	Spiral K-space MR imaging of cortical activation. J Magn Reson Imaging. 1995;5:49–56.	BOLD contrast using spiral EPI sequences.
Scheffler et al. 2001 [6]	Detection of BOLD changes by means of a frequency-sensitive trueFISP technique: preliminary results. NMR Biomed. 2001;14:490–6.	BOLD signal using trueFISP.

References

1. Vaughan JT et al. 7 T whole body imaging: preliminary results. Magn Reson Med. 2009;61:244–8.
2. Vaughan T et al. 9.4 T human MRI: preliminary results. Magn Reson Med. 2006;56:1274–82.
3. Sharma S. 21 Tesla MRI microscopy of mice kidney, heart and skin: quantitation of MRI visible features. Nat Precedings. 2009. doi:10.1038/npre.2009.3484.1.
4. Bandettini PA, Wong EC, Jesmanowicz A, Hinks RS, Hyde JS. Spin-echo and gradient-echo epi of human brain activation using bold contrast: a comparative study at 1.5 T. NMR Biomed. 1994;7:12–20.
5. Oppelt A, Graumann R, Barfuss H. FISP: a new fast MRI sequence. Electromedica. 1986;54:15–8.
6. Scheffler K et al. Detection of BOLD changes by means of a frequency-sensitive trueFISP technique: preliminary results. NMR Biomed. 2001;14:490–6.
7. Ernst RR. Application of Fourier transform spectroscopy to magnetic resonance. Rev Sci Instrum. 1966;37:93.
8. Dale B, Wendt M, Duerk J. A rapid look-up table method for reconstructing MR images from arbitrary K-space trajectories. IEEE Trans Med Imaging. 2001;20:207–17.
9. Meyer C, Hu B, Nishimura D, Macovski A. Fast coronary artery imaging. Magn Reson Imaging. 1992;28: 202–13.
10. Yacoe M, Armstrong K, Cheung L, Meyer C. Spiral spin-echo magnetic resonance imaging of the pelvis with spectrally and spatially selective radiofrequency excitation: comparison with fat-saturated fast spin-echo imaging. Can Assoc Radiol J. 1997;48(4): 247–51.
11. Noll DC, Cohen JD, Meyer CH, Schneider W. Spiral K-space MR imaging of cortical activation. J Magn Reson Imaging. 1995;5:49–56.
12. Cohen JD et al. Temporal dynamics of brain activation during a working memory task. Nature. 1997; 386:604–8.
13. Nishimura DG, Irarrazabal P, Meyer CH. A velocity k-space analysis of flow effects in echo-planar and spiral imaging. Magn Reson Med. 1995;33:549–56.
14. Spielman DM, Pauly JM, Meyer CH. Magnetic resonance fluoroscopy using spirals with variable sampling densities. Magn Reson Med. 1995;34:388–94.

3 Experimental Design and Data Analysis for fMRI

Geoffrey K. Aguirre

Introduction

Functional magnetic resonance imaging (fMRI) methods continue to evolve rapidly. Subtle experimental designs have been joined by more powerful data analysis methods to detect and interpret evoked changes in neural activity. Despite constant development, there are several core principles of fMRI methodology that can be used as a guide to understand both the current state of the field and whatever advance awaits tomorrow. This chapter concerns itself primarily with this core understanding, but considers several specific aspects of fMRI experiments. Along the way, the chapter also notes some of the specific challenges that exist in the fMRI studies of clinical populations, although a detailed consideration of these issues is contained in Chap. 7.

Topics will be raised roughly in the same order as they present themselves in the course of the conception and completion of an fMRI experiment. This order of presentation also moves from general issues in neuroimaging inference to more specific aspects of fMRI and finally to the idiosyncratic properties of blood-oxygen-level-dependent (BOLD) fMRI and their implication for experimental design and analysis. To start, the chapter considers two categories of neuroimaging experiment, each of which examines a different direction of relationship between the brain and behavior. Next, we discuss the different techniques of isolating and manipulating mental operations that might be used in the service of these experimental designs. Regarding experimental design, the chapter considers possible temporal ordering of stimuli within an fMRI experiment, including the paradigmatic "blocked" and "event-related" designs. This section requires us to grapple with two critical properties of BOLD fMRI data: the hemodynamic response function and the temporal autocorrelation of the noise. We then turn our attention to related analysis issues. The steps of data preprocessing that prepare fMRI data for statistical analysis are reviewed, followed by a consideration of univariate analysis of fMRI data.

Basic Types of Neuroimaging Inference

Regardless of the particular neuroimaging methodology employed [e.g., fMRI, positron emission tomography (PET) and event-related potential (ERP)], there are three broad categories of experimental question that might be asked. Each category probes a different direction of relationship between the brain and behavior, and each one makes different assumptions for valid inference. Within these broad categories lie many different experimental designs, each with particular

G.K. Aguirre, MD, PhD (✉)
Department of Neurology, Hospital of the University of Pennsylvania, 3 West Gates Building, 3400 Spruce Street, Philadelphia, PA 19104, USA
e-mail: aguirreg@mail.med.upenn.edu

S.H. Faro and F.B. Mohamed (eds.), *Functional BOLD MRI: Principles and Applications*,
DOI 10.1007/978-1-4939-1995-6_3,

assumptions and inferences. Generally, placing a study within an inferential category can help organize one's thinking about the assumptions that underlie a particular experiment.

Forward Inference

One class of neuroimaging experiments are concerned with *forward inference*, which generally examines the anatomical, neural correlates of a given mental operation. One application of forward inference is to ask *localization* questions. For example, does perception of a face activate a particular area of the brain different from that evoked by perception of other stimuli? Does the cognitive process of "working memory" evoke neural activity within the frontal lobe or somewhere else? In general, these designs present a subject with a task designed to selectively evoke a particular cognitive state of interest, and the neuroimaging method identifies if and where the changes in neural activity accompany the cognitive process. Clearly, this type of experiment requires a way to manipulate the mental state of the subject, isolating the mental operation of interest from the other processes that invariably are present (e.g., button pushing, preparing responses, etc.). The next section discusses several methods that might be used to do so.

If successful, a localization study allows one to conclude that a particular area of the brain is "activated" by a particular cognitive operation. Importantly, neuroimaging methods in general are severely restricted in their ability to make conclusions regarding the *necessity* of a region for a cognitive operation. In other words, the presence of focal activation for a particular mental operation does not imply that a lesion to that area of the brain would impair the subject's ability to perform that mental operation. The reasons for this are manifold. For example, multiple areas of activity might be found, any one of which (perhaps working in parallel, or one serving as a "backup" for the other) would be capable of supporting the process of interest. In this case, the region still plays an interesting role in the cognitive process, although it is not strictly necessary. A second challenge is the lack of perfect control over the mental states of the subject we seek to study. Although stimuli and instructions designed to evoke a particular cognitive process can be presented, there can be no guarantee that the subject has entered that cognitive state and *no other*. The subject may unwittingly engage in confounding cognitive processes in addition to that intended by the experimenter, or alternatively, may fail to differentially engage the process. This is the central challenge of interpretation of most neuroimaging studies of localization – it is difficult to be certain that the experimental variable of interest has been properly manipulated.

Several applications of localization-type neuroimaging studies of patient populations can be conceived. The use of fMRI to identify "eloquent" (or otherwise functionally important) cortex for neurosurgical planning is one example. Importantly, the caveats expressed previously regarding the conclusion of "necessity" using a neuroimaging study are particularly relevant for this application (see Atlas et al. [1] and Chap. 13 for further details).

By contrast, *implementation* studies ask about the computational mechanisms of a cognitive process within a cortical region. This type of study begins with the assumption that a cortical region engages in computations that support a particular cognitive process. The purpose of the study is then to determine the parameters of neural activity that mediate the area's participation in that process. For example, does an area of the prefrontal cortex change its bulk level of neural activity as a function of increasing working memory load (i.e., remember four items instead of two)? Is speed of motion encoded differently from direction of motion within area MT? As is true for all forward inference studies, the key assumption is that the perception or behavior of the subject is controlled by the experiment, permitting conclusions that link neural states to internal mental states.

A related clinical application is the detection of dynamic pathology. The properties of this mode of inference derive from the use of fMRI to detect spontaneous patterns of neural activity that are unlike neural activity evoked by normal mental operations. The prototypical use is the detection of the cortical origin of seizure activity [2]. Unlike many of the other applications of fMRI discussed here, the localization of neural activity does not rely upon a behavioral or stimulus paradigm to create a particular pattern of neural activity, but instead is designed to detect endogenous, pathological neural patterns. This may be done by relating neural imaging signals to the timing of the symptoms or another form of monitoring [e.g., simultaneously acquired scalp electroencephalogram (EEG)]. Alternatively, the study may identify brain areas that demonstrate pathological patterns of neural activity, even when it cannot be specified when those events took place. To do so, it is necessary to specify signal parameters that can distinguish between normal and abnormal neural patterns (e.g., Esteller et al. [3]).

Reverse Inference

A *reverse inference* design probes a different direction of relationship between brain and behavior and asks: What cognitive process does a given task evoke? This type of experiment leverages knowledge about the neural correlates of particular mental states to learn something about an imperfectly understood behavior. One begins by assuming that neural activity in a particular area of the brain is a marker of the presence of a particular mental state and no other. Depending upon the application, this neural activity may be read from local or distributed neural locations.

Focal reverse inference is based upon the presence of neural activity at a particular brain location. For example, neural activity of a certain magnitude at a certain spot in the fusiform gyrus indicates that the subject has the visual perception of a face. The subject then performs a task that may or may not evoke the cognitive process of interest. For example, ambiguous stimuli are presented that can be perceived as a face or a vase. If the specified neural activity is seen, the conclusion is drawn that the subject saw a face at that moment in time. This type of design may therefore be used to test hypotheses regarding the engagement of cognitive processes during a behavioral state in which the cognitive processes need not be under experimental control. This type of experiment has been the basis of the rapidly growing fields of emotional, social, and economic neuroscience, in which activity at certain brain locations is taken as evidence of a particular emotional state or value judgment.

What provides the evidence that a particular region is uniquely activated by a specific cognitive process? Logically, only an exhaustive neuroimaging examination of every possible cognitive process, under every possible circumstance, could provide the necessary evidence. This is obviously practically impossible, so a series of neuroimaging experiments that demonstrate activation of a particular region during a given cognitive process and no other usually suffices to support the assumption (a logical inference termed *enumerative induction*).

Within the clinical realm, this type of inference is used as a surrogate measure of a behavioral state. Some diseases produce symptoms that are subjective, and can only be imperfectly measured by observation or patient report. The experience of pain is an example of this kind. In other cases, patients experience symptoms that they underreport, such as those with drug addiction who minimize their degree of drug craving. Some patients may have important internal cognitive states that are not evident to the clinician, such as patients who are "locked in" from pontine lesions or those who are in a minimally conscious state following more extensive cortical damage [4]. Finally, there are patients who feign neurological deficit either due to psychopathology or due to hope for secondary gain. In each of these cases, fMRI might be used to measure an internal mental state of a subject that is not easily obtained through simple behavioral observation.

A related approach is *distributed reverse inference*. This is the inferential mode behind the enormously powerful and rapidly expanding techniques of multivoxel pattern analysis (MVPA) [5]. In these designs, the pattern of neural activity across voxels is used to classify behavioral or perceptual states. Critically, the process of "decoding" behavior from neural activity is preceded by a training phase, in which the distributed neural response to a particular stimulus is measured. The patterns of response observed during the training period is then used to classify the novel behavioral or perceptual states during the test phase. Therefore, an MVPA experiment effectively includes both a forward inference study (during the training phase) and a reverse inference study (during the test or decoding phase). The result is a uniquely powerful design that provides an inferentially sound basis for prediction and classification.

Connectivity

A third class of experiment examines the relationship between brain states. These approaches obtain the time varying signal from different brain regions and base inferences upon the relationship between these regions. The burgeoning field of resting-state connectivity [6] examines the distribution of phase-locked signal fluctuations across the brain, during a putative rest state, to parcellate cortex and to classify mental states. A related approach quantifies the connectivity between different cortical regions – the extent that one cortical region influences neural activity in another region [7]. These connectivity maps may then be compared across populations (clinical or otherwise) and between different behavioral states. Brain connectivity is detailed in depth in Chap. 6.

Manipulation of the Cognitive Process

As was discussed, many neuroimaging experiments depend upon the isolated manipulation of a cognitive process for study. In particular, localization experiments require that a cognitive process of interest be isolated from other mental operations so that the neural correlates of that process can be observed. In implementation experiments, some aspect of the stimulus or mental operation must be varied so that the neurocomputational correlate of its processing can be studied. Here, we consider several broad classes of experimental manipulation of a cognitive operation. Note that any of these techniques can be coupled with a particular temporal structure of design (e.g., event-related or blocked), described in the next section.

Cognitive subtraction is the prototypical method of isolation of a cognitive process, and is the most problematic. Typically, one condition of an experiment is designed to engage a particular cognitive process, such as face perception, episodic encoding, or semantic recall. This "experimental" condition is contrasted with a "control" condition designed to evoke all of the cognitive processes present in the experimental period, except for the cognitive process of interest. Differences in neural activity between the two conditions can be attributed to the cognitive process of interest. In essence, a cognitive process is isolated in an "all or none" fashion. As discussed previously, there is no direct control over the mental states of the subject, so the danger is always present that the subject might engage in a confounding mental operation in addition to the one of interest. Additionally, cognitive subtraction relies upon the assumption that a cognitive process can be added to a preexisting set of cognitive processes without affecting them (an assumption termed pure insertion). This might fail if, for example, the act of pressing a button to signal a semantic judgment is different from pressing a button in response to a visual cue. Effects upon the imaging signal that result from this difference would be erroneously attributed to semantic judgment per se.

The *cognitive conjunction* design [8] has been proposed to reduce reliance upon the assumption of pure insertion. The method uses a set of paired cognitive subtractions, each of which need not completely isolate the cognitive process of interest. The imaging data are then analyzed to find areas that have a significant, consistent response across subtractions. The identification of the same region across multiple pairs of subtractions strengthens the conclusion that the area is activated by the cognitive process that is isolated in each of the subtraction pairs.

Parametric designs offer an attractive alternative to cognitive subtraction approaches. In a parametric design, the experimenter presents a range of different levels of some parameter, and seeks to identify relationships (linear or otherwise) between imaging signal and the values that the parameter assumes. This can be done to identify the neural correlates of straightforward changes in stimulus properties or manipulations of a cognitive process. As compared to cognitive subtraction methods, failure of the pure-insertion assumption is less plausible for parametric designs as the cognitive process is present during all conditions. This method can be further extended using *factorial* designs, in which multiple parameters are manipulated to identify additive and interactive changes in neural activity [9].

Finally, *carryover* designs examine the effect of stimulus context and history upon neural response [10]. Sequential transitions between stimuli are controlled and the effects examined. The most common application of these designs is for the measurement of neural adaptation or habituation [11]. The approach exploits the well-demonstrated repetition–suppression phenomenon, in which a set of neurons have a reduced response to the repeated presentation of a stimulus. For example, one might hypothesize that the fusiform face area encodes a viewpoint- independent representation of a face. Reduced responses from this cortical area to the second presentation of the same face viewed from a different angle would support this assertion.

Properties of the Bold fMRI System that Impact Experimental Design

The preceding sections have described properties of experimental design that might apply to any neuroimaging method. The next section discusses the ordering of experimental conditions in time, and specifically contrast blocked and event-related designs. To understand the consequences of these experimental design choices, this chapter considers the idiosyncratic properties of one particular neuroimaging method: BOLD fMRI. The chapter focuses on two key properties of BOLD fMRI data that fundamentally impact the design of BOLD fMRI experiments: the hemodynamic response function and the presence of low-frequency noise.

As was described in Chap. 1, changes in neural activity give rise to a series of vascular and hemodynamic changes that ultimately result in changes in the BOLD fMRI signal. While many of the details of this relationship between neural activity and hemodynamic change are still under study, much of the messy details can be conveniently sidestepped by noting that the transformation of neural activity to BOLD fMRI signal is nearly *linear*. This implies, for example, that a doubling in the amplitude of neural activity results in a doubling of the amplitude of the BOLD fMRI signal, and so on. One important property of BOLD fMRI as a linear system is that it can be well characterized by the *hemodynamic response function* (HRF). This is the BOLD fMRI signal that results from a brief (<1 s), intense period of neural activity. Given the shape of the HRF, one can predict the BOLD fMRI signal change that would result from any arbitrary pattern of neural activity.

The HRF itself can be empirically measured from human subjects by studying the BOLD fMRI signal that is evoked by experimentally induced, brief periods of neural activity in known cortical areas (e.g., neural activity in the primary motor cortex in response to a button press). The shape of the HRF reflects its vascular origin, and rises and falls smoothly over a period of about 16 s. While the shape of the HRF varies significantly across subjects, it is very consistent within a subject, even across days to months [12]. The stability of the shape of the HRF proves to be of value in the analysis of fMRI data, as it allows one to predict the pattern of BOLD fMRI signal that might result from an arbitrary pattern of neural activity. One difficulty, however, is that there is some evidence that the shape of the HRF varies from one region of the brain to another (perhaps from variations in neurovascular coupling). This is, however, a difficult notion to test as it is necessary to create evoked patterns of neural activity in disparate areas of the brain that can be guaranteed to be very similar. A further problem is that the properties of the HRF may differ between elderly and young subjects, perhaps as a consequence of vascular disease [13]. The consequences of misspecification of the shape of the HRF will vary depending upon the experimental design used, as elaborated later.

The temporal dynamics of neural activity are quite rapid, in the order of milliseconds, but changes in blood flow take place over the course of seconds. One consequence of this, as demonstrated by the smooth shape of the HRF, is that rapid changes in neural activity are not well represented in the BOLD fMRI signal. The "temporal blurring" induced by the HRF leads to many limitations placed on the types of experiments that can be conducted using BOLD fMRI. Specifically, the smooth shape of the HRF makes it difficult to discriminate closely spaced neural events. Despite this, it is still possible to detect the following: (1) brief periods of neural activity, (2) differences between neural events in a fixed order, spaced as closely as 4 s apart. (3) differences between neural events, *randomly* ordered, closely spaced (e.g., every second or less), and (4) neural-onset asynchronies in the order of 100 ms. The reason that these seemingly paradoxical experimental designs can work is that some patterns of events that occur rapidly or switch rapidly create a low-frequency "envelope": a larger structure of pattern of alternation that can pass through the hemodynamic response function. The next section discusses several types of temporal structures for BOLD fMRI experiments and considers how the shape of the HRF dictates the properties of these designs.

Another important property of BOLD fMRI data is that greater power is present at some temporal frequencies as compared to others under the null hypothesis (i.e., data collected without any experimental intervention). The power spectrum (a frequency representation) of data composed of independent observations (i.e., white noise), should be "flat," with equal power at all frequencies. When calculated for BOLD fMRI, the average power spectrum is found to contain ever increasing power at ever lower frequencies, often termed a 1/frequency distribution. This pattern of noise can also be called "pink," named for the color of light that would result if the corresponding amounts of red, green, blue, etc., of the visible light frequency spectrum were combined. The presence of noise of this type within BOLD fMRI data has two primary consequences. First, traditional parametric and nonparametric statistical tests are invalid for the analysis of BOLD fMRI data, which is why much of the analysis of BOLD fMRI data is conducted using Keith Worsley and Karl Friston's "modified" general linear model [14] and its heirs, as instantiated in statistical parametric mapping (SPM) and other statistical packages. The second impact is upon experimental design. Because of the greater noise at lower frequencies, slow changes in neural activity are more difficult to distinguish from noise.

Interestingly, the consequences for experimental design of the shape of the hemodynamic response function and the noise properties of BOLD fMRI are at odds. Specifically, the shape of the HRF would tend to favor experimental designs that induce slow changes in neural activity, while the presence of low-frequency noise would argue for experimental designs that produce more rapid alterations in neural activity. As it happens, knowledge of the shape of the HRF and the distribution of the noise is sufficient to provide a principled answer as to how best to balance these two conflicting forces.

It is worth noting that other neuroimaging methods have different data characteristics, with different consequences for experimental design. For example, perfusion fMRI provides a noninvasive, quantifiable measure of local cerebral tissue perfusion [15]. Perfusion data do not suffer from the elevated, low-frequency noise present in BOLD and as a result, perfusion fMRI can be used to detect extremely long time-scale changes in neural activity (over minutes to hours to days) that would simply be indistinguishable from noise using BOLD fMRI [16]. This may prove to be very advantageous in studies of clinical populations. Functional changes in patient cognition, either improvement by functional recovery following focal lesions or decline in neurodegenerative disease, evolve over long time scales as well. Perfusion fMRI can be used to obtain stable measurements of evoked neural activity from this dynamic system.

Different Temporal Structures of Bold fMRI Experiments

As BOLD fMRI generally includes multiple task conditions (prototypically, an "experimental" and "control" period), several ways of ordering the presentation of these conditions exist. Different terms are used to describe the pattern of alternation between experimental conditions over time, and include such familiar labels as "blocked" or "event related." While these are often perceived as rather concrete categories, the distinction between blocked, event-related, and other sorts of designs is fairly arbitrary. These may be better considered as extremes along a continuum of arrangements of stimulus order. Consider every period of time during an experiment as a particular experimental condition. This includes the "intertrial interval" or "baseline" periods between stimulus presentations. In this setting, blocked and event-related designs are viewed simply as different ways of arranging periods of "rest" (or no stimulus) with respect to other sorts of conditions. (For a more complete exploration of these concepts, see Friston et al. [17] and Liu [18]).

The prototypical fMRI experiment is a blocked approach, in which two conditions alternate over the course of a scan. For most hypotheses of interest, these periods of time will not be utterly homogeneous, but will consist of several trials of some kind presented together. For example, a given block might present a series of faces to be passively perceived, or a sequence of words to be remembered, or a series of pictures to which the subject must make a living/nonliving judgment and press a button to indicate his response. Blocked designs have the obvious difficulty that the subject can anticipate trial types, which may be undesirable in some settings (e.g., studies of recognition of novel vs. previously learned words). On the other hand, blocked designs have superior statistical power compared to all other experimental designs. This is because the fundamental frequency of the boxcar can be positioned at an optimal location with respect to the filtering properties of the hemodynamic response function and the low frequency noise. For typical shapes of the HRF and distributions of temporal noise, this ideal balancing point occurs with epochs of about 20–30 s in duration.

Event-related designs model signal changes associated with individual trials, as opposed to blocks of trials. This makes it possible to ascribe changes in signal to particular events, allowing one to randomize stimuli, assess relationships between behavior and neural responses, and engage in retrospective assignment of trials. Conceptually, the simplest type of event-related design to consider is one which uses only a single stimulus type, and uses sufficient temporal spacing of trials to permit the complete rise and fall of the hemodynamic response to each trial; a briefly presented picture of a face once every 16 s for example. This is frequently termed a *sparse* event-related design. Importantly, while this prototypical experiment has only one stimulus, it has *two* experimental conditions (the stimulus and the intertrial interval). If one is willing to abandon the fixed ordering and spacing of these conditions, more complex designs become possible. For example, randomly ordered picture presentations and rest periods could be presented once a second (or even more rapidly). The ability to present rapid alternations between conditions initially seems counterintuitive, given the temporal smoothing effects of the hemodynamic response function. While BOLD fMRI is insensitive to the particular high-frequency alternation between one trial and the next, it is still sensitive to the low-frequency "envelope" of the design. In effect, with closely spaced, randomly ordered trials, one is detecting the low frequency consequences of the random assortment of trial types. These rapid event-related designs are fairly sensitive to the accurate specification of the HRF for their success (unless a basis set is used for analysis; see below).

For experimental settings in which one has an unlimited number of trials to present (e.g., flashes of light), but a limited period of scanning time, then rapid, randomly ordered designs are more statistically powerful than "sparse" designs. Alternatively, when the experiment is limited by the number of available trials (e.g., pictures of flightless birds), then maximal statistical power is obtained by presenting the available trials in a sparse manner, and "stretching" the scanning period out as long as possible. In general, provision of stimulus counterbalance is important for valid inference [10]. Counterbalance ensures that each type of stimulus appears equally often before each other stimulus.

The discussion thus far regarding event-related designs has assumed an ability to randomize perfectly the order of presentation of different event types. There are certain types of behavioral paradigms, however, that do not permit a random ordering of the events. For example, the delay period of a working memory experiment always follows the presentation of a stimulus to be remembered. In this case, the different events of the trial cannot be placed arbitrarily close together without risking the possibility of false-positive results that accrue from the hemodynamic response to one trial event (e.g., the stimulus presentation) being interpreted as resulting from neural activity in response to another event (e.g., the delay period). It turns out that, given the shape typically observed for hemodynamic responses, events within a trial as close together as 4 s can be reliably discriminated [19]. Thus, event-related designs can be used to examine directly, for example, the hypothesis that certain cortical areas increase their activity during the delay period of a working memory paradigm without requiring the problematic assumptions traditionally employed in blocked, subtractive designs.

There is a multiplicity of further designs that might be considered that do not fall strictly within "blocked" or "event-related" categories. *Neural-onset asynchrony* designs [20, 21] are used to detect differences in the timing of neural activity evoked by different stimuli. Here, a "sparse" event-related design is used, along with exquisite coupling of the timing of stimulus presentation to image acquisition. A difference in the time of onset of the smooth, BOLD hemodynamic response evoked by two different stimuli within a cortical region is sought. *Traveling wave stimuli* are used to define topographic maps of cortical responses, the most familiar being the retinotopic organization of early visual areas [22]. These designs use stimuli that vary continuously across some sensory space (e.g., retinal eccentricity) and identify for any point within a cortical area the optimal position of the stimulus within the sensory space for the evocation of neural activity. These designs are often combined with cortical flat-map techniques for the display of results [23].

Data Preprocessing

In a perfect world, BOLD fMRI images would be acquired instantaneously from a stationary brain of uniform shape. Unfortunately, this is not the case, and a number of processing steps must be performed prior to the statistical analysis of fMRI data. These steps have two primary goals: (1) to reverse displacements of the data in time or space that may have occurred during acquisition and (2) to enhance the ability to detect spatially extended signals within or across subjects. This section briefly discusses several preprocessing steps that are commonplace in the analysis of BOLD fMRI data.

Distortion Correction

BOLD fMRI data are typically acquired as echo-planar images and as such are likely to be distorted (stretched and pulled) in space to some extent as a result of static magnetic field inhomogeneities produced by concentration of magnetic field lines at (for example) air–tissue interfaces. There are several methods to correct this spatial distortion, and they in most cases use a "map" of the magnetic field within the bore of the magnet to correct distortion. In many cases, this correction is performed by the scanning system itself prior to writing out image data for analysis and does not enter into the routine preprocessing of fMRI data at some institutions.

Slice Acquisition Correction

A single volume of BOLD fMRI data, collected during one repetition time (TR), is assembled from multiple planar acquisitions (slices). One slice is collected at a time, either sequentially or in an interleaved fashion, with the result that each slice samples a slightly different point in time. For a TR of 2 s and 20 axial slices, this would mean that one slice of the brain would be obtained 1 s later than another spatially adjacent slice within the same TR. As a consequence, a neural event that occurs simultaneously on multiple slices within the brain will appear as different, time-delayed BOLD fMRI responses in the data from different slices. Slice acquisition correction compensates for this staggered order of slice acquisition. The correction works by calculating (using sinc interpolation) the BOLD fMRI signal that would have been obtained for a given slice, had that slice been acquired instead at the beginning of the TR. While not of great importance for low-temporal-frequency blocked designs, this preprocessing step is quite important for event-related designs.

Motion Correction

A variety of methods are used to minimize head motion during scanning. These include foam padding around the head; "bite bars," custom-designed, thermo-plastic face masks, and so on. Despite these efforts, subjects nonetheless move their heads during scanning. A common data preprocessing step, therefore, is to attempt to correct the effects of this motion. This is generally done by realigning the image of the brain obtained at each point in time back to the first image acquired at the start of the scanning session. Several methods exist to do so, but most use a "six-parameter" motion correction, in which the brain is treated as a rigid body and the six possible movements (three translations and three rotations) are calculated at each point in time to minimize the image difference between the realigned brain and the brain in its original position. Importantly, motion correction of this kind does not completely remove the effects of movement upon the BOLD fMRI signal. This is because movement of the brain within the exquisitely defined magnetic field gradients created during scanning alters the signal obtained at different points in the slice acquisition. As a result, even after realigning the brain to its original position, movement-induced signal artifacts remain. As a consequence, statistical analysis of BOLD data will often include nuisance covariates that are themselves the six movement parameters measured during realignment. These covariates serve to account for changes in the signal within voxels that are correlated with the movement of the head. (See "Statistical Analysis" section for a further description of nuisance covariates.)

Spatial Normalization

If one wishes to test a hypothesis regarding a certain area of the brain within a population, then it is first necessary to identify that same area of the brain across subjects. This is frequently done by computationally "warping" the anatomical structure of the brain of one subject to match a template brain within a standard, defined space. While there are a variety of sophisticated methods available for registering and aligning the brains of different subjects into a standard space, there are theoretical limits to what such an alignment can achieve. First, there may be intersubject variability in anatomy that cannot be overcome by warping brains to a standard space. For example, the arrangement of the sulci may vary between subjects. Thus, while two subjects may have neural responses at the same "true" cytoarchitectonic location, the position of this site with respect to other landmarks in the brain may differ between subjects, leading to spread of these locations when data are converted to a standard space. Second, even given rigid alignment of anatomy across subjects, there may be variability in the structure–function relationships between subjects. For example, two subjects may truly have distinct face-selective neural regions, but these may be located in different sections of a cortical area as a consequence of differences in experience. Again, when normalized to a standard space, this variability in location will obscure functional dissociations. An alternative to anatomical registration is functional identification. The approach here is to first identify a region across subjects by its functional responses. For example, one might identify a region that responds more to pictures of faces than to general objects. Then, hypotheses regarding the response of this functionally defined region to other types of stimuli can be independently tested across subjects within this area. This powerful approach allows one to make inferences across subjects regarding the responses of some functional area (e.g., the fusiform face area) at the expense of making statements regarding some particular position in a standardized anatomical space.

Spatial Smoothing

It is common practice to digitally smooth BOLD fMRI data in space prior to statistical analysis. There are several reasons for this. First, BOLD fMRI data are typically composed of time-series information from many thousands of individual voxels. Statistical analysis of this data involves application of a statistical test (e.g., *t*-test) at each of these voxels. As there are, therefore, thousands of individual statistical tests being performed, control of the false-positive rate requires a fairly large *t*-result to exceed the chance that random noise will produce a "significant" result in one or more of those thousands of voxels. By smoothing the data in space, one reduces the number of independent statistical tests that are being performed, thus allowing less-stringent control over what *t*-value is considered a significant result. Another motivation for smoothing is that, when analyzing data across a population, spatial smoothing helps to overcome residual differences in anatomy between subjects that might otherwise render common areas of activation nonoverlapping. The amount of spatial smoothing to perform can be difficult to determine, as smoothing too much will decrease statistical sensitivity for small focal areas of activation, while smoothing too little will have the same deleterious effects upon large areas of signal change. A reasonable balance between these two extremes can be obtained by smoothing data with a filter that has a width roughly equal to the size (in voxels) of predicted areas of activity.

Statistical Analysis

Several methods exist to analyze BOLD fMRI data. Some of these are described as "multivariate" techniques, in which latent patterns of spatially coherent activity are identified automatically by the method (e.g., Partial Least Squares, McIntosh et al. [24]). This chapter focuses upon the more commonly implemented "univariate" techniques, in which a statistical model is applied to each voxel independently within a dataset. The discussion concerns in particular the details of the creation of a statistical model for analysis. In many software packages, such as SPM (statistical parametric mapping), some of these details are handled automatically. The purpose of this section is to provide an understanding of what is going on "under the hood."

The centerpiece of the analysis of neuroimaging data is the construction of a model that is composed of one or more "covariates." In general, covariates are predictions regarding patterns of variability in the data, expressed as changes in the BOLD fMRI signal over time within a single voxel. The better the predictions, the more valid and powerful the statistical model becomes. Covariates can be broadly divided into two categories. Covariates of interest describe changes in the signal that are (typically) the result of experimental manipulations and that are the subject of hypothesis testing. Covariates of no-interest describe, instead, changes in the signal that are unintended or undesired, and are not typically the focus of a hypothesis test.

Covariates of interest might be generated in one of two ways. First, covariates might be created to model the expected shape in time of evoked BOLD fMRI signal changes. A principled way to create covariates of this kind is to begin with a prediction regarding the pattern of neural activity that might be evoked by the experiment in a single voxel. For example, a simple "blocked" experimental design might be predicted to produce a uniformly greater amount of bulk neural activity during an experimental condition as compared to a control condition.

The anticipated BOLD fMRI signal under these circumstances can be obtained by applying a model of the hemodynamic response function (HRF) to the predicted pattern of neural activity. As was mentioned before, knowledge of the HRF is sufficient to predict the BOLD fMRI signal that will result from any arbitrary pattern of neural activity, through the mathematical process of convolution. This prediction of BOLD fMRI signal change is then suitable for use as a covariate of interest. The model of the HRF that is used might be obtained from the subject himself during a preliminary experiment (e.g., Aguirre [12]) or an average representation of an HRF across subjects might be employed, as is the case in the SPM (statistical parametric mapping) and other analysis packages.

Alternatively, covariates of interest can represent not a specific pattern of BOLD fMRI response, but instead have the property of flexibly fitting a family of possible responses that might occur. This approach uses a "basis set," which is a collection of covariates that can be scaled and combined to fit any pattern of BOLD fMRI response that might be evoked within a set period of time by a particular experimental condition. In general, the basis set will be composed of multiple covariates, with as many elements as there are points in time to be modeled. For example, in a sparse event-related experiment, in which a stimulus is presented every eight TRs (16 s at a TR of two), then a basis set of eight covariates will be needed to model, in effect, the average evoked BOLD fMRI response across trials. Typically, there is no clear interpretation of any one element of a basis set. Instead, one interprets the explanatory power of the set en mass using an *F*-test. Basis set approaches provide the advantage of flexibility, in that one is sensitive to any pattern of response (or difference between two trial types) that might take place. The price of this flexibility is reduced inferential power. One can no longer say, for example, that a given response was greater in amplitude than another, or longer in duration. Instead, one can only say that some consistent response was present.

As was mentioned, covariates of no-interest model changes in the BOLD fMRI signal that are not thought to be the result of experimental influence. For example, if one was aware of an influence of the room temperature upon the BOLD fMRI signal, and if the pattern of fluctuations of the room temperature were known, a representation of temperature could be included as a covariate to explain variations in the signal that are attributable to temperature fluctuations. Note that some covariates that are not of interest model changes in neural activity and some do not. For example, the experiment may present "instruction" screens occasionally, which would be expected to elicit transient changes in neural activity that are not the subject of any hypothesis. For these types of covariates, which model expected neural effects of no-interest, one would want to convolve the representation of neural change by the hemodynamic response function. For other covariates that are not derived from neural activity (e.g., a measure of subject head motion, or cardiopulmonary variation; Glover et al. [25]), convolution is not indicated.

One can further classify covariates of no-interest as "nuisance" covariates or "confounds." A nuisance covariate is defined as a covariate the inclusion of which is expected to alter only the magnitude of the error term, but not the relationship between the data and covariates of interest. When covariates of no-interest are correlated with covariates about which one wishes to test a hypothesis, they are termed "confounds," and their inclusion will be expected to alter the behavior of the covariates of interest. Under some circumstances, the sign of the relationship between the covariate of interest and the data can be reversed! An example of a covariate that frequently acts as a confounding factor is a *global signal* covariate. A global signal is average signal change over time across the entire brain, obtained by taking a simple average of the voxel-wise time-series. It is common to included a measure of the global signal as a covariate of no-interest (or to scale the data prior to analysis by this measure) to remove changes in blood oxygenation that impact the entire brain (resulting from, for example, changes in heart rate or respiration), which would otherwise obscure regional changes in neural activity. Because of the way in which it is measured, however, the global signal is expected to have some positive correlation with any experimentally evoked signal changes (as the average of all brain voxels will include those voxels responding to the task). As a result, correction for global signal changes can have a confounding effect upon covariates of interest, and greatly change the interpretation of evoked signal changes [26].

The resulting statistical model, composed of covariates of interest and those of no-interest, is then used to evaluate the time-series data from each voxel within the brain. The resulting weights upon the covariates (termed beta values), can then be evaluated alone or in combinations using t and F-statistics. The product is a *statistical map*, in which every voxel in the brain contains a corresponding statistical value for the contrast of the covariates of interest. The final step of analysis involves assigning a level of statistical significance to those values. If the dataset was composed of a single voxel, then this would be a straightforward enterprise: a t-value of greater than 1.96 would be significant at a $p = 0.05$ level (presuming lots of degrees of freedom and a two-tailed test). As there are many voxels, however, corrections must be made for the likelihood that noise alone might render one t-value significant if many are tested. Such a correction attempts to control the false-positive rate at a *map-wise* level, meaning that if 20 statistical maps were produced under null-hypothesis conditions (i.e., in the absence of any actual experimental treatment), only one would on average be expected to contain even a single false-positive voxel. Solutions to perform this correction in the face of spatial smoothness within the statistical map (which yields statistical test in adjacent voxels that are not fully independent) exist within Gaussian Random Field Theory [14] or through permutation [27].

Performing the appropriate, map-wise correction to control the false-positive rate can frequently yield a rather stringent statistical value necessary to label any result as significant. This, in turn, raises concerns about "false-negative" results, in which true experimental effects might be missed because the experiment is underpowered. There are several responses to this concern. Beyond the flippant call for more data, one might choose to relax the p-value that will be accepted as significant. Note that stating that the data were evaluated at a $p = 0.1$ level (corrected for multiple comparisons) is more intellectually honest than reporting results at a $p = 0.00023$ level (uncorrected), the latter tending to lull statistically naïve readers into a false sense of security. It is also preferable, whenever possible, to anatomically narrow one's hypothesis test. Using a predefined region of interest, within which to test hypotheses, can greatly reduce the number of independent statistical tests for which correction is required, thus improving power. In the limit, the number of tests can be reduced to one, by taking the average signal within a region and performing the statistical test upon this representative data. Several methods are available for the definition of regions of interest. They might be defined anatomically, based upon gyral or cytoarchitectonic boundaries, or on the basis of previously reported lesion or functional neuroimaging studies. Regions of interest might also be defined functionally. For example, subjects might participate in an initial scan, the purpose of which is to define a region of cortex that is maximally responsive to faces. Data obtained from this putative "face region" in subsequent experiments could then be studied with the benefits of having focused the hypothesis test. Finally, regions might be defined using a "main effect" contrast, with subsequent, orthogonal "interaction" contrasts tested within the region. For example, an experiment might present pictures of upright faces and inverted faces. A region would be defined as the area that responds more to pictures of faces, in either orientation, as compared to a third baseline condition. Within the defined region, the difference in response between upright and inverted faces could be assessed, without loss of statistical rigor, as the result of the test used to define the region does not prejudice the result of the subsequent orthogonal test of the effect of orientation of the stimulus. Of course, there are inferential consequences (such as loss of generality) of testing hypotheses only within predefined regions of interest. This might be countered by performing in the same experiment focused hypothesis tests within regions of interest, followed by more "exploratory" analyses that evaluate the data from the remainder of the brain, using appropriate map-wise correction for the increased number of voxels.

Yet another approach that has gained popularity is the use of a "false-discovery rate" (FDR) statistical threshold [28]. Instead of controlling the false-positive rate at a map-wise level (allowing, for example, only 1 in 20 maps to have a single false-positive voxel), the FDR method controls the *proportion* of false-positive voxels present within a single map. For example, an FDR threshold of 5% implies that, of the voxels identified as significant within a statistical map, 5% of them are on average expected to be false-positives. This is neither better nor worse than traditional map-wise control of the statistical significance, but is instead a different stance with regard to inference. FDR methods will likely be of considerable use in clinical applications. For example, it may be desirable to express the confidence of results of functional mapping for surgical planning in terms of the specificity of the population of voxels identified.

Conclusion

This chapter summarizes the basic principles underlying analysis of functional neuroimaging data. It also describes the methods that are currently being used in analyzing the functional neuroimaging data as well as new methods that are being developed in this field. (see Table 3.1 for summary of key articles exploring data analysis and experimental designs for fMRI).

Table 3.1 Key articles exploring data analysis and experimental designs for fMRI

Authors	Article title	Significance
Friston K et al. (1995)	The analysis of fMRI time-series revisited. Neuroimage. 1995 Mar;2(1):45–53	A method for detecting activations in fMRI time-series based on the general linear model and a heuristic analysis
Aguirre GK et al. (2002)	Experimental design and the relative sensitivity of BOLD and perfusion fMRI. Neuroimage. 2002 Mar;15(3):488–500	This paper compares the statistical power of BOLD and arterial spin labeling perfusion fMRI for a variety of experimental designs, within and across subjects
Friston K et al. (2010)	Computational and dynamic models in neuroimaging. Neuroimage. 2010 Sep;52(3):752–65. Epub 2009 Dec 28	This article reviews the substantial impact that computational neuroscience has had on neuroimaging over the past years

References

1. Atlas SW, Howard 2nd RS, Maldjian J, Alsop D, Detre JA, Listerud J, et al. Functional magnetic resonance imaging of regional brain activity in patients with intracerebral gliomas: findings and implications for clinical management. Neurosurgery. 1996;38(2):329–38.
2. Detre JA, Alsop DC, Aguirre GK, Sperling MR. Coupling of cortical and thalamic ictal activity in human partial epilepsy: demonstration by functional magnetic resonance imaging. Epilepsia. 1996;37(7): 657–61.
3. Esteller R, Echauz J, D'Alessandro M, et al. Continuous energy variation during the seizure cycle: towards an on-line accumulated energy. Clin Neurophysiol. 2005;116:517–26.
4. Schiff ND, Rodriguez-Moreno D, Kamal A, et al. fMRI reveals large-scale network activation in minimally conscious patients. Neurology. 2005;64(3): 514–23.
5. Haxby JV, Gobbini MI, Furey ML, Ishai A, Schouten JL, Pietrini P. Distributed and overlapping representations of faces and objects in ventral temporal cortex. Science. 2001;293:2425–30.
6. Fox MD, Raichle ME. Spontaneous fluctuations in brain activity observed with functional magnetic resonance imaging. Nat Rev Neurosci. 2007;8:700–11.
7. Buchel C, Friston KJ. Assessing interactions among neuronal systems using functional neuroimaging. Neural Netw. 2000;13:871–82.
8. Price CJ, Friston KJ. Cognitive conjunctions: a new experimental design for fMRI. Neuroimage. 1997; 5:261–70.

9. Sternberg S. Separate modifiability, mental modules, and the use of pure and composite measures to reveal them. Acta Psycholoia. 2001;106:147–246.
10. Aguirre GK, Mattar MG, Magis-Weinberg L. de Bruijn cycles for neural decoding. Neuroimage. 2011;56:1293–300.
11. Grill-Spector K, Malach R. fMR-adaptation: a tool for studying the functional properties of human cortical neurons. Acta Psychol. 2001;107:293–321.
12. Aguirre GK, Zarahn E, et al. The variability of human BOLD hemodynamic responses. Neuroimage. 1998;8:360–9.
13. D'Esposito M, Zarahn E, et al. The effect of normal aging on coupling of neural activity to the BOLD hemodynamic response. Neuroimage. 1999;10(1):6–14.
14. Worsley KJ, Friston KJ. The analysis of fMRI time-series revisted-again. Neuroimage. 1995;2:173–82.
15. Detre JA, Alsop DC. Perfusion fMRI with arterial spin labeling. Functional MRI. In: Bandettini PA, Moonen C. Berlin: Springer Verlag. 1999. p. 47–62.
16. Aguirre GK, Detre JA, Zarahn E, Alsop DC. Experimental design and the relative sensitivity of BOLD and perfusion fMRI. Neuroimage. 2002;15: 488–500.
17. Friston KJ, Zarahn E, et al. Stochastic designs in event-related fMRI. Neuroimage. 1999;10:607–19.
18. Liu T. Efficiency, power, and entropy in event-related fMRI with multiple trial types. Part II: design of experiments. Neuroimage. 2004;21:401–13.
19. Zarahn E, Aguirre GK, et al. A trial-based experimental design for fMRI. Neuroimage. 1997;6(2):122–38.
20. Menon RS, Luknowsky DC, et al. Mental chronometry using latency-resolved functional MRI. Proc Nat Acad science, USA. 1998;95:10902–7.
21. Henson RNA, Price CJ, et al. Detecting latency differences in event-related BOLD responses: application to words versus nonwords and initial versus repeated face presentations. Neuroimage. 2002;15:83–97.
22. Engel SA, Rumelhart DE, et al. fMRI of human visual cortex [letter] [published erratum appears in Nature 1994 Jul 14;370(6485):106]. Nature. 1994; 369(6481):525.
23. Sereno MI, Dale AM, et al. Borders of multiple visual areas in humans revealed by functional magnetic resonance imaging [see comments]. Science. 1995;268(5212):889–93.
24. McIntosh AR, Bookstein FL, et al. Spatial pattern analysis of functional brain images using partial least squares. Neuroimage. 1996;3: 143–57.
25. Glover GH, Li TQ, Ress D. Image-based method for retrospective correction of physiological motion effects in fMRI: RETROICOR. Magn Reson Med. 2000;44:162–7.
26. Aguirre GK, Zarahn E, et al. The inferential impact of global signal covariates in functional neuroimaging analyses. Neuroimage. 1998;8(3):302–6.
27. Nichols TE, Holmes AP. Nonparametric permutation tests for functional neuroimaging: a primer with examples. Hum Brain Mapp. 2002;15:1–25.
28 Nichols T, Hayasaka K. Controlling the familywise error rate in functional neuroimaging: a comparative review. Stat Meth Med Res. 2003;12(5):419–46.

Challenges in fMRI and Its Limitations

4

R. Todd Constable

Introduction

This chapter explores some of the challenges of functional magnetic resonance imaging (fMRI). In particular, the constraints encountered in terms of spatial and temporal resolution and the factors that limit the ability of MRI to detect functional activation are dealt with. Issues of sensitivity and resolution are intimately related and not easily separable. For example, increasing spatial resolution can usually only be achieved at the expense of temporal resolution, spatial coverage, and sensitivity loss. In addition to examining the factors limiting the sensitivity and resolution of fMRI, this chapter also explores some of the trade-offs involved in optimizing one or more of these variables.

There are a number of characteristics that an ideal functional MRI experiment should exhibit. Chief among them is the ability to acquire reliable data in a short period of time, with high spatial and temporal resolution. The ultimate spatial and temporal resolutions of fMRI are in general dictated by the purpose of the study, such as whether the studies are event-related or block design, measuring connectivity of task-based activation, and whether they are single-subject or group investigations.

This chapter reviews the challenges in obtaining reduced acquisition times, with high spatial and temporal resolution. As fMRI experiments are performed at higher field, the limits of temporal and spatial resolution continue to be pushed. Recent experiments have shown that fMRI is capable of sufficient resolution to examine cortical columns in the visual cortex, and activation maps have been presented demonstrating differential activation across cortical layers. It is unlikely, for reasons that are explained, that ultimately all experiments will be performed at very high spatial resolution (at the layer of columns), but continued improvements in fMRI acquisition strategies are bringing this goal closer. Clearly, much more needs to be understood about the brain function at the systems level, at the level of the cortical layers, and ultimately at the neuronal level. Research is underway examining brain function at all of these levels, and as these systems become better understood, the spatial and temporal resolutions required for specific fMRI investigations become clearer.

Most cognitive and many sensory/motor fMRI experiments are limited in terms of spatial and temporal resolution by a wide range of factors. Some of the limitations are imposed by the physics of MR, some are physiological, and others are neuronal systems based. The sections that follow discuss these issues in detail.

R.T. Constable, PhD (✉)
Diagnostic Radiology, Biomedical Engineering, and Neurosurgery, The Anlyan Center, Yale University School of Medicine, 300 Cedar Street, New Haven, CT, 06520, USA
e-mail: todd.constable@yale.edu

S.H. Faro and F.B. Mohamed (eds.), *Functional BOLD MRI: Principles and Applications*, DOI 10.1007/978-1-4939-1995-6_4, © Springer Science+Business Media New York 2015

MR Physics-Based Limitations in FMRI

As explained in Chap. 1, the reader should keep in mind that magnetic resonance imaging, including fMRI, is primarily based on measuring signals from protons (H) on water molecules (H_2O). The local magnetic environment that these protons experience determines, in part, the signal strength obtained from a given tissue region. The magnetic properties of blood are different depending on the oxygenation state of the hemoglobin (Hb), with deoxyhemoglobin (diamagnetic) introducing small local field inhomogenenities, and oxyhemoglobin (paramagnetic) producing a more uniform microscopic field homogeneity. During the echo time (TE), the protons (water molecules) diffuse in and around these Hb molecules. Protons diffusing near deoxyhemoglobin will experience a range of local magnetic fields, leading to rapid dephasing of the signal and hence signal loss. This state typically represents the baseline or control condition in an fMRI experiment. As deoxygenated blood is replaced by oxygenated blood upon neuronal activation, the amount of dephasing is reduced as the local field inhomogeneities are reduced and the water protons experience a more uniform field as they diffuse through the tissue. The signal in the presence of oxygenated blood, therefore, decays more slowly, and thus, at the echo time (TE) stronger signals are recorded in the oxygenated state than in the deoxygenated state. Comparing the signal obtained in the activation state with the control state, a small increase in signal intensity is observed of the order of 4% or less (at 3 T), with the actual amount dependent upon a wide range of factors. This slight change in signal is the chief mechanism exploited in fMRI and forms the basis of blood-oxygenation-level-dependent (BOLD) contrast.

Physics-Based Limitations on Spatial Resolution

Two parameters are of interest in determining the optimum spatial resolution of MRI, and these are image signal and noise. Signal is the signal intensity for any given tissue recorded by the receiver coil. It is dependent upon the amount of magnetization present at the time of the echo. The amount of magnetization present is dependent upon field strength (higher field strength results in higher spin polarization leading to greater initial magnetization), relaxation times (signal decays with two different relaxation times T1, T2, and in the case of gradient echo imaging a third time, T2*), proton density, and the imaging parameters and magnetization history. Proton density refers to how much water is present in a given volume of tissue.

Holding all other imaging parameters constant, the signal varies in direct proportion to the voxel volume. The voxel volume, of course, is directly related to the spatial resolution, and is typically changed by changing the spatial encoding gradient strength (and hence the field of view) and/or by increasing the acquisition matrix size. The relationship between spatial resolution and the signal-to-noise ratio (SNR) is given by:

$$\text{SNR} \propto {}'' x'' y'' z\sqrt{N_x}\sqrt{N_y}\sqrt{N_{\text{ave}}}\,/\sqrt{v},$$

where Δx (delta x) and Δy (delta y) represent the voxel dimensions in x and y, Δz (delta z) is the slice thickness, N_x and N_y represent the sampling matrix size in the x and y directions, N_{ave} is the number of averages, and ν (nu) represents the acquisition bandwidth (one over the sampling rate of the data acquisition).

In general, the noise is unaffected by changes in voxel volume, but the signal intensity is directly proportional to the voxel volume. Voxel volume is determined by the product of slice thickness times the in-plane spatial resolution (volume = $\Delta x \Delta y \Delta z$ [delta x delta y delta z]). The in-plane resolution is determined by dividing the field-of-view (FOV) in the x- and y-directions by the acquisition matrix size in these directions. Consider some typical imaging parameters. For a 200 × 200 mm FOV and an acquisition matrix of (N_x = 64) × (N_y = 64), the in-plane voxel size is 3.125 × 3.125 mm (dividing 200 mm/64). A slice thickness of Δz(delta z) = 5 mm will then result in a voxel volume of 3.125 × 3.125 × 5 = 48.8 mm^3. Changing any of these dimensions can have a dramatic effect on SNR. Decreasing the slice thickness by a factor of 2 will reduce the volume by half, and thus, the SNR will be reduced by a factor of 2. Similarly, doubling the in-plane resolution in the x- and y-directions simultaneously (which will reduce the voxel size in the aforementioned example to 1.56 mm × 1.56 mm) will reduce the voxel volume and hence the SNR by a factor of 4. Clearly, the choice of imaging resolution has a significant impact on the SNR of the images.

If sufficient SNR is present in the raw images of an fMRI experiment, the spatial resolution may be increased by increasing the matrix size, or decreasing the FOV, or both. Ultrahigh resolution MR images have been obtained with in-plane resolutions of the order of tens of μ(mu)m, which is approaching the size of individual neurons. The ultimate constraints on the spatial resolution in MR arise from two phenomena. First, most imaging is performed by collecting an echo, and while this echo is being collected, the signal is decaying across the echo with a relaxation time of T2 in a spin echo, or T2* in a gradient echo, sequence. In most fMRI experiments, the effects of this T2 decay across the echo are minimal, but as the resolution becomes very high, the blurring caused by T2 decay can begin to dominate and limit the resolution achievable. At this extreme, tissues with long T2 will be sharper than tissues with shorter T2, and thus, the resolution throughout the image may vary as a function of tissue T2. The second limiting factor is the diffusion rate of water. Since MR images rely on the signal obtained from freely diffusing water, if a significant amount of water molecules move during data acquisition, this will lead to a blurring, reducing the ability to localize the signal. The localization of this signal is limited to the mean square diffusion distance of water in the amount of time required to spatially localize the signal. At the extremes of spatial resolution in MR, water diffusion is the ultimate limiting factor (see [1]). Functional MRI experiments to date are in a regime well removed from this diffusion effect, and this is, therefore, not a primary limiting factor in fMRI. As we discuss, there are a number of other considerations such as the number of slices acquired, temporal resolution, and image distortion that can influence the choice of spatial resolution. Most studies to date that have used very high spatial resolution tend to focus on one specific cortical area, and studies involving whole-brain coverage are typically performed at much more modest spatial resolutions.

SNR and Field Strength

Increasing field strength leads to increased polarization of spin populations and, therefore, a larger initial magnetization vector. This holds true in fMRI, with the added benefit that the measured change in BOLD amplitude also is larger at a higher field [2–5]. This increase in BOLD signal change and the increase in image SNR can allow for imaging at higher spatial resolutions at high field, allow for imaging at higher temporal resolution (shorter TR), and/or allow shorter imaging sessions. T1s are longer at higher field strength, and thus, smaller flip angles or longer TRs must be used to ensure maximal signal amplitude. By contrast, T2s and T2* in particular are shorter at higher field strength, and thus, the optimum TE for BOLD imaging is shorter at high field strength.

Noise in MR imaging is the term given to any unwanted signal, and these unwanted signals may arise from multiple sources. Thermal noise (random fluctuations of spins aligned with the field) is always present in MR imaging and can only be eliminated by reducing the sample temperature to absolute zero, which is not usually practical in fMRI. Some noise is also generated in the electronics of the MR scanner, and care must be taken when placing electronic equipment, such as projectors for presenting visual stimuli, in the magnet room, as these devices may emit radiofrequency (RF) energy that the receiver coil could sense, leading to significant noise. If the noise from a projector is at a particular frequency then a streak artifact, a line of bright intensity, in the phase encode direction will be clearly visible, whereas if the RF noise is of a broader bandwidth, it will simply decrease the overall SNR of the images (and thus decrease the significance of any activations) without obvious artifacts.

Static Field Inhomogeneities

Also amplified at higher field strengths are the problems of field inhomogeneities that result in signal loss and image distortion. Thus, without compensation methods for BOLD imaging in the presence of field inhomogeneities, moving to higher field strength may not always be advantageous. Medial frontal and medial temporal areas are particularly affected by the amplification of susceptibility effects.

A number of methods have been investigated in an attempt to reduce the impact of macroscopic field inhomogeneities. These are the local field inhomogeneities that arise at air–tissue junctions and, in particular, in brain regions near sinuses [6]. These are referred to as macroscopic static field inhomogeneities, since they alter the main magnetic field in relatively large areas. The challenge in solving this problem is that the BOLD mechanism relies upon differences in local microscopic field inhomogeneities between paramagnetic oxygenated and diamagnetic deoxygenated blood, and therefore, a method that removes the image sensitivity to field inhomogeneities not only will solve the signal loss problem due to static field effects but will also remove sensitivity to BOLD signal changes.

Static field effects are more pronounced along the largest dimension of a voxel, and the source of signal loss is dephasing across this dimension. In most cases, the slice thickness (Δz [delta z]) represents the largest dimension of a voxel, and since the largest dimension is most sensitive to signal loss through dephasing, most of the methods developed have focused on reducing this through-plane dephasing. It should be noted, however, that many of the methods are general and can be applied in any direction. Decreasing the voxel size in any dimension (Δx, Δy, Δz [delta x, delta y, delta z]) will reduce the dephasing across that dimension. The simplest approach to reducing macroscopic susceptibility loss is to move to thinner slices and higher spatial resolution [7, 8]. This involves a significant cost, however, in terms of absolute number of images collected, and the necessarily longer TR required to accommodate the additional slices need to cover the same brain region. With the advent of parallel receiver accelerated imaging approaches [9, 10], however, it is now possible to collect many more slices in a given TR. Without parallel imaging, increasing the TR to accommodate these additional slices leads to a decrease in statistical power [11] and decreases temporal resolution.

Other approaches to solve this problem include z-shimming [12–15] based on original work by Frahm [16], in which multiple acquisitions are collected with different z-refocusing gradient lobes, wherein these gradients are designed to cancel the gradients created by macroscopic susceptibility effects in the body. A minimum of two acquisitions are required (thereby effectively doubling TR) with more acquisitions leading to better compensation. An alternative approach is to design tailored RF pulses [17–19] such that the RF imposes a phase gradient across the slice, which compensates the phase shifts introduced by the local field gradients. Only recently, with the advent of parallel transmit strategies that are rapidly being developed [20, 21], this approach is looking like that it may become more and more feasible, and as more sites obtain the required hardware (multiple RF transmitter channels), and ultimately could become routine [22].

Many of the approaches to static field inhomogeneity compensation are multishot approaches, requiring two or more acquisitions, and thus incur penalties in temporal resolution and statistical power. Two single-shot z-shimming approaches have been presented. Song et al. [23] showed results in which two gradient echo images were collected with different z-shim gradients on each side of an 180° RF pulse. More recently, Yang [24] has published a single-shot approach in which the even echoes in an echo train had 1 z-shim value, while the odd k-space line acquisitions had a second z-shim value, and the phase encode gradient was only incremented on every other echo, rather than on each echo. Such an approach produces two exactly registered (except for distortion effects in the x-direction) z-shim images with equal T2* weighting in a single shot and, therefore, without the usual penalty in TR. This approach, however, doubles the width of the acquisition window, which in turn increases the geometric image distortion in the *y*-direction by a factor of 2, and only half as many slices can be obtained within a given TR. Thus, the ideal solution remains to be found for compensating for these field inhomogeneities while maintaining BOLD sensitivity and temporal resolution.

Moving to high field strength, such as 3 T or greater, provides sufficient BOLD contrast using spin echo techniques or asymmetric spin echo methods wherein microscopic field effects are not refocused by the spin echo but macroscopic effects are refocused. Spin echo-based BOLD imaging has been shown at 1.5 T [25], but the sensitivity at this relatively low field strength is insufficient for most fMRI applications. Sensitivity increases with field strength, and using an asymmetric spin echo EPI acquisition it is possible to tune the sensitivity to field inhomogeneities at different scales [26–28].

The Effect of Acquisition TR

If functional imaging is to be performed in a small, localized brain region, and if subject motion is minimal, then scanning with short TR of the order of 1 s or less provides excellent statistical power relative to the same study performed with a much longer TR [11]. In the limit of decreasing TR, the temporal correlations in the data lead to redundant data collection, and thus, the gain in statistical power as TR is decreased diminishes at very short TR. If subject motion is a problem, however, moving to a longer TR with maximal spatial coverage and very high resolution (both in-plane and through-plane) maximizes the ability of motion correction algorithms to reregister the brain volumes collected over time. In this case then moving to a longer TR and increasing through-plane resolution and coverage, can improve the statistical power in the data. The reader is clearly learning at this point that there are no easy trade-offs in fMRI and many factors must be considered in designing a study and choosing the imaging pulse sequence and parameters. While the discussion so far has focused primarily on MR physics-based challenges in fMRI, the next section discusses a number of physiological phenomena that tend to be the dominant factors limiting the resolution of fMRI.

Physiological Factors Influencing Spatial Resolution

In addition to the standard physics-based factors of signal and noise influencing the spatial resolution of the underlying MR images, a number of physiological factors also impact the resolution that can be obtained with functional MRI.

Physiological-Based Limitations/ Constraints in fMRI

Physiological noise refers to the introduction of unwanted signal changes to the fMRI time-course data as a function of various physiological processes not directly associated with the functional region of the brain that is of interest. The two dominant sources of this noise include signal changes as a function of pulsatile flow through the brain associated with the cardiac cycle, and signal changes associated with respiration. These two primary sources of noise contribute substantially to the need for collecting multiple images per task condition to reliably detect brain activation. In the case of the cardiac cycle, the entire brain pulsates with each beat of the heart, introducing both very small motions and variable vessel flow conditions, which must be averaged out of the data. Respiration changes the susceptibility in the chest as deoxygenated air in the chest is replaced with oxygenated air, and while the chest is obviously some distance from the brain, these changes in susceptibility are detectable in the brain [29].

Blood Oxygenation Changes and Localization

A local change in blood oxygenation in the capillaries does not simply produce a local change in the magnetic field in the capillary. Magnetic field changes are always locally smooth (there are never discontinuities in magnetic field gradients) and thus the field inhomogeneity produced by deoxyhemoglobin extends beyond the wall of the capillary containing the blood. Furthermore, the water, which as we saw previously produces the signal that is recorded, diffuses some distance past these inhomogeneities and can also broaden the effective spatial extent of the field perturbation. Together these factors tend to increase the area in which the signal changes are detectable, and lead to signal changes in the cortical tissue not just the individual capillaries.

The density of the local vasculature may also impact the amplitude of the signal change detected. A change in oxygenation of blood in a capillary dense region (high blood volume) will have a bigger impact on the BOLD signal intensity than the same relative change in oxygenated blood in a region with a sparse capillary network. Work in animal models has demonstrated variable cortical and subcortical capillary densities in several brain regions [30].

The change in blood oxygenation that occurs with activation is over and above the increase in demand for oxygenated blood, and the extent of the region in which a vasculature response is initiated may be larger than the local region where function is increased. This may also contribute to an over estimation of the functional area under investigation. It is currently unclear as to what is the exact relationship between the spatial extent of the cortical tissue activated (and the number or fraction of neurons in the region that is activated) and the spatial extent of the region experiencing a blood flow response.

Functional Spatial Limitations

The question of maximal resolution obtainable with fMRI may be turned around and the question might be posed in terms of the minimum functional unit that can cause a blood flow response upon activation. In fMRI, typically hundreds of thousands of neurons are included in a voxel and it is the mean activity of some part of those neurons that leads to a blood flow response. The relationship between the numbers of neurons that fire and the BOLD response associated with that number is unclear. It is clear, however, that there is a tight coupling between glucose utilization and neuronal spike activity, at least in the sensory/motor cortex. It is not currently feasible to measure by independent methods a significant fraction of the neurons involved in a particular task, and thus to date, investigators have either examined gross electroencephalogram (EEG)-based signals or recorded single neuron spike activity and related magnitude changes in these measures (using either the change in power at a particular frequency in the case of EEG, or the spike rate in the case of single unit recordings) to the BOLD signal change detected [31–36]. Better spike recording methods must be developed before the relationship between the fraction of neurons firing in a voxel can be directly related to a change in oxygenation and/or blood flow.

Brain System Dependent Limitations

As cognitive tasks become more sophisticated in design and more subtle cognitive functions are examined, it will be important to relate the BOLD activation signal to specific networks involved in a task. For example, in a region such as the primary motor cortex wherein the neurons for the digits in the hand are highly interleaved, it has only recently become possible to distinguish activation patterns for the individual digits [37] using high field (7 T) and 1 mm cubed voxel dimensions. There may be many other brain systems that are wired in an even more complicated interleaved sense, in which case it could be very difficult to distinguish between different functional roles for these interleave neurons. Clearly, if neurons are highly interleaved in the cortex then different groups of neurons may be activated by different tasks within a single voxel, but if the same number of neurons is activated by different tasks, no difference in activation will be detectable. This is also related to the issue of the modularity of the brain. To what extent can brain functions be divided into separate modules and what are the neuronal components that make up these modules? Parcellation of the cortex into minimal subunits of activity has recently been shown by Shen [38] using resting-state functional connectivity data, and such an approach may ultimately define the minimal subunits that can be identified in a consistent manner across subjects.

The Draining Vein Problem

A problem that has been discussed since the advent of fMRI is the potential spatial misregistration of functional activity that may occur as a function of the microvasculature. The capillaries, in which the small changes in oxygenation take place upon activation, drain into larger veins downstream from the activation site. Since the amount of blood in a draining vein may be larger than in the upstream capillaries and since the small changes that occur in each capillary may add up to larger BOLD signal changes in the draining veins, this effect could contribute to spatial misregistration of the activation some distance downstream from the true area of cortical activity. A paper by Turner [39] used a quantitative analysis of the geometry of the venous vasculature together with hydrodynamic considerations to calculate upper bounds on the extent of this problem. These calculations revealed that an activated cortical area of 100 mm^2 could generate an oxygenation change in venous blood that extends no more than 4.2 mm beyond the edge of the activated area. While the venous blood obviously drains much greater distances, beyond this limit the oxygenation effect is sufficiently diluted as to be undetectable.

In an attempt to reduce the draining vein problem and produce highly localized functional maps, Menon et al. [40] used the initial increase in the BOLD signal intensity to image ocular dominance columns in the human visual cortex and demonstrated that this use of the initial slope of the BOLD signal increase was effective. More recently, statistical postprocessing methods have been applied to reduce this problem further [41].

Field strength also influences the relative signal change with changes in oxygenation for both tissue and vessels. It has been shown, for example [42], that increasing field strength increases the BOLD sensitivity to tissue changes in oxygenation faster than the increase in vessels. Thus moving to higher field strength reduces the relative contribution of the venous signal changes compared to the true tissue signal changes [43].

The reader should keep in mind that the draining vein problem does not abrogate true BOLD activation in the cortical region activated, but can produce additional, potentially stronger activations further downstream. The fact that the BOLD response in draining veins can be large allows them to be identified by the large percent signal change measured. Excluding signal changes above a certain threshold (in terms of percent signal change), it is possible to produce high resolution maps of cortical function free of this draining vein problem. Cheng [44], for example, produced maps of the cortical columns in the visual cortex, adapting this approach to sustained stimulus presentations. But caution is required with this activation amplitude threshold approach as the signal in draining veins does not necessarily have to be large, and the signal does gradually decrease with distance from the activation site so at some point the threshold approach will fail – and this point is unfortunately at maximal distance from the activation site.

Spin echo imaging is sensitive to microscopic but not macroscopic susceptibility effects [26–28]. At high field strengths (3 T and greater) this approach can achieve sufficient sensitivity for fMRI experiments and can mostly eliminate the draining vein problem [43]. It is well known that spin echo sequences are much less sensitive to the draining vein problem. While most investigators do not like to admit it, the additional relatively large signal changes associated with larger veins can really aid in detecting activation. The sensitivity of gradient echo and spin echo sequences to microscopic susceptibility changes is essentially equal, and thus the choice of gradient echo imaging over spin echo imaging is really made to allow the contribution of larger vessels to the BOLD signal change, to get an added boost from the bigger signal changes associated with these vessels.

Diffusion gradients can also be applied to BOLD imaging sequences to reduce contributions from large vessels [45, 46], and in fact, it is possible to actually use maps of apparent diffusion coefficients to detect activation [47–49].

The Initial Dip

Another method to eliminate the draining vein problem and to possibly provide more precise spatial localization of fMRI activity is to localize activation based on finding regions that exhibit an initial dip in BOLD signal intensity prior to the main signal intensity increase. Following the presentation of a stimulation event, the blood flow response in the cortical region involved in detecting or responding to the event often leads to a complicated pattern of signal changes. Some experiments have shown that there is first a decrease in signal intensity, prior to the increased signal intensity typically observed in BOLD experiments. The initial dip was first observed using optical measures of oxy- and deoxyhemoglobin [50, 51] and has more recently been demonstrated using BOLD sensitive fMRI methods in the visual [52–55] and in the sensory/motor cortex [3]. Since the increased oxygen consumption occurs before the blood flow response has had a chance to compensate, there is a brief decrease in the ratio of oxygenated to deoxygenated blood leading to an initial dip in signal intensity. This initial dip is followed by a signal intensity increase as the blood flow response kicks in and overcompensates for the increased oxygen consumption, leading to an increase in the ratio of oxyhemoglobin to deoxyhemoglobin in the blood and the increase in BOLD contrast that most fMRI experiments typically rely upon. As the blood flow returns to baseline levels after these events, an under-shoot of the signal intensity is also often observed before the intensity finally returns to prestimulus levels.

Theoretically, the initial dip could provide extremely good localization of the activated regions as there is no draining vein problem with this phenomenon, and it directly reflects increased oxygen consumption [3, 55]. Kim et al. [56] exploited this phenomenon to map iso-orientation columns in the rat visual cortex. The initial dip also may be important in understanding the link between changes in cerebral blood flow (CBF), cerebral blood volume (CBV), partial pressure of oxygen (pO_2), and oxygen metabolism under dynamic conditions. However, there are two difficulties associated with the initial dip phenomenon. First, it is controversial in that it is not always observed. As Buxton points out in a commentary on this issue, [57] two papers using optical imaging techniques and whisker barrel stimulation paradigms in a rat model came to opposite conclusions regarding this phenomenon. Lindauer et al. [58] found no evidence for this initial decrease in tissue oxygenation, while Jones et al. [59] did find a reproducible initial increase in deoxyhemoglobin. Many fMRI experiments have also failed to detect the initial dip. However, when dealing with such a small signal change in the presence of significant physiological noise, a negative result does not necessarily mean the phenomena does not exist. Second, the BOLD signal change associated with the initial dip is approximately one tenth that observed with the later BOLD signal increases, and thus, it is very difficult to measure with fMRI and not practical with current methods for the majority of fMRI studies. Encouragingly, however, moving to higher fields such as 7 T appears to make detection of the initial dip more reliable and the results of both optical and fMRI imaging are beginning to converge [60].

Subject Movement

Subject movement is also a constant problem in fMRI experiments; and if human experiments are to move to considerably higher spatial resolution, improved motion correction methods and motion-limiting devices will need to be developed. The trade-off in limiting subject motion is the tension between subject comfort and ability to move. It is possible to position a subject with sufficient padding, tape, and bite bars, such that they cannot move; however, it is not possible to keep such a subject in the magnet for very long due to the discomfort associated with these restraints. Systems designed to track motion and algorithms that allow image registration incorporating geometric distortion correction methods may ultimately improve the ability to correct for any motion, thereby eliminating the need for uncomfortable constraints to be placed on the subjects [61, 62]. Moving to higher field strength may allow for reductions in the overall study time and, therefore, also allow more restraining devices to be used, particularly if the subject is made aware of the fact that the discomfort is only for a brief period of time. In most cases, however, the gain in SNR in moving to higher field strength is used to increase the spatial resolution, or add more tasks, both of which are good choices, but with the result that study time remains fixed.

Other Physiological Changes Associated with Brain Activation

As discussed previously, if CMRO2 (cerebral metabolic rate of oxygen consumption) could be directly measured, or if a BOLD measure of the initial dip does indeed reflect the initial consumption of oxygen, then these approaches would likely provide the maximal spatial resolution. It is unlikely that other MR measures of neural activity such as changes in CBV and CBF will provide higher spatial resolution than the BOLD effect, as these changes also represent rather gross brain responses to increased oxygen demand.

Threshold Effects and Localization

All functional maps are statistical maps of some sort and, therefore, involve the use of a statistical threshold to be chosen to classify tissue(s) as activated or not. However, the actual threshold chosen is arbitrary and the spatial extent of activation varies significantly as a function of this arbitrary statistical threshold. In order to reduce the multiple comparisons problem and reduce the occurrence of spurious single voxel activations arising by chance alone, spatial filtering is also often preformed in the form of a median or cluster filter of some sort. The definition of the size of these filters is also arbitrary and can significantly influence the extent of the activation measured. Thus, spatial resolution of the final activation maps can be significantly influenced by the statistical parameters chosen in the analysis/display software.

Temporal Resolution of the BOLD Response

The previous sections have focused on the issue of spatial resolution in fMRI, but in some cases it may be important to examine the time course of activation for individual events. Action potentials are recorded as electrical spike activity, and these spikes fire over the course of milliseconds. Electrical recordings of ensembles of firing neurons record characteristic peaks and troughs in the form of evoked response potentials (ERPs) in time-scales of the order of hundreds of milliseconds. Functional MR imaging relies on the blood flow response to such neuronal activity, which itself is much, much slower than the activity of individual neurons. From a single event, say for example, a flash of a bright light lasting only 100 ms, the blood flow response in the primary visual cortex may start to increase some 2 s after the event, it may peak between 6 and 8 s and return to baseline by 16–20 s after this single 100 ms flash of light. Since fMRI is usually focused on measuring the response of ensembles of neurons to particular stimuli, it may not be necessary to measure activity with extremely high temporal resolution. But many interesting questions may be probed by examining even this slow blood flow response with high temporal resolution.

There is little evidence to date that within the gross blood flow response typically measured in fMRI, there is detailed information reflecting ERP patterns or specific spike timings. To investigate this further, fMRI experiments will need to be performed with very high temporal resolutions of the order of tens of milliseconds, and such acquisitions are possible, albeit with a very limited number of slices, with the current technology.

The mechanism controlling the blood flow response in the brain is not well understood, nor is the spatial extent of this mechanism clear relative to the actual neuronal activity, and it remains to be seen if there is a meaningful fine-grained temporal modulation of this response with neuronal activity.

Most early fMRI experiments relied upon block designs wherein an activation condition was presented for 30 s or more at a time, and this was alternated with a control condition of equal duration, many times over the course of a study. In such experimental designs many images could be collected over the course of a condition and high temporal resolution was not all that important. (although, as discussed previously, shorter TR acquisitions can have significant benefits in terms of statistical power in the activation maps.) Many experiments are still performed using block designed paradigms because these studies do not require precise timing between the image acquisition and the stimulus presentation and because the statistical power in such studies is maximized, and usually considerably greater than that obtained in event-related designs. Cognitively, however, block design experiments can be of limited value if habituation effects or changes in strategy occur over the course of a long block of similar stimuli, or if the goal is to separate responses to individual stimuli according to some behavioral measure.

To make for much more natural stimulus presentations and to examine the blood flow response to specific stimuli, many experimental designs have moved towards event-related studies. Despite the slow blood flow and oxygenation responses to neuronal activity, many interesting phenomena can be investigated with event-related experimental designs. For example, it is possible to examine the temporal response in a specific region to a wide range of stimuli and quantitatively assess parameters such as time-to-peak, width of response, peak height, and other such factors. For a given brain region it is possible to examine the linearity of the response as stimulus presentation rate is modified, and such studies can provide insight into the coupling of blood flow, oxygenation, and neuronal activity changes.

To properly sample this blood flow response function, short TR acquisitions should be used. The TR should be of the order of 2 s or less, with shorter TR again being better. Alternatively, some investigators have acquired jittered data whereby the time lock between stimuli presentation and image acquisition is varied across events, such that over the course of many events the blood flow response is sampled with high temporal resolution [63]. Increasing the temporal resolution by decreasing the TR necessitates reducing the flip angle of the RF excitation pulse to maintain optimum signal. This reduced flip angle in turn leads to decreased SNR in the individual images, but the gain in statistical power associated with more of these noisier images being collected in a fixed imaging time more than compensates for the slight decrease in SNR of the individual images.

The dependence of the BOLD response on the underlying structure of the microvasculature, however, makes it difficult to compare the blood flow responses across different brain regions. It would be desirable to observe temporal progression of activation patterns moving from one region of the brain to another and thereby obtain a sense of the communication between different brain areas. This is not possible, however, without first characterizing the local variations in the structure of the microvasculature in different cortical regions. Thus while it is difficult to make claims about the progression of activation from region A to B to C as a single task progresses, it is possible to observe differences in the order of this progression across two or more different tasks, assuming the plumbing in a given region remains constant and independent of the task. Event-related paradigms combined with high temporal resolution fMRI acquisition techniques are still in their infancy and much more will be learned from such studies as the field progresses.

Temporal resolution as defined by TR also impacts the ability to filter out, or remove, periodic noise such as that arising from the cardiac or respiratory cycle. Most acquisition strategies sample at a high-enough rate to remove some noise from respiratory effects, but a close look at the noise power spectrum in fMRI reveals components associated with the cardiac cycle, aliased at many different (lower) frequencies due to the relatively low sampling rate of the fMRI data. By low sampling rate it is meant that a slice acquisition is repeated say every second or more, rather than the required sampling rate of at least double the cardiac rate. Sampling at rates that are at least double the periodicity avoids aliasing of noise components to lower frequencies and makes removal of these components much easier in postprocessing.

Pulse Sequences for fMRI: Spatial/ Temporal Resolution

The most common pulse sequences used in fMRI, EPI and spiral imaging, are discussed in detail in Chap. 2. This section will briefly discuss some aspects of these two sequences and alternative strategies that have been investigated to date. If high temporal resolution is desired, most MR imagers are now equipped with the gradient hardware to provide this information with image acquisition times of the order of 40 ms or less. Echo planar imaging (EPI) and single shot spiral methods acquire the entire data set for an image, from a single excitation pulse, and thus within a single TR. In conventional MRI a separate excitation pulse is used for each line of data acquired, allowing a time, TR, to elapse for the magnetization to recover before the next excitation pulse. Thus in conventional scanning an image with 64 phase encoding steps would require 64 × TR seconds to acquire the entire dataset. With a TR of 1.5 s this represents an acquisition time of over 1 min. Echo planar imaging methods, on the other hand, can collect the data for an entire image in as little as 40 ms. Collecting the data in such a rapid manner does have drawbacks. There is a significant decrease in signal-to-noise ratio due to the high bandwidth of the data acquisition that is needed to collect the data rapidly, and there are also significant distortion effects arising from the accumulation of phase errors over the sampling window. These distortion effects arise in the phase encode direction in EPI, and are projected in all directions in spiral scanning. This distortion is not present in the conventionally acquired anatomic scans upon which the activation is usually highlighted. Thus caution must be used in high-resolution work to ensure that the distorted functional image is appropriately registered to the undistorted anatomic image. This is a difficult problem as the distortion in the functional images is locally variable and thus simple rigid body fitting of the two different acquisitions is not sufficient to avoid this problem [64].

One method for reducing the image distortion is to move to a multishot approach, which of course involves a penalty in temporal resolution, but is almost essential when moving to very high field [65]. Another approach is to measure in vivo the image distortion and then use a map of the distortion to correct the final image. Two approaches have been devised to perform this measure and these are field mapping (the image distortion is directly proportional to the distortion in the static magnetic B-field) [66–68] and point spread function mapping (PSF) [69–71]. The field map approach can provide a relatively simple method for correcting image distortions, but it contains no knowledge of the initial distribution of image intensities. This limitation makes it difficult to assign the correct image intensity, and hence functional activation, to the undistorted voxels. The PSF approach, can correctly assign the appropriate image intensities to each voxel in addition to correctly locating each voxel in space.

A field map can be obtained using EPI with only two EPI data acquisitions. However, since the field map is calculated from the phase difference between these two images, phase wrap can be a problem. This problem can be reduced by collecting several acquisitions with different phase-offsets, thereby making unwrapping of the phase errors much easier. PSF maps require a minimum of 16 acquisitions to obtain the PSF in a single direction, but more acquisitions yield higher resolution PSF maps and thus better correction of the image distortion. In summary, with acquisition times of 1 min or less, field maps or PSF maps can be obtained at some point in an fMRI study, allowing correction of the geometric image distortion.

Despite this problem of image distortion, the gain in statistical power in collecting multiple images in a short period of time and the need for activation/control blocks to be short for cognitive reasons necessitates the use of EPI or spiral pulses sequences. Echo planar imaging scans the data space using a raster scan approach and requires state-of-the-art gradients to produce high quality images with minimal image distortion. Spiral scanning, as the name implies, spirals, either in- or out-, from the center of the data space and can be less demanding on the gradient hardware [72]. Most modern magnets now have gradients, which easily ramp as fast as allowed by the US Food and Drug Administration (FDA). The limitations currently encountered are not hardware limitations but are based on subject safety issues. The FDA mandates limitations in dB/dt (the rate at which the gradient can be ramped) because ramping gradients very rapidly can induce current loops in the body that could result in stimulation of muscle groups such as the heart. Small gradient insert coils have been developed that may allow even faster ramping of the gradients as the active length of the gradients may be short enough to minimize the current loops. These gradient insert systems, however, can be physically restricting, limited in terms of FOV, and are not easily moved in and out of the magnet due to the heavy weight of the combined gradients and cooling system. Manufacturers have been reluctant to develop such gradient inserts as the coils are awkward to move, weighing several hundred pounds, and must be properly fastened down each time they are moved lest they torque in the magnet and seriously injure the subject. Going faster also requires faster sampling along the readout gradient, which increases the bandwidth of the data acquisition and negatively impacts the SNR, but with the advantage of decreased geometric distortion.

While EPI and spiral gradient echo acquisitions in their many forms are by far the most commonly used approaches, these sequences are sometimes implemented in three-dimensional (3D) acquisition mode, [15, 73] and it should be noted that there are many other acquisition strategies that can be adapted to fMRI. Other pulse sequences include asymmetric spin echo imaging [74], which combines some gradient echo (T2*) contrast with spin echo (T2) contrast to reduce the signal loss problem associated with static field inhomogeneities, and to reduce the contribution of large vessels, while maintaining sensitivity to the BOLD affect. Inversion recovery asymmetric spin echo [75] has been used to reduce the contribution of cerebrospinal fluid (CSF) to the functional images, reducing the chance of spurious activations arising from pulsatile movement of the CSF.

Fast spin echo imaging [25, 76] has been used in functional MR imaging, but its sensitivity at 1.5 T is too low for most cognitive studies, while at high fields such as 7 T power deposition can become an issue. Variations on the fast spin echo imaging approach, include techniques such as gradient-and spin-echo (GRASE) imaging [77] and ultrafast, low-angle rapid acquisition with relaxation enhancement (RARE) imaging [63], both of which have similar performance to fast spin echo (FSE) but with reduced power deposition. These sequences can be applied with or without inversion recovery pulses to reduce the contribution of CSF. FSE, GRASE, and ultrafast low angle RARE (UFLARE) can all be applied in single shot mode, but because of the large number of additional RF pulses included in these sequences relative to EPI or spiral imaging, the acquisition window can be long. Longer acquisition windows mean fewer slices can be acquired in a TR interval.

A novel technique, first proposed by Scheffler [78], uses a balanced steady-state free precession (SSFP) imaging sequence that is sensitive to activation due to a slight frequency shift associated with local changes in tissue oxygenation. The technique has more recently been refined [79] and has been shown to be effective for producing high resolution fMRI maps free of the image distortions typically observed in EPI BOLD acquisitions.

Single-shot techniques by definition are fast but there are also methods for accelerating multishot techniques. Multishot acquisitions are particularly amenable to multicoil acquisition strategies and the use of sensitivity encoded (SENSE) reconstruction techniques [10]. In this approach, fewer phase encode lines are collected (thereby saving time) but to maintain resolution, the field of view is reduced in direct proportion with the number of phase encode lines. Reducing the field-of-view below approximately 20 cm when imaging the brain usually results in field-of-view wrap artifacts, wherein the structures that extend beyond the FOV are folded back over into the image. With multicoil imaging and SENSE reconstruction, however, the sensitivity profiles of the individual coils making up the multicoil array are used to unwrap the fold-over artifacts and yield high quality images in reduced imaging times. Some decrease in SNR occurs, and as the reduction in the number of phase encode steps becomes large, the reconstruction begins to deteriorate, limiting the reductions to factors of 2 or 3. Collecting fewer phase encode steps with this approach can be used to reduce the imaging time, or it may allow for more slices to be collected within the TR window, thereby increasing spatial coverage without a sacrifice in temporal resolution. As described previously in the discussion on geometric image distortion, increasing the acquisition bandwidth in a multislice two-dimensional (2D) acquisition can also allow an extra slice or two to be acquired within a given TR, since increased bandwidth leads to shorter acquisition windows. This shorter readout time will also reduce image distortion (good) and SNR (bad). For example an acquisition with a bandwidth of 64 kHz may have an SNR of 50. Doubling the acquisition bandwidth to 128 kHz will reduce the image distortion by a factor of 2 and reduce the SNR by $\sqrt{2}$ and allow a few more slices to be squeezed into the TR interval.

State-of-the-art work combining SENSE with a 3D EPI acquisition, to yield 1 mm cubed isotropic voxel dimensions and whole-brain coverage with a temporal resolution of 3.2 s, has just been published by Poser et al. 2010; and this may well be the way forward for achieving high spatial resolution with reasonable temporal resolution.

Imaging Approaches to Other Physiological Measurements

Rather than measuring changes in signal intensity related to relative changes in blood oxygenation as the BOLD contrast mechanism does, it is possible to directly measure changes in cerebral blood flow (CBF) with neuronal activity. As pointed out by Calamante [80] in a review of CBF methods, the sensitivity of MRI to moving spins was noted in the earliest days of nuclear magnetic resonance (NMR) [81]. Today this approach is exploited in imaging applications using both single-slice and multislice acquisition strategies. It is now possible using these MR imaging approaches to measure absolute CBF or, more simply, relative changes in CBF with activation. The techniques for performing such measurements are generally referred to as arterial spin labeling methods.

Arterial Spin Labeling

Arterial spin labeling (ASL) incorporates magnetic labeling of blood flowing into the imaging slice to obtain quantitative information on CBF. The basic strategy of ASL is to acquire two acquisitions, one with and another without labeling of flowing blood, such that subtraction of these acquisitions can yield quantitative perfusion information. This approach makes use of the properties of spins in flowing blood and does not require an exogenous contrast agent. Several papers have been published describing the application of ASL techniques in functional brain imaging [82–87]. For an excellent review, see Yang [2].

There are two categories of methods for approaching spin labeling, and these include continuous ASL and pulsed ASL. Continuous ASL uses a train of RF pulses to continuously saturate protons in the blood upstream from the imaging slice [88, 89]. The saturated spins flow into the imaging slice and establish a steady-state exchange of magnetization with the brain tissue water such that the magnetization measured can be related to the CBF. Pulsed ASL applies a single inversion pulse prior to image acquisition and varies the selectivity of the inversion pulse in successive acquisitions. In pulsed ASL, the inversion pulse is placed upstream of the imaging slice and different images are obtained from acquisitions with and without this labeling pulse.

In both pulsed and continuous ASL methods, there are many factors that can influence the quantification of the CBF. These include slice profile effects, wherein a blurred slice profile can make determination of the arrival time of the tagged spins more difficult to determine. These effects can be minimized with well-designed inversion pulses, which produce very sharp slice profiles, such as some of the longer adiabatic frequency offset corrected inversion (FOCI) pulses [90]. Transit time or path-length effects can also introduce quantification difficulties [91, 92]. Most CBF analysis approaches assume a straight-line trajectory from the tagging plane to the imaging plane; however, this is not necessarily true. Tagged spins can flow obliquely between the two planes and the spins likely will not flow along a straight line, thereby increasing the path length and transit time to the imaging slice. Knowledge of these pathways for all slices and all locations is usually limited, making it difficult to account for this in quantifying the CBF. Minimizing the distance between the labeling slice and the imaging slice can reduce these path-length effects simply by reducing the path length and, therefore, the time allowed for such errors to accumulate. Magnetization transfer (MT) effects can also cause changes in signal intensity in the imaging slice, leading to spurious CBF measures. The MT effect leads to direct signal changes in the imaging slice even in the absence of perfusion. MT effects can also lead to decreases in the apparent T1, which must be taken into account if absolute CBF is to be determined [93]. To avoid such effects, labeling pulses can be applied in a second acquisition, on the opposite, downstream, side of the slice equidistant from where these pulses were applied on the upstream side. Both acquisitions then will have the same MT effect and thus subtraction will eliminate this as a variable.

A final complicating issue in the application of ASL in fMRI is the need for multislice acquisitions. Since all the slices cannot be obtained simultaneously, different slices will have different transit times, and different distances from the labeling pool. This can lead to erroneous differences in the apparent CBF between slices when in fact there may be none. Applying ASL techniques with very fast imaging approaches, and taking the different transit time and path-length effects into consideration, can make multislice imaging more practical [94, 95].

Most ASL approaches used in fMRI have used fast imaging pulse sequences such as EPI [82, 96] or spiral imaging, although modified single-shot RARE and GRASE pulse sequences have been adapted to ASL for fMRI [87]. The advantage of these multishot approaches lies in their reduced sensitivity to field inhomogeneities and, in particular, to the image distortion effect and in increased SNR due to the short effective TEs that can be used (although it should be noted that spiral out sequences can also have very short TEs). These sequences, however, require multiple shots, which increases imaging time, and the imaging time can only be reduced by increasing the echo train length and decreasing the number of slices acquired. As in BOLD imaging, these CBF imaging sequences may be combined with the parallel imaging approaches (multicoil SENSE) [97]. Other approaches have been designed to measure both BOLD and CBF in an interleaved fashion to better characterize the activation observed [24, 86, 98–100]. Finally, just as in BOLD imaging, moving to higher fields with ASL techniques also has advantages. The SNR is generally higher, and because T1 is longer at high field, labeling is better and transit time effects are less significant [24].

Sensitivity

By far, the most commonly used measure of neuronal activation is the BOLD contrast mechanism. There are, however, other contrast mechanisms that can be exploited. Changes in both CBV and CBF can be measured with MR using sequences such as vascular-space occupancy (VASO) [101–103] or venous refocusing for volume estimation (VERVE) [104, 105] for the former measure, and a technique such as arterial spin labeling as described previously for the latter. The change in CBV with activation can be quite large and has been reported to be of the

Table 4.1 Summary of technical challenges in fMRI and some promising solutions

Authors	Challenge	Approach	Pros/cons
Lee et al. 2008 [79]	Static field inhomogeneities: image distortion	Uses a balance SSFP 3D acquisition strategy	Yields distortion free images. Optimization is complex, and 3D acquisition may yield different motion sensitivity.
Deng et al. 2009 [22]	Static field inhomogeneities: signal loss	Parallel transmit RF to compensate for through-plane dephasing	Does not involve a time penalty. Effective, but requires multiple transmitters that most magnets currently do not have.
Qin et al. 2009 [108]	Subject motion	Use external optical devices to track motion	May provide a robust solution to the motion problem. Partial volume effects in low-resolution fMRI acquisitions could still contribute to signal change – this applies to the navigator solution as well.
Poser et al. 2010 [109]	Spatial/temporal resolution at high field (7 T)	Use a 3D EPI approach to obtain isotropic 1 mm voxel sizes and whole-brain coverage.	High isotropic resolution can minimize many problems including static field dephasing and partial volume effects and provide better localization. This is currently very technically challenging, but may become routine in the near future.
White et al. 2010 [107]	Subject motion	Uses navigator echoes to track motion	Potential for high resolution motion tracking. Unclear at this time whether sufficient accuracy to reduce motion sensitivity of fMRI. Potentially differential effects of navigator pulses on selected tissue, decrease in temporal resolution.

order of 30%. In fact, one of the first functional studies in humans was performed using CBV as the measure of activation [106].

As discussed previously, CBF can be measured using arterial spin labeling, but this requires extra hardware and/or pulse sequences that are not usually found as standard equipment on most imagers. This approach is most effective in cases where only a very limited number of slices need to be acquired (one) and in cases where it is acceptable to define the slice orientation based on the anatomy of the arterial vasculature.

Conclusion

It is hoped that this chapter sheds some light on the issues associated with defining the spatial and temporal resolution limits and the sensitivity in functional MRI. New pulse sequences and new imaging hardware are constantly being developed, and combined with a better understanding of the physiological changes that occur with brain activation, the ability to obtain high-resolution fMRI studies in short exam times will continue to improve (Table 4.1). There are many trade-offs to be made in choosing the imaging sequence and parameters to use, and it is hoped that this brief overview sheds some light on the issues involved. Clearly, since many trade-offs must be made, an understanding of these issues will help the investigator to tailor some of these parameters to the specific brain region or study design.

Acknowledgments NIH NS38467, NS40497, EB00473.

References

1. Callaghan PT. Principles of nuclear magnetic resonance microscopy. Oxford: Oxford Science Publications; 1993.
2. Yang Y. Perfusion MR Imaging with pulsed arterial spin-labeling: basic principles and applications in functional brain imaging. Concepts Magn Reson. 2002;14:347–57.
3. Yacoub E, Hu X. Detection of the early decrease in fMRI signal in the motor area. Magn Reson Med. 2001;45:184–90.
4. Yacoub E, Shmuel A, Pfeuffer J, Van De Moortele PF, Adriany G, Ugurbil K, et al. Investigation of the initial dip in fMRI at 7 Tesla. NMR Biomed. 2001;14(7–8):408–12.
5. Yacoub E, Shmuel A, Pfeuffer J, Van De Moortele PF, Adriany G, Andersen P, et al. Imaging brain function in humans at 7 Tesla. Magn Reson Med. 2001;45(4):588–94.

6. Ojemann JG, Akbudak E, Snyder AZ, McKinstry RC, Raichle ME, Conturo TE. Anatomic localization and quantitative analysis of gradient refocused echo-planar fMRI susceptibility artifacts. Neuroimage. 1997;6:156–67.
7. Merboldt KD, Finsterbusch J, Frahm J. Reducing inhomogeneity artifacts in functional MRI of human brain activation – thin sections versus gradient compensation. J Magn Reson. 2000;145(2):184–91.
8. Wadghiri YZ, Johnson G, Turnbull DH. Sensitivity and performance time in MRI dephasing artifact reduction methods. Magn Reson Med. 2001;45:470–6.
9. Sodickson DK, Manning WJ. Simultaneous acquisition of spatial harmonics (SMASH): fast imaging with radiofrequency coil arrays. Magn Reson Med. 1997;38:591–603.
10. Pruessmann KP, Weiger M, Scheidegger MB, Boesiger P. SENSE: sensitivity encoding for fast MRI. Magn Reson Med. 1999;42:952–62.
11. Constable RT, Spencer DD. Repetition time in echo planar functional MR imaging. Magn Reson Med. 2001;46(4):748–55.
12. Constable RT. Functional MR imaging using gradient echo EPI in the presence of large static field inhomogeneities. J Magn Reson Imaging. 1995;5(6):746–52.
13 Constable RT, Spencer DD. Composite image formation in Z-shimmed functional MR imaging. Magn Reson Med. 1999;42(1):110–7.
14. Yang QX, Dardzinski BJ, Li S, Smith MB. Multi-gradient echo with susceptibility inhomogeneity compensation (MGESIC): demonstration of fMRI in the olfactory cortex at 3.0 T. Magn Reson Med. 1997;37:331–5.
15. Glover GH. 3D z-shim method for reduction of susceptibility effects in BOLD fMRI. Magn Reson Med. 1999;42(2):290–9.
16. Frahm J, Merboldt JD, Hanicke W. Direct flash MR imaging of magnetic field inhomogeneities by gradient compensation. Magn Reson Med. 1988;6:474–80.
17. Cho ZH, Ro YM. Reduction of susceptibility artifact in gradient-echo imaging. Magn Reson Med. 1992;23:193–200.
18. Stenger VA, Boada FE, Noll DC. Multishot 3D slice-select tailored RF pulses for MRI. Magn Reson Med. 2002;48(1):157–65.
19. Yip C-Y, Yoon D, Olafsson V, Lee S, Grissom WA, Fessler JA, et al. Spectral-Spatial pulse design for through-plane phase precompensatory slice selection in T2*-weighted functional MRI. Magn Reson Med. 2009;61:1137–47.
20. Katscher U, Bornert P, Leussler C, van den Brink JS. Transmit SENSE. Magn Reson Med. 2003;49(1):144–50.
21. Zhu Y. Parallel excitation with an array of transmit coils. Magn Reson Med. 2004;51(4):775–84.
22. Deng W, Yang C, Alagappan V, Wald LL, Boada FE, Stenger VA. Simultaneous z-shim method for reducing susceptibility artifacts with multiple transmitters. Magn Reson Med. 2009;61:255–9.
23. Song AW. Single-shot EPI with signal recovery from susceptibility induced losses. Magn Reson Med. 2001;46:407–11.
24. Yang Y, Gu H, Zhan W, Xu S, Silbersweig DA, Stern E. Simultaneous perfusion and BOLD imaging using reverse spiral scanning at 3 T: characterization of functional contrast and susceptibility artifacts. Magn Reson Med. 2002;48(2):278–89.
25. Constable RT, Kennan RP, Puce A, McCarthy G, Gore JC. Functional MR imaging using fast spin echo at 1.5 T. Magn Reson Med. 1994;31:686–90.
26. Boxerman JL, Hamberg LM, Rosen BR, Weisskoff RM. MR contrast due to intravascular magnetic-susceptibility perturbations. Magn Reson Med. 1995;34:555–66.
27. Weisskoff RM, Zuo CS, Boxerman JL, Rosen BR. Microscopic susceptibility variation and transverse relaxation: theory and experiment. Magn Reson Med. 1994;31:601–10.
28. Kennan RP, Zhong JH, Gore JC. Intravascular susceptibility contrast mechanisms in tissues. Magn Reson Med. 1994;31:9–21.
29. Raj D, Anderson AW, Gore JC. Respiratory effects in human functional magnetic resonance imaging due to bulk susceptibility changes. Phys Med Biol. 2001;46(12):3331–40.
30. Cavaglia M, Dombrowski SM, Drazba J, Vasanji A, Bokesch PM, Janigro D. Regional variation in brain capillary density and vascular response to ischemia. Brain Res. 2001;910(1–2):81–93.
31. Heeger DJ, Huk AC, Geisler WS, Albrecht DG. Spike versus BOLD: what does neuroimaging tell us about neuronal activity? Nat Neurosci. 2000;3(7):631–3.
32. Rees G, Friston K, Koch C. A direct quantitative relationship between functional properties of human and macaque V5. Nat Neurosci. 2000;3:716–23.
33. Logothetis NK, Guggenberger H, Peled S, Pauls J. Neurophysiological investigation of the basis of the fMRI signal change. Nat Neurosci. 1999;2:555–62.
34 Logothetis NK, Pauls J, Augath M, Trinath T, Oeltermann A. Neurophysiological investigation of the basis of the fMRI signal. Nature. 2001;412:150–7.
35. Hyder F, Rothman DL, Shulman RG. Total neuroenergetics support localized brain activity: implications for the interpretation of fMRI. Proc Natl Acad Sci USA. 2002;99(16):10771–6.
36. Smith AJ, Blumenfeld H, Behar KL, Rothman DL, Shulman RG, Hyder F. Cerebrla energetics and spiking frequency: the neurophysiological basis of fMRI. Proc Natl Acad Sci USA. 2002; 99(16):10765–9770.
37. Sanchez-Panchuelo RM, Francis S, Bowtell R, Schluppeck D. Mapping human somatosensory cortex in individual subjects with 7 T functional MRI, J. Neurophysiol. 2010;103(5):2544–56.
38. Shen X, Papademetris X, Constable RT. Graph-theory based parcellation of functional subunits in the brain from resting-state fMRI data. Neuroimage. 2010;50(3):1027–35.

39. Turner R. How much cortex can a vein drain? Downstream dilution of activation-related cerebral blood oxygenation changes. Neuroimage. 2002;16: 1062–7.
40. Menon RS, Goodyear BG. Submillimeter functional localization in human striate cortex using BOLD contrast at 4 Tesla: implications for the vascular point spread function. Magn Reson Med. 1999;41:230–5.
41. Nencka AS, Rowe DB. Reducing the unwanted draining vein BOLD contribution in fMRI with statistical post-processing methods. Neuroimage. 2007;37:177–88.
42. Gati JS, Menon RS, Ugurbil K, Rutt BK. Experimental determination of the BOLD field strength dependence in vessels and tissue. Magn Reson Med. 1997;38:296–302.
43. Yacoub E, Duong TQ, Van De Moortele P-F, Lindquist M, Adriany G, Kim S-G, et al. Spin-echo fMRI in humans using high spatial resolutions and high magnetic fields. Magn Reson Med. 2003;49:655–64.
44. Cheng K, Waggoner RA, Tanaka K. Mapping human ocular dominance columns with high field (4 T) functional magnetic resonance imaging. Proc Int Soc Magn Reson Med. 2000;8:978.
45. Song AW, Wong EC, Tan SG, Hyde JS. Diffusion weighted fMRI at 1.5 T. Magn Reson Med. 1996;35:155–8.
46. Andersson L, Bolling M, Wirestam R, Holtas S, Stahlberg F. Combined diffusion weighting and CSF suppression in functional MRI. NMR Biomed. 2002;15:235–40.
47. Zhong J, Kennan RP, Gore JC. Effects of susceptibility variations on NMR measurements of diffusion. J Magn Reson. 1991;95:267–80.
48. Lee SP, Silva AC, Ugurbil K, Kim SG. Diffusion-weighted spin-echo fMRI at 9.4 T: microvascular/tissue contribution to BOLD signal changes. Magn Reson Med. 1999;42(5):919–28.
49. Song AW, Woldorff MG, Gangstead S, Mangun GR, McCarthy G. Enhanced spatial localization of neuronal activation using simultaneous apparent-diffusion-coefficient and blood-oxygenation functional magnetic resonance imaging. Neuroimage. 2002;17: 742–50.
50. Frostig RD, Lieke EE, Ts'o DY, Grinvald A. Cortical functional architecture and local coupling between neuronal activity and the microcirculation revealed by in vivo high-resolution imaging of intrinsic signals. Proc Natl Acad Sci USA. 1990;87:6082–6.
51. Malonek D, grinvald A. Interactions between electrical activity and cortical microcirculation revealed by imaging spectroscopy: implications for functional brain mapping. Science. 1996;272:551–4.
52. Ernst T, Hennig J. Observation of a fast response in functional MR. Magn Reson Med. 1994;32:146–9.
53. Menon RS, Ogawa S, Strupp JP, Anderson P, Ugurbil K. BOLD based functional MRI at 4 Tesla includes capillary bed contribution: Echo-planar imaging correlates with previous optical imaging using intrinsic signals. Magn Reson Med. 1995;33:453–9.
54. Hu X, Le TH, Ugurbil K. Evaluation of the early response in fMRI in individual subjects using short stimulus duration. Magn Reson Med. 1997;37: 877–84.
55. Duong TQ, Kim DS, Ugurbil K, Kim SG. Spatiotemporal dynamics of the BOLD fMRI signals: towards mapping submillimeter cortical columns using the early negative response. Magn Reson Med. 2000;44(2):231–42.
56. Kim DS, Duong DQ, Kim S-G. High resolution mapping of iso-orientation columns by fMRI. Nat Neurosci. 2000;3:164–9.
57. Buxton RB. The elusive initial dip. Neuroimage. 2001;13:953–8.
58. Lindauer U, Royl G, Leithner C, Kuhl M, Gold L, Gethmann J, et al. No evidence for early decrease in blood oxygenation in rat whisker cortex in response to functional activation. Neuroimage. 2001;13: 986–99.
59. Jones M, Berwick J, Johnston D, Mayhew J. Concurrent optical imaging spectroscopy and laser-doppler flowmetry: the relationship between blood flow, oxygenation, and volume in rodent barrel cortex. Neuroimage. 2001;13:1000–13.
60. Uludag K, Muller-Bierl B, Ugurbil K. An integrative model for neuronal activity-induced signal changes for gradient and spin echo functional imaging. Neuroimage. 2009;48:150–65.
61. Tremblay M, Tam F, Graham SJ. Retrospective coregistration of functional magnetic resonance imaging data using external monitoring. Magn Reson Med. 2005;53(1):141–9.
62. Speck O, Hennig J, Zaitsev M. Prospective real-time slice-by-slice motion correction for fMRI in freely moving subjects. Magn Reson Mater Phys. 2006;19:55–61.
63. Miezin FM, Maccotta L, Ollinger JM, Petersen SE, Buckner RL, Niendorf T. On the application of susceptibility-weighted ultra-fast low-angle RARE experiments in functional MR imaging. Magn Reson Med. 1999;41:1189–98.
64. Studholme C, Constable RT, Duncan JS. Accurate alignment of functional EPI data to anatomical MRI physics based distortion model. IEEE Trans Med Imaging. 2001;19(11):1115–27.
65. Poser BA, Norris DG. Investigating the benefits of multi-echo EPI for fMRI at 7 T. Neuroimage. 2009;45(4):1162–72.
66. Jezzard P, Balaban RS. Correction for geometric distortion in EPI from B_0 variations. Magn Reson Med. 1995;34:65–73.
67. Jezzard P, Clare S. Sources of distortion in functional MRI data. Hum Brain Mapp. 1999;8(2–3):80–5.
68. Reber PJ, Wong EC, Buxton RB, Frank LR. Correction of off resonance related distortion in echo planar images from Bo field variations. Magn Reson Med. 1995;34:65–73.

69. Robson MD, Gore JC, Constable RT. Measurement of the point spread function in MRI using constant time imaging. Magn Reson Med. 1997;38(5):733–40.
70. Zeng H, Constable RT. Image distortion correction in EPI: Comparison of field mapping with point spread function mapping. Magn Reson Med. 2002;48: 137–46.
71. Zaitsev M, Hennig J, Speck O. Point spread function mapping with parallel imaging techniques and high acceleration factors: fast, robust, and flexible method for echo-planar imaging distortion correction. Magn Reson Med. 2004;52(5):1156–66.
72. Glover GH, Law CS. Spiral in/out BOLD fMRI for increased SNR and reduced susceptibility artifacts. Magn Reson Med. 2001;46:515–22.
73. Yang Y, Wen H, Mattay VS, Balaban RS, Frank JA, Duyn JH. Comparison of 3D BOLD functional MRI with spiral acquisition at 1.5 T and 4.0 T. Neuroimage. 1999;9:446–51.
74. Houston GC, Papadakis NG, Carpenter A, Hall LD, Mukherjee B, James MF, et al. Mapping of the cerebral response to hypoxia measured using graded asymmetric spin echo. Magn Reson Imag. 2000;18:1043–54.
75. Zheng J, Ehrhardt JC, Cizadlo T, Yuh WTC. Comparison of inversion-recovery asymmetric spin-echo EPI and gradient-echo EPI for brain motor activation study. J Magn Reson Imag. 1997;7:843–7.
76. Poser BA, Norris DG. Fast spin echo sequences for BOLD functional MRI. Magma. 2007;20(1):11–7.
77. Jovicich J, Norris DG. Functional MRI of the human brain with GRASE-based BOLD contrast. Magn Reson Med. 1999;41:871–6.
78. Scheffler K, Seifritz E, Bilecen D, Venkatesan R, Hennig J, Deimling M, et al. Detection of BOLD changes by means of a frequency-sensitive trueFISP technique: preliminary results. NMR Biomed. 2001;14:490–6.
79. Lee JH, Dumoulin SO, Saritas EU, Glover GH, Wandell BA, Nishimura DG, et al. Full brain coverage and high-resolution imaging capabilities of passband b-ssfp fMRI at 3 T. Magn Reson Med. 2008;59:1099–110.
80. Calamante F, Thomas DL, Pell GS, Wiersma J, Turner R. Measuring cerebral blood flow using magnetic resonance imaging techniques. J Cereb Blood Flow Metab. 1999;19:701–35.
81. Singer JR. Blood flow rates by nuclear magnetic resonance measurements. Science. 1959;130:1652–3.
82. Edelman RR, Siewert B, Darby DG, Thangaraj V, Nobre AC, Mesulam MM, et al. Quanlitative mapping of cerebral blood flow and functional localization with echo-planar MR imaging and signal targeting with alternating radio frequency. Radiology. 1994;192:513–20.
83. Edelman RR, Chen Q. EPISTAR MRI: multislice mapping of cerebral blood flow. Magn Reson Med. 1998;40:800–5.
84. Kim SG. Quantification of relative cerebral blood flow change by flow-sensitive alternating inversion recovery (FAIR) technique: application to functional mapping. Magn Reson Med. 1995;34:293–301.
85. Yang Y, Frank JA, Hou L, Ye FQ, McLaughlin AC, Duyn JH. Multislice imaging of quantitative cerebral perfusion with pulsed arterial spin-labeling. Magn Reson Med. 1998;39:825–32.
86. Hoge RD, Atkinson J, Gill B, Crelier GR, Marrett S, Pike GB. Investigation of BOLD signal dependence on cerebral blood flow and oxygen consumption: the deoxyhemoglobin dilution model. Magn Reson Med. 1999;42:849–63.
87. Crelier GR, Hoge RD, Munger P, Pike GB. Perfusion based functional magnetic resonance imaging with single shot RARE and GRASE acquisitions. Magn Reson Med. 1999;41:132–6.
88. Detre JA, Leigh JS, Williams DS, Koretsky AP. Perfusion imaging. Magn Reson Med. 1992;23: 37–45.
89. Gonzalez-At JB, Alsop DC, Detre JA. Cerebral perfusion and arterial transit time changes during task activation determined with continuous arterial spin labeling. Magn Reson Med. 2000;43:739–46.
90. Yongbi MN, Yang Y, Frank JA, Duyn JH. Multislice perfusion imaging in human brain using the C-FOCI inversion pulse: comparison with hyperbolic secant. Magn Reson Med. 1999;42:1098–105.
91. Alsop DC, Detre JA. Reduced transit-time sensitivity in noninvasive magnetic resonance imaging of human cerebral blood flow. J Cereb Blood Flow Metab. 1996;16:1236–49.
92. Qiu M, Maguire P, Arora J, Planeta-Wilson B, Weinzimmer D, Wang J, et al. Arterial transit time effects in pulsed arterial spin labeling CBF mapping: insight from a PET and MR study in normal human subjects. Magn Reson Med. 2010;63(2):374–84.
93. Zhang W, Williams DS, Koretsky AP. Measurement of brain perfusion by volume-localized NMR spectroscopy using inversion of arterial water spins: accounting for transit time and cross-relaxation. Magn Reson Med. 1992;25:362–71.
94. Wong EC, Buxton RB, Frank LR. Implementation of quantitative perfusion imaging techniques for functional brain mapping using pulsed arterial spin labeling. NMR Biomed. 1997;10(4–5):237–49.
95. Ye FQ, Yang Y, Duyn J, Mattay VS, Frank JA, Weinberger DR, et al. Quantitation of regional cerebral blood flow increases during motor activation: a multislice, steady-state, arterial spin tagging study. Magn Reson Med. 1999;42:404–7.
96. Darby DG, Nobre AC, Thangaraj V, Edelman R, Mesulam MM, Warach S. Cortical activation in the human brain during lateral saccades using EPISTAR functional magnetic resonance imaging. Neuroimage. 1996;3:53–62.
97. Perthen JE, Bydder M, Restom K, Liu TT. SNR and functional sensitivity of BOLD and perfusion-based

fMRI using arterial spin labeling with spiral SENSE at 3 T. Magn Reson Imaging. 2008;26(4):513–22.
98. Lai S, Wang J, Jahng G-H. FAIR exempting separate T1 measurement (FAIREST): a novel technique for online quantitative perfusion imaging and multi-contrast fMRI. NMR Biomed. 2001;14:507–16.
99. Luh W-M, Wong EC, Bandettini PA, Ward D, Hyde JS. Comparison of simultaneously measured perfusion and BOLD signal increases during brain activation with T1-based tissue identification. Magn Reson Med. 2000;44:137–43.
100. Aguirre GK, Detre JA, Zarahn E, Alsop DC. Experimental design and the relative sensitivity of BOLD and perfusion fMRI. Neuroimage. 2002;15: 488–500.
101. Lu H, Golay X, Pekar JJ, van Zijl PCM. Functional magnetic resonance imaging based on changes in vascular space occupancy. Magn Reson Med. 2003;50:263–74.
102. Scouten A, Constable RT. Applications and limitations of whole-brain MAGIC VASO functional imaging. Magn Reson Med. 2007;58(2):306–15.
103. Scouten A, Constable RT. VASO-based calculations of CBV change: accounting for the dynamic CSF volume. Magn Reson Med. 2008;59(2):308–15.
104. Stefanovic B, Pike GB. Venous refocusing for volume estimation: VERVE functional magnetic resonance imaging. Magn Reson Med. 2005;53(2): 339–47.
105. Chen JJ, Pike GB. BOLD-specific cerebral blood volume and blood flow changes during neuronal activation in humans. NMR Biomed. 2009;22(10): 1054–62.
106. Belliveau JW, Kennedy DN, McKinstry RC, Buchbinder BR, Weisskoff RM, Cohen MS, et al. Functional mapping of the human visual cortex by magnetic resonance imaging. Science. 1991; 254(4):716.
107. White N, Roddey C, Shankaranarayanan A, Han E, Rettman D, Santos J, et al. PROMO: real-time prospective motion correction in MRI using image-based tracking. Magn Reson Med. 2010;63:91–105.
108. Qin L, van Gelderen P, Derbyshire JA, Jin F, Lee J, de Zwart JA, et al. Prospective head-movement correction for high-resolution MRI using an in-bore optical tracking system. Magn Reson Med. 2009; 62:924–34.
109. Poser BA, Koopmans PJ, Witzel T, Wald LL, Barth M. Three dimensional echo-planar imaging at 7 Tesla. NeuroImage. 2010;51(1):261–6.

5 Neurovascular Uncoupling in Functional MR Imaging

Jorn Fierstra and David John Mikulis

Definition of Terms

Terms referring to cerebrovascular autoregulation are often used interchangeably and have been assigned different meanings according to different users and groups. Although we are not claiming to be the final authority on this issue, we would like to establish the following definitions to inform the reader in order to minimize uncertainty.

Cerebrovascular autoregulation refers to the mechanism that maintains constant blood flow in the brain under varying day-to-day physiological conditions (e.g., changes in blood pressure and changes in the partial pressure of arterial carbon dioxide ($PaCO_2$). It is achieved through control of resistance in precapillary blood vessels (either by relaxation or contraction of smooth muscle). It is believed that this mechanism also accounts for flow augmentation during neuronal activity [1, 2].

Cerebrovascular reserve is the remaining capacity to augment blood flow by decreasing vascular resistance (vasodilatation). Cerebrovascular reactivity (CVR) can be used as an indicator of how much cerebrovascular reserve is left in a given vascular bed. CVR is defined as the percent change in cerebral blood flow/percent change in flow stimulus. For blood oxygen level-dependent (BOLD) magnetic resonance imaging (MRI), CVR is the percentage change in BOLD signal per mmHg change in end-tidal PCO_2 ($P_{ET}CO_2$). With severe chronic vascular disease (e.g., a vascular occlusion or high-grade stenosis), this reserve capacity can reach its limit. The vascular bed downstream of the affected vessel is maximally dilated in order to maintain sufficient blood flow to the brain tissue at baseline. Here the autoregulatory mechanism is still intact (vasodilatation occurred) but is operating at its maximum endpoint. The reserve capacity for additional augmentation of blood flow is, therefore, exhausted.

Arterial "steal" physiology refers to a brain region where blood flow paradoxically drops when a vasodilatory stimulus is applied. Two conditions must be met for this to happen. The first is that cerebrovascular reserve must be exhausted. The second is that sufficient reserve capacity exists in surrounding tissue such that flow resistance can drop in response to the vasoactive stimulus.

J. Fierstra, PhD Candidate
Rudolf Magnus Institute of Neuroscience, University Medical Center Utrecht, Utrecht, The Netherlands

Division of Neuroradiology, Division of Neurosurgery, Toronto Western Hospital, University Health Network, 399 Bathurst Street, Toronto, ON, M5T 2S8, Canada
e-mail: jornfierstra@gmail.com

D.J. Mikulis, MD (✉)
Division of Neuroradiology, University Health Network: Toronto Western Hospital, University of Toronto, 399 Bathurst Street, Toronto, ON, M5T 2S8, Canada
e-mail: mikulis@uhnres.utoronto.ca

S.H. Faro and F.B. Mohamed (eds.), *Functional BOLD MRI: Principles and Applications*,
DOI 10.1007/978-1-4939-1995-6_5,

Introduction

Twenty percent of the baseline cardiac output is directed toward the brain, which only accounts for 2% of the body weight, underscoring the high metabolic requirements of neurons and glia. In addition, a considerable increase in cerebral blood flow (CBF) occurs during neuronal activation [3]. This high demand for blood flow is associated with a flow control pathway that is not fully understood but appears to act through the same final common effector as the cerebrovascular autoregulatory mechanism. This effector is arterial vascular resistance mediated by smooth muscle tone of the pre-capillary sphincter in arteries and arterioles [1, 2]. The manner in which active neurons signal for augmentation of blood flow, and the reason that such a considerable flow increase is needed are not completely understood and continue to be actively investigated.

If we can assume that the final common pathway for blood flow modulation occurs through vascular resistance and arterial smooth muscle tone, than there are clinically relevant issues that arise in patients with chronic cerebrovascular disease; i.e., a vascular stenosis or occlusion.

First of all, functional imaging of neuronal networks using techniques that measure blood flow augmentation during activation of neuronal networks may be compromised leading to false-negative results. The second issue, and one that is just beginning to emerge as a potentially new disease entity, relates to chronic exposure of neuronal networks to the impending adverse effects of vascular beds that have already responded to proximal vascular stenosis with maximal smooth muscle relaxation; i.e., vascular beds that are already operating at the extreme of the autoregulatory reserve capacity. In effect, these vascular beds are unable to respond to a neuronal signal for augmentation of blood flow. This chapter will therefore address how the state of the flow control mechanism can be investigated using imaging, how functional imaging of neuronal activation may be compromised, and will open the investigation of the adverse effects of chronically compromised blood flow control on the health of regional neuronal networks.

Control of Cerebral Blood Flow

Modulation of vascular resistance is the mechanism for controlling blood flow at the pre-capillary level. CBF is modulated via control of the luminal diameter of the supplying arteries and arterioles. Smooth muscle tone in these vessels directly affects blood vessel diameter and therefore vascular resistance. Also, vascular resistance can be affected by capillary bed outflow resistance. Therefore, resistance in sinovenous outflow pathways can also have an impact on capillary blood flow, but the discussion of venous outflow disorders is beyond the scope of this chapter. Modulation of arterial vascular resistance is the underlying mechanism responsible for the brain's ability to control blood flow and has been termed cerebrovascular autoregulation. This mechanism is responsive to many different physiological stimuli. The first of these is a pressure responsive mechanism that maintains constant blood flow in the microcirculation through a wide range of perfusion pressures [4]. It is a smooth muscle reflex mechanism where an increase in pressure produces a rapid reflex increase in smooth muscle tone increasing vascular resistance and vice versa. The second is a response to metabolic vasoactive molecules such as CO_2, O_2, potassium, calcium, serotonin, and endothelin [5]. The third is a vasoactive response to local neuronal activity, termed the neurovascular unit [6, 7]. As indicated previously, the final common response pathway to these stimuli is thought to be smooth muscle tone in the arterial system, including the pre-capillary arterioles, where the pre-capillary sphincter is thought to reside [1, 2]. The sphincter represents a "valve" at the interface between the arterioles and capillary bed.

The cerebrovascular autoregulation serves to maintain metabolic homeostasis by ensuring adequate blood flow, and thus constant delivery of oxygen and glucose to the brain. The mechanism also serves to remove metabolic "waste" products, under varying physiological conditions and states of neuronal activity. The coupling between neuronal activation and blood flow was first described by Roy and Sherrington [8].

Neurovascular Coupling and Functional Magnetic Resonance Imaging

Following the increase in neuronal activity in the brain, the local cerebral blood flow increases much more than the cerebral metabolic rate of oxygen ($CMRO_2$), resulting in a decrease in the oxygen extraction fraction (OEF) [8–10]. The increase in the amount of oxygen consumed is only about one-third of the amount delivered [11]. This effect has been termed "neurovascular uncoupling" [10]. The increase in the concentration of oxyhemoglobin and the decrease in deoxyhemoglobin appearing in draining venules underlies the basic mechanism of blood oxygen level-dependent (BOLD) functional magnetic resonance imaging (fMRI) for distinguishing active from stable neuronal networks.

The first application of fMRI with BOLD acquisitions was performed in an animal model by Ogawa et al. in 1990 [12], followed by Kwong et al. in humans in 1992 [13]. Their work reported that changes in the activity of the brain affected the local MR signal and provided an intrinsic mechanism for detecting brain activation. The change in signal occurs due to changes in local magnetic field strength induced by the paramagnetic effects of deoxyhemoglobin. Application of this effect using BOLD-fMRI has revolutionized the detection and analysis of neuronal networks. Clinical applications are now being used routinely for preoperative assessment of eloquent network components in relation to resectable brain lesions.

However, the underlying assumption, upon which these clinical techniques is based, is that the cerebrovascular autoregulatory mechanism is intact. The remainder of this discussion will focus on the affect on brain mapping and the consequences on the health and integrity of the brain itself when this condition is not met.

Assessing the Cerebrovascular Autoregulatory Reserve by Performing Cerebrovascular Reactivity Measurements

Cerebrovascular autoregulatory compensation fails when smooth muscle in the pre-capillary sphincter cannot either further relax or constrict in response to a vasoactive stimulus. The ability to interrogate the existing "setpoint" of smooth muscle tone would be very useful in determining how much of an additional response is present within the vascular system. This "reactivity" assessment can be performed by determining how much of an increase or decrease in blood flow occurs in response to a given vasoactive stimulus. This is termed cerebrovascular reactivity (CVR), and is defined as the percent change in cerebral blood flow/percent change in flow stimulus. There are numerous imaging methodologies available for making this measurement, including ultrasound, MRI, computed tomography (CT), single photon emission CT (SPECT), and positron emission tomography (PET) using different stimuli and different imaging contrast agents. Since it is beyond the scope of this chapter to fully elaborate on each of these imaging modalities, we will focus on the quantitative BOLD-MRI CVR method that we have pioneered in association with precise and independent control of end-tidal CO_2 and O_2 ($P_{ET}CO_2$ and $P_{ET}O_2$). This technique enables a method of end-inspiratory rebreathing [14] that allows precise iso-oxic pseudo-square wave changes in $P_{ET}CO_2$ (RespirAct, Thornhill Research Inc., Toronto, Canada), while acquiring BOLD-MR imaging sequences. Maintaining oxygen at a normal level decreases the T1-inflow effects that might alter the BOLD signal during the acquisition [15]. The near-square wave changes in $P_{ET}CO_2$ result in a robust response of the brain vasculature that can easily be detected in the BOLD signal and can be mapped spatially (Fig. 5.1a) [16, 17]. CVR is defined as percent change in BOLD signal/mmHg change in $P_{ET}CO_2$. The relationship of CVR as a measure of cerebrovascular reserve capacity against changes in cerebral blood flow has been validated using arterial spin labeling (ASL) techniques [18].

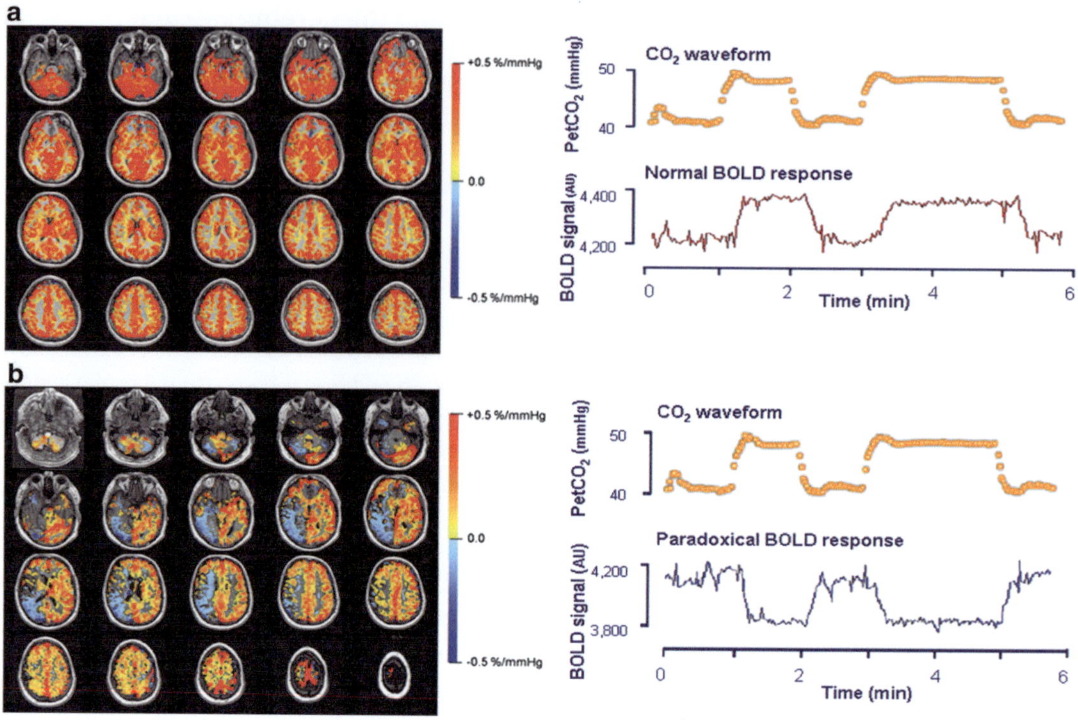

Fig. 5.1 Spatial CVR maps acquired with BOLD-MRI and precise control of $P_{ET}CO_2$. Near square wave changes in end-tidal CO_2 ($P_{ET}CO_2$) induce robust increases in the raw BOLD signal (arbitrary units) enabling fMRI type signal analysis. (**a**) Shows a normal increase in BOLD signal during a hypercarbic stimulus, resulting in a spatial CVR map showing normal reactivity. Note the diminished response in the white matter compared to the gray matter. This is a normal finding [17]. (**b**) An example of a paradoxical decreased in BOLD signal during hypercarbia demonstrating an area with exhausted autoregulatory reserve on the spatial CVR map (*blue area*), indicating disease

Exhausted Cerebrovascular Reserve Associated with Steal Physiology

In general, vascular diseases impair the ability of the feeding vasculature to deliver adequate flow to the microcirculation. Cerebrovascular autoregulation can compensate for supply deficits through vasodilatation decreasing the vascular resistance. However, in the case of severe chronic cerebrovascular disease, arterial smooth muscle is maximally relaxed in order to maintain sufficient blood flow at baseline. With maximal smooth muscle relaxation of the pre-capillary sphincter, the reserve capacity has reached its limit, the vascular resistance is at a minimum, and further flow augmentation is not possible. However, normal surrounding vascular beds are still able to lower vascular resistance. The overall effect is a diversion of blood toward the lower resistance vascular bed. Under these conditions a flow stimulus such as carbon dioxide (CO_2) will increase flow to the normal territory and decrease flow to the territory with exhausted autoregulatory reserve ("steal physiology").

Using the term *impaired* autoregulation to describe this process may be erroneous since the autoregulatory mechanism itself is not defective. The cerebrovascular reserve, however, has reached its limit and therefore the autoregulatory mechanism can no longer drop the vascular resistance when further flow augmentation is needed. This process may be more appropriately named "exhaustion of cerebrovascular reserve."

With BOLD-MRI assessment of CVR, brain areas with exhausted cerebrovascular reserve can be mapped (Fig. 5.1b, Table 5.1). These areas show a paradoxical response in BOLD signal during hypercarbia and a decrease in CBF [18].

Table 5.1 Summary of key BOLD-MRI CVR research demonstrating exhausted cerebrovascular reserve associated with steal physiology and its impact on normal appearing brain tissue on conventional MR imaging

Authors	Subjects	Findings
Mandell et al. (2008) [17]	28 young healthy subjects (age range 22–42)	Young healthy subjects exhibit steal physiology in the deep white matter
Mandell et al. (2008) [18]	38 patients with severe cerebrovascular steno-occlusive disease	Brain areas exhibiting steal physiology demonstrate a decrease in CBF
Fierstra et al. (2010) [19]	17 patients with severe unilateral cerebrovascular steno-occlusive disease	Patients exhibiting unilateral steal physiology with normal appearing brain tissue on conventional MRI, demonstrate an 8% thinner cerebral cortex as compared to the contralateral, unaffected hemipshere
Conklin et al. (2010) [31]	22 Moyamoya patients with unilateral steal physiology, 12 age-matched healthy controls	Normal appearing white matter exhibiting steal physiology is spatially correlated with elevated ADC in patients with Moyamoya disease

Abbreviations: *CBF* cerebral blood flow, *ADC* apparent diffusion coefficient, *MRI* magnetic resonance imaging

The Consequences of Exhausted Cerebrovascular Reserve Associated with Steal Physiology on Neuronal Network Mapping Using BOLD-MRI

Functional MRI depends on an adequate response of the cerebrovascular autoregulatory mechanism to augment blood flow when a vasodilatory stimulus is applied. The increase in blood flow results in washout of deoxyhemoglobin that can be detected in the BOLD signal. In chronic cerebrovascular disease, with progressive stenosis, cerebrovascular reserve gets progressively smaller resulting in a parallel decrease in BOLD signal, eventually leading to a paradoxical (negative) BOLD signal when the autoregulatory reserve is exhausted (Fig. 5.1b) [19]. Under these conditions, augmentation of flow under any stimulus including neuronal activation is theoretically not possible. If there is no awareness of this flow-limiting condition, analysis of fMRI data can be erroneous. Analysis of the BOLD signal response to neuronal activation eventually requires application of a threshold to distinguish active neuronal network components from inactive tissue. If the threshold is decreased, more activation is observed. In fact, thresholds can be lowered enough to show virtually any anatomical site as a component of the network map (Fig. 5.2) [20]. This bias can lead to inclusion of a false-positive activation in the fMRI map. In addition, false-negative errors may also occur, leading to erroneous conclusion of adaptive plasticity as an explanation for the pattern of neuronal activation. The case summarized in Figs. 5.3 and 5.4 highlight the importance of these issues. It is also important to recognize that other disorders can have a secondary affect on brain blood flow that can impair the flow response to neuronal activation. For example, brain tumors or arteriovenous malformations (AVMs), either by virtue of local mass effect or from arterial-venous shunting, can alter CVR and local flow dynamics. False-negative activation of eloquent tissue in the vicinity of such a lesion can occur, potentially increasing the risk of an adverse surgical outcome. The solution is to map CVR using BOLD-MRI either with precision control of CO_2 or using a breath-hold to elevate CO_2 (Fig. 5.5). The CVR map can then be compared to the fMRI map for confirmation that blood flow increases are possible in the area of interest distal to a stenosis, in the vicinity of a tumor, or near an AVM, thus validating the fMRI response. The breath-hold CVR method can be performed using the same BOLD sequence as the fMRI acquisition and analyzed using the same software. Just as in fMRI, the "task" consists of a 25-s breath-hold each minute for 4–5 min. Although not quantitative, the method is robust enough to determine whether steal physiology is present (Fig. 5.5).

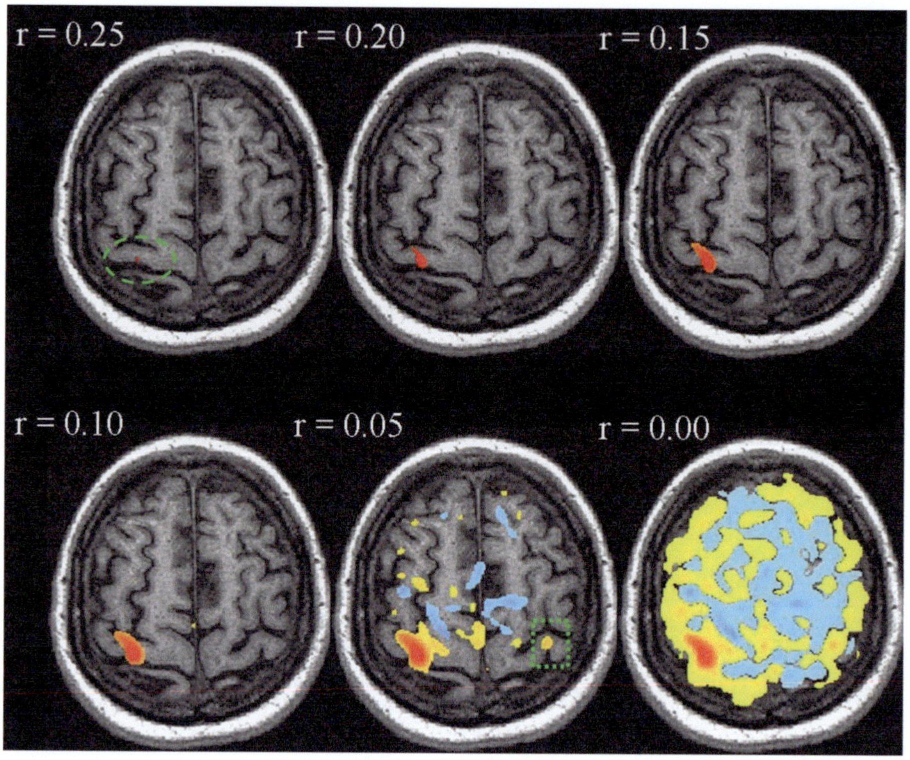

Fig. 5.2 Influence of thresholding on the fMRI map of a finger tapping task. Functional MRI maps generated following the acquisition of a left hand finger tapping fMRI paradigm. The *upper left* image shows voxels with the highest *r*-correlation (*green dashed circle*) during the task. This was obtained by increasing the threshold until only one final group of voxels remained. Not surprisingly, these voxels were in the expected location of the hand homunculus in the primary motor cortex controlling left hand function. Lowering the activation threshold reveals greater spatial activity, eventually leading to visible activity in the left primary motor cortex (*green dashed square*). It is common to see activation in both motor cortices during unilateral hand tasks [20]. Lowering the threshold even further to zero reveals "activation" (or "deactivation" in *blue*) of the whole brain. Care must be taken when interpreting patterns of functional networks since the number and extent of constituents are threshold dependent

Distinguishing Hemodynamic from Embolic Neurological Events

Ischemia can be the result of embolic occlusion of arteries distal to an embolic source such as clot within the heart or an atherosclerotic plaque in the cervical carotid artery. The ability to distinguish between these possibilities is important since treatment will vary accordingly. For example, medical management is usually indicated in symptomatic patients with carotid plaques associated with low-grade stenoses. High-grade stenoses in excess of 90% can produce symptoms by embolic, hemodynamic, or combined mechanisms. If there is a hemodynamic component with steal physiology, there is a higher risk of disabling ischemic stroke than if the condition is purely embolic [21]. The only effective treatment for steal physiology is revascularization. CVR is clearly capable of identifying the presence of steal physiology, although the application of this technique in patients is not generally practiced primarily because of the overall low incidence of steal physiology in patients with cerebrovascular diseases and because of technical challenges in implementing CVR analysis.

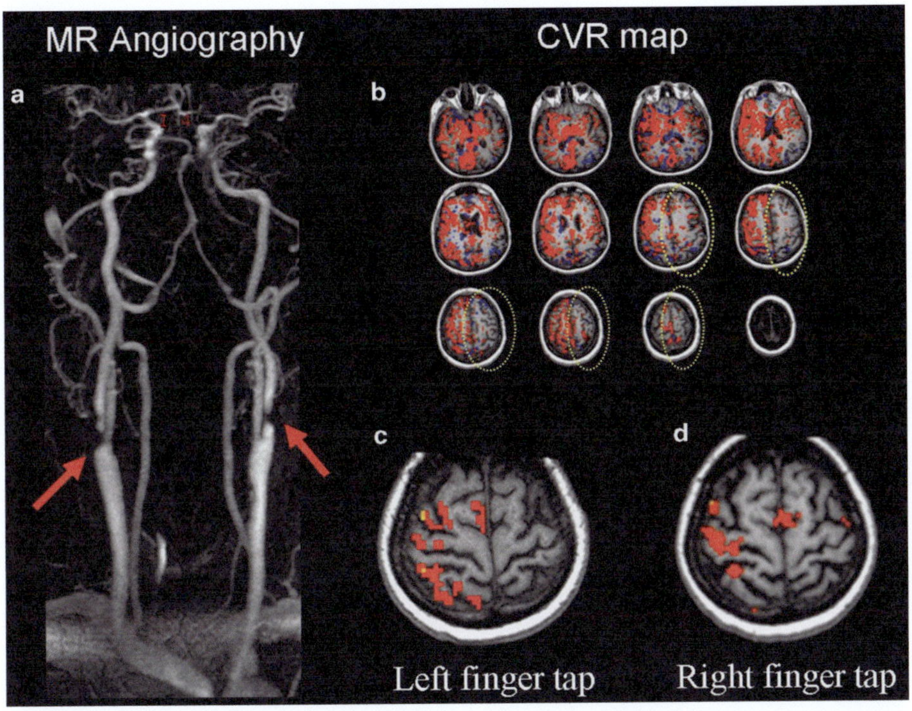

Fig. 5.3 Plasticity vs. absence of neurovascular response? A 70-year-old man with shaking hand syndrome. His right hand became uncontrollable during use such that the latter part of his signature became progressively illegible. (**a**) Shows bilateral high-grade stenosis (>90%) of the internal carotid arteries (*red arrows*). Interestingly, despite similar stenoses, autoregulatory reserve on the CVR map was exhausted only on the left side (*yellow dashed circles* in (**b**)). (**c**) Functional MRI map shows the expected right motor cortex activation during left finger tapping. A right finger tapping paradigm in (**d**) showed no activation in the left hemisphere. However, there was considerable activation in the ipsilateral hemisphere. This was initially felt to be the result of a shift in control of the right hand to the right hemisphere until the CVR map revealed an absence of the neurovascular response. The fMRI map was therefore deemed unreliable in this case. Interestingly, validation of the neurovascular response has not been performed in most fMRI research studies of patients with ischemic stroke, who by definition would have a high probability of neurovascular uncoupling

The Long-Term Consequences of Chronic Steal Physiology on the Brain: "The Neurovascular Uncoupling Syndrome"

The brain areas demonstrating exhausted cerebrovascular reserve with steal physiology are at high risk for developing a future acute ischemic event [22–24]. However, steal physiology can occur episodically and can exist over a long period of time without ictal signs of ischemia, but may still affect the integrity of both gray and white matter.

The pathological effects of acute ischemia are well characterized. Acute severe reduction of blood flow in the core of an infarct results in complete loss of neurons. Surrounding the infarct core is the penumbra suffering from reduced blood flow where viable neurons are at risk of death if blood flow is not restored in a timely fashion. However, in brain regions thought to represent tissue with reversible injury, selective neuronal necrosis has been observed despite timely restoration of blood flow [25].

Less well understood is the chronic brain exposure to episodes of sublethal hypoperfusion. This question of whether chronic episodic isch-

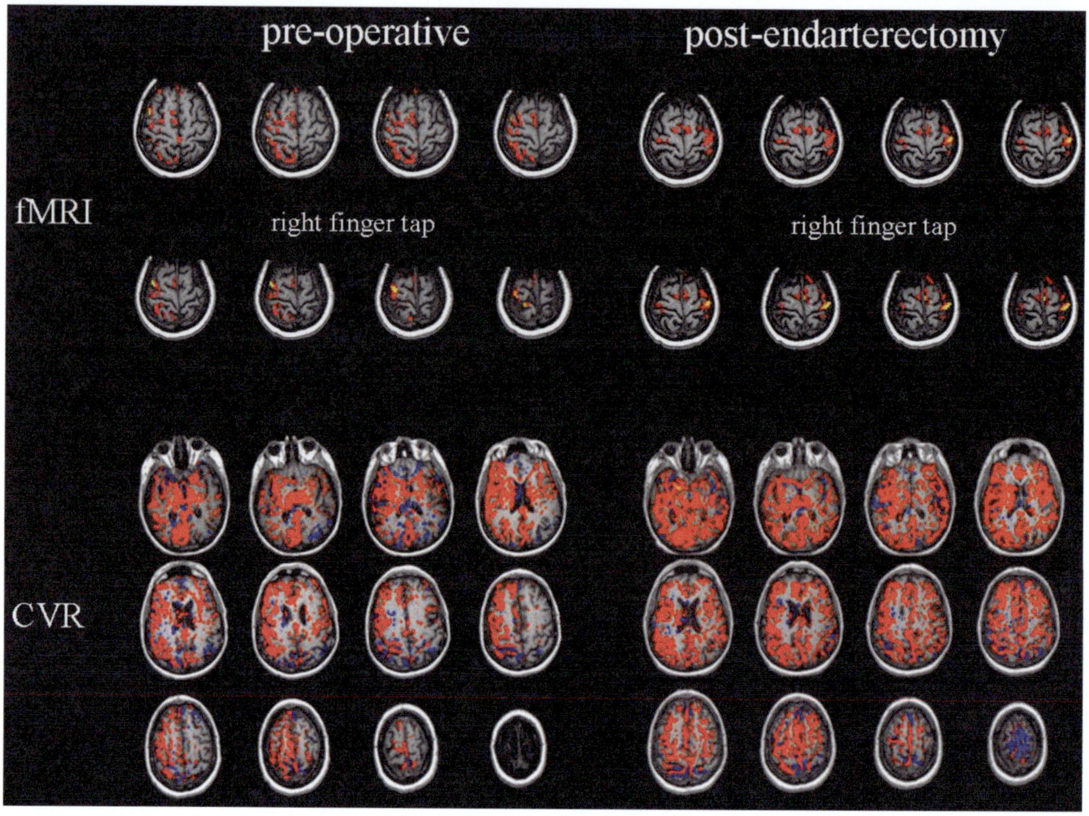

Fig. 5.4 Motor cortex activation before and after revascularization. These are pre-and post-endarterectomy fMRI and CVR maps of the same patient in Fig. 5.3. Postoperatively, neurovascular coupling has been restored to the left hemisphere and control of the right upper extremity has "shifted" back to the left hemisphere according to the fMRI map. Shifting of motor control as seen on the fMRI maps is more likely the result of re-established neurovascular coupling rather than plastic changes in the brain

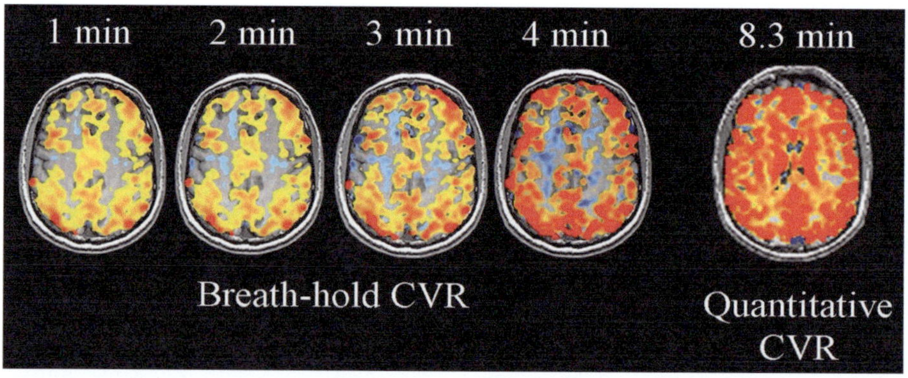

Fig. 5.5 Efficacy of breath-hold BOLD-MRI for establishing the presence of normal neurovascular coupling. Hypercarbia is inducible during breath-holding and can be used to generate nonquantitative maps of CVR. These maps are sufficient to establish the presence of positive vs. absent vs. paradoxical reactivity. Twenty-five second breath-holds per minute for 4 min can yield high quality CVR maps similar to that obtained using precision control of end-tidal CO_2. Since the end-tidal values of CO_2 are not available during breath-hold (unless arterial blood gases are monitored continuously), the breath-hold CVR maps are not quantitative

emia can produce pathological effects short of frank infarction in humans has been a longstanding question and difficult to document. We have addressed this question by studying patients who have chronic steno-occlusive disease with unilateral exhausted cerebrovascular reserve associated with steal physiology. Patients showing normal cortex without evidence of visible ischemic injury on conventional MRI were investigated. The thickness of the cortex in the region of steal physiology was compared with the cortical thickness in the normal hemisphere and was found to be 8% thinner [19]. Although the reasons for this reduction in thickness have not been verified with histology, the following are possible explanations. Hypoperfusion might lead to selective loss of neurons, or a decrease in cerebral blood volume (CBV). It is, however, more likely that CBV would be normal or even increased since maximal vasodilatation is present. Furthermore, decreased CBV is thought to occur only in the setting of stage III ischemia [26, 27], which is seen in the core of an acute infarct. Another explanation is the loss of neuroglial complexity with loss of volume in the neuropil. Chronic exposure of neurons to flow insufficiency during activation may result in a loss of synaptic density and decreased dendritic arborization. Under these conditions neurons divert metabolic resources toward survival over function [28, 29]. Another possible mechanism is that these episodes of hypoperfusion during activation may cause inhibition of protein synthesis resulting in delayed neuronal death [30].

White matter is not immune to these effects although the mechanism may be different. Conklin et al. [31] performed apparent diffusion coefficient (ADC) measurements in the white matter of subjects with unilateral steal physiology and cortical thinning, but without structural abnormalities on conventional imaging. ADC values in the steal hemisphere were significantly elevated compared to the normal hemisphere, suggesting the presence of chronic injury. It remains to be determined if the findings represent degeneration secondary to injury of neuronal cell bodies on the side of the thinner cortex, or due to the direct effects of steal physiology and episodic ischemia on the axons themselves.

The vascular deficit may also have a direct effect on glial cells. Astrocytes play a supporting role in the neurovascular unit [32]. When the autoregulatory reserve is exhausted, astrocyte metabolism may be impaired, increasing vulnerability of the neurons to injury. Inversely, or more likely in tandem, is the potential loss of these supporting cells due to pruning of neuronal complexity. Metabolic stress on oligodendrocytes resulting in "decay" of myelin may be an alternative explanation for elevated white matter water diffusion.

Follow-up work by our group has been performed [33] employing cortical thickness measurements in patients previously identified with cortical thinning who underwent successful surgical revascularization and normalization of CVR. Thirty of 30 hemispheres showed increased cortical thickness, indicating that revascularization can reverse cortical thinning. This observation would favor a reversible cause of neuroglial injury as selective neuronal necrosis would not be expected to recover. Perhaps restoration of flow augmentation following revascularization restored metabolic balance and reversed degeneration in the neural networks and supporting cells.

Overall, the underlying pathophysiology is complex and not well understood. Nevertheless, these studies demonstrate the first indication that areas with steal physiology show structural changes in brain tissue. Neurons in the affected brain regions are operating in an environment where inadequate blood flow is present during activation, leading to diminished delivery of nutrients and diminished removal of waste products. We now believe that this condition should be referred to as true neurovascular uncoupling since the normal increase in blood flow during neuronal activation is no longer occurring. If cortical thinning and increased white matter diffusion correlate with deterioration in neurocognitive and functional performance measures specific to the affected vascular territory, it would be appropriate to consider defining the disorder as "*neurovascular uncoupling syndrome*."

Conclusion

The considerable increase in cerebral blood flow that occurs during increases in neuronal activity can be mapped using fMRI. Pulse sequences sensitive to blood flow such as arterial spin labeling, or sequences sensitive to magnetic field inhomogeneities (produced by deoxyhemoglobin) such as long echo time gradient echoes (BOLD imaging) can be used to create functional maps of neuronal activity. The ability to show the relationship between resectable brain lesions and eloquent cortex with these maps has become the standard of practice for presurgical planning. Interpretation of the fMRI maps must take into consideration the integrity of neurovascular coupling. If there is doubt, then assessment of CVR can be performed either quantitatively using tight control of CO_2 or with a breath-hold CVR analysis. This can also be performed in the research setting to validate fMRI studies in subjects with vascular diseases who, for example, may be undergoing plasticity analysis following acute ischemic stroke.

Another important potential clinical application of BOLD CVR MRI is in distinguishing embolic from hemodynamic ischemic events, especially for identification and referral of patients with steal physiology for revascularization either via endarterectomy, angioplasty with stenting, or even extracranial-intracranial (EC-IC) bypass in the case of the occluded carotid or middle cerebral artery (MCA).

In the future, detection and treatment of steal physiology in patients who do not have discrete ischemic events but have evidence of cortical thinning and increased white matter water diffusion ("neurovascular uncoupling syndrome") may be important in order to prevent accelerated neurological deterioration within the affected vascular territory via elective revascularization.

References

1. Martini FH. Anatomy and physiology. 2007 ed. Pearson Education Inc: Singapore; 2007. p. 531–76.
2. Johnson LR, Byrne JH. Essential medical physiology. 2nd ed. Philadelphia: Lippincott-Raven; 1998. p. 225–33.
3. Ye OF, Yang Y, Duyn J, et al. Quantitation of regional cerebral blood flow increases during motor activation: a multislice, steady-state, arterial spin tagging study. Magn Reson Med. 1999;42:404–7.
4. Edvinsson L, MacKenzie ET, McCulloch J, et al. Cerebral blood flow and metabolism. New York: Raven Press; 1993. p. 57–91.
5. Squire LR, Bloom FE, Spitzer LE, et al. Fundamental neuroscience. 3rd ed. London: Elsevier Inc; 2008. p. 41–296.
6. Koehler RC, Roman RJ, Harder DR. Astrocytes and the regulation of cerebral blood flow. Trends Neurosci. 2009;32:160–9.
7. Hamel E. Perivascular nerves and the regulation of cerebrovascular tone. J Appl Physiol. 2006;100: 1059–64.
8. Roy CS, Sherrington CS. On the regulation of the blood supply of the brain. J Physiol. 1890;11: 85–108.
9. Buxton RB, Uludag K, Dubowitz DJ, Liu TT. Modeling the hemodynamic response to brain activation. Neuroimage. 2004;23:S220–33.
10. Fox PT, Raichle ME. Focal physiological uncoupling of cerebral blood flow and oxidative metabolism during somatosensory stimulation in human subjects. Proc Natl Acad Sci USA. 1986;83:1140–44.
11. Davis TL, Kwong KK, Weisskoff RM, Rosen BR. Calibrated functional MRI: mapping the dynamics of oxidative metabolism. Proc Natl Acad Sci USA. 1998;95(4):1834–39.
12. Ogawa S, Lee TM, Kay AR, Tank DW. Brain magnetic resonance imaging with contrast dependent on blood oxygenation. Proc Natl Acad Sci USA. 1990;87:9868–72.
13. Kwong KK, Belliveau JW, Chesler DA, et al. Dynamic magnetic resonance imaging of human brain activity during primary sensory stimulation. Proc Natl Acad Sci USA. 1992;89:5675–79.
14 Slessarev M, Prisman E, Han J, et al. Prospective targeting and control of end-tidal CO_2 and O_2 concentrations. J Physiol. 2007;581(3):1207–19.
15. Prisman E, Slessarev M, Han J, et al. Comparison of the effects of independently controlled end-tidal PCO_2 and PO_2 on blood oxygen level-dependent (BOLD) MRI. J Magn Reson Im. 2008;27:185–91.
16. Vesely A, Sasano H, Volgyesi G, et al. MRI mapping of cerebrovascular reactivity using square wave changes in end-tidal PCO_2. Magn Reson Med. 2001;45:1011–3.
17. Mandell DM, Han JS, Poublanc J, et al. Selective reduction of blood flow to white matter during hypercapnia corresponds with leukoaraiosis. Stroke. 2008;39:1993–98.
18. Mandell DM, Han JS, Poublanc J, et al. Mapping cerebrovascular reactivity using blood oxygen level-dependent MRI in patients with arterial steno-occlusive disease: comparison with arterial spin labeling. Stroke. 2008;39(7):2021–8.
19. Fierstra J, Poublanc J, Han J, et al. Steal physiology is spatially correlated with cortical thinning. J Neurol Neurosurg Psych. 2010;81:290–93.

20. Horenstein C, Lowe MJ, Koening KA, Phillips MD. Comparison of unilateral and bilateral complex finger tapping-related activation in premotor and primary motor cortex. Hum Brain Mapp. 2009;30(4): 1397–412.
21. Yokota C, Hasegawa Y, Minematsu K, Yamaguchi T. Effect of acetazolamide reactivity and long-term outcome in patients with major cerebral artery occlusive diseases. Stroke. 1998;29:640–44.
22. Silvestrini M, Vernieri F, Pasqualetti P, et al. Impaired cerebral vasoreactivity and risk of stroke in patients with asymptomatic carotid artery stenosis. JAMA. 2000;283:2122–7.
23. Schoof J, Lubahn W, Baeumer M, et al. Impaired cerebral autoregulation distal to carotid stenosis/occlusion is associated with increased risk of stroke at cardiac surgery with cardiopulmonary bypass. J Thorac Cardiovasc Surg. 2007;134:690–6.
24. Yonas H, Smith HA, Durham SR, et al. Increased stroke risk predicted by compromised cerebral blood flow reactivity. J Neurosurg. 1993;79:483–9.
25. Guadagno JV, Jones PS, Aigbirhio FI, et al. Selective neuronal loss in rescued enumbra relates to initial hypoperfusion. Brain. 2008;131(Pt 10):2666–78.
26. Derdeyn CP, Videen TO, Yundt KD, et al. Variability of cerebral blood volume and oxygen extraction: stages of cerebral haemodynamic impairment revisited. Brain. 2002;125(Pt 3):595–607.
27. Powers WJ. Cerebral hemodynamics in ischemi cerebrovascular disease. Ann Neurol. 1991;29:231–40.
28. Garcia JH, Lassen NA, Weiller C, et al. Ischemic stroke and incomplete infarction. Stroke. 1996;27: 761–65.
29. Nakagawara J, Sperling B, Lassen NA. Incomplete brain infarction of reperfused cortex may be quantitated with iomazenil. Stroke. 1997;28:124–32.
30. Yamauchi H, Kudoh T, Kishibe Y, et al. Selective neuronal damage and borderzone infarction in carotid artery occlusive disease: a 11 C-flumazenil PET study. J Nucl Med. 2005;46:1973–9.
31. Conklin J, Fierstra J, Crawley A, et al. Impaired cerebrovascular reactivity with steal phenomenon is associated with increased diffusion in white matter of patients with Moyamoya disease. Stroke. 2010;41:1610–16.
32. Blanco VM, Stern JE, Filosa JA. Tone-dependent vascular responses to astrocyte-derived signals. Am J Physiol Heart Circ Physiol. 2008;294:2855–63.
33. Fierstra J, MacLean DB, Fisher JA, et al. Surgical revascularization reverses cerebral cortical thinning in patients with chronic cerebrovascular steno-occlusive disease. Stroke. 2011 April 14.

Functional Connectivity MR Imaging

6

Michelle Hampson, Xilin Shen, and R. Todd Constable

Introduction

Brain function arises out of interactions between brain areas. Neuroimaging studies of brain function are, therefore, concerned not only with activity in discrete brain areas but also with the interactions between areas. A variety of approaches have been developed to study these interactions. The simplest of these is to examine *functional connectivity*, defined as "temporal correlations between spatially remote neurophysiological events" [1, 2]. Because functional connectivity is defined as a correlation, it does not imply causal effects. The term *effective connectivity* is used to describe the "influence that one neural system exerts over another." [1] This chapter is focused on the methods and applications of functional connectivity analyses. The reader is referred elsewhere for information about current approaches for inferring effective connectivity [3–6].

Functional connectivity can be (and has been) assessed in many different ways in functional MRI studies [7]. A variety of mathematical models have been used, including, but not limited to, correlation [2], coherence [8], regression [9], principal coordinates analysis [3], and independent components analysis [10]. Despite their differences, these methods all share the fundamental property that they reveal covariance in activity between brain areas. We describe the most common of these methods in the next subsection. In addition to variability in the methods used to assess functional connectivity, there are differences in the types of data to which the methods are applied. Studies have examined functional connectivity across scans in which different tasks were performed during different periods of time [11], across event-related paradigms [12], and across scans in which subjects performed one task consistently throughout the scan [13–15]. Using a looser definition of functional connectivity that includes correlations between brain areas that are not necessarily temporal, some fMRI studies have also correlated activation patterns across subjects [16, 17]. All of these approaches can yield interesting views of human brain function, but interpretation of the results and comparisons across studies must take into account these methodological differences.

Recently, there has been growing interest in the assessment of functional connectivity during

M. Hampson, PhD (✉)
Department of Diagnostic Radiology, Yale University, MRRC, TAC-N121, 300 Cedar Street, 208043, New Haven, CT 06520-8043, USA
e-mail: michelle.hampson@yale.edu

X. Shen, PhD
Associate Research Scientist, Department of Diagnostic Radiology, Yale University, 300 Cedar Street, New Haven, CT 06520, USA
e-mail: xilin.shen@yale.edu

R.T. Constable, PhD
Diagnostic Radiology, Biomedical Engineering, and Neurosurgery, The Anlyan Center, Yale University School of Medicine, 300 Cedar Street, New Haven, CT 06520, USA
e-mail: todd.constable@yale.edu

S.H. Faro and F.B. Mohamed (eds.), *Functional BOLD MRI: Principles and Applications*, DOI 10.1007/978-1-4939-1995-6_6,

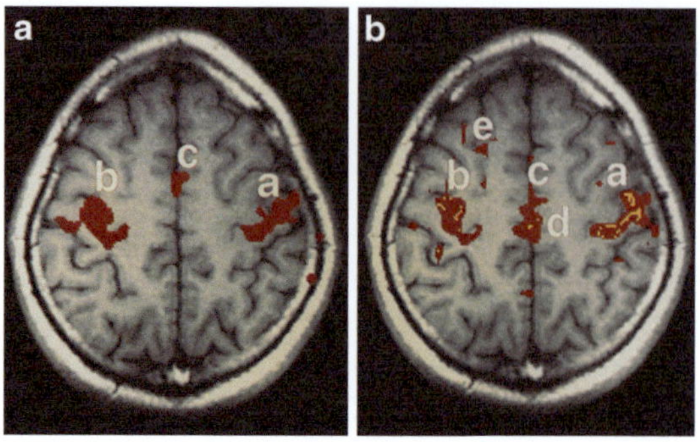

Fig. 6.1 Brain activation during finger-tapping task (panel **a**) compared to a map of resting state correlations to a seed region in left motor cortex (panel **b**, seed in region **b**). A striking similarity is apparent illustrating how resting correlations can delineate functional networks. Reproduced with permission from [2]

scans in which subjects are resting. The first fMRI study of resting state functional connectivity reported high functional connectivity between motor regions when subjects were not executing (or expecting to execute) a motor task, as shown in Fig. 6.1 [2]. Although that study examined only a single slice of brain and, thus, was able to employ a sample rate high enough to filter out cardiac and respiratory noise, similar findings were reported with multislice acquisitions [18]. The effect was found to be reversibly suppressed by hypercapnia [19], to be more pronounced in blood-oxygenation-dependent (BOLD) maps than in maps of blood flow [20], and to be T2* dependent [21]. Other brain systems were soon found to have similar patterns of elevated resting-state connectivity between component regions [18, 22, 23], even when those component regions were distal and nonhomologous [24, 25]. A comparison between resting state functional connectivity within the motor system and the known patterns of anatomical connectivity as established by anatomical, histochemical, and physiological techniques revealed close correspondence [26]. In addition, patterns of resting state functional connectivity in the motor system resembled the patterns of activation during a motor task, both in terms of the precise locations of peak activations/correlations, and the degree of lateralization present across subjects in those activations/correlations [27]. Finally, measures of resting state functional connectivity between homologous cortices were reduced in patients with agenesis of the corpus collosum [28]. These early findings supported the possibility that resting state functional connectivity could provide information about the functional architecture of the brain.

Thus, researchers began examining resting-state connectivity for information about the structure and basic organization of the brain. At the same time, studies of interregional connectivity during cognitive or perceptual tasks were utilized to gain information about the functional organization needed for specific types of mental processes [29, 30]. Studies examining both resting and task-related connectivity patterns yielded a dynamic view of connectivity as modified by a variety of mental functions including motor activity [31, 32], language perception [24], visual perception [13, 15], reading [33], and working memory [14, 34]. In general, functional connectivity between brain areas involved in a task tended to increase or remain strong during task performance, while connectivity of a region involved in a task with other regions not involved in the same task tended to decrease during task performance [13–15, 24]. These studies supported the notion that functional connectivity measurements reflect, to some degree, the cognitive activity occurring during the measurement period.

If functional connectivity provides information about ongoing cognitive processes, then it can also be used as a window into processes occurring in the resting state. This exciting possibility was illustrated by a study investigating resting-state connectivity in the so-called default mode network [9]. "Default mode network" is a term that has become associated with a set of brain areas identified via meta-analyses as having higher blood flow at rest than during cognition [35, 36]. It has been suggested that these brain areas may engage in baseline (or "default mode") functions of the brain such as monitoring of the environment and evaluating the salience of incoming information [37]. In support of the view that these regions function together as a network, they were found to be highly functionally connected at rest [9]. In a departure from the typical interpretation of resting-state functional connectivity data, this finding was also interpreted as evidence that the so-called default mode network is tonically active at rest.

The degree to which functional connectivity measures reflect mental activities occurring during the measurement period and the degree to which they reflect the basic architecture of the brain, independent of the ongoing mental activity, are currently open questions. Given that functional connectivity can be manipulated by assigning different mental tasks, there is clearly a component of the measurement that depends on the ongoing mental function. However, there also appears to be a strong component of resting-state functional connectivity that is not dependent on the current mental activity. A recent study examining correlations between brain areas in the anaesthetized monkey has reported similar patterns of connectivity as seen in conscious, resting humans in the oculomotor, somatomotor, visual, and so-called default mode circuitry [38]. In addition, patterns of connectivity in healthy subjects at various levels of consciousness, including light sleep [39] and coma [40], are similar to those seen in conscious, resting subjects. Furthermore, significant resting-state connections are reproducible across scan sessions from the same subject [41], suggesting that transient thought patterns are not dominating these measurements. Finally, there is a growing literature reporting correspondence between anatomical connectivity, as measured with diffusion tensor imaging, and resting-state functional connectivity patterns [42–47]. These findings suggest that resting-state connectivity measures can reveal the basic functional architecture of the brain, independent of the ongoing conscious cognitive processes. However, they do not rule out the possibility that resting-state mental activity is influencing our measures of resting correlations to some degree. Therefore, it may be possible that we can also gain information regarding baseline mental processes via studies of resting-state functional connectivity.

Standard Methods

In this section, several of the most popular types of analyses used in functional connectivity studies are described. We begin by describing the processing steps involved in computing seed-based connectivity maps. We then describe the related and very simple approach in which region-to-region correlations are computed directly (without a seed map). Third, data-driven methods that do not require a priori definition of regions of interest, such as independent components analysis, are described. Finally, we describe network analyses that can be applied to connectivity data. We emphasize that this section is intended as an introduction to the basic and most common functional connectivity analyses, not a comprehensive summary.

Seed-To-Whole Brain Connectivity Maps

Whole-brain maps of correlations to specific seed regions are in theory very simple. The time course of the region is first computed, usually by averaging the time course of all the pixels in that region. This time course is then correlated with time course of every pixel in the brain, and the resulting *r*-values are transformed to Gaussian variables via Fisher's transform. These basic steps yield a map of the strength of correlation to the seed region in terms of Gaussian variables. Some optional steps and design decisions are discussed below.

Preprocessing

In addition to the standard preprocessing steps used in conventional fMRI analyses – such as motion correction, slice timing adjustment, spatial smoothing, etc. – there are several preprocessing steps commonly adopted in functional connectivity analyses, particularly resting-state functional connectivity analyses.

Removal of Physiologic Noise

Physiologic noise, such as fluctuations in BOLD signal due to cardiac pulsation and respiration, is a general concern in functional imaging [48–51]. This concern is particularly salient for functional connectivity studies because physiologic fluctuations can cause elevated correlations between brain areas in BOLD signal that are unrelated to neural activity. Collecting high sample rate recordings of the cardiac and respiratory cycles (using, for example, a pulse oximeter and respiratory belt) during the functional imaging session is recommended. There are a variety of techniques for removing the effects of cardiac and respiration from the imaging data when high sample rate recordings of these physiologic cycles are available [52–55]. If high-sample rate recordings of cardiac and respiration are not collected during the imaging session, a method has been proposed for estimating them that makes use of spatial templates representing regions in the brain with large amounts of cardiac and respiratory noise [56]. The effects of cardiac and respiratory noise may also be reduced by processing steps such as regressing out global signal changes, or regressing out the average time course in the white matter [52, 57] (see later text for more about these processing steps).

Temporal Filtering

Low-pass filtering with a cutoff of 0.08 Hz was used in the first fMRI resting-state functional connectivity study [2], and many subsequent resting-state functional connectivity studies have used low-pass filtering with similar or less stringent cutoff frequencies. It has been shown that the interregional correlations identified in functional connectivity studies are driven by low frequency fluctuations below 0.1 Hz [58]. Therefore, low-pass filtering at this frequency tends to increase the signal-to-noise ratio. In order to also remove very low frequencies associated with drift (<0.01 Hz), some studies use a band-pass rather than a low-pass filter, typically retaining frequencies in a range around 0.01–0.1 Hz.

Removal of Time Courses Believed to Be Associated with Noise Sources

A set of time courses believed to capture potential sources of spurious correlation are often removed from the data via regression or orthogonalization during preprocessing. These time courses include the motion parameters, a time course of the signal in white matter regions, a time course of the signal in the ventricles, and a time course of the global signal (or the mean slice time course). In addition to removing these time courses, some studies also remove the first temporal derivatives of them. If these time courses are not removed during preprocessing, they may be removed later when the data are correlated with the seed region time course by using a partial correlation model, or by including them as a covariate in a regression model. It should be noted that the practice of removing global time course has been criticized as potentially distorting the data and forcing negative correlations to exist between brain areas [59] (see also [60]).

Seed Region Definition

One of the most critical decisions in seed map analyses is how to define the seed region. There are many possible ways to define a seed region and the precise definition used will affect not only the power of the study but also the interpretation of the results. The seed region can be defined anatomically, based on a predefined atlas, or functionally.

Anatomically Defined or Atlas-Based Seed Regions

A seed region defined anatomically can be drawn on each subject based on their individual brain structure or can be drawn on a standardized reference brain to which each subject's data has been mapped. The latter approach is dependent on the quality of registration across subjects in the area of the seed. The former provides greater specificity and, thus, is likely to increase power, but is more labor-intensive. Another method for defining seeds based on brain anatomy that does not depend on the existence of a clearly delineated structure is to select a single point on a reference brain (e.g., a Talairach coordinate) and to include a volume of a fixed size around that coordinate in each subject [61]. Once again, this approach is dependent on the quality of registration across subjects in the area of the seed. Atlas-based approaches use atlases that have predefined anatomic structures already in a reference space, such as the one available freely online at http:\\www.bioimagesuite.org.

Task-Based Functionally Defined Seed Regions

A seed region can be defined functionally based on task activations in specific subjects, based on composite activations of all subjects in the study, or based on activations in prior studies that are mapped to this group of subjects via transformations to/from a reference brain. One popular approach is to take the Talairach coordinate of activation from a prior study and create a volume in each subject centered on that coordinate [62]. Defining the seed region functionally in each subject based on individual activation patterns is potentially quite a powerful approach and is the only approach that adjusts for differences in the anatomic location of a functional area across subjects (e.g., if a functional area is located farther along a sulcus in some subjects than others). When the seed region is defined functionally in each subject based on individual activation patterns, it is often defined as the *n* most activated pixels in each subject, rather than using a fixed threshold across subjects [34]. This practice ensures that the seed region is a similar size across subjects, rather than covering a huge swath of cortex in one subject and a tiny region in another.

An additional approach to defining seed regions (and in fact partitioning the entire cortex into functional subunits) is described in the subsection titled "Data-Driven Approaches." There are a variety of methods described there for using functional connectivity data to define individual subunits with coherent activity that could, in theory, be used in seed-to-whole-brain or seed-to-seed analyses.

Postprocessing

After correlating the seed-region time courses with each pixel in the brain, the *r*-values are typically transformed to Gaussian values via Fishers transform. However, Fishers transform does not transform the data to a standard normal Gaussian distribution. If the global time course has been removed, the mean of the distribution will be around zero (if not, the mean of the distribution will tend to be positive), but the standard deviation is unknown. It is related to the degrees of freedom in the data, which is influenced by the temporal autocorrelation of the fMRI data. In order to adjust the data to a standard normal distribution – which can be useful, for example, to evaluate significance of specific connections in an individual subject – postprocessing normalization can be applied [18]. This step also provides a final check on the quality of the individual subjects' data by verifying that it does indeed have a Gaussian distribution after the Fisher's transform (a non-Gaussian distribution can be an indicator of too much motion or scanner instability).

Direct Correlation of Regional Time Courses (Seed-to-Seed)

An even simpler approach to functional connectivity analysis does not produce whole-brain maps at all. Instead, a set of regions in the brain are defined, based on a priori interests, and the time course for each of those regions is computed for each subject (typically by averaging across all pixels in the region). The regional time courses are then correlated in a pair-wise manner and the *r*-values are converted to Gaussian variables via Fisher's transform. A variant of this approach involves partial correlation of each pair of regions, so as to remove the effects of all the other brain regions [63].

Directly correlating regional time courses has the advantage that all the regions of interest are treated in a similar manner. For example, when computing connectivity between region A and region B, results from the single-seed-region-to-whole-brain approach can depend on whether A or B is used as the seed. Direct correlation of the regional time courses does not have this problem. Furthermore, many different regions can be correlated directly in a single analysis, so connectivity throughout the brain can be computed, not just connectivity to the seed region [64–67]. Of course, the seed region approach can be extended to examine more connections by creating multiple seed maps, but this becomes computationally expensive when many are needed.

On the other hand, direct correlation of regional time courses has the drawbacks that whole-brain maps are not created for visualizing connectivity patterns, and postprocessing of the whole-brain distribution is not possible (so, for example, it is difficult to evaluate significance of a connection in a single subject). Because these two related methods have different strengths, they are sometimes used in conjunction [34, 68, 69].

Data-Driven Approaches

These approaches allow the investigation of functional connectivity without any a priori assumptions regarding regions of interest.

Independent Components Analysis

This popular approach decomposes the data into a set of statistically independent components [70]. Whether the components are spatially or temporally independent depends upon the type of independent components analysis (ICA) applied. For functional imaging, spatially independent components are typically extracted [71]. The components, therefore, correspond to statistically independent spatial maps each with an associated time course. The value each voxel takes in the component map reflects how much that voxel expresses the associated time course. Thus, each component represents pixels that share a temporal pattern of activity (i.e., that covary together). These components are typically interpreted as either brain networks or noise sources.

There are several advantages of using ICA. First, ICA is a data-driven approach that examines the whole brain. Therefore, it is not dependent upon the selection of a priori regions of interest and is not limited to examining the connections to prespecified regions. Second, ICA has the potential to capture noise sources in separate components, and thus has built-in noise removal without special preprocessing steps [10, 52], although it does not always do a good job of separating noise sources from the signals of interest [52].

On the other hand, there are some major challenges in the use of ICA in functional connectivity studies. First, the results of ICA are dependent upon the number of components extracted. A couple of methods for addressing this problem have been described in the imaging literature [72, 73]. Second, ICA does not lend itself naturally to multisubject analyses. If ICA is simply applied to each subject separately, the result will be a unique set of components for each subject and it is not obvious what common variable can be extracted for comparisons across subjects. Several approaches have been developed to allow multisubject analyses of imaging data using ICA. A simple approach that is somewhat popular is to match ICA components in each subject to a template representing a network of interest; the best-matching component is then used for the multisubject analysis [74]. However, adoption of this approach results in an analysis that is no longer whole-brain or data-driven and, thus, sacrifices some of the key advantages of ICA. Other approaches that do not sacrifice these qualities have been described [75–78]. Another challenge in the use of ICA is that decisions regarding which components do or do not represent noise can be difficult, requiring subjective judgments or arbitrary matching criteria to be employed.

Despite the challenges inherent in implementing ICA, it has great potential for studying the organization of networks throughout the brain. For example, a recent meta-analysis comparing activation patterns across many different paradigms with functional networks extracted from resting data using ICA revealed close correspondence between the brain systems identified in these two different types of data [79]. This illustrates the power of resting connectivity to reveal the functional architecture of the entire brain.

Other Data-Driven Methods for Parcellation of the Brain

ICA is the most popular of many data-driven analyses for parcellating the brain, but a wide variety of other algorithms exist with different strengths and weaknesses. These include Gaussian mixture models [80], hierarchical clustering [63, 81], k-means [82–84], and edge-finding methods [85]. ICA and other data-driven parcellation algorithms have typically been used to identify networks in the brain, but, extending data-driven analyses to a finer parcellation, they can be also used for the identification of subunits of uniform activity within a region.

The Gaussian mixture model and the *k*-means algorithm are two robust unsupervised techniques that are commonly used for cluster analysis and have been applied to isolate distinct cortical systems in the brain [80, 82–84, 86]. A stable partition of the human cortex into two global systems has been shown by Golland [86] based on resting-state fMRI using the Gaussian mixture model. Consistent functional delineation of regions of interest, for example the subdivision between SMA and pre-SMA, has been obtained by several groups [83, 84] based on both task and resting-state data using the *k*-means algorithm.

Correlation maps based on spontaneous BOLD signals have also proven useful in defining finer functional boundaries [85, 87]. A surface-based approach has been described [85] where a selected part of the cortical surface is inflated and seed points are placed on the inflated surface. For each seed, a correlation map to the entire region of interest is generated and the difference between correlation maps is converted to form an image. Standard edge detection algorithms are then applied to identify the boundaries of different functional areas. Another approach was introduced for parcellating the human thalamus [87]. In this study, the cortex was divided into five regions based on anatomical landmarks, and the mean time course of each region was computed. The partial correlations between voxels in the thalamus and the five cortical regions were computed, yielding maps showing distinctive divisions within the thalamus.

Parcellation algorithms based on graph theory have also become popular in brain network analysis. Graph theory is a common methodology for the study of complex networks and has long been exploited by investigators in social network studies [88–91]. There are two levels of graph theory to consider. In the section at the end of this chapter, we consider graph theory as it is applied to analyze the network properties, such as the wiring architecture and efficiency. Most of the literature on graph theory and its application to brain network analysis is focused on that problem and uses predefined regions as network nodes. In this section, however, we consider a different branch of graph theory that can be used to subdivide a network into smaller components where the intranetwork connections are maximized.

The normalized cut algorithm [92] and the modularity detection algorithm [93] are two graph-based partitioning approaches that have been introduced to examine resting-state brain networks [94–96]. The graph-based algorithms are designed to maximize the association within subgroups. It was reported that seven consistent functionally connected networks were identified based on a group clustering result [96]. Another approach that maximizes the modularity of the graph [94] successfully delineated seed regions with anatomically meaningful structures in rat brain. We have recently shown that a normalized cut approach could be used to isolate seed regions from resting-state data [97]. To illustrate this type of approach, we depict in Fig. 6.2 a parcellation of the whole brain using a graph-based algorithm.

While many of the techniques described in this section are still under development, they represent a category of methods that can potentially produce meaningful seed regions anywhere in the brain without the need for clear anatomic landmarks or for task-based fMRI activations in that region, hence providing excellent flexibility for studies of connectivity and functional networks.

Assessment of Network Properties After Node Identification

The function of brain networks is an emergent property of the entire network structure. Although some information can be gleaned by examining individual functional connections, a more holistic understanding of complex brain networks is ultimately needed. There are several approaches to this issue. Computational models have been developed that attempt to reproduce in some

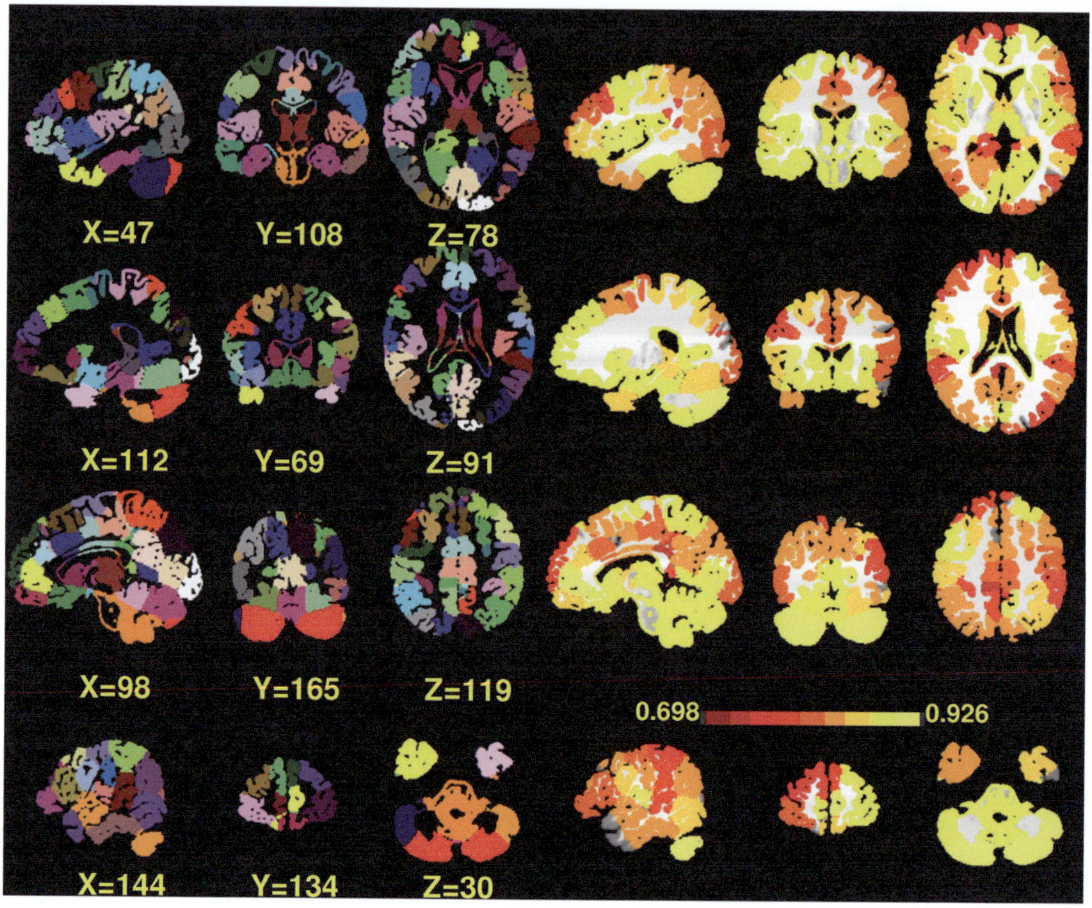

Fig. 6.2 A whole-brain segmentation into 200 subunits based on resting-state fMRI from 43 subjects. The segmentation was obtained using a graph-based parcellation approach. Each subunit is shown in a unique color on the *left half* of the figure. The *right half* of the figure shows the reproducibility of each corresponding subunit, with *yellow* indicating high reproducibility, and *red* indicating low reproducibility. The reproducibility measures the invariance of a subunit definition across subjects, in other words, subunits of high reproducibility are considered more stable and consistent

simplified manner the function and dynamics of brain networks [98–102]. One of the challenges in creating such models is that many details must be specified in a model, such as which nodes in the network are anatomically connected, what kinds of conduction delays exist between nodes, etc. Unfortunately, there is not always sufficient data available to specify this information with confidence, and assumptions typically need to be made upon which the model behavior depends. Thus, computational network modeling is a challenging, but important, field of brain research.

In this subsection, we describe an alternative approach to studying brain networks that is based on network theory. In network theory, a network is defined as a mathematical object comprised of a set of n vertices $V = \{v_1, v_2, \ldots v_n\}$ and a set of m edges $E = \{e(i, j)\}$ that connect the vertices: $e(i, j) = 1$ if there is an edge connecting v_i and v_j, and $e(i, j) = 0$ if there is not an edge. A network can be built using either structural or functional connectivity data. The vertices represent nodes, and the presence or absence of an edge is determined by the connectivity measures, such as the existence of a neural tract or the degree of covariation in the BOLD signal.

A number of measures have been derived to characterize properties of networks and properties of nodes within those networks. These measures include degree, characteristic path length, clustering coefficient, betweenness centrality, and global/local efficiency, to name a few. One of the simplest network measures of connectivity of a node is degree. The degree d_i of a vertex v_i is defined as the total number of edges with v_i as one end. In other words, the degree d_i is the number of neighbors of vertex v_i. Assuming that a network is connected, then a path can be found connecting one vertex to any other vertex in the network, and the path length is the number of edges along the path. The characteristic path length of the network is the average of the shortest path length between all pairs of vertices in the network. It is a global measure of connections in the network. The clustering coefficient, in contrast, is a local measure. Suppose vertex v_i has degree d_i, thus it has d_i neighbors. The largest number of connections that can exist between the d_i neighbors is $d_i(d_i - 1)/2$ when every neighbor is connected to every other neighbor. The clustering coefficient is the ratio of the number of edges that actually exist in the network to the maximum possible. The characteristic path length and the clustering coefficient are two useful quantities in identifying "small-world" networks [91]. Another useful measure, betweenness centrality, is defined for each single vertex. It measures the fraction of all shortest paths that pass through that vertex. For a comprehensive review of network measures, see the recent paper by Rubinov and colleagues [103].

Vertices with high degree or betweenness centrality are usually referred to as "hubs." They play an important role in controlling information flow, and a number of brain hubs have been discovered by analyzing network properties [104–106]. In the work of Sporns and colleagues [106], structural connectivity data were acquired for both cat and macaque brain. Based on multiple network properties, a number of "hub" regions were identified that had been previously classified as polysensory or multimodal regions. These hub regions were then divided, based on network properties, into two different classes of hubs that, when lesioned, had opposite effects on the small-world index. In another study, regional characteristic path length was used to define 20 hubs in the resting human brain based on functional connectivity data [104]. It was shown that the network was in general resilient to random attacks; however, the most damaging attacks were on hub regions. Most recently, the relationship between the topography of cortical hubs and the patterns of vulnerability in Alzheimer's disease was explored [105]. Similarities between the regions of high amyloid deposition and hub locations were identified, suggesting that cortical hubs are preferentially affected in Alzheimer's disease. For more information about the use of network analyses to understand complex brain systems, we refer the reader to a recent review paper [107].

One of the limitations in using network analyses is that they can be very sensitive to the definition of the nodes. A simple approach that incorporates minimal assumptions regarding brain structure and organization is to compute network measures at the level of voxels. This allows computation of network properties for each tissue element in the brain [105, 108, 109]. For example, degree can be computed for each voxel as the sum of the connections above a specific correlation threshold (typically something like $r > 0.25$) between a reference voxel and all the other gray matter voxels in the brain. This measure provides a single number for each voxel in the brain that reflects its total direct connectivity. Whole-brain voxel based maps of network properties can identify cortical regions with certain properties, such as high intrinsic connectivity, or these maps can be contrasted across populations or correlated with behavioral measures. Some of the potentially powerful uses of voxel-based measures of intrinsic connectivity include: providing a functional brain phenotype for genetic studies, examining functional organization of the brain across a wide range of neuronal disorders (unbiased by a priori region selection), and characterizing pharmaceutical effects on brain function.

Relating Function to Connectivity

The ability to assess functional connectivity for individual subjects allows the examination of individual differences in functional connectivity.

This is one of the exciting advances made possible by the improved temporal resolution functional magnetic resonance imaging (fMRI) provides relative to positron emission tomography (PET). PET studies examining interregional correlations typically computed them as correlations across subjects, because they did not have the temporal resolution to allow estimates of functional connectivity for each subject (although there were exceptions to this [110]).

Several of the earliest fMRI studies to examine connectivity–behavior correlations illustrate the power and broad utility of this approach. In a remarkable study relating genetics to functional connectivity and behavior, functional connectivity between the amygdala and the rostral anterior cingulate cortex during a task involving processing of fearful stimuli was shown to be both related to genetic variant and responsible for approximately 30% of variation across subjects in temperamental anxiety [111]. More studies of this nature, linking genetics to behavior and imaging, are needed.

In another study, resting state functional connectivity between the angular gyrus and Broca's area (a connection known to be disrupted in dyslexia [16, 112]) was found to be correlated with reading comprehension [33], underscoring the functional relevance of individual differences in resting brain patterns. When functional connectivity was evaluated in the same subjects during a sentence reading task, correlations between this functional connection and reading abilities increased dramatically [33]. Thus, although resting data may contain information regarding individual differences in capacity, tasks that drive the networks of interest may have more power to highlight disparities in specific circuits.

In some cases, the information provided by connectivity–behavior correlations can challenge popular theories of brain function. In a study of connectivity between component regions of the default mode network, we found that functional connectivity between default mode regions was stronger for individuals who performed better on a working memory task [34]. This was true whether connectivity was assessed at rest or during performance of the task. This was a surprising finding given the popular view that the default mode network distracts from focused cognition, and must be shut down to properly focus on the desired task. If disengagement of the default network is necessary for good performance on cognitive tasks, functional connectivity between regions in the default network would be expected to be lowest for those high performers who are most successful at shutting it down. That is, a negative relationship would be expected between connectivity in this network and working memory performance. By contrast, the positive correlation found suggests this network facilitates cognition. As shown in Fig. 6.3, the positive relationship between default network connectivity and working memory performance has now been reproduced and extended to older adult populations [113, 114]. Although incongruent with the currently popular view that the default network distracts from cognition, this finding is consistent with the growing literature reporting that the default mode network is disrupted for a range of disorders involving cognitive dysfunction including autism [115], mild cognitive impairment [116], Alzheimer's disease [74], schizophrenia [117], and attention deficit hyperactivity disorder [118].

Interest in the default mode network has been increased by studies reporting that this network is anticorrelated with a set of regions that typically activate during attention-demanding cognitive tasks, including dorsolateral prefrontal cortex, premotor areas, and the intraparietal sulcus, in the resting state [62, 119]. However, the studies reporting these anticorrelations used global regression, which forces anticorrelations to exist in the data [59]. The question of whether these anticorrelations reflect a true relationship, or simply a processing artifact is a matter of debate [59, 62, 120]. Whether default mode regions are oscillating in antiphase to classic cognitive regions or not, the functional relationships between cognitive and default mode regions appear to be related to cognitive function [121], even when global regression is not used in the analysis [122]. Recent modeling work has illustrated that anticorrelations between networks in the brain can arise without any long-range inhibitory connections, but their emergence can be sensitive to parameters such as conduction delay, coupling strength, and noise level [101, 102]. This raises

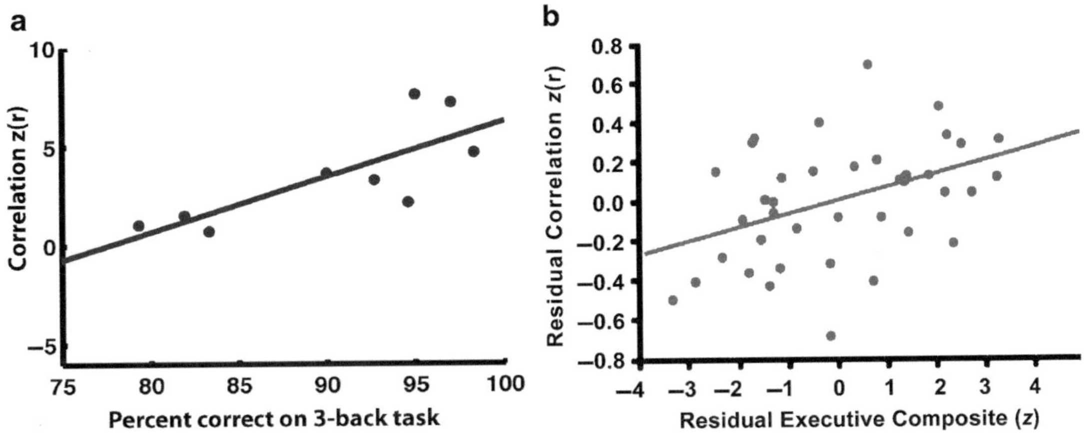

Fig. 6.3 Functional connectivity between medial frontal cortex and posterior cingulate/precuneus plotted against measures of cognitive function for adults aged 28–45 in panel (**a**) and for older adults aged 60–93 in panel (**b**). Units of functional connectivity on the *y*-axis are not comparable across studies due to differences in normalization applied. Data from panel (**a**) was reported in [34] and panel (**b**) is reproduced with permission from [113]

the question of whether variation across subjects in one of the corresponding neural characteristics, such as conduction delay, could give rise to differences in cognitive function.

A variety of other early studies illustrate how connectivity–behavior relationships can inform our understanding of brain function [123, 124], but we will just highlight two here. First, correlations between resting state functional connectivity patterns and two different behavioral measures (representing anxiety and executive functioning) were used to dissociate the function of distinct, but commonly coactivated attentional networks [125]. Second, an inverse correlation between symptom severity and functional connectivity between homologous posterior parietal areas in patients with spatial neglect was reported [126]. Remarkably, recovery of function was also associated with increased connectivity between the same parietal regions.

Functional MRI studies of connectivity–behavior correlations are now used ubiquitously to help interpret the function of different brain connections. They have become a particularly popular tool in clinical studies, in which they are often used to clarify the aspects of a complex psychiatric disorder that relate to a particular aberrant connection.

Clinical Applications

Correlations between brain areas have been studied extensively in psychiatric populations. Before fMRI came into widespread use, there were a number of PET studies investigating how activity patterns in different regions of the brain were correlated in patient groups [112, 127–134]. Building on this research, fMRI studies of functional connectivity in psychiatric populations have recently exploded in popularity. In particular, resting state functional connectivity has been recognized as a valuable tool in psychiatry, because it allows the study of brain networks without requiring subjects to perform tasks to activate those networks. Thus, it avoids confounds related to differences in performance level and effort between groups that traditional functional MRI studies must address. Furthermore, resting state functional connectivity can be used to study brain function in patients who are incapable of cognitive tasks (such as comatose patients). In this section, we provide a brief overview of the contributions of fMRI-based functional connectivity mapping to psychiatry.

A disruption of integration of information across the brain has been hypothesized to underlie autism [135]. There have been a range of studies examining functional connectivity in autistic subjects (or subjects with autism spectrum disorders) during a variety of task paradigms involving language [135], biological motion processing [136], executive function [137–140], working memory [141, 142], mental imagery [143], visuomotor coordination [144–146], theory of mind [147], episodic memory [148], and processing of faces [142, 149, 150], as well as a few resting-state connectivity studies [151–153]. On the whole, disconnection between brain areas that are strongly connected in healthy subjects appears to characterize the disorder [135–137, 139, 140, 142–144, 147, 149, 151, 152]. However, a few studies have reported increased or more extensive connectivity [146, 148], or a combination of increases and decreases in connectivity for autistic subjects [141, 145, 153]. It has been suggested that autism is associated with more diffuse (less focal) connectivity that is not appropriately localized to functional circuits, resulting in overall reduced signal to noise in networks important for healthy cognitive function [148].

Another disorder that has long been hypothesized to result from disrupted functional connectivity is schizophrenia [154–156]. Various theories regarding the specific form of dysconnection underlying this disorder have been proposed. Many early imaging studies reported disrupted communication within networks incorporating frontal and temporal regions of the brain [154, 157, 158] and support for disrupted frontotemporal circuitry has come from both resting state [159] and task-based [160–162] functional connectivity MR imaging. A theory of disruption in corticothalamocerebellar networks has also been proposed [163] and supported by subsequent functional connectivity studies [164, 165]. In fact, disturbed connectivity across a multitude of different brain networks has been associated with schizophrenia [166–170]. There is particularly large and growing literature on aberrant connectivity in the default mode network of schizophrenic subjects [117, 171–179]. While some of these studies have reported increases in connectivity within the default-mode network [175, 176], others have reported decreases [172] or a combination of increases and decreases [117, 174, 178]. Conflicting reports on functional connectivity in schizophrenia are not limited to the default mode network, but are a more general problem in this extensive, complicated literature [180], possibly due to the heterogeneous nature of this disorder, as well as differences in methodologies used.

Mood and anxiety disorders have been less extensively studied with functional connectivity MR imaging. Studies of anxiety disorders [181–184], bipolar disorder [185–187], and depression [168, 188–190] have reported aberrant connectivity with the amygdala. Depression has also been associated with disrupted patterns of connectivity to subregions of the anterior cingulate cortex [187, 191–195] and within the default mode network [195–198]. Similar circuitry has been examined in post-traumatic stress disorder (PTSD), and disturbed connectivity reported with anterior cingulate, amygdalae, and default mode regions across a variety of PTSD subgroups [199–203].

As noted in the preceding paragraphs, there is a recently emerging focus in the clinical literature on the role of the default mode network in brain dysfunction. Aberrant connectivity in this network has been reported across a wide range of disorders, suggesting its importance across many domains of cognitive function. Recent research has suggested that a key default mode region, the precuneus/posterior cingulate cortex, represents a major connector "hub" of the brain [42, 204], possibly accounting for the ubiquitous associations found between default mode dysfunction and mental illness.

Interest in the default mode network is perhaps most pronounced in the study of age-related disorders of cognitive function. Even in healthy subjects, connectivity in the default mode network is related to cognitive function [34] and has been shown to be lower in older adults than younger ones [114]. Thus, deterioration of this network may play a role in the cognitive decline associated with healthy aging. Disruptions in the default mode network have also been implicated in age-related dementias, particularly mild cognitive impairment [205] and Alzheimer's disease [74]. High amyloid deposition has been reported in default mode areas [206], and the density of amyloid deposition is correlated with connectivity in

Table 6.1 Summary of key functional connectivity studies

Authors	fMRI paradigm	Functional connectivity method	Result
Biswal et al. 1995 [2]	Rest	Seed-to-whole brain	Resting state correlations in BOLD signal revealed motor network
Lowe et al. 1998 [18]	Rest	Seed-to-whole brain	Biswal's findings extended to multislice acquisitions and other brain systems
Grecius et al. 2003 [9]	Rest	Seed-to-whole brain	Default mode regions correlated at rest
Just et al. 2004 [135]	Sentence comprehension	Seed-to-seed	Decreased long-range connections in autism
Pezawas et al. 2005 [111]	Object and emotional face matching blocks	Seed-to-whole brain	Cingulate–amygdala functional connectivity related to genetics and temperament
Hampson et al. 2006 [34]	Rest and working memory (assessed separately)	Seed-to-whole brain, seed-to-seed	Default mode connectivity related to working memory performance
Fransson, 2005 [119]; Fox et al. 2005 [62]	Rest	Seed-to-whole brain	Default mode regions anticorrelated at rest with regions activated during attention demanding cognitive tasks
Smith et al. 2009 [79]	Resting fcMRI compared with task activation networks	Independent components analysis	Strong correspondence between networks identified by resting state functional connectivity analysis and task activation protocols
Biswal et al. 2010 [233]	Rest	Seed-to-whole brain, independent components analysis	Publicly available, multicenter database of resting data introduced and used to examine age, gender, and site related resting connectivity effects

the default network [207, 208]. Thus, the default network has become a major focus in Alzheimer's research, in addition to a long-standing interest in the role of the medial temporal lobe in this disorder [209, 210].

These clinical conditions are only a few of the most highly studied using functional connectivity MR imaging. Disturbances in functional connectivity have been reported across a wide range of other clinical conditions including, but not limited to, multiple sclerosis [211, 212], addiction [213–216], obsessive–compulsive disorder [217], Tourette syndrome [218], premature birth [219, 220], epilepsy [221–224], and attention-deficit disorder [118, 225].

Conclusion

Studies investigating functional connectivity in the human brain are opening up new avenues of research and providing novel insights into brain organization and function (Table 6.1). However, the biological bases of interregional correlations in functional MRI data are still not well understood. Basic research relating these synchronous, low-frequency fluctuations to measurements in other modalities, such as electroencephalography [226, 227] or electrophysiology [120, 228], has made some progress, but more work is needed.

Important avenues for future clinical research include investigating changes in the brain connectivity that may be associated with compensation [67, 229] or recovery [126] of function. Studies of the effects of interventions on brain networks, such as pharmaceutical drugs [193, 230–232], may also shed light on the neural mechanisms underlying improvements in symptoms. Ultimately, a better understanding of these mechanisms may facilitate the development of more effective interventions.

References

1. Friston KJ, Frith CD, Frackowiak RSJ. Time-dependent changes in effective connectivity measured with PET. Hum Brain Mapp. 1993;1:69–79.

2. Biswal BB, Yetkin FZ, Haughton VM, Hyde JS. Functional connectivity in the motor cortex of the resting human brain using echo-planar MRI. Magn Reson Med. 1995;34:537–41.
3. Friston KJ, Harrison L, Penny W. Dynamic causal modelling. Neuroimage. 2003;19(4):1273–302.
4. Goebel R, Roebroeck A, Kim DS, Formisano E. Investigating directed cortical interactions in time-resolved fMRI data using vector autoregressive modeling and Granger causality mapping. Magn Reson Imaging. 2003;21(10):1251–61.
5. Marrelec G, Daunizeau J, Pélégrini-Issac M, Doyon J, Benali H. Conditional correlation as a measure of mediated interactivity in fMRI and MEG/EEG. IEEE Trans Signal Process. 2005;53:3505–16.
6. McIntosh AR, Gonzalez-Lima F. Network interactions among limbic cortices, basal forebrain, and cerebellum differentiate a tone conditioned as a Pavlovian excitor or inhibitor: fluorodeoxyglucose mapping and covariance structural modeling. J Neurophysiol. 1994;72(4):1717–33.
7. Horwitz B. The elusive concept of brain connectivity. Neuroimage. 2003;19:466–70.
8. Sun FT, Miller LM, D'Esposito M. Measuring interregional functional connectivity using coherence and partial coherence analyses of fMRI data. Neuroimage. 2004;21(2):647–58.
9. Greicius MD, Krasnow B, Reiss AL, Menon V. Functional connectivity in the resting brain: a network analysis of the default mode hypothesis. Proc Natl Acad Sci USA. 2003;100(1):253–8.
10. Kiviniemi V, Kantola JH, Jauhiainen J, Hyvarinen A, Tervonen O. Independent component analysis of nondeterministic fMRI signal sources. Neuroimage. 2003;19(2 Pt 1):253–60.
11. Callicott JH, Straub RE, Pezawas L, Egan MF, Mattay VS, Hariri AR, et al. Variation in DISC1 affects hippocampal structure and function and increases risk for schizophrenia. Proc Natl Acad Sci USA. 2005;102(24):8627–32.
12. Roth JK, Courtney SM. Neural system for updating object working memory from different sources: sensory stimuli or long-term memory. Neuroimage. 2007;38(3):617–30.
13. Hampson M, Olson IR, Leung H-C, Skudlarski P, Gore JC. Changes in functional connectivity of human MT/v5 with visual motion input. Neuroreport. 2004;15(8):1315–9.
14. Lowe MJ, Dzemidzic M, Lurito JT, Mathews VP, Phillips MD. Correlations in low-frequency BOLD fluctuations reflect cortico-cortical connections. Neuroimage. 2000;12(5):582–7.
15. Nir Y, Hasson U, Levy I, Yeshurun Y, Malach R. Widespread functional connectivity and fMRI fluctuations in human visual cortex in the absence of visual stimulation. Neuroimage. 2006;30:1313–24.
16. Pugh KR, Mencl EW, Shaywitz BA, Shaywitz SE, Fulbright RK, Constable RT, et al. The angular gyrus in developmental dyslexia: task-specific differences in functional connectivity within posterior cortex. Psychol Sci. 2000;11(1):51–6.
17. Schafer RJ, Lacadie C, Vohr B, Kesler SR, Katz KH, Schneider KC, et al. Alterations in functional connectivity in language in prematurely born adolescents. Brain. 2009;132(Pt 3):661–70. Epub ahead of print.
18. Lowe MJ, Mock BJ, Sorenson JA. Functional connectivity in single and multislice echoplanar imaging using resting-state fluctuations. Neuroimage. 1998;7:119–32.
19. Biswal B, Hudetz AG, Yetkin FZ, Haughton VM, Hyde JS. Hypercapnia reversibly suppresses low-frequency fluctuations in the human motor cortex during rest using echo-planar MRI. J Cereb Blood Flow Metab. 1997;17:301–8.
20. Biswal BB, Van Kylen J, Hyde JS. Simultaneous assessment of flow and BOLD signals in resting-state functional connectivity maps. NMR Biomed. 1997;10:165–70.
21. Peltier SJ, Noll DC. T2* dependence of low frequency functional connectivity. Neuroimage. 2002;16:985–92.
22. Cordes D, Haughton VM, Arfanakis K, Wendt GJ, Turski PA, Moritz CH, et al. Mapping functionally related regions of brain with functional connectivity MR imaging. AJNR Am J Neuroradiol. 2000;21:1636–44.
23. Stein T, Moritz C, Quigley M, Cordes D, Haughton V, Meyerand E. Functional connectivity in the thalamus and hippocampus studied with functional MR imaging. AJNR Am J Neuroradiol. 2000;21:1397–401.
24. Hampson M, Peterson BS, Skudlarski P, Gatenby JC, Gore JC. Detection of functional connectivity using temporal correlations in MR images. Hum Brain Mapp. 2002;15:247–62.
25. van de Ven VG, Formisano E, Prvulovic D, Roeder CH, Linden DE. Functional connectivity as revealed by spatial independent component analysis of fMRI measurements during rest. Hum Brain Mapp. 2004;22(3):165–78.
26. Xiong J, Parsons LM, Gao J-H, Fox PT. Interregional connectivity to primary motor cortex revealed using MRI resting state images. Hum Brain Mapp. 1999;8:151–6.
27. DeLuca M, Smith S, DeStefano N, Federico A, Matthews PM. Blood oxygenation level dependent contrast resting state networks are relevant to functional activity in the neocortical sensorimotor system. Exp Brain Res. 2005;167:587–94.
28. Quigley M, Cordes D, Moritz C, Haughton V, Seth R, Meyerand ME. Role of the corpus callosum in functional connectivity. AJNR Am J Neuroradiol. 2003;24:208–12.
29. Husain FT, McKinney CM, Horwitz B. Frontal cortex functional connectivity changes during sound categorization. Neuroreport. 2006;17(6):617–21.
30. Bokde AL, Tagamets MA, Friedman RB, Horwitz B. Functional interactions of the inferior frontal cortex during the processing of words and word-like stimuli. Neuron. 2001;30(2):609–17.
31. Jiang T, He Y, Zang Y, Weng X. Modulation of functional connectivity during the resting state and the motor task. Hum Brain Mapp. 2004;22(1):63–71.

32. Morgan VL, Price RR. The effect of sensorimotor activation on functional connectivity mapping with MRI. Magn Reson Imaging. 2004;22:1069–75.
33. Hampson M, Tokoglu F, Sun Z, Schafer RJ, Skudlarski P, Gore JC, et al. Connectivity–behavior analysis reveals that functional connectivity between left BA39 and Broca's area varies with reading ability. Neuroimage. 2006;31:513–9.
34. Hampson M, Driesen NR, Skudlarski P, Gore JC, Constable RT. Brain connectivity related to working memory performance. J Neurosci. 2006;26(51): 13338–43.
35. Mazoyer B, Zago L, Mellet E, Bricogne S, Etard O, Houdé O, et al. Cortical Networks for working memory and executive functions sustain the conscious resting state in man. Brain Res Bull. 2001;54(3): 287–98.
36. Shulman GL, Fiez JA, Corbetta M, Buckner RL, Miezin FM, Raichle ME, et al. Common blood flow changes across visual tasks: II. Decreases in cerebral cortex. J Cogn Neurosci. 1997;9(5):648–63.
37. Raichle ME, MacLeod AM, Snyder AZ, Powers WJ, Gusnard DA, Shulman GL. A default mode of brain function. Proc Natl Acad Sci USA. 2001;98(2): 676–82.
38. Vincent JL, Patel GH, Fox MD, Snyder AZ, Baker JT, Essen DCV, et al. Intrinsic functional architecture in the anaesthetized monkey brain. Nature. 2007;447:83–6.
39. Horovitz SG, Fukunaga M, Zwart JAd, Gelderen Pv, Fulton SC, Balkin TJ, et al. Low frequency BOLD fluctuations during resting wakefulness and light sleep: a simulataneous EEG-fMRI study. Hum Brain Mapp. 2008;29:671–82.
40. Boly M, Tshibanda L, Vanhaudenhuyse A, Noirhomme Q, Schnakers C, Ledoux D, et al. Functional connectivity in the default network during resting state is preserved in a vegetative but not in a brain dead patient. Hum Brain Mapp. 2009;30(8): 2393–400.
41. Shehzad Z, Kelly AM, Reiss PT, Gee DG, Gotimer K, Uddin LQ, et al. The resting brain: unconstrained yet reliable. Cereb Cortex. 2009;19(10):2209–29.
42. Hagmann P, Cammoun L, Gigandet X, Meuli R, Honey CJ, Wedeen VJ, et al. Mapping the structural core of human cerebral cortex. PLoS Biol. 2008;6(7):e159.
43. Honey CJ, Sporns O, Cammoun L, Gigandet X, Thiran JP, Meuli R, et al. Predicting human resting-state functional connectivity from structural connectivity. Proc Natl Acad Sci USA. 2009;106(6): 2035–40.
44. Koch MA, Norris DG, Hund-Georgiadis M. An investigation of functional and anatomical connectivity using magnetic resonance imaging. Neuroimage. 2002;16:241–50.
45. Skudlarski P, Jagannathan K, Calhoun VD, Hampson M, Skudlarska BA, Pearlson G. Measuring brain connectivity: diffusion tensor imaging validates resting state temporal correlations. Neuroimage. 2008; 43(3):554–61.
46. Greicius MD, Supekar K, Menon V, Dougherty RF. Resting-state functional connectivity reflects structural connectivity in the default mode network. Cereb Cortex. 2009;19(1):72–8.
47. Lowe MJ, Beall EB, Sakaie KE, Koenig KA, Stone L, Marrie RA, et al. Resting state sensorimotor functional connectivity in multiple sclerosis inversely correlates with transcallosal motor pathway transverse diffusivity. Hum Brain Mapp. 2008;29(7): 818–27.
48. Dagli MS, Ingleholm JE, Haxby JV. Localization of cardiac-induced signal change in fMRI. Neuroimage. 1999;9:407–15.
49. Raj D, Anderson AW, Gore JC. Respiratory effects in human functional magnetic resonance imaging due to bulk susceptibility changes. Phys Med Biol. 2001;46:3331–40.
50. Shmueli K, van Gelderen P, de Zwart JA, Horovitz SG, Fukunaga M, Jansma JM, et al. Low-frequency fluctuations in the cardiac rate as a source of variance in the resting-state fMRI BOLD signal. Neuroimage. 2007;38(2):306–20.
51. Wise RG, Ide K, Poulin MJ, Tracey I. Resting fluctuations in arterial carbon dioxide induce significant low frequency variations in BOLD signal. Neuroimage. 2004;21(4):1652–64.
52. Birn RM, Diamond JB, Smith MA, Bandettini PA. Separating respiratory-variation-related fluctuations from neuronal-activity-related fluctuations in fMRI. Neuroimage. 2006;31:1536–48.
53. Chang C, Cunningham JP, Glover GH. Influence of heart rate on the BOLD signal: the cardiac response function. Neuroimage. 2009;44(3):857–69.
54. Glover GH, Li T-Q, Ress D. Image-based method for retrospective correction of physiological motion effects in fMRI: RETROICOR. Magn Reson Med. 2000;44:162–7.
55. Hu X, Le TH, Parrish T, Erhard P. Retrospective estimation and correction of physiological fluctuation in functional MRI. Magn Reson Med. 1995;34:201–12.
56. Beall EB, Lowe MJ. Isolating physiologic noise sources with independently determined spatial measures. Neuroimage. 2007;37(4):1286–300.
57. Giove F, Gili T, Iacovella V, Macaluso E, Maraviglia B. Images-based suppression of unwanted global signals in resting-state functional connectivity studies. Magn Reson Imaging. 2009;27(8):1058–64.
58. Cordes D, Haughton VM, Arfanakis K, Carew JD, Turski PA, Moritz CH, et al. Frequencies contributing to functional connectivity in the cerebral cortex in "resting-state" data. AJNR Am J Neuroradiol. 2001;22(7):1326–33.
59. Murphy K, Birn RM, Handwerker DA, Jones TB, Bandettini PA. The impact of global signal regression on resting state correlations: are anti-correlated networks introduced? Neuroimage. 2008;44(3): 893–905.
60. Fox MD, Raichle ME. Spontaneous fluctuations in brain activity observed with functional magnetic resonance imaging. Nat Rev Neurosci. 2007;8: 000–711.

61. Di Martino A, Scheres A, Margulies DS, Kelly AM, Uddin LQ, Shehzad Z, et al. Functional connectivity of human striatum: a resting state FMRI study. Cereb Cortex. 2008;18(12):2735–47.
62. Fox MD, Snyder AZ, Vincent JL, Corbetta M, Essen DCV, Raichle ME. The human brain is intrinsically organized into dynamic, anticorrelated functional networks. Proc Natl Acad Sci USA. 2005;102(27): 9673–8.
63. Salvador R, Suckling J, Coleman MR, Pickard JD, Menon D, Bullmore E. Neurophysiological architecture of functional magnetic resonance images of human brain. Cereb Cortex. 2005;15:1332–42.
64. Fair DA, Cohen AL, Power JD, Dosenbach NU, Church JA, Miezin FM, et al. Functional brain networks develop from a "local to distributed" organization. PLoS Comput Biol. 2009;5(5):e1000381.
65. Fair DA, Dosenbach NU, Church JA, Cohen AL, Brahmbhatt S, Miezin FM, et al. Development of distinct control networks through segregation and integration. Proc Natl Acad Sci USA. 2007;104(33): 13507–12.
66. Liang M, Zhou Y, Jiang T, Liu Z, Tian L, Liu H, et al. Widespread functional disconnectivity in schizophrenia with resting-state functional magnetic resonance imaging. Neuroreport. 2006;17(26):209–13.
67. Liu Y, Yu C, Liang M, Li J, Tian L, Zhou Y, et al. Whole brain functional connectivity in the early blind. Brain. 2007;130:2085–96.
68 Dosenbach NU, Fair DA, Miezin FM, Cohen AL, Wenger KK, Dosenbach RA, et al. Distinct brain networks for adaptive and stable task control in humans. Proc Natl Acad Sci USA. 2007;104(26):11073–8.
69. Wang K, Liang M, Wang L, Tian L, Zhang X, Li K, et al. Altered functional connectivity in early Alzheimer's disease: a resting-state fMRI study. Hum Brain Mapp. 2007;28(10):967–78.
70. Bell AJ, Sejnowski TJ. An information-maximization approach to blind separation and blind deconvolution. Neural Comput. 1995;7(6):1129–59.
71. McKeown MJ, Makeig S, Brown GG, Jung TP, Kindermann SS, Bell AJ, et al. Analysis of fMRI data by blind separation into independent spatial components. Hum Brain Mapp. 1998;6(3):160–88.
72. Beckmann CF, Smith SM. Probabilistic independent component analysis for functional magnetic resonance imaging. IEEE Trans Med Imaging. 2004; 23(2):137–52.
73. Li YO, Adali T, Calhoun VD. Estimating the number of independent components for functional magnetic resonance imaging data. Hum Brain Mapp. 2007;28(11):1251–66.
74. Greicius MD, Srivastava G, Reiss AL, Menon V. Default-mode network activity distinguishes Alzheimer's disease from healthy aging: evidence from functional MRI. Proc Natl Acad Sci USA. 2004;101(13):4637–42.
75. Beckmann CF, Smith SM. Tensorial extensions of independent component analysis for multisubject FMRI analysis. Neuroimage. 2005;25(1):294–311.
76. Calhoun VD, Adali T, Pearlson GD, Pekar JJ. A method for making group inferences from functional MRI data using independent component analysis. Hum Brain Mapp. 2001;14(3):140–51.
77. Calhoun VD, Adali T, Pekar JJ. A method for comparing group fMRI data using independent component analysis: application to visual, motor and visuomotor tasks. Magn Reson Imaging. 2004;22(9):1181–91.
78. Guo Y, Pagnoni G. A unified framework for group independent component analysis for multi-subject fMRI data. Neuroimage. 2008;42(3):1078–93.
79. Smith SM, Fox PT, Miller KL, Glahn DC, Fox PM, Mackay CE, et al. Correspondence of the brain's functional architecture during activation and rest. Proc Natl Acad Sci USA. 2009;106(31):13040–5.
80. Golland Y, Golland P, Bentin S, Malach R. Data-driven clustering reveals a fundamental subdivision of the human cortex into two global systems. Neuropsychologia. 2008;46(2):540–53.
81. Cordes D, Haughton V, Carew JD, Arfanakis K, Maravilla K. Hierarchical clustering to measure connectivity in fMRI resting-state data. Magn Reson Imaging. 2002;20(4):305–17.
82. Mezer A, Yovel Y, Pasternak O, Gorfine T, Assaf Y. Cluster analysis of resting-state fMRI time series. Neuroimage. 2009;45(4):1117–25.
83. Kim JH, Lee JM, Jo HJ, Kim SH, Lee JH, Kim ST, et al. Defining functional SMA and pre-SMA subregions in human MFC using resting state fMRI: functional connectivity-based parcellation method. Neuroimage. 2010;49(3):2375–86.
84. Klein JC, Behrens TE, Robson MD, Mackay CE, Higham DJ, Johansen-Berg H. Connectivity-based parcellation of human cortex using diffusion MRI: Establishing reproducibility, validity and observer independence in BA 44/45 and SMA/pre-SMA. Neuroimage. 2007;34(1):204–11.
85. Cohen AL, Fair DA, Dosenbach NU, Miezin FM, Dierker D, Van Essen DC, et al. Defining functional areas in individual human brains using resting functional connectivity MRI. Neuroimage. 2008; 41(1):45–57.
86. Golland P, Golland Y, Malach R. Detection of spatial activation patterns as unsupervised segmentation of fMRI data. Med Image Comput Comput Assist Interv. 2007;10(Pt 1):110–8.
87. Zhang D, Snyder AZ, Fox MD, Sansbury MW, Shimony JS, Raichle ME. Intrinsic functional relations between human cerebral cortex and thalamus. J Neurophysiol. 2008;100(4):1740–8.
88. Boccaletti S, Latora V, Moreno Y, Chavez M, Hwang D-U. Complex networks: structure and dynamics. Phys Rep. 2006;424(4–5):175–308.
89. Eguiluz VM, Hernandez-Garcia E, Piro O, Klemm K. Effective dimensions and percolation in hierarchically structured scale-free networks. Phys Rev E Stat Nonlin Soft Matter Phys. 2003;68(5 Pt 2):055102.
90. Newman ME. Modularity and community structure in networks. Proc Natl Acad Sci USA. 2006; 103(23):8577–82.

91. Watts DJ, Strogatz SH. Collective dynamics of 'small-world' networks. Nature. 1998;393(6684):440–2.
92. Shi J, Malik J. Normalized cuts and image segmentation. IEEE Trans Pattern Anal Mach Intell. 2000;22(8):888–905.
93. Newman ME. Finding community structure in networks using the eigenvectors of matrices. Phys Rev E Stat Nonlin Soft Matter Phys. 2006;74(3 Pt 2):036104.
94. Schwarz AJ, Gozzi A, Bifone A. Community structure and modularity in networks of correlated brain activity. Magn Reson Imaging. 2008;26(7):914–20.
95. Thirion B, Dodel S, Poline JB. Detection of signal synchronizations in resting-state fMRI datasets. Neuroimage. 2006;29(1):321–7.
96. van den Heuvel M, Mandl R, Hulshoff Pol H. Normalized cut group clustering of resting-state FMRI data. PLoS ONE. 2008;3(4):e2001.
97. Shen X, Papademetris X, Constable RT. Graph-theory based parcellation of functional subunits in the brain from resting-state fMRI data. Neuroimage. 2010;50(3):1027–35.
98. Golfinopoulos E, Tourville JA, Guenther FH. The integration of large-scale neural network modeling and functional brain imaging in speech motor control. Neuroimage. 2010;52(3):862–74.
99. Horwitz B, Glabus MF. Neural modeling and functional brain imaging: the interplay between the data-fitting and simulation approaches. Int Rev Neurobiol. 2005;66:267–90.
100. Husain FT, Tagamets MA, Fromm SJ, Braun AR, Horwitz B. Relating neuronal dynamics for auditory object processing to neuroimaging activity: a computational modeling and an fMRI study. Neuroimage. 2004;21(4):1701–20.
101. Deco G, Jirsa V, McIntosh AR, Sporns O, Kotter R. Key role of coupling, delay, and noise in resting brain fluctuations. Proc Natl Acad Sci USA. 2009;106(25):10302–7.
102. Honey CJ, Kotter R, Breakspear M, Sporns O. Network structure of cerebral cortex shapes functional connectivity on multiple time scales. Proc Natl Acad Sci USA. 2007;104(24):10240–5.
103. Rubinov M, Sporns O. Complex network measures of brain connectivity: uses and interpretations. Neuroimage. 2010;52(3):1059–69.
104. Achard S, Salvador R, Whitcher B, Suckling J, Bullmore E. A resilient, low-frequency, small-world human brain functional network with highly connected association cortical hubs. J Neurosci. 2006;26(1):63–72.
105. Buckner RL, Sepulcre J, Talukdar T, Krienen FM, Liu H, Hedden T, et al. Cortical hubs revealed by intrinsic functional connectivity: mapping, assessment of stability, and relation to Alzheimer's disease. J Neurosci. 2009;29(6):1860–73.
106. Sporns O, Honey CJ, Kotter R. Identification and classification of hubs in brain networks. PLoS One. 2007;2(10):e1049.
107. Bullmore E, Sporns O. Complex brain networks: graph theoretical analysis of structural and functional systems. Nat Rev Neurosci. 2009;10(3):186–98.
108. Constable RT, Hara Y, Tokoglu F, Papademetris X. Intrinsic connectivity contrast: a novel contrast mechanism for investigating a wide range of brain disorders. Proceedings of the ISMRM Annual Meeting 2009:4493.
109. Constable RT, Hara Y, Tokoglu F, Papademetris X. Intrinsic connectivity contrast: a voxel level summary of tissue connectivity. Proceedings of the OHBM Annual Meeting 2009:275-M.
110. Glabus MF, Horwitz B, Holt JL, Kohn PD, Gerton BK, Callicott JH, et al. Interindividual differences in functional interactions among prefrontal, parietal and parahippocampal regions during working memory. Cereb Cortex. 2003;13(12):1352–61.
111. Pezawas L, Meyer-Lindenberg A, Drabant EM, Verchinski BA, Munoz KE, Kolachana BS, et al. 5-HTTLPR polymorphism impacts human cingulate-amygdala interactions: a genetic susceptibility mechanism for depression. Nat Neurosci. 2005;8(6):828–34.
112. Horwitz B, Rumsey JM, Donohue BC. Functional connectivity of the angular gyrus in normal reading and dyslexia. Proc Natl Acad Sci USA. 1998;95:8939–44.
113. Andrews-Hanna JR, Snyder AZ, Vincent JL, Lustig C, Head D, Raichle ME, et al. Disruption of large-scale brain systems in advanced aging. Neuron. 2007;56(5):924–35.
114. Sambataro F, Murty VP, Callicott JH, Tan HY, Das S, Weinberger DR, et al. Age-related alterations in default mode network: impact on working memory performance. Neurobiol Aging. 2010;31(5):839–52.
115. Kennedy DP, Redcay E, Courchesne E. Failing to deactivate: resting functional abnormalities in autism. Proc Natl Acad Sci USA. 2006;103(21):8275–80.
116. Rombouts SA, Barkhof F, Goekoop R, Stam CJ, Scheltens P. Altered resting state networks in mild cognitive impairment and mild Alzheimer's disease: an fMRI study. Hum Brain Mapp. 2005;26(4):231–9.
117. Garrity AG, Godfrey DP, McKiernan K, Lloyd D, Kiehl KA, Calhoun VD. Aberrant "default mode" functional connectivity in schizophrenia. Am J Psychiatry. 2007;164:450–7.
118. Castellanos FX, Margulies DS, Kelly C, Uddin LQ, Ghaffari M, Kirsch A, et al. Cingulate-precuneus interactions: a new locus of dysfunction in adult attention-deficit/hyperactivity disorder. Biol Psychiatry. 2008;63(3):332–7.
119. Fransson P. Spontaneous low-frequency BOLD signal fluctuations: an fMRI investigation of the resting-state default mode of brain function hypothesis. Hum Brain Mapp. 2005;26:15–29.
120. Popa D, Popescu AT, Pare D. Contrasting activity profile of two distributed cortical networks as a function of attentional demands. J Neurosci. 2009;29(4):1191–201.

121. Kelly AMC, Uddin LQ, Biswal BB, Castellanos FX, Milham MP. Competition between functional brain networks mediates behavioral variability. Neuroimage. 2008;39:527–37.
122. Hampson M, Driesen NR, Roth JK, Gore JC, Constable RT. Functional connectivity between task-positive and task-negative brain areas and its relation to working memory performance. Magn Reson Imaging. 2010;28(8):1051–7.
123. Schmithorst VJ, Holland SK. Functional MRI evidence for disparate developmental processes underlying intelligence in boys and girls. Neuroimage. 2006;31(3):1366–79.
124. Schmithorst VJ, Holland SK, Plante E. Cognitive modules utilized for narrative comprehension in children: a functional magnetic resonance imaging study. Neuroimage. 2006;29(1):254–66.
125. Seeley WW, Menon V, Schatzberg AF, Keller J, Glover GH, Kenna H, et al. Dissociable intrinsic connectivity networks for salience processing and executive control. J Neurosci. 2007;27(9):2349–56.
126. He BJ, Snyder AZ, Vincent JL, Epstein A, Shulman GL, Corbetta M. Breakdown of functional connectivity in frontoparietal networks underlies behavioral deficits in spatial neglect. Neuron. 2007;53:905–18.
127. Horwitz B, Grady CL, Schlageter NL, Duara R, Rapoport SI. Intercorrelations of regional cerebral glucose metabolic rates in Alzheimer's disease. Brain Res. 1987;407:294–306.
128. Horwitz B, Rumsey JM, Grady CL, Rapoport SI. The cerebral metabolic landscape in autism. Intercorrelations of regional glucose utilization. Arch Neurol. 1988;45(7):749–55.
129. Horwitz B, Schapiro MB, Grady CL, Rapoport SI. Cerebral metabolic pattern in young adult Down's syndrome subjects: altered intercorrelations between regional rates of glucose utilization. J Ment Defic Res. 1990;34(3):237–52.
130. Horwitz B, Swedo SE, Grady CL, Pietrini P, Schapiro MB, Rapaport JL, et al. Cerebral metabolic pattern in obsessive–compulsive disorder: altered intercorrelations between regional rates of glucose utilization. Psychiatry Res Neuroimaging. 1991;40:221–37.
131. Metter EJ, Riege WH, Hanson WR, Phelps ME, Kuhl DE. Local cerebral metabolic rates of glucose in movement and language disorders from positron tomography. Am J Physiol. 1984;246(6 Pt 2): R897–900.
132. Metter EJ, Riege WH, Kameyama M, Kuhl DE, Phelps ME. Cerebral metabolic relationships for selected brain regions in Alzheimer's, Huntington's, and Parkinson's diseases. J Cereb Blood Flow Metab. 1984;4(4):500–6.
133. Volkow ND, Brodie JD, Wolf AP, Gomez-Mont F, Cancro R, Van Gelder P, et al. Brain organization in schizophrenia. J Cereb Blood Flow Metab. 1986; 6(4):441–6.
134. Mallet L, Mazoyer B, Martinot JL. Functional connectivity in depressive, obsessive–compulsive, and schizophrenic disorders: an explorative correlational analysis of regional cerebral metabolism. Psychiatry Res. 1998;82(2):83–93.
135. Just MA, Cherkassky VL, Keller TA, Minshew NJ. Cortical activation and synchronization during sentence comprehension in high-functioning autism: evidence of underconnectivity. Brain. 2004;127 (Pt 8):1811–21.
136. Castelli F, Frith C, Happe F, Frith U. Autism, Asperger syndrome and brain mechanisms for the attribution of mental states to animated shapes. Brain. 2002;125(Pt 8):1839–49.
137. Just MA, Cherkassky VL, Keller TA, Kana RK, Minshew NJ. Functional and anatomical cortical underconnectivity in autism: evidence from an FMRI study of an executive function task and corpus callosum morphometry. Cereb Cortex. 2007;17(4):951–61.
138. Lee PS, Yerys BE, Della Rosa A, Foss-Feig J, Barnes KA, James JD, et al. Functional connectivity of the inferior frontal cortex changes with age in children with autism spectrum disorders: a fcMRI study of response inhibition. Cereb Cortex. 2009;19(8):1787–94.
139. Solomon M, Ozonoff SJ, Ursu S, Ravizza S, Cummings N, Ly S, et al. The neural substrates of cognitive control deficits in autism spectrum disorders. Neuropsychologia. 2009;47(12):2515–26.
140. Kana RK, Keller TA, Minshew NJ, Just MA. Inhibitory control in high-functioning autism: decreased activation and underconnectivity in inhibition networks. Biol Psychiatry. 2007;62(3):198–206.
141. Koshino H, Carpenter PA, Minshew NJ, Cherkassky VL, Keller TA, Just MA. Functional connectivity in an fMRI working memory task in high-functioning autism. Neuroimage. 2005;24(3):810–21.
142. Koshino H, Kana RK, Keller TA, Cherkassky VL, Minshew NJ, Just MA. fMRI investigation of working memory for faces in autism: visual coding and underconnectivity with frontal areas. Cereb Cortex. 2008;18(2):289–300.
143. Kana RK, Keller TA, Cherkassky VL, Minshew NJ, Just MA. Sentence comprehension in autism: thinking in pictures with decreased functional connectivity. Brain. 2006;129(Pt 9):2484–93.
144. Villalobos ME, Mizuno A, Dahl BC, Kemmotsu N, Muller RA. Reduced functional connectivity between V1 and inferior frontal cortex associated with visuomotor performance in autism. Neuroimage. 2005; 25(3):916–25.
145. Turner KC, Frost L, Linsenbardt D, McIlroy JR, Muller RA. Atypically diffuse functional connectivity between caudate nuclei and cerebral cortex in autism. Behav Brain Funct. 2006;2:34.
146. Mizuno A, Villalobos ME, Davies MM, Dahl BC, Muller RA. Partially enhanced thalamocortical functional connectivity in autism. Brain Res. 2006; 1104(1):160–74.
147. Mason RA, Williams DL, Kana RK, Minshew N, Just MA. Theory of Mind disruption and recruitment of the right hemisphere during narrative comprehension in autism. Neuropsychologia. 2008;46(1): 269–80.

148. Noonan SK, Haist F, Muller RA. Aberrant functional connectivity in autism: evidence from low-frequency BOLD signal fluctuations. Brain Res. 2009;1262: 48–63.
149. Kleinhans NM, Richards T, Sterling L, Stegbauer KC, Mahurin R, Johnson LC, et al. Abnormal functional connectivity in autism spectrum disorders during face processing. Brain. 2008;131(Pt 4):1000–12.
150. Welchew DE, Ashwin C, Berkouk K, Salvador R, Suckling J, Baron-Cohen S, et al. Functional disconnectivity of the medial temporal lobe in Asperger's syndrome. Biol Psychiatry. 2005;57(9):991–8.
151. Cherkassky VL, Kana RK, Keller TA, Just MA. Functional connectivity in a baseline resting-state network in autism. Neuroreport. 2006;17:1687–90.
152. Kennedy DP, Courchesne E. The intrinsic functional organization of the brain is altered in autism. Neuroimage. 2008;39(4):1877–85.
153. Monk CS, Peltier SJ, Wiggins JL, Weng SJ, Carrasco M, Risi S, et al. Abnormalities of intrinsic functional connectivity in autism spectrum disorders. Neuroimage. 2009;47(2):764–72.
154. Friston KJ, Frith CD. Schizophrenia: a disconnection syndrome? Clin Neurosci. 1995;3(2):89–97.
155. Hoffman RE, McGlashan TH. Parallel distributed processing and the emergence of schizophrenic symptoms. Schizophr Bull. 1993;19(1):119–40.
156. Weinberger DR, Aloia MS, Goldberg TE, Berman KF. The frontal lobes and schizophrenia. J Neuropsychiatry Clin Neurosci. 1994;6(4):419–27.
157. Fletcher P, McKenna PJ, Friston KJ, Frith CD, Dolan RJ. Abnormal cingulate modulation of fronto-temporal connectivity in schizophrenia. Neuroimage. 1999;9(3):337–42.
158. Weinberger DR, Lipska BK. Cortical maldevelopment, anti-psychotic drugs, and schizophrenia: a search for common ground. Schizophr Res. 1995;16(2):87–110.
159. Vercammen A, Knegtering H, den Boer JA, Liemburg EJ, Aleman A. Auditory hallucinations in schizophrenia are associated with reduced functional connectivity of the temporo-parietal area. Biol Psychiatry. 2010;67(10):912–8.
160. Crossley NA, Mechelli A, Fusar-Poli P, Broome MR, Matthiasson P, Johns LC, et al. Superior temporal lobe dysfunction and frontotemporal dysconnectivity in subjects at risk of psychosis and in first-episode psychosis. Hum Brain Mapp. 2009;30(12):4129–37.
161. Jeong B, Wible CG, Hashimoto R, Kubicki M. Functional and anatomical connectivity abnormalities in left inferior frontal gyrus in schizophrenia. Hum Brain Mapp. 2009;30(12):4138–51.
162. Lawrie SM, Buechel C, Whalley HC, Frith CD, Friston KJ, Johnstone EC. Reduced frontotemporal functional connectivity in schizophrenia associated with auditory hallucinations. Biol Psychiatry. 2002;51(12):1008–11.
163. Andreasen NC, O'Leary DS, Cizadlo T, Arndt S, Rezai K, Ponto LL, et al. Schizophrenia and cognitive dysmetria: a positron-emission tomography study of dysfunctional prefrontal–thalamic–cerebellar circuitry. Proc Natl Acad Sci USA. 1996; 93(18):9985–90.
164. Honey GD, Pomarol-Clotet E, Corlett PR, Honey RA, McKenna PJ, Bullmore ET, et al. Functional dysconnectivity in schizophrenia associated with attentional modulation of motor function. Brain. 2005;128(Pt 11):2597–611.
165. Shen H, Wang L, Liu Y, Hu D. Discriminative analysis of resting-state functional connectivity patterns of schizophrenia using low dimensional embedding of fMRI. Neuroimage. 2010;49(4):3110–21.
166. Benetti S, Mechelli A, Picchioni M, Broome M, Williams S, McGuire P. Functional integration between the posterior hippocampus and prefrontal cortex is impaired in both first episode schizophrenia and the at risk mental state. Brain. 2009;132(Pt 9): 2426–36.
167. Henseler I, Falkai P, Gruber O. A systematic fMRI investigation of the brain systems subserving different working memory components in schizophrenia. Eur J Neurosci. 2009;30(4):693–702.
168. Friedel E, Schlagenhauf F, Sterzer P, Park SQ, Bermpohl F, Strohle A, et al. 5-HTT genotype effect on prefrontal-amygdala coupling differs between major depression and controls. Psychopharmacology (Berl). 2009;205(2):261–71.
169. Gavrilescu M, Rossell S, Stuart GW, Shea TL, Innes-Brown H, Henshall K, et al. Reduced connectivity of the auditory cortex in patients with auditory hallucinations: a resting state functional magnetic resonance imaging study. Psychol Med. 2010;40(7):1149–58.
170. Hoptman MJ, D'Angelo D, Catalano D, Mauro CJ, Shehzad ZE, Kelly AM, et al. Amygdalofrontal functional disconnectivity and aggression in schizophrenia. Schizophr Bull. 2010;36(5):1020–8.
171. Bluhm RL, Miller J, Lanius RA, Osuch EA, Boksman K, Neufeld RW, et al. Retrosplenial cortex connectivity in schizophrenia. Psychiatry Res. 2009;174(1): 17–23.
172. Bluhm RL, Miller J, Lanius RA, Osuch EA, Boksman K, Neufeld RWJ, et al. Spontaneous low-frequency fluctuations in BOLD signal in schizophrenic patients: anomalies in the default network. Schizophr Bull. 2007;33(4):1004–12.
173. Camchong J, Macdonald AW, III, Bell C, Mueller BA, Lim KO, Altered functional and anatomical connectivity in schizophrenia. Schizophr Bull. 2011;37(3):640–50.
174. Mannell MV, Franco AR, Calhoun VD, Canive JM, Thoma RJ, Mayer AR. Resting state and task-induced deactivation: a methodological comparison in patients with schizophrenia and healthy controls. Hum Brain Mapp. 2010;31(3):424–37.
175. Whitfield-Gabrieli S, Thermenos HW, Milanovic S, Tsuang MT, Faraone SV, McCarley RW, et al. Hyperactivity and hyperconnectivity of the default network in schizophrenia and in first-degree relatives of persons with schizophrenia. Proc Natl Acad Sci USA. 2009;106(4):1279–84.

176. Zhou Y, Liang M, Tian L, Wang K, Hao Y, Liu H, et al. Functional disintegration in paranoid schizophrenia using resting-state fMRI. Schizophr Res. 2007;97:194–205.
177. Meda SA, Stevens MC, Folley BS, Calhoun VD, Pearlson GD. Evidence for anomalous network connectivity during working memory encoding in schizophrenia: an ICA based analysis. PLoS ONE. 2009;4(11):e7911.
178. Sambataro F, Blasi G, Fazio L, Caforio G, Taurisano P, Romano R, et al. Treatment with olanzapine is associated with modulation of the default mode network in patients with schizophrenia. Neuropsychopharmacology. 2010;35(4):904–12.
179. Wolf RC, Vasic N, Sambataro F, Hose A, Frasch K, Schmid M, et al. Temporally anticorrelated brain networks during working memory performance reveal aberrant prefrontal and hippocampal connectivity in patients with schizophrenia. Prog Neuropsychopharmacol Biol Psychiatry. 2009;33(8):1464–73.
180. Greicius M. Resting-state functional connectivity in neuropsychiatric disorders. Curr Opin Neurol. 2008;21(4):424–30.
181. Etkin A, Prater KE, Schatzberg AF, Menon V, Greicius MD. Disrupted amygdalar subregion functional connectivity and evidence of a compensatory network in generalized anxiety disorder. Arch Gen Psychiatry. 2009;66(12):1361–72.
182. Goldin PR, Manber-Ball T, Werner K, Heimberg R, Gross JJ. Neural mechanisms of cognitive reappraisal of negative self-beliefs in social anxiety disorder. Biol Psychiatry. 2009;66(12):1091–9.
183. Guyer AE, Lau JY, McClure-Tone EB, Parrish J, Shiffrin ND, Reynolds RC, et al. Amygdala and ventrolateral prefrontal cortex function during anticipated peer evaluation in pediatric social anxiety. Arch Gen Psychiatry. 2008;65(11):1303–12.
184. Monk CS, Telzer EH, Mogg K, Bradley BP, Mai X, Louro HM, et al. Amygdala and ventrolateral prefrontal cortex activation to masked angry faces in children and adolescents with generalized anxiety disorder. Arch Gen Psychiatry. 2008;65(5):568–76.
185. Rich BA, Fromm SJ, Berghorst LH, Dickstein DP, Brotman MA, Pine DS, et al. Neural connectivity in children with bipolar disorder: impairment in the face emotion processing circuit. J Child Psychol Psychiatry. 2008;49(1):88–96.
186. Wang F, Kalmar JH, He Y, Jackowski M, Chepenik LG, Edmiston EE, et al. Functional and structural connectivity between the perigenual anterior cingulate and amygdala in bipolar disorder. Biol Psychiatry. 2009;66(5):516–21.
187. Anand A, Li Y, Wang Y, Lowe MJ, Dzemidzic M. Resting state corticolimbic connectivity abnormalities in unmedicated bipolar disorder and unipolar depression. Psychiatry Res. 2009;171(3):189–98.
188. Dannlowski U, Ohrmann P, Konrad C, Domschke K, Bauer J, Kugel H, et al. Reduced amygdala-prefrontal coupling in major depression: association with MAOA genotype and illness severity. Int J Neuropsychopharmacol. 2009;12(1):11–22.
189. Hamilton JP, Gotlib IH. Neural substrates of increased memory sensitivity for negative stimuli in major depression. Biol Psychiatry. 2008;63(12):1155–62.
190. Irwin W, Anderle MJ, Abercrombie HC, Schaefer SM, Kalin NH, Davidson RJ. Amygdalar interhemispheric functional connectivity differs between the non-depressed and depressed human brain. Neuroimage. 2004;21(2):674–86.
191. Anand A, Li Y, Wang Y, Gardner K, Lowe MJ. Reciprocal effects of antidepressant treatment on activity and connectivity of the mood regulating circuit: an FMRI study. J Neuropsychiatry Clin Neurosci. 2007;19(3):274–82.
192. Anand A, Li Y, Wang Y, Wu J, Gao S, Bukari L, et al. Activity and connectivity of brain mood regulating circuit in depression: a functional magnetic resonance study. Biol Psychiatry. 2005;57:1079–88.
193. Anand A, Li Y, Wang Y, Wu J, Gao S, Bukhari L, et al. Antidepressant effect on connectivity of the mood-regulating circuit: an fMRI study. Neuropsychopharmacology. 2005;30:1334–44.
194. Cullen KR, Gee DG, Klimes-Dougan B, Gabbay V, Hulvershorn L, Mueller BA, et al. A preliminary study of functional connectivity in comorbid adolescent depression. Neurosci Lett. 2009;460(3):227–31.
195. Greicius MD, Flores BH, Menon V, Glover GH, Solvason HB, Kenna H, et al. Resting-state functional connectivity in major depression: abnormally increased contributions from subjenual cingulate cortex and thalamus. Biol Psychiatry. 2007;62(5):429–37. epub ahead of print.
196. Bluhm R, Williamson P, Lanius R, Theberge J, Densmore M, Bartha R, et al. Resting state default-mode network connectivity in early depression using a seed region-of-interest analysis: decreased connectivity with caudate nucleus. Psychiatry Clin Neurosci. 2009;63(6):754–61.
197. Vasic N, Walter H, Sambataro F, Wolf RC. Aberrant functional connectivity of dorsolateral prefrontal and cingulate networks in patients with major depression during working memory processing. Psychol Med. 2009;39(6):977–87.
198. Zhou Y, Yu C, Zheng H, Liu Y, Song M, Qin W, et al. Increased neural resources recruitment in the intrinsic organization in major depression. J Affect Disord. 2010;121(3):220–30.
199. Lanius RA, Williamson PC, Bluhm RL, Densmore M, Boksman K, Neufeld RW, et al. Functional connectivity of dissociative responses in posttraumatic stress disorder: a functional magnetic resonance imaging investigation. Biol Psychiatry. 2005;57(8):873–84.
200. Lanius RA, Williamson PC, Densmore M, Boksman K, Neufeld RW, Gati JS, et al. The nature of traumatic memories: a 4-T FMRI functional connectivity analysis. Am J Psychiatry. 2004;161(1):36–44.

201. Simmons AN, Paulus MP, Thorp SR, Matthews SC, Norman SB, Stein MB. Functional activation and neural networks in women with posttraumatic stress disorder related to intimate partner violence. Biol Psychiatry. 2008;64(8):681–90.
202. Bluhm RL, Williamson PC, Osuch EA, Frewen PA, Stevens TK, Boksman K, et al. Alterations in default network connectivity in posttraumatic stress disorder related to early-life trauma. J Psychiatry Neurosci. 2009;34(3):187–94.
203. Lanius RA, Bluhm RL, Coupland NJ, Hegadoren KM, Rowe B, Theberge J, et al. Default mode network connectivity as a predictor of post-traumatic stress disorder symptom severity in acutely traumatized subjects. Acta Psychiatr Scand. 2010;121(1):33–40.
204. Achard S, Salvador R, Whitcher B, Suckling J, Bullmore E. A resilient, low-frequency, small-world human brain functional network with highly connected association cortical hubs. J Neurosci. 2006;26(1):63–72.
205. Bai F, Watson DR, Yu H, Shi Y, Yuan Y, Zhang Z. Abnormal resting-state functional connectivity of posterior cingulate cortex in amnestic type mild cognitive impairment. Brain Res. 2009;1302:167–74.
206. Buckner RL, Snyder AZ, Shannon BJ, LaRossa G, Sachs R, Fotenos AF, et al. Molecular, structural, and functional characterization of Alzheimer's disease: evidence for a relationship between default activity, amyloid, and memory. J Neurosci. 2005;25(34):7709–17.
207. Hedden T, Van Dijk KR, Becker JA, Mehta A, Sperling RA, Johnson KA, et al. Disruption of functional connectivity in clinically normal older adults harboring amyloid burden. J Neurosci. 2009;29(40):12686–94.
208. Sheline YI, Raichle ME, Snyder AZ, Morris JC, Head D, Wang S, et al. Amyloid plaques disrupt resting state default mode network connectivity in cognitively normal elderly. Biol Psychiatry. 2010;67(6):584–7.
209. Allen G, Barnard H, McColl R, Hester AL, Fields JA, Weiner MF, et al. Reduced hippocampal functional connectivity in Alzheimer disease. Arch Neurol. 2007;64(10):1482–7.
210. Wang L, Zang Y, He Y, Liang M, Zhang X, Tian L, et al. Changes in hippocampal connectivity in the early stages of Alzheimer's disease: evidence from resting state fMRI. Neuroimage. 2006;31(2):496–504.
211. Lowe MJ, Phillips MD, Lurito JT, Mattson D, Dzemidzic M, Mathews VP. Multiple sclerosis: low-frequency temporal blood oxygen level-dependent fluctuations indicate reduced functional connectivity – initial results. Radiology. 2002;224(1):184–92.
212. Au Duong MV, Audoin B, Boulanouar K, Ibarrola D, Malikova I, Confort-Gouny S, et al. Altered functional connectivity related to white matter changes inside the working memory network at the very early stage of MS. J Cereb Blood Flow Metab. 2005;25(10):1245–53.
213. Hong LE, Gu H, Yang Y, Ross TJ, Salmeron BJ, Buchholz B, et al. Association of nicotine addiction and nicotine's actions with separate cingulate cortex functional circuits. Arch Gen Psychiatry. 2009;66(4):431–41.
214. Liu J, Liang J, Qin W, Tian J, Yuan K, Bai L, et al. Dysfunctional connectivity patterns in chronic heroin users: an fMRI study. Neurosci Lett. 2009;460(1):72–7.
215. Ma N, Liu Y, Li N, Wang CX, Zhang H, Jiang XF, et al. Addiction related alteration in resting-state brain connectivity. Neuroimage. 2010;49(1):738–44.
216. Zhang X, Chen X, Yu Y, Sun D, Ma N, He S, et al. Masked smoking-related images modulate brain activity in smokers. Hum Brain Mapp. 2009;30(3):896–907.
217. Harrison BJ, Soriano-Mas C, Pujol J, Ortiz H, Lopez-Sola M, Hernandez-Ribas R, et al. Altered corticostriatal functional connectivity in obsessive–compulsive disorder. Arch Gen Psychiatry. 2009;66(11):1189–200.
218. Church JA, Fair DA, Dosenbach NU, Cohen AL, Miezin FM, Petersen SE, et al. Control networks in paediatric Tourette syndrome show immature and anomalous patterns of functional connectivity. Brain. 2009;132(Pt 1):225–38.
219. Gozzo Y, Vohr B, Lacadie C, Hampson M, Katz KH, Maller-Kesselman J, et al. Alterations in neural connectivity in preterm children at school age. Neuroimage. 2009;48(2):458–63.
220. Schafer RJ, Lacadie C, Vohr B, Kesler SR, Katz KH, Schneider KC, et al. Alterations in functional connectivity for language in prematurely born adolescents. Brain. 2009;132(Pt 3):661–70.
221. Addis DR, Moscovitch M, McAndrews MP. Consequences of hippocampal damage across the autobiographical memory network in left temporal lobe epilepsy. Brain. 2007;130(Pt 9):2327–42.
222. Liao W, Zhang Z, Pan Z, Mantini D, Ding J, Duan X, et al. Altered functional connectivity and small-world in mesial temporal lobe epilepsy. PLoS One. 2010;5(1):e8525.
223. Morgan VL, Gore JC, Abou-Khalil B. Functional epileptic network in left mesial temporal lobe epilepsy detected using resting fMRI. Epilepsy Res. 2010;88(2–3):168–78.
224. Waites AB, Briellmann RS, Saling MM, Abbott DF, Jackson GD. Functional connectivity networks are disrupted in left temporal lobe epilepsy. Ann Neurol. 2006;59(2):335–43.
225. Tian L, Jiang T, Wang Y, Zang Y, He Y, Liang M, et al. Altered resting-state functional connectivity patterns of anterior cingulate cortex in adolescents with attention deficit hyperactivity disorder. Neurosci Lett. 2006;400:39–43.
226. He BJ, Snyder AZ, Zempel JM, Smyth MD, Raichle ME. Electrophysiological correlates of the brain's intrinsic large-scale functional architecture. Proc Natl Acad Sci USA. 2008;105(41):16039–44.

227. Mantini D, Perrucci MG, Del Gratta C, Romani GL, Corbetta M. Electrophysiological signatures of resting state networks in the human brain. Proc Natl Acad Sci USA. 2007;104(32):13170–5.
228. Leopold DA, Murayama Y, Logothetis NK. Very slow activity fluctuations in monkey visual cortex: implications for functional brain imaging. Cereb Cortex. 2003;13(4):422–33.
229. Cader S, Cifelli A, Abu-Omar Y, Palace J, Matthews PM. Reduced brain functional reserve and altered functional connectivity in patients with multiple sclerosis. Brain. 2006;129(Pt 2):527–37.
230. Rubia K, Halari R, Cubillo A, Mohammad AM, Brammer M, Taylor E. Methylphenidate normalises activation and functional connectivity deficits in attention and motivation networks in medication-naive children with ADHD during a rewarded continuous performance task. Neuropharmacology. 2009;57(7–8):640–52.
231. Wink AM, Bernard F, Salvador R, Bullmore E, Suckling J. Age and cholinergic effects on hemodynamics and functional coherence of human hippocampus. Neurobiol Aging. 2006;27:1395–404.
232. Martuzzi R, Ramani R, Qiu M, Rajeevan N, Constable RT. Functional connectivity and alterations in baseline brain state in humans. Neuroimage. 2010;49(1):823–34.
233. Biswal BB, Mennes M, Zuo XN, Gohel S, Kelly C, Smith SM, et al. Toward discovery science of human brain function. Proc Natl Acad Sci USA. 2010; 107(10):4734–9.

7 Clinical Challenges of Functional MRI

Nader Pouratian and Susan Y. Bookheimer

Introduction

Functional magnetic resonance imaging (fMRI) has revolutionized clinical brain mapping by allowing relatively rapid and noninvasive assessment of brain activity. Because of its relative ease, it has become the predominant functional neuroimaging technique since its original report by Belliveau et al. [1]. The appeal of fMRI is attributable to several advantages that it offers over other functional neuroimaging techniques. Perhaps the most important advantages, especially in clinical populations, relate to the safety of fMRI: it is noninvasive, in contrast to either the Wada test or electrical stimulation mapping, and does not require exposure to ionizing radiation (as with positron emission tomography [PET]). The other major advantage of fMRI is that it offers the opportunity for reliable, repeated measurements of the same task to investigate response consistency, to compare activations across tasks, and to measure change over time. Above all, fMRI is sufficiently powerful to produce maps of cognitive and motor functions that are reliable and valid at the single-subject level. This has made possible the transition of fMRI from a research tool into a practical, approved, and reimbursable clinical procedure.

Despite its advantages, fMRI presents several unique challenges, especially in the clinical setting. One of these challenges arises from the fact that fMRI does not directly measure neuronal activity. Instead, fMRI detects coupled perfusion-related signals that serve as a proxy for neuronal activity. Functional MRI analysis typically makes assumptions about the characteristics of neurovascular coupling and, therefore, the significance of fMRI activations; these assumptions are more suspect in a clinical setting when pathology may alter normal coupling mechanisms.

Clinical fMRI is also complicated by factors not normally encountered in a healthy population (Tables 7.1 and 7.2).

For example, the presence of intracerebral pathologies (e.g., arteriovenous malformations [AVMs]) can induce field inhomogeneities and may also alter neurovascular coupling mechanisms, both of which may hamper measurement of reliable hemodynamic-based fMRI signals. Surgical clips from prior procedures can create patches of signal loss, and often these are in the very regions in which mapping is needed.

Other important challenges of clinical fMRI include the ability of patients to comply with imaging protocols and perform cognitive tasks. For example, imaging in clinical populations is

N. Pouratian, MD, PhD (✉)
Department of Neurosurgery, University of California, 10945 Le Conte Avenue, Suite 2120, Los Angeles, CA 90095, USA
e-mail: npouratian@mednet.ucla.edu

S.Y. Bookheimer, PhD
Department of Psychiatry and Biobehavioral Sciences, David Geffen School of Medicine at UCLA, 760 Westwood Plaza, Suite 17-369, Los Angeles, CA 90095, USA
e-mail: Sbook@ucla.edu

S.H. Faro and F.B. Mohamed (eds.), *Functional BOLD MRI: Principles and Applications*,
DOI 10.1007/978-1-4939-1995-6_7,

Table 7.1 Potential limitations of fMRI in clinical populations

Field inhomogeneities in ROI
Movement artifacts
Altered baseline intelligence
Impaired task compliance
Impaired motivation
Sensitivity to certain stimuli (e.g., flickering lights)

often associated with increased head movement; in one study [2] nearly 30% of subjects with intracranial masses were excluded from the final analysis due to gross motion artifact. This is a particularly difficult problem if one wishes to study patients with movement disorders such as Parkinson's and Tourette's. Impairments in cognition may also alter patients' abilities to com-

Table 7.2 Summary of key literature

Authors	Article title	Summary
Ojemann 1989 [17]	Cortical language localization in left, dominant hemisphere. An electrical stimulation mapping investigation in 117 patients. J Neurosurg 1989; 71:316–326	Substantial individual variability in the exact location of language function among the patients showed that language cannot be reliably localized on anatomic criteria alone
Stark and Squire 2001 [37]	When zero is not zero: The problem of ambiguous baseline conditions in fMRI. Proc Natl Acad Sci USA 2001; 98:12760–12765	Periods of rest are associated with significant cognitive activity and, therefore, provide a nonoptimal baseline for memory tasks. The findings have important implications for the design and interpretation of a wide range of fMRI studies of cognition
Greicius 2003 [40]	Functional connectivity in the resting brain: a network analysis of the default mode hypothesis. Proc Natl Acad Sci USA. 2003 Jan 7;100(1):253–8	Functional imaging studies have shown that certain brain regions, including posterior cingulate cortex (PCC) and ventral anterior cingulate cortex (vACC), consistently show greater activity during resting states than during cognitive tasks. This finding led to the hypothesis that these regions constitute a network supporting a default mode of brain function
Gaillard 2004 [54]	fMRI language task panel improves determination of language dominance. Neurology. 2004 Oct 26;63(8):1403–8	A panel of fMRI language paradigms may be more accurate for evaluating partial epilepsy patients than a single task
Ruff et al. 2008 [53]	Assessment of the language laterality index in patients with brain tumor using functional MR imaging: effects of thresholding, task selection, and prior surgery. AJNR Am J Neuroradiol. 2008 Mar; 29(3):528–35. Epub 2008 Jan 9	The study sought to determine whether changing the statistical threshold for different language tasks influences the language laterality index (LI) for a group of controls, patients with tumor without prior surgery, and patients with tumor and prior surgery. The resulting data suggest that the LI may be threshold- and task-dependent
Binder et al. 1980 [57]	A comparison of five fMRI protocols for mapping speech comprehension systems. Epilepsia 2008 Dec;49(12):1980–97	Brain regions involved in semantic processing were identified only when an active, nonlinguistic task was used as a baseline, supporting the notion that semantic processing occurs whenever attentional resources are not controlled. Identification of these lexical–semantic regions is particularly important for predicting language outcome in patients undergoing temporal lobe surgery
Sanai et al. 2008 [86]	Mapping the horizon: techniques to optimize tumor resection before and during surgery. Clin Neurosurg. 2008;55:14–9	The article reviews current and future imaging modalities as well as state of the art intraoperative techniques that can facilitate extent of tumor resection while minimizing the associated neurological morbidity profile
Giussani et al. 2010 [72]	DTI fiber tracking to differentiate demyelinating diseases from diffuse brain stem glioma. Neuroimage. 2010 Aug 1;52(1):217–23	Diffuse brainstem tumors and demyelinating diseases can share common clinical and radiological features, sometimes making diagnosis difficult. DTI fiber tracking of the pyramid tracts in patients with suspected intrinsic brainstem tumor or demyelinating disease presents two clearly different patterns that may help in differentiating between these two pathologies when conventional MRI and clinical data are inconclusive

plete tasks, both with respect to motivation and task difficulty (i.e., the presumed difficulty of a task may be different in various populations due to differences in baseline skills).

Finally, clinical brain mapping emphasizes results for the individual rather than for a group, impacting strongly on the choice of analysis methods. Moreover, altered anatomy due to intracerebral lesions may prohibit spatial registration and normalization tools commonly used in group statistics, making it difficult to directly compare results from patients with those from a normative sample [3].

This chapter will elaborate on some of the most salient points, including study and task design, data analysis, and reproducibility, in applying fMRI to clinical planning. Although there are a large number of clinical fMRI studies being published, few have tackled these challenges fully. Ultimately, our ability to derive clinical benefit from functional MRI will depend upon finding appropriate solutions to these challenges.

Mapping Cognitive Function with Activation Versus Disruption

Until the advent of fMRI and other perfusion-based brain mapping techniques, our understanding of the functional organization of the brain largely stemmed from studying the effects of brain lesions. Although brain lesions were limited to strokes and other "accidents of nature" initially, Penfield recognized in 1937 that temporary brain lesions could also be induced to study brain function by applying electrical stimulations directly on the cortex [4]. More recently, transcranial magnetic stimulation has been introduced as a means of inducing temporary lesions noninvasively [5]. By mapping the effects of lesions, these disruption-based techniques identify parts of the brain that are essential and critical for executing a given task; in essence, those regions which, when disrupted, result in catastrophic loss of function for which other brain regions cannot compensate. These disruption-based techniques of mapping the brain have emerged as the gold standard of clinical brain mapping, especially in the neurosurgical arena.

Functional MRI differs fundamentally from the classic lesion-based approach to clinical brain mapping in that instead of only identifying areas of the brain that are essential for performing a task, fMRI indicates all brain areas that demonstrate activity-related changes during a given task, regardless of whether a given brain area is in fact critical for task performance (i.e., both "essential" and supplemental cortical areas). Because of this fundamental difference in methodology, fMRI maps and lesion maps will inevitably differ. Both maps are probably clinically relevant, but one must be aware of the different data produced, their implications, and the types of conclusions that can be drawn from each.

As discussed in earlier chapters, fMRI offers an indirect measure of brain function: instead of directly measuring neuronal activity, fMRI maps the brain by detecting functional hemodynamic responses that are coupled to neuronal activity. To establish clinical validity of the instrument assumes both that MRI signal changes reflect underlying neural activity, and, assuming we accept this relationship, that a particular patient has a normal fMRI response (e.g., the blood flow response is unaffected by their clinical condition). This complexity can be illustrated by conceptualizing brain mapping as a series of mathematical functions (adapted from Villringer and Dirnagl [6]) (Fig. 7.1).

Given a stimulus x, there is a given neuronal response $f(x)$, which represents the "true" brain map. The neuronal response is coupled to a functional hemodynamic response by a neurovascular coupling function, p. The uncertainty of this neurovascular coupling function introduces one of the biggest challenges and one of the most significant sources of error in interpreting clinical fMRI studies. What ultimately matters about the neurovascular relationship is the degree and precision of spatial coupling between neuronal activities. As discussed later, the spatial coupling between fMRI activation signals and electrophysiologically active cortex may not be as precise as most would like it to be.

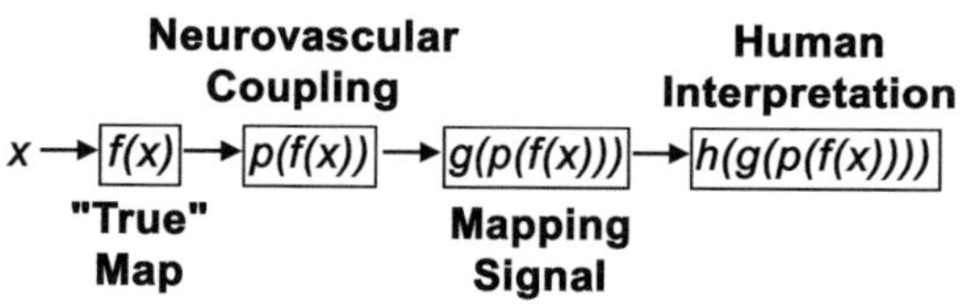

Fig. 7.1 Cascade of functional brain mapping functions. The mapping signal observed and reported is actually not a "true" map of neuronal activity. Rather, it is a product of a series of complex functions, including, for example, the coupling of neuronal activity and local cerebral perfusion, or neurovascular coupling (*p*). In order to better understand how functional brain maps relate to underlying "true" maps, it is critical to characterize the robustness of neurovascular coupling under different stimulus conditions, in different cortices, and in the presence of different pathologies

Several studies indicate that hemodynamic responses can be significantly different across brain regions, especially when adjacent to major pathology. In a study of 98 patients, Krings and colleagues showed that the distance of a central mass from the motor region significantly influenced the magnitude of activation, even in patients without paresis [7]. Other studies have found similar suppression of the hemodynamic response adjacent to pathology [8, 9]. Conversely, in a study of 14 patients, Schlosser and colleagues suggest that fMRI activation patterns in patients with frontal lobe tumors when mapped using a verbal fluency paradigm were comparable to signals in normal controls [10]. Similarly, Righini and colleagues studied 17 patients with frontoparietal masses and found little difference in motor activations between the affected and unaffected hemispheres [2]. The contradiction in these studies highlights the need to be aware of the possibility that adjacent pathologies may alter cerebral hemodynamics, but that this alteration is most likely pathology and location dependent and, possibly, task dependent. Finally, different physiological states (e.g., hypercapnia, hypoxia, and hypertension) and different disease states (e.g., vasculitis and angiopathies) can differentially impact the relationship between neuronal activity and functional perfusion [11, 12]. Schmitz and colleagues have shown, in a rodent model, that brief exposure to hypercapnia may potentiate the hemodynamic response without affecting the underlying electrophysiological response [13, 14]. In fact, highlighting the effect that hypercapnia may have on signals, in normal subjects, hypercapnia can be used in a normal subject as a means of contrast enhancement [15]. The age of the subject may also affect the magnitude of the hemodynamic response and the coupling mechanism itself [7]. Understanding the underlying coupling dynamics is essential to interpreting fMRI results. It is this uncertainty that continues to motivate continued investigation of neurovascular coupling dynamics.

Assuming neurovascular coupling is intact, several more functions are still applied before arriving at any conclusions from fMRI data. The functional perfusion response produces a brain mapping signal, g: $g(p(f(x)))$. The function g is determined not only by the physics behind fMRI signals sources (i.e., field strengths, scan sequences), but also by the recording capabilities of the particular scanner, including, but not limited to, resolution limitations, data filtering, and artifacts that may be introduced by different disease processes or medical interventions (e.g., coils, clips, AVMs, air cavities after neurosurgical resections).

Finally, yet another function is introduced into the formula, h, for the introduction of human study design, human interpretation, and statistics. Human interpretation of mapping signals, when not quantitative, is always susceptible to bias. The bias may be inadvertent and may be as subtle as in selecting an inappropriate control for comparison or measuring inappropriate signal parameters from which to draw conclusions. However, strict adherence to automated and quantitative analysis has its own problems. Base rates, for instance, can and should influence how we interpret findings. As an example, the incidence of right hemisphere language in a right-handed individual without a developmental disorder is extremely low – may be a few percent, based on studies of patients with strokes. An apparent finding of greater right than left hemisphere activation on language tasks in a patient with a space occupying lesion near the language cortex creates a dilemma: does one give greater weight to the actual data, or to the base rates? Simply reporting the data in this case is insufficient; one has to know and report the base rates, the degree of uncertainty, and recommendations for alternative approaches to verification (an invasive procedure). The statistics and thresholds commonly used in fMRI also introduce error and misinterpretations, presenting yet another challenge to clinical interpretation scans. Where does one set a threshold in a clinical study: strictly, as in typical research studies, or liberally, in order to avoid false negatives? What are the potential implications of making a false-positive versus a false-negative error? Simply showing the data may not convey the information necessary to allow surgeons to make an informed decision.

Although many studies compare "blobs" across groups, there are a number of assumptions that underlie those blobs. In order to better understand the underlying map, or $f(x)$, we must deconvolve this complex function by characterizing the factors that influence all of these functions. Alternatively, the investigator can pay special attention to study design and analysis in order to minimize assumptions and to strengthen their conclusions. Many of these issues of study design and analysis are discussed as follows.

Technical Considerations

Field Strength

Magnetic field strength is an important consideration in clinical fMRI study design. Increasing field strength provides a greater dynamic range of data collection and, ultimately, a greater signal-to-noise ratio (SNR) and contrast-to-noise ratio (CNR) (e.g., Kruger et al. 2001 [16]). This is discussed in detail in Chap. 4. While the greater SNR biases one toward higher field strength, they also pose problems which, in some brain regions or in some clinical conditions, may prove insurmountable. The most difficult complication arising from increased field strength is the associated increase in susceptibility artifact, especially near tissue interfaces. This is a particular problem in the inferior temporal lobes and the inferior medial frontal lobes, which are adjacent to the air-filled sinuses. These areas of susceptibility artifact produce both spatial distortion and MR signal loss, which make it difficult or impossible to identify activity-related changes in fMR images. This is of particular importance for language mapping, in which investigators expect to find several temporal lobe language areas (e.g., Ojemann et al. [17]). Lack of signal in these regions does not indicate lack of activity, but may be due to lack of sensitivity to identify appropriate signals. Devlin and colleagues have proposed alternate strategies when imaging these regions of high susceptibility but also acknowledge that these artifacts can only be partially overcome and that alternative data acquisition paradigms are necessary to address this issue [18]. Appropriate selection of scan sequence, in some cases, may help overcome some susceptibility artifacts, especially when imaging adjacent to pathology.

Scan Sequence and Susceptibility

The most commonly used fMRI pulse sequence is the gradient echo echo-planar (EPI) sequence. EPI is the fast scanning technique that acquires all slice locations with a single TR, and which has made fMRI practical [19] The gradient echo sequence is optimized to maximize susceptibility due to blood oxygenation-level dependent (BOLD) contrast. An unfortunate but necessary side effect is that it also maximizes unwanted susceptibility artifacts at tissue interfaces, especially at high field. In certain brain regions, particularly the amygdala, basal temporal region, and orbitofrontal cortex, the susceptibility artifacts may make imaging these regions impossible.

Clinical fMRI in patients who have had prior brain surgery may be complicated by the presence of implanted devices, such as plates and screws. While most of these devices are considered "magnet compatible," that is, they are not ferromagnetic and do not pose a safety concern, susceptibility artifacts can generate profound distortions around these objects, including massive signal loss and spatial distortion. It should also be noted that many of these devices have not been tested at high field and could pose a safety risk that does not exist at lower field strength. Typically, these objects will be implanted close to or on top of the precise regions the clinician would like to have mapped.

There is a wide variety of simple approaches to reducing susceptibility artifacts at air–tissue interfaces and around objects during functional imaging. Reducing voxel size is one. In the amygdala, for instance, Merboldt et al. [20] calculated that voxel sizes of 4–8 μL or less are necessary to recover sufficient signal. Fransson et al. [21] used a high resolution acquisition method to receiver signal in the hippocampus using coronal acquisitions and in-plane resolution of 2 mm^2 and slice thickness of 1 mm. For most centers, this approach is impractical, both to a lack of non-standard sequences on clinically oriented machines and because for many systems the associated reduction on field of view (FOV) is not acceptable. However, for patients with a focal lesion in which a small FOV is all that is necessary, small voxel studies may be appropriate. The loss of CNR within small voxels may also prohibit the practical use of this approach.

To some extent, use of alternative pulse sequences can improve, but not wholly overcome, these artifacts. Port et al. [22] performed a series of imaging studies on titanium screws embedded in gel to determine parameters that would decrease susceptibility artifacts in EP images. They reported three factors that can reduce artifacts: reducing the TE, increasing the frequency matrix, and reducing slice thickness. The latter two approaches are identical to those reported by Merboldt and colleagues [20] for imaging at air–tissue boundaries. However, the effects of reducing TE on susceptibility are controversial. Susceptibility artifacts due to signal loss at air–tissue interfaces are greater with longer TEs. Gorno-Tempini et al. [23] used a double echo EPI sequence to compare susceptibility artifacts and BOLD signal changes at tissue interfaces, comparing TEs of 27 and 40 ms. They used a face-processing task, which is known to activate the fusiform gyrus in the base of the temporal lobe, an area likely to suffer from susceptibility-induced signal loss. While the lower TE did not change their ability to detect BOLD signals in those regions unaffected by susceptibility artifacts, the lower TE was not sufficient to recover the BOLD signal in the problem areas. Spiral in–out sequences have also shown benefits in reducing artifacts in fMRI [24].

Various pulse sequences have differential effects on susceptibility artifacts. One alternative to the commonly used gradient echo EPI scan is the asymmetric spin echo. Both spin echo and gradient echo sequences base their signals on magnetic susceptibility contrast as described previously. The spin-echo sequence, however, refocuses the spin dephasing caused by field inhomogeneity. The consequence is that a spin echo sequence reduces susceptibility artifacts at air–tissue boundaries, but will also result in CNR loss due to reduced BOLD contrast. At high field, this loss may be an acceptable trade-off. Spin-echo sequences tend to recover signal from larger, rather than smaller boundaries and, thus, have been thought to affect unwanted susceptibility artifacts preferentially, including effects in larger blood vessels, while preserving signal changes in the capillaries. The *asymmetric* spin echo sequence shifts the time differential between the image acquisition and readout, allowing the signal to decay; thus, the amount of reversible dephasing that occurs can be varied by adjusting the length of this shift. The longer the asymmetry, the more the spin echo images resemble a gradient echo image. Stables et al. [25] have demonstrated that varying these parameters can optimize for a particular perturbation size (i.e., a small or large blood vessel). Several fMRI studies have used a spin echo sequence effectively in high susceptibility areas such as the hippocampus and amygdala (e.g., [26–28]). Figure 7.2 shows examples of a gradient echo and asymmetric spin echo EPI images using otherwise identical parameters in the same subject. The recovery of signal in high susceptibility areas, especially around a lesion, is quite apparent, though not complete.

Other modifications to the EPI sequence may reduce susceptibility artifacts. Cordes et al. [29] advocate using a second refocusing gradient in the slice selection orientation to reduce susceptibility artifacts. A more complicated approach offered by

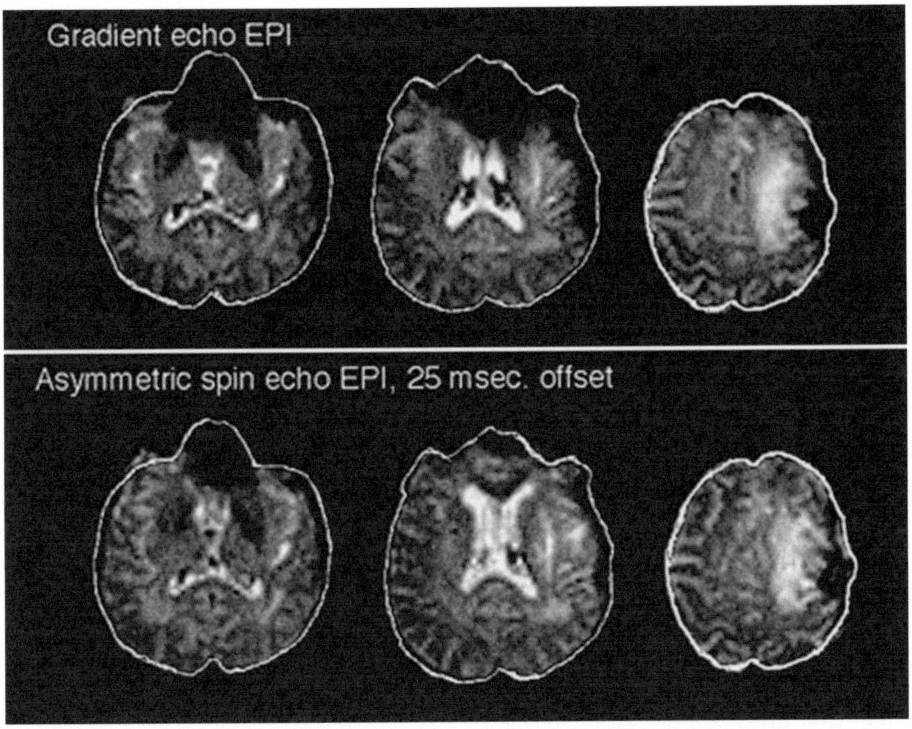

Fig. 7.2 Gradient echo versus Asymmetric Spin Echo EPI: Gradient echo (TR = 2.5, TE = 45, 64 × 64 matrix, FOV = 20, 1 NEX) and asymmetric spin echo (TR = 2.5, TE = 45, offset = 25 ms, 64 × 64 matrix, FOV = 20, 1 NEX) EPI scans in two areas of high susceptibility (*left*) at air–tissue interfaces in basal temporal and orbitofrontal cortex (*right*) near the lesion with prior resection. The outlines are derived from a high-resolution spin echo EPI (TR = 4,000; TE = 54, 128 × 128 matrix, 20 mm FOV, 5 mm thick, 4 NEX). Note reduced susceptibility in ASE scans in both regions of high susceptibility

Stenger et al. [30] uses three-dimensional tailored radiofrequency (RF) pulses to refocus regions where the susceptibility is greatest, using a modified spiral k-space trajectory.

In spiral scanning, k-space is traversed in a spiral pattern emanating either from the center to the exterior (spiral-in), the reverse (spiral-out), or in some combination (e.g., dual-echo in-out). Glover and Law [31] reported that a spiral-in trajectory or a combination of in and out trajectories can both increase SNR while reducing susceptibility. Yang et al. [32] developed a reverse spiral scanning technique simultaneous with perfusion imaging with arterial spin labeling. Comparisons of susceptibility artifacts between forward and reverse spiral scanning suggested less susceptibility in the reverse sequence, with adequate BOLD signal in high susceptibility regions. Other techniques to reduce susceptibility artifacts in spiral scans include a sensitivity encoding sequencing [33], which shortens the readout duration, thus minimizing signal loss. However, the effects of BOLD signal recovery were less dramatic.

Study and Task Design

Issues in task design, particularly, choice of activation and control tasks, as well as difficulty level, are important considerations in all fMRI studies; however, in the clinical arena, these difficulties take on special significance, as errors in task design can lead to false conclusions that may harm patients. Here, we discuss three issues of particular importance in clinical fMRI: choice of control conditions, the effect of practice on observed fMRI activations, and the appropriate level of difficulty given the population to be studied.

Task Selection

Functional MRI activations represent a contrast between two conditions; in the earliest fMRI studies, this contrast was identified by simply subtracting rest or control condition images from those acquired during a task [34, 35]. This simple subtraction approach assumes the following: (1) a hierarchical organization of brain function; (2) that the investigator can accurately decompose a complex task; and (3) cognitive activity and brain function are insignificant during rest conditions.

The assumption that an investigator can accurately decompose a task into its components is a challenge in itself. Not all subjects will always use the same strategy to perform a task, nor can we easily deduce all the cognitive processes that are required to complete a given task function. This challenge may be even more difficult in a clinical population in which there may be subclinical or overt cognitive deficits that may alter the strategies used to perform a task. That is to say, tasks that have been shown to be suitable for brain mapping in the general healthy population cannot necessarily be applied blindly to a sick population. Finally, this approach assumes cognitive functions linearly summate to produce the observed fMRI signals and that there is no interaction between cognitive functions that may produce a unique output based on the combination of tasks.

To test the assumptions of linearity of hierarchical structure, Sidtis and colleagues compared activation maps using "simple subtraction" (maps were generated by subtracting a rest condition from a task condition) and "complex subtractions" (maps were generated by subtracting two tasks that were presumed to only differ with respect to a single parameter) [36]. The three tasks used were syllable repetition, phonation, and lip closure; syllable repetition was assumed to be a combination of phonation and lip closure for the purposes of this study. Lip closure maps were generated by "simple subtraction" of the rest condition from the lip closure condition and "complex subtraction" maps were generated by subtracting the phonation condition from the syllable repetition condition. The simple and complex subtraction maps were different both with respect to signal intensities and distribution, suggesting that the condition of additivity necessary to decompose complex tasks by subtraction was not present in the data, calling into serious question subtraction methodology and the assumption that we can accurately decompose tasks.

Stark and Squire examined activation patterns associated with rest conditions (used as a baseline) to determine if "rest" is necessarily an appropriate control or baseline, with particular attention to memory tasks looking at the medial temporal lobe [37]. The authors measured fMRI signals during seven different tasks: novel pictures, familiar pictures, noise detection, odd/even discrimination, arrow discrimination, moving fixation, and rest; the first two tasks were considered memory tasks while the last five were considered to be various controls. Not surprisingly, the authors demonstrate that identifying activity in the medial temporal lobe (including hippocampal and parahippocampal structures) varied depending on the control condition used. In fact, the authors report that activity within these structures was *higher* during the rest condition than during other control conditions. Consequently, identifying activity in the region of interest (ROI) intimately depended on the control condition used. This study highlights two important points. First, fMRI activations represent contrasts between two conditions and do not indicate whether a part of the brain was active. Rather, it means there was not a significant enough change in neuronal activity *relative to baseline* to evoke a functional hemodynamic response. This highlights the need for careful selection of baseline tasks and even more careful interpretation of observed activation patterns. Second, "rest" does not mean that the brain is quiescent; the brain is cognitively active even during rest. Indeed a recent surge in interest in resting state connectivity indicates at least one functional network that is more active at rest than during task performance. Gusnard and Raichle review the concept of a "physiological baseline," suggesting that in fact the brain has a high level of activity at baseline and that this must be considered when using rest as a control condition and when interpreting functional activation studies [38]. Importantly, they provide a thorough discussion of task-related *decreases* in activation and argue that while some of these decreases may represent a task-dependent decrease in cerebral activity, many decreases seem to be task-independent, representing an "organized mode of brain function, which is attenuated during various goal-directed behaviors" [38]. This so called "default mode network" [39, 40] involves several regions including medial parietal cortex, hippocampus, and temporal cortex which typically are reduced in blood flow during task performance across a wide range of tasks. As several of these regions are frequent targets for clinical mapping, hippocampus and dominant temporal lobe, understanding how they respond during task engagement and how these responses compare to disruption methods is completely unstudied.

Practice Effects

Paradigm design is not only important with respect to selection of tasks, but also with respect to task timing. Several studies now indicate that practicing a task can significantly alter activation patterns, revealing different maps that may represent alternative strategies for performing the given task, such as automatization [41–44]. Raichle and associates were the first to report that functional activation patterns can be altered by relatively brief periods of practice [41]. Comparing a novel verbal response selection task with reading visually presented nouns, they found a practice-related decrease in cortical activation of those regions mediating performance at the beginning of the task after only 15 min of practice. Moreover, other brain regions increased activity, such that, with practice, the verbal response task more resembled the reading task. This practice effect was reversed by introducing a novel list of words, allowing the authors to conclude that the activation patterns associated with practice represented an automatization of the task that was reversible. Van Mier et al. [43] and Petersen et al. [42] report similar findings of shifts in activation patterns, or change in functional neuroanatomy, from one part of the brain to another with practice, which is thought to represent an activity-dependent shift in effortful task performance to skilled, automatic task performance.

Similarly, Madden and colleagues [44] reported a decrease in functional activation with practice in the two populations they studied, young adults (20–29 years) and older adults (62–79 years). Using a verbal recognition memory task, this group characterized activation patterns during encoding, baseline, and retrieval, and found that activation patterns were different (both increased magnitude and different spatial distribution) between these populations for each task. Interestingly, despite differences initially, both groups demonstrated practice-related effects, showing decreased activation magnitude, although the practice effects were greater in the younger population than in the elderly. The authors concluded that older adults required a more distributive network of brain activation in order to perform the given task and, while task performance improved with practice, the smaller practice effect observed in the older group represents a continual recruitment of cognitive processes and attention to support task execution that is not required in the younger population, who can learn and automate more quickly and effectively.

Not all groups, however, have reported activation of additional areas with practice. Garavan and associates argued that if the core task is unchanged by practice, then practice may cause a decreased magnitude of activation but will not necessarily recruit additional areas of the brain [45]. Using a visuospatial working memory (VSWM) task, they reported decreased fMRI activations in the four areas of interest with activation, but did not report seeing additional areas of activation with practice. They suggested that their observations were consistent with the fact that the task used continues to tax the VSWM system and cannot be automated completely, regardless of amount of practice. This raises an interesting consideration that not all cognitive tasks are equally susceptible to practice effects.

The existence of practice effects and relative rapidity of onset are important technical considerations in implementing a functional brain mapping study, especially if one wishes to identify those brain regions that are actively involved in and essential to task performance. Most fMRI studies take approximately 1 h to complete, during which time brain activation patterns may be modified secondary to practice. It is, therefore, critical to plan experiments efficiently and to continually provide novel stimuli and tasks in order to assure that practice-related changes do not taint the results (unless, of course, it is the practice-related effects that are being investigated in the first place).

Task Difficulty

Another important consideration that is intimately related to the concept of practice is task difficulty. It is hypothesized that the changes seen due to practice are largely due to decreases in task difficulty with practice and therefore automatization of task performance. If a task is too easy, the task may activate brain areas involved with performing automatic activities without taxing the appropriate cognitively critical areas of interest. On the contrary, if a task is too difficult, it may recruit additional attentional areas and supplementary areas (areas that a task may not normally activate) to help execute a task.

The paradigm of mapping a paretic or plegic patient offers an excellent means of discussing task difficulty and its effects on fMRI activations. For these patients, the effort and difficulty to complete a motor task is undoubtedly greater than for a healthy volunteer. The source of the paresis (i.e., intracerebral versus spinal) will influence the fMRI activation pattern. In a study of patients with central masses near the motor strip, fMRI activations of primary motor cortex decreased with increasing paresis, independent of the distance of the central mass from the motor strip, although the degree of paresis did not correlate with the magnitude of the observed fMRI signal [3, 7]. The observed decrease in primary motor activation cannot be unambiguously attributed to a decreased number of functional neurons in the motor strip, compression due to mass effect (although the observation was independent of distance of the mass from the central strip), tumor-mediated changes in local cerebral hemodynamics, changes in global perfusion due to the presence of a neoplasm, or a combination of these factors [3]. It is critically important from the perspective of clinical brain mapping to consider if a better primary motor strip mapping signal could have been obtained by changing the level of difficulty of the given motor task. Could a more significant signal be elicited from the primary motor strip if the motor task is made more complex and drives the remaining primary motor neurons harder? What if the motor task is made simpler? Could a simpler task induce greater activation by giving the remaining primary motor neurons a task they are fully capable of executing? These may be important points of consideration in interpreting clinical data.

In the same study, the investigators report larger secondary motor activations in patients with paresis than without paresis. This is likely attributable to the difficulty of the task for the paretic patients [3]. Similar to the case of elderly patients recruiting a broader network of neurons than younger controls in order to execute a memory task [45], the paretic patients may be recruiting additional cortical areas in order to execute a task that is relatively difficult for them given their current medical condition. Krings and colleagues therefore conclude, "With increasing task complexity (or with decreasing motor skills), this network must increase its excitatory output, resulting in a higher neuronal activity, more pronounced regional cerebral blood flow changes" [3].

In tasks of higher cognitive functioning, the problem of task difficulty may be even more complex. For instance, in our work with patients who have a genetic risk for Alzheimer's, older volunteers with normal memory but who carried the APO-4 allele (which conveys a strong risk of AD) had an increase in the magnitude and spatial extent of brain activation on fMRI in comparison to age- and memory-matched controls [46]. Among subjects who have mild AD, however, there is a significant decrease in fMRI activation [47, 48].

In parametric studies of memory load in normal volunteers, increased memory load was associated with increased activation that varied parametrically [49]. Thus, the relationship between task difficulty and activation magnitude is complex, and performance level must be considered a critical factor in interpreting fMRI results.

Patients with aphasia due to brain lesions show similar alterations in brain activity. For instance, Sonty et al. [50] showed that patients with primary progressive aphasia had activation like normals in primary language areas and also additional language activation in regions outside language cortices, suggesting the use of compensatory strategies. Kim et al. [51] found that the pattern of reorganization in patients with focal lesions varied across individuals, and appeared related to whether the lesions were cortical or subcortical. Calvert et al. [52] found that patterns of fMRI activation during language tasks in a frontal lobe CVA patient depended upon the task; increased right hemisphere Broca's analog was activated during the most difficult task, whereas the left hemisphere Broca's was active for a matched control subject.

Together, the existing data suggest that patients with deficits tend to utilize compensatory strategies that engage additional brain regions to accomplish the task. The pattern of fMRI activation during compensation may give a false impression about localization of function, for instance, increased compensatory RH activation may incorrectly suggest the patient has right hemisphere speech dominance. Thus, clinical use of fMRI for localization of function must take into account the patient's level of cognitive performance. Impaired performance can easily lead to false conclusions about functional localization, particularly in language tasks.

Ultimately, it is important to consider whether differences in activation patterns across conditions or groups represent differences in brain organization and function or an artifact of differential capability to cope with task difficulty. We suggest investigators pay close attention to task difficulty in designing, interpreting, and drawing conclusions from their clinical studies, especially when the general medical condition of one group is significantly different than the comparison group.

Task Choice

In clinical imaging for surgical planning, the functions most commonly mapped are motor and language. Motor mapping is relatively straightforward when the clinical questions center around preserving the motor strip. While many studies have reported results of cerebellar and basal ganglia activation during motor task performance for groups of individuals, we are aware of no studies designed specifically for mapping these regions. As deep brain stimulation surgery for Parkinson's disease and other movement disorders have developed, there may ultimately arise a demand for subcortical motor mapping, though at present these surgeries are performed on anatomical grounds, and based on response to stimulation during the procedure.

Language mapping is a more complex evaluation and there are many approaches to task choice. Early studies focused on a single paradigm: word generation, which has been found to be reliable across sites in indicating frontal language areas in particular (e.g., Rutten et al. [55]). However, the language system is complex, and different tasks may be best suited to map different brain regions, such as naming for the basal temporal language area, semantic decision tasks for Wernicke's area, and reading for inferior temporal and inferior parietal regions.

An alternative strategy is to assess function using a "panel of tasks." Gaillard and colleagues described using a panel of language tasks (verbal fluency, reading comprehension, and auditory comprehension) to assess hemispheric lateralization rather than a single task (e.g., Gaillard et al. [54]). They found that using a panel of tasks resulted in superior inter-rater reliability than relying on a single task, reduces the likelihood of having "nondiagnostic findings," and improves concordance between laterality assessments based of fMRI and Wada testing.

Deciding on the baseline tasks for language has been a very controversial subject; while some have argued against using activation controls, which may induce activity in language areas unintentionally (e.g., Bookheimer [56]), others have argued in favor of tailored baseline, sensory activation controls (e.g., Binder et al. [57]). In a study examining the magnitude of activation and degree of lateralization during a series of comprehension tasks, Binder et al. [57] found that using a tone control task produced stronger laterality effects than using a rest comparison, and argued that semantic processing may occur at rest, obscuring possible LH language areas during language tasks. However, the location of their results is not consistent with the loci of Wernicke's area as reported by other investigators, and their results have not been validated with a gold standard measure of intrahemispheric localization of function. In our view, the potential for false-negative errors is greatest when there are sensory activation controls that may inadvertently activate "eloquent" cortex, or which, when containing nonlinguistic sensory information, may produce task-related decreases in language areas. In such a scenario, use of these tasks as controls may falsely indicate task-related activation, which is rather due to deactivation of the control task. Clearly the issue of how to choose both activation and control tasks remains of extreme importance, and regardless of theoretical reasons for choosing an approach, any combination of task and control conditions requires confirmation with a gold standard – Wada tests for laterality, ESM for intrahemispheric localization – to fully validate the approach.

Special Task Considerations

An additional complication in choosing language tasks concerns whether the patient is bilingual and how (and whether) to map native versus nonnative languages. Though results vary depending upon language proficiency and age of second language acquisition, there is consensus that second languages may have unique representations in the brain that can be measured with fMRI as well as with electrocorticography. ESM studies have consistently found areas of unique representations for different languages in bilingual patients (e.g., Lucas et al. [58]) and fMRI studies of normal control, bilingual subjects show differences in language representations based on age of onset [59] as well as proficiency [60], language-specific differences in organization (e.g., reading in phonological versus pictographic based languages [61]). Therefore, it is typically necessary to map both native and second languages in bilingual patients.

Head Motion

Excessive head motion is always a problem in fMRI studies but is of particular concern in clinical studies. While in group-average research studies subjects with too much motion can be removed from analysis, or at least will just add error; in clinical fMRI examinations, a single valid study, often in a limited time window, may be all that is possible. Further, cognitive compromise makes it more difficult for many patients to stay still voluntarily. Typically, head motion is managed by registration of all images in a time series, or by mathematically removing variance due to motion (e.g., Jenkinson et al. [62], Grootoonk et al. [63]), or even removing images from the time series that are affected by head motion. However, there is consensus that too much motion is uncorrectable through such means; further, the potential effects of head motion may add noise that obscures true signal, or may create artifacts that appear as activation, particularly when the motion is correlated with the task (e.g., Desmond et al. [64]). For these reasons, obtaining motion-free, high-quality data from patients is of particular importance, and the raw data must be carefully examined for the presence of motion.

Analysis

Adequate study and task design are not sufficient to be able to draw strong conclusions from a clinical fMRI study. Careful selection of analysis techniques and attention to the particular challenges of analysis limitations is necessary in order to accurately interpret mapping data. Analysis in clinical studies differs from other studies most significantly in that analysis is done "within subjects" rather than at a group level. Moreover, one must also be cognizant of the methods used to quantify fMRI activations and the techniques that can be used to optimize the sensitivity and specificity of the derived functional maps.

Within Subject Versus Group Analysis

The vast corpus of data in functional imaging relies almost exclusively on group-averaged data. Early efforts in PET, and later fMRI research, focused on developing superior tools for registering and ultimately warping brains from different subjects into a common space in order to increase SNR through subject averaging. While these efforts have been extremely useful in making it possible to answer broad questions about human cognition, these approaches have limited clinical utility for the individual patient. Here, we differentiate between clinical research studies, which have and will continue to use group averaging procedures, from true clinical fMRI, in which a clinician will attempt to make a diagnosis or decision for an individual based on their fMRI results. First, we consider the broad nature of the question to be answered.

Why will patients be referred for fMRI? Common current applications are to make a decision relevant to surgical intervention, such as, in what hemisphere is language located or where within a hemisphere does a particular functional reside. Future applications may include diagnosis: Does a particular pattern of activation indicate a diagnosis of dyslexia, autism, obsessive compulsive disorder, or even malingering? The optimal analytic technique will depend upon the specific question being asked and the desired balance between sensitivity and specificity. The derived fMRI maps must also prove to be reliable and reproducible. It is conceivable that in the future fMRI maps can be used as an imaging biomarker, in which an individual's brain activation pattern could be compared to a probabilistic functional atlas in order to determine the statistical likelihood that a patient belongs to a particular diagnostic class. While this approach is not currently available, new attempts to find functional landmarks, such as the International Consortium for Human Brain Mapping, should further such efforts. Here, we focus on reliability of methods for within-subject analysis in the common current applications.

Given an experimental design that includes at least one activation and one control condition, several approaches to analysis may reveal "active" brain regions. Statistical approaches – including correlation coefficients between MR signal and a predicted response curve, *t*-tests comparing activation versus control voxel intensities, and Komogorov-Smirnov tests, which show differences not only in mean but also in variance – produce a statistical value for which an investigator must determine a threshold of statistical significance (often arbitrarily). Current controversies include how to threshold data, whether to use a statistical value or magnitude measure (percent signal change) or to count "volume of activation," i.e., the number of voxels exceeding a statistical threshold as a dependent variable. Each technique has advantages and disadvantages, but few studies have carefully examined the reliability and validity of various approaches.

Dependent Measures

Functional MRI activations can be quantified broadly in two dimensions: spatial extent and magnitude of activation. Calculating activation size, by means of voxel counting, has become the most common approach to quantifying fMRI activity, especially in the clinical arena. This approach has several limitations, which must be thoroughly understood prior to relying on such data for clinical management. To illustrate these limitations, we review the application of voxel counting to studies of language lateralization.

When studying language lateralization, the extent of fMRI activation is quantified by counting the number of voxels exceeding a statistical threshold of correlation with a predetermined hemodynamic function. These voxel counts are then used to compute laterality indices (LI), defined as:

$$[V_L - V_R]/[V_L + V_R] \times 100]$$

where V_L and V_R are activation volumes for the left and right hemispheres, respectively. A similar index can be calculated for the intracarotid amobarbital procedure (IAP, the Wada test) using the error rates for each hemisphere injected.

In an early study analyzing the concordance of fMRI and Wada testing for determining laterality, Binder and colleagues found a strong correlation between the two procedures despite using a relatively simple single-task whole-brain fMRI design [65]. The high concordance rate reported is striking considering their use of a single language task, the lack of trial-to-trial reliability of voxel counting, and the methodological differences between disruption-based mapping (i.e., Wada testing) and activation-based mapping (i.e., fMRI). While the Wada test identifies areas that are essential for language function, fMRI identifies *all* areas that are involved with language processing (essential or not), including networks that are not specifically related to language such as motor, sensory, and attentional systems. The authors propose that their use of a control paradigm (a perceptual discrimination task) in part controls for these factors, which is probably in fact true, but unlikely to account for all the aforementioned differences. In the subsequent sections, we will explore these limitations and review methodological developments that help overcome these obstacles and make clinical fMRI more reliable.

Despite the common assumption that all voxels exceeding threshold carry identical weight, studies indicate that fMRI-based LI determinations vary according to the statistical threshold applied [55, 66]. For example, Gaillard and colleagues found in one patient that using a threshold of $t = 2$ resulted in bilateral dominance, whereas using a threshold of $t = 3$ demonstrated left-hemisphere dominance. A potential solution to this problem was proposed by Ramsey and colleagues who reported that maps created using conjunction analysis (see discussion that follows) are less susceptible to such thresholding effects [67]. Besides the susceptibility to the threshold applied, maps created using a predefined statistical threshold do not account for differences in activation magnitude (or percent signal change from baseline). It is conceivable that LI (which is based on voxel counts) can be 0, implying equal hemispheric activation, but that the average magnitude of activation in one hemisphere is significantly greater than the other. In such a scenario there is clear hemispheric asymmetry, although voxel counts (and LI) do not reflect the underlying differences in activation. Suarez and colleagues have recently proposed a "threshold-independent" method of determining LI that is based upon integrated weighted t-scores for all positively correlated voxels [68]. These authors found that using this threshold-independent model produced superior concordance rates between fMRI and Wada testing, although the number of patients studies was modest ($N = 14$).

Determination of LI based on voxel counts is also significantly dependent upon the ROI used for the analysis. In most cases, whole brain analysis is used to determine LI, which can be problematic because it includes activations in areas that are not normally expected to have lateralized function (e.g., occipital lobe and other midline regions) and excludes the possibility that specific brain regions may be differentially lateralized (e.g., Broca's versus Wernicke's areas). In fact, recent analyses have indicated that exclusion of midline structures from fMRI-based LI determinations improves concordance with Wada-based laterality assessments [66]. Likewise, ROI based analyses of Broca's and Wernicke's area (based on canonical anatomical boundaries) can often demonstrate differential lateralization of distinct language networks, especially in the setting of chronic intracranial pathologies such as AVMs [69]. Lehericy and associates similarly reported region-specific concordances [70]. Having employed multiple language tasks, they found that the only statistically significant relationships identified were between the asymmetry of frontal lobe fMRI activations for semantic verbal fluency and covert sentence repetition and Wada asymmetry indices.

On the contrary, fMRI asymmetry in the temporal lobes (regardless of language task) and fMRI asymmetries noted while story listening did not correlate with Wada asymmetries. By using region-specific analyses, Lhericy and colleagues were trying to address one of the major limitations of current analytic techniques. The weakness of the study was in comparing single-task activations with Wada results rather than looking at conjunction analyses or the entire panel of tasks to create a more robust and reproducible fMRI-based map of laterality.

Reproducibility

Obtaining reproducible and reliable fMRI maps in the clinical setting is complicated by patient-specific and disease-related challenges that are not encountered in the controlled scientific setting. Developing methods to improve the reliability of these maps are of paramount importance, especially now that functional brain mapping is being used increasingly for clinical decision making [65, 71, 73].

Functional MRI signals can demonstrate marked instability from trial-to-trial [72]. Differences in noise due to both artifacts and physiological factors can produce striking differences in *perceived* extent of activation, even though the actual magnitude of activation is likely the same across trials. The noise variance propagates through to statistical calculations and produces a widely varying number of voxels that exceed statistical threshold. Accordingly, the number of significantly activated voxels can vary by up to 750% between trials. On the contrary, the slope of the regression line, which is essentially the percent signal change, is much more stable across trials and subjects, with less than 20% variability across trials. Monte Carlo simulations support the assertion that even in very poor CNR conditions, the percent signal change can be determined with relatively good accuracy and precision [73].

A simple approach to improve the SNR is to average numerous trials. When using voxel-counting as a means of measuring activation size, SNR and activation size only begin to plateau only after averaging 150 trials [74]. In most studies, particularly in the clinical setting, the number of trials averaged is usually far less, on the order of 5–10. It is, therefore, critical to be mindful of sources of noise and to employ other strategies (both with respect to task design, data acquisition, and analysis) that maximize signal-to-noise and minimize the effect of trial-to-trial variations. One such strategy is to measure response magnitude within a statistically defined ROI across trials or tasks rather than comparing changes in the number of voxels that exceed a statistical threshold.

Conjunction Analysis

Considering the intrinsic noise associated with fMRI data acquisition (both physiological and equipment-related), strategies such as conjunction analysis have been devised to extract mapping signals that are clinically significant and consistent across tasks [56, 66, 71] (see Fig. 7.3). Conjunction analysis identifies all voxels that consistently exceed statistical threshold for two or more independent, yet related, tasks. By Bayes theorem, the probability of observing significant voxels by chance on multiple scans is equal to the product of the prior probability of chance for each. By using a low statistical threshold for each individual scan, the probability of eliminating functionally significant voxels is minimized, effectively reducing the chance of a false-negative result. Conversely, by requiring that the same voxel be active across multiple tasks, this analysis minimizes false-positive results.

The power of this technique was demonstrated by Pouratian and colleagues in a study comparing language-related fMRI activations with intraoperative ESM [71]. The authors created conjunction fMRI maps of expressive language (conjunction of two out of three expressive language tasks: visual object naming, word generation, and auditory response naming) and receptive language (conjunction of visual responsive naming and sentence comprehension) and compared these fMRI activations with intraoperative ESM (Fig. 7.3).

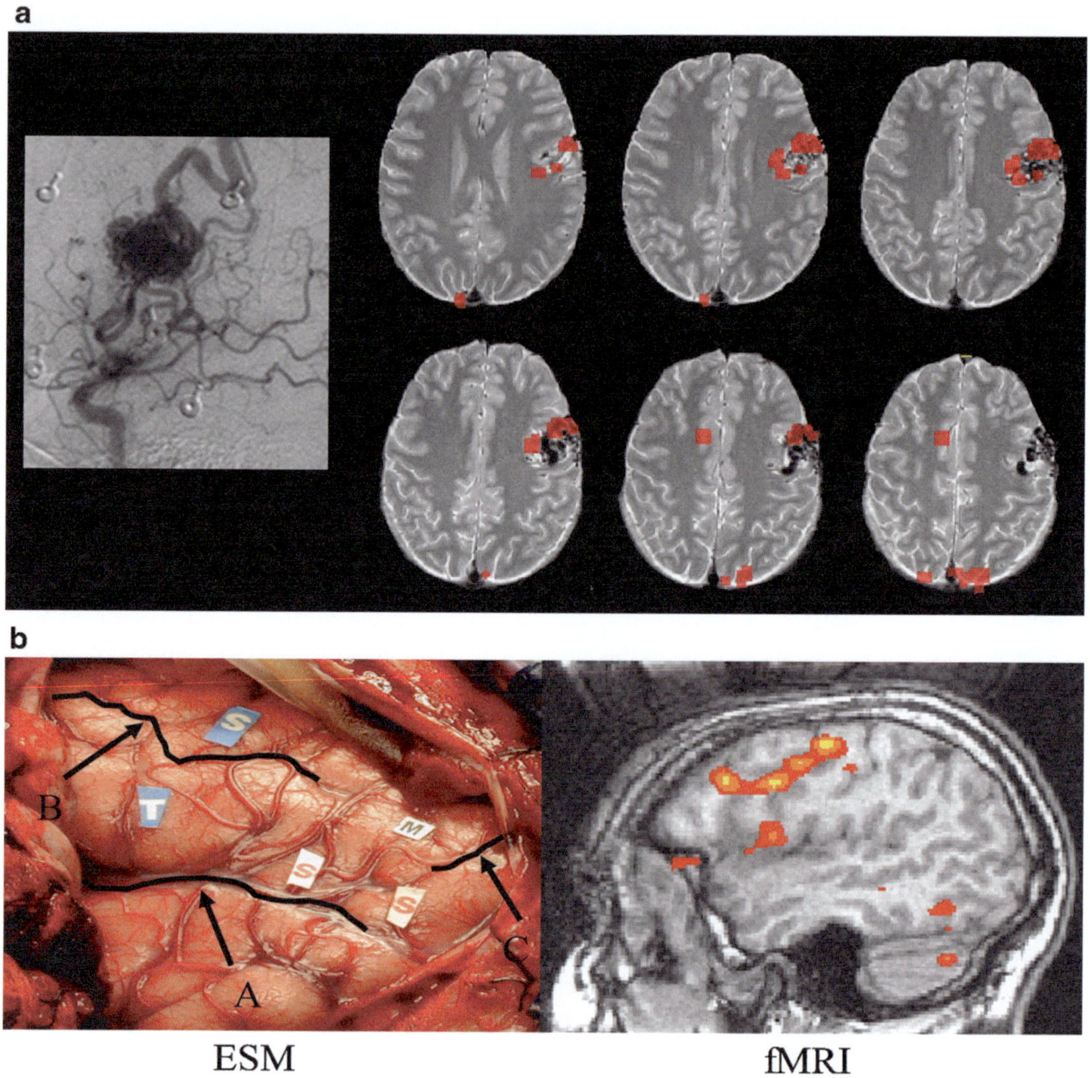

Fig. 7.3 Functional MRI activations adjacent to AVM. Significant fMRI activations are commonly identified adjacent to AVMs. (**a**) In this image, fMRI activations of language expression (created by conjunction analysis) are seen adjacent to a frontal AVM, identifying Broca's Area. Note that activations are not identified within the vascular malformation. (**b**) Functional MRI activations were both qualitatively and quantitatively similar to the intraoperative electrocortical stimulation maps. Figure illustrates correlation of ESM and fMRI with some areas on nonessential activation. Adapted from Pouratian et al. [71]

For the population studied, the authors report sensitivity and specificity values of expression fMRI activations of up to 100 and 66.7%, respectively, in the frontal lobe and of comprehension fMRI activations of up to 96.2 and 69.8%, respectively, in the parietal/temporal lobes.

Conjunction analysis has also been shown to improve the concordance between fMRI assessment of laterality and Wada testing [66, 67]. Ramsey and colleagues initially reported that in contrast to mapping responses to a single language task, conjunction analysis yields a high LI, which paralleled neuropsychological assessment of hemispheric dominance [67]. Moreover, they found that conjunction analysis results in LI that are more consistent across statistical thresholds than individual task analysis. To better understand the reliability of fMRI to assess language laterality, Arora and colleagues [66] performed a comprehensive comparison of fMRI and Wada testing for laterality assessment. The authors investigated the effect of language tasks employed, varying statistical thresholds, and other analytic techniques such as the conjunction analysis. By using conjunction analysis, the authors found the concordance between fMRI and Wada-based assessment of laterality increased from 77–83% to 91% [66].

Based on methodological differences between ESM and fMRI, false positives (i.e., imperfect specificity) are expected. Functional MRI is an activation-based technique and will, therefore, identify all activated brain regions regardless of whether they are "essential" or supplementary. On the other hand, ESM and the Wada test will only identify areas that are essential to language processing. Conjunction analyses minimize the discrepancy between these techniques by only identifying those areas that are consistently activated across language tasks.

Applying FMRI to Clinical Planning

Significance of Signal Localization

The precise relationship between observed fMRI signals and the underlying electrophysiological activity of the brain is still not well defined. The relationship is even more uncertain in the setting of intracranial pathology (especially vascular pathology), further complicating the interpretation of fMRI studies in the clinical setting. Depending on the scan sequence used, the BOLD fMRI signals can even center in adjacent sulci [75–77] and be up to 1 cm away from electrophysiologically active cortex [77]. Despite the imprecision, fMRI mapping signals demonstrate a consistent spatial relationship with cortical stimulation-based maps and are, therefore, still clinically relevant (see Giussani et al. [73] for comprehensive review) [71, 73]. In most cases, to achieve clinically useful levels of sensitivity and specificity (up to 100% and ~70%, respectively), a "sphere of influence" of fMRI activity of approximately 0.5–1.0 cm must be assumed and multiple tasks must be mapped and interpreted using a conjunction analysis [71, 78–81]. Because of the spatial imprecision of fMRI, especially when doing whole head imaging, it is important not to overinterpret small differences in spatial extent or lack of difference in spatial extent as representing a clear difference in activation patterns or a lack of difference in activation patterns, respectively.

Reliability of Signal Adjacent to Pathology

The reliability of fMRI signals in the setting of intracranial pathology is often questioned because of the introduction of susceptibility artifact into the intracranial space (e.g., AVMs, cavernous angiomas, and surgical clips) and because of the uncertain impact of the intracranial pathology on the normal physiology of the brain.

Susceptibility artifact due to intracranial pathology such as an AVM prevents mapping within the area of susceptibility. Therefore, physicians must be cognizant of areas of signal "drop-out" in which the lack of mapping signal may be due to an inability to detect activity-related MR signal changes rather than due to lack of activity. The question remains, however, as to whether reliable signals can be obtained from adjacent to the pathologies. In a study of 14 patients, Schlosser and colleagues report that fMRI signals in patients with frontal lobe tumors were comparable to signals in normal controls [10]. Similarly, Righini and colleagues found little difference in motor activations between the affected and unaffected hemispheres in 17 patients with frontoparietal masses [2]. Pouratian and colleagues also reported that functional activations, which correlate with intraoperative cortical stimulation mapping, can consistently and reliably be measured adjacent to vascular malformations (i.e., AVMs and cavernous hemangiomas) [71]. These reports are consistent with our findings at UCLA, in which we regularly and successfully map motor and language cortices, in patients scheduled for neurosurgical intervention, near eloquent cortices (Fig. 7.4).

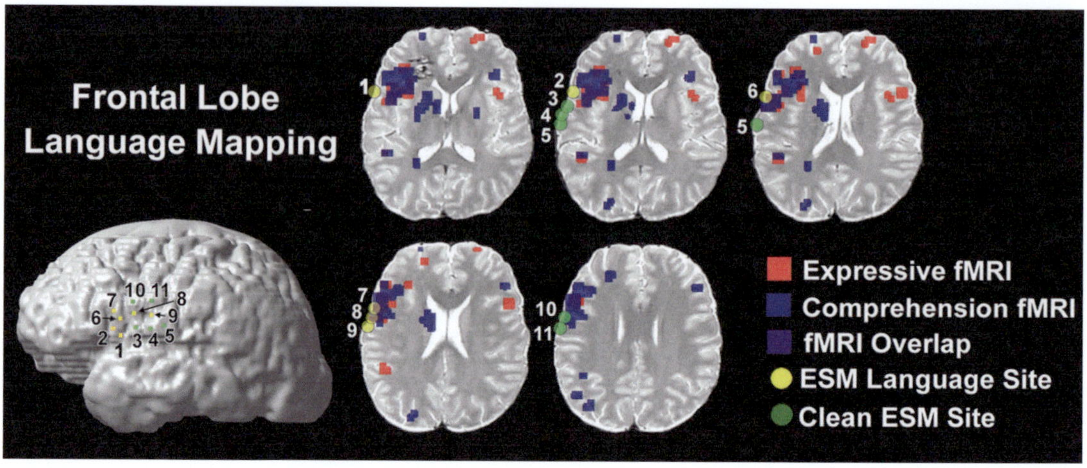

Fig. 7.4 Frontal lobe language mapping using fMRI with conjunction analysis. Yellow circles are areas essential for language as determined by ESM. Green circles are areas that when stimulated did not disrupt language function. Red activations are conjunction fMRI maps of language expression. Blue activations are conjunction fMRI maps of language comprehension. ESM sites are shown with a 5-mm radius (determined to produce the highest sensitivity with the least cost to specificity) and parietal/temporal. Red (expression) activations tend to overlap with, or are adjacent to, essential (*yellow*) ESM sites but avoid nonessential (*green*) ESM sites. Blue activations in the frontal lobe also appear predictive but with lower specificity in this subject than the expression fMRI activations. Adapted from Pouratian et al. [71]

Reports of abnormal fMRI activations adjacent to pathology likely represent cases in which the pathology has infiltrated the cortex of interest and, therefore, altered normal cortical function, cerebral hemodynamics, or both. Because of the importance of preserving eloquent function, if fMRI maps are being using for neurosurgical guidance, it is imperative to verify preoperative fMRI maps intraoperatively with intraoperative direct cortical stimulation mapping in order to ensure preservation of eloquent function.

Relationship to Outcomes

Although many studies have investigated the relationship between fMRI and electrophysiological maps [78–80, 82, 84], very few studies have quantified the sensitivity and specificity of fMRI activations relative to electrophysiological maps and no studies have vigorously assessed the relationship between fMRI maps and clinical outcomes. While it is helpful to understand the relationship between fMRI and ESM (the gold standard), the relationship between fMRI maps, extent of resection, and clinical outcomes is ultimately the most important determinant of the clinical utility and reliability of fMRI.

To date, ESM remains the gold standard with respect to intraoperative brain mapping because it is the only functional brain mapping technique that has been rigorously evaluated with respect to clinical outcomes. Haglund and colleagues, who were the first to characterize postoperative clinical outcomes relative to distance of resection from ESM-defined language sites, reported that maintenance of a 1 cm margin around ESM-defined language sites prevents postoperative dysphasia [85]. Sanai and colleagues recently published a follow-up study reporting a 1.6% rate of dysphasia when tumor resections were restricted to greater than 1 cm away from cortical areas where intraoperative stimulation produced language disruption [86]. Besides confirming the original report, they demonstrate that ESM is also reliable in patients with gliomas and not only in epilepsy patients (who were the subject of Haglund and colleague's report).

Outcomes studies such as this need to be done to better understand the clinical utility and reliability of fMRI, especially as an increasing number of centers have begun to build sufficient confidence in fMRI mapping to obviate the need for intraoperative mapping in some patients [87]. In light of mounting evidence that extensive tumor removal imparts a survival and quality-of-life advantage, there is a growing need and demand to develop superior and more reliable mapping methods to aid physicians and surgeons in providing safe avenues to resect intracranial pathologies [88].

Conclusion

Functional MRI is a powerful brain mapping tool whose use has grown exponentially over the last decade. Despite formal approval of fMRI as a clinical tool for presurgical planning, there remains no single established and accepted protocol for task presentation, analysis, or interpretation of results. Further, there remain few studies that have carefully validated a consistent fMRI approach with objective and quantitative measures in established gold-standard techniques, particularly intraoperative corticography. Of particular concern is the use of fMRI "packages" that present experiments and analyze data blindly, without careful review of image quality, artifacts, subject performance, and individual patient needs and deficits. As fMRI becomes more widely available in clinical settings lacking experienced staff in functional imaging, it is important to acknowledge and address many of the limitations that continue to challenge this modality. Moreover, as with any clinical test, it will be important to quantify its sensitivity, specificity, and relationship to outcomes in the future. Different clinical applications, experimental paradigms, analysis approach, and even equipment can produce different results; valid application of fMRI to clinical cases will have to demonstrate reliability and validity for each application separately. The field should move rapidly toward developing uniform approaches to clinical fMRI that are valid, reliable, and replicable across centers, while establishing professional standards for clinicians who wish to perform these studies. Currently, no such standards exist. We believe that for most applications, clinical decisions should not rest solely on fMRI results. Rather, fMRI may augment existing clinical tools as validation of the techniques continues [88].

References

1. Belliveau JW, Kennedy Jr DN, McKinstry RC, Buchbinder BR, Weisskoff RM, Cohen MS, et al. Functional mapping of the human visual cortex by magnetic resonance imaging. Science. 1991; 254(5032):716–9.
2. Righini A, de Divitiis O, Prinster A, Spagnoli D, Appollonio I, Bello L, et al. Functional MRI: primary motor cortex localization in patients with brain tumors. J Comput Assist Tomogr. 1996;20:702.
3. Krings T, Topper R, Willmes K, Reinges MHT, Gilsbach JM, Thron A (2002a) Activation in primary and secondary motor areas in patients with CNS neoplasms and weakness. Neurology 58.
4. Penfield W, Boldrey E. Somatic motor and sensory representation in the cerebral cortex of man as studied by electrical stimulation. Brain. 1937;60:389–443.
5. Jahanshahi M, Rothwell J. Transcranial magnetic stimulation studies of cognition: an emerging field. Exp Brain Res. 2000;131:1–9.
6. Villringer A, Dirnagl U. Coupling of brain activity and cerebral blood flow: basis of functional neuroimaging. Cerebrovasc Brain Metab Rev. 1995;7:240–76.
7. Krings T, Reinges MHT, Willmes K, Nuerk HC, Meister IG, Gilsbach JM, et al. Factors related to the magnitude of T2* MR signal changes during functional imaging. Neuroradiology. 2002;44:459–66.
8. Holodny AI, Schulder M, Liu WC, Wolko J, Maldjian JA, Kalnin AJ. The effect of brain tumors on BOLD functional MR imaging activation in the adjacent motor cortex: implications for image-guided neurosurgery. Am J Neuroradiol. 2000;21:1415–22.
9. Schreiber A, Hubbe U, Ziyeh S, Hennig J. The influence of gliomas and nonglial space-occupying lesions on blood-oxygen-level-dependent contrast enhancement. Am J Neuroradiol. 2000;21:1055–63.
10. Schlosser R, Husche S, Gawehn J, Grunert P, Vucurevic G, Geserich T, et al. Characterization of BOLD-fMRI signal during a verbal fluency paradigm in patients with intracerebral tumors affecting the frontal lobe. Magn Reson Imaging. 2002;20:7–16.
11. Chen JJ, Pike GB. Global cerebral oxidative metabolism during hypercapnia and hypocapnia in humans: implications for BOLD fMRI. J Cereb Blood Flow Metab. 2010 Jun;30(6):1094–9. Epub 2010 Apr 7.
12. An H, Liu Q, Chen Y, Lin W. Evaluation of MR-derived cerebral oxygen metabolic index in experimental

hyperoxic hypercapnia, hypoxia, and ischemia.Stroke. 2009 Jun;40(6):2165–72. Epub 2009 Apr 9.
13. Schmitz B, Bettiger BW, Hossmann KA. Brief hypercapnia enhances somatosensory activation of blood flow in rat. J Cereb Blood Flow Metab. 1996;16: 1307–11.
14. Bock C, Schmitz B, Kerskens CM, Gyngell ML, Hossmann KA, Hoehn-Berlage M. Functional MRI of somatosensory activation in rat: effect of hypercapnic up-regulation on perfusion and BOLD-imaging. Magn Reson Med. 1998;39:457–61.
15. Bandettini PA, Wong EC. A hypercapnia-based normalization method for improved spatial localization of human brain activation with fMRI. NMR Biomed. 1997;10:197–203.
16. Kruger G, Kastrup A, Glover GH. Neuroimaging at 1.5 T and 3.0 T: comparison of oxygenation-sensitive magnetic resonance imaging. Magn Reson Med. 2001;45(4):595–604.
17. Ojemann G, Ojemann J, Lettich E, Berger M. Cortical language localization in left, dominant hemisphere. An electrical stimulation mapping investigation in 117 patients. J Neurosurg. 1989;71:316–26.
18. Devlin JT, Russell RP, Davis MH, Price CJ, Wilson J, Moss HE, et al. Susceptibility-induced loss of signal: comparing PET and fMRI on a semantic task. Neuroimage. 2000;11:589–600.
19. Cohen MS, Weisskoff RM. Ultra-fast imaging. Magn Reson Imaging. 1991;9:1–37.
20. Merboldt KD, Fransson P, Bruhn H, Frahm J. Functional MRI of the human amygdala? Neuroimage. 2001;14(2):253–7.
21. Fransson P, Merboldt KD, Ingvar M, Petersson KM, Frahm J. Functional MRI with reduced susceptibility artifact: high-resolution mapping of episodic memory encoding. Neuroreport. 2001;12(7):1415–20.
22. Port JD, Pomper MG. Quantification and minimization of magnetic susceptibility artifacts on GRE images. J Comput Assist Tomogr. 2000;24(6): 958–64.
23. Gorno-Tempini ML, Hutton C, Josephs O, Deichmann R, Price C, Turner R. Echo time dependence of BOLD contrast and susceptibility artifacts. Neuroimage. 2002;15(1):136–42.
24. Glover GH, Thomason ME. Improved combination of spiral-in/out images for BOLD fMRI. Magn Reson Med. 2004;51(4):863–8.
25. Stables LA, Kennan RP, Gore JC. Asymmetric spin-echo imaging of magnetically inhomogeneous systems: theory, experiment, and numerical studies. Magn Reson Med. 1998;40(3):432–42.
26. Stern CE, Corkin S, Gonzalez RG, Guimaraes AR, Baker JR, Jennings PJ, et al. The hippocampal formation participates in novel picture encoding: evidence from functional magnetic resonance imaging. Proc Natl Acad Sci USA. 1996;93(16):8660–5.
27. Hariri A, Bookheimer SY, Mazziotta J. A neural network for modulating the emotional response to faces. Neuroreport. 2000;11(1):43–8.
28. LaBar KS, Gatenby JC, Gore JC, LeDoux JE, Phelps EA. Human amygdala activation during conditioned fear acquisition and extinction: a mixed-trial fMRI study. Neuron. 1998;20(5):937–45.
29. Cordes D, Turski PA, Sorenson JA. Compensation of susceptibility-induced signal loss in echo-planar imaging for functional applications. Magn Reson Imaging. 2000;18(9):1055–68.
30. Stenger VA, Boada FE, Noll DC. Three-dimensional tailored RF pulses for the reduction of susceptibility artifacts in T (*)(2)-weighted functional MRI. Magn Reson Med. 2000;44(4):525–31.
31. Glover GH, Law CS. Spiral-in/out BOLD fMRI for increased SNR and reduced susceptibility artifacts. Magn Reson Med. 2001;46(3):515–22.
32. Yang Y, Gu H, Zhan W, Xu S, Silbersweig DA, Stern E. Simultaneous perfusion and BOLD imaging using reverse spiral scanning at 3T: characterization of functional contrast and susceptibility artifacts. Magn Reson Med. 2002;48(2):278–89.
33. Weiger M, Pruessmann KP, Osterbauer R, Bornert P, Boesiger P, Jezzard P. Sensitivity-encoded single-shot spiral imaging for reduced susceptibility artifacts in BOLD fMRI. Magn Reson Med. 2002;48(5):860–6.
34. Kwong KK, Belliveau JW, Chesler DA, Goldberg IE, Weisskoff RM, Poncelet BP, et al. Dynamic magnetic resonance imaging of human brain activity during primary sensory stimulation. Proc Natl Acad Sci USA. 1992;89:5675–9.
35. Ogawa S, Tank DW, Menon R, Ellermann JM, Kim SG, Merkle H, et al. Intrinsic signal changes accompanying sensory stimulation: functional brain mapping with magnetic resonance imaging. Proc Natl Acad Sci USA. 1992;89:5951–5.
36. Sidtis JJ, Strother SC, Anderson JR, Rottenberg DA. Are brain functions really additive? Neuroimage. 1999;9:490–6.
37. Stark CEL, Squire LR. When zero is not zero: the problem of ambiguous baseline conditions in fMRI. Proc Natl Acad Sci USA. 2001;98:12760–5.
38. Gusnard DA, Raichle ME. Searching for a baseline: functional imaging and the resting human brain. Nat Rev Neurosci. 2001;2:685–94.
39. Fox MD, Zhang D, Snyder AZ, Raichle ME. The global signal and observed anticorrelated resting state brain networks. J Neurophysiol. 2009;101(6):3270–83.
40. Greicius MD, Krasnow B, Reiss AL, Menon V. Functional connectivity in the resting brain: a network analysis of the default mode hypothesis. Proc Natl Acad Sci USA. 2003;100(1):253–8.
41. Raichle ME, Fiez JA, Videen TO, MacLeod AK, Pardo JV, Fox PT, et al. Practice-related changes in human brain functional anatomy during nonmotor learning. Cerebral Cortex. 1994;4:8–26.
42. Petersen SE, van Mier H, Fiez JA, Raichle ME. The effects of practice on the functional anatomy of task performance. Proc Natl Acad Sci USA. 1998;95: 853–60.
43. van Mier H, Tempel LW, Perlmutter JS, Raichle ME, Petersen SE. Changes in brain activity during motor

learning measured with PET: effects of hand of performance and practice. J Neurophysiol. 1998;80: 2177–99.
44. Madden DJ, Turkington TG, Provenzale JM, Denny LL, Hawk TC, Gottlob LR, et al. Adult age differences in the functional neuroanatomy of verbal recognition memory. Hum Brain Map. 1999;7:115–35.
45. Garavan H, Kelley D, Rosen A, Rao SR, Stein EA. Practice-related functional activation changes in a working memory task. Microsc Res Tech. 2000;51:54–63.
46. Bookheimer SY, Strojwas MH, Cohen MS, Saunders AM, Pericak-Vance MA, Mazziotta JC, et al. Patterns of brain activation in people at risk for Alzheimer's disease. N Engl J Med. 2000;343(7):450–6.
47. O'Brien JL, O'Keefe KM, Laviolette PS, Deluca AN, Blacker D, Dickerson BC. Sperling RA. Neurology: Longitudinal fMRI in elderly reveals loss of hippocampal activation with clinical decline; 2010 [Epub ahead of print].
48. Rombouts SA, Barkhof F, Veltman DJ, Machielsen WC, Witter MP, Bierlaagh MA, Lazeron RH, Valk J, Scheltens P. Functional MR imaging in Alzheimer's disease during memory encoding. AJNR Am J Neuroradiol. 2000 Nov-Dec;21(10):1869–75.
49. Jaeggi SM, Seewer R, Nirkko AC, Eckstein D, Schroth G, Groner R, et al. Does excessive memory load attenuate activation in the prefrontal cortex? Load-dependent processing in single and dual tasks: functional magnetic resonance imaging study. Neuroimage. 2003;19(2 Pt 1):210–25.
50. Sonty SP, Mesulam MM, Thompson CK, Johnson NA, Weintraub S, Parrish TB, et al. Primary progressive aphasia: PPA and the language network. Ann Neurol. 2003;53(1):35–49.
51. Kim DS, Duong TQ, Kim SG. High-resolution mapping of iso-orientation columns by fMRI. Nat Neurosci. 2000;3:164–9.
52. Calvert GA, Brammer MJ, Morris RG, Williams SC, King N, Matthews PM (2000). Using fMRI to study recovery from acquired dysphasia. Brain Lang. 2000 Feb 15;71(3):391–9.
53. Ruff IM, Petrovich Brennan NM, Peck KK, Hou BL, Tabar V, Brennan CW, Holodny AI. Assessment of the language laterality index in patients with brain tumor using functional MR imaging: effects of thresholding, task selection, and prior surgery. AJNR Am J Neuroradiol. 2008 Mar;29(3):528–35. Epub 2008 Jan 9.
54. Gaillard WD, Balsamo L, Xu B, McKinney C, Papero PH, Weinstein S, et al. fMRI language task panel improves determination of language dominance. Neurology. 2004;63(8):1403–8.
55. Rutten GJ, Ramsey NF, van Rijen PC, van Veelen CW. Reproducibility of fMRI-determined language lateralization in individual subjects. Brain Lang. 2002;80(3):421–37.
56. Bookheimer SY, Zeffiro TA, Blaxton T, Malow BA, Gaillard WD, Sato S, et al. A direct comparison of PET activation and electrocortical stimulation mapping for language localization. Neurology. 1997;48: 1056–65.
57 Binder JR, Swanson SJ, Hammeke TA, Sabsevitz DS. A comparison of five fMRI protocols for mapping speech comprehension systems. Epilepsia. 1980;49(12):1980–97.
58 Lucas 2nd TH, McKhann 2nd GM, Ojemann GA. Functional separation of languages in the bilingual brain: a comparison of electrical stimulation language mapping in 25 bilingual patients and 117 monolingual control patients. J Neurosurg. 2004;101(3):449–57.
59 Bloch C, Kaiser A, Kuenzli E, Zappatore D, Haller S, Franceschini R, Luedi G, Radue EW, Nitsch C. The age of second language acquisition determines the variability in activation elicited by narration in three languages in Broca's and Wernicke's area. Neuropsychologia. 2009 Feb;47(3):625–33. Epub 2008 Nov 17.
60. Chee MW, Hon N, Lee HL, Soon CS. Relative language proficiency modulates BOLD signal change when bilinguals perform semantic judgments. Blood oxygen level dependent. Neuroimage. 2001;13 (6 Pt 1):1155–63.
61. Tan LH, Spinks JA, Feng CM, Siok WT, Perfetti CA, Xiong J, et al. Neural systems of second language reading are shaped by native language. Hum Brain Mapp. 2003;18(3):158–66.
62. Jenkinson M, Bannister P, Brady M, Smith S. Improved optimization for the robust and accurate linear registration and motion correction of brain images. Neuroimage. 2002;17(2):825–41.
63. Grootoonk S, Hutton C, Ashburner J, Howseman AM, Josephs O, Rees G, et al. Characterization and correction of interpolation effects in the realignment of fMRI time series. Neuroimage. 2000;11(1):49–57.
64. Desmond JE, Atlas SW. Task-correlated head movement in fMR imaging: false activations can contaminate results despite motion correction. AJNR Am J Neuroradiol. 2000;21(8):1370–1.
65. Binder JR, Swanson SJ, Hammeke TA, Morris GL, Mueller WM, Fischer M. Determination of language dominance using functional MRI: a comparison with the Wada test. Neurology. 1996;46:978–84.
66. Arora J, Pugh K, Westerveld M, Spencer S, Spencer DD, Todd Constable R. Language lateralization in epilepsy patients: fMRI validated with the Wada procedure. Epilepsia. 2009 Oct;50(10):2225–41.
67. Ramsey NF, Sommer IE, Rutten GJ, Kahn RS. Combined analysis of language tasks in fMRI improves assessment of hemispheric dominance for language functions in individual subjects. Neuroimage. 2001;13(4):719–33.
68. Suarez RO, Whalen S, Nelson AP, Tie Y, Meadows ME, Radmanesh A, Golby AJ. Threshold-independent functional MRI determination of language dominance: a validation study against clinical gold standards.Epilepsy Behav. 2009 Oct;16(2):288–97. Epub 2009 Sep 4.
69. Lee DJ, Pouratian N, Bookheimer SY. Martin NA. J Neurosurg: Factors predicting language lateralization in patients with perisylvian vascular malformations; 2010 [Epub ahead of print].

70. Lehéricy S, Cohen L, Bazin B, Samson S, Giacomini E, Rougetet R, Hertz-Pannier L, Le Bihan D, Marsault C, Baulac M (2000) Functional MR evaluation of temporal and frontal language dominance compared with the Wada test. Neurology 54.
71. Pouratian N, Bookheimer SY, Rex DE, Martin NA, Toga AW. Utility of preoperative functional magnetic resonance imaging for identifying language cortices in patients with vascular malformations. J Neurosurg. 2002;97:21–32.
72. Giussani C, Poliakov A, Ferri RT, Plawner LL, Browd SR, Shaw DW, et al. DTI fiber tracking to differentiate demyelinating diseases from diffuse brain stem glioma. Neuroimage. 2010;52(1):217–23.
73. Cohen MS, DuBois RM. Stability, repeatability, and the expression of signal magnitude in functional magnetic resonance imaging. J Magn Reson Imaging. 1999;10:33–40.
74. Huettel SA, McCarthy G. The effects of single-trial averaging upon the spatial extent of fMRI activation. Neuroreport. 2001;12:2411–6.
75. Lai S, Hopkins AL, Haacke EM, Li D, Wasserman BA, Buckley P, et al. Identification of vascular structures as a major source of signal contrast in high resolution 2D and 3D functional activation imaging of the motor cortex at 1.5T: preliminary results. Magn Reson Med. 1993;30:387–92.
76. Pouratian N, Bookheimer SY, O'Farrell AM, Sicotte NL, Cannestra AF, Becker D, et al. Optical imaging of bilingual cortical representations: case report. J Neurosurg. 2000;93:686–91.
77. Cannestra AF, Pouratian N, Bookheimer SY, Martin NA, Becker D, Toga AW. Temporal spatial differences observed by functional MRI and human intraoperative optical imaging. Cerebral Cortex. 2001;11:773–82.
78. Roux FE, Boulanouar K, Ranjeva JP, Manelfe C, Tremoulet M, Sabatier J, et al. Cortical intraoperative stimulation in brain tumors as a tool to evaluate spatial data from motor functional MRI. Invest Radiol. 1999;34:225–9.
79. Corina DP, Poliakov A, Steury K, Martin R, Mulligan K, Maravilla K, et al. Correspondences between language cortex identified by cortical stimulation mapping and fMRI. NeuroImage. 2000; 11:S295.
80 Lurito JT, Lowe MJ, Sartorius C, Mathews VP. Comparison of fMRI and intraoperative direct cortical stimulation in localization of receptive language areas. J Comput Assist Tomogr. 2000;24:99–105.
81 Pouratian N, Sicotte N, Rex D, Martin NA, Becker D, Cannestra AF, et al. Spatial/temporal correlation of BOLD and optical intrinsic signals in humans. Magn Reson Med. 2002;47:766–76.
82 Mueller WM, Yetkin FZ, Hammeke TA, Morris GL, 3rd, Swanson SJ, Reichert K, Cox R, Haughton VM (1996) Functional magnetic resonance imaging mapping of the motor cortex in patients with cerebral tumors. Neurosurgery 39:515–520; discussion 520–511.
83. Roux FE, Boulanouar K, Ranjeva JP, Tremoulet M, Henry P, Manelfe C, et al. Usefulness of motor functional MRI correlated to cortical mapping in Rolandic low-grade astrocytomas. Acta Neurochirurgica. 1999;141:71–9.
84. Rutten GJ, van Rijen PC, van Veelen CW, Ramsey NF. Language area localization with three-dimensional functional magnetic resonance imaging matches intrasulcal electrostimulation in Broca's area. Ann Neurol. 1999;46:405–8.
85. Haglund MM, Berger MS, Shamseldin M, Lettich E, Ojemann GA (1994) Cortical localization of temporal lobe language sites in patients with gliomas. Neurosurgery 34:567–576; discussion 576.
86. Sanai N, Berger MS. Mapping the horizon: techniques to optimize tumor resection before and during surgery. Clin Neurosurg. 2008;55:14–9.
87. Cannestra AF, Pouratian N, Forage J, Bookheimer SY, Martin NA, Toga AW. Functional magnetic resonance imaging and optical imaging for dominant-hemisphere perisylvian arteriovenous malformations. Neurosurgery. 2004;55(4):804–12.
88. Asthagiri AR, Pouratian N, Sherman J, Ahmed G, Shaffrey ME. Advances in brain tumor surgery. Neurol Clin. 2007;25(4):975–1003.

Part II

Neuroanatomical Atlas

Neuroanatomical Atlas of Key Presurgical and Cognitive Eloquent Cortex Regions

8

Feroze B. Mohamed, Michael Yannes, Muhammed Malik, and Scott H. Faro

Introduction

In this chapter, we have displayed several important areas of normal functioning adult brain using functional magnetic resonance imaging (fMRI) blood oxygen level-dependent (BOLD) imaging. These images may serve as a reference or template for users of fMRI for brain mapping. The fMR images shown here highlight areas of brain activation arising from simple motor, language, visual, auditory tasks, and cognitive paradigms. An illustration of the key clinical Brodmann areas and corresponding neuroanatomical correlates is presented. Basic functional descriptions of these areas are also included. A somatotopic fMRI mapping of the human motor cortex was created for the tongue, face, hand, wrist, trunk, and foot. A review of the basic functional role of these cortices and potential clinical deficits are also presented.

The fMRI experiments in these conditions were carried out by simple box-car type block design experiments on a 3-Tesla scanner. These included a rest condition where no activity was performed, followed by an activation period where the subject was asked to perform a specific task. The representation of visual function as well as language and auditory areas were also obtained using a block design. In these experiments, a crosshair display was used as a rest condition.

The images shown here are represented in radiological coordinates and are presented in three different orientations: axial (left), sagittal (middle), and coronal (right). The color map overlying the images are statistical maps and the graded change in color from yellow to white represent varying statistical value (*t*-score) from low to high statistical significance. A composite display showing the motor homunculus with corresponding fMRI activation maps is shown at the end of the chapter. The postprocessing of the fMRI data was performed with SPM8 software (Statistical Parametric Mapping, Wellcome Department of Cognitive Neurology, University

F.B. Mohamed, PhD (✉)
Department of Radiology, Functional Brain Imaging Center, Temple University School of Medicine, 3401 North Broad Street, Philadelphia, PA 19140-5103, USA
e-mail: feroze@temple.edu

M. Yannes, BS
Department of Radiology, Temple University School of Medicine, 1316 W. Ontario Street, Philadelphia, PA 19140, USA
e-mail: michael.yannes@gmail.com

M. Malik, BS
Department of Radiology, Temple University School of Medicine, 3401 North Broad Street, Philadelphia, PA 19140, USA
e-mail: muhammed.malik@gmail.com

S.H. Faro, MD
Department of Radiology, Functional Brain Imaging Center, Temple University School of Medicine, 3401 North Broad Street, Philadelphia, PA 19140-5103, USA
e-mail: faros@tuhs.temple.edu

S.H. Faro and F.B. Mohamed (eds.), *Functional BOLD MRI: Principles and Applications*, DOI 10.1007/978-1-4939-1995-6_8,

College of London) [1] running under the Matlab (The Mathworks, Inc.) environment. A Pentium-based PC was used to generate all the images shown in this section (Fig. 8.1).

Key Clinical Brodmann Areas: Neuroanatomical and Cognitive Correlates

- 1, 2, 3 = postcentral gyrus, sensory cortex
- 4 = precentral gyrus, motor cortex
- 6 = supplemental motor area (SMA). Involved in planning of complex coordinated movements
- 7 = parietal, posterior, to postcentral sensory cortex. Involved in visual motor coordination
- 8 = superior frontal gyrus, anterior to premotor cortex. Involved in frontal eye field (control of eye movements), and planning of complex movements
- 9/10/46 = dorsolataral prefrontal cortex. Involved in executive functions
- 10/11/47 = orbitofrontal cortex. Involved in decision-making processes
- 17 = posterior medial occipital, primary visual cortex
- 22/42 = Wernicke's language region (posterior portion of 22). Also includes small portions of 39 and 40
- 23/29/30/31 = posterior cingulate. Involved in memory, spatial awareness, proprioception
- 32/33 = anterior cingulate. Involved in coordinating cognitive functions of the frontal lobe with motor cortex, involved in reward anticipation, motivation as well as decision making
- 39 = inferior parietal lobule, angular gyrus. Involved in word comprehension and arithmetic functions
- 40 = inferior parietal lobule, supramarginal gyrus. Involved in word recognition
- 41/42 = superior mid lateral temporal, primary auditory cortex
- 44/45 = inferior lateral frontal lobe, Broca's language region

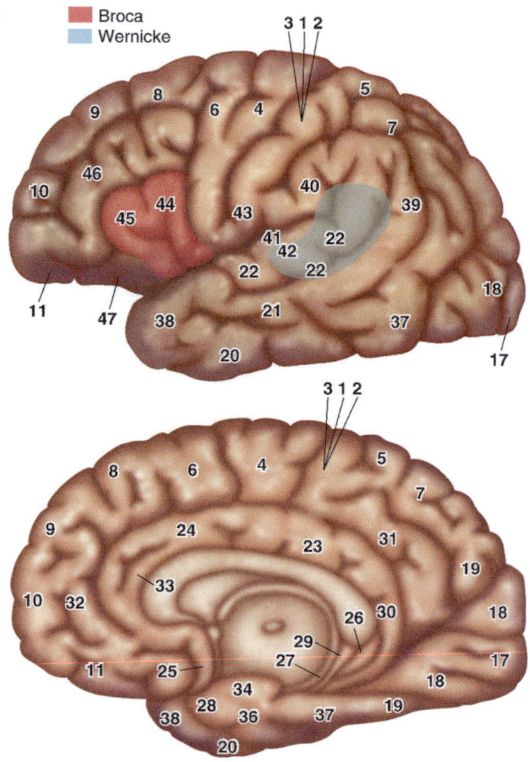

Fig. 8.1 Broca's and Wernicke's areas of the brain

Inferior Frontal Gyrus

Functional role: The inferior frontal gyrus is subdivided into three main areas: the pars opercularis, the pars triangularis, and the pars orbitalis (Brodmann's areas 44, 45, 47). The left inferior frontal gyrus, specifically the pars opercularis and pars triangularis, are considered to be part of Broca's area. Broca's area, in contrast to Wernicke's area, is a major language production center of the brain. Language programs and comprehension is produced in Wernicke's area, and sent anteriorly along the arcuate fasciculus before entering the production centers of Broca's area. Patients with focal lesions to the left inferior frontal gyrus present with symptoms of nonfluent aphasia. In contrast to Wernicke's aphasia, these patients can understand speech, but have difficulty with speech production. Their speech is slowed, yet contains relatively concrete and appropriate nouns, verbs, and adjectives [2] (Fig. 8.2).

Superior Temporal Gyrus

Functional role: In 90% of right-handed people, the left superior temporal gyrus is colloquially called "Wernicke's area." Wernicke's area is considered to be a part of Brodmann areas 22, 39, and 40. Although modern neuroimaging has started to ammend old viewpoints, Wernicke's area is still commonly known as the "language comprehension" center. More specifically, Wernicke's area is believed to be the center that associates sounds and words with concepts and concrete ideas. In Wernicke's area lesions, speech has a relatively normal syntax and rhythm, but its content is unintelligible. The speech has relatively few intelligible nouns, verbs, and adjectives. This presents as a jargon aphasia, in which many phonemic and semantic paraphasias are present [2] (Fig. 8.3).

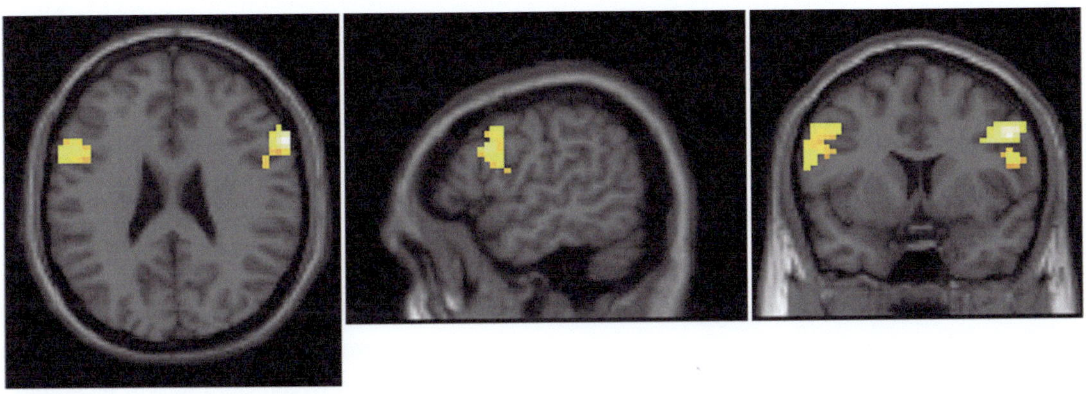

Fig. 8.2 Inferior frontal gyrus: axial (*left*), sagittal (*middle*), and coronal (*right*). *Task description:* Patient was asked to perform a sentence completion task. Designed in a "boxcar" format, with 30 s of fill-in-the-blank sentences and 30 s of gibberish sentences. The action of sentence completion activates many areas of the brain; this scan was masked to only show activation of the inferior frontal gyrus activity (statistical threshold: $P < 0.01$)

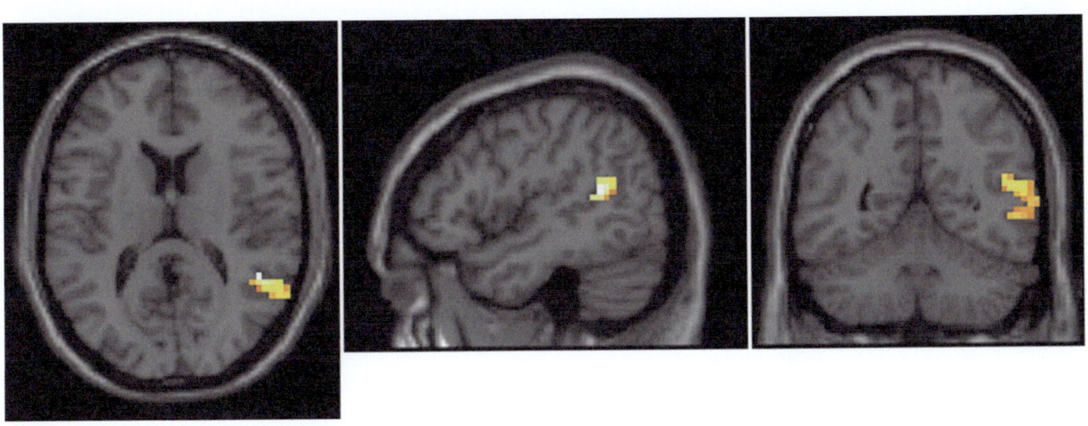

Fig. 8.3 Superior temporal gyrus: axial (*left*), sagittal (*middle*), and coronal (*right*). *Task description:* Patient was asked to perform a sentence completion task. Designed in a "boxcar" format, with 30 s of fill-in-the-blank sentences and 30 s of gibberish sentences. The action of sentence completion activates many areas of the brain; this scan was masked to only show activation of the superior temporal gyrus (statistical threshold: $P < 0.01$)

Middle Frontal Gyrus/Dorsolateral Prefrontal Cortex

Functional role: The middle frontal gyrus roughly correlates to Brodmann's area 46 and parts of Brodmann's area 9 and 10, which is a small part of the dorsolateral prefrontal cortex (DLPFC) The DLPFC is one of the last of all brain regions to develop and myelinate (along with the orbitofrontal cortex), and serves a critical role in executive functioning. These functions include integration of sensory and motor information, and the regulation of intellectual function and action, including concentration, planning, judgment, and problem solving. Perhaps most importantly, the DLPFC has a vital role in regulating working memory, and thus, attention. The DLPFC is closely connected with other areas of the prefrontal cortex, so it is difficult to attribute simply one disease manifestation. However, patients with bilateral lesions to the DLPFC can present with symptoms ranging from abulia to "dysexecutive syndrome." Patient with abulia often have the drive and will to carry out objectives, but lack the attention and drive to follow those through with those objectives [3] (Fig. 8.4).

Superior Frontal Gyrus

Functional role: The superior frontal gyrus is diffusely considered to be part of Brodmann's area 8, and part of 4, 6, and 9. These regions have diffuse functional capabilities. Brodmann area 8 is responsible for initiation of eye movements, and is part of the premotor cortex (Brodmann area 6). The premotor cortex is primarily responsible for the initiation and planning of motor control. This activity is different from stimulation of the primary motor cortex, because it usually elicits more complex movement of multiple joints, resembling natural coordinated movement. Focal lesions to the superior frontal gyrus would cause many far-reaching deficits, including both motor and executive functioning [2] (Fig. 8.5).

Precentral Gyrus

Functional role: The precentral gyrus contains the primary motor cortex. The primary motor cortex corresponds to Brodmann's area 4. Its primary function is the execution, as well as some planning, of movement. The primary motor cortex receives parallel input from the supplementary

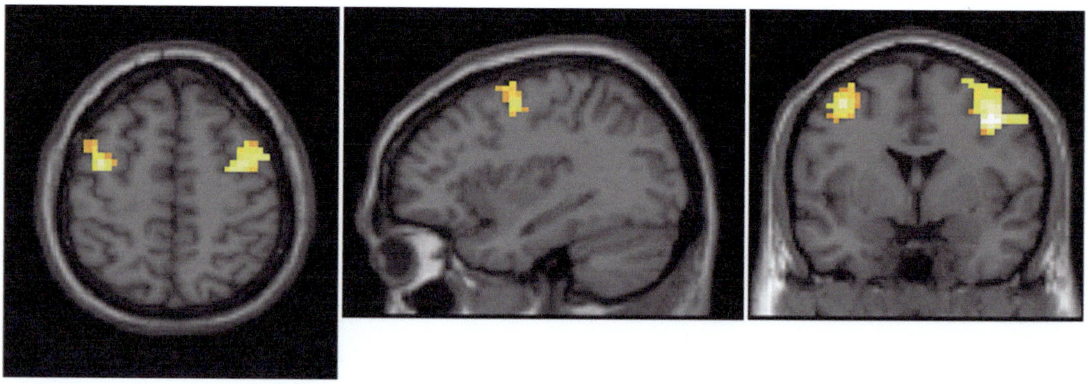

Fig. 8.4 Middle frontal gyrus/dorsolateral prefrontal cortex: axial (*left*), sagittal (*middle*), and coronal (*right*). *Task description:* Patient was asked to perform a sentence completion task. Designed in a "boxcar" format, 30 s of fill-in-the-blank sentences and 30 s of gibberish sentences. The action of sentence completion activates many areas of the brain; this scan was masked to only show activation of the middle frontal gyrus activity (statistical threshold: $P < 0.01$)

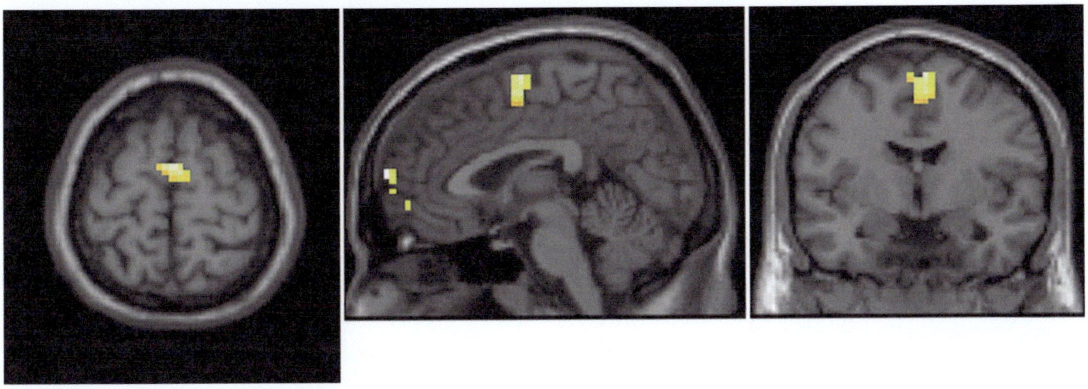

Fig. 8.5 Superior frontal gyrus: axial (*left*), sagittal (*middle*), and coronal (*right*). *Task description:* Patient was asked to perform a sentence completion task. Designed in a "boxcar" format, 30 s of fill-in-the-blank sentences and 30 s of gibberish sentences. The action of sentence completion activates many areas of the brain; this scan was masked to only show activation of the superior frontal gyrus activity (statistical threshold: $P < 0.01$)

motor areas (SMAs), premotor areas, the basal ganglia, as well as the cerebellum to execute fluid, appropriate motor activity. The axons of the primary motor cortex descend down the spinal cord as a major motor tract in the human body (Fig. 8.6a–f).

The primary motor cortex, like the somatosensory cortex posterior to it (Fig. 8.7), is organized somatotopically. This organization is colloquially called a homunculus. The head representation is located more lateral within the gyrus, while the knees and feet hook over the superior aspect of the hemisphere and descend medially. Both motor and sensory homunculi have a disproportionate amount of area corresponding to the face and hands, reflecting the extent of both tactile sensation and manual dexterity given to those areas.

Lesions to one hemisphere's premotor cortex cause contralateral hemiparesis or hemiplegia to the corresponding area of the body represented on the somatotopic representation [2].

Supplementary Motor Area

Functional role: The SMA corresponds to Brodmann's area 6. The SMA is partially responsible for the planning of complex motor activities and bimanual control of those motor activities. While the premotor cortex generates complex motor plans in response to externally generated cues, the SMA generates complex motor plans in response to internally generated cues. An example of this would be performing a motor response by memory, or having a volitional motor response. When motor plans are simply thought about, there is activity in the SMA (Fig. 8.8).

Patients with focal lesions to the SMA most commonly present with motor apraxia, or the inability to perform volitional motor actions, even in the absence of physical paralysis. When asked to do a motor task volitionally, these patients cannot do so (e.g., extending their arm); however, these patients can move spontaneously in response to a stimulus (e.g., using their arm to scratch an itch) [4].

Orbitofrontal Cortex

Functional role: The orbitofrontal cortex corresponds to Brodmann areas 10, 11, and 47. The orbitofrontal cortex works in concert with the anterior cingulate cortex to generate a representation of reward, and importantly, to adjust that concept of reward over time. While the anterior cingulate gyrus generates a more moment-to-moment cost–benefit

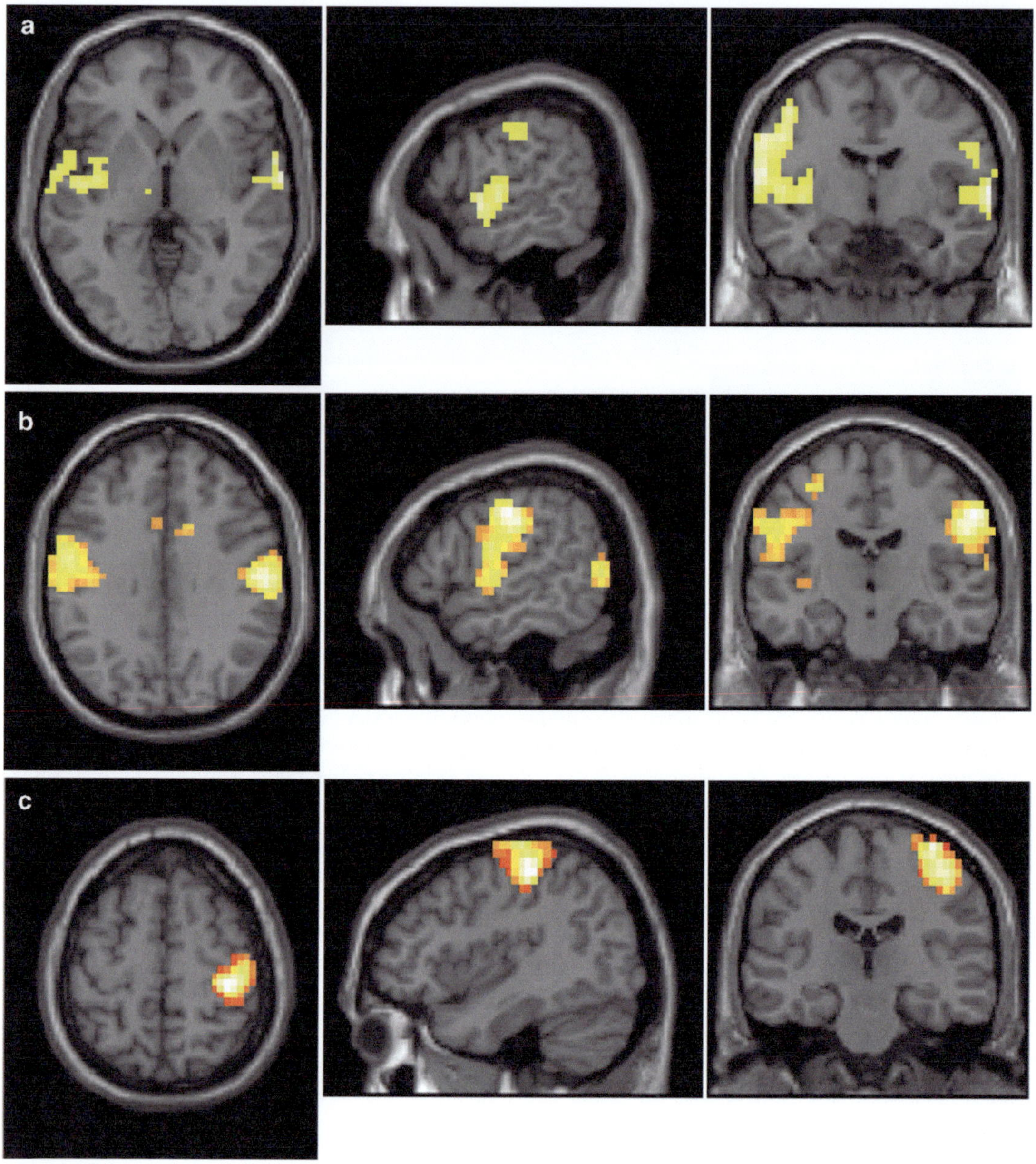

Fig. 8.6 Precentral gyrus: (**a**) Tongue; (**b**) face; (**c**) right hand motor task; (**d**) right wrist; (**e**) trunk; (**f**) foot; axial (*left*), sagittal (*middle*), and coronal (*right*). *Task description:* Patient was asked to move various areas of body. Designed in "boxcar" format, with 10 s of movement and 10 s of inactivity (statistical threshold: $P < 0.01$)

analysis of situations, the orbitofrontal cortex seems to have more of a role in basing decisions on expected outcomes, and modulating those decisions to increase wanted effects in the future. The orbitofrontal cortex provides cognitive flexibility in the face of changing contexts [5] (Fig. 8.9).

The orbitofrontal cortex is one of the later parts of the brain to reach maturity. This may help to biologically explain the impulsive behavior and lack of foresight of teenage youth. Patients with lesions to the oribitofrontal cortex commonly present with "dysexecutive syndrome." In this syndrome, patients often present with poor judgment and foresight, the inability to learn from experiences, emotional lability, and poor interpersonal skills. Interestingly, patients often perform poorly on gambling tasks, situations that require quick cognitive flexibility and assessment of situations.

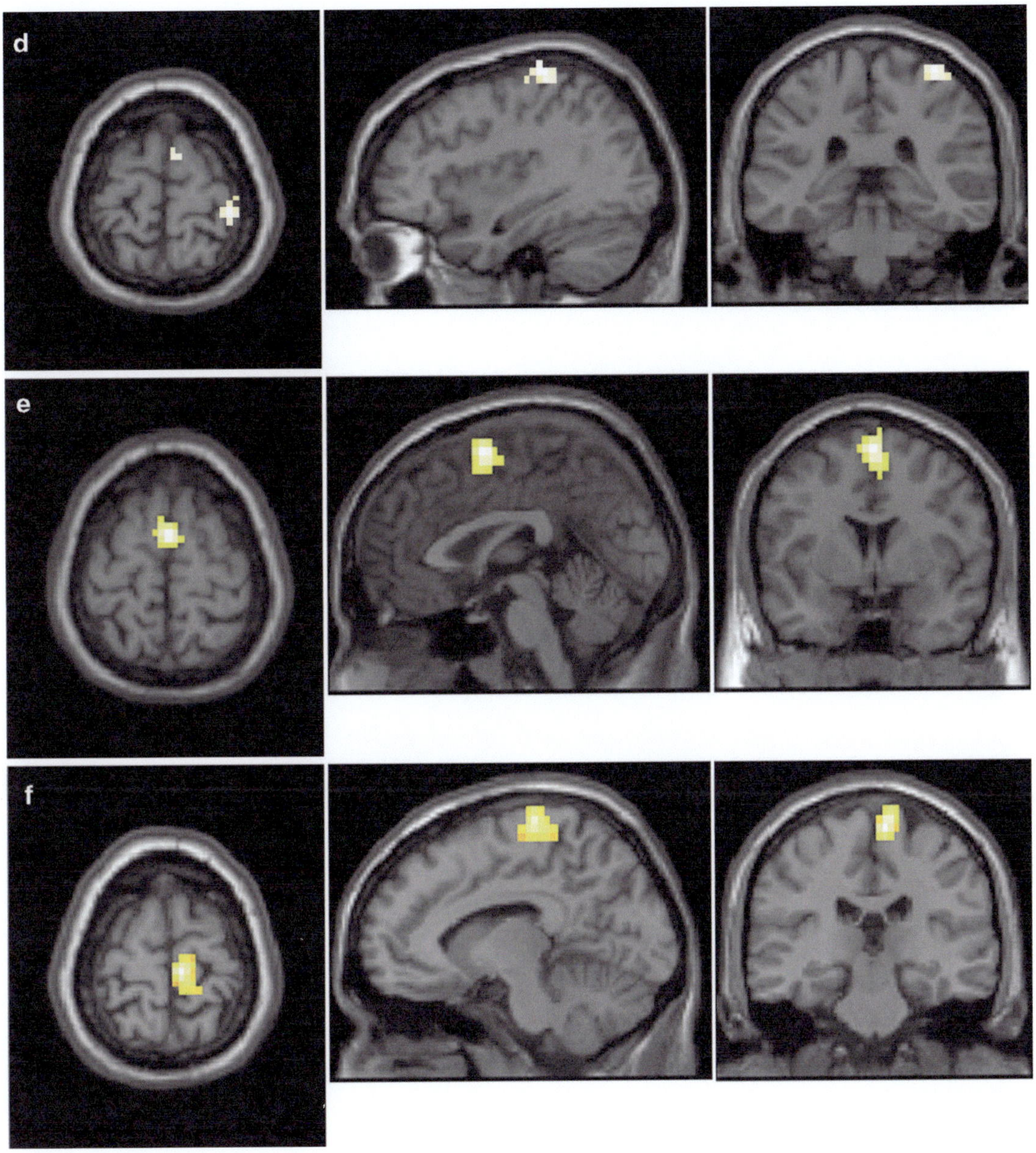

Fig. 8.6 (continued)

Posterior Cingulate Cortex

Functional role: The posterior cingulate cortex corresponds to Brodmann's area 23, 29, 30, and 31. Brodmann's areas 29 and 30 include the retrosplenial cortex, a functionally different area from areas 23 and 31. The retrosplenial cortex has diffuse connections with the anterior thalamus and the hippocampus, leading to its importance in the recall of episodic memory and spatial navigation. The rest of the posterior cingulate cortex is believed to function in proprioception and visuospatial function. Focal lesions to the retrosplenium cortex contribute to anterograde amnesia (Fig. 8.10).

Anterior Cingulate

Functional role: The anterior cingulate cortex correlates to Brodmann's area 32 and 33. The dorsal region of the anterior cingulate cortex helps to

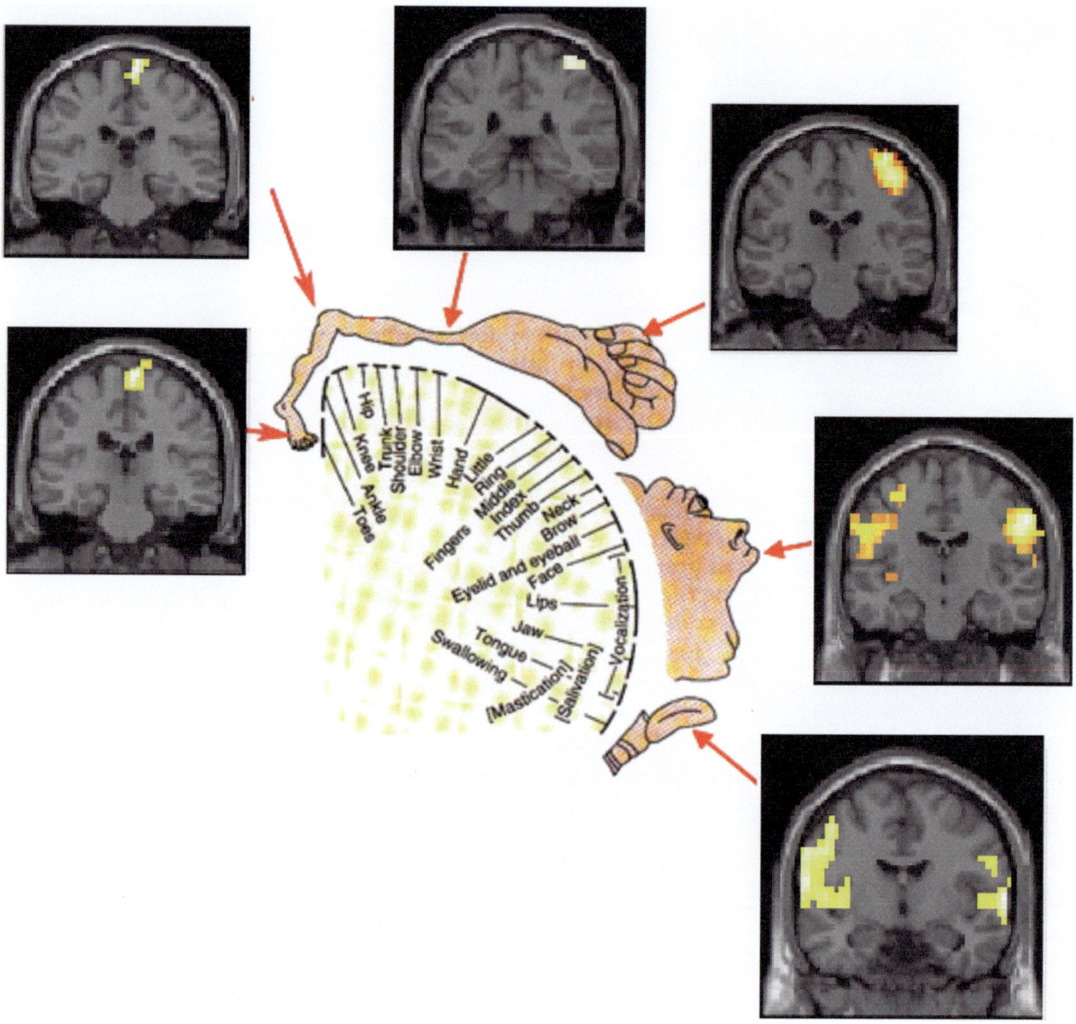

Fig. 8.7 Somatotopic mapping in the human somatosensory motor cortex along with corresponding functional MRI activation patterns

connect cognitive function of the frontal cortices with motor control of the parietal cortices. In this function, it processes and filters stimuli and directs input to different cortical regions. The ventral region of the anterior cingulate cortex has diffuse connections with the amygdala, hypothalamus, nucleus accumbens, and insula. It is part of the circuit involved in reward anticipation and motivation, as well as decision making. The anterior cingulate is the region of the brain that is important in maintaining goals to tasks, as well as the rules to carry them out. In addition, it is important in generating a moment-to-moment cost–benefit analysis of situations. Finally, it is part of the circuit involved in error detection and modulation of emotional responses [6] (Fig. 8.11).

Because of its role in error detection, various psychological tasks elicit anterior cingulate activation. Most notably, these include the Stroop test and Wisconsin Card Sorting Task.

Patients with lesions to the anterior cingulate region thus present with problems in error detection. In addition, the most notable symptom of a lesion to the anterior cingulate is akinetic mutism, or the loss of ability to speak and move. Patients with unilateral lesions to one

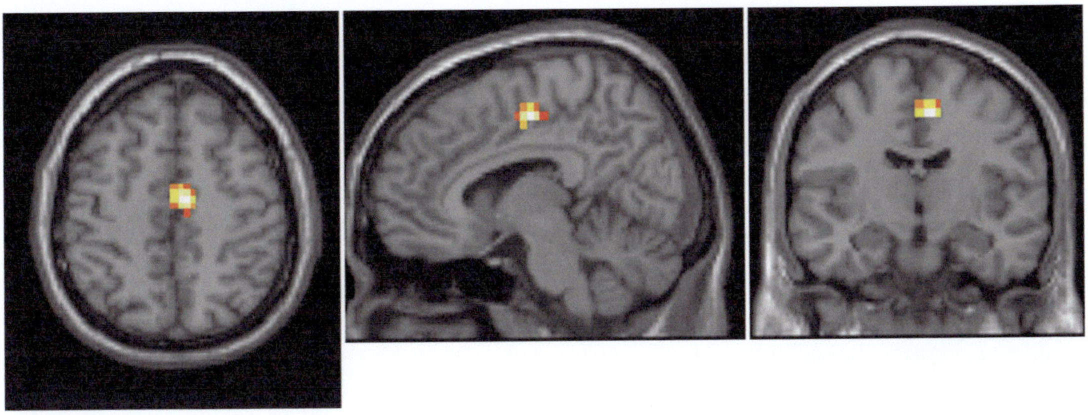

Fig. 8.8 Supplementary motor area: axial (*left*), sagittal (*middle*), and coronal (*right*). *Task description:* Patient was asked to move the foot. Designed in "boxcar" format, with 10 s of movement and 10 s of inactivity. The action of foot movement activates many areas of the brain; this scan was masked to only show activation of the supplementary motor area (statistical threshold: $P < 0.01$)

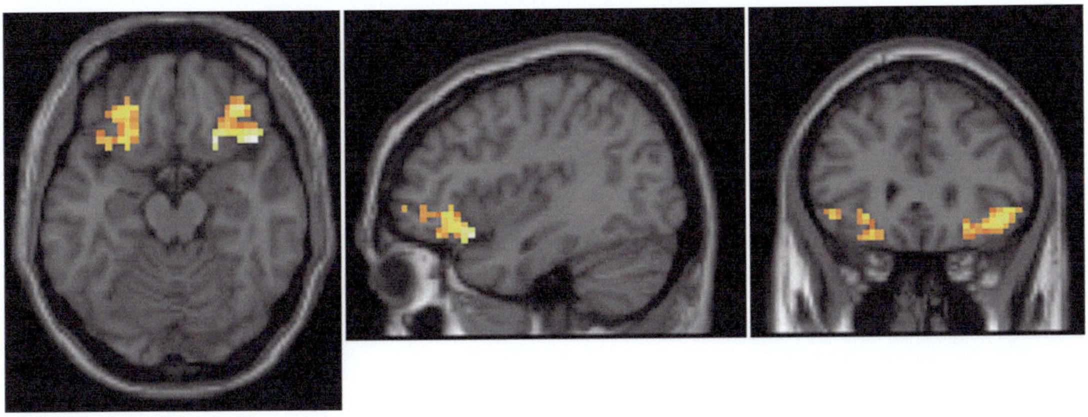

Fig. 8.9 Orbitofrontal cortex: axial (*left*), sagittal (*middle*), and coronal (*right*). *Task description:* Patient was asked to perform a sentence completion task. Designed in a "boxcar" format, 30 s of fill-in-the-blank sentences and 30 s of gibberish sentences. The action of sentence completion activates many areas of the brain; this scan was masked to only show activation of the orbitofrontal cortex (statistical threshold: $P < 0.01$)

hemisphere's anterior cingulated cortex can present with symptoms of "Alien Hand Syndrome," which is categorized by a lack of agency on one side of the body [7].

Cerebellum (Hand Movement)

Functional role: The cerebellum's most understandable role is in motor control. Notedly, the cerebellum does not initiate movement, but rather, is responsible for timing, precision, and coordination of movement. These functions collectively contribute to the role of the cerebellum in fine motor control. Additionally, medial regions of the cerebellum serve as effectors of vestibular input and as controllers of gait. The cerebellum contains a greater number of neurons than any other subdivision in the brain. It is of metencephalic origin, and its defining histological characteristics are that of an extensively branching dendritic system of Purkinje cells. Deficits in cerebellar activity can elicit symptoms of ataxia [2] (Fig. 8.12).

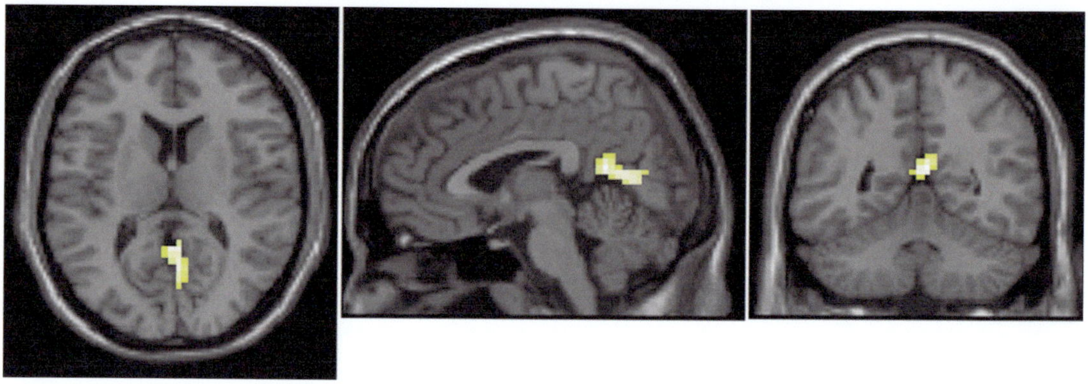

Fig. 8.10 Posterior cingulate cortex: axial (*left*), sagittal (*middle*), and coronal (*right*). *Task description:* Patient was asked to perform a sentence completion task. Designed in a "boxcar" format, 30 s of fill-in-the-blank sentences and 30 s of gibberish sentences. The action of sentence completion activates many areas of the brain; this scan was masked to only show activation of the posterior cingulate (statistical threshold: $P < 0.01$)

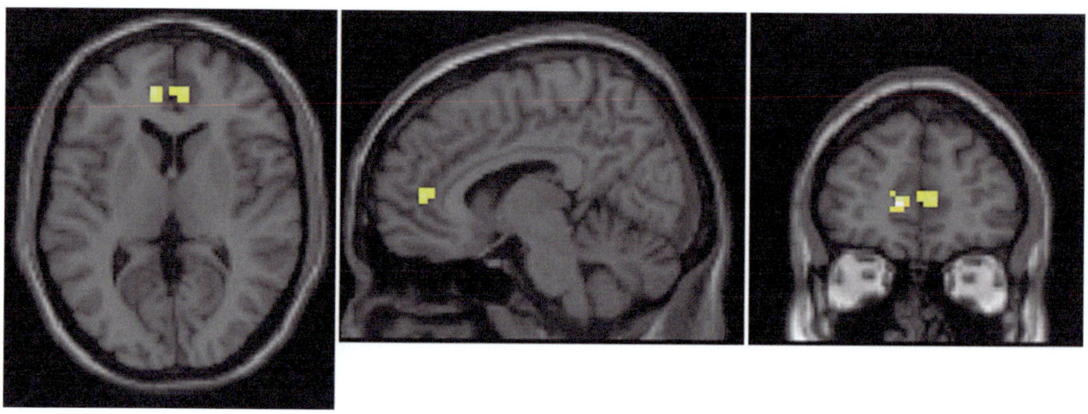

Fig. 8.11 Anterior cingulate: axial (*left*), sagittal (*middle*), and coronal (*right*). *Task description:* Patient was asked to perform a sentence completion task. Designed in a "boxcar" format, 30 s of fill-in-the-blank sentences and 30 s of gibberish sentences. The action of sentence completion activates many areas of the brain; this scan was masked to only show activation of the anterior cingulate (statistical threshold: $P < 0.01$)

Inferior Parietal Lobule

Functional role: The inferior parietal lobule has two subdivisions: the supramarginal gyrus [8] (Brodmann area 40) and the angular gyrus [9] (Brodmann area 39). The supramarginal gyrus has the function of visual word recognition, in regards to both meaning and phonology. The angular gyrus has been found to be involved in understanding metaphors, perhaps underlying its functioning in giving words meaning. Additionally, the angular gyrus appears to have some function in arithmetic. Both of these areas are important in the orderly or sequential performance of tasks (Fig. 8.13).

Inferior parietal lobule focal lesions can be one cause of asteroeognosis, or the inability to identify an object by touch. Additionally, lesions to this region in the non-dominant hemisphere can be one cause of "neglect syndrome," in which the patient fails to recognize the opposite side of the body (usually left) and its surroundings. Lesions to the inferior parietal lobule have most consistently led to the constellation of symptoms known as Gerstmann syndrome,

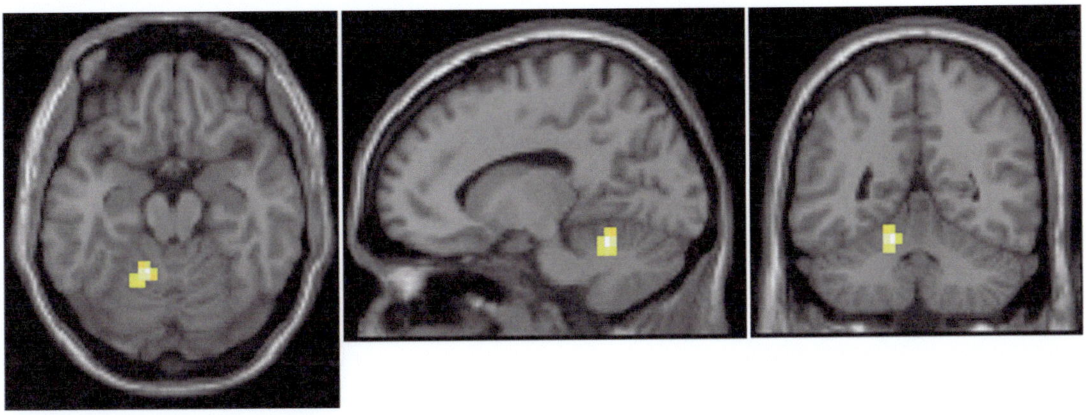

Fig. 8.12 Cerebellum (hand movement): axial (*left*), sagittal (*middle*), and coronal (*right*). *Task description:* Patient was asked to move left hand at radiocarpal (wrist) joint. Designed in a "boxcar" format, 30 s of fill-in-the-blank sentences and 30 s of gibberish sentences. The action of hand movement activates many areas of the brain; this scan was masked to only show activation of the depict cerebellar activity (statistical threshold: $P < 0.01$)

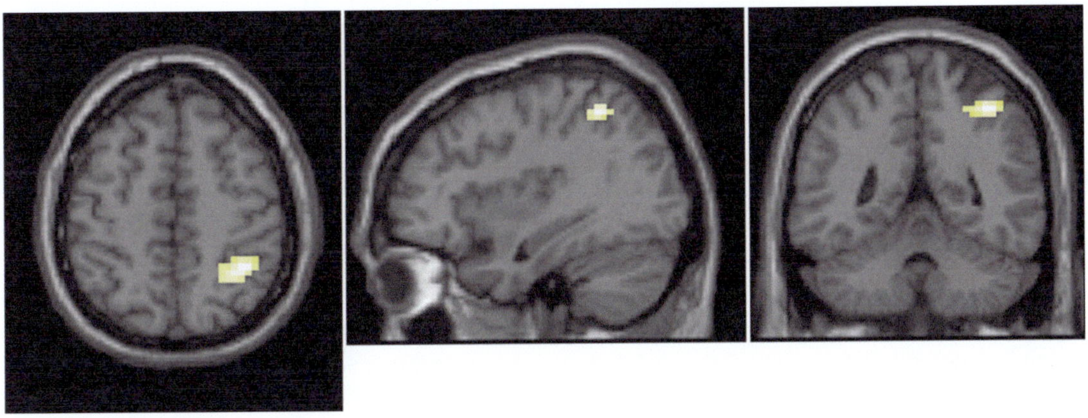

Fig. 8.13 Inferior parietal lobule: axial (*left*), sagittal (*middle*), and coronal (*right*). *Task description:* Patient was asked to perform a sentence completion task. Designed in a "boxcar" format, 30 s of fill-in-the-blank sentences and 30 s of gibberish sentences. The action of sentence completion activates many areas of the brain; this scan was masked to only show activation of the inferior parietal lobule (statistical threshold: $P < 0.01$)

which includes the symptoms of finger agnosia, acalculia, right–left confusion, agraphia, and sometimes alexia [10].

Hippocampus: Medial Middle Temporal Gyrus

Functional role: The hippocampus' most important function is the consolidation of memory and learning, specifically concerning episodic and semantic memories. Interestingly, patients with bilateral lesions to the hippocampus still have the ability to process procedural memories (such as how to ride a bicycle or play an instrument), as well as implicit memory, or recalling information without conscious recollection of knowing it. This suggests that although the hippocampus is critical in memory formation, there are other auxiliary circuits for memory formation (Fig. 8.14).

The mechanism through which the hippocampus "forms" memories is under intense study. However, the leading theory is that stimulating neuronal circuits simultaneously enhances signal

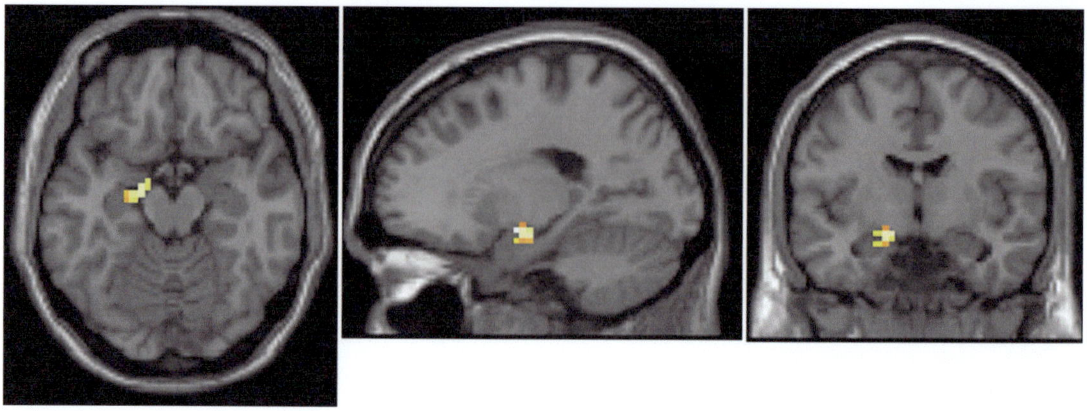

Fig. 8.14 Hippocampus: medial middle temporal gyrus: axial (*left*), sagittal (*middle*), and coronal (*right*). *Task description:* Patient was asked to perform a sentence completion task. Designed in a "boxcar" format, with 30 s of fill-in-the-blank sentences and 30 s of gibberish sentences. The action of sentence completion activates many areas of the brain; this scan was masked to only show activation of the hippocampus (statistical threshold: $P < 0.01$)

transmission through those circuits. This type of activity is called long-term potentiation, or LTP. It is best observed in neurons that have NMDA glutamate receptors; since these receptors are densely found in the hippocampus, this corroborates its function in learning and memory. Having the ability to change synaptic strength with changes in input underlies the concept of synaptic plasticity.

Bilateral lesions to the hippocampal regions result in anterograde amnesia, or the inability to form new memories, and to a lesser extent, retrograde amnesia, or the inability to remember past memories. It is unclear whether hippocampal degeneration is responsible for Alzheimer's disease and dementia in the elderly, although there is evidence suggesting that elderly people who show hippocampal atrophy perform poorly on memory tasks [4].

Transverse Temporal Gyrus

Functional role: The transverse temporal gyrus contains the primary auditory cortex. The primary auditory cortex corresponds to Brodmann's area 41 and 42. Its primary function is in the perception of frequency, sound intensity, and duration. Additionally, one hemisphere's primary auditory cortex functions in the localizing of contralaterally originating sounds. The primary auditory cortex is not the only area that is responsible for localizing sounds; the superior olivary nuclear complex and inferior colliculus also help in this task (Fig. 8.15a, b).

The primary auditory cortex, much like the primary motor and somatosensory cortices, is organized in a predictable manner. Lower frequencies project to more ventral regions of the gyrus, while higher frequencies project to more dorsal regions.

The auditory system has complex bilateral connections, beginning as low as the cochlear nuclei. Thus, lesions to one primary auditory cortex rarely cause difficulty with audition. However, for a short time before the other auditory cortex compensates, there may be a small auditory deficit from the contralateral side [2].

Fusiform Gyrus

Functional role: The fusiform gyrus corresponds to Brodmann's area 37. Located within the inferior temporal gyrus, it is part of the ventral stream of visual processing. More specifically, the fusiform gyrus has been implicated in the processing of faces. In addition, it may be responsible for the differentiation of very closely related objects and

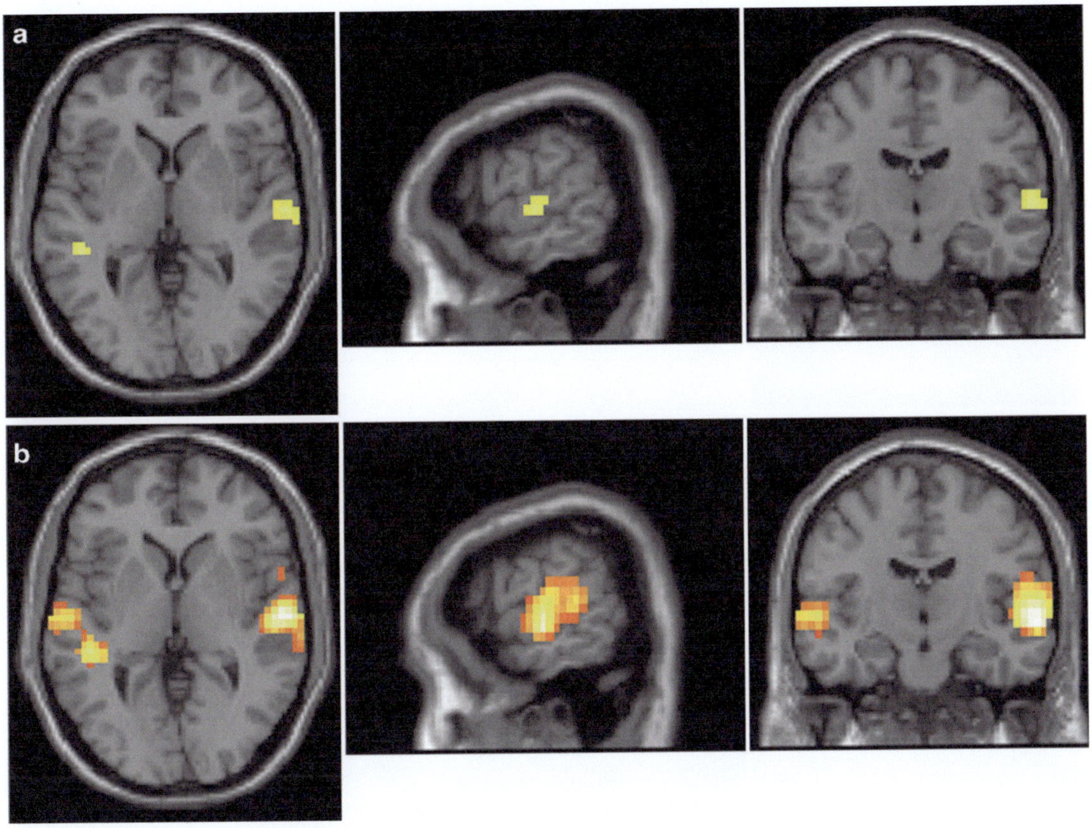

Fig. 8.15 Transverse temporal gyrus: (**a**) audio tone (500 Hz); (**b**) audio tone (1,000 Hz); axial (*left*), sagittal (*middle*), and coronal (*right*). *Task description:* Patient listened to audio tones of (**a**) 500 Hz, and (**b**) 1,000 Hz. Designed in "boxcar" format, with 10 s of audio and 10 s of silence (statistical threshold: $P < 0.01$)

familiar objects, as well as the processing of colors and words [11] (Fig. 8.16).

Patients with bilateral lesions to the fusiform gyrus, in addition to the expected deficits in ventral stream processing, would present with an inability to recognize faces, known as prosopagnosia. In this disease state, patients are able to correctly identify other objects, but cannot identify individual faces. Capgras delusion may be a related disorder to prosopagnosia. In this disorder, patients claim that familiar persons members and loved ones are not real, but rather, imposters. This delusion is believed to be a result of a disconnect of the fusiform gyrus with the limbic system, responsible for associating objects with emotional responses [12].

Visual Cortex

Functional role: The visual cortex is represented by Brodmann's area 17, 18, and 19. It is composed of both the striate cortex (V1), as well as the extrastriate cortex (V2–V5). V1 receives information from the optic radiations projecting back from the lateral geniculate nucleus, and is a well-defined map of spatial information in the visual field. V2–V5 are areas of the visual cortex dedicated to different perception of visual modalities such as form and motion (Fig. 8.17).

There are two pathways from which the visual pathway projects information, a dorsal and a ventral pathway. The dorsal pathway is

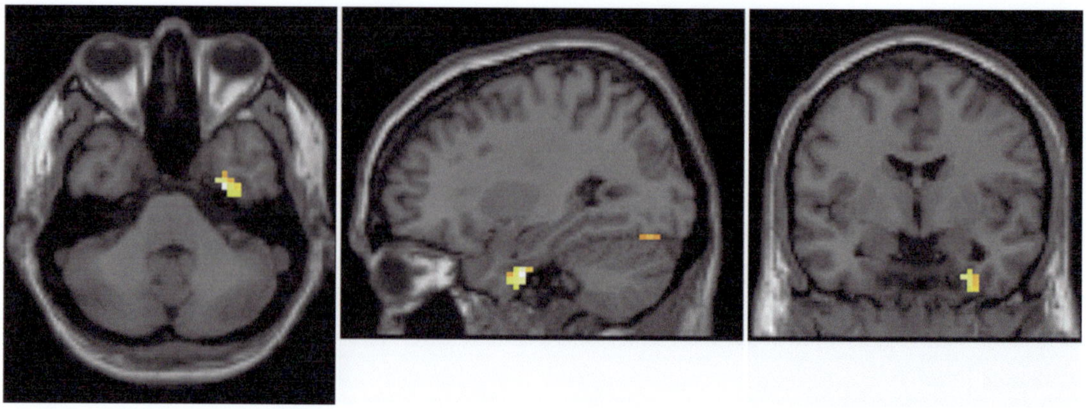

Fig. 8.16 Fusiform gyrus: axial (*left*), sagittal (*middle*), and coronal (*right*). *Task description:* Patient was asked to perform a sentence completion task. Designed in a "boxcar" format, with 30 s of fill-in-the-blank sentences and 30 s of gibberish sentences. The action of sentence completion activates many areas of the brain; this scan was masked to only show activation of the fusiform gyrus (statistical threshold: $P < 0.01$)

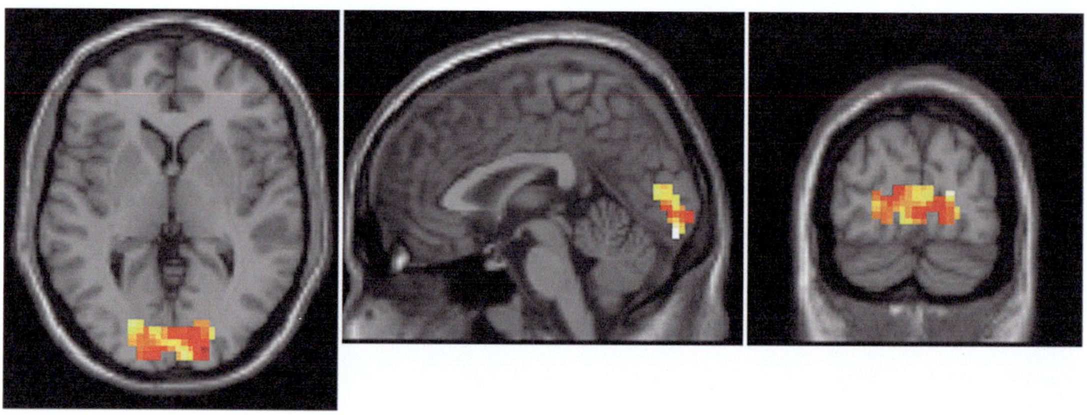

Fig. 8.17 Visual cortex: axial (*left*), sagittal (*middle*), and coronal (*right*). *Task description:* Patient presented with paradigm of alternating checkerboard and crosshair. Designed in "boxcar" format, with 10 s of checkerboard and 10 s of crosshair (statistical threshold: $P < 0.01$)

commonly termed the "where" pathway, and conveys motion information to the heteromodal associative cortex in the posterior parietal lobe. The ventral pathway is commonly termed the "what" pathway, and conveys color and form information to the heteromodal associative cortex in the inferior temporal lobe.

The visual cortex and its associative areas represent a large portion of the cortex. Discreet lesions to different parts of the cortex can lead to a complete loss of vision, homonymous anopsias (loss of a field of vision), deficits in processing motion or object information, or a combination of those functions [2].

Ventral Occipito-Temporal Cortex

Functional role: The ventral occipito-temporal cortex (VOTC) is a relatively newly discovered functional area. It is found roughly in Brodmann area 37. Recent evidence suggests that the VOTC is necessary for object recognition. Interestingly, this activation is adjacent to, and may overlap with the visual word-form area. It may serve as a functional role in higher level unimodal processing of visual information. Interestingly, VOTC activation patterns may vary based on content in the images, suggesting

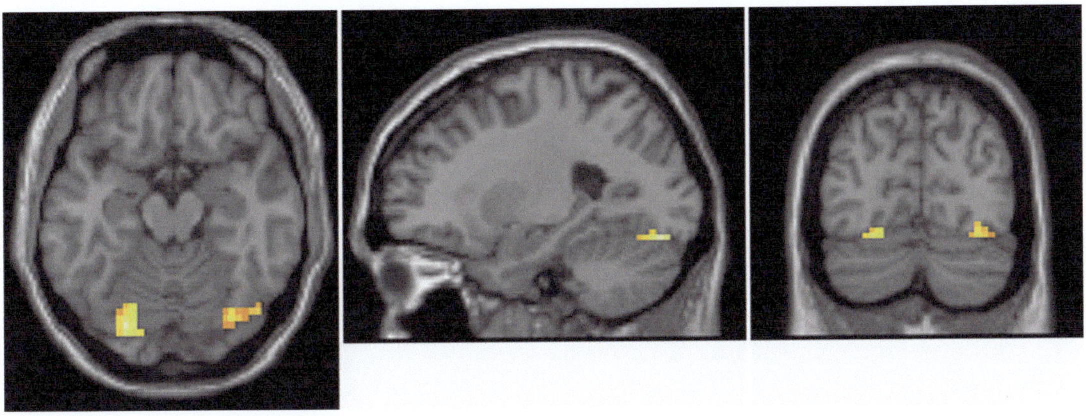

Fig. 8.18 Ventral occipito-temporal cortex (VOTC): axial (*left*), sagittal (*middle*), and coronal (*right*). *Task description:* Patient was asked to perform a sentence completion task. Designed in a "boxcar" format, with 30 s of fill-in-the-blank sentences and 30 s of gibberish sentences. The action of sentence completion activates many areas of the brain; this scan was masked to only show activation of the VOTC (statistical threshold: $P < 0.01$)

other input to this area. Recently, evidence suggests that auditory and visual information are combined additively to sharpen visual category-selective responses. Patients with lesions to VOTC will present with a unimodal associative agnosia [13] (Fig. 8.18).

References

1. Frackowiak RSJ, Friston KJ, Frith CD, Dolan RJ, Mazziotta JC, editors. Human brain function. San Diego: Academic; 1997.
2. Young PA, Young PH, Torbert DL. Basic clinical neuroscience. 2nd ed. Philadelphia, PA: Lippincott Williams & Wilkins; 2008.
3. Blumenfeld H. Neuroanatomy through clinical cases. New York: Sinauer Associates; 2002.
4. Kandel ER, Schwartz JH, Jessell TM. Principles of neural science. 4th ed. New York: McGraw-Hill; 2000.
5. Kringelbach ML. The orbitofrontal cortex: linking reward to hedonic experience. Nat Rev Neurosci. 2005;6(9):691–702.
6. Allman J, Hakeem A, Erwin J. The anterior cingulate cortex: the evolution of an interface between emotion and cognition. Ann N Y Acad Sci. 2001; 935:107–17.
7. Goldberg G. When aliens invade: multiple mechanisms for dissociation between will and action. J Neurol Neurosurg Psychiatry. 2000;68(1):7.
8. Celsis P, Boulanouar K, Doyon B. Differential fMRI responses in the left posterior superior temporal gyrus and left supramarginal gyrus to habituation and change detection in syllables and tones. Neuroimage. 1999;9(1):135–44.
9. Ramachandran VS, Hubbard EM. Synaesthesia – a window into perception, thought and language. J Conscious Stud. 2001;8(12):3–34.
10. National Institute of Neurological Disorders and Stroke. NINDS Gerstmann's Syndrome Information Page. Gerstmann's Syndrome Information Page. NINDS, 2 July 2008. http://www.ninds.nih.gov///.htm. Accessed 18 May 2010.
11. Kanwisher N, McDermott J, Chun M. The fusiform face area: a module in human extrastriate cortex specialized for face perception. J Neurosci. 1997;17(11):4302–11.
12. Ellis H, Lewis M. Capgras delusion: a window on face recognition. Trends Cogn Sci. 2001;5(4): 149–56.
13. Adam R, Noppeney U. Prior auditory information shapes visual category-selectivity in ventral occipito-temporal cortex. Neuroimage. 2010;52(4):1592–602.

Part III

BOLD Functional MRI: Clinical Applications

fMRI of Language Systems: Methods and Applications

9

Jeffrey R. Binder

Introduction

Language functions were among the first to be ascribed a specific location in the human brain [1] and have been the subject of intense research for more than a century. Many researchers across the globe, working in disciplines as varied as linguistics, psychology, neurology, anthropology, and philosophy, have devoted entire careers to understanding language processes and their biological bases, resulting in thousands of books and tens of thousands of research articles on this topic. This overwhelming volume of research attests to the complexity of language and its central importance to human society.

Scientific investigation of the neural basis of language began in earnest with the work of Broca, Wernicke, and other 19th century neurologists [1, 2], leading to the classical *Wernicke–Lichtheim* model of language and aphasia [3, 4]. Regrettably, this already incomplete model has been further simplified by generations of clinical practitioners and general neurology textbooks, to the point where understanding of language processing is often reduced to a simple "expressive/receptive" dichotomy that bears little resemblance to the original model or to the facts at hand [5–7]. Only recently, with the advent of functional imaging methods and particularly their application in clinical situations, has this large gap between scientific knowledge and clinical practice become problematic. Language is best understood as a general term for several distinct cognitive and sensory association processes, each with its own somewhat distinct neural representation. The interpretation of activated areas on fMRI maps requires an understanding of these component processes and how they are differentially engaged by tasks, as well as an understanding of how extralinguistic task factors modulate brain activation, producing activated areas on fMRI maps that are not indicative of language processes.

This chapter provides a very brief overview of some of this information and surveys some hemodynamic imaging techniques for identifying brain regions involved in language processing. The primary goal is to build a common vocabulary and shared knowledge base so that functional imagers might communicate more effectively with language scientists in jointly designing and interpreting fMRI studies.

Some Proposed Clinical Applications of FMRI Language Mapping

Some current techniques used for language mapping include the intracarotid amobarbital (Wada) test [8], electrical stimulation mapping (ESM) with implanted grids or intraoperative electrodes

J.R. Binder, MD (✉)
Department of Neurology, Medical College of Wisconsin, 8701 Watertown Plank Road, MEB Room 4670, Milwaukee, WI, 53226, USA
e-mail: jbinder@mcw.edu

S.H. Faro and F.B. Mohamed (eds.), *Functional BOLD MRI: Principles and Applications*, DOI 10.1007/978-1-4939-1995-6_9, © Springer Science+Business Media New York 2015

[9, 10], positron emission tomography (PET) [11], and magnetic source imaging (MEG) [12]. These methods, while extremely useful, are generally invasive (Wada, ESM), lacking in spatial precision (Wada), costly, or not widely available (PET, MEG). Major advantages of fMRI include excellent spatial resolution, low risk, and wide availability. In addition, fMRI can be performed repeatedly in the same subject within and across scanning sessions, providing improved statistical power, measures of test–retest reliability, the ability to monitor changes in activation serially over time, and the potential for exploring a wide range of cognitive processes.

Presurgical Applications

The primary application for language mapping with fMRI is in identifying critically important language areas prior to brain tumor removal or epilepsy surgery. Optimal presurgical evaluation includes estimation and minimization of the surgical risks. Functional brain mapping techniques can contribute to this process in several ways. By determining the location of important brain functions, mapping techniques might help predict the risk of postoperative language deficits. During the surgical procedure itself, functional maps might be used to minimize such deficits by avoiding important functional areas.

A very large number of fMRI studies and reviews pertaining to this application have been published [13–53]. Recent studies have suggested that fMRI language lateralization is at least as good as the Wada test at predicting postoperative language and verbal memory outcomes [54–56]. One hotly debated issue, which can only be touched on briefly in this chapter, is whether fMRI will ever be able to completely replace more invasive "lesion" methods such as ESM [53]. Whether or not this goal ever comes to pass, however, it seems almost certain that fMRI has the potential to provide valuable adjunctive information concerning localization of language. At least, this information will be useful for identifying patients who require more invasive mapping, such as ESM, because of planned surgery in potentially sensitive regions.

Prediction of Outcome in Aphasia

FMRI language activation measures might be useful in predicting long-term outcome in the acute or subacute phase of acquired aphasia. Long-term outcome is known to be predictable from lesion size, severity of the initial deficit, and regional patterns of resting glucose metabolism [57–64]. FMRI might conceivably offer independent predictive value by detecting residual functional capacity in perilesional or contralateral homologous brain regions. Aside from the intrinsic value of prognostic information for patients and caregivers, such information might also be useful for cost-effective allocation of resources in the rehabilitation setting. No systematic studies of this potential application have as yet been published, although a large number of fMRI studies have investigated chronic patterns of neural reorganization in aphasia [65–77].

Diagnosis

FMRI might prove useful for diagnosis of brain illnesses that perturb language processing but do not cause gross structural changes, such as developmental dyslexia and aphasia, milder forms of autism, schizophrenia, and early dementia. The neurobiological basis for many of these disorders is still not known, and in many cases it remains unclear whether the disease represents a single entity or a group of distinct subtypes. With careful study, it may be possible to define "signature" activation patterns that are highly characteristic of particular illnesses or illness subtypes [78–80]. This information could lead to an improved understanding of such illnesses and how they disrupt normal language processes. These patterns could also be followed over time as an additional indicator of disease progression or stability.

Monitoring Treatment Effects

A small number of studies have shown changes in language-related activation patterns after remediation or rehabilitation therapy for language disorders [81]. While the primary measure of treatment efficacy will always be improvement in behavioral performance, such physiological measures may offer new insights into the mechanisms by which behavioral performance improves, possibly enabling selection of more specific and effective therapeutic strategies.

Language and Language Processes

What is language? One definition often cited is that language processes are those that enable communication. This definition is overly inclusive, however, in that many bodily functions (e.g., cardiac, pulmonary, general arousal, and sustained attention functions) are necessary for communication to occur but are not linguistic in nature. Many linguistic and nonlinguistic tasks require neural systems that process auditory or visual sensory information, hold such information in a short-term store, direct attention to specific features or aspects of the information, perform comparative and other operations on the information, select a response based on such operations, and carry out the response. Careful consideration of these general purpose functions is especially relevant for interpreting and designing language studies, which often employ relatively complex tasks involving motor, sensory, attention, memory, and "central executive" functions in addition to language. Should these other processes be considered part of the language system because they are so necessary for adequate task performance, or should they be delineated from language processes per se? In choosing a control task against which a language task is to be contrasted, investigators tacitly establish which components of the task are not, by their definition, part of the language process in which they are interested. In this chapter, I assume that the goal of language mapping is to identify neural systems involved specifically in language processes, i.e., to distinguish these brain networks from early sensory, motor, and general executive systems.

A more meaningful definition of language is that it is a system of communication based on the symbolic representation and manipulation of information. Languages are also, by definition, *generative*, in that the symbols of a language can be productively combined to make a virtually limitless number of new expressions. In formulating a general definition of this kind, however, it is critical to keep in mind that language is not a unitary process, but rather a collection of processes operating at distinct levels and on distinct types of information. These processes include the following: *phonetics*, the processes governing production and perception of speech sounds; *phonology*, the processes by which speech sounds are represented and manipulated in abstract form; *orthography*, the processes by which written characters are represented and manipulated in abstract form; *semantics*, the processing of word meanings, names, and other declarative knowledge about the world; and *syntax*, the processes by which words are combined to make sentences and sentences analyzed to reveal underlying relationships between words. A basic assumption of language mapping is that activation tasks can be designed to make varying demands on these processing subsystems. For example, a task requiring careful listening to word-like nonwords (often called pseudowords, e.g., "nurdle") would make strong demands on phonetic perception (and on pre-phonetic auditory processing and attention) but very little demand on semantic or syntactic processing, given that the stimuli have no (or very little) meaning. On the contrary, a task requiring semantic categorization of printed words (e.g., Is it an animal or not?) would make great demands on orthographic and semantic processing but relatively little on phonetic, phonological, or syntactic processing.

On the other hand, the processing subcomponents of language often act together. The extent to which each component can be examined in isolation remains a major methodological issue, as it is not yet clear to what extent the systems responsible for these processes become active "automatically" when presented with linguistic stimuli [82]. One familiar example of this is the Stroop effect, in which orthographic and phonological processing of printed words occurs even when subjects are instructed to attend to the color of the print, and even when this processing interferes with task performance [83]. Other examples include semantic priming effects during word recognition, picture–word interference effects, lexical effects on phonetic perception, orthographic effects on letter perception, and semantic–syntactic interactions during sentence comprehension [84–92]. If linguistic stimuli such as words and pictures evoke obligatory, automatic language processing, these effects need to be considered in the design and interpretation of language activation experiments. Use of such stimuli in a baseline condition could result in undesirable subtraction (or partial subtraction) of language-related activation. Because investigators frequently try to match stimuli in control and language tasks very closely, such inadvertent subtraction is relatively commonplace in functional imaging studies of language processing. One example is the widely employed "word generation" task, which is sometimes paired with a control task involving repetition or reading of words [93–95]. In most of these studies, which were aimed at detecting activation related to semantic processing, there has been relatively little activation in temporal and parietal areas that are known to be involved in semantic processing. In contrast, subtractions involving control tasks that use nonlinguistic stimuli generally reveal a much more extensive network of left hemisphere temporal, parietal, and frontal language processing areas [5, 82, 96, 97].

A final crucial theoretical issue is the extent to which language processes occur during "resting" states or states with minimal task requirements (e.g., visual fixation or passive stimulation). Language involves interactive systems for manipulating *internally stored knowledge* about words and word meanings. In examining these systems, we typically use familiar stimuli or cues to engage processing, yet it seems likely that activity in these systems could occur independently of external stimulation and task demands. The idea that the conscious mind can be internally active independent of external events has a long history in psychology and neuroscience [98–103]. When asked, subjects in experimental studies frequently report experiencing seemingly unprovoked thoughts (including words and recognizable images) that are unrelated to the task at hand [101, 104, 105]. The precise extent to which such "mind wandering" engages linguistic knowledge remains unclear [106, 107], but many researchers have demonstrated close parallels between behavior and language content, suggesting that at least some internal thought processes make use of verbally encoded semantic knowledge and other linguistic representations [106, 108, 109]. Recent functional imaging studies have made it abundantly clear that "rest" and similar conditions are actually active states in which subjects frequently are engaged in processing linguistic and other information [110–118]. Use of such states as control conditions for language imaging studies may thus obscure similar processes that occur during the language task of interest. This is a difficult problem because the internal processes in question cannot be directly measured or precisely controlled.

Some Common Pitfalls in Language Mapping

Many different language and control tasks are in use at different imaging centers (see, for example, http://www.asfnr.org/paradigms.html), and there has been very little standardization or validation of these protocols. The typical activation patterns resulting from these various protocols, to the extent that they are known with any certainty, are often strikingly different. Many include unexpected activation in early visual or auditory areas, motor areas, or dorsal parietal regions. Others show similar patterns of activation despite being designed to elicit entirely different functions (see, for example, the "Auditory Responsive Naming" and "Semantic Decision" paradigms at http://www.asfnr.org/paradigms.html). The reasons for this variability and lack of control are not mysterious – they are the product of inadequate consideration of the cognitive processes involved in the language and baseline conditions being compared. A few concrete examples to illustrate some of these problems are given as follows.

Inadequate Analysis of Language Tasks

As was mentioned earlier, clinicians have been taught for generations to categorize language functions as "expressive" or "receptive." Leaving aside the widespread misuse of these terms (any patient in an emergency room who has trouble speaking is now labeled "expressive aphasia" even if their speech is fluent jargon), these terms have very limited utility for analyzing or predicting the results of fMRI language studies. A standard "expressive" task such as word production (e.g., word generation, picture naming, spontaneous speech) relies on a number of component language processes that are similar or identical to components underlying a standard "receptive" task such as word comprehension. Word production begins with retrieval of a concept from a store of semantic knowledge (semantic processing), followed by activation of a sound-based representation of the target word (phonological processing) [119]. Both of these processes are required for word comprehension as well, thus there is considerable overlap in the brain regions activated by production and comprehension tasks [120]. In most word production tasks, the subject is given a cue of some kind, whether an experimental stimulus, picture, or question, which requires comprehension of the cue using phonetic or orthographic analysis, phonological processing, and semantic processing. Thus a simple expressive/receptive classification scheme is entirely inadequate for characterizing the processes elicited by a given task, potentially leading to misinterpretation of activation responses, erroneous predictions, and general confusion about the utility of a task in a given clinical situation.

Inadequate Control Tasks

It is well known that blood oxygen level dependent (BOLD) fMRI signals are not absolute measures of neural activity, but reflect a complex combination of neurovascular coupling, blood flow, and oxygen extraction. Equally important to remember is that activation maps do not represent the signal in a single condition, but rather the *difference* in signal between two (or more) conditions. Thus, the control (or baseline) condition is as important as the language condition in determining an activation pattern. Extremely different patterns can result from the same language task when contrasted with different control conditions [121]. Conversely, very similar patterns can result from very different language tasks when these are contrasted with different control conditions. If the aim is to identify regions specifically involved in language processes, then the baseline condition must control for any early auditory or visual sensory processing, as well as any "general executive" (arousal, attention, working memory, decision) and motor response requirements of the language task. One unfortunately very common example of inadequate control is the use of a resting or visual fixation baseline (see, for example, http://www.asfnr.org/paradigms.html). When this baseline is used with a language task consisting of listening to words or sentences, the activation pattern is dominated by bilateral activation of the superior temporal gyrus and Heschl's gyrus. Many authors refer to this bilateral activation as "Wernicke's area," implying that it represents critical language comprehension zones. In fact, however, this region consists of early auditory and auditory association cortex [122–126]. Isolated unilateral damage to this region, even on the left side, rarely causes speech or language comprehension deficits [127, 128], and the lesions that cause Wernicke aphasia are posterior and ventral to this region, in the middle temporal gyrus and inferior parietal lobe [129, 130].

To the inexperienced eye, discussion of such problems may seem at first to be nothing more than academic exercises, designed perhaps to needlessly complicate the situation or exclude the uninitiated. But consider the real consequences of labeling bilateral auditory cortex as "Wernicke's area" in a patient about to undergo left temporal lobe surgery. First, because the activation is likely to be bilateral, the surgeon may believe, probably inaccurately, that the patient has "bilateral language." In fact, the activation produced by this passive listening fMRI paradigm, which mainly represents auditory processing, is not correlated with language lateralization measured by the Wada test [30]. Second, the surgeon might needlessly avoid activated areas in the HG and STG, leading to incomplete resection of a mass or epileptic focus. Third, and perhaps most importantly, the use of a resting baseline has prevented the surgeon from seeing language areas in the middle temporal gyrus and inferior parietal lobe that play a more central role in lexical–semantic processing, because these regions are also active during the resting state [6, 112, 121, 130, 131]. Resection of these regions, declared "safe to remove" by the fMRI test, is likely to produce language comprehension and production deficits.

Lack of Behavioral Data

Many fMRI language paradigms do not include collection of measureable behavioral responses from the subject. In some cases, as in the widely used "silent word generation" paradigm, measurement of vocal responses is felt to be too technically difficult or likely to produce artifacts (but see numerous examples of vocal responses used in fMRI [132–135]). In other cases, as in the passive listening task, there is no actual task specified for the subject to perform. The weakness of such paradigms is that there is no objective evidence of what cognitive state the subject was in during the scan. If the subject was given a task, there is no verification that the subject performed the task or how well it was performed. If no task was given, there is no knowledge of whether the subject attended to the stimuli at all. These are not major problems when the subjects are highly motivated and healthy volunteers. The situation is quite different, however, when studying cognitively impaired neurological patients whose attention and motivation may be in question. Without behavioral data, it is usually impossible to tell whether abnormal activation is the result of brain disease, inattention, or poor compliance with task instructions.

Survey of Common Language Activation Protocols

This section describes some of the task contrasts that have been used in language activation studies and the results that can be expected. A schematic model of some of the major left hemisphere regions involved in language is shown in Fig. 9.1, color-coded according to their putative functional roles. The variety of possible stimuli and tasks that could be used to engage these language processes is vast, and a coherent, concise discussion is difficult. Table 9.1 lists some of the broad categories of stimuli that have been used and some of the brain systems they tend to engage.

"Auditory Nonspeech" refers to noises or tones that are not perceived as speech. Such stimuli can be variably complex in their temporal or spectral features, and possess to varying degrees the acoustic properties of speech (see [123, 136–139]). They activate primary and association auditory cortex to varying degrees depending on their precise acoustic characteristics. "Auditory Phonemes" are speech sounds that do not comprise words in the listener's language; these may be simple consonant–vowel monosyllables or longer sequences. In addition to early auditory cortex, speech phonemes activate "auditory word-form" systems that are relatively specialized for the perception of speech sounds, whether presented in the form of nonwords, words, or sentences [123, 136, 138–143].

"Visual Nonletter" refers here to any visual stimulus not recognized by the subject. Examples include characters from unfamiliar alphabets, nonsense signs, and false font. Such stimuli can be variably complex and possess to varying degrees the visual properties of familiar letters. They activate primary and association visual cortex to varying degrees depending on their visual characteristics. "Visual Letter Strings" are random strings of letters that do not form familiar or easily pronounceable letter combinations (e.g., FCJVB). "Visual Pseudowords" are letter strings that are not words but possess the orthographic and phonological characteristics of real words (e.g., SNADE). Letter strings are claimed to activate a "visual word-form area" located in the left posterior occipitotemporal sulcus; this area responds more strongly to pseudowords and words than to random letter strings [144–146].

The degree to which these stimuli engage the processes listed in Table 9.1 may depend partly on the task that the subject is asked to perform, although the processes in Table 9.1 seem to be

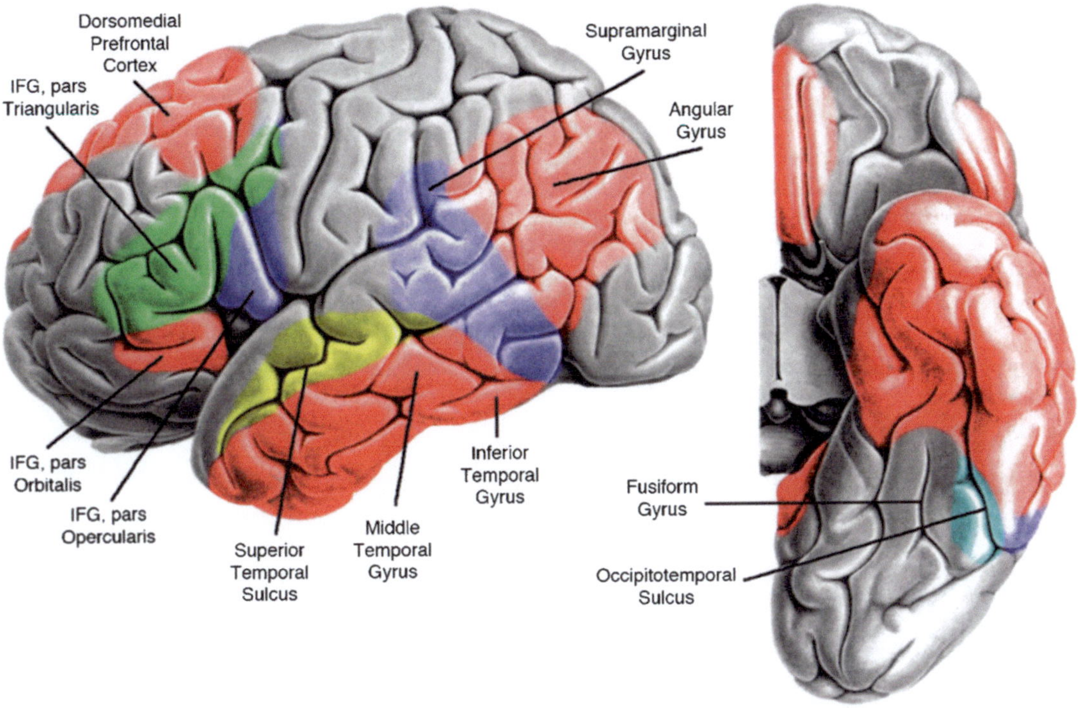

Fig. 9.1 Schematic drawing of some putative language areas in the dominant hemisphere. Yellow = phoneme and auditory word form perception area. Red = semantic storage and retrieval systems. Blue = phonological access and phonological output systems. Light blue = visual word form perception area. Green = general verbal retrieval, selection, and working memory functions

Table 9.1 Stimulus effects on sensory and linguistic processing systems

Stimuli	Early sensory	Auditory word form	Visual word form	Object recognition	Syntax
Auditory nonspeech	Aud	–	–	–	–
Auditory phonemes	Aud	+	–	–	–
Auditory words	Aud	+	–	–	–
Auditory sentences	Aud	+	–	–	+
Visual nonletters	Vis	–	–	–	–
Visual letter strings	Vis	–	+/–	–	–
Visual pseudowords	Vis	–	+	–	–
Visual words	Vis	–	+	–	–
Visual sentences	Vis	–	+	–	+
Visual objects	Vis	–	–	+	–

activated relatively automatically even when subjects are given no explicit task. This is less true for the processing systems listed in Table 9.2, which are more strongly task-dependent. The semantic system makes up a large part of the "default mode network" active during "rest" and similar states with low attentional demands [111, 112, 114, 116–118, 121, 131]. Nonsemantic tasks can suppress this ongoing semantic processing by requiring a focusing of attention on perceptual, orthographic, or phonological properties of stimuli [112, 115–117, 121, 131]. Examples include "Sensory Discrimination" tasks (e.g., intensity, size, color, frequency, or more complex

Table 9.2 Effects of task states on some linguistic processing systems

Tasks	Semantics	Phonological Access	Speech Articulation	Working Memory	Other Language
Rest or "Passive"	+	–	–	–	–
Sensory discrimination	–	–	–	+/–	–
Read or repeat covert	+	+	–	+/–	–
Read or repeat overt	+	+	+	+/–	–
Phonetic decision	–	+	–	+	–
Phonological decision	–	+	–	+	–
Orthographic decision	–	+/–	–	–	–
Semantic decision	+	+/–	–	+	Semantic search
Word generation covert	+	+	–	+	Lexical search
Word generation overt	+	+	+	+	Lexical search
Naming covert	+	+	–	–	Lexical search
Naming overt	+	+	+	–	Lexical search

feature-based discriminations), "Phonetic Decision" tasks in which the subject must detect a target phoneme or phonemes, "Phonological Decision" tasks requiring a decision based on the phonological structure of a stimulus (e.g., detection of rhymes, judgment of syllable number), and "Orthographic Decision" tasks requiring a decision based on the letters in the stimulus (e.g., case matching, letter identification). Other tasks, such as reading and repeating, make no overt demands on semantic systems but may elicit automatic semantic processing. The extent to which this occurs probably depends on how meaningful the stimulus is: sentences likely elicit more semantic processing than isolated words, which in turn elicit more than pseudowords. Finally, many tasks make overt demands on retrieval and use of semantic knowledge. These include "Semantic Decision" tasks requiring a decision based on the meaning of the stimulus (e.g., "Is it living or nonliving?"), "Word Generation" tasks requiring retrieval of a word or series of words related in meaning to a cue word, and "Naming" tasks requiring retrieval of a verbal label for an object or object description.

"Phonological Access" refers to the processes engaged in retrieving a phonological (sound-based) representation of a word. These processes are required for both overt and covert reading, repeating, naming, and word generation. In addition, any task that engages reading, such as an orthographic or semantic decision on printed words or pseudowords, will automatically engage phonological access processes to some degree [82, 83, 90]. In contrast, "Speech Articulation" processes are engaged fully only when an overt spoken response is produced [147]. Verbal "Working Memory" is required whenever a written or spoken stimulus must be held in memory. This applies to repetition tasks if the stimulus to be repeated is relatively long, to auditory decision tasks if the auditory stimulus must be remembered while the decision is being made, and to most word generation tasks, since the cue must be maintained in memory while the response is retrieved. Finally, semantic decision, word generation, and naming tasks make strong demands on frontal mechanisms involved in searching for and retrieving information associated with a stimulus.

With these somewhat oversimplified stimulus and task characterizations, it is possible to make some general predictions about the processing systems whose level of activation will differ when two task conditions are contrasted, and thus the likely pattern of brain activation that will be observed in a subtraction analysis. Some commonly encountered examples are listed as follows and in Table 9.3.

Table 9.3 Some task contrasts used for language mapping and the regions in which robust activations are typically observed

	Ventrolateral prefrontal	Dorsal prefrontal	Superior temporal	Ventrolateral temporal	Ventral occipital	Angular gyrus
Hearing words vs. rest			B			
Hearing words vs. nonspeech sounds			L > R			
Word generation vs. rest	L > R			L > R	B	
Word generation vs. reading	L					
Object naming vs. rest	B			L > R	B	
Semantic decision vs. sensory discrimination	L	L	L > R	L		L
Semantic decision vs. phonological decision		L		L		L
Reading sentences vs. letter strings	L > R		L > R	L > R		

L left hemisphere, *R* right hemisphere, *B* bilateral

Language Task: Passively Listening to Words or Sentences

Control Task: Rest

As shown in Table 9.1, auditory words activate early auditory cortices and auditory word-form areas. Because both rest and passive stimulation are accompanied by spontaneous semantic processes and make no other overt cognitive demands, no other language systems should appear in the contrast. These predictions are confirmed by many studies employing this contrast, which results primarily in activation of the superior temporal gyrus auditory cortex bilaterally (Fig. 9.2a) [123, 148–150]. The activation is relatively symmetrical and is unrelated to language dominance as measured by Wada testing [30].

Language Task: Passively Listening to Words or Sentences

Control Task: Passively Listening to Nonspeech

Because there are no differences in task requirements in this contrast, and because semantic processing occurs in all passive conditions, the activation pattern depends mainly on acoustic differences between the speech and nonspeech stimuli. Studies employing such contrasts reliably show stronger activation by words in the middle and anterior superior temporal sulcus, with some leftward lateralization, and little or no activation elsewhere (Fig. 9.2b) [123, 136, 151–153]. Similar patterns are observed whether the speech stimuli are words or pseudowords [123].

Language Task: Word Generation

Control Task: Rest or Fixation

The word generation task requires the subject to think of a word in response to a cue of some kind. In some protocols, a single cue (e.g., a letter, word, or semantic category) is provided only at the beginning of an activation period; in others, a different cue is provided every few seconds. Because the rest state includes no control for sensory processing, early auditory or visual cortices may be activated bilaterally depending on the sensory modality of the cue stimulus (Table 9.1), though the strength of this activation depends on the rate of cue presentation. Unlike rest, word generation makes demands on phonological access, verbal working memory, and lexical search systems (Table 9.2). Speech articulation systems will also be activated if an overt spoken response is used. These predictions are confirmed by many studies employing this contrast, which mainly activates the left inferior frontal gyrus and left greater than right premotor cortex, systems thought to be involved in phonological production, verbal working memory, and lexical search [22, 23, 30, 36, 148, 154–157]. There may be weak activation of left posterior temporal or ventral temporal regions, possibly due to engagement of auditory or visual word form systems.

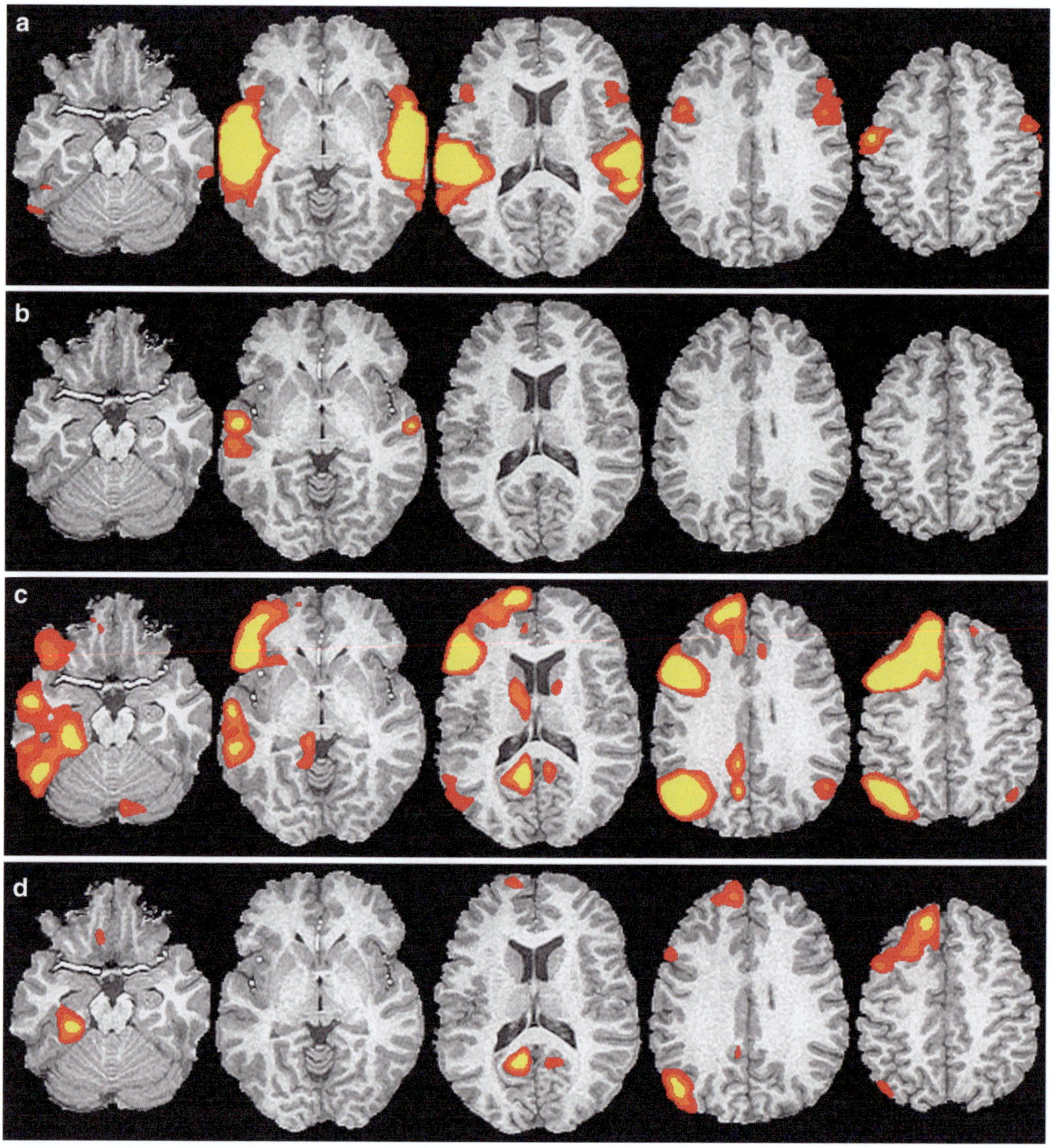

Fig. 9.2 Group average fMRI activation patterns in neurologically normal, right-handed volunteers during four language paradigms. (**a**) Passive listening to spoken words contrasted with resting (28 subjects). Superior temporal activation occurs bilaterally. (**b**) Passive listening to spoken words contrasted with passive listening to tones (same 28 subjects as in *panel A*). Superior temporal sulcus activation occurs bilaterally, more prominent on the left. (**c**) Semantic decision on auditory words contrasted with a tone decision control task (30 subjects). Activation is strongly left-lateralized in inferior frontal, dorsomedial prefrontal, lateral and ventral temporal, angular, and posterior cingulate cortices. (**d**) Semantic decision on auditory words contrasted with a phonological task using pseudowords (same 30 subjects as in *panel C*). Activation is strongly left-lateralized in dorsomedial prefrontal, angular, ventral temporal, and posterior cingulate cortices. There is no activation of Broca's or Wernicke's area. The images are serial axial sections spaced at 15-mm intervals through stereotaxic space, starting at $z = -15$. The left hemisphere is on the reader's left (neurologic coordinate)

Language Task: Word Generation

Control Task: Reading or Repeating

This protocol is similar to the previous one, but with a control task using words in the same stimulus modality. The matched control stimuli remove any activation of sensory or word-form systems. Both tasks are accompanied by semantic processing (automatic semantic access in the case of the control task, effortful semantic retrieval in the case of word generation) and phonological access processes. The word generation task makes greater demands on lexical search and on working memory; consequently, greater activation is expected in left inferior frontal areas associated with these processes. These predictions match findings in many studies using this contrast [93, 94, 155, 158].

Language Task: Visual Object Naming

Control Task: Rest or Fixation

Compared to rest, visual objects activate early visual sensory cortices and object recognition systems bilaterally (Table 9.1) [159–161]. There may be additional, left-lateralized activation in semantic systems of the ventrolateral posterior temporal lobe [162–166]. Unlike rest, naming requires lexical search and phonological access, and, when overt, speech articulation (Table 9.2). These predictions match findings in several studies using this contrast, which show extensive bilateral visual system activation and modest left-lateralized inferior frontal activation [23, 166–168].

Language Task: Semantic Decision

Control Task: Sensory Discrimination

These tasks can be given in either the visual or auditory modality. If the stimuli used for the sensory discrimination task are nonlinguistic (e.g., tones or nonsense shapes), then the semantic decision task will produce relatively greater activation in auditory or visual word-form systems, depending on the sensory modality. In addition, there will be greater activation of phonological access, semantics, and semantic search mechanisms in the semantic decision task. Working memory systems may or may not be activated, depending on whether or not the sensory task also has a working memory demand. These predictions match findings in studies using this contrast, which show left-lateralized activation of auditory (middle and anterior superior temporal sulcus) or visual (mid-fusiform gyrus) word-form regions and extensive activation of left prefrontal, lateral and ventral left temporal, and left posterior parietal systems involved in semantic processing (Fig. 9.2c) [5, 32, 96, 169, 170].

Language Task: Semantic Decision

Control Task: Phonological Decision

This protocol is similar to the previous one but incorporates a phonological control to isolate semantic processing. The stimuli used for phonological decision are either words or pseudowords. Thus, there are no physical differences between the stimuli, and no difference in activation of sensory or word-form systems is expected. There will be greater activation of semantic systems and semantic search mechanisms in the semantic decision task. These predictions match findings in many studies using this contrast, which show activation of left prefrontal, lateral and ventral left temporal, and left posterior parietal systems in semantic retrieval (Fig. 9.2d) [96, 112, 131, 171–175].

Language Task: Sentence or Word Reading

Control Task: Passively Viewing Letter strings

Compared to letter strings, sentences engage visual word-form, syntactic, and phonological access systems, and probably working memory if the words are presented one at a time. Both reading and passive viewing probably involve semantic processing. There should be relative left-lateralized activation of the occipitotemporal (visual word-form) region, posterior superior temporal gyrus and STS (phonological access), and inferior frontal gyrus (phonology, working memory, syntax). These predictions are consistent with several studies using this contrast [82, 176–179].

These examples cover but a small sample of the possible language activation protocols. There are also numerous published studies employing designs that do not fit neatly into the schema provided here. Many of these represent attempts to further define or fractionate a particular language process, or to define further the functional role of a specific brain region. The reader should appreciate that the review given here is merely a coarse outline of some of the most commonly used types of stimuli and tasks. Above all, it is important to note that activations in a particular part of the language system are seldom "all or none," but vary in a graded way depending on the particular stimuli and tasks used.

In many clinical settings, the main goal of language mapping is simply to identify as many language-related areas as possible and to assess hemispheric lateralization of language. A review of Table 9.3 suggests that the "Semantic Decision versus Sensory Discrimination" paradigm may offer advantages for this purpose in terms of the sheer number of regions activated and leftward lateralization of activation. Binder et al. put this prediction to a quantitative test by comparing the extent and lateralization of activation produced by five language-related task contrasts, conducted on the same 26 participants during a single scanning session [121]. These contrasts included the following: (1) passively listening to words versus resting, (2) passively listening to words versus passively listening to tones, (3) performing a semantic decision task with words versus resting, (4) performing a semantic decision task with words versus a sensory discrimination task with tones, and (5) performing a semantic decision task with words versus a phonological task with pseudowords. As shown in Fig. 9.3, the Semantic Decision–Tone Decision contrast produced by far the largest activation volume in the left hemisphere, as well as an optimal combination of extensive activation and strong left lateralization.

Language Lateralization: Normative, Reliability, and Validation Studies

As with any clinical test, the applicability of language mapping techniques to clinical patients depends on the reliability and validity of the results. It goes without saying that any imaging protocol applied to patients should first be tested in a sample of healthy volunteers. The initial aims of gathering normative data in this case are the following: (1) to verify the feasibility of the procedure and estimate the likelihood of obtaining uninterpretable results (i.e., test failures), (2) to verify that activation occurs in the expected brain regions and is lateralized to the left hemisphere in right-handed subjects, (3) to estimate the range of intersubject variability that occurs in the normal population, and (4) to determine the average test–retest reproducibility of the results. If significant variability in results is observed, a secondary aim is to determine some of the factors (e.g., age, sex, handedness) associated with this variability.

Normative Studies

Several language mapping protocols have been carried out in relatively large samples of normal subjects [180–185]. All of these protocols produced left-lateralized activation patterns in right-handed subjects. Lateralization has been quantified in most of these studies using some type of left-right difference score. One commonly used version is based on the left-right difference in the number of activated voxels (activation volume), normalized by the total number of activated voxels (i.e., $[L - R]/[L + R]$). This index varies from -1 (all activated voxels in the right hemisphere) to $+1$ (all activated voxels in the left hemisphere). This type of index depends on the statistical threshold used to classify voxels as "active" and tends to increase with increasingly stringent thresholds due to the elimination of false-positive voxels in both hemispheres [39, 41]. Others have advocated measures based on

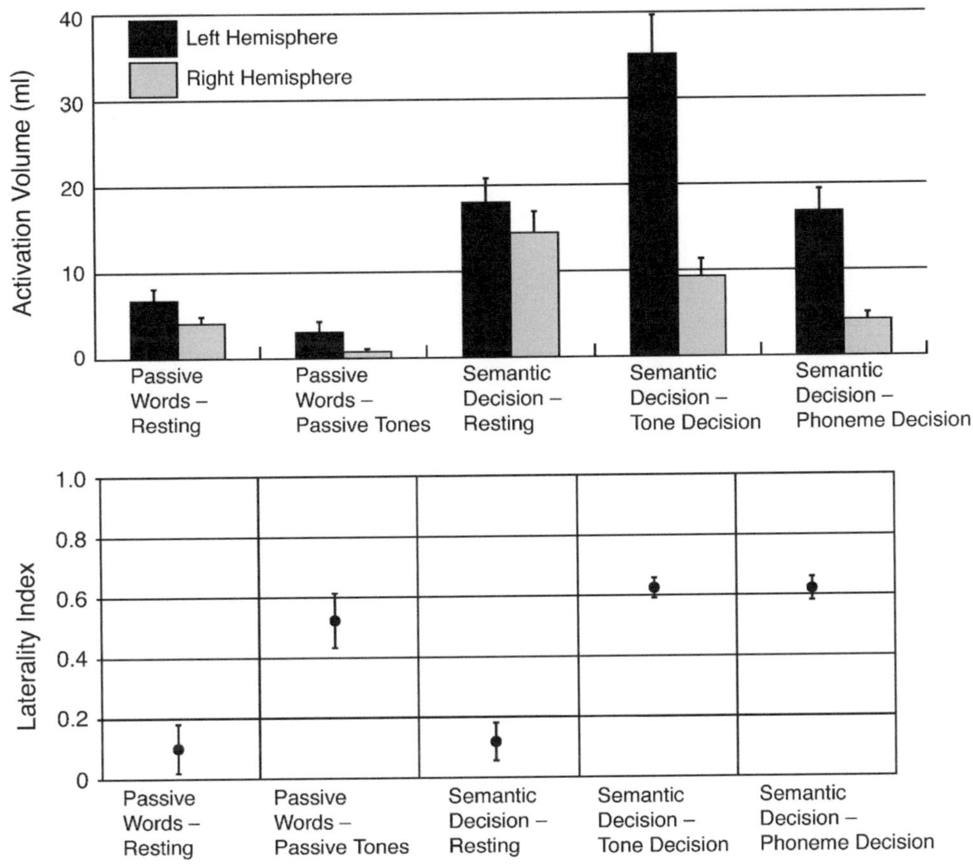

Fig. 9.3 Group average activation volumes (top graph) and laterality indexes (bottom graph) for five fMRI language paradigms [121]. Laterality indexes can vary from −1 (all activation in the right hemisphere) to +1 (all activation in the left hemisphere). Error bars represent standard error. The Semantic Decision – Tone Decision paradigm produces the greatest left hemisphere activation as well as a strongly left-lateralized pattern

magnitude rather than volume of activation [23, 36, 41, 168]. Lateralization indexes (LI) can be computed for the entire hemisphere or for homologous regions of interest (ROIs). Focusing on language-related ROIs avoids the problem of nonspecific or non-language activation in bilateral sensory, motor, and executive systems, which is characteristic of some task contrasts [39, 168].

Figure 9.4 shows the intersubject variability observed for one such LI. The subjects were 100 right-handed healthy adults; they were scanned during a block-design fMRI protocol contrasting an auditory word semantic decision task with an

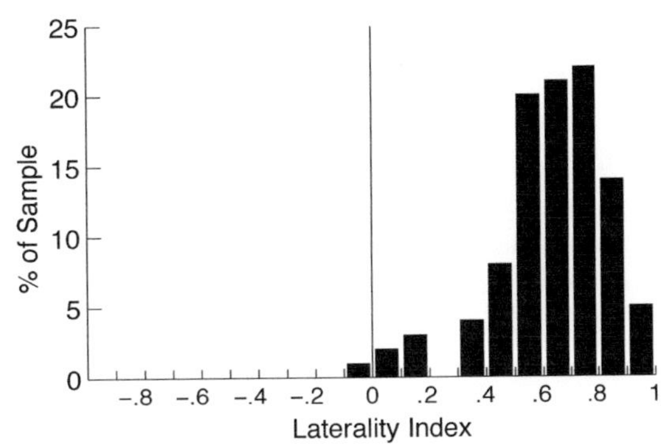

Fig. 9.4 Frequency distribution of language LI in 100 healthy subjects. (Adapted from [180])

auditory nonspeech sensory discrimination task [180]. LIs in this group ranged from strong left dominance (LI = 0.97) to roughly symmetrical representation (LI = −0.05), with a group median LI of 0.66. Using a dominance classification scheme based on a cutoff LI value of ±0.20, 94% of subjects were classified as left-dominant, 6% were symmetrical, and none had right dominance. Thus, although LI values ranged widely, the vast majority of subjects were left-hemisphere dominant. Similar variability in lateralization among normal, right-handed subjects was observed in two other large studies [181, 186].

Several studies have attempted to identify subject variables associated with language lateralization. One group of investigators, using fMRI to contrast a visual phonological decision task with a visual letter string orthographic decision task (a contrast likely to activate visual word-form and phonological access systems), found significant effects of gender on lateralization, particularly in the frontal lobe, with women showing relative symmetry of activation and men showing leftward lateralization [187, 188]. Other PET [95, 189], fMRI [181, 183, 185, 190–192], and functional transcranial Doppler [186] studies, together involving more than 1,500 healthy subjects, have failed to find differences between men and women in terms of lateralization of language functions [193, 194]. Several large series have documented a relative rightward shift of language functions in left-handed and ambidextrous subject samples compared to right-handed subjects [181, 183, 195]. It is important to note, however, that this difference reflects a group tendency only, due to the fact that a larger minority (20–25%) is symmetrical or right dominant. Most left-handed and ambidextrous subjects are, like right-handers, left-dominant for language. These estimates of language dominance and handedness effects in normal subjects agree very well with earlier Wada language studies in patients with late-onset seizures [180, 196, 197].

Two studies reported age effects on language dominance, manifested as a decline in the LI (greater symmetry of language processing) with increasing age [180, 183]. Similar declines in hemispheric specialization have been observed for other cognitive domains [198, 199], and may reflect recruitment of homologous functional regions as compensation for age-related declines in neural functional capacity. Level of education had no effect on LI in the one study in which it was assessed [180].

Two fMRI studies directly compared LIs from a sample of normal subjects with those from patients with epilepsy [41, 180]. Both studies included only right-handed individuals to avoid confounding effects of handedness. Patients with epilepsy had a higher incidence of atypical (symmetric or right-lateralized) language dominance; this was particularly true for patients with left-sided seizure foci [41]. In one study, there was a clear relationship between LI and age of onset of seizures ($r = 0.50$, $p < 0.001$), with language tending to shift more toward the right hemisphere with earlier onset [180]. These effects are in agreement with Wada studies showing effects of side of seizure focus and age at onset on language lateralization [196, 197, 200, 201].

Test–Retest Reliability

Test–retest reliability of language activation procedures has not been sufficiently studied. There are two clinical issues to consider, the first being the reliability of activation of specific voxels across different testing sessions, which is an obvious concern if the goal is to identify specific brain regions that are potentially critical for language. Several authors mention good test–retest reproducibility in a few subjects, though without quantitative analyses [23, 181, 202]. In one of the first quantitative studies of this issue, Rutten et al. measured the overlap of activated voxels across two test sessions as the proportion activated in both sessions relative to the minimum number activated in either the first or second session [39]. Functional data from the two sessions were registered to a common anatomical image and apparently were not spatially smoothed. The results were somewhat disappointing: the best overlap, achieved by combining data from three different activation paradigms and thereby maximizing statistical power, was only 40%. This implies that, for any given activated voxel, there is less than a 50% chance that the same voxel will be activated on retesting with the same protocol. A very similar result (approximately 45% overlap between sessions) was reported in another study using very similar methods [42].

There are, however, several reasons why these estimates may be overly pessimistic. First, accurate measurement of reproducibility at the single voxel level requires exquisitely precise spatial registration of voxels across sessions, as well as identical placement of the voxel grid relative to brain tissue across sessions to achieve identical partial-volume averaging effects; neither of these goals seems practically possible. A more realistic measure of reproducibility, therefore, might be based on spatially smoothed versions of the activation maps or on activation in anatomically defined ROIs. Second, it is clear that reproducibility depends on how accurately the level of activation is estimated within each session, i.e., on the statistical power, which is determined largely by the number of image volumes acquired [203]. The data of Rutten et al. show this effect clearly: when data from any one of the three activation paradigms was analyzed alone, thereby reducing two-thirds the number of image volumes included in the activation analysis for each session, reproducibility dropped to 25% or less. Thus, it seems reasonable to expect that test–retest reproducibility (i.e., reliability of the activation map) can be optimized simply by increasing the number of image volumes acquired at each session. This increase in reliability will, however, be a decelerating exponential function of image volume number; thus, there will be a point at which significant improvement in reliability cannot be attained without exceeding the practical limits on image acquisition in a single session. These limitations have yet to be worked out for any fMRI language protocols.

The second clinical issue concerns the reliability of language lateralization measurements. Two large studies (with 54 patients [204] and 34 patients [42]) examined this question from the point of view of reliability within a testing session. Both studies involved epilepsy patients performing a Semantic Decision versus Sensory Discrimination paradigm; both examined the correlation between a language LI based on data from the first half of an imaging session and LI based on the second half of the session (intrasession reliability). Results were remarkably similar, showing correlations of 0.89 [204] and 0.90 [42]. Other investigators measured reliability of the language LI across sessions [39, 41, 42, 168]. Rutten et al. found a correlation of approximately 0.80 across sessions in 9 healthy control subjects using the combined data from three activation tasks. Interestingly, the correlation did not change across different activation thresholds. This indicates that, although the LI in any given session is affected by the stringency of the activation threshold, LI in relation to the LIs of other subjects will not change as long as the same threshold is applied to all subjects. Adcock et al. [41] found a correlation of 0.65 between LIs from two different sessions in 31 subjects (a mix of healthy controls and epilepsy patients). This value seems somewhat low, though the authors state that "in all cases the categorical definitions of laterality on the first and second examinations were in agreement." Fernández et al. reported a correlation of 0.82 in a sample of 12 epilepsy patients scanned in two different sessions on the same day [42]. Finally, Jansen et al. reported a correlation of 0.66 in 10 healthy controls scanned in two different sessions on the same day. They stressed the strong dependence of this correlation on choice of LI method, ROI, and task, with the optimal reproducibility associated with a magnitude-based LI measure, a frontal ROI, and a word generation task. Collectively, these results suggest a relatively high degree of reproducibility of fMRI language LIs. In addition to the factors identified in these studies, the stability of the LI probably depends to a large degree on the statistical power of each measurement (i.e., number of images acquired), and the group correlation probably increases with the range of LI values in the subject sample.

Wada Comparisons

Demonstration that a language mapping procedure produces left-lateralized activation, and that this functional lateralization varies in the expected direction with handedness and seizure focus, provides good preliminary validation that the activated regions are truly related to language. Further evidence is available from at least three sources: (1) comparison of fMRI results with Wada language lateralization testing in the same patients, (2) comparison of fMRI results with ESM of language in the same patients, and (3) correlation with language outcomes after brain surgery. Other potential sources of validation, which are not discussed further here, include comparisons with language lateralization and localization measures derived from PET [205], magnetoencephalography [12], EEG [206], transcranial magnetic stimulation [207], functional transcranial Doppler [208], dichotic listening [184], and MRI structural morphometry [209].

Results from a now large number of published studies (Table 9.4) suggest a relatively high level of agreement between fMRI and Wada tests on measures of language lateralization (Table 9.4) [13–15, 18, 22, 23, 30, 32, 37, 40, 41, 43, 45–47, 50–52, 210]. A variety of language tasks have been employed in these studies, the most common by far being covert word generation. Other tasks included semantic decision with auditory or visual words, passive listening to sentences or stories, phonological (rhyme) decision, covert object naming, and passive reading. These language tasks have been paired with a variety of baseline conditions, most commonly rest, fixation, a passive sensory control, or an active sensory discrimination task.

While semantic decision and word generation paradigms generally produce high (70–100%) rates of concordance with the Wada, results obtained with Sentence Listening versus Rest [30], Object Naming versus Rest [23], and Object Naming versus Sensory Discrimination [37] protocols were not correlated with Wada results. This lack of concordance probably stems from the fact that these contrasts produce strong activation in auditory and visual sensory systems that are not strongly lateralized and only weak activation in prefrontal language areas. Word generation tasks produce strong frontal activation but relatively weak temporal and parietal activation. The most concordant results obtained with these tasks are based on activation in a frontal ROI. This characteristic of the word generation tasks is potentially problematic for clinical applications in patients with temporal lobe pathology, for several reasons. First, it is possible that language lateralization in such cases could differ for the frontal and temporal lobes, and it would be preferable to know the dominance pattern in the region in which surgery is to be undertaken. Second, if the goal is not simply to determine language dominance but rather to detect language-related cortex with optimal sensitivity for surgical planning, then lack of dominant temporal or parietal lobe activation represents a clear failure of the task paradigm. As discussed earlier, another major limitation of covert word generation tasks is that they do not allow monitoring or assessment of task performance.

Comparisons with ESM

A number of studies have compared fMRI language maps with language maps obtained using ESM [17, 19, 20, 23–26, 31, 32, 38, 211–214]. These studies are of great potential interest because they permit a test of whether fMRI activation foci represent "critical" language areas. Some regions activated during language tasks may play a minor, supportive role rather than a critical role, and resection of these active foci may not necessarily produce clinically relevant deficits. It is vital to distinguish these noncritical areas from those that are critical to normal function. The assumption underlying the ESM technique is that the temporary deactivation induced by electrical interference will identify any such critical areas.

The published studies comparing fMRI and cortical stimulation report encouraging results. These reports have involved relatively small samples (<15 patients). Methods for comparing the activation maps have tended to be qualitative and subjective rather than quantitative and objective, with a few exceptions [17, 38, 211, 212, 214]. Fitzgerald et al. reported, in 11 patients, an average sensitivity of 81% and specificity of 53% when using fMRI to predict "critical" language sites on intraoperative ESM, employing a criterion that the fMRI focus in question spatially

Table 9.4 Wada-fMRI language lateralization comparisons

Lead author, year	*N*	Language task	Control task	Result
Desmond (1995)	7	Semantic decision (vis words)	Orthographic decision	100% concordance
Binder (1996)	22	Semantic decision (aud words)	Tone decision	100% conc., $r = 0.96$
Bahn (1997)	7	Covert phonological word gen	Rest	100% conc.
Hertz-Pannier (1997)	6	Covert or overt word gen	Rest	100% conc.
Worthington (1997)	12	Covert phonological word gen	Rest	56% conc.
Yetkin (1998)	13	Covert phonological word gen	Rest	100% conc., $r = 0.91$
Benson (1999)	12	Covert verb gen.	Fixation	100% conc.
		Covert object naming	Fixation	n.s. lateralization
		Covert word reading	Fixation	n.s. lateralization
Lehéricy (2000)	10	Covert semantic word gen	Rest	$r = 0.88$ for a frontal ROI
		Covert sentence repetition	Rest	n.s. correlation
		Passive story listening	Nonword listening	n.s. correlation
Baciu (2001)	8	Rhyme decision (vis words)	Shape decision	100% concordance
Binder (2001)	49	Semantic decision (aud words)	Tone decision	98% conc.
Carpentier (2001)	10	Semantic/syntactic decision	Sensory discrimination	90% conc.
Gaillard (2002)	18	Covert responsive naming	Passive dot patterns	83% conc.
Spreer (2002)	13	Semantic matching (vis words)	Color matching	100% conc. for frontal ROI
Rutten (2002)	18	Covert verb gen	Shape detection	72% conc. for verb gen
		Covert semantic word gen	Rest	83% combining all tasks
		Covert object naming	Shape detection	n.s. conc. for others
		Covert sentence reading	Shape detection	
Adcock (2003)	19	Covert phonological word gen	Rest	100% conc.
Sabbah (2003)	20	Covert semantic word gen	Rest	95% conc.
Woermann (2003)	94	Covert phonological word gen	Rest	91% conc.
Gaillard (2004)	25	Visual rating of maps from 3 language paradigms		84% conc.
Deblaere (2004)	17	Covert phonological word gen	Covert counting	100% conc. for frontal ROI
Benke (2006)	68	Semantic decision	Tone decision	79% conc. for frontal ROI
Szaflarski (2008)	28	Semantic decision (aud words)	Tone decision	$r = 0.74$
		Covert verb gen	Sequential finger tap	$r = 0.65$
Suarez (2009)	14	Covert semantic word gen	Fixation	86% conc. for frontal ROI
Arora (2009)	38	Visual sentence judgment	Shape matching	66% conc.
	37	Auditory sentence judgment	Tone matching	70% conc.
	31	Covert word gen	Shape matching	65% conc.
	28	Conjunction analysis of all 3 activation maps		71% conc.

overlaps the stimulation site [17]. When the criterion was loosened to include instances in which the fMRI focus was within 2 cm of the stimulation site, sensitivity improved to 92% but specificity was 0%. Sensitivity and specificity were highly variable across subjects. Rutten et al. reported an average sensitivity of 92% and specificity of 61%, but this analysis was performed after removing 3 patients (out of 11) in whom ESM showed *no* language sites [38]. Moreover, the fMRI data appear to have been used during surgery to select the sites for cortical stimulation, so the measurements being compared were not made independently. Similar results were reported in three other small series [211, 212, 214].

Several factors make these comparisons particularly difficult to carry out. One problem is in matching the task characteristics across the two modalities. FMRI studies usually employ controls for nonlinguistic aspects of task performance, whereas this is typically not true of stimulation mapping studies. For example, stimulation studies often focus on speech arrest, which can result from disruption of motor or attentional systems as well as language systems [21]. A second difficulty is the fact that many fMRI activation foci lie buried in the depths of sulci, which are not available for stimulation mapping. Thus, it is reasonable to expect that many foci of activation observed by fMRI simply will not be tested adequately during ESM. On the other hand, edema and angiogenesis associated with mass lesions and hemodynamic abnormalities near vascular malformations may alter neurovascular coupling, compromising the sensitivity of fMRI in these regions [212, 215, 216]. Finally, the assumptions forming the basis for the ESM technique have yet to be adequately tested. There is, for example, very little evidence that resection of "critical" areas detected by cortical stimulation necessarily leads to postoperative language deficits. One study, in fact, showed that the likelihood of finding "critical" foci in the left anterior temporal lobe was higher among patients with poor language function, even though these patients are less likely to show language decline after left anterior temporal lobectomy (ATL) [217, 218]. Moreover, there is very little evidence that ESM has any effect on preventing language decline [219], suggesting that there are critical language areas that may not be detected by focal electrical interference. This lack of sensitivity might occur, for example, if language functions were redundantly distributed across a number of nearby zones, several of which fell within the resection area but none of which produced a language deficit when deactivated in isolation.

Outcome Prediction Studies

It could be argued that neither the Wada test nor cortical stimulation mapping constitute an ideal "gold standard" against which to judge fMRI language maps. Both of these tests have recognized limitations, and both differ sufficiently from fMRI in terms of methodology and level of spatial detail that it is probably unreasonable to expect strong concordance with fMRI maps. A more meaningful measure of the validity of fMRI language maps is how well they predict postoperative deficits. The purpose of preoperative language mapping, after all, is to assess the risk of such deficits and (in the case of cortical stimulation mapping) to minimize their severity. If fMRI can predict postoperative deficits as well as, or better than, the Wada test, then what need is there to compare fMRI directly with the Wada?

Prediction of Language Outcome

Sabsevitz et al. [44] assessed the ability of preoperative fMRI to predict naming decline in 24 consecutively encountered patients undergoing left ATL. FMRI employed a Semantic Decision versus Tone Decision protocol (Fig. 9.2c). All left ATL patients also underwent Wada testing and intraoperative cortical stimulation mapping, and surgeries were performed blind to the fMRI data. Compared to a control group of 32 right ATL patients, the left ATL group declined postoperatively on the 60-item Boston Naming Test ($p < 0.001$). Within the left ATL group, however, there was considerable variability, with 13 patients (54%) showing significant declines relative to the control group and the remainder no decline. A laterality index based on fMRI activation in a temporal lobe region of interest was strongly correlated with outcome ($r = -0.64$, $p < 0.001$), such that the degree of language lateralization toward the surgical (left) hemisphere was related to poorer naming outcome, whereas language lateralization toward the nonsurgical (right) hemisphere was associated with less or no decline (Fig. 9.5). Of note, an LI based on a frontal lobe ROI was considerably less predictive ($r = -0.47$, $p < 0.05$), suggesting that an optimal LI is one that indexes lateralization near the surgical resection area. The fMRI temporal lobe LI showed 100% sensitivity, 73% specificity, and a positive predictive value of 81% for predicting significant decline. By comparison, the Wada language LI showed a somewhat weaker correlation with decline ($r = -0.50$, $p < 0.05$), 92% sensitivity, 43% specificity, and a positive predictive value of 67%.

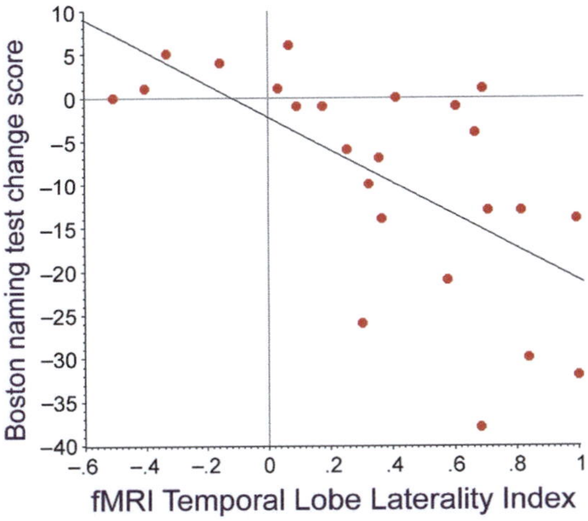

Fig. 9.5 Scatterplot depicting the relationship between preoperative lateralization of language-related brain activation in a temporal lobe region of interest and postoperative decline in confrontation naming performance. (Adapted from Sabsevitz DS, Swanson SJ, Hammeke TA, Spanaki MV, Possing ET, Morris GL 3rd, et al. Use of preoperative functional neuroimaging to predict language deficits from epilepsy surgery. *Neurology* 2003;60(11):1788–92)

These results suggest that preoperative fMRI could be used to stratify patients in terms of risk for language decline, allowing patients and physicians to more accurately weigh the risks and benefits of surgery. It is crucial to note, however, that these results hold only for the particular methods used in the study and may not generalize to other fMRI protocols, analysis methods, patient populations, or surgical procedures. Future studies should not only confirm these results using larger patient samples but also test their generalizability to other protocols.

Prediction of Verbal Memory Outcome

Verbal memory decline is observed in 30–60% of patients who undergo left anterior temporal lobe resection for epilepsy [220–225]. The Wada memory test is used at many centers to assess the risk of memory decline, though its predictive capability has been called into question [226–232]. Several small studies examined whether hippocampal functional asymmetry measured with fMRI can predict memory outcome [233–237], with some encouraging initial results. Given the technical difficulty of measuring robust BOLD signals in the hippocampus, the present author and colleagues tested an alternative strategy of using the language lateralization index to predict memory outcome [55].

The study involved 60 patients who underwent left ATL resection, with language lateralization measured preoperatively using a Semantic Decision versus Tone Decision paradigm (Fig. 9.2c). Verbal memory was measured preoperatively and 6 months after surgery. All patients also underwent preoperative Wada language and memory testing. Verbal memory decline was observed in roughly half of the patients. Preoperative measures that predicted verbal memory outcome included the preoperative memory score (more decline in patients with higher scores, $r = 0.662$), the fMRI language lateralization index (more decline in patients with stronger leftward lateralization, $r = 0.432$), the Wada language asymmetry score (more decline in patients with stronger leftward lateralization, $r = 0.398$), the age at onset of epilepsy (more decline in patients with later age at onset, $r = 0.341$), and the Wada memory asymmetry score ($r = 0.331$). These variables were entered into a stepwise multivariate regression model. The preoperative score, fMRI language LI, and age at onset all contributed independent significant predictive value and collectively accounted for about 50% of the variance in outcome (Fig. 9.6). Addition of the Wada variables did not improve the model. When patients were categorized as showing decline or no decline, the model showed sensitivity of 90% and specificity of 80% for predicting decline.

These results are interesting for several reasons. Most intriguing is the finding that *language* lateralization, whether measured by fMRI or the Wada test, is a better predictor of verbal memory outcome than Wada memory testing. The underlying problem with Wada memory testing is that it uses visual objects that can be encoded both verbally as object names and as nonverbal images. Wada memory asymmetry thus reflects overall lateralization of hippocampal function rather than specifically verbal memory. On the contrary, language lateralization indicates which hippocampus

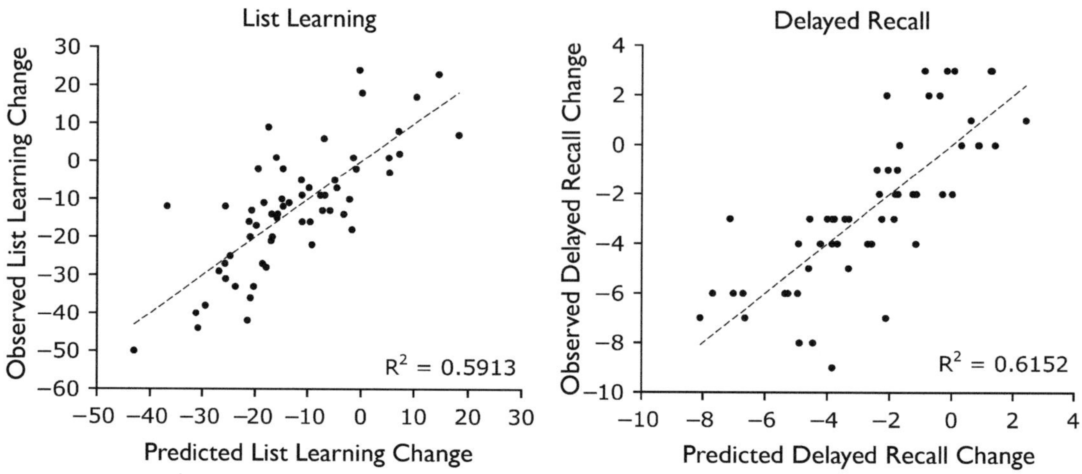

Fig. 9.6 Predicted versus observed individual memory change scores in 60 left ATL surgery patients on tests of word list learning and delayed recall. Predicted list learning change scores were computed from the formula: 17.67–0.704 (Preoperative Score) – 0.280 (Age at Onset) – 12.19 (fMRI LI). Predicted delayed recall change scores were computed from the formula: 3.76–0.688 (Preoperative Score) – 0.093 (Age at Onset) – 2.14 (fMRI LI). (Adapted from [55])

is likely to be most involved in verbal memory encoding. These data also have direct implications for clinical practice, in that they confirm the utility of fMRI for predicting verbal memory outcome in patients undergoing left temporal lobe resection. The fMRI language LI is a safe, noninvasive measure that improves prediction accuracy relative to other noninvasive measures. The finding that Wada memory lateralization is not a strong predictor of verbal memory outcome and adds no predictive value beyond these noninvasive measures confirms several previous studies that also examined multivariate prediction models [227, 230–232, 238]. These results call into question the routine use of the Wada test for predicting material-specific verbal memory outcome, particularly if a validated fMRI measure of language lateralization is available.

Illustrative Cases Using Language FMRI for Quantitative Outcome Prediction

Several examples are presented of quantitative outcome prediction using preoperative fMRI language lateralization. Figure 9.7 illustrates preoperative language activation patterns in two patients who subsequently underwent left ATL complicated by significant declines in object naming performance. Figure 9.8, in contrast, illustrates preoperative language activation patterns in two patients who subsequently underwent left ATL without any decline in object naming. Figure 9.9 shows preoperative language activation patterns in three patients who subsequently underwent left ATL. Verbal memory change scores were accurately predicted by a multivariate model that includes the fMRI language lateralization index, age at onset of epilepsy, and preoperative test score.

Conclusion and Future Applications: Use of FMRI Language Maps in Surgical Planning

It remains to be established how useful fMRI language activation maps will be for more precise planning of surgical resections. At least three significant problems complicate progress: (1) inconsistencies in language maps produced by different activation protocols, (2) the failure to date to find an activation protocol that reliably activates the

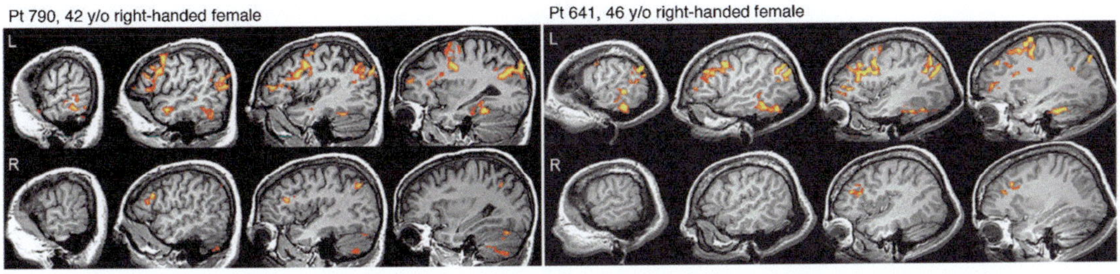

Fig. 9.7 Presurgical language mapping (Semantic Decision vs. Tone Decision) in two patients with intractable left temporal lobe epilepsy. Maps are thresholded at $p < 0.001$. Both patients had strong leftward lateralization of temporal lobe activity (Patient 790 temporal LI = 0.84, Patient 641 temporal LI = 0.82), and both declined on the Boston Naming Test after left anterior temporal lobectomy (Patient 790 BNT change = −30, Patient 641 BNT change = −13)

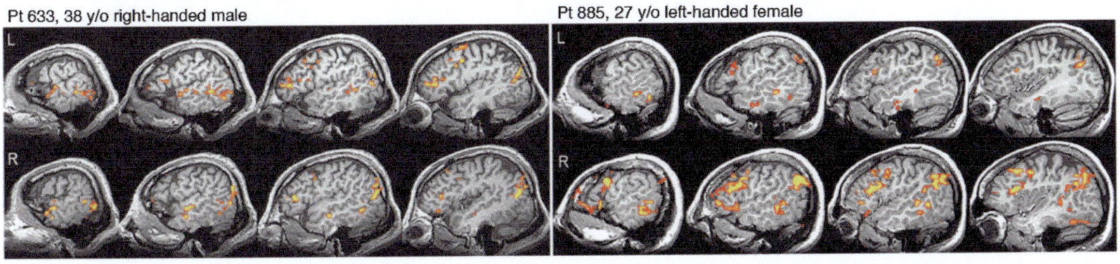

Fig. 9.8 Presurgical language mapping (Semantic Decision versus Tone Decision) in two more patients with intractable left temporal lobe epilepsy. Both had clear bilateral temporal lobe activation (Patient 633 temporal LI = 0.03, Patient 885 temporal LI = −0.33), and neither patient declined on the Boston Naming Test after left anterior temporal lobectomy (Patient 633 BNT change = +1, Patient 885 BNT change = +5). In Patient 633, the Wada language asymmetry was strongly left lateralized (Wada LI = 0.87), incorrectly predicting language decline. These cases illustrate the utility of quantitative presurgical fMRI of the temporal lobes for predicting language decline from left temporal lobe surgery

anterior temporal lobe where the majority of epilepsy surgeries are performed, and (3) an inadequate understanding of the meaning of fMRI activations.

As indicated earlier, different fMRI language activation protocols in current clinical use produce markedly different patterns of activation [27, 33, 121, 239]. While it is plausible to anticipate minor variance in activation profiles due to differential demands on separate subcomponents of language functions by different activation tasks, it is unlikely that this accounts for the full range of variance in these studies. Rather, these findings suggest that activation maps are strongly dependent on the specific contrast made between language and control tasks used in the activation protocol (see previous discussion). Of note, none of the language activation protocols currently in common use are associated with robust anterior temporal lobe activation. Because the dominant anterior temporal lobe is known to contribute to language processes [97, 130, 136, 149, 240–245], and left ATL not infrequently results in language decline [246–249], it follows that these protocols are not detecting crucial language areas. Clearly, further language activation task development is necessary. It may also be necessary, as some have suggested [27, 37], to incorporate multiple activation protocols before a complete picture of language zones in an individual can be discerned.

In addition to these issues concerning sensitivity of the activation protocol, it is conceivable that some regions activated during language tasks may play a minor or nonspecific role rather

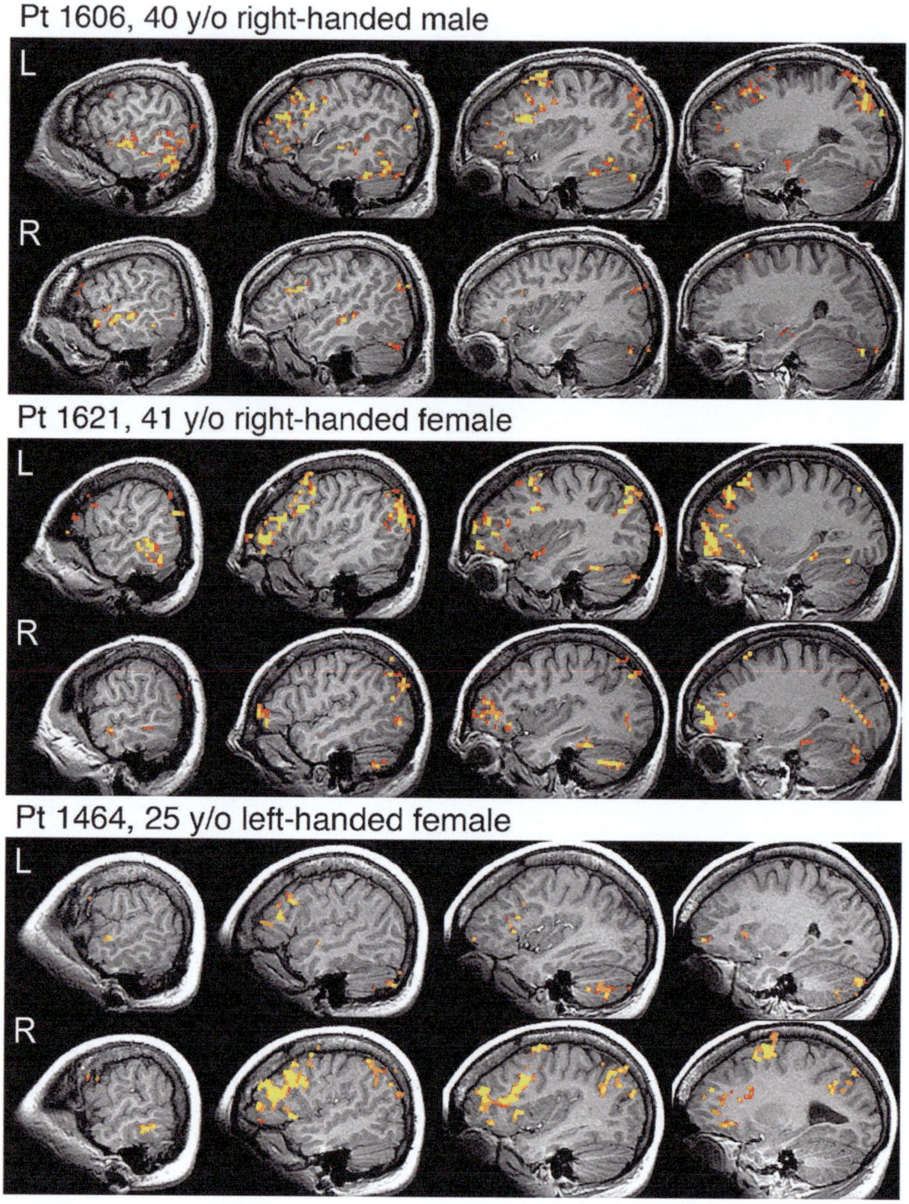

Fig. 9.9 Prediction of verbal memory outcome in three patients with intractable left temporal lobe epilepsy. Presurgical language fMRI in Patient 1606 showed whole hemisphere LI = 0.58. Together with late epilepsy onset (age 36) and very high preoperative memory scores, the patient was predicted to have a large decline of −43 on word-list learning. The actual change score was −50. FMRI in Patient 1,621 showed whole hemisphere LI = 0.47. With late epilepsy onset (age 28) and moderately high preoperative memory scores, the patient was predicted to have a decline of −24 on word-list learning. The actual change score was −25. FMRI in Patient 1,464 showed LI = −0.68, indicating right-lateralized language. With moderately late onset (age 12) and high preoperative scores, the patient was predicted to have a small decline of −10 on word-list learning. The actual change score was −7. These cases illustrate how presurgical language fMRI can be integrated into a multivariate model to predict verbal memory outcome in left temporal lobe surgery

than a critical role in language. Resection of these "active" foci may not necessarily produce clinically relevant or persisting deficits. Thus, those who would use fMRI activation maps to decide which brain regions can be resected in an individual patient run two risks: (1) resection of critical language zones that are "not activated" due to insensitivity of the particular language activation protocol employed, resulting in post-operative language decline, and (2) sparing of "activated" regions that are actually not critical for language, resulting in suboptimal seizure control. Only through very carefully designed studies – in which resections are performed blind to the fMRI data, standardized procedures are used for assessing outcome, and quantitative measures are made of the anatomical and functional lesion – will the usefulness of fMRI language maps for planning surgical resections be determined (Table 9.5).

Table 9.5 Further suggested reading on language mapping

Grabowski et al. 2000 [6]	Investigating language with functional neuroimaging. In: Toga AW, Mazziotta JC, eds. Brain mapping: The systems. San Diego, CA: Academic Press, 2000: 425–461	The authors provide a thorough review of early PET and fMRI language studies and interpret these in the context of a modern, large-scale neuroanatomical model
McCandliss et al. 2003 [250]	The visual word form area: expertise for reading in the fusiform gyrus. Trends in Cognitive Sciences 2003;7:293–299	A concise review of early work on the "visual word form area," a region in ventral left occipitotemporal cortex that plays a crucial role in efficient recognition of written words
Scott et al. 2003 [126]	The neuroanatomical and functional organization of speech perception. Trends in Neurosciences 2003;26:100–107	A detailed but compact summary of the anatomical and functional organization of superior temporal regions implicated in audition and speech perception
Indefrey et al. 2004 [119]	The spatial and temporal signatures of word production components. Cognition 2004;92:101–144	This review article describes the multiple processing stages involved in word production and summarizes a wealth of PET, fMRI, MEG, and ERP data linking these stages with probable anatomical substrates
Novick et al. 2005 [251]	Cognitive control and parsing: Reexamining the role of Broca's area in sentence comprehension. Cognitive, Affective, & Behavioral Neuroscience 2005;5:263–281	This in-depth discussion reviews evidence regarding the role of the left inferior frontal gyrus in sentence comprehension and more general cognitive control processes
Price et al. 2006 [252]	Design and analysis of fMRI studies with neurologically impaired patients. Journal of Magnetic Resonance Imaging 2006;23:816–826	This paper discusses some of the key methodological issues involved in functional imaging of patients with neurological damage, especially aphasia
Patterson et al. 2007 [243]	Where do you know what you know? The representation of semantic knowledge in the human brain. Nature Reviews Neuroscience 2007;8:976–987	This wide-ranging review makes the case for a central role of the anterior temporal lobe in semantic processing, based on neuropsychological and neuroimaging data
Binder et al. 2009 [131]	Where is the semantic system? A critical review and meta-analysis of 120 functional neuroimaging studies. Cerebral Cortex 2009;19:2767–2796	This review and voxel-based meta-analysis summarizes a large body of fMRI and PET studies of semantic processing, with discussion of the key brain regions involved and relationship to the "default mode" network
Richlan et al. 2009 [253]	Functional abnormalities in the dyslexic brain: A quantitative meta-analysis of neuroimaging studies. Human Brain Mapping 2009;10:3299–3308	This voxel-based meta-analysis summarizes the results of 17 functional imaging studies of developmental dyslexia, highlighting involvement of the posterior lateral temporal lobe
Graves et al. 2010 [135]	Neural systems for reading aloud: A multiparametric approach. Cerebral Cortex 2010;20:1799–1815	This paper reviews the effects of a number of lexical variables (including word frequency, spelling-sound consistency, and imageability) on brain systems involved in reading and provides new data on distinct networks that support reading with and without semantic mediation

References

1. Broca P. Remarques sur le siège de la faculté du langage articulé; suivies d'une observation d'aphemie. Bull Soc Anatomique Paris. 1861;6:330–57.
2. Wernicke C. Der aphasische Symptomenkomplex. Breslau: Cohn & Weigert; 1874.
3. Lichtheim L. On aphasia. Brain. 1885;7:433–84.
4. Geschwind N. Aphasia. N Engl J Med. 1971;284: 654–6.
5. Binder JR, Frost JA, Hammeke TA, Cox RW, Rao SM, Prieto T. Human brain language areas identified by functional MRI. J Neurosci. 1997;17: 353–62.
6. Grabowski TJ, Damasio AR. Investigating language with functional neuroimaging. In: Toga AW, Mazziotta JC, editors. Brain mapping: The systems. San Diego, CA: Academic Press; 2000. p. 425–61.
7. Démonet J-F, Thierry G, Cardebat D. Renewal of the neurophysiology of language: functional neuroimaging. Physiol Rev. 2005;85:49–95.
8. Loring DW, Meador KJ, Lee GP, King DW. Amobarbital effects and lateralized brain function: The Wada Test. New York: Springer-Verlag; 1992.
9. Lesser RP, Lueders H, Klem G, et al. Extraoperative cortical functional localization in patients with epilepsy. J Clin Neurophysiol. 1987;4:27–53.
10. Ojemann G, Ojemann J, Lettich E, Berger M. Cortical language localization in left, dominant hemisphere: An electrical stimulation mapping investigation in 117 patients. J Neurosurg. 1989;71:316–26.
11. Pardo JV, Fox PT. Preoperative assessment of the cerebral hemispheric dominance for language with CBF PET. Hum Brain Mapp. 1993;1:57–68.
12. Breier JI, Simos PG, Zouridakis G, et al. Language dominance determined by magnetic source imaging: a comparison with the Wada procedure. Neurology. 1999;53:938–45.
13. Binder JR, Swanson SJ, Hammeke TA, et al. Determination of language dominance using functional MRI: A comparison with the Wada test. Neurology. 1996;46:978–84.
14. Desmond JE, Sum JM, Wagner AD, et al. Functional MRI measurement of language lateralization in Wada-tested patients. Brain. 1995;118:1411–9.
15. Bahn MM, Lin W, Silbergeld DL, et al. Localization of language cortices by functional MR imaging compared with intracarotid amobarbital hemispheric sedation. Am J Radiol. 1997;169:575–9.
16. Binder J. FMRI: Language mapping. Neurosurg Clin N Am. 1997;8:383–92.
17. Fitzgerald DB, Cosgrove GR, Ronner S, et al. Location of language in the cortex: A comparison between functional MR imaging and electrocortical stimulation. Am J Neuroradiol. 1997;18:1529–39.
18. Hertz-Pannier L, Gaillard WD, Mott S, et al. Noninvasive assessment of language dominance in children and adolescents with functional MRI: a preliminary study. Neurology. 1997;48:1003–12.
19. Stapleton SR, Kiriakipoulos E, Mikulis D, et al. Combined utility of functional MRI, cortical mapping, and frameless stereotaxy in the resection of lesions in eloquent areas of brain in children. Pediatr Neurosurg. 1997;26:68–82.
20. Yetkin FZ, Mueller WM, Morris GL, et al. Functional MR activation correlated with intraoperative cortical mapping. Am J Neuroradiol. 1997;18:1311–5.
21. Benbadis SR, Binder JR, Swanson SJ, et al. Is speech arrest during Wada testing a valid method for determining hemispheric representation of language? Brain Lang. 1998;65:441–6.
22. Yetkin FZ, Swanson S, Fischer M, et al. Functional MR of frontal lobe activation: Comparison with Wada language results. Am J Neuroradiol. 1998;19: 1095–8.
23. Benson RR, FitzGerald DB, LeSeuer LL, et al. Language dominance determined by whole brain functional MRI in patients with brain lesions. Neurology. 1999;52:798–809.
24. Ruge MI, Victor JD, Hosain S, et al. Concordance between functional magnetic resonance imaging and intraoperative language mapping. Stereotact Funct Neurosurg. 1999;72:95–102.
25. Rutten GJM, van Rijen PC, van Veelen CWM, Ramsey NF. Language area localization with three-dimensional functional magnetic resonance imaging matches intrasulcal electrostimulation in Broca's area. Ann Neurol. 1999;46:405–8.
26. Schlosser MJ, Luby M, Spencer DD, Awad IA, McCarthy G. Comparative localization of auditory comprehension by using functional magnetic resonance imaging and cortical stimulation. J Neurosurg. 1999;91:626–35.
27. Gaillard WD, Theodore WH. Mapping language in epilepsy with functional neuroimaging. Neuroscientist. 2000;6:391–401.
28. Hammeke TA, Bellgowan PSF, Binder JR. FMRI methodology: Cognitive function mapping. Adv Neurol. 2000;83:221–33.
29. Hirsch J, Ruge MI, K.H.S. K, et al. An integrated functional magnetic resonance imaging procedure for preoperative mapping of cortical areas associated with tactile, motor, language, and visual functions. Neurosurgery. 2000;47:711–22.
30. Lehéricy S, Cohen L, Bazin B, et al. Functional MR evaluation of temporal and frontal language dominance compared with the Wada test. Neurology. 2000;54:1625–33.
31. Lurito JT, Lowe MJ, Sartorius C, Mathews VP. Comparison of fMRI and intraoperative direct cortical stimulation in localization of receptive language areas. J Comput Assist Tomogr. 2000;24:99–105.
32. Carpentier A, Pugh KR, Westerveld M, et al. Functional MRI of language processing: dependence on input modality and temporal lobe epilepsy. Epilepsia. 2001;42:1241–54.
33. Detre JA, Floyd TF. Functional MRI and its applications to the clinical neurosciences. Neuroscientist. 2001;7:64–79.

34. Spreer J, Quiske A, Altenmüller DM, et al. Unsuspected atypical hemispheric dominance for language as determined by fMRI. Epilepsia. 2001; 52:957–9.
35. Binder JR, Achten E, Constable RT, et al. Functional MRI in epilepsy. Epilepsia. 2002;43 Suppl 1:51–63.
36. Liégois F, Connelly A, Salmond CH, Gadian DG, Vargha-Khadem F, Baldeweg T. A direct test for lateralization of language activation using fMRI: Comparison with invasive assessments in children with epilepsy. Neuroimage. 2002;17:1861–7.
37. Rutten G-J, Ramsey N, van Rijen P, Alpherts W, van Veelen C. fMRI-determined language lateralization in patients with unilateral or mixed language dominance according to the Wada test. Neuroimage. 2002;17:447–60.
38. Rutten GJM, Ramsey NF, van Rijen PC, Noordmans HJ, van Veelen CW. Development of a functional magnetic resonance imaging protocol for intraoperative localization of critical temporoparietal language areas. Ann Neurol. 2002;51:350–60.
39. Rutten GJ, Ramsey N, van Rijen P, van Veelen C. Reproducibility of fMRI-determined language lateralization in individual subjects. Brain Lang. 2002;80:421–37.
40. Spreer J, Arnold S, Quiske A, et al. Determination of hemisphere dominance for language: comparison of frontal and temporal fMRI activation with intracarotid amytal testing. Neuroradiology. 2002;44: 467–74.
41. Adcock JE, Wise RG, Oxbury JM, Oxbury SM, Matthews PM. Quantitative fMRI assessment of the differences in lateralization of language-related brain activation in patients with temporal lobe epilepsy. Neuroimage. 2003;18:423–38.
42. Fernández G, Specht K, Weis S, et al. Intrasubject reproducibility of presurgical language lateralization and mapping using fMRI. Neurology. 2003;60: 969–75.
43. Sabbah P, Chassoux F, Leveque C, et al. Functional MR imaging in assessment of language dominance in epileptic patients. Neuroimage. 2003;18:460–7.
44. Sabsevitz DS, Swanson SJ, Hammeke TA, et al. Use of preoperative functional neuroimaging to predict language deficits from epilepsy surgery. Neurology. 2003;60:1788–92.
45. Woermann FG, Jokeit H, Luerding R, et al. Language lateralization by Wada test and fMRI in 100 patients with epilepsy. Neurology. 2003;61:699–701.
46. Gaillard WD, Balsamo L, Xu B, et al. fMRI language task panel improves determination of language dominance. Neurology. 2004;63:1403–8.
47. Benke T, Koylu B, Visani P, et al. Language lateralization in temporal lobe epilepsy: a comparison between fMRI and the Wada Test. Epilepsia. 2006;47: 1308–19.
48. Abou-Khalil B. An update on determination of language dominance in screening for epilepsy surgery: teh Wada test and newer non-invasive alternatives. Epilepsia. 2007;48:442–55.
49. Pelletier I, Sauerwein HC, Lepore F, Saint-Amour D, Lassonde M. Non-invasive alternatives to the Wada test in the presurgical evaluation of language and memory functions in epilepsy patients. Epileptic Disord. 2007;9:111–26.
50. Szaflarski JP, Holland SK, Jacola LM, Lindsell C, Privitera MD, Szaflarski M. Comprehensive presurgical functional MRI language evaluation in adult patients with epilepsy. Epilepsy Behav. 2008;12: 74–83.
51. Arora J, Pugh K, Westerveld M, Spencer S, Spencer DD, Constable RT. Language lateralization in epilepsy patients: fMRI validated with the Wada procedure. Epilepsia. 2009;50:2225–41.
52. Suarez RO, Whalen S, Nelson AP, et al. Threshold-independent functional MRI determination of language dominance: A validation study against clinical gold standards. Epilepsy Behav. 2009;16:288–97.
53. Giussani C, Roux F-E, Ojemann J, Sganzerla EP, Pirillo D, Papagno C. Is preoperative functional magnetic resonance imaging reliable for language areas mapping in brain tumor surgery? Review of language functional magnetic resonance imaging and direct cortical stimulation correlation studies. Neurosurgery. 2010;66:113–20.
54. Sabsevitz DS, Swanson SJ, Morris GL, Mueller WM, Seidenberg M. Memory outcome after left anterior temporal lobectomy in patients with expected and reversed Wada memory asymmetry scores. Epilepsia. 2001;42:1408–15.
55. Binder JR, Sabsevitz DS, Swanson SJ, Hammeke TA, Raghavan M, Mueller WM. Use of preoperative functional MRI to predict verbal memory decline after temporal lobe epilepsy surgery. Epilepsia. 2008;49:1377–94.
56. Binder JR, Swanson SJ, Sabsevitz DS, Hammeke TA, Raghavan M, Mueller WM. A comparison of two fMRI methods for predicting verbal memory decline after left temporal lobectomy: Language lateralization vs. hippocampal activation asymmetry. Epilepsia. 2010;51:618–26.
57. Kertesz A, Harlock W, Coates R. Computer tomographic localization, lesion size, and prognosis in aphasia and nonverbal impairment. Brain Lang. 1979;8:34–50.
58. Porch BE, Collins M, Wertz RT, Friden TP. Statistical prediction of change in aphasia. J Speech Hear Res. 1980;23:312–21.
59. Selnes OA, Knopman DS, Niccum N, Rubens AB, Larson D. Computed tomographic scan correlates of auditory comprehension deficits in aphasia: A prospective recovery study. Ann Neurol. 1983;13: 558–66.
60. Metter EJ, Jackson CA, Kempler D, Hanson WR. Temporoparietal cortex and the recovery of language comprehension in aphasia. Aphasiology. 1992;6: 349–58.
61. Ferro JM. The influence of infarct location on recovery from global aphasia. Aphasiology. 1992;6: 415–30.

62. Code C, Rowley D, Kertesz A. Predicting recovery from aphasia with connectionist networks: Preliminary comparisons with multiple regression. Cortex. 1994;30:527–32.
63. Karbe H, Kessler J, Herholz K, Fink GR, Heiss W-D. Long-term prognosis of poststroke aphasia studied with positron emission tomography. Arch Neurol. 1995;52:186–90.
64. Pedersen PM, Jorgensen HS, Nakayama H, Raaschou HO, Olsen TS. Aphasia in acute stroke: Incidence, determinants, and recovery. Ann Neurol. 1995;38:659–66.
65. Cao Y, Vikingstad EM, George KP, Johnson AF, Welch KMA. Cortical language activation in stroke patients recovering from aphasia with functional MRI. Stroke. 1999;30:2331–40.
66. Calvert GA, Brammer MJ, Morris RG, Williams SCR, King N, Matthews PM. Using fMRI to study recovery from acquired dysphasia. Brain Lang. 2000;71:391–9.
67. Rosen HJ, Petersen SE, Linenweber MR, et al. Neural correlates of recovery from aphasia after damage to left inferior frontal cortex. Neurology. 2000;55:1883–94.
68. Perani D, Cappa SF, Tettamanti M, et al. A fMRI study of word retrieval in aphasia. Brain Lang. 2003;85:357–68.
69. Fernandez B, Cardebat D, Demonet JF, et al. Functional MRI follow-up study of language processes in healthy subjects and during recovery in a case of aphasia. Stroke. 2004;35:2171–6.
70. Meinzer M, Elbert T, Wienbruch C, Djundja D, Barthel G, Rockstroh B. Intensive language training enhances brain plasticity in chronic aphasia. BMC Biology. 2004;2:http://www.biomedcentral.com/1741-7007/1742/1720.
71. Naeser MA, Martin PI, Baker EH, et al. Overt propositional speech in chronic nonfluent aphasia studied with the dynamic susceptibility contrast fMRI method. Neuroimage. 2004;22:29–41.
72. Zahn R, Drews E, Specht K, et al. Recovery of semantic word processing in global aphasia: a functional MRI study. Cogn Brain Res. 2004;18:322–36.
73. Fridriksson J, Morrow L. Cortical activation and language task difficulty in aphasia. Aphasiology. 2005;19:239–50.
74. Crosson B, McGregor K, Gopinath KS, et al. Functional MRI of language in aphasia: a review of the literature and the methodological challenges. Neuropsychol Rev. 2007;17:157–77.
75. Meinzer M, Flaisch T, Breitenstein C, Wienbruch C, Elbert T, Rockstroh B. Functional re-recruitment of dysfunctional brain areas predicts language recovery in chronic aphasia. Neuroimage. 2008;39:2038–46.
76. Leonard B, de Partz M-P, Grandin C, Pillon A. Domain-specific reorganization of semantic processing after extensive damage to the left temporal lobe. Neuroimage. 2009;45:572–86.
77 Postman-Caucheteux WA, Birn RM, Pursley RH, et al. Single-trial fMRI shows contralesional activity linked to overt naming errors in chronic aphasic patients. Journal of Cognitive Neuroscience. 2010;in press.
78 Eden GF, VanMeter JW, Rumsey JM, Maisog JM, Woods RP, Zeffiro TA. Abnormal processing of visual motion in dyslexia revealed by functional brain imaging. Nature. 1996;382:66–9.
79 Demb JB, Boynton GM, Heeger DJ. Brain activity in visual cortex predicts individual differences in reading performance. Proc Natl Acad Sci USA. 1997;94:13363–6.
80. Shaywitz SE, Shaywitz BA, Pugh KR, et al. Functional disruption in the organization of the brain for reading in dyslexia. Proc Natl Acad Sci USA. 1998;95:2636–41.
81. Temple E, Deutsch GK, Poldrack RA, et al. Neural deficits in children with dyslexia ameliorated by behavioral remediation: Evidence from functional MRI. Proc Natl Acad Sci USA. 2003;100:2860–5.
82. Price CJ, Wise RSJ, Frackowiak RSJ. Demonstrating the implicit processing of visually presented words and pseudowords. Cereb Cortex. 1996;6:62–70.
83. Macleod CM. Half a century of research on the Stroop effect: an integrative review. Psychol Bull. 1991;109:163–203.
84. Reicher GM. Perceptual recognition as a function of meaningfulness of stimulus material. J Exp Psychol. 1969;81:274–80.
85. Warren RM, Obusek CJ. Speech perception and phonemic restorations. Percept Psychophys. 1971;9:358–62.
86. Ganong WF. Phonetic categorization in auditory word perception. J Exp Psychol Hum Percept Perform. 1980;6:110–5.
87. Marslen-Wilson WD, Tyler LK. Central processes in speech understanding. Philos Trans R Soc Lond B. 1981;295:317–32.
88. Carr TH, McCauley C, Sperber RD, Parmalee CM. Words, pictures, and priming: On semantic activation, conscious identification, and the automaticity of information processing. J Exp Psychol Hum Percept Perform. 1982;8:757–77.
89. Marcel AJ. Conscious and unconscious perception: Experiments on visual masking and word recognition. Cogn Psychol. 1983;15:197–237.
90. Van Orden GC. A ROWS is a ROSE: Spelling, sound, and reading. Mem Cogn. 1987;15:181–98.
91. Burton MW, Baum SR, Blumstein SE. Lexical effects on phonetic categorization of speech: The role of acoustic structure. J Exp Psychol Hum Percept Perform. 1989;15:567–75.
92. Glaser WR. Picture naming. Cognition. 1992;42:61–105.
93. Petersen SE, Fox PT, Posner MI, Mintun M, Raichle ME. Positron emission tomographic studies of the cortical anatomy of single-word processing. Nature. 1988;331:585–9.

94. Raichle ME, Fiez JA, Videen TO, et al. Practice-related changes in human brain functional anatomy during nonmotor learning. Cereb Cortex. 1994;4:8–26.
95. Buckner RL, Raichle ME, Petersen SE. Dissociation of human prefrontal cortical areas across different speech production tasks and gender groups. J Neurosci. 1995;74:2163–73.
96. Démonet J-F, Chollet F, Ramsay S, et al. The anatomy of phonological and semantic processing in normal subjects. Brain. 1992;115:1753–68.
97. Damasio H, Grabowski TJ, Tranel D, Hichwa RD, Damasio AR. A neural basis for lexical retrieval. Nature. 1996;380:499–505.
98. James W. Principles of psychology. New York: Dover Publications; 1890.
99. Hebb DO. The problem of consciousness and introspection. In: Adrian ED, Bremer F, Jasper HH, eds. Brain mechanisms and consciousness. A symposium. Springfield, IL: Charles C. Thomas, 1954: 402–421.
100. Miller GA, Galanter E, Pribram K. Plans and the structure of behavior. New York: Holt; 1960.
101. Pope KS, Singer JL. Regulation of the stream of consciousness: Toward a theory of ongoing thought. In: Schwartz GE, Shapiro D, editors. Consciousness and self-regulation. New York: Plenum Press; 1976. p. 101–35.
102. Aurell CG. Perception: a model comprising two modes of consciousness. Percept Mot Skills. 1979;49:431–44.
103. Picton TW, Stuss DT. Neurobiology of conscious experience. Curr Opin Neurobiol. 1994;4:256–65.
104. Antrobus JS, Singer JL, Greenberg S. Studies in the stream of consciousness: Experimental enhancement and suppression of spontaneous cognitive processes. Percept Mot Skills. 1966;23:399–417.
105. Teasdale JD, Proctor L, Lloyd CA, Baddeley AD. Working memory and stimulus-independent thought: Effects of memory load and presentation rate. Eur J Cogn Psychol. 1993;5:417–33.
106. Révész G, editor. Thinking and speaking: A symposium. Amsterdam: North Holland Publishing; 1954.
107. Weiskrantz L, editor. Thought without language. Oxford: Clarendon; 1988.
108. Vygotsky LS. Thought and language. New York: Wiley; 1962.
109. Karmiloff-Smith A. Beyond modularity: A developmental perspective on cognitive science. Cambridge, MA: MIT Press; 1992.
110. Andreasen NC, O'Leary DS, Cizadlo T, et al. Remembering the past: Two facets of episodic memory explored with positron emission tomography. Am J Psychiatry. 1995;152:1576–85.
111. Shulman GL, Fiez JA, Corbetta M, et al. Common blood flow changes across visual tasks: II. Decreases in cerebral cortex. J Cogn Neurosci. 1997;9:648–63.
112. Binder JR, Frost JA, Hammeke TA, Bellgowan PSF, Rao SM, Cox RW. Conceptual processing during the conscious resting state: a functional MRI study. J Cogn Neurosci. 1999;11:80–93.
113 Mazoyer B, Zago L, Mellet E, et al. Cortical networks for working memory and executive functions sustain the conscious resting state in man. Brain Res Bull. 2001;54:287–98.
114 Raichle ME, McLeod AM, Snyder AZ, Powers WJ, Gusnard DA, Shulman GL. A default mode of brain function. Proc Natl Acad Sci USA. 2001;98:676–82.
115 Stark CE, Squire LR. When zero is not zero: The problem of ambiguous baseline conditions in fMRI. Proc Natl Acad Sci U S A. 2001;98:12760–6.
116 McKiernan KA, Kaufman JN, Kucera-Thompson J, Binder JR. A parametric manipulation of factors affecting task-induced deactivation in functional neuroimaging. J Cogn Neurosci. 2003;15:394–408.
117. McKiernan KA, D'Angelo BR, Kaufman JN, Binder JR. Interrupting the "stream of consciousness": An fMRI investigation. Neuroimage. 2006;29:1185–91.
118. Mason MF, Norton MI, Van Horn JD, Wegner DM, Grafton ST, Macrae CN. Wandering minds: the default network and stimulus-independent thought. Science. 2007;315:393–5.
119. Indefrey P, Levelt WJM. The spatial and temporal signatures of word production components. Cognition. 2004;92:101–44.
120. Awad M, Warren JE, Scott SK, Turkheimer FE, Wise RJS. A common system for the comprehension and production of narrative speech. J Neurosci. 2007;27:11455–64.
121. Binder JR, Swanson SJ, Hammeke TA, Sabsevitz DS. A comparison of five fMRI protocols for mapping speech comprehension systems. Epilepsia. 2008;49:1980–97.
122. Binder JR, Frost JA, Hammeke TA, Rao SM, Cox RW. Function of the left planum temporale in auditory and linguistic processing. Brain. 1996;119: 1239–47.
123. Binder JR, Frost JA, Hammeke TA, et al. Human temporal lobe activation by speech and nonspeech sounds. Cereb Cortex. 2000;10:512–28.
124. Kaas JH, Hackett TA. Subdivisions of auditory cortex and processing streams in primates. Proc Natl Acad Sci USA. 2000;97:11793–9.
125. Poremba A, Saunders RC, Sokoloff L, Crane A, Cook M, Mishkin M. Functional mapping of the primate auditory system. Science. 2003;299:568–72.
126. Scott SK, Johnsrude IS. The neuroanatomical and functional organization of speech perception. Trends Neurosci. 2003;26:100–7.
127. Buchman AS, Garron DC, Trost-Cardamone JE, Wichter MD, Schwartz D. Word deafness: one hundred years later. J Neurol Neurosurg Psychiatry. 1986;49:489–99.
128. Poeppel D. Pure word deafness and the bilateral processing of the speech code. Cogn Sci. 2001;25: 679–93.
129. Binder JR. Wernicke aphasia: A disorder of central language processing. In: D'Esposito ME, editor. Neurological foundations of cognitive neuroscience. Cambridge, MA: MIT Press; 2002. p. 175–238.

130. Dronkers NF, Wilkins DP, Van Valin RD, Redfern BB, Jaeger JJ. Lesion analysis of the brain areas involved in language comprehension. Cognition. 2004;92:145–77.
131. Binder JR, Desai R, Conant LL, Graves WW. Where is the semantic system? A critical review and meta-analysis of 120 functional neuroimaging studies. Cereb Cortex. 2009;19:2767–96.
132. Birn RM, Bandettini PA, Cox RW, Shaker R. Event-related FMRI of tasks involving brief motion. Hum Brain Mapp. 1999;7:106–14.
133. Binder JR, Medler DA, Desai R, Conant LL, Liebenthal E. Some neurophysiological constraints on models of word naming. Neuroimage. 2005;27: 677–93.
134. Desai R, Conant LL, Waldron E, Binder JR. FMRI of past tense processing: The effects of phonological complexity and task difficulty. J Cogn Neurosci. 2006;18:278–97.
135. Graves WW, Desai R, Humphries C, Seidenberg MS, Binder JR. Neural systems for reading aloud: A multiparametric approach. Cereb Cortex. 2010;20: 1799–815.
136. Scott SK, Blank C, Rosen S, Wise RJS. Identification of a pathway for intelligible speech in the left temporal lobe. Brain. 2000;123:2400–6.
137. Davis MH, Johnsrude IS. Hierarchical processing in spoken language comprehension. J Neurosci. 2003; 23:3423–31.
138. Liebenthal E, Binder JR, Spitzer SM, Possing ET, Medler DA. Neural substrates of phonetic perception. Cereb Cortex. 2005;15:1621–31.
139. Benson RR, Richardson M, Whalen DH, Lai S. Phonetic processing areas revealed by sinewave speech and acoustically similar non-speech. Neuroimage. 2006;31:342–53.
140. Belin P, Zatorre RJ, Ahad P. Human temporal-lobe response to vocal sounds. Cogn Brain Res. 2002;13: 17–26.
141. Dehaene-Lambertz G, Pallier C, Serniclaes W, Sprenger-Charolles L, Jobert A, Dehaene S. Neural correlates of switching from auditory to speech perception. Neuroimage. 2005;24:21–33.
142. Mottonen R, Calvert GA, Jaaskelainen IP, et al. Perceiving identical sounds as speech or non-speech modulates activity in the left posterior superior temporal sulcus. Neuroimage. 2006;30:563–9.
143. Desai R, Liebenthal E, Waldron E, Binder JR. Left posterior temporal regions are sensitive to auditory categorization. J Cogn Neurosci. 2008;20: 1174–88.
144. Cohen L, Dehaene S, Naccache L, et al. The visual word form area. Spatial and temporal characterization of an initial stage of reading in normal subjects and posterior split-brain patients. Brain. 2000; 123:291–307.
145. Cohen L, Lehéricy S, Chochon F, Lemer C, Rivaud S, Dehaene S. Language-specific tuning of visual cortex? Functional properties of the Visual Word Form Area. Brain. 2002;125:1054–69.
146. Binder JR, Medler DA, Westbury CF, Liebenthal E, Buchanan L. Tuning of the human left fusiform gyrus to sublexical orthographic structure. Neuroimage. 2006;33:739–48.
147. Wise RSJ, Scott SK, Blank SC, Mummery CJ, Murphy K, Warburton EA. Separate neural subsystems within "Wernicke's area". Brain. 2001; 124:83–95.
148. Wise R, Chollet F, Hadar U, Friston K, Hoffner E, Frackowiak R. Distribution of cortical neural networks involved in word comprehension and word retrieval. Brain. 1991;114:1803–17.
149. Mazoyer BM, Tzourio N, Frak V, et al. The cortical representation of speech. J Cogn Neurosci. 1993;5: 467–79.
150. Price CJ, Wise RJS, Warburton EA, et al. Hearing and saying. The functional neuro-anatomy of auditory word processing. Brain. 1996;119:919–31.
151. Zatorre RJ, Evans AC, Meyer E, Gjedde A. Lateralization of phonetic and pitch discrimination in speech processing. Science. 1992;256:846–9.
152. Mummery CJ, Ashburner J, Scott SK, Wise RJS. Functional neuroimaging of speech perception in six normal and two aphasic subjects. J Acoust Soc Am. 1999;106:449–57.
153. Belin P, Zatorre RJ, Lafaille P, Ahad P, Pike B. Voice-selective areas in human auditory cortex. Nature. 2000;403:309–12.
154. Eulitz C, Elbert T, Bartenstein P, Weiller C, Müller SP, Pantev C. Comparison of magnetic and metabolic brain activity during a verb generation task. Neuroreport. 1994;6:97–100.
155. Warburton E, Wise RJS, Price CJ, et al. Noun and verb retrieval by normal subjects. Studies with PET. Brain. 1996;119:159–79.
156. Ojemann JG, Buckner RL, Akbudak E, et al. Functional MRI studies of word-stem completion: Reliability across laboratories and comparison to blood flow imaging with PET. Hum Brain Mapp. 1998;6:203–15.
157. Palmer ED, Rosen HJ, Ojemann JG, Buckner RL, Kelley WM, Petersen SE. An event-related fMRI study of overt and covert word stem completion. Neuroimage. 2001;14:182–93.
158. Thompson-Schill SL, D'Esposito M, Kan IP. Effects of repetition and competition on activity in left prefrontal cortex during word generation. Neuron. 1999;23:513–22.
159. Malach R, Reppas JB, Benson RR, et al. Object-related activity revealed by functional magnetic resonance imaging in human occipital cortex. Proc Natl Acad Sci USA. 1995;92:8135–9.
160. Kanwisher N, Woods R, Iacoboni M, Mazziotta J. A locus in human extrastriate cortex for visual shape analysis. J Cogn Neurosci. 1996;91:133–42.
161. Grill-Spector K, Kushnir T, Edelman S, Avidian-Carmel G, Itzchak Y, Malach R. Differential processing of objects under various viewing conditions in the human lateral occipital complex. Neuron. 1999;24:187–203.

162. Bookheimer SY, Zeffiro TA, Blaxton T, Gaillard T, Theodore W. Regional cerebral blood flow during object naming and word reading. Hum Brain Mapp. 1995;3:93–106.
163. Martin A, Wiggs CL, Ungerleider LG, Haxby JV. Neural correlates of category-specific knowledge. Nature. 1996;379:649–52.
164. Price CJ, Moore CJ, Humphreys GW, Frackowiak RSJ, Friston KJ. The neural regions sustaining object recognition and naming. Proc R Soc Lond B. 1996;263:1501–7.
165. Zelkowicz BJ, Herbster AN, Nebes RD, Mintun MA, Becker JT. An examination of regional cerebral blood flow during object naming tasks. J Int Neuropsychol Soc. 1998;4:160–6.
166. Murtha S, Chertkow H, Beauregard M, Evans A. The neural substrate of picture naming. J Cogn Neurosci. 1999;11:399–423.
167. Kiasawa M, Inoue C, Kawasaki T, et al. Functional neuroanatomy of object naming: A PET study. Graefes Arch Clin Exp Ophthalmol. 1996;234:110–5.
168. Jansen A, Menke R, Sommer J, et al. The assessment of hemispheric lateralization in functional MRI—Robustness and reproducibility. Neuroimage. 2006; 33:204–17.
169. Vandenberghe R, Price C, Wise R, Josephs O, Frackowiak RSJ. Functional anatomy of a common semantic system for words and pictures. Nature. 1996;383:254–6.
170. Müller R-A, Kleinhans N, Courchesne E. Linguistic theory and neuroimaging evidence: an fMRI study of Broca's area in lexical semantics. Neuropsychologia. 2003;in press.
171. Price CJ, Moore CJ, Humphreys GW, Wise RJS. Segregating semantic from phonological processes during reading. J Cogn Neurosci. 1997;9:727–33.
172. Mummery CJ, Patterson K, Hodges JR, Price CJ. Functional neuroanatomy of the semantic system: divisible by what? J Cogn Neurosci. 1998;10:766–77.
173. Roskies AL, Fiez JA, Balota DA, Raichle ME, Petersen SE. Task-dependent modulation of regions in the left inferior frontal cortex during semantic processing. J Cogn Neurosci. 2001;13:829–43.
174. Devlin JT, Matthews PM, Rushworth MFS. Semantic processing in the left inferior prefrontal cortex: A combined functional magnetic resonance imaging and transcranial magnetic stimulation study. J Cogn Neurosci. 2003;15:71–84.
175. Scott SK, Leff AP, Wise RJS. Going beyond the information given: a neural system supporting semantic interpretation. Neuroimage. 2003;19:870–6.
176. Bavelier D, Corina D, Jezzard P, et al. Sentence reading: a functional MRI study at 4 tesla. J Cogn Neurosci. 1997;9:664–86.
177. Herbster AN, Mintun MA, Nebes RD, Becker JT. Regional cerebral blood flow during word and nonword reading. Hum Brain Mapp. 1997;5:84–92.
178. Indefrey P, Kleinschmidt A, Merboldt K-D, et al. Equivalent responses to lexical and nonlexical visual stimuli in occipital cortex: a functional magnetic resonance imaging study. Neuroimage. 1997;5:78–81.
179. Chee MW, Caplan D, Soon CS, et al. Processing of visually presented sentences in Mandarin and English studied with fMRI. Neuron. 1999;23:127–37.
180. Springer JA, Binder JR, Hammeke TA, et al. Language dominance in neurologically normal and epilepsy subjects: a functional MRI study. Brain. 1999;122:2033–45.
181. Pujol J, Deus J, Losilla JM, Capdevila A. Cerebral lateralization of language in normal left-handed people studied by functional MRI. Neurology. 1999;52: 1038–43.
182. Vikingstad EM, George KP, Johnson AF, Cao Y. Cortical language lateralization in right handed normal subjects using functional magnetic resonance imaging. J Neurol Sci. 2000;175:17–27.
183. Szaflarski JP, Binder JR, Possing ET, McKiernan KA, Ward DB, Hammeke TA. Language lateralization in left-handed and ambidextrous people: fMRI data. Neurology. 2002;59:238–44.
184. Hund-Georgiadis M, Lex U, Friederici AD, von Cramon DY. Non-invasive regime for language lateralization in right- and left-handers by means of functional MRI and dichotic listening. Exp Brain Res. 2002;145:166–76.
185. Plante E, Schmithorst VJ, Holland SK, Byars AW. Sex differences in the activation of language cortex during childhood. Neuropsychologia. 2006;44:1210–21.
186. Knecht S, Deppe M, Dräger B, et al. Language lateralization in healthy right-handers. Brain. 2000;123:74–81.
187. Shaywitz BA, Shaywitz SE, Pugh KR, et al. Sex differences in the functional organization of the brain for language. Nature. 1995;373:607–9.
188. Pugh KR, Shaywitz BA, Shaywitz SE, et al. Cerebral organization of component processes in reading. Brain. 1996;119:1221–38.
189. Price CJ, Moore CJ, Friston KJ. Getting sex into perspective. Neuroimage. 1996;3:S586.
190. Frost JA, Binder JR, Springer JA, et al. Language processing is strongly left lateralized in both sexes: Evidence from FMRI. Brain. 1999;122:199–208.
191. Szaflarski JP, Holland SK, Schmithorst VJ, Byars AW. fMRI study of language lateralization in children and adults. Hum Brain Mapp. 2006;27: 202–12.
192. Ihnen SKZ, Church JA, Petersen SE, Schlaggar BL. Lack of generalizability of sex differences in the fMRI BOLD activity associated with language processing in adults. Neuroimage. 2009;45:1020–32.
193. Sommer IEC, Aleman A, Bouma A, Kahn RS. Do women really have more bilateral language representation than men? A meta-analysis of functional imaging studies. Brain. 2004;127:1845–52.
194. Sommer IE, Aleman A, Somers M, Boks MP, Kahn RS. Sex differences in handedness, asymmetry of the planum temporale and functional language lateralization. Brain Res. 2008;1206:76–88.

195. Knecht S, Dräger B, Deppe M, et al. Handedness and hemispheric language dominance in healthy humans. Brain. 2000;123:2512–8.
196. Rasmussen T, Milner B. The role of early left-brain injury in determining lateralization of cerebral speech functions. Ann NY Acad Sci. 1977;299:355–69.
197. Loring DW, Meador KJ, Lee GP, et al. Cerebral language lateralization: Evidence from intracarotid amobarbital testing. Neuropsychologia. 1990;28:831–8.
198. Grady CL, Maisog JM, Horwitz B, et al. Age-related changes in cortical blood flow activation during visual processing of faces and location. J Neurosci. 1994;14:1450–62.
199. Grady CL, McIntosh AR, Bookstein F, Horwitz B, Rapoport SI, Haxby JV. Age-related changes in regional cerebral blood flow during working memory for faces. Neuroimage. 1998;8:409–25.
200. Woods RP, Dodrill CB, Ojemann GA. Brain injury, handedness, and speech lateralization in a series of amobarbital studies. Ann Neurol. 1988;23:510–8.
201. Risse GL, Gates JR, Fangman MC. A reconsideration of bilateral language representation based on the intracarotid amobarbital procedure. Brain Lang. 1997;33:118–32.
202. Binder JR, Rao SM, Hammeke TA, et al. Lateralized human brain language systems demonstrated by task subtraction functional magnetic resonance imaging. Arch Neurol. 1995;52:593–601.
203. Cohen MS, Dubois RM. Stability, repeatability, and the expression of signal magnitude in functional magnetic resonance imaging. J Magn Reson Imaging. 1999;10:33–40.
204. Binder JR, Hammeke TA, Possing ET, et al. Reliability and validity of language dominance assessment with functional MRI. Neurology. 2001;56 Suppl 3:A158.
205. Xiong J, Rao S, Gao JH, Woldorff M, Fox PT. Evaluation of hemispheric dominance for language using functional MRI: a comparison with positron emission tomography. Hum Brain Mapp. 1998;6: 42–58.
206. Altenmüller DM, Kriechbaum W, Helber U, Moini S, Dichgans J, Petersen D. Cortical DC-potentials in identification of the language dominant hemisphere: linguistical and clinical aspects. Acta Neurochirurgica. 1993;56 (Suppl.):20–33.
207. Khedr EM, Hamed E, Said A, Basahi J. Handedness and language cerebral lateralization. Eur J Appl Physiol. 2002;87:469–73.
208. Deppe M, Knecht S, Papke K, et al. Assessment of hemispheric language lateralization: A comparison between fMRI and fTCD. J Cereb Blood Flow Metab. 2000;20:263–8.
209. Eckert MA, Leonard CM, Possing ET, Binder JR. Uncoupled leftward asymmetries for planum morphology and functional language processing. Brain Lang. 2006;98:102–11.
210. Deblaere K, Boon PA, Vandemaele P, et al. MRI language dominance assessment in epilepsy patients at 1.0 T: region of interest analysis and comparison with intracarotid amytal testing. Neuroradiology. 2004; 46:413–20.
211. Pouratian N, Bookheimer SY, Rex DE, Martin NA, Toga AW. Utility of preoperative functional magnetic resonance imaging for identifying language cortices in patients with vascular malformations. J Neurosurg. 2002;97:21–32.
212. Roux FE, Boulanouar K, Lotterie JA, Mejdoubi M, LeSage JP, Berry I. Language functional magnetic resonance imaging in preoperative assessment of language areas: Correlation with direct cortical stimulation. Neurosurgery. 2003;52:1335–47.
213. Signorelli F, Guyotat J, Schneider F, Isnard J, Bret P. Technical refinements for validating functional MRI-based neuronavigation data by electrical stimulation during cortical language mapping. Minim Invasive Neurosurg. 2003;46:265–8.
214. Bizzi A, Blasi V, Falini A, et al. Presurgical functional MR imaging of language and motor functions: Validation with intraoperative electrocortical mapping. Radiology. 2008;2:579–89.
215. Håberg A, Kvistad KA, Unsgård G, Haraldseth O. Preoperative blood oxygen level dependent functional magnetic resonance imaging in patients with primary brain tumors: Clinical application and outcome. Neurosurgery. 2004;54:902–15.
216. Ulmer JL, Hacein-Bey L, Mathews VP, et al. Lesion-induced pseudo-dominance at functional magnetic resonance imaging: Implications for preoperative assessments. Neurosurgery. 2004;55:569–81.
217. Chelune GJ. Using neuropsychological data to forecast postsurgical cognitive outcome. In: Lüders H, editor. Epilepsy Surgery. New York: Raven Press; 1991. p. 477–85.
218. Schwartz TH, Devinsky O, Doyle W, Perrine K. Preoperative predictors of anterior temporal language areas. J Neurosurg. 1998;89:962–70.
219. Hermann BP, Perrine K, Chelune GJ, et al. Visual confrontation naming following left anterior temporal lobectomy: A comparison of surgical approaches. Neuropsychology. 1999;13:3–9.
220. Hermann BP, Seidenberg M, Haltiner A, Wyler AR. Relationship of age at onset, chronologic age, and adequacy of preoperative performance to verbal memory change after anterior temporal lobectomy. Epilepsia. 1995;36:137–45.
221. Helmstaedter C, Elger CE. Cognitive consequences of two-thirds anterior temporal lobectomy on verbal memory in 144 patients: a three-month follow-up study. Epilepsia. 1996;37:171–80.
222. Martin RC, Sawrie SM, Roth DL, et al. Individual memory change after anterior temporal lobectomy: a base rate analysis using regression-based outcome methodology. Epilepsia. 1998;39:1075–82.
223. Lee TMC, Yip JTH, Jones-Gotman M. Memory deficits after resection of left or right anterior temporal lobe in humans: A meta-analytic review. Epilepsia. 2002;43:283–91.
224. Gleissner U, Helmstaedter C, Schramm J, Elger CE. Memory outcome after selective amygdalohippocampectomy in patients with temporal lobe epilepsy: One-year follow-up. Epilepsia. 2004;45:960–2.
225. Baxendale S, Thompson P, Harkness W, Duncan J. Predicting memory decline following epilepsy

surgery: A multivariate approach. Epilepsia. 2006; 47:1887–94.

226. Lee GP, Loring DW, Smith JR, Flanigin HF. Intraoperative hippocampal cooling and Wada memory testing in the evaluation of amnesia risk following anterior temporal lobectomy. Arch Neurol. 1995;52:857–61.

227. Chelune GJ, Najm IM. Risk factors associated with postsurgical decrements in memory. In: Luders HO, Comair Y, editors. Epilepsy surgery. 2nd ed. Philadelphia: Lippincott; 2000. p. 497–504.

228. Kubu CS, Girvin JP, McLachlan RS, Pavol M, Harnadek MC. Does the intracarotid amobarbital procedure predict global amnesia after temporal lobectomy? Epilepsia. 2000;41:1321–9.

229. Simkins-Bullock J. Beyond speech lateralization: a review of the variability, reliability, and validity of the intracarotid amobarbital procedure and its nonlanguage uses in epilepsy surgery candidates. Neuropsychol Rev. 2000;10:41–74.

230. Stroup E, Langfitt JT, Berg M, McDrmott M, Pilcher W, Como P. Predicting verbal memory decline following anterior temporal lobectomy (ATL). Neurology. 2003;60:1266–73.

231. Kirsch HE, Walker JA, Winstanley FS, et al. Limitations of Wada memory asymmetry as a predictor of outcomes after temporal lobectomy. Neurology. 2005;65:676–80.

232. Lineweaver TT, Morris HH, Naugle RI, Najm IM, Diehl B, Bingaman W. Evaluating the contributions of state-of-the-art assessment techniques to predicting memory outcome after unilateral anterior temporal lobectomy. Epilepsia. 2006;47:1895–903.

233. Rabin ML, Narayan VM, Kimberg DY, et al. Functional MRI predicts post-surgical memory following temporal lobectomy. Brain. 2004;127:2286–98.

234. Richardson MP, Strange BA, Thompson PJ, Baxendale SA, Duncan JS, Dolan RJ. Pre-operative verbal memory fMRI predicts post-operative memory decline after left anterior temporal lobe resection. Brain. 2004;127:2419–26.

235. Richardson MP, Strange BA, Duncan JS, Dolan RJ. Memory fMRI in left hippocampal sclerosis. Optimizing the approach to predicting postsurgical memory. Neurology. 2006;66:699–705.

236. Frings L, Wagner K, Halsband U, Schwarzwald R, Zentner J, Schulze-Bonhage A. Lateralization of hippocampal activation differs between left and right temporal lobe epilepsy patients and correlates with postsurgical verbal learning decrement. Epilepsy Res. 2008;78:161–70.

237. Powell HWR, Richardson MP, Symms MR, et al. Preoperative fMRI predicts memory decline following anterior temporal lobe resection. J Neurol Neurosurg Psychiatry. 2008;79:686–93.

238. Lacruz ME, Alarcon G, Akanuma N, et al. Neuropsychological effects associated with temporal lobectomy and amygdalohippocampectomy depending on Wada test failure. J Neurol Neurosurg Psychiatry. 2004;75:600–7.

239. Binder JR, Price CJ. Functional imaging of language. In: Cabeza R, Kingstone A, editors. Handbook of functional neuroimaging of cognition. Cambridge, MA: MIT Press; 2001. p. 187–251.

240. Grabowski TJ, Damasio H, Tranel D, Ponto LL, Hichwa RD, Damasio AR. A role for left temporal pole in the retrieval of words for unique entities. Hum Brain Mapp. 2001;13:199–212.

241. Hamberger MJ, Goodman RR, Perrine K, Tamny TR. Anatomic dissociation of auditory and visual naming in the lateral temporal cortex. Neurology. 2001;56:56–61.

242. Humphries C, Willard K, Buchsbaum B, Hickok G. Role of anterior temporal cortex in auditory sentence comprehension: an fMRI study. Neuroreport. 2001; 12:1749–52.

243. Patterson K, Nestor PJ, Rogers TT. Where do you know what you know? The representation of semantic knowledge in the human brain. Nat Rev Neurosci. 2007;8:976–87.

244. Pobric GG, Jefferies E, Lambon Ralph MA. Anterior temporal lobes mediate semantic representation: mimicking semantic dementia by using rTMS in normal participants. Proc Natl Acad Sci USA. 2007; 104:20137–41.

245. Schwartz MF, Kimberg DY, Walker GM, et al. Anterior temporal involvement in semantic word retrieval: voxel-based lesion-symptom mapping evidence from aphasia. Brain. in press.

246. Hermann BP, Wyler AR, Somes G, Clement L. Dysnomia after left anterior temporal lobectomy without functional mapping: frequency and correlates. Neurosurgery. 1994;35:52–7.

247. Langfitt JT, Rausch R. Word-finding deficits persist after left anterotemporal lobectomy. Arch Neurol. 1996;53:72–6.

248. Davies KG, Bell BD, Bush AJ, Hermann BP, Dohan FC, Jaap AS. Naming decline after left anterior temporal lobectomy correlates with pathological status of resected hippocampus. Epilepsia. 1998; 39:407–19.

249. Bell BD, Davies KG, Hermann BP, Walters G. Confrontation naming after anterior temporal lobectomy is related to age of acquisition of the object names. Neuropsychologia. 2000;38:83–92.

250. McCandliss BD, Cohen L, Dehaene S. The visual word form area: expertise for reading in the fusiform gyrus. Trends Cogn Sci. 2003;7:293–9.

251. Novick JM, Trueswell JC, Thompson-Schill SL. Cognitive control and parsing: Reexamining the role of Broca's area in sentence comprehension. Cogn Affect Behav Neurosci. 2005;5:263–81.

252. Price CJ, Crinion JT, Friston KJ. Design and analysis of fMRI studies with neurologically impaired patients. J Magn Reson Imaging. 2006;23: 816–26.

253. Richlan F, Kronbichler M, Wimmer H. Functional abnormalities in the dyslexic brain: A quantitative meta-analysis of neuroimaging studies. Hum Brain Mapp. 2009;10:3299–308.

Functional MRI Studies of Memory in Aging, Mild Cognitive Impairment, and Alzheimer's Disease

10

Shannon L. Risacher, Heather A. Wishart, and Andrew J. Saykin

Introduction

In the human brain, functionally and anatomically defined systems exist for encoding, consolidating, and retrieving memories of experiences (episodic memory); accumulating and accessing factual information in a body of knowledge (semantic memory); and actively processing and manipulating information (working memory). These three memory systems can be distinguished from other nondeclarative memory systems such as procedural learning and priming [1–4]. Brain-behavior studies using a variety of approaches from lesion-based research to functional magnetic resonance imaging (fMRI) demonstrate distinct though highly interrelated neural circuitry for episodic, semantic, and working memory [3, 5]. Each of these memory systems, despite their close interaction, is affected somewhat differently by aging and dementia.

In this chapter, the episodic, semantic, and working memory systems will be considered in turn, with special attention to changes associated with normal aging and with age-related memory disorders such as Alzheimer's disease (AD) and mild cognitive impairment (MCI). The first section explores the neuroanatomical substrates of episodic memory, as characterized by fMRI studies in healthy young adults. Next, we discuss fMRI studies of the changes in episodic memory that occur in healthy aging, as well as in MCI and AD. We also discuss functional and resting-state connectivity studies of episodic memory. In the final portion of the episodic memory section, we highlight studies in which fMRI techniques of episodic memory have been used as biomarkers of preclinical changes in memory and after pharmacological intervention. In the second section of the chapter, we explore fMRI studies of semantic memory in healthy young adults, aging, and in patients with MCI and AD. Similar to the previous episodic section, we then highlight further application of fMRI studies of semantic memory, including functional and resting-state connectivity and use of this technique as a biomarker. In the third section, we discuss fMRI studies of working memory in healthy young adults, older adults, and patients with MCI and AD. We also discuss functional and resting-state

S.L. Risacher, BS
Department of Radiology and Imaging Sciences, Indiana University School of Medicine, IU Center for Neuroimaging, 950 West Walnut Street, R2, E124, Indianapolis, IN 46202, USA
e-mail: srisache@iupui.edu

H.A. Wishart, PhD
Brain Imaging Laboratory, Department of Psychiatry, Dartmouth Medical School, One Medical Center Drive, Lebanon, NH 03756, USA
e-mail: Heather.A.Wishart@dartmouth.edu

A.J. Saykin, PsyD, ABPP/CN (✉)
Center for Neuroimaging, Department of Radiology and Imaging Sciences, Indiana University School of Medicine, 950 West Walnut Street, R2 E124, Indianapolis, IN 46202, USA
e-mail: asaykin@iupui.edu

S.H. Faro and F.B. Mohamed (eds.), *Functional BOLD MRI: Principles and Applications*,
DOI 10.1007/978-1-4939-1995-6_10, © Springer Science+Business Media New York 2015

connectivity studies of working memory and use of working memory fMRI techniques as biomarkers. Next, we briefly discuss some methodological considerations that are important for using fMRI techniques, particularly in older adults and patients with MCI and AD. Finally, we explore future directions of fMRI research, including applications to genomic studies of memory, advancements in technology, and potential for combining fMRI with other multimodal imaging techniques.

Episodic Memory

Episodic memory refers to memory for events or information encoded with respect to a particular temporal or spatial context [4]. Originally defined to encompass memory for specific information presented, for example, during a testing session, the concept has been reformulated to have at its core the conscious recollection of previous experiences. The emphasis is on memory for experience itself, not knowledge about the world derived from experience [6]. Episodic memory can be broadly defined as three separate cognitive processes: encoding, consolidation, and retrieval. Episodic encoding and retrieval processes can be studied using fMRI, due to the limited and definable nature of the response time-course. In other words, neural responses associated with episodic encoding occur upon or shortly after the presentation of a stimulus to be encoded, while responses associated with episodic retrieval occur upon or shortly after a request for recall or recognition of previously encoded information. However, consolidation of information is less easily studied due to the ill-defined nature of the response (i.e., time of occurrence and length of response). Other important distinctions pertaining to episodic memory function include the success with which the processes are performed (i.e., whether they result in the formation of an accurate, inaccurate, or no memory trace); the sensory modality in which the information is received (i.e., auditory and/or visual), and the nature of the material (i.e., verbal, spatial, and pictorial). There are a variety of episodic memory fMRI probes, many of which are specifically designed to address or manipulate certain of these aspects of episodic memory processing; sample tasks for episodic encoding and retrieval are shown in Table 10.1a.

fMRI Studies of Episodic Memory

Both episodic encoding and retrieval processes are thought to be subserved by a similar broad network of brain regions, including the prefrontal cortex (PFC), medial temporal lobe (MTL), and parietal and temporal cortices. For more detail on episodic memory circuitry, the reader is referred to several review articles (Table 10.2) [7–21].

fMRI of Episodic Encoding: The Role of the PFC

Episodic encoding studies have identified primarily left PFC activations during verbal encoding tasks (novel words versus previously presented material, association encoding of word pairs, encoding of words versus control conditions) [22–25], while nonverbal encoding tasks (similar task paradigms with encoding of objects, faces, patterns, and spatial information) show activation of the bilateral PFC [22, 24–29] (Fig. 10.1). The lateralization by content type is confirmed in direct comparisons of encoding of verbal and nonverbal stimuli, with greater activation of the left PFC during word encoding relative to scene, pattern, and texture encoding [22, 25] and greater activation of the right PFC during texture encoding relative to word encoding [25]. The left-lateralized nature of the signal associated with episodic encoding of verbal or easily verbalized material suggests an underlying association with semantic working memory systems in Broca's area (BA45) [30, 31]. This theory is supported by results from a study by Otten and Rugg, which found that words encoded with semantic associations show significantly greater activation in the left PFC than those encoded with phonological associations [32].

Table 10.1 Sample fMRI task characteristics for episodic, semantic, and working memory

Study	Memory domain	Modality	Design	Stimuli	Control condition	Performance monitoring
(A) Episodic memory						
Kelly et al. 1998 [24]	Episodic encoding	Visual	Block	Verbal (words)	Fixation	Recognition after scan
Kelly et al. 1998 [24]	Episodic encoding	Visual	Block	Object (line drawings)	Fixation	Recognition after scan
Wagner et al. 1998 [53]	Episodic retrieval	Visual	Block	Verbal (words)	Reading	Part of task
(B) Semantic memory						
Saykin et al. 1999 [254]	Semantic: category matching	Auditory	Block	Word pairs: category–example and category–function pairs	Nonword matching	Part of task
(C) Working memory						
Rypma and D'Esposito 2000 [390]	Working: delayed response	Visual	Event-related	Series of targets (letters, or objects and locations) encoded and retained over an unfilled interval; after interval participants respond whether target was part of retained sequence		Part of task
Wishart et al. 2006 [321]	Working: constant monitoring	Auditory	Block	"*N*-back" task: target letters are presented in sequence; participant must respond when a target letter is the same as a target letter either 1-back, 2-back, or 3-back in sequence		Part of task

Table 10.2 Selected review articles and meta-analyses of episodic memory for further reading

Episodic memory		
Authors	Study subjects	Article title
Fletcher et al. 1997 [8]	Young adults	The functional neuroanatomy of episodic memory. *Trends Neurosci.* May 1997;20(5):213–218
Desgranges et al. 1998 [13]	Young adults	The functional neuroanatomy of episodic memory: The role of the frontal lobes, the hippocampal formation, and other areas. *NeuroImage.* 1998;8: 198–213
Lepage et al. 1998 [42]	Young adults	Hippocampal PET activations of memory encoding and retrieval: The HIPER model. *Hippocampus.* 1998;8:313–322
Schacter et al. 1999 [9]	Young adults	Medial temporal lobe activations in fMRI and PET studies of episodic encoding and retrieval. *Hippocampus.* 1999;9(1):7–24
Wagner et al. 1999 [10]	Young adults	When encoding yields remembering: insights from event-related neuroimaging. *Philosophical Transactions of the Royal Society of London - Series B: Biological Sciences.* 1999;354(1387):1307–1324
Cabeza et al. 2000 [7]	Young adults	Imaging cognition II: An empirical review of 275 PET and fMRI studies. *Journal of Cognitive Neuroscience.* 2000;12(1):1–47
Davachi 2006 [12]	Young adults	Item, context, and relational episodic encoding in humans. *Curr Opin Neurobiol.* Dec 2006; 16(6):693–700
Eichenbaum et al. 2007 [14]	Young adults	The medial temporal lobe and recognition memory. *Annu Rev Neurosci.* 2007;30:123–152
Vilberg et al. 2008 [71]	Young adults	Memory retrieval and the parietal cortex: a review of evidence from a dual-process perspective. *Neuropsychologia.* 2008;46(7):1787–1799
Spaniol et al. 2009 [21]	Young adults	Event-related fMRI studies of episodic encoding and retrieval: meta-analyses using activation likelihood estimation. *Neuropsychologia.* Jul 2009; 47(8–9):1765–1779

(continued)

Table 10.2 (continued)

Episodic memory		
Authors	Study subjects	Article title
Kim 2010 [18]	Young adults	Dissociating the roles of the default-mode, dorsal, and ventral networks in episodic memory retrieval. *Neuroimage.* May 1 2010;50(4):1648–1657
Grady et al. 2000 [91]	Healthy aging	Changes in memory processing with age. *Current Opinion in Neurobiology.* 2000;10:224–231
Langley et al. 2000 [378]	Healthy aging	Functional neuroimaging of memory: implications for cognitive aging. *Microsc Res Tech.* Oct 1 2000;51(1):75–84
Cabeza 2001 [122]	Healthy aging	Cognitive neuroscience of aging: contributions of functional neuroimaging. *Scand J Psychol.* Jul 2001;42(3):277–286
Cabeza 2002 [105]	Healthy aging	Hemispheric asymmetry reduction in old adults: The HAROLD model. *Psychol. Aging.* 2002;17:85–100
Cabeza et al. 2002 [106]	Healthy aging	Aging gracefully: Compensatory brain activity in high-performing older adults. *NeuroImage.* 2002;17:1394–1402
Hedden et al. 2005 [377]	Healthy aging	Healthy and pathological processes in adult development: new evidence from neuroimaging of the aging brain. *Curr Opin Neurol.* Dec 2005; 18(6):740–747
Rajah et al. 2005 [116]	Healthy aging	Region-specific changes in prefrontal function with age: a review of PET and fMRI studies on working and episodic memory. *Brain.* Sep 2005;128(Pt 9):1964–1983
Grady 2000 [376]	Healthy aging	Cognitive neuroscience of aging. *Ann N Y Acad Sci.* Mar 2008;1124:127–144
Wagner 2000 [198]	MCI and AD	Early detection of Alzheimer's disease: An fMRI marker for people at risk? *Nature Neuroscience.* 2000;3(10):973–974
Zakzanis et al. 2003 [145]	MCI and AD	A meta-analysis of structural and functional brain imaging in dementia of the Alzheimer's type: a neuroimaging profile. *Neuropsychol Rev.* Mar 2003;13(1):1–18.
Wierenga et al. 2003 [385]	MCI and AD	Use of functional magnetic resonance imaging in the early identification of Alzheimer's disease. *Neuropsychol Rev.* Jun 2007;17(2):127–143
Dickerson et al. 2008 [379]	MCI and AD	Functional abnormalities of the medial temporal lobe memory system in mild cognitive impairment and Alzheimer's disease: insights from functional MRI studies. *Neuropsychologia.* 2008;46(6):1624–1635.
Drzezga 2008 [381]	MCI and AD	Concept of functional imaging of memory decline in Alzheimer's disease. *Methods.* Apr 2008; 44(4):304–314
Han et al. 2009 [382]	MCI and AD	Functional magnetic resonance imaging of compensatory neural recruitment in aging and risk for Alzheimer's disease: review and recommendations. *Dement Geriatr Cogn Disord.* 2009;27(1):1–10
Dickerson et al. 2009 [380]	MCI and AD	Large-scale functional brain network abnormalities in Alzheimer's disease: insights from functional neuroimaging. *Behav Neurol.* 2009;21(1):63–75
Ries et al. 2008 [383]	MCI and AD	Magnetic resonance imaging characterization of brain structure and function in mild cognitive impairment: a review. *J Am Geriatr Soc.* May 2008;56(5):920–934
Sperling et al. 2010 [384]	MCI and AD	Functional alterations in memory networks in early Alzheimer's disease. *Neuromolecular Med.* Mar 2010;12(1):27–43

Although the precise role of the PFC in episodic encoding has not been established, a number of reports have suggested that it plays a key role in top-down processing. The PFC likely plays a strategic role by organizing incoming information to allow for more efficient episodic storage [19, 20]. The PFC may also allow for encoding of new information through associations with semantic

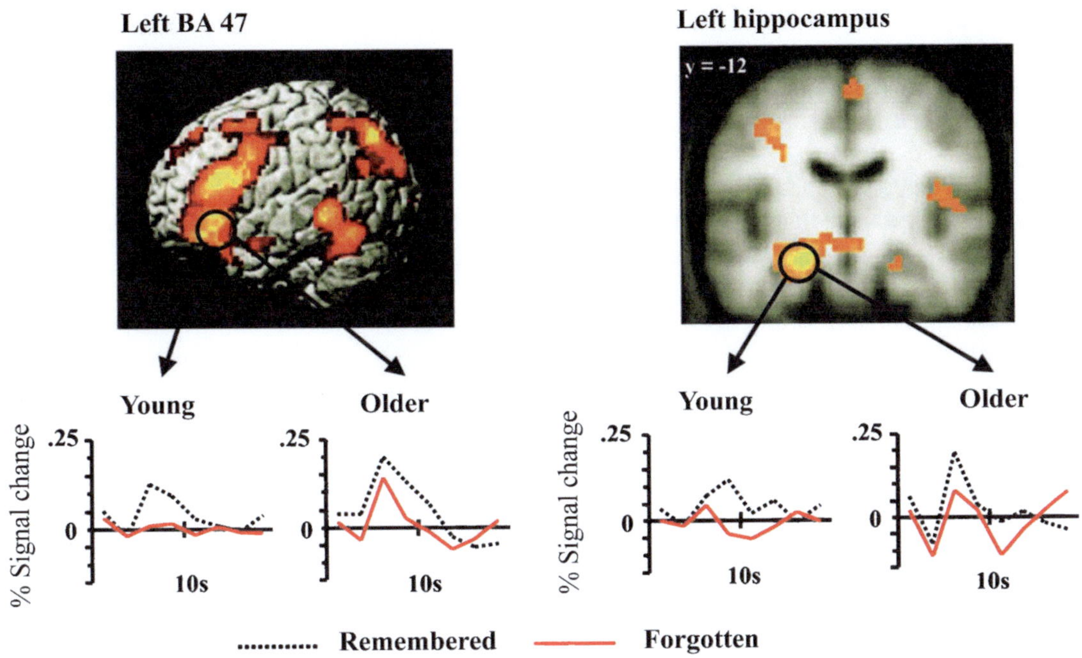

Fig. 10.1 Brain regions showing activation during episodic encoding. A broad pattern of brain regions including the left PFC (BA47) and hippocampus (B) were activated by both young and older adults during an fMRI study of episodic encoding of verbal material. Additionally, young adults but not older adults showed increased activation on subsequently remembered items relative to forgotten items. Reproduced with permission from Morcom AM, Good CD, Frackowiak RS, Rugg MD. Age effects on the neural correlates of successful memory encoding. *Brain.* 2003;126(Pt 1):213–229

knowledge [33, 34]. Other reports have suggested that the PFC may provide a filter for episodic encoding by modulating the input of sensory information from sensory cortical regions to the MTL [15, 35–37]. By monitoring and selecting the sensory information with the greatest relevance to the goal or task, the PFC can provide top-down control of which information is ultimately incorporated into an episodic memory trace.

fMRI of Episodic Encoding: The Role of the MTL

In addition to the PFC, the MTL has been routinely implicated in fMRI studies of episodic encoding [9, 21, 26, 27, 38–44]. The MTL is defined by a circuit of regions including the hippocampal formation (dentate gyrus, CA1, CA2, and CA3 fields, and subiculum), entorhinal cortex, perirhinal cortex, parahippocampal complex, and the amygdala [7, 13, 45, 46]. Hippocampal activation seems to be particularly sensitive to new information and demonstrates decreasing activation with repeated exposure to a stimulus [27, 44, 47]. Similar to activations in the PFC, episodic encoding activations in the MTL show content-based laterality [48]. Episodic encoding of verbal material shows activation in the left MTL [24, 47, 49], while encoding of nonverbal material demonstrates bilateral MTL activation [24, 27, 43, 44, 50]. Furthermore, the presence and extent of MTL activation is associated with successful memory formation. Studies have shown high association between activation in the hippocampal formation and subsequent successful retrieval, such as increased hippocampal activation during encoding of accurately retrieved items relative to forgotten items [10, 26, 49].

fMRI Studies of Episodic Retrieval

Episodic retrieval has also been shown to involve many of the same brain regions as those activated during episodic encoding, including the PFC, MTL, and temporal and parietal cortices. Episodic retrieval paradigms traditionally test two main types of verbal or nonverbal information retrieval, including free or cued recall and recognition. When an area of fMRI activation is measured in response to an episodic retrieval task, a number of additional questions emerge regarding the "meaning" of this activation, including but not limited to:

1. Are measured fMRI activations due to the actual recall/recognition of items or the process by which memory retrieval is monitored or searched for accuracy?
2. Do activations vary based on the information content (i.e., verbal or nonverbal) or on the nature of the requested response (content versus contextual)?
3. Are responses in recognition tasks due to actual recollection or familiarity judgment?

fMRI Studies of Episodic Retrieval: The Role of the PFC

Verbal and nonverbal episodic retrieval tasks demonstrate significant activation in the right and/or bilateral PFC, including regions of the posterior ventrolateral (BA45/47), frontopolar (BA10), and dorsal PFC (BA8/9) [25, 51–53]. The predominately right-lateralized nature of this response, relative to the previously discussed left-lateralized PFC responses during episodic encoding led to the development of a general theory called the "hemispheric encoding and retrieval asymmetry" (HERA) model [54, 55]. Specifically, the HERA model posits that left PFC regions are involved primarily in retrieval from semantic memory and encoding into episodic memory, and right PFC regions are involved in retrieval of information from episodic memory [7, 34, 55, 56]. Although initially proposed in response to functional positron emission tomography (PET) imaging studies, results supporting the HERA model have repeatedly been observed in studies using fMRI [16, 21, 24, 25, 39, 57–59].

fMRI Studies of Episodic Retrieval: The Role of the MTL

Regions of the MTL, including the hippocampus, and parahippocampal and perirhinal cortices, have been implicated in episodic retrieval [14, 17, 38, 60]. Studies using fMRI have identified bilateral hippocampal activations during episodic retrieval, with retrieval of verbal information primarily showing left hippocampal activation and nonverbal retrieval demonstrating right-lateralized or bilateral hippocampal activations [9, 21, 27, 57, 61–64]. This asymmetry is superimposed on a historical, lesion-based, material-specificity model, [65] which posits a left MTL specialization for verbal memory, and a right MTL specialization for material that is not readily verbally coded. Early brain insults also appear to modulate this model [66–68]. Additional fMRI studies have also attempted to parse whether subdivisions within the MTL mediate separate episodic memory functions. Initial studies of hippocampal activation in episodic memory using functional PET imaging techniques suggested a rostrocaudal gradient of hippocampal activity during episodic encoding and retrieval [42]. However, this hippocampal encoding/retrieval model (HIPER) has been refuted by studies employing event-related fMRI techniques, which have suggested a more complex set of findings regarding hippocampal organization for episodic memory processes [9, 38]. Other studies have investigated whether different structures within the MTL have separate functions in episodic encoding and retrieval [12, 38]. A number of studies have suggested that the hippocampal formation is specifically involved in the encoding of contextual or relational memories [41, 69], while the perirhinal cortex is activated during the encoding of memories for specific learned items [40, 41, 70].

fMRI Studies of Episodic Retrieval: The Role of the Parietal Cortex

In addition to MTL and prefrontal regions, activations in the lateral and medial parietal lobe are often observed during episodic retrieval paradigms [71]. These activations have been posited to reflect sensory and perceptual processes associated with recollection [72, 73]. Studies designed to characterize the specific role of the parietal lobe in episodic memory have resulted in the delineation of three functionally distinct subregions of the parietal lobe, including the lateral superior parietal cortex, the lateral inferior parietal cortex, and the medial parietal cortex. Recent fMRI studies implicate the activation of the superior parietal cortex during episodic retrieval tasks, including greater activation for "familiar" or "old" items relative to "new" items [74, 75]. However, the signal is unaffected by modality or task difficulty. Therefore, the bilateral superior parietal regions are thought to be involved in attentional processing and focus on behaviorally relevant stimuli rather than playing a specific role in episodic memory per se [71, 76]. On the other hand, activations in the lateral inferior parietal cortex show a specific association with successful recollection and greater activation during "remembered" relative to "known" items [63, 64]. Thus, studies suggest that the inferior parietal cortex plays a specific role in episodic memory processing, possibly representing a neural station for coordination between episodic and working memory [71, 77–79]. Although the medial parietal lobe has routinely been implicated in memory disorders, with degeneration in the precuneus reported in early stages of AD, fMRI activation in this region during an episodic memory task is thought to represent a "familiarity" signal rather than "recollection" [71]. In other words, the medial parietal cortex may not play a role in successful episodic retrieval, but instead is thought to mediate the familiarity of target stimuli.

fMRI Studies to Identify the Neural Correlates of the Steps of Episodic Retrieval

To evaluate the various roles of regions that show activation in episodic retrieval studies, the steps of episodic retrieval must be defined. Retrieval of episodic information can be broadly divided into three general functions, including (1) preparation and attention to the task requests and probes (i.e., "retrieval preparation"); (2) search and accuracy monitoring of retrieved information ("retrieval mode"); and (3) successful recollection of content or context ("retrieval success"). These separate steps appear to be neurally represented in both overlapping and distributed anatomic locations. Using high temporal resolution task paradigms such as jittering of probes and null trials, the bilateral frontopolar regions have been shown to mediate "retrieval preparation" [80–83]. Specifically, a study by Dobbins and Han used variable delays between task initiation and presentation of the target recognition probe to demonstrate that right frontopolar activation occurred prior to the presentation of the delayed probes [80]. Frontopolar regions, along with the dorsal PFC, have also been implicated in "retrieval mode" functions [29, 84]. A number of reports suggest that the left frontopolar and bilateral dorsal PFC are activated regardless of the type of retrieval task (item/content retrieval versus contextual retrieval) or the content of the retrieved information (verbal or nonverbal) [85, 86]. Furthermore, this activation has a sustained and tonic pattern of response during retrieval blocks, suggesting involvement in the general process of episodic retrieval instead of activation in response to specific retrieval probes [84, 86]. Finally, "retrieval success" has been primarily linked to the activation of the MTL, suggesting that this region is important for the recall of specific item and contextual information associated with successful retrieval [87].

Age-Related Changes in Episodic Memory

A large body of literature suggests that episodic memory processes, particularly encoding and retrieval, decline with age [88–93]. Whether this is related to "normal aging" of the brain or to an accumulation of age-related diseases remains a topic of debate [94–96]. There is some evidence to suggest relatively selective age-related atrophy of prefrontal cortical areas involved in episodic memory circuitry [97], with preservation of medial temporal lobe structures [97–99], though this too is debatable [100–102]. Furthermore, regenerative processes and reorganization in the adult human brain may help allay development of cognitive problems despite structural brain changes [103, 104]. Therefore, significant questions remain as to the neural and cognitive basis of episodic memory decline in aging. For reviews of episodic memory processes in aging, see Table 10.2.

fMRI Studies of Episodic Encoding and Retrieval in Normal Aging

A number of functional neuroimaging, electrophysiological, and behavioral studies suggest that the prefrontal functional asymmetries for memory processes present in young adults are diminished or absent in older adults. Healthy older adults demonstrate reduced left PFC activation and increased right PFC activation during intentional and incidental encoding [105–107] (Fig. 10.2). Additionally, older adults show diminished right PFC activation and enhanced left PFC activation in episodic retrieval [105–112]. In other words, research suggests that the HERA model does not hold in normal aging. This concept has been articulated in the HAROLD (*H*emispheric *A*symmetry *R*eduction in *Old* Adults) model [105]. The HAROLD model has repeatedly been shown in fMRI studies utilizing a wide variety of both verbal and nonverbal episodic encoding and retrieval tasks in older adults. Interestingly, the decreasing asymmetry of PFC responses to episodic encoding and retrieval in older adults is at least somewhat dependent on cognitive strategy. In fact, a few studies have shown that older adults have PFC responses similar to young adults during successful encoding and retrieval when taught to use deep encoding strategies [113–115]. These findings suggest that the regional deficit in activation in older adults during encoding is related to inefficient recruitment of available brain resources, rather than an irreversible loss of the underlying tissue due to cell death or dysfunction.

Two main theories have been created to explain the reduced lateralization in older adults, including the "compensatory" hypothesis and the "dedifferentiation" hypothesis [106, 110]. The compensatory hypothesis posits that increased bilateral representation of cognitive functions in older adults may reflect a form of compensatory brain reorganization that helps support normal cognitive function [105, 106, 116]. In fact, increased task complexity leads to bilateral activation in young adults, suggesting that bilateral representation assists with difficult processing [117]. Furthermore, increased bilateral PFC activation has been associated with better performance in older adults [104–106], although not all studies support this association [118]. The compensatory nature of bilateral PFC activation would parallel findings on brain functional reorganization following acquired brain damage. For example, in the case of unilateral focal acquired brain damage, recovery of function can be associated with bilateral hemispheric representation (among other types of reorganization) for functions such as language and movement [119, 120]. However, some studies found that decreased activation does not always occur in conjunction with increased activation in other areas, which does not support the compensation hypothesis and suggests that this pattern of decreased and increased activation may not necessarily be linked [115].

On the other hand, bilateral hemispheric representation may simply reflect diminished selectivity or "dedifferentiation" of the neural substrate of cognition in older adults [106, 115]. Previous reports have demonstrated a strong intercorrelation among different measures of cognitive ability in older adults, even across cognitive domains [121]. The dedifferentiation hypothesis suggests that decreased functional specialization may occur across the brain with normal aging, including decreased PFC asymmetry. The dedifferentiation and compensation theories may not be mutually exclusive, with the dedifferentiation theory sometimes reflecting a type of compensation, depending on investigators' use of these terms [122].

Structural degeneration of the PFC has been reported in healthy aging, while the MTL is relatively spared [97]. However, some studies have suggested alterations in MTL activation during episodic encoding and retrieval tasks in older individuals relative to young controls, including a decreased magnitude and extent of hippocampal activation during episodic encoding and retrieval tasks (Fig. 10.2a) [109, 111, 123–125]. Small and colleagues used the BOLD fMRI signal obtained at rest to estimate regional basal metabolism and examine the integrity of hippocampal subregions in healthy controls and individuals with dementia [126, 127]. This method rests on the assumption that basal deoxyhemoglobin levels reflect hemodynamic variables, such as oxygen extraction, that are related to basal metabolism. Using this method, Small examined hippocampal circuitry activity at rest in 70 individuals ranging in age from 20 to 88 years. In two hippocampal subregions, the subiculum and the dentate gyrus, an apparent decline in resting BOLD fMRI occurred as a linear function of age. However, decline in the entorhinal cortex was more variable, present only in a subset of older adults. This variability was interpreted as evidence that the entorhinal change was not a normal age-related change but rather an indicator of a pathological process.

In addition to decreased PFC asymmetry and altered MTL activation, older adults may also show a posterior to anterior shift in activation during episodic retrieval called the "posterior–

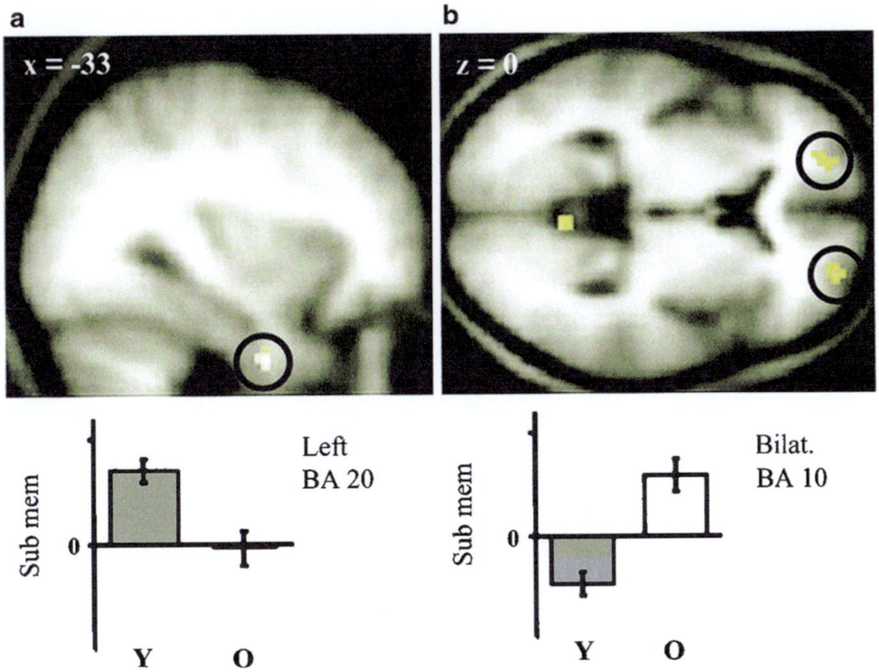

Fig. 10.2 Brain regions demonstrating age-related differences in activity during successful episodic encoding of verbal information. (**a**) Young adults showed greater activation than older adults in left anterior inferior temporal cortex (BA 20). (**b**) Older adults showed greater activation than young adults in bilateral anterior prefrontal cortex, supporting the HAROLD model of increased bilateral representation of episodic memory. Reproduced with permission Morcom AM, Good CD, Frackowiak RS, Rugg MD. Age effects on the neural correlates of successful memory encoding. *Brain.* 2003;126(Pt 1):213–229

anterior shift in aging" (PASA) [128, 129]. This pattern is proposed to result from a shift in processing in which the PFC is increasingly engaged to compensate for deficits in sensory processing mediated by the occipital cortex. The PASA has been shown to be a specific effect of aging rather than task difficulty and occurs in many different types of cognitive tasks, including episodic retrieval [128].

Though structural brain changes likely play a role in inducing age-related changes in activity of episodic memory circuitry, studies comparing deep and shallow encoding strategies offer preliminary evidence that age-related differences in the approach to a task may also contribute to the extent and location of brain activation [39, 115]. This underscores the importance of incorporating both structural and functional brain imaging methods in studies of cognition and aging, and of carefully monitoring participants' cognitive strategy use or approach to the task in addition to other aspects of their task performance.

Episodic Memory in Alzheimer's Disease and Related Conditions

Impairment of episodic memory is a core feature of age-related dementias, including AD and amnestic MCI, which is considered to be a prodromal stage of AD. Amnestic MCI is the most commonly studied subtype of MCI and is characterized by a relatively isolated impairment of episodic memory in the context of otherwise normal daily functioning and an absence of dementia [130–133]. For reviews and diagnostic criteria for MCI, see [130–134]. MCI and mild AD patients show significant structural neurodegeneration, with the earliest atrophic changes occurring in the hippocampus and entorhinal cortex, followed by progressive atrophy of the frontal, parietal, and temporal lobes [135–139]. Patients with amnestic MCI are significantly more likely to progress to mild AD, with an annualized conversion rate of 10–15%, relative to only 1–2% annual conversion of healthy elders to AD [133]. Neurodegenerative changes assessed using structural MRI techniques have been shown to accurately predict the rate of MCI to AD progression, suggesting that these measures may provide sensitive biomarkers for therapeutic trials [140–143]. For additional information regarding the role of structural MRI in MCI and AD, the reader is directed to a number of review articles [144–154].

fMRI Studies of Episodic Memory in Patients with AD

In addition to the structural changes associated with AD, patients also show altered brain function during cognitive tasks, including episodic encoding and retrieval. Studies utilizing fMRI have shown that patients with AD show reduced medial temporal activation relative to healthy elderly, including decreased activation of the hippocampus, entorhinal cortex, and parahippocampal gyri during episodic memory encoding of verbal and nonverbal material [125, 155–161] (Fig. 10.3). The extent of hippocampal activation is associated with successful encoding in healthy elders and patients with AD, suggesting that the reduced MTL activation is related to the observed impairments in encoding in AD [155, 162]. Furthermore, entorhinal cortex activation patterns have been shown to be particularly useful in discriminating AD patients from healthy elderly controls [159]. In addition to the reduced MTL activation, AD patients show increased activation in frontal and parietal cortical areas relative to age-matched controls during episodic encoding tasks [125, 156, 161, 163]. These regions of increased activation may suggest compensatory changes, dedifferentiation, or altered strategies for encoding in patients with AD. Patients with AD also show reduced PFC and MTL activations during episodic retrieval [164, 165]. The extent of PFC activation has been shown to be directly associated with retrieval success in AD patients [162]. Additionally, the extent of PFC activation during episodic retrieval within the AD patients was significantly associated with hippocampal volume, a marker of disease severity [165]. This finding is also consistent with the notion that medial temporal and frontal regions form an integrated circuit underlying episodic memory, and that damage in one part of the circuitry may be reflected in altered activation of other regions.

fMRI Studies of Episodic Memory in Patients with MCI

In contrast to the relatively consistent findings from fMRI studies of AD patients, studies of episodic encoding and retrieval in patients with MCI have been equivocal. Some reports have demonstrated increased MTL activation in MCI patients relative to healthy elderly during episodic tasks [166–169] (Figs. 10.3 and 10.4), while other studies have demonstrated significantly reduced MTL activations [160, 166, 170]. Further inspection of the results from these studies, as well as longitudinal follow-up studies of patients with MCI, has led to the formulation of a general pattern of MTL activation along the spectrum from healthy aging to AD [155, 166, 171]. Very mild early MCI patients show increased MTL activation during episodic tasks, which may reflect functional compensatory effects in an attempt to maintain normal

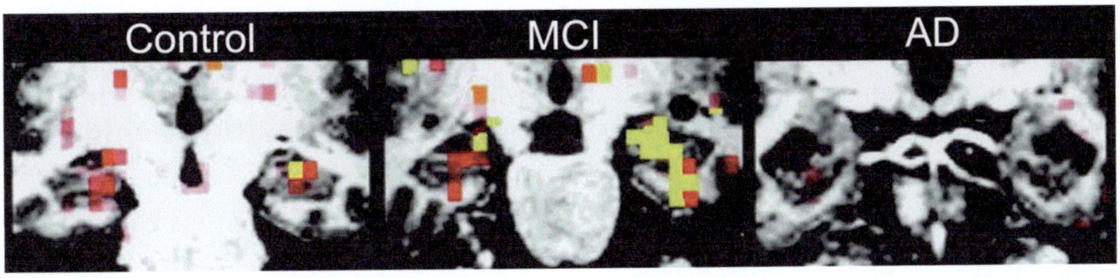

Fig. 10.3 Alterations in fMRI activations during episodic encoding in patients with MCI and AD. Patients with AD show significantly reduced hippocampal activation relative to healthy elderly controls and patients with MCI during an fMRI study of episodic encoding using a face-name association task. Patients with MCI show increased activation relative to healthy elderly. Reproduced with permission from Dickerson BC, Salat DH, Greve DN, et al. Increased hippocampal activation in mild cognitive impairment compared to normal aging and AD. *Neurology*. Aug 9 2005;65(3):404–411

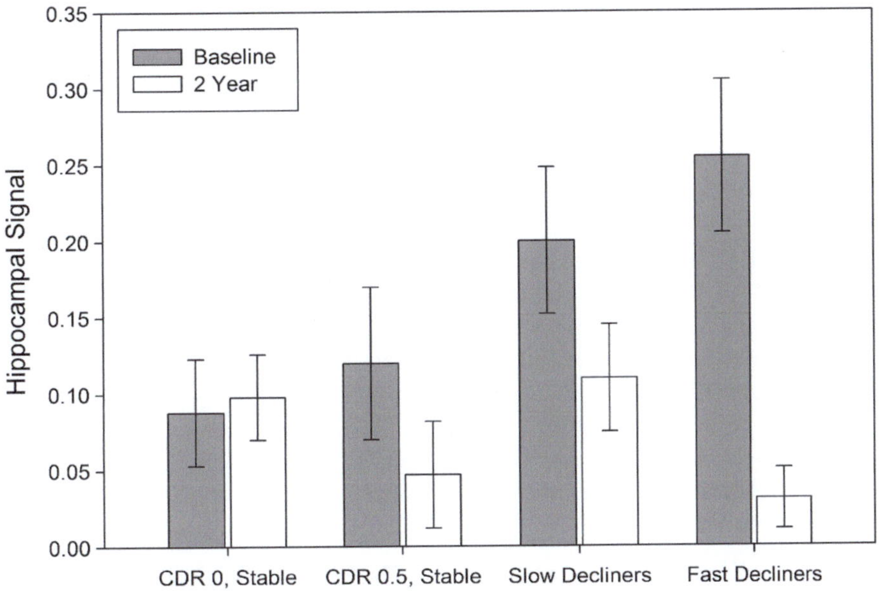

Fig. 10.4 Increased hippocampal activation at baseline is associated with faster decline in cognition over 2 years. A longitudinal study of healthy older adults and older adults with mild impairment demonstrated that increased hippocampal activation in an fMRI study of episodic encoding at baseline is associated with faster decline in cognition over 2 years. Furthermore, the difference between baseline and 2-year hippocampal activation was significantly greater in participants who demonstrated the greatest decline in cognition, relative to participants who remained stable or had a slower decline. Adapted from data presented in O'Brien JL, O'Keefe KM, LaViolette PS, et al. Longitudinal fMRI in elderly reveals loss of hippocampal activation with clinical decline. *Neurology*. Jun 15 2010;74(24):1969–1976

memory performance and overcome abnormal pathology and neurodegeneration. In fact, fMRI studies of these mild MCI patients often show near-normal levels of performance on episodic tasks. However, later stage MCI patients show significantly reduced MTL activation and impaired memory performance on episodic tasks. Late MCI participants also show a reduced "adaptation" response to repeated presentation of stimuli during encoding [172]. The increased MTL activation observed in mild MCI patients may be a sensitive predictor of future progression to AD, as early MCI patients with the highest baseline level of MTL activation during an episodic encoding task demonstrate a faster rate of decline over 2–6 years [171, 173]. For example, as shown in Fig. 10.4, patients who progressed most quickly or "fast decliners" had significantly greater hippocampal activity during an episodic encoding task at baseline relative to healthy elderly, stable early MCI patients, and even MCI patients who progressed at a slower rate ("slow decliners") [171]. Furthermore, fast decliners showed a significantly greater loss of hippocampal activation during an episodic memory task longitudinally and thus demonstrated significantly reduced hippocampal activation during episodic encoding at the 2-year follow-up visit relative to healthy elderly, stable MCI patients, and slow decliners [171]. In addition to the variable MTL responses across the spectrum of MCI severity, differences in response may also be evident within the MTL substructures. A recent high-resolution fMRI study suggested that patients with mild MCI show increased activation in the CA3 and dentate gyrus of the hippocampal formation and decreased activation in the entorhinal cortex [174].

Functional and Resting-State Connectivity Associated with Episodic Memory

Traditionally, fMRI and other types of functional neuroimaging studies have focused on specific and independent regions of activation associated with a task. However, complex cognitive tasks usually require a network of regions working together [175, 176]. Therefore, a number of recent reports have focused on the connection between fMRI signals in anatomically distinct regions during task-induced activations ("functional connectivity") [176] and during "resting" periods in the absence of functional tasks ("resting-state connectivity") [38, 177]. Functional connectivity analyses, along with other new fMRI analysis techniques, provide an opportunity to better understand the complex neural processes underlying memory in healthy young and older adults, as well as in patients with AD.

fMRI Studies of Episodic Associated Connectivity in Healthy Young Adults

Studies of functional connectivity have implicated neural networks linking the PFC, parietal and temporal cortices, and the MTL in episodic encoding tasks [178–180]. Specifically, successful episodic encoding activates a functional network that includes the hippocampus and other MTL regions, the medial and lateral parietal lobe, lateral temporal cortical regions, and the PFC [179]. Additionally, a recent study by Burianova and colleagues suggested that a common functional network that includes the MTL, lateral temporal cortex, PFC, and cingulate underlies autobiographical, episodic, and semantic memory systems [180]. Functional connectivity analyses have also identified a functional network associated with episodic retrieval. A network including frontal and parietal cortical regions has been implicated in successful episodic retrieval [181, 182], although the activity of this network may be dependent on the depth of episodic encoding [182].

Resting-state connectivity investigations have reported a network of anatomically distinct brain regions referred to as the "default mode network" (DMN), which is active during rest conditions and deactivates upon task initiation [183, 184]. This distributed network includes the medial parietal cortex/precuneus, posterior cingulate, medial PFC, and MTL [38, 183, 184]. The DMN has been shown to activate slightly to task cues and then deactivate significantly upon task initiation, suggesting that these regions may be involved in attentiveness and internal readiness.

fMRI Studies of Episodic Associated Connectivity in Healthy Older Adults

Functional and resting connectivity techniques have also been utilized to investigate episodic memory function in older adults. Older adults show greater prefrontal connectivity, inferior parietal connectivity, and decreased hippocampal connectivity during episodic encoding and retrieval relative to younger adults using structural equation modeling of fMRI and PET data [3, 185–187]. Daselaar and colleagues suggested similar alterations in functional connectivity during a verbal episodic memory task, including a reduction in the hippocampal–parietotemporal functional network and an increase in the rhinal–frontal network in older adults relative to younger participants [123]. The strength of hippocampal–medial parietal connectivity is associated with episodic retrieval performance in older adults [188].

Alterations in the DMN or "resting-state" network have also been reported in older participants [189–191]. Specifically, older adults show reduced deactivation of the DMN upon episodic task initiation relative to young controls, including impaired deactivation of the precuneus and posterior cingulate. Furthermore, older adults with high performance on a post-scan recognition test demonstrated significantly greater deactivation of the precuneus relative to older adults who performed poorly, suggesting that the deactivation of the DMN is important in successful encoding [192]. Overall, the DMN and functional networks associated with episodic memory demonstrate age-related alterations, which may lead to memory dysfunction and/or serve as biomarkers for future cognitive decline.

fMRI Studies of Episodic Associated Connectivity in Patients with MCI and AD

In addition to alterations in regional activations during episodic tasks, patients with MCI and AD show altered functional and resting-state connectivity. Patients with AD show impaired functional connectivity between the left and right hippocampus [193], as well as impairment in connectivity of an episodic encoding network that includes the hippocampus, inferior prefrontal cortex, fusiform gyrus, and visual-association cortex [166]. On the other hand, impairment of connectivity in patients with MCI may be dependent on stage of disease, with late-stage MCI patients showing impairment and early-stage MCI patients showing increased connectivity of the hippocampal-PFC-parietal network (Fig. 10.5a). Patients with AD may also engage additional alternative networks to accomplish tasks relative to those used by healthy elderly [163].

A number of studies have also shown impaired deactivation of the DMN upon task initiation in patients with MCI and AD [166, 194–197]. Specifically, AD and late-stage MCI patients showed impaired deactivation of the DMN, including deficits in deactivation of the precuneus, posterior cingulate, lateral parietal cortex, temporal cortices, anterior cingulate, and medial frontal cortices. However, early-stage MCI patients showed an enhanced deactivation of the DMN upon task initiation relative to late-stage MCI, AD, and healthy elderly (Fig. 10.5b). The greatest differences between patients and healthy elderly occurred in the earliest phase of deactivation in the anterior frontal cortex, including the anterior cingulate and medial frontal lobe [195]. Furthermore, the extent of deactivation in the anterior frontal cortex could successfully classify healthy elderly versus MCI patients and MCI versus AD patients, while the extent of deactivation in the precuneus successfully classified healthy elderly from both patient groups [195]. Alterations in the DMN function have also been shown to be highly associated with alterations in MTL activity and connectivity, suggesting an association between these impairments and episodic memory function [166, 173, 194].

fMRI of Episodic Memory Function as a Biomarker: Patients At-Risk for AD and after Therapeutic Intervention

Evidence is emerging that functional neuroimaging is sensitive to the earliest stages of dementia, even before marked clinical symptoms of AD or

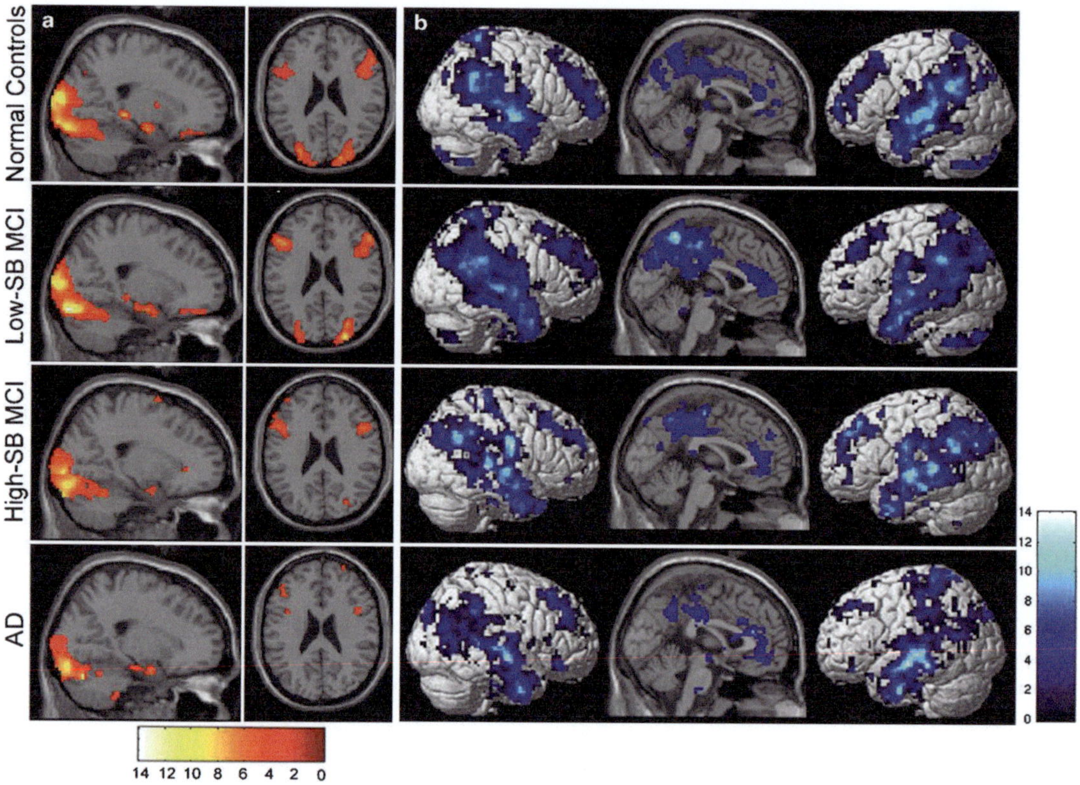

Fig. 10.5 Functional and resting-state connectivity associated with episodic memory is altered in MCI and AD relative to healthy elderly. A functional network (A, *yellow-red*) between the visual cortex, hippocampus, and inferior PFC was observed during an episodic encoding task in all participants. Deactivation of the resting-state network (B, *blue*), including the medial parietal, lateral temporal, and PFC, was also observed upon task initiation in all participants. However, MCI and AD patients demonstrated altered activation and deactivation of both of these networks. Early (Low-SB) MCI patients demonstrated increased connectivity of both the functional and resting-state networks. However, late (High-SB) MCI and AD patients showed decreased functional and resting-state connectivity relative to early MCI and healthy elderly. Adapted with permission from Celone KA, Calhoun VD, Dickerson BC, et al. Alterations in memory networks in mild cognitive impairment and Alzheimer's disease: an independent component analysis. *J Neurosci.* Oct 4 2006;26(40):10222–10231

MCI are evident [198]. Participants who express subjective cognitive complaints but no clinically significant memory impairment, a group which is at higher risk for developing MCI and AD, show significant alterations in brain activity during episodic encoding relative to age-matched controls. In a recent report by Rodda and colleagues, patients with cognitive complaints showed significantly increased activation of the left PFC during an episodic encoding task relative to age-matched controls without complaints [199]. Furthermore, the magnitude of the left PFC response was significantly positively associated with successful retrieval both within the group with complaints and across all participants. These results may reflect a compensation of the PFC to counteract a subclinical memory decline, although additional studies are needed to further characterize this population cross-sectionally and longitudinally.

Cognitively intact, middle-aged to older individuals who are at-risk for AD by virtue of their genetic [apolipoprotein E (ApoE), ε4 (epsilon 4) allele] status [200] also show altered fMRI activation during episodic tasks. In an early study, Bookheimer and colleagues found increased intensity and spatial extent of activation in temporal, parietal, and prefrontal regions during episodic

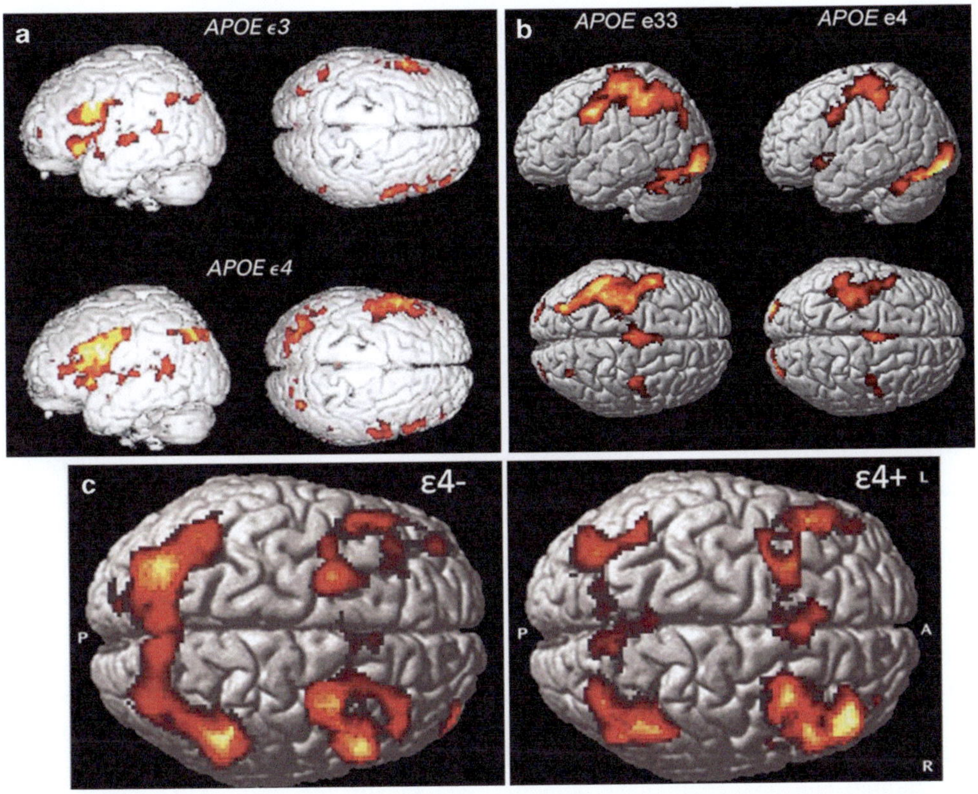

Fig. 10.6 Functional MRI activation during episodic, semantic, and working memory paradigms as a function of ApoE ε4 (epsilon 4) genotype. Functional MRI techniques have been used as biomarkers in studies of cognitively healthy older adults to examine the effect of ApoE ε4 (epsilon 4) genotype on task-induced activation. (**a**) Activation in the PFC was significantly greater in ApoE ε4 (epsilon 4) positive participants relative to ApoE ε4 (epsilon 4) negative participants in an fMRI study of episodic memory. On the other hand, ApoE ε4 (epsilon 4) positive participants demonstrated significantly reduced activation during (**b**) semantic and (**c**) working memory tasks relative to ApoE ε4 (epsilon 4) negative participants. Figure adapted with permission from: (A) Bookheimer SY, Strojwas MH, Cohen MS, et al. Patterns of brain activation in people at risk for Alzheimer's disease. *The New England Journal of Medicine.* 2000;343(7):450–456. Copyright ©2000 Massachusetts Medical Society. All rights reserved; (B) Lind J, Persson J, Ingvar M, et al. Reduced functional brain activity response in cognitively intact apolipoprotein E epsilon4 carriers. *Brain.* May 2006;129(Pt 5):1240–1248.; and (C) Wishart HA, Saykin AJ, Rabin LA, et al. Increased brain activation during working memory in cognitively intact adults with the APOE epsilon4 allele. *Am J Psychiatry.* Sep 2006;163(9): 1603–1610

encoding and retrieval in individuals who were ε4 (epsilon 4) positive compared with those without the ε4 (epsilon 4) allele (see Fig. 10.6a) [201]. Baseline activation patterns predicted memory decline over the next 2 years. The fact that these individuals were recruiting broader areas to accomplish the episodic memory task suggests that changes in activation may occur very early during the course of memory disorders such as AD. These changes may play a compensatory role and may represent an early marker for subsequent cognitive decline. Subsequently, a follow-up study reported no differences between ε4 (epsilon 4) positive and negative groups in fMRI brain activation patterns on an attention/working memory task [202]. This was interpreted as evidence that compensatory brain activation in ε4 (epsilon 4) carriers is specific to the episodic memory system. Similar results were also reported in older adults, with ApoE ε4 (epsilon 4) positive participants demonstrating greater brain response during novel picture encoding in the bilateral fusiform gyri, superior parietal lobe, and the frontal cortex relative to ApoE ε4 (epsilon 4) negative participants [203]. In contrast, other studies have shown reduced MTL and PFC activation in ApoE ε4 (epsilon 4) positive participants at-risk for AD during episodic memory tasks [204, 205].

In addition to potential utility as an early marker of disease, activations during episodic encoding tasks have been used in studies to evaluate the effect of acetylcholinesterase inhibitor (AChEI) treatments on brain function in patients with MCI and AD. In a preliminary study of seven patients with mild AD, Rombouts and colleagues investigated the effects of rivastigmine, a cholinesterase inhibitor, on brain activity patterns during episodic memory performance (and working memory, as described later) [206]. A single dose of the medication led to a bilateral increase in activation in the fusiform gyrus during face encoding, suggesting that rivastigmine affects task-related brain activity in regions associated with cholinergic circuitry. Additional studies to investigate other AChEI treatments, including galantamine and donepezil, have demonstrated similar increased activation in medicated patients with MCI and AD [207, 208]. The effects of anticholinergic medications such as scopolamine and/or mecamylamine have also been investigated using fMRI studies of episodic memory [209, 210]. A recent study by Dumas and colleagues demonstrated modulation of MTL and cortical activations after administration of scopolamine or mecamylamine, including decreased activation in the left parietal and occipital cortices, insula, and parahippocampal gyrus, but increased activation in the right hippocampus [209]. Overall, these studies suggest that activation measured using fMRI is sensitive to the effects of pharmacological treatments, and thus, may be useful in therapeutic trials to assess both efficacy and mechanism of action.

Summary

Functional MRI studies of episodic memory have implicated a network of brain regions involved with both episodic encoding and retrieval, including bilateral PFC, MTL, and parietal and lateral temporal cortices. In young adults, episodic encoding and retrieval appear to be lateralized in the frontal cortex, with encoding localized to the left PFC and retrieval localized in the right PFC. However, in older adults, this hemispheric lateralization appears to be reduced or absent. Patients with MCI and AD show altered activation during episodic encoding and retrieval, which may be dependent on disease stage. Early MCI patients show increased MTL activation during episodic tasks, while late MCI and AD patients show decreased activation in the MTL. Furthermore, increased hippocampal activation at baseline may be a biomarker of progression. Functional MRI studies of task-related connectivity studies have implicated networks that include frontal, parietal, and temporal cortices in episodic memory function. Resting-state networks that include the medial parietal and frontal cortex have also been identified in fMRI studies of episodic memory. Both functional and resting-state networks are altered in normal aging, as well as MCI and AD. Finally, the use of fMRI studies of episodic memory as a biomarker have shown promise in detecting preclinical altered activation patterns in individuals at-risk for dementia and in pharmacological intervention studies.

Semantic Memory

Semantic memory is broadly defined as knowledge about the world and includes the set of ideas, words, and symbols that are generally shared by individuals within a culture [7, 211]. Unlike episodic memories, semantic memories are not context dependent. Semantic memory consists of knowledge about the meaning of words, the properties of objects, and general facts. For example, remembering the movie you saw last week depends on episodic memory, but remembering the meaning of the word "movie," the knowledge that "movies are often made in Hollywood," and the fact that "Hollywood is in the state of California in the USA" are examples of semantic memory. For selected reviews of fMRI studies of semantic memory, see Table 10.3.

Table 10.3 Selected review articles of semantic memory for further reading

Semantic memory		
Authors	Study subjects	Article title
Binder et al. 2009 [213]	Young adults	Where is the semantic system? A critical review and meta-analysis of 120 functional neuroimaging studies. *Cereb Cortex.* Dec 2009;19(12):2767–2796
Cappa 2008 [386]	Young adults	Imaging studies of semantic memory. *Curr Opin Neurol.* Dec 2008;21(6):669–675
Cabeza et al. 2000 [7]	Young adults	Imaging cognition II: An empirical review of 275 PET and fMRI studies. *Journal of Cognitive Neuroscience.* 2000;12(1):1–47
Vigneau et al. 2006 [216]	Young adults	Meta-analyzing left hemisphere language areas: phonology, semantics, and sentence processing. *Neuroimage.* May 1 2006;30(4):1414–1432
Cabeza 2001 [122]	Healthy aging	Cognitive neuroscience of aging: contributions of functional neuroimaging. *Scand J Psychol.* Jul 2001;42(3):277–286
Grady et al. 2000 [91]	Healthy aging	Changes in memory processing with age. *Current Opinion in Neurobiology.* 2000;10:224–231
Grady 2008 [376]	Healthy aging	Cognitive neuroscience of aging. *Ann N Y Acad Sci.* Mar 2008;1124:127–144
Hedden et al. 2005 [377]	Healthy aging	Healthy and pathological processes in adult development: new evidence from neuroimaging of the aging brain. *Curr Opin Neurol.* Dec 2005;18(6):740–747
Langley et al. 2000 [378]	Healthy aging	Functional neuroimaging of memory: implications for cognitive aging. *Microsc Res Tech.* Oct 1 2000;51(1):75–84
Wingfield et al. 2006 [387]	Healthy aging	Language and the aging brain: patterns of neural compensation revealed by functional brain imaging. *J Neurophysiol.* Dec 2006;96(6):2830–2839
Drzezga 2008 [381]	MCI and AD	Concept of functional imaging of memory decline in Alzheimer's disease. *Methods.* Apr 2008;44(4):304–314
Wierenga and Bondi 2007 [385]	MCI and AD	Use of functional magnetic resonance imaging in the early identification of Alzheimer's disease. *Neuropsychol Rev.* Jun 2007;17(2):127–143

fMRI of the Neuroanatomical Substrates of Semantic Memory

As might be expected given the rich associative and inferential processes that can be invoked for the recollection of even simple factual information and words, studies of semantic memory suggest a broad neural circuitry underlying semantic processing [7, 212–216]. The first studies regarding the neural networks associated with semantic memory were in patients with brain damage, neurodegenerative disorders, and brain lesions. More recently, functional neuroimaging techniques have been utilized in patients with selective deficits in semantic memory, as well as healthy participants engaging in semantic memory retrieval (Fig. 10.7). Functional semantic memory studies primarily assess the semantic network through tasks focused on naming, categorization, or generation of concepts, words, or objects. Sample fMRI measures of semantic memory are presented in Table 10.1b.

A recent meta-analysis was conducted by Binder and colleagues exploring the results from numerous functional neuroimaging studies of semantic memory to identify brain regions involved in semantic processing [213]. This report highlighted the seven most commonly reported regions involved in semantic memory from functional neuroimaging studies with healthy young adults. The most commonly reported regions showing activation included: (1) the posterior inferior parietal lobe, including the angular gyrus and supramarginal gyrus; (2) the lateral temporal lobe, including the middle and inferior temporal gyri; (3) the ventromedial temporal lobe, including the fusiform gyrus and the parahippocampal gyrus; (4) the dorsomedial PFC, including the superior frontal gyrus and middle frontal gyrus; (5) the inferior frontal lobe, particularly the pars orbitalis; (6) the ventromedial and orbital PFC; and (7) the

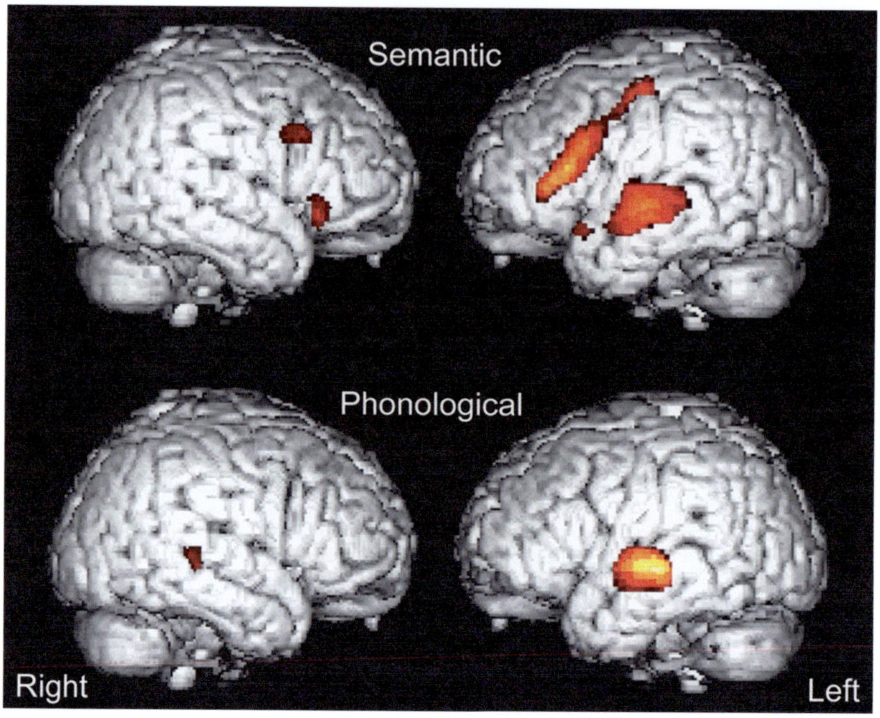

Fig. 10.7 Functional MRI activations during semantic processing in young and older healthy controls. Overlapping activations during a semantic decision task (*top*) were observed in young and older healthy controls in the left lateral temporal cortex and the inferior PFC (*left* > *right*). Only a limited cluster in the posterior lateral temporal cortex was observed during a phonological only task (*bottom*), suggesting that the activations in the PFC and anterior lateral temporal lobe were specific to semantic processing (*top*). Reproduced with permission from Johnson SC, Saykin AJ, Flashman LA, et al. Similarities and differences in semantic and phonological processing with age: Patterns of functional MRI activation. *Aging, Neuropsychology, and Cognition.* 2001;8(4):307–320. Taylor & Francis

posterior cingulate gyrus and ventral precuneus. Although activations in these regions were significantly more likely to be left-lateralized in right-handed individuals, bilateral activations were also reported [213].

Studies of patients with focal lesions and carefully designed functional studies have provided evidence about the function of each of these locations in semantic processing. The seven regions listed have a variety of functions that fall into three basic categories: (a) regions that are involved in long-term storage of specific semantic knowledge, often by category; (b) regions that are involved in the integration of semantic knowledge from multiple domains into a coherent understanding and/or expression of overall concepts; and (c) regions that primarily connect semantic memory processing with other memory and cognitive networks [217].

Long-term storage of semantic knowledge is thought to be category-specific and linked to the sensory-perceptual features that best represent category examples. For example, living things may be associated with visual-shape perceptual features, while tools or implements may be more associated with visual-motion perceptual features [213, 214, 217]. The major neuroanatomic regions thought to mediate long-term storage of semantic knowledge include the lateral temporal cortex, including the middle and inferior temporal gyri, the ventral temporal cortex, including the fusiform gyrus, and the ventral-medial PFC [213]. The lateral and ventral temporal regions are primarily involved in storage and retrieval of perceptual features and knowledge about objects, facts, and words [213]. Regional specificity within the temporal cortex by category and perceptual features has also been observed. The posterior temporal cortex is particularly implicated in long-term storage of tool and action concepts [221], while the fusiform gyrus is thought to have a role in storage of visual attributes of semantic knowledge [222]. Semantic dementia, a progressive neurodegenerative form of frontotemporal dementia (FTD), is associated with extensive atrophy of the lateral and ventral temporal cortex [218–220]. Patients with semantic dementia often show significant deficits in semantic knowledge with relative sparing of other types of memory (i.e., episodic, working, and procedural) [219]. Additionally, patients with damage to the anterior temporal cortex often show greater impairment for semantic knowledge about "living things" [223]. The ventral medial PFC, including the rostral and subgenual cingulate gyrus, gyrus rectus, and medial orbitofrontal cortex are thought to be involved in storage and retrieval of the emotional attributes of semantic concepts [213, 224]. The ventral medial PFC has also been linked with motivation, the affective nature of semantic concepts, reward processing, and self-knowledge or semantic self-awareness [225, 226].

Processing and integration of semantic knowledge appears to involve a number of neuroanatomic regions, including the posterior inferior parietal lobe, including the angular gyrus and supramarginal gyrus, the dorsal medial PFC, including the middle and superior frontal gyri, and regions of the inferior frontal lobe, particularly the pars orbitalis [213]. The posterior inferior parietal lobe is thought to be particularly involved in comprehension and expression of overall concepts [213, 227]. For example, a recent fMRI study with healthy young adults indicated that the activation of this region occurred at the end of sentence presentation and was only present when the stimulus conveyed a coherent meaning [228]. The inferior parietal lobe is also thought to be involved in other types of complex semantic processing, including sentence comprehension, discourse, problem-solving, and planning [213]. The dorsal medial PFC is also thought to play a role in semantic integration and is particularly implicated in self-guided and -motivated retrieval [229] and formulation of semantic concepts [213]. Patients with damage to this area have difficulty with the generation of new speech (i.e., category lists) and unique responses during discourse [213, 230]. The inferior frontal lobe, including the pars orbitalis, is thought to play a similar role to the dorsal medial PFC and is associated with task difficulty and complex planning of semantic articulations. Interestingly, damage to this area does not affect the accuracy of semantic processing but instead impairs processing "efficiency" or "speed" [213, 231].

In addition to long-term storage and semantic integration, selected regions of the semantic network implicated in Binder et al. [214] are likely to mediate connections between the semantic memory and other memory systems. The parahippocampal gyrus is thought to be a direct interface between the semantic and episodic memory systems, connecting semantic knowledge stored in the lateral temporal cortex with episodic memory processing in the MTL [213, 215]. The posterior cingulate and ventral precuneus have also been implicated in the integration of semantic and episodic memory, as well as emotion processing, spatial attention, and visual imagery [232–234]. Activation of the parahippocampal gyrus and the posterior cingulate or precuneus by semantic processing may reflect episodic and/or emotional experiences associated with specific semantic concepts [213, 235].

fMRI of Semantic Memory in Normal Aging

An important component of semantic memory, knowledge or "crystallized intellect," is thought to be preserved and possibly even enhanced in normal aging [94, 236]. However, the efficiency and accuracy with which information is retrieved from semantic memory can be affected in older adults [237–239]. Functional neuroimaging studies exploring changes in semantic memory processing in normal aging have found similar alterations as observed in studies of episodic memory in older adults (see "fMRI of Episodic Encoding and Retri-eval in Normal Aging" section). Specifically, older adults show reduced lateralization of semantic retrieval, which has been posited in the "HAROLD" model, as previously discussed [105, 107]. This reduction in hemispheric asymmetry may represent compensation, reductions in processing efficacy, or dedifferentiation of cognitive function. Functional MRI studies of semantic memory have demonstrated increased bilateral activations in older adults relative to young adults using a variety of semantic paradigms, including naming tasks with multiple semantic categories, semantic memory for famous people, as well as sentence processing and comprehension [240–245]. Despite having equivalent performance to the younger participants, older adults show a significant positive association between greater bilateral activation and performance on the semantic tasks [244]. In a recent study, Tyler and colleagues also demonstrated a significant association between greater atrophy in the left inferior frontal gyrus, as measured by reduced gray matter density, and increased activation in the right inferior and middle frontal gyri during a sentence comprehension task [246]. These authors suggested that the bilateral activation in older adults during semantic processing compensates for reduced GM density in the frontal lobe associated with aging.

In addition to reduced lateralization, older adults demonstrated other alterations in activation relative to young controls during fMRI studies of semantic memory. Studies utilizing both naming and semantic processing tasks suggested a greater magnitude and extent of activation in older adults relative to young adults [243, 245, 246]. Specifically, older adults showed greater activation in the bilateral medial, inferior, and dorsal lateral PFC, lateral temporal cortex, posterior lateral temporoparietal regions, and fusiform gyrus than young adults. Additionally, a study by Wierenga and colleagues demonstrated an altered hemodynamic response (HDR) during semantic tasks in older adults relative to younger controls [244]. Specifically, older adults had a different HDR time-course in regions of interest (ROIs) in the frontal and temporal lobes with a delayed rise to peak activation and return to baseline.

fMRI Studies of Semantic Memory in MCI and AD

As in episodic memory, semantic memory is affected in MCI and AD, although the more profound changes typically occur later in the disease. Eventually, significant deficits in identification and knowledge can emerge [95]. AD patients can show category-specific impairments (i.e., "living things" more impaired than "artifacts") and category-independent deficits [247–249]. MCI patients often show minimal or no deficits in semantic memory [250]. Functional MRI studies of patients with MCI and AD have shown significant alterations in activations associated with semantic memory paradigms, including semantic classification, category-matching, naming, and other semantic tasks [251–255]. In simple semantic tasks where performance of AD patients and healthy elderly is similar, AD patients show primarily reduced activation in the lateral frontal and temporoparietal cortices relative to healthy controls [251–253, 255]. These regions are primarily implicated in category-independent processing and integration of semantic knowledge, thus suggesting particular impairment in higher-level semantic processing in patients with AD [255]. On the other hand, other studies have found increased activations in patients with MCI and AD relative to healthy elderly in both the frontal and temporal lobes during both simple and more difficult semantic tasks [253, 254]. For example, in an early study examining these issues, Saykin and colleagues demonstrated that two semantic category-matching tasks activated left lateral prefrontal and temporal regions, whereas a phonologic control task activated only temporal areas [254]. In patients with mild AD, the spatial extent of left frontal activation on the semantic task was greater than in elderly controls, though accuracy was lower in the patient group. Figure 10.8 shows a surface render of brain activation during a semantic decision-making task for category-function pairs (e.g. match: beverage-sip and mismatch: vehicle-sip). Similar to the increased activation seen in older adults during semantic tasks, this increased activation was thought to be compensatory. In fact, the extent of

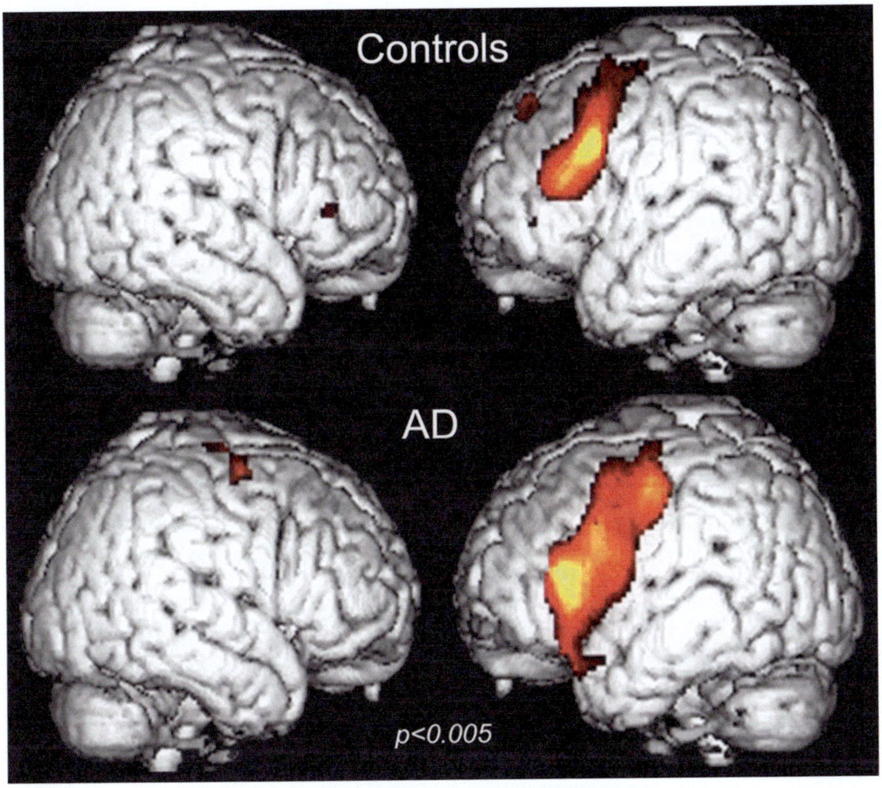

Fig. 10.8 Expanded region of activation in the PFC in semantic decision task in AD patients. Surface render of fMRI brain activation during semantic decision making (match vs. mismatch) for category–function pairs (e.g., match: beverage-sip, mismatch: vehicle-sip). *Upper panel* is activation for the healthy elderly control group; *bottom panel* is mild AD group. Note the expanded spatial extent of activation in the patient group in the left frontal region in the AD patients. Figure based on a further analysis of data published in Saykin AJ, Flashman LA, Frutiger SA, et al. Neuroanatomic substrates of semantic memory impairment in Alzheimer's disease: patterns of functional MRI activation. *J Int Neuropsychol Soc.* Jul 1999;5(5):377–392

increased activation in the lateral frontal cortex during semantic processing was significantly associated with the extent of atrophy in the frontal lobe in AD patients [252]. This finding offers support for the compensatory recruitment hypothesis in semantic memory in AD, suggesting that an increased extent and amplitude of brain activation may help to offset disease-related structural changes in the brain, which are evident in AD patients in widespread regions throughout the brain [256]. However, other reasons for the alterations in activation are also possible.

The conflicting results from different studies may result from the different semantic tasks employed and differences in performance between patients with AD and healthy elderly controls. Additionally, the extent and magnitude of activation during semantic memory tasks may depend on disease stage and clinical severity, similar to the results from patients with MCI and AD in episodic memory studies [251, 253]. In fact, patients with MCI show increased activation during semantic memory tasks, particularly in the dorsolateral PFC, inferior parietal lobe, and temporoparietal regions [250, 251].

fMRI Studies of Semantic Memory Associated Connectivity in Healthy Young Adults

To determine the functional networks involved in semantic memory processing, recent studies have employed fMRI functional connectivity analysis techniques to assess networks associated with semantic task performance in healthy young adults. One study utilized an independent component analysis (ICA) technique to analyze fMRI activations during a semantic decision task and identified seven unique and independent networks [257]. Two of these networks were left- and right-lateralized hemispheric networks connecting the inferior and middle frontal gyri, inferior parietal lobule, middle temporal, as well as other regions. These networks were thought to be involved in task-specific semantic processing. The remaining five functional networks included two additional task-specific networks, the "pre-supplementary motor area (SMA)-thalamus" network and the "parietal-frontal" network, which are involved in the integration of multiple features and mental imagery, respectively; two networks involved in basic sensory processing, the "temporal-frontal" network for auditory processing, and the "occipital-motor" network, which is involved in visual functioning; and the resting-state DMN. The DMN, which included the angular gyri, posterior cingulate, ventromedial PFC, and dorsomedial PFC, was also shown in a separate study to be "deactivated" upon initiation of a perceptual task but not a semantic task [258]. These results suggest that the lack of "deactivation" of the DMN upon initiation of a semantic task may be due to on-going semantic processing as part of the "at-rest" activity.

A study by Vitali and colleagues examined whether different semantic categories showed separate or overlapping functional networks [259]. The results from healthy young adults demonstrated the presence of different functional networks for the processing of tools and animals. Semantic processing of tools demonstrated increased activation in three functional networks, which included: (1) a left-lateralized network including the dorsolateral PFC, pre-motor regions (including the pre-SMA), inferior parietal lobule, and temporoparietal regions; (2) a connection between the inferior frontal and superior occipital gyri; (3) a network including the inferior frontal gyri, lateral fusiform gyri, and the temporoparietal junction. On the other hand, semantic processing of animals showed a much more limited left-lateralized functional network connecting the visual association areas (lateral and medial fusiform gyri with the superior and inferior occipital gyri), as well as a network connecting the inferior frontal gyri and medial fusiform gyri, and a network connecting the inferior frontal gyri and inferior occipital gyri. The results of this study suggest independent and minimally overlapping functional networks are involved in the processing of separate semantic categories (tools and animals), with overlap in only the inferior frontal and fusiform gyri.

fMRI of Semantic Memory in Patients At-Risk for AD and after Therapeutic Intervention

Some studies have suggested minimal deficits in semantic memory performance in early stage MCI and AD patients [250, 251], while others show measurable impairments in MCI and AD patients [260–262]. However, alterations in brain activation during semantic memory tasks have been observed in patients with MCI and AD, as well as patients at-risk for developing AD due to genetic status and/or a family history of illness. A number of recent studies have shown increased activation in frontal and temporoparietal regions during semantic memory task performance in participants at-risk for AD due to ApoE genotype and/or family history of AD, even in the absence of performance deficits [244, 263] (Fig. 10.6b). However, reduced activations in the inferior parietal and bilateral anterior cingulate during semantic categorization in ApoE ε4 (epsilon4) positive participants have also been reported [264]. Owing to the presence of alterations observed in brain activation in the absence of clinical deficits in performance, fMRI studies of semantic memory may provide a useful biomarker for early AD.

Pharmacological intervention studies utilizing fMRI techniques have also been performed to assess pharmacological alterations of brain activation associated with semantic memory in patients with AD. A study by McGeown and colleagues measured fMRI activation patterns during a semantic association task in AD patients before and after treatment with rivastigmine, a cholinesterase inhibitor and treatment for AD [265]. These results were also compared with fMRI results during the same task in healthy elderly. After treatment with a cholinesterase inhibitor, patients with AD showed a "more normal" activation pattern as defined by patterns of activation in healthy elderly. Specifically, treatment with rivastigmine resulted in increased activation in the temporal and frontal lobes, as well as the bilateral fusiform gyri, relative to pretreatment baseline in patients with AD. These results support the potential use of semantic memory fMRI activation changes as a biomarker for early diagnosis and treatment efficacy in AD patients.

Summary

Semantic memory retrieval has primarily been linked to activations of the PFC, lateral temporal cortex, and posterior inferior parietal lobe in fMRI studies of semantic processing in young adults. In young adults, PFC activations associated with semantic retrieval are primarily left-lateralized, while healthy older adults show decreased PFC lateralization. Similar to reports utilizing episodic memory tasks, patients with MCI and AD show altered activation patterns in fMRI studies of semantic memory. The direction and magnitude of the alterations associated with MCI and AD may be dependent on disease stage and severity. Functional connectivity studies in young adults have implicated a variety of functional semantic networks connecting the frontal, temporal, and parietal cortices. Functional MRI studies of semantic memory have also been utilized as biomarkers, with alterations in brain activation reported in patients at-risk for AD and after pharmacological interventions.

Working Memory

Working memory can be defined as the maintenance of small amounts of information in active stores, while other cognitive operations are performed. These other operations may include such processes as language comprehension, problem-solving, memory encoding, and many others. The ability to hold information in working memory is fundamental to executing cognitive processes efficiently and accurately [1, 2, 266]. Baddeley and colleagues proposed a model in which the working memory system has a central executive that, together with an episodic buffer, allocates attentional resources to separate subsystems for verbal and nonverbal information, referred to as the "phonological loop" and "visuospatial sketchpad," respectively [1, 2, 267]. Working memory subsystems, including the "phonological loop" and "visuospatial sketchpad" are thought to include two basic mechanisms: (1) a phonological or visuospatial store where the information in working memory is stored during use and (2) an articulatory or coordinate system rehearsal process through which information in the storage is repeatedly updated and refreshed to maintain accurate and necessary details. For detailed reviews of models of working memory, see [2, 268, 269] and Table 10.4.

Table 10.4 Selected review articles of working memory

Working memory		
Authors	Study subjects	Article title
Baddeley 2010 [270]	Young adults	Working memory. *Curr Biol.* Feb 23 2010; 20(4):R136–140
Cabeza et al. 2000 [7]	Young adults	Imaging cognition II: An empirical review of 275 PET and fMRI studies. *Journal of Cognitive Neuroscience.* 2000;12(1):1–47
D'Esposito 2007 [275]	Young adults	From cognitive to neural models of working memory. *Philos Trans R Soc Lond B Biol Sci.* May 29 2007;362(1481):761–772
Smith et al. 1998 [283]	Young adults	Neuroimaging analyses of human working memory. *Proc Natl Acad Sci USA.* Sep 29 1998;95(20):12061–12068

(continued)

Table 10.4 (continued)

Working memory		
Authors	Study subjects	Article title
Smith et al. 1998 [284]	Young adults	Components of verbal working memory: evidence from neuroimaging. *Proc Natl Acad Sci USA*. Feb 3 1998;95(3):876–882
Wager et al. 2003 [287]	Young adults	Neuroimaging studies of working memory: a meta-analysis. *Cogn Affect Behav Neurosci*. Dec 2003;3(4):255–274
Cabeza 2001 [122]	Healthy aging	Cognitive neuroscience of aging: contributions of functional neuroimaging. *Scand J Psychol*. Jul 2001;42(3):277–286
Grady et al. 2000 [91]	Healthy aging	Changes in memory processing with age. *Current Opinion in Neurobiology*. 2000;10:224–231
Grady 2008 [376]	Healthy aging	Cognitive neuroscience of aging. *Ann N Y Acad Sci*. Mar 2008;1124:127–144
Hedden et al. 2005 [377]	Healthy aging	Healthy and pathological processes in adult development: new evidence from neuroimaging of the aging brain. *Curr Opin Neurol*. Dec 2005;18(6):740–747
Langley et al. 2000 [378]	Healthy aging	Functional neuroimaging of memory: implications for cognitive aging. *Microsc Res Tech*. Oct 1 2000;51(1):75–84
Rajah et al. 1983 [116]	Healthy aging	Region-specific changes in prefrontal function with age: a review of PET and fMRI studies on working and episodic memory. *Brain*. Sep 2005;128(Pt 9):1964–1983
Drzezga 2008 [381]	MCI and AD	Concept of functional imaging of memory decline in Alzheimer's disease. *Methods*. Apr 2008;44(4):304–314
Han et al. 2009 [382]	MCI and AD	Functional magnetic resonance imaging of compensatory neural recruitment in aging and risk for Alzheimer's disease: review and recommendations. *Dement Geriatr Cogn Disord*. 2009;27(1):1–10

fMRI Studies of the Neural Basis of Working Memory

Although lesion studies provided the earliest mapping of the neural representations of working memory, functional neuroimaging studies have provided convincing evidence for the involvement of a broad network of brain areas in working memory processes. A number of different tasks are employed to measure working memory in functional neuroimaging studies, including paradigms featuring continuous monitoring of information (e.g., "n-back" tasks), delayed response, temporal ordering of material, and manipulation of information. Sample working memory fMRI probes that contrast or emphasize different processing demands are presented in Table 10.1c.

One theory of the neural representations of the subsystems of working memory proposes that the central executive, phonological loop, visuospatial sketchpad, and episodic buffer may exist in unique and separate brain regions that are specific to these processes [270–272]. Alternatively, the storage of verbal and nonverbal material in working memory may occur in regions responsible for perceptual processing of this material and connections with the central executive may provide selective attention on these sources of information during working memory tasks [273, 274]. Studies have recently provided evidence supporting the latter of these theories, although debate about the neural seat of working memory continues [275].

Initial functional imaging studies of healthy young adults engaging in working memory tasks has suggested that a number of regions are involved in the various subsystems (Fig. 10.9). Storage and maintenance of spatial material in working memory has primarily been mapped to the frontal eye fields (FEF), superior frontal sulcus, and intraparietal sulcus [276–278], which are regions known to be involved in the motor and functional aspects of eye movement. Activations of the primary visual cortex have also been reported in studies of spatial working memory [279]. Studies suggest that the representation of saccade eye movements and occulomotor coordi-

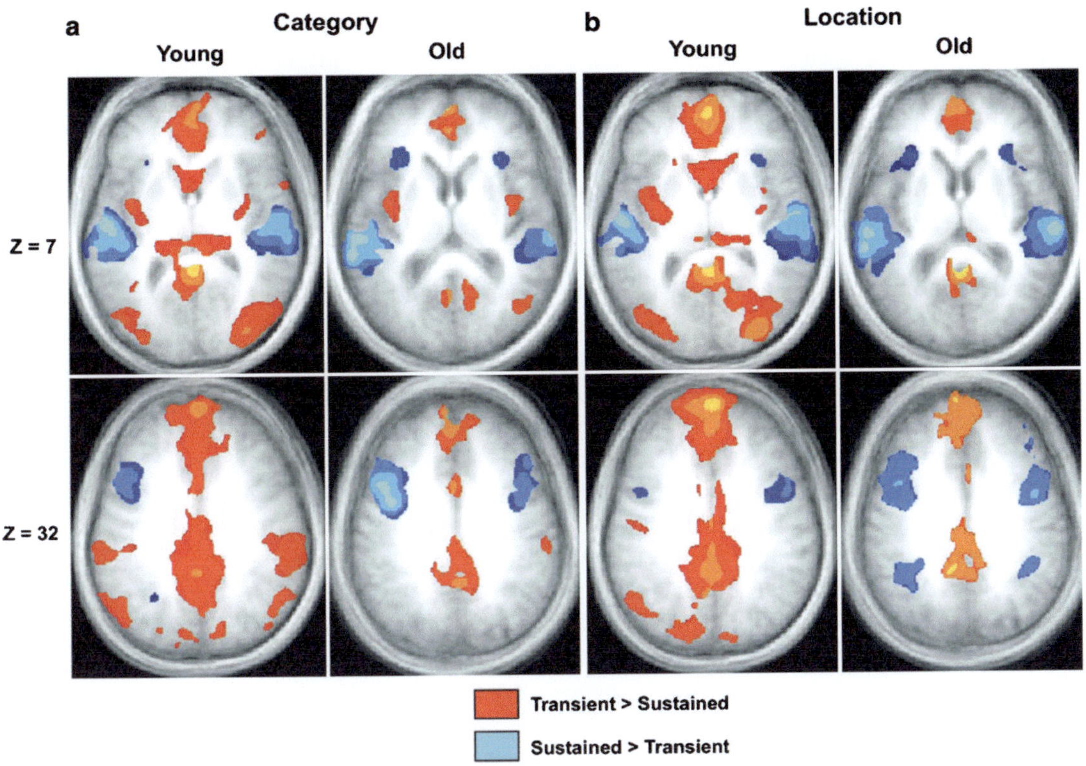

Fig. 10.9 Altered patterns of activation in spatial and nonspatial working memory tasks with normal aging. Pattern of activation during auditory working memory (A; category) nonspatial and (B; location) spatial tasks were observed in bilateral frontal, parietal, and temporal cortices. Extent and magnitude of both transient (item specific) and sustained (item independent) activation was significantly reduced in healthy older adults relative to young controls for both spatial and nonspatial working memory. Reproduced with permission from Grady CL, Yu H, Alain C. Age-related differences in brain activity underlying working memory for spatial and nonspatial auditory information. *Cereb Cortex.* Jan 2008;18(1): 189–199

nates may be stored in the FEF. Maintenance of spatial information results from the rehearsal of the spatial saccade vector to the spatial target location, which involves communication between the FEF and intraparietal sulcus [278].

In contrast, the storage and maintenance of verbal working memory information involves activity in the inferior posterior parietal cortex, precuneus, the lateral PFC (Broca's area), regions involved in the motor aspects of speech production [supplementary motor area (SMA) and cerebellum], and subcortical regions (thalamus and striatum) [280–284]. Functional imaging studies have suggested that the inferior parietal cortex may be the site of phonological storage with maintenance of the verbal information in working memory resulting from a subvocal rehearsal process involving coordination between the lateral PFC and SMA.

Nonspatial and nonverbal (i.e., objects, faces, etc.) information has been proposed to be stored primarily in posterior cortical areas, including the inferior temporal lobe, during working memory processing [285–287]. For example, working memory processing of faces has been shown to be specifically associated with activations in the fusiform gyrus [288].

Finally, the frontal lobe, including the anterior PFC, dorsolateral PFC, and ventrolateral PFC, as well as the lateral and medial superior parietal lobe have been implicated as the neural seat of the central executive during working memory tasks [37, 275, 289]. Other types of executive processing have also been associated with activation in the PFC and other regions. For example, selective attention is associated with activation in the medial PFC and inferior temporal lobe.

Overall, the broad network of frontal and parietal lobar regions involved in working memory has been theorized to be divided into separate streams of information processing by the material type and/or the type and amount of executive functioning. Functional imaging studies have suggested material-specific hemispheric specialization in both the parietal cortex and the PFC, with left lateralization for processing of verbal information and right lateralization for processing of both object and spatial information [7, 287, 290]. However, the lateralization by material type in the PFC is dependent on the amount of executive processing, as tasks with greater executive demand show more bilateral representation for all types of material. General divisions by material type based on dorsal/ventral information streams have also been proposed [287, 291]. For example, separate though overlapping neural representations for visual working memory processes have been observed in functional imaging studies. Spatial ("where") information is thought to follow a dorsal stream of processing in the superior parietal lobe, while object ("what") information follows a ventral stream of processing in the inferior parietal temporal lobes [276]. This separation of neural representations in working memory is analogous to the dissociation in the visual system between dorsal occipitoparietal pathways thought to be involved in the processing of spatial locations and relations among objects, and ventral occipitotemporal pathways that are involved in the processing of the perceptual characteristics that are important for recognition of objects [292, 293].

Finally, subdivisions within the frontal lobe by material type and/or type of executive processing have also been reported in functional neuroimaging studies of working memory [287, 290, 294]. The ventral/ventrolateral PFC has been suggested to be particularly involved in the processing of nonspatial information and in relatively simple executive tasks such as information maintenance. On the other hand, dorsal/dorsolateral PFC regions process spatial information and are activated during more complex executive tasks requiring maintenance and/or manipulation. Other conceptualizations hold that it is the type of processing rather than the type of information that is related to the dorsal/ventral division of PFC activity during working memory [290]. For example, the dorsal PFC may be primarily involved in temporal order memory and continuous monitoring executive tasks, while the ventral PFC is involved in continuous monitoring, temporal ordering, and manipulation of information [287].

fMRI Studies of Working Memory in Healthy Aging

Behavioral and functional neuroimaging studies indicate age-related changes in working memory [295, 296]. Many of the functional neuroimaging studies of working memory in normal aging have reported increased activity in older adults relative to younger controls, as well as increased bilateral activations, similar to that seen in other types of memory (i.e., "HAROLD" model in episodic memory) [104, 297]. Studies in older adults utilizing working memory paradigms with all material types (spatial, verbal, nonverbal, nonspatial) have reported increased activity in the PFC, parietal lobe, and other regions relative to young adults [91, 112, 116, 297, 298]. Age-related deficiencies in hippocampal activation have also been reported for feature-binding in working memory, the process whereby individual elements of experience are bound together [299].

A meta-analysis by Rajah and D'Esposito suggests that age-related changes in PFC activity are region specific [116]. The ventral PFC shows conflicting results, with some studies showing greater activation in older adults relative to young controls and others showing the reverse [245, 300]. However, activity in the dorsal PFC during working memory tasks has consistently been reported to be greater in healthy older adults relative to young adults [109, 245]. Finally, the anterior PFC shows bilateral activation during working memory tasks in older adults, while young adults show only unilateral activation [245, 299]. The increased activity and bilateral representation may be a compensatory change in older adults, as there are age-associated structural changes in the PFC [97]. Interestingly, increased activation appears to be selective for paradigms in which the performance of older adults is equivalent to young controls [112, 301]. Studies in which older adults show impaired task performance relative to young controls demonstrate a different pattern in which older adults show equal or less activation in the PFC relative to younger participants [298] (Fig. 10.9).

fMRI Studies of Working Memory in MCI and AD

In addition to assessing changes in older adults, fMRI studies have been used to measure alterations in brain activity during working memory tasks in patients with MCI and AD. Patients with AD show marked deficits in working memory [302], while patients with MCI show more subtle changes in working memory, particularly in early stages of the disease. Functional MRI studies of working memory in patients with AD have shown conflicting results, which may be due to varying severities of the working memory task deficit [303–305]. A study by Yetkin and colleagues demonstrated that patients with AD have increased activation during a working memory task in the right superior frontal gyrus, bilateral middle frontal gyri, bilateral anterior cingulate, bilateral middle temporal gyri, and bilateral fusiform gyri relative to age-matched controls [305]. However, in this study, AD patients did not show significantly impaired performance. In another fMRI study of verbal working memory in patients with AD, patients showed significantly impaired performance, along with reduced activation in the left frontal pole, left ventrolateral PFC, left insula, as well as the right premotor cortex, and increased activation only in the left precuneus [303]. These results suggest that the extent and level of activation during working memory tasks is associated with the level of performance in AD patients and support a compensatory role for the observed increases in activation.

Patients with MCI also show alterations in activation during verbal working memory tasks relative to healthy elderly controls. Some studies demonstrate increased activity during working memory tasks in MCI patients, primarily in frontal and parietal regions, including the right superior frontal gyri, as well as bilateral middle frontal gyri, anterior cingulate, middle temporal gyri, and fusiform gyri [305, 306]. Furthermore, MCI patients show significantly greater activation than patients with AD during a verbal working memory task, even in the presence of equivalent levels of performance, in the right parahippocampal gyrus, left inferior frontal gyrus, bilateral cingulate and lingual gyri, right lentiform nucleus, right fusiform gyrus, and the left supramarginal gyrus [305]. Relative to healthy elderly, MCI patients may also show recruitment of alternative processing techniques and brain regions to perform working memory tasks. However, other studies show decreased activity in MCI patients relative to healthy elderly [307].

Functional neuroimaging studies of working memory have also been shown to be useful in contrasting different types of dementia and may assist in differential diagnosis of dementia type. In a study comparing patients with AD to individuals with early FTD on a working memory task, both groups showed activation of frontal, parietal, and thalamic regions [308]. However, patients with FTD showed less frontal and parietal activation than those with AD and greater cerebellar activation. The authors suggested that fMRI may be useful for differentiating AD and FTD early in the disease course, even when the structural changes are minimal.

Investigations of working memory function in patients with AD have also been useful in characterizing the brain regions that are involved in working memory subsystems. Patients with AD often show a particularly significant impairment in the episodic buffer subsystem of working memory, as proposed by Baddeley and colleagues. To investigate the neural substrate of the episodic memory buffer, Berlingeri and colleagues compared atrophy on structural MRI between AD patients showing significant impairments in the episodic buffer and patients with AD who show relative sparing of this subsystem [309]. Patients with impaired episodic buffer processing showed significantly greater atrophy of the left anterior hippocampus relative to those with intact episodic buffer processing. The authors suggest that the anterior hippocampus may be an important region for this working memory subsystem, given the role of the MTL in episodic memory processing. Results from a recent fMRI study by Luck and colleagues also support the importance of the MTL as the neural seat of the episodic buffer. In healthy young adults, activation in the MTL was observed during encoding and maintenance of episodic material in working memory but not for retrieval [310].

fMRI Studies of Working Memory Associated Connectivity in Healthy Young Adults

The distributed neural activity associated with working memory tasks represents a set of functionally connected networks that include multiple brain regions. A number of recent reports have addressed the functional connectivity of fMRI activations in anatomically distinct brain regions during working memory tasks in healthy young adults [311–313]. Using a delayed face recognition working memory task, two functional networks connecting the fusiform gyrus and right inferior frontal gyrus, as well as the fusiform gyrus and hippocampus were identified [313]. The strength of these connections was dependent on working memory load. Protzner and colleagues investigated whether the sensory modality of working memory input would activate different functional networks [312]. Three unique functional networks were identified, including: (1) a modality-independent network, which included the ventrolateral PFC, dorsolateral PFC, occipitoparietal cortex, and temporal pole; (2) an auditory-input-specific network connecting the left superior temporal gyrus, frontal operculum, and bilateral superior parietal cortex; and (3) a visual-input-specific network including the primary visual cortex and right anterior PFC. A number of studies have also implicated associations between the DMN and working memory tasks [311, 314, 315]. Deactivation of this network, which includes the posterior cingulate and medial frontal cortex, was significantly associated with performance on working memory tasks, as well as task difficulty.

fMRI Studies of Working Memory Associated Connectivity in Healthy Aging, MCI, and AD

Alterations in working memory-associated functional connectivity have also been reported in cognitively healthy older adults, as well as in patients with MCI and AD. Healthy older adults show increased functional connectivity in working memory task-related networks, including a functional network connecting the superior and inferior parietal cortex, inferior frontal gyri, dorsolateral PFC, premotor cortex, and occipital cortex [316]. However, other data suggests reduced functional connectivity of working memory networks in older adults, particularly reduced activity of parietal-PFC networks [317]. The DMN also shows decreased connectivity in healthy older adults relative to younger controls, suggesting altered resting-state activity with aging [190, 316, 318]. Furthermore, patients with MCI and AD show more significant impairment of the DMN [195, 319].

fMRI Studies of Working Memory in Patients At-risk for AD and After Pharmacological Intervention

Similar to reports utilizing episodic and semantic memory paradigms, fMRI studies of working memory have been performed in patients at increased risk for developing AD due to genetic background (i.e., ApoE ε4 [epsilon4] positive) and/or family history of dementia. Young adults with an increased risk for AD due to the presence of an ApoE ε4 (epsilon4) allele show greater activity in widespread frontal, parietal, temporal, and other regions during an fMRI working memory challenge than those who are ApoE ε4 (epsilon4) negative [320]. Similar results have been shown in older adults who are cognitively healthy but ApoE ε4 (epsilon4) positive [321], although some conflicting reports have emerged [202]. Wishart and colleagues found that ApoE ε4 (epsilon4) positive older adults show greater activation during an *n*-back working memory task in the bilateral medial frontal gyri, bilateral medial parietal regions, right dorsolateral PFC, and right anterior cingulate gyrus relative to older adults without an ApoE ε4 (epsilon4) allele [321] (Fig. 10.6c). The identification of fMRI patterns of altered activation during working memory tasks provides an early biomarker of functional changes, which may be predictive of future progression to dementia, but longitudinal studies are needed.

Similar to fMRI studies of episodic memory, anticholinergic therapies have been investigated using fMRI of working memory tasks in healthy young adults [322, 323]. Reduced extent and amplitude of PFC activation after administration of scopolamine or mecamylamine was reported in studies with young and older women [322, 323]. Several studies have also investigated working memory-related activation patterns on fMRI in response to cholinergic interventions in patients with MCI and AD. Goekoop and colleagues, in a single group design, evaluated whether an 8-week treatment with galantamine could cause alterations in fMRI activation patterns and magnitude in patients with MCI [324]. Relative to baseline, patients with MCI showed increased activation after galantamine treatment in the right precuneus and middle frontal gyrus in response to a working memory task. Furthermore, the extent of increased activation was significantly associated with increased performance on the working memory task. Saykin and colleagues examined the effects of a 10-week treatment with donepezil on patients with MCI relative to untreated but rescanned healthy elderly controls and found similar treatment-induced increases in activation during a working memory task relative to pretreatment baseline [307]. In this study, patients with MCI showed reduced frontal and parietal activation during a working memory task at baseline relative to healthy elderly controls, despite similar performance. However, after treatment, MCI patients demonstrated a significant increase in activation in the left superior frontal gyrus, dorsolateral PFC, temporal lobe, and occipital lobe. After treatment with donepezil, patients with MCI demonstrated nearly equivalent brain activation and performance to controls, suggesting a "normalization" of working memory processes after treatment. The extent of increased activity in the frontal lobe was also significantly associated with both increased performance and baseline hippocampal volume, suggesting different treatment responsiveness based on severity of baseline MTL atrophy.

Other studies have assessed the effects of cholinergic therapies on working memory-related activations in patients with AD. Rombouts and colleagues examined the effect of acute cholinergic enhancement on brain activity during working memory in a sample of patients with mild AD [206]. After a single dose of rivastigmine, activity in the PFC cortex, including the left middle and superior frontal gyri, was enhanced during a basic working memory condition. When the working memory demands were increased, both increases and decreases in activation in different regions were seen. Specifically, increased working memory load led to rivastigmine-related increased activation in the left middle frontal gyrus, as well as the right inferior and superior frontal gyri. However, increased working memory load was also associated with decreased activation in other locations of the right superior frontal gyrus and the right middle frontal gyrus. McGeown and colleagues assessed the effects of chronic administration (20-weeks) of rivastigmine on working memory-associated brain activation in patients with mild AD, as well as brain activation in untreated age-matched controls [265]. Patients with AD showed increased activation during a working memory task in the right inferior, middle, and superior frontal gyri, as well as the right medial frontal and precentral gyri after chronic treatment with rivastigmine relative to pretreatment baseline. Treatment with rivastigmine also led to decreased activation in the left middle frontal, precentral, and cingulate gyri, as well as the left insula and thalamus in AD patients after treatment relative to pretreatment baseline activation. Elderly controls demonstrated primarily right frontal and insular activation during this working memory task. These results suggest that chronic treatment with rivastigmine leads to increased right lateralization of working memory activation in patients with AD, which is a more "normal" pattern of activation. However, the extent to which these changes are task-dependent remains to be determined.

The results of studies with cognitively healthy individuals with high-genetic risk for AD suggest that fMRI studies of working memory may be a particularly sensitive biomarker for subclinical alterations in cognitive functioning and future disease progression. Additionally, studies assessing the effects of acute and chronic treatment with cholinergic interventions in healthy elders and patients with MCI and AD indicate that fMRI techniques can be useful in determining the brain regions in which a medication exerts its primary functional effects. Overall, fMRI studies of working memory are well suited for measuring changes in brain function even in the absence of measurable behavioral and cognitive deficits. These techniques may also be useful when employed before and after drug treatment to monitor mechanisms and efficacy.

Summary

Functional MRI studies of working memory in young adults have shown a pattern of bilateral frontal, parietal, and temporal activation, although the particular regions identified vary with the type of information being processed (i.e., verbal, object, spatial, etc.). Older adults show increased activation and increased bilateral representation, while patients with MCI and AD show either increased or decreased activations depending on the severity of working memory impairment. Connectivity studies in young adults have shown that activation of functional networks connecting the parietal, frontal, and temporal cortices, as well as deactivation of the DMN, are associated with working memory tasks. Healthy older adults and patients with MCI and AD show alterations in working memory-related functional and resting-state connectivity. Functional MRI studies of working memory have also shown altered activation patterns in individuals at-risk for dementia and after pharmacological interventions, suggesting utility of this measure as a biomarker.

Methodological Issues in the Use of fMRI in Aging and Dementia Research

A number of methodological considerations must be addressed when conducting and interpreting fMRI research in healthy aging and dementia. For example, there is evidence to suggest that normal aging affects some aspects of the coupling of the hemodynamic response (HDR) with neural activity [325, 326]. Using a simple reaction time task (one known to evoke similar electrical potentials in young and old adults), D'Esposito and colleagues found in excess of four times more activated voxels in sensorimotor cortex in young adults relative to older participants [327]. Other aspects of the HDR, such as the shape of the curve and the within-group variance, did not significantly differ as a function of age. In contrast, Huettel and colleagues found age differences in the shape of the HDR, within-group variability, and the number of activated voxels on a visual task [328]. The younger adults showed a later time to peak, less variability, and twice as many activated voxels as the older adults, though both groups activated similar regions of the visual cortex. Age-related prolongation of the time lag in signal change on fMRI has also been reported [329]. Other groups have observed smaller areas [330, 331] or larger areas [332] of activation in older adults compared with younger individuals, or no significant differences between groups [242]. Buckner and colleagues observed similar summation between young and older adults of the HDR across brain regions examined with a sensorimotor task, and suggested that even if absolute measurement differences exist between age groups, there should be preservation of relative task-related changes in activation [333]. These issues indicate the need for sophisticated experimental design, post-processing, and interpretation of fMRI data in aging research in relation to performance, strategy, reaction time, and other variables to ensure that reported findings are not spurious effects of basic physiological or artifactual signal differences between young and older groups.

Many fMRI studies in young and older controls, as well as patients with MCI and AD, utilize subtraction methods to determine regions of activation associated with a task. In other words, activation patterns during a cognitive task of interest are compared with those elicited by a control task. The control task can take a wide variety of forms, including other attention or cognitive tasks that are not of interest (i.e., episodic memory task versus reading words), responding to a similar task paradigm but with pseudo-stimuli (i.e., semantic task versus pseudo-words), or a resting state (i.e., fixation). However, it is a very large assumption to consider the difference between a task of interest and even a well-designed control task to result only in activations that are specific to the cognitive process of interest [334, 335]. Event-related fMRI designs may be useful in addressing some of these concerns.

Further technical and scientific issues are encountered when using fMRI to study patients with disease, including MCI and AD. Currently, the conditions and importance of alterations in brain activity in patients with AD are not well understood. For example, does increased activation in patients relative to controls reflect compensation, de-differentiation, or both? Could expanded activation represent a disinhibition in some cases? If patients perform abnormally on an activation task, how should the resulting activation maps be compared with those of healthy controls with no performance deficits? How should atrophy and lesions be taken into account when interpreting fMRI data? Approaches that integrate structural neuroimaging, carefully designed activation tasks, as well as close monitoring of in-scanner task performance will likely help address such questions [134]. Additionally, the use of well-designed event-related fMRI techniques can help to address issues of performance by allowing comparison of only successful task responses as well as an analysis of errors.

Future Directions

Recent creative applications of functional neuroimaging have been successfully used to study a range of biological and psychological processes. Functional imaging has provided new insights into the role of genetic variation resulting in a new transdisciplinary field referred to as "Imaging Genetics." The multimodal combination of fMRI with other imaging techniques is another direction that permits characterization of multiple aspects of memory and memory-associated disease. Finally, technological advances in MRI, such as ultra-high field strength, coils, and software, may also open a path to new understanding of the neuroanatomical and physiological correlates of memory function and mechanisms of memory dysfunction.

fMRI Studies of Imaging Genetics

The goal of imaging genetic studies is to use neuroimaging data as an endophenotype with which to analyze genetic variation, including single nucleotide polymorphisms (SNPs), insertions, deletions, and gene copy number variations (CNVs), as well as specific mutations. SNPs are common genetic variations in which a single base pair at a specific chromosomal location is altered. Current microarray technology can assay 1–2 million SNPs and CNVs on a single chip. Using structural, functional, and molecular imaging, the influence of genetic variation on normal brain structure and function, as well as pathology in disease states can be assessed.

Functional neuroimaging techniques have been used to map the effects of genetic variants on memory performance in healthy young adults, older adults, and in people at-risk for dementia (i.e., ApoE ε4 [epsilon4] positive). Studies have suggested up to 50% of memory performance is hereditary [336] and thus, identification of genetic variants may help to elucidate the basis of normal memory processing, as well as memory dysfunction. A recent review on imaging genomic studies of episodic memory highlighted five genetic polymorphisms associated with episodic memory function that have been investigated using functional neuroimaging techniques, including genes encoding for: (1) brain-derived neurotrophic factor (*BDNF*); (2) the dopamine catalyzing enzyme, catechol-O-methyltransferase (*COMT*); (3) calmodulin-binding transcription activator 1 (*CAMTA1*); (4) prion protein (*PRNP*); and (5) a protein called "WW, C2, and coil-coiled domain containing 1" (*KIBRA*) [337].

A genetic polymorphism in the *BDNF* gene that results in a valine (val) to methionine (met) substitution has been associated with altered episodic memory performance, as well as altered brain activations during memory tasks, in healthy young adults and in aging [338–340]. Specifically, participants who are met/met homozygous show lower accuracy on episodic retrieval tasks in some studies. Furthermore, carriers of the met polymorphism show reduced MTL activations during episodic encoding and retrieval, even in the absence of performance differences as a function of genotype. A recent study by Sambataro and colleagues suggested an interaction between the *BDNF Val66Met* polymorphism and aging, with met/met participants showing a more significant age-related decline in hippocampal activation during episodic encoding and retrieval [341].

A genetic polymorphism in the *COMT* gene, which also results in a valine to methionine substitution, has been shown to alter enzymatic activity leading to increased dopamine levels [342], as well as to affect episodic, semantic, and working memory performance and associated brain activation [343–348]. Participants with the met/met genotype show better performance on all types of memory. Imaging genomic studies have shown a dose-dependent association between the met allele and increased hippocampal activation, as well as decreased ventrolateral PFC activation, during episodic encoding and retrieval [343]. Functional connectivity analyses have also shown changes in hippocampal-PFC connectivity associated with *COMT* genotype [348]. An interaction between the *COMT* polymorphism and normal aging has also been reported, with val/val homozygous older adults showing greater functional connectivity during a working memory task in the frontal lobe relative to met/met homozygotes [347].

Genetic variations in the *CAMTA1* and *PRNP* genes have also shown associations with episodic memory performance, as well as altered brain activation during functional tasks. Participants with the *CAMTA1* T-allele show poor episodic performance and increased MTL activation during episodic retrieval [349]. A polymorphism in the *PRNP* gene causing a valine to methionine substitution has been associated with poorer memory performance in young adults [350]. Met/met homozygotes gene also show increased activation during episodic retrieval in the medial and lateral temporal lobe, as well as the middle and inferior frontal gyri. Polymorphisms in the *KIBRA* gene have also been implicated in altered episodic memory function and associated brain activations. A study by Papassotiropoulos and colleagues suggested that an SNP resulting in a C to T intronic substitution was associated with episodic memory performance [351]. Specifically, C/C homozygous participants had decreased episodic recall relative to participants with a T-allele, as well as increased activation during episodic retrieval in the MTL, medial frontal gyri, and inferior parietal gyri.

Two additional genetic variants, the gene encoding dystrobrevin-binding protein 1 (*DTNBP1*) and the gene encoding neuregulin 1 (*NRG1*), have been identified as risk factors for schizophrenia and recently have also been associated with alterations in brain activation during episodic and working memory tasks. A recent study by Thimm and colleagues reported alterations in brain activation in the frontal, parietal, and occipital lobe during episodic memory encoding and retrieval in carriers of the *DTNBP1* A-allele [352], which has been associated with an increased risk of schizophrenia [353]. Despite the activation differences, no differences were reported in episodic memory performance as a function of genotype. Another recent report showed increased activation during an episodic memory task in the cingulate gyrus, left middle frontal gyrus, bilateral fusiform gyri, and left middle occipital gyrus in participants homozygous for the *NRG1* C/C allele [354], which is also associated with an increased risk of schizophrenia [355]. Similar to the results seen with the *DTNBP1* risk allele, no significant difference in performance was observed as a function of *NRG1* genotype.

To date, the majority of fMRI genetic studies of memory have focused on memory function in healthy young and older adults. Although the findings have been mixed, allelic variations that are associated with decreased performance appear to be more commonly associated with increased brain activation. These results may suggest decreased neural efficiency in these individuals resulting in a need for an increased magnitude and extent of activation to maintain "normal" memory function. Future studies with more sophisticated paradigms and longitudinal follow-up may help to more conclusively characterize genetic differences in memory-related brain activations.

The combination of imaging and genetics may also provide useful predictors of future cognitive decline and/or disease progression. As previously discussed, fMRI studies of carriers of the ApoE ε4 (epsilon4) allele, which is a significant risk factor for the development of AD [356], have demonstrated significant alterations in brain activity in cognitively normal young and older adults. Therefore, future studies of additional genetic variations, further characterization of genetic factors associated with disease, and longitudinal fMRI studies may allow for early identification of individuals at a high risk for disease.

Future developments in imaging genetic studies with fMRI are likely to build on emerging structural imaging genetic studies of MCI and AD that incorporate biological pathway-based and genome-wide association approaches. Present and future genome-wide association studies (GWAS) employing imaging techniques may discover new genes or loci relevant to structure/function relationships important for memory in healthy young and older adults and in patients with MCI and AD. Some recent examples of imaging GWAS reports include those using data from the Alzheimer's Disease Neuroimaging Initiative (ADNI) [357–361].

Multimodal Imaging Studies and Technological Advancements in MRI

Approaches that will likely see increasing use in future research involve combining fMRI with other imaging techniques. By evaluating each participant with two or more types of imaging, multimodal approaches promise improved characterization of the neural substrates of memory in health and in disease states. Recent studies have begun to implement multimodal imaging, including reports combining fMRI with PET, arterial spin labeling (ASL), which is an MR-based technique to measure changes in blood flow, and diffusion tensor imaging (DTI), which is a technique to measure white matter integrity [362–366]. For example, studies combining fMRI with targeted molecular imaging using PET have demonstrated a significant anatomical overlap between the DMN and amyloid deposition, as measured by Pittsburgh compound B (PiB) [367]. Furthermore, cognitively normal elders with significant amyloid burden (i.e., "PiB positive" PET scans) have significant disruption of the DMN relative to PiB negative healthy elderly participants, similar to that reported in AD patients [362, 364, 365].

Another important advance for future fMRI studies is the increased availability of ultra-high magnetic field strength scanners operating at 7 Tesla (7T) and above. To date, a few fMRI studies have been done with humans using a 7T magnet, including visual field and somatosensory cortex mapping [368, 369]. However, due to the increased resolution and sensitivity afforded by 7T or higher magnets, and major efforts to solve technical challenges at these field strengths, fMRI studies of cognition will likely be forthcoming in the near future.

Conclusion

Episodic, semantic, and working memory processes are mediated by widely distributed cortical and subcortical networks. Frontal, parietal, and temporal cortices are functionally connected as part of multiple networks essential for successful memory encoding and retrieval. Many age-related changes in neural functions associated with memory have been reported, including reduced prefrontal asymmetry, altered MTL and frontal activations during memory tasks, and changes in connectivity between frontal, parietal, and temporal lobe functional and resting-state networks (Table 10.5). These changes may be a direct effect of structural and physiological changes in the aging brain and/or may reflect age-related differences in cognitive strategy or approach to task performance. In individuals with MCI and AD, further disease stage-dependent alterations in brain activation/deactivation are observed. Early MCI and other prodromal stages often are associated with increased activation during memory tasks, which has been conceptualized as a compensatory response. However, late-stage MCI and AD patients show significantly reduced activations, likely resulting from neurodegeneration of MTL and PFC regions involved in memory processing. MCI and AD patients also show significantly disrupted functional and resting-state memory networks reflecting degeneration and disconnection of key regions.

Despite significant technical challenges, research using fMRI and other neuroimaging techniques is advancing knowledge of the effects of aging and dementia on memory circuitry. These findings have major potential implications for early detection of dementia and treatment monitoring, especially if used in combination with genetic testing and PET-based methods for in vivo detection of amyloid plaque burden in AD [202, 370–373]. New PET tracers are needed for neurofibrillary tangle pathology but are not yet available. Functional MRI has already demonstrated promise in imaging genomic studies of memory-related variants, reflecting its unique sensitivity and applicability to subtle alterations in memory function. Advances in MRI technology and combining fMRI with other multimodal imaging techniques will permit enhanced characterization of the neuroanatomic and physiological substrates of memory both in healthy individuals and in disease processes. Early detection of disease and treatment monitoring are especially important at this time because many disease modifying medications to slow the progression of neurodegeneration and cognitive decline are under development [374, 375]. As fMRI research progresses, trials of therapeutic agents could greatly benefit from more sensitive and disease-specific functional techniques for detecting and monitoring the progression of disease, as well as treatment response.

Acknowledgements Supported in part by the following grants from: the National Institutes of Health (CTSI Training Grant, TL1 RR025759 to SLR; NIA R01 AG19771 and NIH R01 CA101318 to AJS; Indiana Alzheimer's Disease Center, P30 AG10133-18S1 Core Supplement to Drs. B. Ghetti and AJS); the Alzheimer's

Table 10.5 Additional selected review articles and meta-analyses for further reading

Authors	Article title	Significance
D'Esposito et al. 2003 [325]	Alterations in the BOLD fMRI signal with aging and disease: a challenge for neuroimaging. *Nat Rev Neurosci.* Nov 2003;4(11):863–872	Alterations in BOLD with aging
Dickerson 2006 [388]	Functional magnetic resonance imaging of cholinergic modulation in mild cognitive impairment. *Curr Opin Psychiatry.* May 2006;19(3):299–306	Function MRI of cholinergic alterations
Greicius 2008 [389]	Resting-state functional connectivity in neuropsychiatric disorders. *Curr Opin Neurol.* Aug 2008;21(4):424–430	Functional and resting-state connectivity
Rasch et al. 2010 [337]	Imaging genetics of cognitive functions: Focus on episodic memory. *Neuroimage.* Jan 11 2010	Imaging genetics of memory

Disease Neuroimaging Initiative (NIH U01 AG024904 and RC2 AG036535-01); the Indiana Economic Development Corporation (IEDC #87884 to AJS); and the Alzheimer's Association.

References

1. Baddeley A. Working Memory. In: Gazzaniga MS, editor. The cognitive neurosciences. Cambridge, MA: MIT Press; 1995.
2. Baddeley A. Recent developments in working memory. Curr Opin Neurobiol. 1998;8(2):234–8.
3. Krause JB, Taylor JG, Schmidt D, Hautzel H, Mottaghy FM, Muller-Gartner HW. Imaging and neural modeling in episodic and working memory processes. Neural Netw. 2000;13(8–9):847–59.
4. Tulving E, Donaldson W. The organization of memory. New York: Academic Press; 1972.
5. Nyberg L, Marklund P, Persson J, et al. Common prefrontal activations during working memory, episodic memory, and semantic memory. Neuropsychologia. 2003;41:371–7.
6. Tulving E, Markowitsch HJ. Episodic and declarative memory: role of the hippocampus. Hippocampus. 1998;8(3):198–204.
7. Cabeza R, Nyberg L. Imaging cognition II: An empirical review of 275 PET and fMRI studies. J Cogn Neurosci. 2000;12(1):1–47.
8. Fletcher PC, Frith CD, Rugg MD. The functional neuroanatomy of episodic memory. Trends Neurosci. 1997;20(5):213–8.
9. Schacter DL, Wagner AD. Medial temporal lobe activations in fMRI and PET studies of episodic encoding and retrieval. Hippocampus. 1999;9(1):7–24.
10. Wagner AD, Koutstaal W, Schacter DL. When encoding yields remembering: insights from event-related neuroimaging. Philos Trans R Soc Lond B Biol Sci. 1999;354(1387):1307–24.
11. Cabeza R. Role of parietal regions in episodic memory retrieval: the dual attentional processes hypothesis. Neuropsychologia. 2008;46(7):1813–27.
12. Davachi L. Item, context and relational episodic encoding in humans. Curr Opin Neurobiol. 2006;16(6):693–700.
13. Desgranges B, Baron JC, Eustache F. The functional neuroanatomy of episodic memory: The role of the frontal lobes, the hippocampal formation, and other areas. Neuroimage. 1998;8:198–213.
14. Eichenbaum H, Yonelinas AP, Ranganath C. The medial temporal lobe and recognition memory. Annu Rev Neurosci. 2007;30:123–52.
15. Fletcher PC, Henson RN. Frontal lobes and human memory: insights from functional neuroimaging. Brain. 2001;124(Pt 5):849–81.
16. Gilbert SJ, Spengler S, Simons JS, et al. Functional specialization within rostral prefrontal cortex (area 10): a meta-analysis. J Cogn Neurosci. 2006;18(6):932–48.
17. Henson R. A mini-review of fMRI studies of human medial temporal lobe activity associated with recognition memory. Q J Exp Psychol B. 2005;58(3–4):340–60.
18. Kim H. Dissociating the roles of the default-mode, dorsal, and ventral networks in episodic memory retrieval. Neuroimage. 2010;50(4):1648–57.
19. Milner B, Petrides M, Smith ML. Frontal lobes and the temporal organization of memory. Hum Neurobiol. 1985;4(3):137–42.
20. Shimamura AP. Memory and the prefrontal cortex. Ann NY Acad Sci. 1995;769:151–9.
21. Spaniol J, Davidson PS, Kim AS, Han H, Moscovitch M, Grady CL. Event-related fMRI studies of episodic encoding and retrieval: meta-analyses using activation likelihood estimation. Neuropsychologia. 2009;47(8–9):1765–79.
22. Harrington GS, Tomaszewski Farias S, Buonocore MH, Yonelinas AP. The intersubject and intrasubject reproducibility of FMRI activation during three encoding tasks: implications for clinical applications. Neuroradiology. 2006;48(7):495–505.
23. Shallice T, Fletcher P, Frith CD, Grasby P, Frackowiak RS, Dolan RJ. Brain regions associated with acquisition and retrieval of verbal episodic memory. Nature. 1994;368(6472):633–5.
24. Kelley WM, Miezin FM, McDermott KB, et al. Hemispheric specialization in human dorsal frontal cortex and medial temporal lobe for verbal and nonverbal memory encoding. Neuron. 1998;20(5):927–36.
25. Wagner AD, Poldrack RA, Eldridge LL, Desmond JE, Glover GH, Gabrieli JD. Material-specific lateralization of prefrontal activation during episodic encoding and retrieval. Neuroreport. 1998;9(16):3711–7.
26. Brewer JB, Zhao Z, Desmond JE, Glover GH, Gabrieli JD. Making memories: brain activity that predicts how well visual experience will be remembered. Science. 1998;281(5380):1185–7.
27. Gabrieli JD, Brewer JB, Desmond JE, Glover GH. Separate neural bases of two fundamental memory processes in the human medial temporal lobe. Science. 1997;276(5310):264–6.
28. Roland PE, Zilles K. Structural divisions and functional fields in the human cerebral cortex. Brain Res Brain Res Rev. 1998;26(2–3):87–105.
29. McDermott KB, Buckner RL, Petersen SE, Kelley WM, Sanders AL. Set- and code-specific activation in frontal cortex: an fMRI study of encoding and retrieval of faces and words. J Cogn Neurosci. 1999;11(6):631–40.
30. Busatto G, Howard RJ, Ha Y, et al. A functional magnetic resonance imaging study of episodic memory. Neuroreport. 1997;8(12):2671–5.
31. Otten LJ, Henson RN, Rugg MD. Depth of processing effects on neural correlates of memory encoding: relationship between findings from across- and within-task comparisons. Brain. 2001;124(Pt 2):399–412.

32. Otten LJ, Rugg MD. Task-dependency of the neural correlates of episodic encoding as measured by fMRI. Cereb Cortex. 2001;11(12):1150–60.
33. Gabrieli JD, Poldrack RA, Desmond JE. The role of left prefrontal cortex in language and memory. Proc Natl Acad Sci USA. 1998;95(3):906–13.
34. Tulving E, Kapur S, Craik FI, Moscovitch M, Houle S. Hemispheric encoding/retrieval asymmetry in episodic memory: positron emission tomography findings. Proc Natl Acad Sci USA. 1994;91(6):2016–20.
35. Buckner RL. Functional-anatomic correlates of control processes in memory. J Neurosci. 2003;23(10):3999–4004.
36. Simons JS, Spiers HJ. Prefrontal and medial temporal lobe interactions in long-term memory. Nat Rev Neurosci. 2003;4(8):637–48.
37. Miller EK, Cohen JD. An integrative theory of prefrontal cortex function. Annu Rev Neurosci. 2001;24:167–202.
38. Greicius MD, Krasnow B, Boyett-Anderson JM, et al. Regional analysis of hippocampal activation during memory encoding and retrieval: fMRI study. Hippocampus. 2003;13(1):164–74.
39. Daselaar SM, Veltman DJ, Rombouts SA, Raaijmakers JG, Jonker C. Neuroanatomical correlates of episodic encoding and retrieval in young and elderly subjects. Brain. 2003;126(Pt 1):43–56.
40. Davachi L, Mitchell JP, Wagner AD. Multiple routes to memory: distinct medial temporal lobe processes build item and source memories. Proc Natl Acad Sci USA. 2003;100(4):2157–62.
41. Davachi L, Wagner AD. Hippocampal contributions to episodic encoding: insights from relational and item-based learning. J Neurophysiol. 2002;88(2):982–90.
42. Lepage M, Habib R, Tulving E. Hippocampal PET activations of memory encoding and retrieval: The HIPER model. Hippocampus. 1998;8:313–22.
43. Rombouts SA, Machielsen WC, Witter MP, Barkhof F, Lindeboom J, Scheltens P. Visual association encoding activates the medial temporal lobe: a functional magnetic resonance imaging study. Hippocampus. 1997;7(6):594–601.
44. Stern CE, Corkin S, Gonzalez RG, et al. The hippocampal formation participates in novel picture encoding: evidence from functional magnetic resonance imaging. Proc Natl Acad Sci USA. 1996;93(16):8660–5.
45. Braak H, Braak E, Yilmazer D, Bohl J. Functional anatomy of human hippocampal formation and related structures. J Child Neurol. 1996;11(4):265–75.
46. Van Hoesen GW. Anatomy of the medial temporal lobe. Magn Reson Imaging. 1995;13(8):1047–55.
47. Dolan RJ, Fletcher PC. Dissociating prefrontal and hippocampal function in episodic memory encoding. Nature. 1997;388(6642):582–5.
48. Golby AJ, Poldrack RA, Brewer JB, et al. Material-specific lateralization in the medial temporal lobe and prefrontal cortex during memory encoding. Brain. 2001;124(Pt 9):1841–54.
49. Wagner AD, Schacter DL, Rotte M, et al. Building memories: remembering and forgetting of verbal experiences as predicted by brain activity. Science. 1998;281(5380):1188–91.
50. Aguirre GK, Detre JA, Alsop DC, D'Esposito M. The parahippocampus subserves topographical learning in man. Cereb Cortex. 1996;6(6):823–9.
51. Buckner RL, Koutstaal W, Schacter DL, Dale AM, Rotte M, Rosen BR. Functional-anatomic study of episodic retrieval. II. Selective averaging of event-related fMRI trials to test the retrieval success hypothesis. Neuroimage. 1998;7(3):163–75.
52. Buckner RL, Koutstaal W, Schacter DL, Wagner AD, Rosen BR. Functional-anatomic study of episodic retrieval using fMRI. I. Retrieval effort versus retrieval success. Neuroimage. 1998;7(3):151–62.
53. Wagner AD, Desmond JE, Glover GH, Gabrieli JD. Prefrontal cortex and recognition memory. Functional-MRI evidence for context-dependent retrieval processes. Brain. 1998;121(Pt 10):1985–2002.
54. Lepage M, Ghaffar O, Nyberg L, Tulving E. Prefrontal cortex and episodic memory retrieval mode. Proc Natl Acad Sci USA. 2000;97(1):506–11.
55. Nyberg L, Cabeza R, Tulving E. PET studies of encoding and retrieval: The HERA Model. Psychol Bull Rev. 1996;3:135–48.
56. Nyberg L, McIntosh AR, Cabeza R, Habib R, Houle S, Tulving E. General and specific brain regions involved in encoding and retrieval of events: what, where, and when. Proc Natl Acad Sci USA. 1996;93(20):11280–5.
57. Wagner K, Frings L, Quiske A, et al. The reliability of fMRI activations in the medial temporal lobes in a verbal episodic memory task. Neuroimage. 2005;28(1):122–31.
58. Henson RN, Shallice T, Dolan RJ. Right prefrontal cortex and episodic memory retrieval: a functional MRI test of the monitoring hypothesis. Brain. 1999;122(Pt 7):1367–81.
59. McDermott KB, Ojemann JG, Petersen SE, et al. Direct comparison of episodic encoding and retrieval of words: an event-related fMRI study. Memory. 1999;7(5–6):661–78.
60. Henson RN, Hornberger M, Rugg MD. Further dissociating the processes involved in recognition memory: an FMRI study. J Cogn Neurosci. 2005;17(7):1058–73.
61. Daselaar SM, Fleck MS, Cabeza R. Triple dissociation in the medial temporal lobes: recollection, familiarity, and novelty. J Neurophysiol. 2006;96(4):1902–11.
62. Dolcos F, LaBar KS, Cabeza R. Remembering one year later: role of the amygdala and the medial temporal lobe memory system in retrieving emotional memories. Proc Natl Acad Sci USA. 2005;102(7):2626–31.
63. Montaldi D, Spencer TJ, Roberts N, Mayes AR. The neural system that mediates familiarity memory. Hippocampus. 2006;16(5):504–20.

64. Yonelinas AP, Otten LJ, Shaw KN, Rugg MD. Separating the brain regions involved in recollection and familiarity in recognition memory. J Neurosci. 2005;25(11):3002–8.
65. Milner B. Psychological aspects of focal epilepsy and its neurosurgical management. Adv Neurol. 1975;8:299–321.
66. Hermann BP, Seidenberg M, Haltiner A, Wyler AR. Relationship of age at onset, chronologic age, and adequacy of preoperative performance to verbal memory change after anterior temporal lobectomy. Epilepsia. 1995;36(2):137–45.
67. Saykin AJ, Gur RC, Sussman NM, O'Connor MJ, Gur RE. Memory deficits before and after temporal lobectomy: Effect of laterality and age of onset. Brain Cogn. 1989;9:191–200.
68. Saykin AJ, Robinson LJ, Stafiniak P, et al. Neuropsychological effects of temporal lobectomy: Acute changes in memory, language, and music. In: Bennett T, editor. Neuropsychology of Epilepsy. New York: Plenum Press; 1992.
69. Sperling RA, Bates JF, Cocchiarella AJ, Schacter DL, Rosen BR, Albert MS. Encoding novel face-name associations: a functional MRI study. Hum Brain Mapp. 2001;14(3):129–39.
70. Ranganath C, Yonelinas AP, Cohen MX, Dy CJ, Tom SM, D'Esposito M. Dissociable correlates of recollection and familiarity within the medial temporal lobes. Neuropsychologia. 2004;42(1):2–13.
71. Vilberg KL, Rugg MD. Memory retrieval and the parietal cortex: a review of evidence from a dual-process perspective. Neuropsychologia. 2008;46(7): 1787–99.
72. Kahn I, Davachi L, Wagner AD. Functional-neuroanatomic correlates of recollection: implications for models of recognition memory. J Neurosci. 2004;24(17):4172–80.
73. Gottfried JA, Smith AP, Rugg MD, Dolan RJ. Remembrance of odors past: human olfactory cortex in cross-modal recognition memory. Neuron. 2004;42(4):687–95.
74. Henson RN, Rugg MD, Shallice T, Josephs O, Dolan RJ. Recollection and familiarity in recognition memory: an event-related functional magnetic resonance imaging study. J Neurosci. 1999;19(10):3962–72.
75. Woodruff CC, Johnson JD, Uncapher MR, Rugg MD. Content-specificity of the neural correlates of recollection. Neuropsychologia. 2005;43(7): 1022–32.
76. Corbetta M, Kincade JM, Shulman GL. Neural systems for visual orienting and their relationships to spatial working memory. J Cogn Neurosci. 2002;14(3):508–23.
77. Herron JE, Henson RN, Rugg MD. Probability effects on the neural correlates of retrieval success: an fMRI study. Neuroimage. 2004;21(1):302–10.
78. Ravizza SM, Delgado MR, Chein JM, Becker JT, Fiez JA. Functional dissociations within the inferior parietal cortex in verbal working memory. Neuroimage. 2004;22(2):562–73.
79. Shannon BJ, Buckner RL. Functional-anatomic correlates of memory retrieval that suggest nontraditional processing roles for multiple distinct regions within posterior parietal cortex. J Neurosci. 2004;24(45):10084–92.
80. Dobbins IG, Han S. Cue- versus probe-dependent prefrontal cortex activity during contextual remembering. J Cogn Neurosci. 2006;18(9):1439–52.
81. Dobbins IG, Han S. Isolating rule- versus evidence-based prefrontal activity during episodic and lexical discrimination: a functional magnetic resonance imaging investigation of detection theory distinctions. Cereb Cortex. 2006;16(11):1614–22.
82. Simons JS, Owen AM, Fletcher PC, Burgess PW. Anterior prefrontal cortex and the recollection of contextual information. Neuropsychologia. 2005;43(12):1774–83.
83. Simons JS, Gilbert SJ, Owen AM, Fletcher PC, Burgess PW. Distinct roles for lateral and medial anterior prefrontal cortex in contextual recollection. J Neurophysiol. 2005;94(1):813–20.
84. Velanova K, Jacoby LL, Wheeler ME, McAvoy MP, Petersen SE, Buckner RL. Functional-anatomic correlates of sustained and transient processing components engaged during controlled retrieval. J Neurosci. 2003;23(24):8460–70.
85. Dobbins IG, Foley H, Schacter DL, Wagner AD. Executive control during episodic retrieval: multiple prefrontal processes subserve source memory. Neuron. 2002;35(5):989–96.
86. Dobbins IG, Wagner AD. Domain-general and domain-sensitive prefrontal mechanisms for recollecting events and detecting novelty. Cereb Cortex. 2005;15(11):1768–78.
87. Cabeza R, Rao SM, Wagner AD, Mayer AR, Schacter DL. Can medial temporal lobe regions distinguish true from false? An event-related functional MRI study of veridical and illusory recognition memory. Proc Natl Acad Sci USA. 2001;98(8):4805–10.
88. Anderson ND, Craik FIM. Memory in the aging brain. In: Craik FIM, editor. The Oxford Handbook of Memory. New York: Oxford; 2000. p. 411–25.
89. Balota DA, Dolan PO, Duchek JM. Memory changes in healthy older adults. In: Craik FIM, editor. The Oxford Handbook of Memory. New York: Oxford; 2000. p. 395–409.
90. Nyberg L, Backman L, Erngrund K, Olofsson U, Nilsson LG. Age differences in episodic memory, semantic memory, and priming: relationships to demographic, intellectual, and biological factors. J Gerontol B Psychol Sci Soc Sci. 1996;51(4): P234–240.
91. Grady C, Craik FI. Changes in memory processing with age. Curr Opin Neurobiol. 2000;10:224–31.
92. Park DC, Smith AD, Lautenschlager G, et al. Mediators of long-term memory performance across the lifespan. Psychol Aging. 1996;11:621–37.
93. Zacks RT, Hasher L, Li KZH. Human memory. In: Salthouse TA, editor. The Handbook of Aging and Cognition. Mahwah, NJ: Erlbaum; 1999. p. 200–30.

94. Baltes PB. The aging mind: potential and limits. Gerontologist Eng. 1993;33(5):580–94.
95. Flashman LA, Wishart HA, Saykin AJ. Boundaries Between Normal Aging and Dementia: Perspectives from Neuropsychological and Neuroimaging Investigations. In: Oxman TE, editor. Dementia: Presentations, Differential Diagnosis and Nosology. 2nd ed. Baltimore: Johns Hopkins University Press; 2003.
96. Schroots JJF, Birren JE. Theoretical issues and basic questions in the planning of longitudinal studies of health and aging. In: Schroots JJF, editor. Aging, health and competence: The next generation of longitudinal studies. Amsterdam: Elsevier; 1993. p. 4–34.
97. Raz N, Gunning FM, Head D, et al. Selective aging of the human cerebral cortex observed in vivo: Differential vulnerability of the prefrontal gray matter. Cereb Cortex. 1997;7(3):268–82.
98. Bigler ED, Blatter DD, Anderson CV, et al. Hippocampal volume in normal aging and traumatic brain injury. AJNR Am J Neuroradiol. 1997;18(1): 11–23.
99. DeCarli C, Murphy DG, Gillette JA, et al. Lack of age-related differences in temporal lobe volume of very healthy adults. AJNR Am J Neuroradiol Eng. 1994;15(4):689–96.
100. Greenwood PM. The frontal aging hypothesis evaluated. J Int Neuropsychol Soc. 2000;6:705–26.
101. Greenwood PM. Reply to west. J Int Neuropsychol Soc. 2000;6:730.
102. West R. In defense of the frontal lobe hypothesis of cognitive aging. J Int Neuropsychol Soc. 2000;6: 727–9.
103. Kempermann G, Gage FH. New nerve cells for the adult brain. Sci Am. 1999;280:48–53.
104. Reuter-Lorenz PA, Stanczak L, Miller AC. Neural recruitment and cognitive aging: Two hemispheres are better than one, especially as you age. Psychol Sci. 1999;10(6):494–500.
105. Cabeza R. Hemispheric asymmetry reduction in old adults: The HAROLD model. Psychol Aging. 2002; 17:85–100.
106. Cabeza R, Anderson ND, Locantore JK, McIntosh AR. Aging gracefully: Compensatory brain activity in high-performing older adults. Neuroimage. 2002; 17:1394–402.
107. Stebbins GT, Carrillo MC, Dorfman J, et al. Aging effects on memory encoding in the frontal lobes. Psychol Aging. 2002;17(1):44–55.
108. Anderson KE, Perera GM, Hilton J, Zubin N, Paz Dela R, Stern Y. Functional magnetic resonance imaging study of word recognition in normal elders. Prog Neuropsychopharmacol Biol Psychiatry. 2002;26(4):647–50.
109. Cabeza R, Daselaar SM, Dolcos F, Prince SE, Budde M, Nyberg L. Task-independent and task-specific age effects on brain activity during working memory, visual attention and episodic retrieval. Cereb Cortex. 2004;14(4):364–75.
110. Grady CL. Age-related differences in face processing: a meta-analysis of three functional neuroimaging experiments. Can J Exp Psychol. 2002;56(3): 208–20.
111. Morcom AM, Good CD, Frackowiak RS, Rugg MD. Age effects on the neural correlates of successful memory encoding. Brain. 2003;126(Pt 1):213–29.
112. Morcom AM, Li J, Rugg MD. Age effects on the neural correlates of episodic retrieval: increased cortical recruitment with matched performance. Cereb Cortex. 2007;17(11):2491–506.
113. Grady CL, McIntosh AR, Rajah MN, Beig S, Craik FI. The effects of age on the neural correlates of episodic encoding. Cereb Cortex. 1999;9(8):805–14.
114. Mandzia JL, Black SE, McAndrews MP, Grady C, Graham S. fMRI differences in encoding and retrieval of pictures due to encoding strategy in the elderly. Hum Brain Mapp. 2004;21(1):1–14.
115. Logan JM, Sanders AL, Snyder AZ, Morris JC, Buckner RL. Under-recruitment and nonselective recruitment: dissociable neural mechanisms associated with aging. Neuron. 2002;33(5):827–40.
116. Rajah MN, D'Esposito M. Region-specific changes in prefrontal function with age: a review of PET and fMRI studies on working and episodic memory. Brain. 2005;128(Pt 9):1964–83.
117. Belger A, Banich MT. Costs and benefits of integrating information between the cerebral hemispheres: a computational perspective. Neuropsychology. 1998;12(3):380–98.
118. Erickson KI, Colcombe SJ, Wadhwa R, et al. Training-induced plasticity in older adults: effects of training on hemispheric asymmetry. Neurobiol Aging. 2007;28(2):272–83.
119. Fawcett JW, Rosser AE, Dunnett SB. Brain Damage, Brain Repair. New York: Oxford U.P; 2001.
120. Muller RA, Rothermel RD, Behen ME, Muzik O, Mangner TJ, Chugani HT. Differential patterns of language and motor reorganization following early left hemisphere lesion: a PET study. Arch Neurol. 1998;55(8):1113–9.
121. Baltes PB, Lindenberger U. Emergence of a powerful connection between sensory and cognitive functions across the adult life span: a new window to the study of cognitive aging? Psychol Aging. 1997;12(1): 12–21.
122. Cabeza R. Cognitive neuroscience of aging: contributions of functional neuroimaging. Scand J Psychol. 2001;42(3):277–86.
123. Daselaar SM, Fleck MS, Dobbins IG, Madden DJ, Cabeza R. Effects of healthy aging on hippocampal and rhinal memory functions: an event-related fMRI study. Cereb Cortex. 2006;16(12):1771–82.
124. Dennis NA, Daselaar S, Cabeza R. Effects of aging on transient and sustained successful memory encoding activity. Neurobiol Aging. 2007;28(11):1749–58.
125. Sperling RA, Bates JF, Chua EF, et al. FMRI studies of associative encoding in young and elderly controls and mild Alzheimer's disease. J Neurol Neurosurg Psychiatry. 2003;74(1):44–50.

126. Small SA, Tsai WY, DeLaPaz R, Mayeux R, Stern Y. Imaging hippocampal function across the human life span: is memory decline normal or not? Ann Neurol. 2002;51(3):290–5.
127. Small SA, Wu EX, Bartsch D, et al. Imaging physiologic dysfunction of individual hippocampal subregions in humans and genetically modified mice. Neuron. 2000;28(3):653–64.
128. Davis SW, Dennis NA, Daselaar SM, Fleck MS, Cabeza R. Que PASA? The posterior-anterior shift in aging. Cereb Cortex. 2008;18(5):1201–9.
129. Dennis NA, Hayes SM, Prince SE, Madden DJ, Huettel SA, Cabeza R. Effects of aging on the neural correlates of successful item and source memory encoding. J Exp Psychol Learn Mem Cogn. 2008; 34(4):791–808.
130. Petersen RC. Aging, mild cognitive impairment, and Alzheimer's disease. Neurol Clin. 2000;18(4): 789–806.
131. Petersen RC, Doody R, Kurz A, et al. Current concepts in mild cognitive impairment. Arch Neurol. 2001;58(12):1985–92.
132. Petersen RC, Stevens JC, Ganguli M, Tangalos EG, Cummings JL, DeKosky ST. Practice parameter: Early detection of dementia: Mild cognitive impairment (an evidence-based review). Report of the Quality Standards Subcommittee of the American Academy of Neurology. Neurology. 2001;56: 1133–42.
133. Petersen RC, Roberts RO, Knopman DS, et al. Mild cognitive impairment: ten years later. Arch Neurol. 2009;66(12):1447–55.
134. Saykin AJ, Wishart HA. Mild Cognitive Impairment: Conceptual issues and structural and functional brain correlates. In: Ovsiew F, editor. Seminars in clinical neuropsychiatry. 2003.
135. Braak H, Braak E, Bohl J. Staging of Alzheimer-related cortical destruction. Eur Neurol. 1993;33(6): 403–8.
136. Chetelat G, Desgranges B, de la Sayette V, Viader F, Eustache F, Baron JC. Mapping gray matter loss with voxel-based morphometry in mild cognitive impairment. Neuroreport. 2002;13:1939–43.
137. de Leon MJ, Convit A, DeSanti S, et al. The hippocampus in aging and Alzheimer's disease. Neuroimaging Clin N Am Eng. 1995;5(1):1–17.
138. de Leon MJ, Convit A, George AE, et al. In vivo structural studies of the hippocampus in normal aging and in incipient Alzheimer's disease. Ann NY Acad Sci Eng. 1996;777:1–13.
139. Jack Jr CR, Petersen RC, O' Brien PC, Tangalos EG. MR-based hippocampal volumetry in the diagnosis of Alzheimer's disease. Neurol Eng. 1992;42(1): 183–8.
140. Jack Jr CR, Shiung MM, Gunter JL, et al. Comparison of different MRI brain atrophy rate measures with clinical disease progression in AD. Neurology. 2004;62(4):591–600.
141. Jack Jr CR, Shiung MM, Weigand SD, et al. Brain atrophy rates predict subsequent clinical conversion in normal elderly and amnestic MCI. Neurology. 2005;65(8):1227–31.
142. Risacher SL, Saykin AJ, West JD, Shen L, Firpi HA, McDonald BC. Baseline MRI predictors of conversion from MCI to probable AD in the ADNI cohort. Curr Alzheimer Res. 2009;6(4):347–61.
143. Devanand DP, Liu X, Tabert MH, et al. Combining early markers strongly predicts conversion from mild cognitive impairment to Alzheimer's disease. Biol Psychiatry. 2008;64(10):871–9.
144. Risacher SL, Saykin AJ. Neuroimaging of Alzheimer's Disease, Mild Cognitive Impairment and Other Dementias. In: Sweet LH, Cohen RA, editors. Brain imaging in behavioral medicine and clinical neuroscience. New York: Springer; 2011.
145. Zakzanis KK, Graham SJ, Campbell Z. A meta-analysis of structural and functional brain imaging in dementia of the Alzheimer's type: a neuroimaging profile. Neuropsychol Rev. 2003;13(1):1–18.
146. de Leon MJ, DeSanti S, Zinkowski R, et al. MRI and CSF studies in the early diagnosis of Alzheimer's disease. J Intern Med. 2004;256(3):205–23.
147. de Leon MJ, Mosconi L, Blennow K, et al. Imaging and CSF studies in the preclinical diagnosis of Alzheimer's disease. Ann NY Acad Sci. 2007;1097:114–45.
148. DeCarli C. The role of neuroimaging in dementia. Clin Geriatr Med. 2001;17(2):255–79.
149. Good CD. Dementia and ageing. Br Med Bull. 2003;65:159–68.
150. Weiner MW. Imaging and biomarkers will be used for detection and monitoring progression of early Alzheimer's disease. J Nutr Health Aging. 2009;13:332.
151. Whitwell JL, Jack CR, Jr. Neuroimaging in dementia. Neurol Clin. 2007;25(3):843–857, viii.
152. Wolf H, Hensel A, Kruggel F, et al. Structural correlates of mild cognitive impairment. Neurobiol Aging. 2004;25(7):913–24.
153. Wolf H, Jelic V, Gertz HJ, Nordberg A, Julin P, Wahlund LO. A critical discussion of the role of neuroimaging in mild cognitive impairment. Acta Neurol Scand Suppl. 2003;179:52–76.
154. Wolk DA, Price JC, Saxton JA, et al. Amyloid imaging in mild cognitive impairment subtypes. Ann Neurol. 2009;65:557–68.
155. Dickerson BC, Salat DH, Greve DN, et al. Increased hippocampal activation in mild cognitive impairment compared to normal aging and AD. Neurology. 2005;65(3):404–11.
156. Pariente J, Cole S, Henson R, et al. Alzheimer's patients engage an alternative network during a memory task. Ann Neurol. 2005;58(6):870–9.
157. Kato T, Knopman D, Liu H. Dissociation of regional activation in mild AD during visual encoding: A functional MRI study. Neurology. 2001;57:812–6.
158. Rombouts SA, Barkhof F, Veltman DJ, et al. Functional MR imaging in Alzheimer's disease during memory encoding. AJNR Am J Neuroradiol. 2000;21(10):1869–75.

159. Small SA, Perera GM, DeLaPaz R, Mayeux R, Stern Y. Differential regional dysfunction of the hippocampal formation among elderly with memory decline and Alzheimer's disease. Ann Neurol. 1999; 45(4):466–72.
160. Machulda MM, Ward HA, Borowski B, et al. Comparison of memory fMRI response among normal, MCI, and Alzheimer's patients. Neurology. 2003;61(4):500–6.
161. Gron G, Bittner D, Schmitz B, Wunderlich AP, Riepe MW. Subjective memory complaints: objective neural markers in patients with Alzheimer's disease and major depressive disorder. Ann Neurol. 2002;51(4):491–8.
162. Corkin S, Functional MRI. for studying episodic memory in aging and Alzheimer's disease. Geriatrics. 1998;53 Suppl 1:S13–15.
163. Grady CL, McIntosh AR, Beig S, Keightley ML, Burian H, Black SE. Evidence from functional neuroimaging of a compensatory prefrontal network in Alzheimer's disease. J Neurosci. 2003;23(3):986–93.
164. Golby A, Silverberg G, Race E, et al. Memory encoding in Alzheimer's disease: an fMRI study of explicit and implicit memory. Brain. 2005;128(Pt 4): 773–87.
165. Saykin AJ, Flashman LA, Johnson S, et al. Frontal and hippocampal memory circuitry in early Alzheimer's disease: Relation of structural and functional MRI changes. Neuroimage. 2000;11(5):S123.
166. Celone KA, Calhoun VD, Dickerson BC, et al. Alterations in memory networks in mild cognitive impairment and Alzheimer's disease: an independent component analysis. J Neurosci. 2006;26(40): 10222–31.
167. Trivedi MA, Murphy CM, Goetz C, et al. fMRI activation changes during successful episodic memory encoding and recognition in amnestic mild cognitive impairment relative to cognitively healthy older adults. Dement Geriatr Cogn Disord. 2008;26(2): 123–37.
168. Dickerson BC, Salat DH, Bates JF, et al. Medial temporal lobe function and structure in mild cognitive impairment. Ann Neurol. 2004;56(1):27–35.
169. Hamalainen A, Pihlajamaki M, Tanila H, et al. Increased fMRI responses during encoding in mild cognitive impairment. Neurobiol Aging. 2007; 28(12):1889–903.
170. Johnson SC, Schmitz TW, Moritz CH, et al. Activation of brain regions vulnerable to Alzheimer's disease: the effect of mild cognitive impairment. Neurobiol Aging. 2006;27(11):1604–12.
171. O'Brien JL, O'Keefe KM, LaViolette PS, et al. Longitudinal fMRI in elderly reveals loss of hippocampal activation with clinical decline. Neurology. 2010;74(24):1969–76.
172. Johnson SC, Baxter LC, Susskind-Wilder L, Connor DJ, Sabbagh MN, Caselli RJ. Hippocampal adaptation to face repetition in healthy elderly and mild cognitive impairment. Neuropsychologia. 2004; 42(7):980–9.
173. Miller SL, Fenstermacher E, Bates J, Blacker D, Sperling RA, Dickerson BC. Hippocampal activation in adults with mild cognitive impairment predicts subsequent cognitive decline. J Neurol Neurosurg Psychiatry. 2008;79(6):630–5.
174. Yassa MA, Stark SM, Bakker A, Albert MS, Gallagher M, Stark CE. High-resolution structural and functional MRI of hippocampal CA3 and dentate gyrus in patients with amnestic Mild Cognitive Impairment. Neuroimage. 2010;51(3): 1242–52.
175. McIntosh AR. Towards a network theory of cognition. Neural Netw. 2000;13(8–9):861–70.
176. Friston KJ, Buechel C, Fink GR, Morris J, Rolls E, Dolan RJ. Psychophysiological and modulatory interactions in neuroimaging. Neuroimage. 1997; 6(3):218–29.
177. Greicius MD, Menon V. Default-mode activity during a passive sensory task: uncoupled from deactivation but impacting activation. J Cogn Neurosci. 2004;16(9):1484–92.
178. Nyberg L, Persson J, Habib R, et al. Large scale neurocognitive networks underlying episodic memory. J Cogn Neurosci. 2000;12(1):163–73.
179. Ranganath C, Heller A, Cohen MX, Brozinsky CJ, Rissman J. Functional connectivity with the hippocampus during successful memory formation. Hippocampus. 2005;15(8):997–1005.
180. Burianova H, McIntosh AR, Grady CL. A common functional brain network for autobiographical, episodic, and semantic memory retrieval. Neuroimage. 2010;49(1):865–74.
181. Takahashi E, Ohki K, Kim DS. Dissociated pathways for successful memory retrieval from the human parietal cortex: anatomical and functional connectivity analyses. Cereb Cortex. 2008;18(8): 1771–8.
182. Iidaka T, Matsumoto A, Nogawa J, Yamamoto Y, Sadato N. Frontoparietal network involved in successful retrieval from episodic memory. Spatial and temporal analyses using fMRI and ERP. Cereb Cortex. 2006;16(9):1349–60.
183. Gusnard DA, Raichle ME. Searching for a baseline: functional imaging and the resting human brain. Nat Rev Neurosci. 2001;2(10):685–94.
184. Raichle ME, MacLeod AM, Snyder AZ, Powers WJ, Gusnard DA, Shulman GL. A default mode of brain function. Proc Natl Acad Sci USA. 2001;98(2): 676–82.
185. Cabeza R, Grady CL, Nyberg L, et al. Age-related differences in neural activity during memory encoding and retrieval: a positron emission tomography study. J Neurosci. 1997;17(1):391–400.
186. Achard S, Bullmore E. Efficiency and cost of economical brain functional networks. PLoS Comput Biol. 2007;3(2):e17.
187. Grady CL, McIntosh AR, Craik FI. Age-related differences in the functional connectivity of the hippocampus during memory encoding. Hippocampus. 2003;13(5):572–86.

188. Wang L, Laviolette P, O'Keefe K, et al. Intrinsic connectivity between the hippocampus and posteromedial cortex predicts memory performance in cognitively intact older individuals. Neuroimage. 2010;51(2):910–7.
189. Andrews-Hanna JR, Snyder AZ, Vincent JL, et al. Disruption of large-scale brain systems in advanced aging. Neuron. 2007;56(5):924–35.
190. Damoiseaux JS, Beckmann CF, Arigita EJ, et al. Reduced resting-state brain activity in the "default network" in normal aging. Cereb Cortex. 2008; 18(8):1856–64.
191. Lustig C, Snyder AZ, Bhakta M, et al. Functional deactivations: change with age and dementia of the Alzheimer type. Proc Natl Acad Sci USA. 2003; 100(24):14504–9.
192. Daselaar SM, Prince SE, Cabeza R. When less means more: deactivations during encoding that predict subsequent memory. Neuroimage. 2004;23(3):921–7.
193. Li SJ, Li Z, Wu G, Zhang MJ, Franczak M, Antuono PG. Alzheimer disease: evaluation of a functional MR imaging index as a marker. Radiology. 2002; 225(1):253–9.
194. Greicius MD, Srivastava G, Reiss AL, Menon V. Default-mode network activity distinguishes Alzheimer's disease from healthy aging: evidence from functional MRI. Proc Natl Acad Sci USA. 2004;101(13):4637–42.
195. Rombouts SA, Barkhof F, Goekoop R, Stam CJ, Scheltens P. Altered resting state networks in mild cognitive impairment and mild Alzheimer's disease: an fMRI study. Hum Brain Mapp. 2005;26(4):231–9.
196. Sorg C, Riedl V, Muhlau M, et al. Selective changes of resting-state networks in individuals at risk for Alzheimer's disease. Proc Natl Acad Sci USA. 2007;104(47):18760–5.
197. Wang L, Zang Y, He Y, et al. Changes in hippocampal connectivity in the early stages of Alzheimer's disease: evidence from resting state fMRI. Neuroimage. 2006;31(2):496–504.
198. Wagner AD. Early detection of Alzheimer's disease: An fMRI marker for people at risk? Nat Neurosci. 2000;3(10):973–4.
199. Rodda JE, Dannhauser TM, Cutinha DJ, Shergill SS, Walker Z. Subjective cognitive impairment: increased prefrontal cortex activation compared to controls during an encoding task. Int J Geriatr Psychiatry. 2009;24(8):865–74.
200. Smith JD. Apolipoproteins and aging: emerging mechanisms. Ageing Res Rev. 2002;1(3):345–65.
201. Bookheimer SY, Strojwas MH, Cohen MS, et al. Patterns of brain activation in people at risk for Alzheimer's disease. N Engl J Med. 2000; 343(7):450–6.
202. Burggren AC, Small GW, Sabb FW, Bookheimer SY. Specificity of brain activation patterns in people at genetic risk for Alzheimer disease. Am J Geriatr Psychiatry. 2002;10(1):44–51.
203. Bondi MW, Houston WS, Eyler LT, Brown GG. fMRI evidence of compensatory mechanisms in older adults at genetic risk for Alzheimer disease. Neurology. 2005;64(3):501–8.
204. Elgh E, Larsson A, Eriksson S, Nyberg L. Altered prefrontal brain activity in persons at risk for Alzheimer's disease: an fMRI study. Int Psychogeriatr. 2003;15(2):121–33.
205. Trivedi MA, Schmitz TW, Ries ML, et al. Reduced hippocampal activation during episodic encoding in middle-aged individuals at genetic risk of Alzheimer's disease: a cross-sectional study. BMC Med. 2006;4:1.
206 Rombouts SA, Barkhof F, Van Meel CS, Scheltens P. Alterations in brain activation during cholinergic enhancement with rivastigmine in Alzheimer's disease. J Neurol Neurosurg Psychiatry. 2002;73(6): 665–71.
207. Kircher TT, Erb M, Grodd W, Leube DT. Cortical activation during cholinesterase-inhibitor treatment in Alzheimer disease: preliminary findings from a pharmaco-fMRI study. Am J Geriatr Psychiatry. 2005;13(11):1006–13.
208. Goekoop R, Scheltens P, Barkhof F, Rombouts SA. Cholinergic challenge in Alzheimer patients and mild cognitive impairment differentially affects hippocampal activation – a pharmacological fMRI study. Brain. 2006;129(Pt 1):141–57.
209. Dumas JA, McDonald BC, Saykin AJ, et al. Cholinergic modulation of hippocampal activity during episodic memory encoding in postmenopausal women: a pilot study. Menopause. 2010;17(4):852–9.
210. Bozzali M, MacPherson SE, Dolan RJ, Shallice T. Left prefrontal cortex control of novel occurrences during recollection: a psychopharmacological study using scopolamine and event-related fMRI. Neuroimage. 2006;33(1):286–95.
211. Budson AE. Understanding memory dysfunction. Neurologist. 2009;15(2):71–9.
212. Martin A. Functional neuroimaging of semantic memory. In: Kingstone A, editor. Handbook of Functional Neuroimaging of Cognition. Cambridge, MA: Bradford; 2001. p. 153–86.
213. Binder JR, Desai RH, Graves WW, Conant LL. Where is the semantic system? A critical review and meta-analysis of 120 functional neuroimaging studies. Cereb Cortex. 2009;19(12):2767–96.
214. Grossman M, Smith EE, Koenig P, et al. The neural basis for categorization in semantic memory. Neuroimage. 2002;17(3):1549–61.
215. Levy DA, Bayley PJ. Squire LR. The anatomy of semantic knowledge: medial vs. lateral temporal lobe. Proc Natl Acad Sci USA. 2004;101(17):6710–5.
216. Vigneau M, Beaucousin V, Herve PY, et al. Meta-analyzing left hemisphere language areas: phonology, semantics, and sentence processing. Neuroimage. 2006;30(4):1414–32.
217. Grossman M, Koenig P, DeVita C, et al. The neural basis for category-specific knowledge: an fMRI study. Neuroimage. 2002;15(4):936–48.
218. Jefferies E, Lambon Ralph MA. Semantic impairment in stroke aphasia versus semantic dementia: a case-series comparison. Brain. 2006;129(Pt 8):2132–47.

219. Warrington EK. The selective impairment of semantic memory. Q J Exp Psychol. 1975;27(4):635–57.
220. Mummery CJ, Patterson K, Wise RJ, Vandenberghe R, Price CJ, Hodges JR. Disrupted temporal lobe connections in semantic dementia. Brain. 1999; 122(Pt 1):61–73.
221. Wallentin M, Lund TE, Ostergaard S, Ostergaard L, Roepstorff A. Motion verb sentences activate left posterior middle temporal cortex despite static context. Neuroreport. 2005;16(6):649–52.
222. Simmons WK, Ramjee V, Beauchamp MS, McRae K, Martin A, Barsalou LW. A common neural substrate for perceiving and knowing about color. Neuropsychologia. 2007;45(12):2802–10.
223. Gainotti G. What the locus of brain lesion tells us about the nature of the cognitive defect underlying category-specific disorders: a review. Cortex. 2000;36(4):539–59.
224. Kuchinke L, Jacobs AM, Grubich C, Vo ML, Conrad M, Herrmann M. Incidental effects of emotional valence in single word processing: an fMRI study. Neuroimage. 2005;28(4):1022–32.
225. Bechara A, Damasio H, Damasio AR. Emotion, decision making and the orbitofrontal cortex. Cereb Cortex. 2000;10(3):295–307.
226. Bechara A, Tranel D, Damasio H. Characterization of the decision-making deficit of patients with ventromedial prefrontal cortex lesions. Brain. 2000;123(Pt 11):2189–202.
227. Ni W, Constable RT, Mencl WE, et al. An event-related neuroimaging study distinguishing form and content in sentence processing. J Cogn Neurosci. 2000;12(1):120–33.
228. Humphries C, Binder JR, Medler DA, Liebenthal E. Time course of semantic processes during sentence comprehension: an fMRI study. Neuroimage. 2007;36(3):924–32.
229. Lehmann S, Murray MM. The role of multisensory memories in unisensory object discrimination. Brain Res Cogn Brain Res. 2005;24(2):326–34.
230. Robinson G, Blair J, Cipolotti L. Dynamic aphasia: an inability to select between competing verbal responses? Brain. 1998;121(Pt 1):77–89.
231. Price CJ, Mummery CJ, Moore CJ, Frakowiak RS, Friston KJ. Delineating necessary and sufficient neural systems with functional imaging studies of neuropsychological patients. J Cogn Neurosci. 1999; 11(4):371–82.
232. Epstein RA, Parker WE, Feiler AM. Where am I now? Distinct roles for parahippocampal and retrosplenial cortices in place recognition. J Neurosci. 2007;27(23):6141–9.
233. Maddock RJ. The retrosplenial cortex and emotion: new insights from functional neuroimaging of the human brain. Trends Neurosci. 1999;22(7):310–6.
234. Hassabis D, Kumaran D, Maguire EA. Using imagination to understand the neural basis of episodic memory. J Neurosci. 2007;27(52):14365–74.
235. O'Reilly RC, Rudy JW. Conjunctive representations in learning and memory: principles of cortical and hippocampal function. Psychol Rev. 2001;108(2): 311–45.
236. Salthouse TA. Speed and knowledge as determinants of adult age differences in verbal tasks. J Gerontology Eng. 1993;48(1):29–36.
237. Albert MS, Heller HS, Milberg W. Changes in naming ability with age. Psychol Aging. 1988;3(2): 173–8.
238. Au R, Joung P, Nicholas M, Obler LK. Naming ability across the adult life span. Aging Cognition. 1995;2(4):300–11.
239. Rich JB, Park NW, Dopkins S, Brandt J. What do Alzheimer's disease patients know about animals? It depends on task structure and presentation format. J Int Neuropsychol Soc. 2002;8(1):83–94.
240. Cooke A, Grossman M, DeVita C, et al. Large-scale neural network for sentence processing. Brain Lang. 2006;96(1):14–36.
241. Gold BT, Andersen AH, Jicha GA, Smith CD. Aging influences the neural correlates of lexical decision but not automatic semantic priming. Cereb Cortex. 2009;19(11):2671–9.
242. Johnson SC, Saykin AJ, Flashman LA, et al. Similarities and differences in semantic and phonological processing with age: Patterns of functional MRI activation. Aging Neuropsychol Cognition. 2001;8(4):307–20.
243. Nielson KA, Douville KL, Seidenberg M, et al. Age-related functional recruitment for famous name recognition: an event-related fMRI study. Neurobiol Aging. 2006;27(10):1494–504.
244. Wierenga CE, Benjamin M, Gopinath K, et al. Age-related changes in word retrieval: role of bilateral frontal and subcortical networks. Neurobiol Aging. 2008;29(3):436–51.
245. Grossman M, Cooke A, DeVita C, et al. Age-related changes in working memory during sentence comprehension: an fMRI study. Neuroimage. 2002;15(2):302–17.
246. Tyler LK, Shafto MA, Randall B, Wright P, Marslen-Wilson WD, Stamatakis EA. Preserving syntactic processing across the adult life span: the modulation of the frontotemporal language system in the context of age-related atrophy. Cereb Cortex. 2010;20(2): 352–64.
247. Garrard P, Patterson K, Watson PC, Hodges JR. Category specific semantic loss in dementia of Alzheimer's type. Functional-anatomical correlations from cross-sectional analyses. Brain. 1998; 121(Pt 4):633–46.
248. Grossman M. Not all words are created equal. Category-specific deficits in central nervous system disease. Neurology. 1998;50(2):324–5.
249. Grossman M, Robinson K, Biassou N, White-Devine T, D'Esposito M. Semantic memory in Alzheimer's disease: representativeness, ontologic category, and material. Neuropsychology. 1998;12(1):34–42.
250. Woodard JL, Seidenberg M, Nielson KA, et al. Semantic memory activation in amnestic mild cognitive impairment. Brain. 2009;132(Pt 8):2068–78.

251. Gigi A, Babai R, Penker A, Hendler T, Korczyn AD. Prefrontal compensatory mechanism may enable normal semantic memory performance in mild cognitive impairment (MCI). J Neuroimaging. 2010; 20(2):163–8.
252. Johnson SC, Saykin AJ, Baxter LC, et al. The relationship between fMRI activation and cerebral atrophy: comparison of normal aging and alzheimer disease. Neuroimage. 2000;11(3):179–87.
253. McGeown WJ, Shanks MF, Forbes-McKay KE, Venneri A. Patterns of brain activity during a semantic task differentiate normal aging from early Alzheimer's disease. Psychiatry Res. 2009;173(3): 218–27.
254. Saykin AJ, Flashman LA, Frutiger SA, et al. Neuroanatomic substrates of semantic memory impairment in Alzheimer's disease: patterns of functional MRI activation. J Int Neuropsychol Soc. 1999;5(5):377–92.
255. Grossman M, Koenig P, Glosser G, et al. Neural basis for semantic memory difficulty in Alzheimer's disease: an fMRI study. Brain. 2003;126(Pt 2): 292–311.
256. Taler V, Risacher SL, West JD, et al. Differential neuroanatomical substrates of language performance by diagnostic group and task in the ADNI cohort. J Int Neuropsychol Soc. Submitted for publication.
257. Assaf M, Jagannathan K, Calhoun V, Kraut M, Hart Jr J, Pearlson G. Temporal sequence of hemispheric network activation during semantic processing: a functional network connectivity analysis. Brain Cogn. 2009;70(2):238–46.
258. Binder JR, Frost JA, Hammeke TA, Bellgowan PS, Rao SM, Cox RW. Conceptual processing during the conscious resting state. A functional MRI study. J Cogn Neurosci. 1999;11(1):80–95.
259. Vitali P, Abutalebi J, Tettamanti M, et al. Generating animal and tool names: an fMRI study of effective connectivity. Brain Lang. 2005;93(1):32–45.
260. Adlam AL, Bozeat S, Arnold R, Watson P, Hodges JR. Semantic knowledge in mild cognitive impairment and mild Alzheimer's disease. Cortex. 2006; 42(5):675–84.
261. Duong A, Whitehead V, Hanratty K, Chertkow H. The nature of lexico-semantic processing deficits in mild cognitive impairment. Neuropsychologia. 2006;44(10):1928–35.
262. Mickes L, Wixted JT, Fennema-Notestine C, et al. Progressive impairment on neuropsychological tasks in a longitudinal study of preclinical Alzheimer's disease. Neuropsychology. 2007;21(6):696–705.
263. Smith JA, Knight RG. Memory processing in Alzheimer's disease. Neuropsychologia. 2002;40(6): 666–82.
264. Lind J, Persson J, Ingvar M, et al. Reduced functional brain activity response in cognitively intact apolipoprotein E epsilon4 carriers. Brain. 2006;129(Pt 5):1240–8.
265. McGeown WJ, Shanks MF, Venneri A. Prolonged cholinergic enrichment influences regional cortical activation in early Alzheimer's disease. Neuropsychiatr Dis Treat. 2008;4(2):465–76.
266 Mencl WE, Pugh KR, Shaywitz SE, et al. Network analysis of brain activations in working memory: behavior and age relationships. Microsc Res Tech. 2000;51(1):64–74.
267. Baddeley AD. Is working memory still working? Am Psychol. 2001;56(11):851–64.
268. Becker JT, Morris RG. Working memory(s). Brain Cogn. 1999;41:1–8.
269. Curtis CE, D'Esposito M. Persistent activity in the prefrontal cortex during working memory. Trends Cogn Sci. 2003;7(9):415–23.
270. Baddeley A. Working memory. Curr Biol. 2010;20(4):R136–140.
271. Baddeley A. Working memory. C R Acad Sci III. 1998;321(2–3):167–73.
272. Baddeley A. Working memory. Science. 1992; 255(5044):556–9.
273. Cowan N. Evolving conceptions of memory storage, selective attention, and their mutual constraints within the human information-processing system. Psychol Bull. 1988;104(2):163–91.
274. Cowan N, Nugent LD, Elliott EM, Ponomarev I, Saults JS. The role of attention in the development of short-term memory: age differences in the verbal span of apprehension. Child Dev. 1999;70(5): 1082–97.
275. D'Esposito M. From cognitive to neural models of working memory. Philos Trans R Soc Lond B Biol Sci. 2007;362(1481):761–72.
276. Courtney SM, Petit L, Maisog JM, Ungerleider LG, Haxby JV. An area specialized for spatial working memory in human frontal cortex. Science. 1998;279(5355):1347–51.
277. Awh E, Jonides J. Overlapping mechanisms of attention and spatial working memory. Trends Cogn Sci. 2001;5(3):119–26.
278. Curtis CE, Rao VY, D'Esposito M. Maintenance of spatial and motor codes during oculomotor delayed response tasks. J Neurosci. 2004;24(16):3944–52.
279. Klein C, Fischer B, Hartnegg K, Heiss WH, Roth M. Optomotor and neuropsychological performance in old age. Exp Brain Res. 2000;135(2):141–54.
280. Chein JM, Fiez JA. Dissociation of verbal working memory system components using a delayed serial recall task. Cereb Cortex. 2001;11(11):1003–14.
281. Davachi L, Maril A, Wagner AD. When keeping in mind supports later bringing to mind: neural markers of phonological rehearsal predict subsequent remembering. J Cogn Neurosci. 2001;13(8): 1059–70.
282. Jonides J, Schumacher EH, Smith EE, et al. The role of parietal cortex in verbal working memory. J Neurosci. 1998;18(13):5026–34.
283. Smith EE, Jonides J. Neuroimaging analyses of human working memory. Proc Natl Acad Sci USA. 1998;95(20):12061–8.
284. Smith EE, Jonides J, Marshuetz C, Koeppe RA. Components of verbal working memory: evidence

from neuroimaging. Proc Natl Acad Sci USA. 1998;95(3):876–82.

285. Druzgal TJ, D'Esposito M. Dissecting contributions of prefrontal cortex and fusiform face area to face working memory. J Cogn Neurosci. 2003;15(6): 771–84.

286. Linden DE, Bittner RA, Muckli L, et al. Cortical capacity constraints for visual working memory: dissociation of fMRI load effects in a fronto-parietal network. Neuroimage. 2003;20(3):1518–30.

287. Wager TD, Smith EE. Neuroimaging studies of working memory: a meta-analysis. Cogn Affect Behav Neurosci. 2003;3(4):255–74.

288. Ranganath C, DeGutis J, D'Esposito M. Category-specific modulation of inferior temporal activity during working memory encoding and maintenance. Brain Res Cogn Brain Res. 2004;20(1):37–45.

289. Gazzaley A, Cooney JW, McEvoy K, Knight RT, D'Esposito M. Top-down enhancement and suppression of the magnitude and speed of neural activity. J Cogn Neurosci. 2005;17(3):507–17.

290. D'Esposito M, Aguirre GK, Zarahn D, Ballard RK, Shin JL. Functional MRI studies of spatial and nonspatial working memory. Cogn Brain Res. 1998; 7:1–13.

291. Smith EE, Jonides J. Storage and executive processes in the frontal lobes. Science. 1999;283(5408): 1657–61.

292. Levy R, Goldman-Rakic PS. Segregation of working memory functions within the dorsolateral prefrontal cortex. Exp Brain Res. 2000;133(1):23–32.

293. Sala JB, Rama P, Courtney SM. Functional topography of a distributed neural system for spatial and nonspatial information maintenance in working memory. Neuropsychologia. 2003;41:341–56.

294. D'Esposito M, Postle BR, Jonides J, Smith EE. The neural substrate and temporal dynamics of interference effects in working memory as revealed by event-related functional MRI. Proc Natl Acad Sci USA. 1999;96(13):7514–9.

295. Anders TR, Fozard JL, Lillyquist TD. Effects of age upon retrieval from short-term memory. Dev Psychol. 1972;6:214–7.

296. VanderLinden M, Bredart S, Beerten A. Age-related differences in updating working memory. Br J Psychol Eng. 1994;85(Pt 1):145–52.

297. Grady CL. Brain imaging and age-related changes in cognition. Exp Gerontol. 1998;33(7–8):661–73.

298. Mattay VS, Fera F, Tessitore A, et al. Neurophysiological correlates of age-related changes in working memory capacity. Neurosci Lett. 2006;392(1–2):32–7.

299. Mitchell KJ, Johnson MK, Raye CL, D'Esposito M. fMRI evidence of age-related hippocampal dysfunction in feature binding in working memory. Cogn Brain Res. 2000;10(1–2):197–206.

300. Park DC, Welsh RC, Marshuetz C, et al. Working memory for complex scenes: age differences in frontal and hippocampal activations. J Cogn Neurosci. 2003;15(8):1122–34.

301. Grady CL, Yu H, Alain C. Age-related differences in brain activity underlying working memory for spatial and nonspatial auditory information. Cereb Cortex. 2008;18(1):189–99.

302. Baddeley AD, Baddeley HA, Bucks RS, Wilcock GK. Attentional control in Alzheimer's disease. Brain. 2001;124:1492–508.

303. Lim HK, Juh R, Pae CU, et al. Altered verbal working memory process in patients with Alzheimer's disease: an fMRI investigation. Neuropsychobiology. 2008;57(4):181–7.

304. Peters JC, Goebel R, Roelfsema PR. Remembered but unused: the accessory items in working memory that do not guide attention. J Cogn Neurosci. 2009;21(6):1081–91.

305. Yetkin FZ, Rosenberg RN, Weiner MF, Purdy PD, Cullum CM. FMRI of working memory in patients with mild cognitive impairment and probable Alzheimer's disease. Eur Radiol. 2006;16(1): 193–206.

306. Bokde AL, Karmann M, Born C, et al. Altered brain activation during a verbal working memory task in subjects with amnestic mild cognitive impairment. J Alzheimers Dis. 2010;21(1):103–118.

307. Saykin AJ, Wishart HA, Rabin LA, et al. Cholinergic enhancement of frontal lobe activity in mild cognitive impairment. Brain. 2004;127(Pt 7):1574–83.

308. Rombouts SA, van Swieten JC, Pijnenburg YA, Goekoop R, Barkhof F, Scheltens P. Loss of frontal fMRI activation in early frontotemporal dementia compared to early AD. Neurology. 2003;60(12): 1904–8.

309. Berlingeri M, Bottini G, Basilico S, et al. Anatomy of the episodic buffer: a voxel-based morphometry study in patients with dementia. Behav Neurol. 2008;19(1–2):29–34.

310. Luck D, Danion JM, Marrer C, Pham BT, Gounot D, Foucher J. The right parahippocampal gyrus contributes to the formation and maintenance of bound information in working memory. Brain Cogn. 2010;72(2):255–63.

311. Hampson M, Driesen NR, Skudlarski P, Gore JC, Constable RT. Brain connectivity related to working memory performance. J Neurosci. 2006;26(51): 13338–43.

312. Protzner AB, Cortese F, Alain C, McIntosh AR. The temporal interaction of modality specific and process specific neural networks supporting simple working memory tasks. Neuropsychologia. 2009;47(8–9): 1954–63.

313. Rissman J, Gazzaley A, D'Esposito M. Dynamic adjustments in prefrontal, hippocampal, and inferior temporal interactions with increasing visual working memory load. Cereb Cortex. 2008;18(7):1618–29.

314. Anticevic A, Repovs G, Shulman GL, Barch DM. When less is more: TPJ and default network deactivation during encoding predicts working memory performance. Neuroimage. 2010;49(3):2638–48.

315. Esposito F, Aragri A, Latorre V, et al. Does the default-mode functional connectivity of the brain

correlate with working-memory performances? Arch Ital Biol. 2009;147(1–2):11–20.
316. Grady CL, Protzner AB, Kovacevic N, et al. A multivariate analysis of age-related differences in default mode and task-positive networks across multiple cognitive domains. Cereb Cortex. 2010;20(6):1432–47.
317. Li Z, Moore AB, Tyner C, Hu X. Asymmetric connectivity reduction and its relationship to "HAROLD" in aging brain. Brain Res. 2009;1295:149–58.
318. Sambataro F, Murty VP, Callicott JH, et al. Age-related alterations in default mode network: impact on working memory performance. Neurobiol Aging. 2010;31(5):839–52.
319. Saunders NL, Summers MJ. Attention and working memory deficits in mild cognitive impairment. J Clin Exp Neuropsychol. 2010;32(4):350–7.
320. Filbey FM, Slack KJ, Sunderland TP, Cohen RM. Functional magnetic resonance imaging and magnetoencephalography differences associated with APOEepsilon4 in young healthy adults. Neuroreport. 2006;17(15):1585–90.
321. Wishart HA, Saykin AJ, Rabin LA, et al. Increased brain activation during working memory in cognitively intact adults with the APOE epsilon4 allele. Am J Psychiatry. 2006;163(9):1603–10.
322. Craig MC, Brammer M, Maki PM, et al. The interactive effect of acute ovarian suppression and the cholinergic system on visuospatial working memory in young women. Psychoneuroendocrinology. 2010;35(7):987–1000.
323. Dumas JA, Saykin AJ, McDonald BC, McAllister TW, Hynes ML, Newhouse PA. Nicotinic versus muscarinic blockade alters verbal working memory-related brain activity in older women. Am J Geriatr Psychiatry. 2008;16(4):272–82.
324. Goekoop R, Rombouts SA, Jonker C, et al. Challenging the cholinergic system in mild cognitive impairment: a pharmacological fMRI study. Neuroimage. 2004;23(4):1450–9.
325. D'Esposito M, Deouell LY, Gazzaley A. Alterations in the BOLD fMRI signal with ageing and disease: a challenge for neuroimaging. Nat Rev Neurosci. 2003;4(11):863–72.
326. Tekes A, Mohamed MA, Browner NM, Calhoun VD, Yousem DM. Effect of age on visuomotor functional MR imaging. Acad Radiol. 2005;12(6):739–45.
327. D'Esposito M, Zarahn E, Aguirre GK, Rympa B. The effect of normal aging on the coupling of neural activity to the BOLD hemodynamic response. Neuroimage. 1999;10:6–14.
328. Huettel SA, Singerman JD, McCarthy G. The effects of aging upon the hemodynamic response measured by functional MRI. Neuroimage. 2001;13(1):161–75.
329. Taoka T, Iwasaki S, Uchida H, et al. Age correlation of the time lag in signal change on EPI-fMRI. J Comput Assist Tomogr. 1998;22(4):514–7.
330. Mehagnoul-Schipper DJ, van der Kallen BF, Colier WN, et al. Simultaneous measurements of cerebral oxygenation changes during brain activation by near-infrared spectroscopy and functional magnetic resonance imaging in healthy young and elderly subjects. Hum Brain Mapp. 2002;16(1):14–23.
331. Ross MH, Yurgelun-Todd DA, Renshaw PF, et al. Age-related reduction in functional MRI response to photic stimulation. Neurology. 1997;48(1):173–6.
332. Ward NS, Frackowiak RS. Age-related changes in the neural correlates of motor performance. Brain. 2003;126(Pt 4):873–88.
333. Buckner RL, Snyder AZ, Sanders AL, Raichle ME, Morris JC. Functional brain imaging of young, nondemented, and demented older adults. J Cogn Neurosci. 2000;12 Suppl 2:24–34.
334. Price CJ, Friston KJ. Cognitive conjunction: a new approach to brain activation experiments. Neuroimage. 1997;5(4 Pt 1):261–70.
335. Price CJ, Moore CJ, Friston KJ. Subtractions, conjunctions, and interactions in experimental design of activation studies. Hum Brain Mapp. 1997;5(4):264–72.
336. McClearn GE, Johansson B, Berg S, et al. Substantial genetic influence on cognitive abilities in twins 80 or more years old. Science. 1997;276(5318):1560–3.
337. Rasch B, Papassotiropoulos A, de Quervain DF. Imaging genetics of cognitive functions: focus on episodic memory. Neuroimage. 2010;53(3):870–7.
338. Egan MF, Kojima M, Callicott JH, et al. The BDNF val66met polymorphism affects activity-dependent secretion of BDNF and human memory and hippocampal function. Cell. 2003;112(2):257–69.
339. Hariri AR, Goldberg TE, Mattay VS, et al. Brain-derived neurotrophic factor val66met polymorphism affects human memory-related hippocampal activity and predicts memory performance. J Neurosci. 2003;23(17):6690–4.
340. Hashimoto R, Moriguchi Y, Yamashita F, et al. Dose-dependent effect of the Val66Met polymorphism of the brain-derived neurotrophic factor gene on memory-related hippocampal activity. Neurosci Res. 2008;61(4):360–7.
341. Sambataro F, Murty VP, Lemaitre HS, et al. BDNF modulates normal human hippocampal ageing [corrected]. Mol Psychiatry. 2010;15(2):116–8.
342. Lachman HM, Morrow B, Shprintzen R, et al. Association of codon 108/158 catechol-O-methyltransferase gene polymorphism with the psychiatric manifestations of velo-cardio-facial syndrome. Am J Med Genet. 1996;67(5):468–72.
343. Bertolino A, Blasi G, Latorre V, et al. Additive effects of genetic variation in dopamine regulating genes on working memory cortical activity in human brain. J Neurosci. 2006;26(15):3918–22.
344. Bertolino A, Rubino V, Sambataro F, et al. Prefrontal-hippocampal coupling during memory processing is modulated by COMT val158met genotype. Biol Psychiatry. 2006;60(11):1250–8.
345. de Frias CM, Annerbrink K, Westberg L, Eriksson E, Adolfsson R, Nilsson LG. COMT gene polymorphism is associated with declarative memory in

adulthood and old age. Behav Genet. 2004; 34(5):533–9.
346. Reuter M, Montag C, Peters K, Kocher A, Kiefer M. The modulatory influence of the functional COMT Val158Met polymorphism on lexical decisions and semantic priming. Front Hum Neurosci. 2009;3:20.
347. Sambataro F, Reed JD, Murty VP, et al. Catechol-O-methyltransferase valine(158)methionine polymorphism modulates brain networks underlying working memory across adulthood. Biol Psychiatry. 2009;66(6):540–8.
348. Schott BH, Seidenbecher CI, Fenker DB, et al. The dopaminergic midbrain participates in human episodic memory formation: evidence from genetic imaging. J Neurosci. 2006;26(5):1407–17.
349. Huentelman MJ, Papassotiropoulos A, Craig DW, et al. Calmodulin-binding transcription activator 1 (CAMTA1) alleles predispose human episodic memory performance. Hum Mol Genet. 2007;16(12): 1469–77.
350. Buchmann A, Mondadori CR, Hanggi J, et al. Prion protein M129V polymorphism affects retrieval-related brain activity. Neuropsychologia. 2008;46(9):2389–402.
351. Papassotiropoulos A, Stephan DA, Huentelman MJ, et al. Common Kibra alleles are associated with human memory performance. Science. 2006; 314(5798):475–8.
352. Thimm M, Krug A, Markov V, et al. The impact of dystrobrevin-binding protein 1 (DTNBP1) on neural correlates of episodic memory encoding and retrieval. Hum Brain Mapp. 2010;31(2):203–9.
353. Owen MJ, Williams NM, O'Donovan MC. Dysbindin-1 and schizophrenia: from genetics to neuropathology. J Clin Invest. 2004;113(9):1255–7.
354. Krug A, Markov V, Krach S, et al. The effect of Neuregulin 1 on neural correlates of episodic memory encoding. Neuroimage. 2010;53(3):985–91.
355. Stefansson H, Sigurdsson E, Steinthorsdottir V, et al. Neuregulin 1 and susceptibility to schizophrenia. Am J Hum Genet. 2002;71(4):877–92.
356. Kim J, Basak JM, Holtzman DM. The role of apolipoprotein E in Alzheimer's disease. Neuron. 2009; 63(3):287–303.
357. Saykin AJ, Shen L, Foroud TM, et al. Alzheimer's Disease Neuroimaging Initiative biomarkers as quantitative phenotypes: Genetics core aims, progress, and plans. Alzheimers Dement. 2010;6(3): 265–73.
358. Stein JL, Hua X, Morra JH, et al. Genome-wide analysis reveals novel genes influencing temporal lobe structure with relevance to neurodegeneration in Alzheimer's disease. Neuroimage. 2010;51(2): 542–54.
359. Stein JL, Hua X, Lee S, et al. Voxelwise genome-wide association study (vGWAS). Neuroimage. 2010;53(3):1160–74.
360. Shen L, Kim S, Risacher SL, et al. Whole genome association study of brain-wide imaging phenotypes for identifying quantitative trait loci in MCI and AD: A study of the ADNI cohort. Neuroimage. 2010;53(3):1051–63.
361. Potkin SG, Guffanti G, Lakatos A, et al. Hippocampal atrophy as a quantitative trait in a genome-wide association study identifying novel susceptibility genes for Alzheimer's disease. PLoS ONE. 2009; 4(8):e6501.
362. Hedden T, Van Dijk KR, Becker JA, et al. Disruption of functional connectivity in clinically normal older adults harboring amyloid burden. J Neurosci. 2009;29(40):12686–94.
363. Restom K, Bangen KJ, Bondi MW, Perthen JE, Liu TT. Cerebral blood flow and BOLD responses to a memory encoding task: a comparison between healthy young and elderly adults. Neuroimage. 2007;37(2):430–9.
364. Sheline YI, Raichle ME, Snyder AZ, et al. Amyloid plaques disrupt resting state default mode network connectivity in cognitively normal elderly. Biol Psychiatry. 2010;67(6):584–7.
365. Sperling RA, Laviolette PS, O'Keefe K, et al. Amyloid deposition is associated with impaired default network function in older persons without dementia. Neuron. 2009;63(2):178–88.
366. Zhang K, Johnson B, Pennell D, Ray W, Sebastianelli W, Slobounov S. Are functional deficits in concussed individuals consistent with white matter structural alterations: combined fMRI & DTI study. Exp Brain Res. 2010;204(1):57–70.
367. Buckner RL, Snyder AZ, Shannon BJ, et al. Molecular, structural, and functional characterization of Alzheimer's disease: evidence for a relationship between default activity, amyloid, and memory. J Neurosci. 2005;25(34):7709–17.
368. Hoffmann MB, Stadler J, Kanowski M, Speck O. Retinotopic mapping of the human visual cortex at a magnetic field strength of 7T. Clin Neurophysiol. 2009;120(1):108–16.
369. Sanchez-Panchuelo RM, Francis S, Bowtell R, Schluppeck D. Mapping human somatosensory cortex in individual subjects with 7T functional MRI. J Neurophysiol. 2010;103(5):2544–56.
370. Bondi MW. Genetic and brain imaging contributions to neuropsychological functioning in preclinical dementia. J Int Neuropsychol Soc. 2002;8:915–7.
371. Shoghi-Jadid K, Small GW, Agdeppa ED, et al. Localization of neurofibrillary tangles and beta-amyloid plaques in the brains of living patients with Alzheimer disease. Am J Geriatr Psychiatry. 2002;10(1):24–35.
372. Klunk WE, Lopresti BJ, Ikonomovic MD, et al. Binding of the positron emission tomography tracer Pittsburgh compound-B reflects the amount of amyloid-beta in Alzheimer's disease brain but not in transgenic mouse brain. J Neurosci. 2005;25(46): 10598–606.
373. Klunk WE, Engler H, Nordberg A, et al. Imaging brain amyloid in Alzheimer's disease with Pittsburgh Compound-B. Ann Neurol. 2004;55(3):306–19.

374. Burggren AC, Bookheimer SY. Structural and functional neuroimaging in Alzheimer's disease: an update. Curr Top Med Chem. 2002;2(4):385–93.
375. Citron M. Alzheimer's disease: strategies for disease modification. Nat Rev Drug Discov. 2010;9(5):387–98.
376. Grady CL. Cognitive neuroscience of aging. Ann NY Acad Sci. 2008;1124:127–44.
377. Hedden T, Gabrieli JD. Healthy and pathological processes in adult development: new evidence from neuroimaging of the aging brain. Curr Opin Neurol. 2005;18(6):740–7.
378. Langley LK, Madden DJ. Functional neuroimaging of memory: implications for cognitive aging. Microsc Res Tech. 2000;51(1):75–84.
379. Dickerson BC, Sperling RA. Functional abnormalities of the medial temporal lobe memory system in mild cognitive impairment and Alzheimer's disease: insights from functional MRI studies. Neuropsychologia. 2008;46(6):1624–35.
380. Dickerson BC, Sperling RA. Large-scale functional brain network abnormalities in Alzheimer's disease: insights from functional neuroimaging. Behav Neurol. 2009;21(1):63–75.
381. Drzezga A. Concept of functional imaging of memory decline in Alzheimer's disease. Methods. 2008;44(4):304–14.
382. Han SD, Bangen KJ, Bondi MW. Functional magnetic resonance imaging of compensatory neural recruitment in aging and risk for Alzheimer's disease: review and recommendations. Dement Geriatr Cogn Disord. 2009;27(1):1–10.
383. Ries ML, Carlsson CM, Rowley HA, et al. Magnetic resonance imaging characterization of brain structure and function in mild cognitive impairment: a review. J Am Geriatr Soc. 2008;56(5):920–34.
384. Sperling RA, Dickerson BC, Pihlajamaki M, et al. Functional alterations in memory networks in early Alzheimer's disease. Neuromolecular Med. 2010;12(1):27–43.
385. Wierenga CE, Bondi MW. Use of functional magnetic resonance imaging in the early identification of Alzheimer's disease. Neuropsychol Rev. 2007;17(2):127–43.
386. Cappa SF. Imaging studies of semantic memory. Curr Opin Neurol. 2008;21(6):669–75.
387. Wingfield A, Grossman M. Language and the aging brain: patterns of neural compensation revealed by functional brain imaging. J Neurophysiol. 2006;96(6):2830–9.
388. Dickerson BC. Functional magnetic resonance imaging of cholinergic modulation in mild cognitive impairment. Curr Opin Psychiatry. 2006;19(3):299–306.
389. Greicius M. Resting-state functional connectivity in neuropsychiatric disorders. Curr Opin Neurol. 2008;21(4):424–30.
390. Rypma B, D'Esposito M. Isolating the neural mechanisms of age-related changes in human working memory. Nat Neurosci. 2000;3(5):509–15.

fMRI Wada Test: Prospects for Presurgical Mapping of Language and Memory

11

Brenna C. McDonald, Jacob Kean, and Andrew J. Saykin

Introduction

Since the inception of functional magnetic resonance imaging (fMRI) in the early 1990s, clinicians and researchers have been interested in the potential utility of this technology for replacement of and intracarotid amobarbital test (IAT). The IAT, or Wada test, is an invasive angiographic procedure, with some potential risks, that has long served as the conventional procedure for preoperative lateralization of language and memory. The IAT is used primarily in patients under consideration for neurosurgery to treat epilepsy but also in other neurosurgical populations (e.g., motor cortex tumor, arteriovenous malformation in language association cortex, etc.). With a validated assessment paradigm, there would be significant advantages of fMRI assessment of memory and language functions in place of the IAT. Functional MRI is a repeatable, noninvasive procedure with no significant known health risks for most individuals. It is also very flexible and can be readily modified to assess the clinical questions at issue for a particular patient. Furthermore, cost analysis has demonstrated considerable savings of total direct costs for fMRI over IAT [1].

While some patients (e.g., those with ferromagnetic metal in their bodies or those who are moderately or severely claustrophobic) may be unable or ineligible to undergo fMRI, the number of those who meet these exclusion criteria is no greater than for the IAT. Furthermore, while the IAT can provide information regarding predominant hemispheric lateralization of language functions, and to a lesser degree memory, it cannot provide information regarding the spatial location of brain regions critical for these tasks. By contrast, fMRI, with typical spatial resolution of 2–4 mm, can provide much more precise information regarding localization of brain regions that are active during memory and language tasks.

Both the IAT and fMRI are potentially useful techniques for representing the location of important cognitive functions that are considered as part of surgery planning. The IAT was developed first and has a long history of use, and therefore

B.C. McDonald, PsyD, MBA (✉)
Department of Radiology and Imaging Sciences, Indiana University School of Medicine, 950 West Walnut Street, R2 E124, Indianapolis, IN 46202, USA
e-mail: mcdonalb@iupui.edu

J. Kean, PhD
Department of Physical Medicine and Rehabilitation, Indiana University Center for Neuroimaging, Rehabilitation Hospital of Indiana, Indiana University School of Medicine, 4141 Shore Drive, Indianapolis, IN 46254, USA
e-mail: jakean@indiana.edu

A.J. Saykin, PsyD, ABPP/CN
Center for Neuroimaging, Department of Radiology and Imaging Sciences, Indiana University School of Medicine, 950 West Walnut Street, R2 E124, Indianapolis, IN 46202, USA
e-mail: asaykin@iupui.edu

S.H. Faro and F.B. Mohamed (eds.), *Functional BOLD MRI: Principles and Applications*, DOI 10.1007/978-1-4939-1995-6_11,

became a "gold standard" to which fMRI language and memory localization paradigms have been compared. Many basic aspects of the IAT's validity and reliability have never been systematically investigated, however, due to the nature of the procedure and the lack of alternative techniques available for this purpose. This chapter stresses the contrast between these methods. It is clear, however, that the same standards of measurement should be applied to both tests. For example, it is possible that both techniques adequately measure the lateralization of language. In contrast, both may not adequately assess the location of memory abilities. The focus of much of the research literature and other discussions has been on replacing the IAT with fMRI, which would be a worthy goal if possible, given factors noted throughout this chapter, including the increased time, risk, and cost of the IAT. This focus may, however, at times overlook basic measurement issues that apply to both techniques; in the end, the overarching goal is clearly to obtain the most reliable and valid data possible to meet the stated need of localization of language and memory functions.

The conclusions of several empirical studies and reviews of the literature to date strongly suggest that fMRI paradigms can be successfully used to replace the IAT in terms of language lateralization. Indeed, since the first edition of this volume, clinical practice has shifted in many medical centers [2, 3] with fMRI being used for language localization in cases where memory is not a primary concern (e.g., frontal lobe lesions or seizure foci, resections in the hemisphere nondominant for language), and IAT not being conducted unless fMRI cannot be obtained or results are inconclusive. While the status of appropriately reliable and valid memory assessment paradigms is not as advanced, significant progress has been made in this area as well. Despite the apparent advantages of fMRI in such presurgical assessment, there remain methodological challenges and issues of interpretation that have thus far prevented its widespread use in place of the IAT. This chapter will briefly discuss the background of the IAT and its risks and benefits compared to fMRI. The body of literature examining the capacity of fMRI to lateralize and localize expressive and receptive language functions effectively is reviewed, as well as more recent advances in utilizing fMRI findings to predict postsurgical outcome. These factors are critical in consideration of instances when fMRI may be appropriately used instead of IAT, and also for recognition of cases where complementary data from both procedures is likely to be clinically important.

The IAT: History and Background

As noted by other authors [4, 5], the first use of selective anesthetization to localize human language function was reported by Gardner in 1941 [6]. Gardner utilized intracranial injection of procaine hydrochloride to unilaterally anesthetize frontal brain regions in two left-handed brain tumor patients, to assess lateralization of hemispheric dominance for language prior to resective surgery and prevent surgically induced aphasia. The model for modern IAT procedures, however, is the work of Juhn Wada [7], who established the feasibility of selective hemispheric anesthetization using intracarotid injection of sodium amobarbital.

Wada's original work in the 1940s was designed to attempt to minimize the cognitive side effects of electroconvulsive shock therapy (ECT) by preventing bilateral generalization of ECT-related seizure activity through temporary anesthetization of the language-dominant hemisphere [5]. The utility of this technique for presurgical evaluation of epilepsy quickly became apparent, and Wada pioneered this approach both in Japan and later with his colleagues at the Montreal Neurological Institute. While significant variations can currently be encountered across surgical epilepsy centers in terms of IAT procedures, several standardized methodologies have been published ([4, 5, 8–12], for review see [13]), and the IAT is considered an important component of presurgical evaluation of patients with epilepsy, along with clinical neuropsychological assessment, which is important for providing a context within which to interpret IAT results [14–17]. IAT may also be used much as Gardner originally proposed, to assess the lateralized integrity of cognition prior to resection of nonepileptogenic lesions (e.g., brain tumors, vascular malformations, etc.) located in frontal or temporal cortex presumed to be critical to language and/or memory functions.

The need for lateralization and localization of cognitive functions such as language and memory is self-evident. For patients under consideration for resective surgery to treat medically refractory seizures, particularly in the case of temporal lobe epilepsy (TLE), the seizure focus that is likely to be resected includes brain regions potentially critical to the support of language and memory. It therefore becomes vital to provide as much information as possible regarding the potential deficits that might occur as a result of surgery, should the seizure focus (e.g., a sclerotic hippocampus) also be supporting one or more critical cognitive functions. For patients whose presumed seizure focus lies adjacent to or within language cortex, detailed presurgical localization of eloquent tissue is needed to assess the feasibility of surgery and define the potential resection margin. The IAT is typically used for hemispheric lateralization of language functioning, while intracranial electrocortical stimulation mapping (ESM) can provide more precise mapping of language cortex, either prior to or during epilepsy surgery (and therefore serve as another "gold standard" for comparison with IAT or fMRI results in cases where ESM data is available). An increasing literature is also demonstrating a potential for fMRI to take on a similar role in terms of intraoperative evaluation, and studies have shown promising concordance between ESM and fMRI.

While the left hemisphere is the dominant hemisphere for language in the great majority of healthy right-handed individuals, the neurodevelopmental abnormalities that can be associated with epilepsy make atypical language lateralization (right hemisphere dominance or bilateral participation in language) more likely in epileptic patients [18–26], particularly those with left hemispheric seizure onset [27]. Atypical language dominance has been demonstrated in 20–30% of epilepsy patients [25, 28], and has been linked to handedness, age at seizure onset, type of MRI abnormality, and both higher [29] and lower [21, 30] verbal abilities. For left-handed individuals, the issue of hemispheric language dominance is particularly important, given the increased prevalence of right hemisphere dominance for language in those who are left-handed [31, 32]. Right hemisphere language dominance has been shown to be strongly correlated with handedness in healthy individuals, with one study showing right hemisphere dominance in 4% of strongly right-handed, 15% of ambidextrous, and 27% of left-handed participants [33]. Even in right-handed individuals some studies have shown a higher rate of right hemisphere dominance than previously suspected [34], and many fMRI studies show some degree of bilateral activation in right-handed individuals from normal as well as clinical samples [10, 35–38], though most language-related activation is observed in the dominant hemisphere. Such nondominant hemisphere activation may relate to linguistic task complexity or to nonverbal aspects of language, such as prosody, narrative organization, inference, or language pragmatics [20, 39–45].

Assessment of hemispheric support of memory functioning is particularly important in TLE patients, given the critical role of medial temporal lobe (MTL) structures, including the hippocampus, entorhinal cortex, and amygdala, in encoding of new information. The IAT does not lateralize memory per se, but rather assesses the potential for unilateral hemispheric support of memory encoding, to prevent an iatrogenic postsurgical amnestic syndrome such as that exhibited in the classic case of patient H.M. [46]. In TLE the presence of mesial temporal sclerosis or other hippocampal disease may preclude effective support of memory functions by the region to be resected. Some patients, however, demonstrate memory functioning using the diseased hemisphere on IAT, indicating the potential for acquired postoperative cognitive deficits. This issue becomes an even greater concern in TLE patients with normal MRI scans, who may be more likely to have MTL tissue supporting memory in the presumed epileptogenic region.

Limitations in the use of the IAT include its invasive nature and attendant risk of potential medical complications, such as infarction, carotid artery dissection, potentiation of seizures, and adverse reaction to contrast or anesthetizing agents [47, 48], though surveys have indicated that such IAT morbidity is rare. For high volume epilepsy centers, the typical risk of IAT-related complication is <1% [49]. Certain patient risk factors can also increase the risk of angiography and therefore contraindicate use of the IAT. For example, individuals with significant vascular risk factors or other major medical problems may not be appropriate candidates for such a procedure. Additionally, very young children are also often not considered for IAT, given the cognitive demands and medical risks involved in the test. Other limitations of the IAT include invalidation of studies due to aberrant vasculature (e.g., arteriovenous malformations) or to normal neurodevelopmental vascular variations such as persistent fetal circulation or significant cortical cross-flow. Given the short-acting nature of sodium amobarbital and the other drugs typically used to anesthetize the cerebral hemispheres, the IAT is a very time-sensitive procedure that can be invalidated by individual variation in sensitivity to the anesthetic agent used (e.g., obtundation in some patients versus failure of anesthetization due to the presence of anticonvulsant medications [50]), as well as to related delays and nonstandardized administration of test stimuli. IAT studies can also be nondiagnostic due to failure to adequately lateralize language or memory functioning in a given individual. Finally, though some standardized IAT protocols are available [4, 5, 8–12], comparison of IAT studies across epilepsy surgery centers can be challenging, as methodology and interpretation of the IAT procedure vary considerably from site to site.

Description of a Standardized IAT Protocol

As noted previously, a number of standardized IAT procedures have been developed and disseminated among surgical epilepsy centers, while other facilities may use unique site-specific techniques. In the late 1980s, a coauthor of this chapter (AJS) developed a standardized IAT protocol at Graduate Hospital in Philadelphia [9, 51], which continues to be in use at a number of epilepsy centers in the US. A catheter is positioned under fluoroscopy into the internal carotid artery (ICA). Following cerebral angiography the patient is available for cognitive testing. All patients receive studies ipsilateral and contralateral to the seizure focus on the same day with 30–45 min between injections, unless patient-specific factors (e.g., a persistent trigeminal artery on one side) preclude assessment of either hemisphere.

The procedure is begun on the presumed side of surgery, then repeated on the contralateral side. The neuropsychological protocol [51] was designed for rapid speech and memory assessment. Emphasis is placed on quantitative memory evaluation for verbal and nonverbal material, and for material that can be encoded either verbally or nonverbally (common objects). This provides a continuum of verbal–nonverbal material for encoding. Two forms of equivalent task difficulty were developed by randomization of the original item pool. The standard dosage is 125 mg of sodium amobarbital in 5 cc saline with slow hand injection over 5 s in each ICA, with injections separated by at least 30 min. Occasionally it is necessary to titrate the dosage of sodium amobarbital up or down (usually in 25 mg increments) to achieve the goal of unilateral anesthesia as indicated by hemiparesis or electroencephalogram (EEG) without causing global sedation or obtundation.

Language testing begins immediately after injection until speech normalizes, and includes: (1) automatic speech (counting, recitation of the alphabet); (2) comprehension (following simple commands, Modified Token Test); (3) word and sentence repetition; (4) visual confrontation naming (three objects); and (5) reading (three words). Memory testing commences about 2 min after injection, and overlaps with the language protocol (naming and word reading). During the registration and encoding phase, the patient is shown three common objects (e.g., spoon, glove, cup) one at a time and asked to name and remember them. Each stimulus is exposed for approximately 5–10 s with emphasis placed on ensuring that the patient is attending to the stimuli. Special care must be taken to present the stimuli in the intact visual field. The same procedure is followed for three low-imagery words (e.g., random, enough, prefer) and three abstract designs (after Kimura [52]).

At 10 min after injection, if language and motor functioning have returned to baseline, the free and cued recall phase is begun. Progressively structured recall testing is initiated by asking the patient to recall "everything that you remember from the test." Responses are recorded verbatim. Cued recall is then initiated (e.g., "Did I show you any objects?"). Paper and felt-tip pen are provided for drawings of the abstract designs. During the recognition phase, the patient is shown a series of nine stimuli (separately for objects, words, and designs). Three of the nine are target stimuli and six are distractors, fixing the probability of a chance correct response at 33%. For each item the patient must determine whether he/she has seen the item during the test. Patients are also asked to provide a confidence rating so that signal detection analysis can be applied for determination of sensitivity and bias in responses [53]. Response alternatives are: "Definitely No" (nontarget); "Probably No"; "Probably Yes" (target); "Definitely Yes." Responses are recorded; outcome is total number of targets correct and subscores for each type of material. False-positive responses are considered in the interpretation of the test results. For the designs a second recognition task is administered, in which all nine designs are shown simultaneously, and the patient is asked to "Select the three that you think you might have seen earlier during the test." To assess emotional change during the IAT, behavioral observations are made regarding affective changes following injection. All patients are interviewed by the attending neuropsychologist after the procedure to elicit any subjective reactions. Interpretation of IAT data includes conclusions regarding language laterality based on the comprehensive language assessment. Memory performance is compared for each injection following adjustment for false-positive responses. Any atypical features of the examination (e.g., cortical cross-flow, obtundation) are also noted.

Replacement of the IAT with Functional Neuroimaging

Given the limitations of the IAT, suggestions for alternative technologies for gathering presurgical data regarding brain regions supporting cognitive functions have included event-related potentials [54], transcranial magnetic stimulation [55–57], functional transcranial Doppler ultrasonography [58–63], magnetoencephalography (MEG) [64] in combination with fMRI, and near-infrared spectroscopy [65–67]. Functional MRI and ^{15}O-water or ^{18}F-fluorodeoxyglucose positron emission tomography (PET) [68–74] have been specifically proposed as alternatives to the IAT to localize language and memory cortex more precisely. Disadvantages of PET include invasiveness, lower availability and repeatability than fMRI, and lower spatial resolution. In this chapter we focus on fMRI studies of memory and language functioning as related to the IAT, although we address aspects of other functional imaging methodologies where appropriate.

The IAT demonstrates functional lateralization through unilateral hemispheric suppression of neuronal activity by anesthetization of the anterior and middle cerebral arterial distribution, followed by assessment of the cognitive functions of interest. By contrast, as described elsewhere in this volume, fMRI detects blood oxygen level dependent (BOLD) signal during cognitive processing in an unsedated patient. This BOLD signal serves as an endogenous contrast agent, and as a marker of task-related neuronal activity. As with the IAT, fMRI paradigms designed to assess language and memory functioning vary considerably. Although some language tasks (e.g., verbal fluency paradigms) have been more widely used, specific task and scan parameters are rarely consistent across studies, making direct comparison of fMRI activation patterns difficult. Despite this concern, some broad conclusions regarding the status of fMRI assessment of language and memory can be made.

fMRI Language Paradigms and the IAT

Significant progress has been made in the past 15 years with regard to the development of language-based fMRI paradigms. While replicating IAT language results would require only establishing hemispheric dominance for language, most groups designing fMRI language paradigms to replace the IAT are interested in achieving activation of the broad neural networks subserving various language functions, not only to lateralize language at the hemispheric level, but to localize specific aspects of language functioning to more focal brain regions, particularly in the frontal and temporal lobes. In studies of epilepsy patients and healthy control participants, activation in inferior frontal regions approximating Broca's area has been readily elicited using a number of language paradigms, most commonly naming or word generation tasks. Auditory language paradigms have been shown to activate temporal lobe receptive language cortex (i.e., Wernicke's area). Such tasks often also activate primary auditory cortex bilaterally, and may show additional activation in posterior superior temporal gyrus. As bilateral primary auditory cortex activation is of less utility in assessing hemispheric language dominance, some tasks use auditory control conditions to allow for subtraction of primary auditory cortex activation. Such strategies may, however, also remove from analysis activation of brain regions important in language processing, potentially resulting in a reduction of the laterality asymmetry (commonly referred to as asymmetry indices [AIs] or laterality indices [LIs]; this abbreviation will be used here across studies for consistency, though terminology used in source citations varies) many studies use as a measure of language dominance, and thus making dominance appear less marked. Reading-based tasks offer an alternative for localization of middle and superior temporal lobe receptive language areas involved in reading decoding and comprehension, as well as frontal regions involved in grammatical language processing or verbal working memory. Semantic retrieval aspects of these tasks are thought to engage anterior language regions. However, such tasks may not be appropriate in populations with limited reading skills (e.g., young children or cognitively impaired individuals), and require the availability of additional equipment to display visual stimuli.

Though different tasks have been used to elicit language-related activation – including word generation, naming, and reading paradigms – most studies have found near-perfect agreement between lateralization based on fMRI activation patterns and that based on IAT. In the few studies where discrepancies between fMRI and IAT have been noted, these more typically reflect a nondiagnostic study in one modality or bilateral language participation in one study but not in the other, rather than frank disagreement regarding hemispheric language dominance.

Early Studies

Desmond and colleagues [75] were the first to publish findings in epilepsy patients in whom language dominance was studied with both IAT and fMRI. In their series of seven patients, 100% concordance was observed between the two methods with regard to language lateralization. In addition, they provided data on intrahemispheric localization, namely activation of frontal lobe language regions (Brodmann's areas 45, 46, and 47), when patients were asked to make semantic as compared to perceptual judgments about visually presented words. While seminal, the use of a reading task precluded more general conclusions about localization of speech and aural comprehension, also critical aspects of language for surgical planning. In an early study addressing the issue of language comprehension, Binder and colleagues [10] likewise found complete agreement between IAT and fMRI language lateralization in a series of 22 consecutive epilepsy surgery patients, as well as high concordance (r = 0.96) between IAT and fMRI LIs. These authors also demonstrated intrahemispheric activation of lateral frontal and heteromodal temporoparietooccipital cortex during a single-word semantic decision-making task, using a baseline tone discrimination task to control for activation of auditory and attentional systems. This task design permitted elegant localization of areas involved in speech comprehension, but, it could be argued, prevented examination of language as a multidimensional ability intimately related to both hearing and attention. In a later study, Benbadis et al. [76] reanalyzed fMRI and IAT data from the Binder et al. [10] sample to determine whether IAT speech arrest alone constitutes sufficient criteria for determination of language dominance, in comparison to the comprehensive language evaluation cited in Binder et al. [10] They found that an LI calculated solely based on speech arrest did not significantly correlate with either the comprehensive IAT LI or with fMRI language lateralization. Categorical classification of language dominance as right, left, or bilateral was likewise discordant in several cases when using the speech arrest index, as compared to the complete agreement between IAT and fMRI reported by Binder et al. [10] when IAT lateralization was based on comprehensive speech assessment. Benbadis et al. [76] therefore concluded that IAT speech arrest alone is not a valid indicator of language lateralization, highlighting the importance of the consideration of assessment techniques in the evaluation of IAT and fMRI concordance, as an inappropriate strategy (e.g., a nonspecific measure such as speech arrest), in either modality may lead to spurious conclusions regarding concordance (or lateralization).

In the first extension of this type of research to pediatric populations, Hertz-Pannier et al. [38] used fMRI to assess language dominance in 11 children and adolescents with complex partial seizures using word generation tasks. In seven cases where IAT, ESM, or surgical outcome results were available for comparison, findings regarding language dominance were concordant with fMRI LIs. All patients demonstrated highest activation in the vicinity of Broca's area (inferior frontal gyrus), as well as in the middle and superior frontal gyri, and cingulate gyrus activation was observed in all but two patients. These authors noted that second studies were successful in four children whose initial studies were uninterpretable due to noncompliance or motion artifact. Studies were also repeated in two other children to assess reproducibility of the fMRI findings; language lateralization and spatial extent of activation were comparable across studies. These findings offered promising preliminary evidence that fMRI is a feasible technique for assessing language dominance in pediatric epilepsy surgery candidates without the potential risks of IAT or ESM. Another potential advantage of fMRI in studying language functions in young patients is the potential to observe intrahemispheric reorganization in cases of early brain injury and recovery, which could not be visualized with the IAT.

Regional Activation and Assessment of Laterality

Since these early studies a number of groups have published findings demonstrating high concordance between fMRI and IAT language lateralization or ESM [11, 27, 64, 77–92], even in individuals with atypical language representation. Such studies generally find 90–100% agreement between fMRI and IAT language lateralization techniques, though lower rates have occasionally been reported [18, 20, 93–96] (see Table 11.1 for summary of studies comparing language lateralization using fMRI and IAT).

In the largest sample reported to date, 91% concordance between IAT and fMRI language lateralization was found in 94 epilepsy patients [28]. In general, activation of frontal lobe language regions (i.e., Broca's area) tends to be more reliably demonstrated and more consistently lateralizing than activation of temporal language areas (i.e., Wernicke's area) and tends to correlate best with IAT language lateralization [84, 85]. This is particularly true for individuals with strongly lateralized language functioning (to either hemisphere) and is likely in part due to the nature of commonly used fMRI language probes (i.e., word generation), which rely heavily on expressive language functions. For individuals with significant bilateral language representation, however, LIs based primarily on the frontal regions activated by word generation tasks have

Table 11.1 Summary of concordance between IAT and fMRI language lateralization results and regions of fMRI activation

Authors	Sample (age range, years)[a]	IAT language tasks	fMRI language tasks	IAT/fMRI concordance	fMRI language regions activated
Desmond et al. 1995 [75]	*n* = 7 (20–53)	Presence of speech arrest, paraphasic errors, and errors in naming, repetition, reading, and aural comprehension	Visually presented words 1. Semantic encoding: Abstract vs. Concrete 2. Perceptual encoding: Upper vs. Lower case	100%	Frontal
Binder et al. 1996 [10]	*n* = 22 (17–64)	Numerical rating of speech arrest, ability to follow commands, paraphasic errors, naming, repetition, reading, and comprehension	Aurally presented noun categorization task	100%	Frontal, temporal, temporo-parieto-occipital junction
Bahn et al. 1997 [81]	*n* = 7 (mean = 29)	Assessment of naming, reading, and recall	Covert word generation to a target letter and to rhyme with a target word (aural stimuli)	100%	Frontal, temporal
Hertz-Pannier et al. 1997 [38]	*n* = 6 (10–18)	Not reported	Covert and overt word generation to a target letter and to a target semantic category (aural stimuli)	100%	Frontal, temporal
Worthington et al. 1997 [96]	*n* = 12 (12–56)	Assessment of naming, repetition, reading, and comprehension	Covert word generation to a target letter	42%[b]	Not reported
Benbadis et al. 1998 [76] (subset of patients from Binder et al. 1996 [10])	*n* = 21 (17–64)	Numerical rating of speech arrest, ability to follow commands, paraphasic errors, naming, repetition, reading, and comprehension	Aurally presented noun categorization task	71–100%[c]	Frontal, temporal, temporo-parieto-occipital junction
Yetkin et al. 1998 [11]	*n* = 13 (22–43)	Numerical rating of speech arrest, ability to follow commands, paraphasic errors, naming, repetition, reading, and comprehension	Covert word generation to a target letter (aural stimuli)	100%	Frontal
Benson et al. 1999 [82]	*n* = 12 (19–70)	Assessment of speech arrest, paraphasic errors, naming, comprehension, and reading	Visually presented verb generation task	92%[d]	Not reported[e]
Lehéricy et al. 2000 [89]	*n* = 10 (18–55)	Assessment of serial speech, naming, reading, spelling, and ability to follow commands	Covert word generation to semantic category, covert sentence repetition, and story listening (all aural stimuli)	100%[f]	Frontal, temporal
Brockway et al. 2000 [83]	*n* = 11 (mean = 34.1)	Language comprehension and naming	Inferential discourse and covert naming in response to an aurally presented definition	100%	Frontal, temporal, temporo-parieto-occipital junction
Hirsch et al. 2000 [87]	*n* = 13 (11–79)	Not reported	Picture naming by internal (silent) speech and listening to recordings of spoken names	100%	Frontal
Baciu et al. 2001 [79]	*n* = 10 (20–48)	Presence/absence of speech arrest followed by transient aphasia	Visually presented rhyming/visual detection task	80–100%[g]	Frontal, temporal
Carpentier et al. 2001 [18]	*n* = 10 (24–51)	Assessment of speech arrest, paraphasic errors, comprehension, repetition, and naming	Identification of syntactic and semantic errors in sentences (aural and visual stimuli)	80–90%[h]	Frontal, temporal
Gao et al. 2001 [86]	*n* = 4 (25–44)	Not reported	Reciting poems	100%	Temporal

Gaillard et al. 2002 [20]	n = 20 (8–56)	Not reported	Covert naming in response to reading	75%[i]	Frontal, temporal
Rutten et al. 2002 [95]	n = 18 (20–54)	Assessment of naming, expressive language, and paraphasic errors	Visually presented verb generation, verbal fluency, picture naming, and sentence comprehension	83%[j]	Frontal, temporoparietal
Sabbah et al. 2003 [27]	n = 20 (9–48)	Assessment of speech arrest, oral and written comprehension, naming, repetition, and reading	Phonemic and semantic fluency	95%	Frontal, temporal
Woermann et al. 2003 [28]	n = 94 (mean ≈ 31)[k]	Not reported	Verbal fluency	91%	Frontolateral, temporoposterior, parietal, frontomesial
Gaillard et al. 2004 [94]	n = 25 (11–55)	Auditory comprehension, counting, spelling, naming, repetition, and reading	Semantic and phonemic fluency, covert one-word responses, reading stories, and listening to stories	84%	Frontal, temporal
Kamada et al. 2007 [64]	n = 29 (mean = 34.6)	Auditory comprehension, counting, naming, and reading	Covert verb generation to aurally presented noun	90%[l]	Frontal, temporal
Kamada et al. 2007 [88]	n = 22 (18–71)	Not reported	Covert verb generation to aurally presented noun	100%	Frontal
Kesavadas et al. 2007 [2]	n = 5 (12–15)	Not reported	Covert verbal fluency tasks and verb generation tasks	80%	Reported as "eloquent cortex," but not further specified

[a]Excluding healthy control subjects and epilepsy patients who did not receive IAT, when information was reported for this subpopulation
[b]Five patients demonstrated identical language laterality on IAT and fMRI. Three patients had disagreement between IAT and fMRI, one patient had bilateral IAT but lateralized fMRI, and three patients had a nondiagnostic fMRI study
[c]71% agreement was found between fMRI lateralization and IAT lateralization based solely on speech arrest; 100% concordance was found when IAT lateralization incorporated comprehensive language assessment
[d]Eleven patients demonstrated identical language laterality on IAT and fMRI. One patient had equivocal findings on IAT and lateralized fMRI
[e]While images are presented highlighting activation patterns in selected subjects, discussion of specific language regions activated is not included
[f]Nine patients demonstrated left hemisphere dominance on both IAT and fMRI language measures, though strength of lateralization varied. One patient showed bilateral IAT, with strong right hemisphere fMRI lateralization of frontal language regions, but weak left lateralization of temporal areas
[g]fMRI and IAT were entirely consistent in eight patients with conclusive IAT studies. Two patients had inconclusive IAT studies. In one of these, VEEG findings confirmed fMRI language lateralization. In the other, no other data was conclusive with regard to language lateralization
[h]IAT and fMRI findings were concordant in eight patients when the whole brain was considered in fMRI analysis, and in nine patients when Brodmann's area 41/42 was excluded from analysis
[i]Five patients demonstrated concordant laterality on IAT and fMRI. One patient had a nondiagnostic IAT study, and one had a nondiagnostic fMRI study. One patient with left hemisphere language dominance on IAT showed bilateral language representation on fMRI and two patients with bilateral language functioning on IAT showed left hemisphere dominance on fMRI. In no case was there frank disagreement between IAT and fMRI
[j]Of the three patients in whom fMRI and IAT were discordant, one was left dominant on fMRI but mixed dominant on IAT, one was mixed dominant on fMRI but left dominant on IAT, and one was right dominant on fMRI but left dominant on IAT
[k]Mean ages were reported separately for left (mean = 32.5) and right (mean = 29.9) language lateralization
[l]Concordance was reported for all patients, who had a variety of lesions, but not separately for the subgroup (n = 29) of patients with epilepsy

been less consistent with IAT results (i.e., one modality suggesting more bilateral language representation, while the other suggests unilateral language dominance). For TLE in particular, the advantages of more reliable elicitation of temporal lobe language-related activation are readily evident, given the surgical target. To elicit more posterior language-related activation and address the concern regarding accurately identifying individuals with bilateral language representation, a few groups have utilized multiple fMRI language paradigms, with analytic approaches to LI creation incorporating data across tasks.

For example, Rutten et al. [95] used four language tasks (verb generation, verbal fluency, picture naming, and sentence comprehension) to attempt reliable localization of language regions in 18 TLE patients, with a focus on distinguishing between patients with unilateral and bilateral language dominance. Through the use of a combined task analysis (CTA) technique previously validated in healthy control subjects [97], they found more robust and reliable results than with any single task, reporting lateralization concordance in 10 of 11 patients with left-dominant language by IAT, 3 of 4 with bilateral IAT dominance, and 2 of 3 right-dominant by IAT. Activation in posterior (temporoparietal) language regions was observed in all patients. Verb generation was the most useful single task in terms of concordance with the IAT, consistent with the overall finding in the literature to date (i.e., that verbal fluency tasks are particularly robust for this purpose), though it was not found to be as effective in patients with bilateral hemispheric participation in language.

Of note, Rutten et al. [95] used a fixed, user-independent approach to statistical analysis, which did not allow for individual variability in the threshold set for significant activation, a method that has both strengths and limitations for clinical practice. This method provides an objective strategy for analyzing such data in clinical decision-making, and use of a less stringent threshold maximizes power to detect task-related activation. As the authors note, however, the threshold chosen can have a marked effect on the LI achieved. More stringent thresholds at times produce more strongly lateralized results, particularly in individuals who demonstrate relatively higher degrees of brain activation during fMRI tasks, while less stringent thresholds can sometimes allow more effective detection of lateralization in individuals with lesser magnitude of activation. In a validation study of a different approach for threshold-independent LI calculation, Suarez et al. [91] found that their threshold-independent method produced unambiguous lateralization in all 14 epilepsy patients evaluated, and greatly reduced disagreement with "gold standard" measures (IAT, ESM, and/or clinical outcome), compared to more traditional threshold-dependent means of calculating LIs.

Other groups have likewise used multiple fMRI tasks to localize language-critical brain regions, but have utilized patient- and task-specific thresholds to maximize utility for surgical planning purposes [94, 98]. Gaillard et al. [20] assessed hemispheric language dominance in children and adults with partial epilepsy of presumed temporal or frontotemporal origin using a covert naming in response to reading fMRI paradigm, in which individuals silently named an object after reading a sentence describing the object. This task activated both frontal and temporal language regions in the majority of cases. As discussed previously, as most prior work reliably demonstrated activation in frontal but not posterior language regions (unless multiple language tasks were used), consistent activation of broader language networks with a single task would be a clinical advantage. However, inclusion of multiple language tasks in the fMRI protocol provides redundancy that can be highly beneficial in cases where data from one task proves unusable for any reason (e.g., subject motion, occurrence of a seizure, etc.) or where there is reason to suspect a participant may be better able to complete some types of tasks than others. The approach of including multiple tasks to assess a particular cognitive function can therefore also be seen to have clinical advantages [92].

As noted previously, task modality can also affect language lateralization results, again highlighting the importance of consideration of task-related factors. Carpentier et al. [18] utilized visual and aural language comprehension fMRI tasks to lateralize language functioning in ten epilepsy surgery candidates with left hemisphere seizure foci in or near presumed language cortex and ten healthy controls. While fMRI activation was observed in a wide neural network of brain regions involved in language comprehension, Broca's area was the most consistently activated region, demonstrating activation in all subjects for both tasks, with controls demonstrating more robust LIs than epilepsy patients. Functional MRI language lateralization scores demonstrated greater agreement with IAT and neuropsychological testing for the visual versus the auditory task. Strongest agreement was found using an fMRI LI including only Brodmann's areas 44/45 and 22, and the conjunction analysis of both fMRI tasks (see Table 11.2 for summary of studies comparing IAT and fMRI language LIs).

Discordance Between fMRI and IAT

Overall, fMRI paradigms designed to lateralize and localize language functions have typically been successful in demonstrating activation patterns that are concordant with IAT results. Such agreement has been found for individuals with both typical and atypical language dominance, as noted previously (though with some caveats) and illustrated by Biega et al. [99] in a case study of an individual with right TLE who showed bilateral independent Broca's area representation on both fMRI and IAT. In studies with lower concordance rates, typically discrepancies involve technically inadequate or nondiagnostic IAT or fMRI studies, or bilateral representation on one study and unilateral hemispheric dominance on the other. Surgery or ESM have at times confirmed the functional imaging findings [71, 73, 100] in the small percentage of studies that have shown only partial agreement or conflicting language lateralization findings from IAT and fMRI (or PET). In very few cases has frank disagreement between fMRI and IAT been noted. These infrequent instances in which IAT and fMRI language lateralization disagree highlight the importance of consideration of all available clinical data in presurgical epilepsy cases, including scalp and intracranial EEG recordings, seizure semiology, neuropsychological assessment, structural MRI, ESM, and other functional neuroimaging techniques such as PET and single photon emission computed tomography (SPECT). It is also important to recognize that this caveat likewise applies to IAT, where results can be nondiagnostic for language dominance for a number of technical and patient-specific reasons, as noted previously.

Such discrepancies may reflect difficulties in sensitivity to functional reorganization in individuals with atypical dominance, or hemispheric dissociation of receptive and expressive language [64, 101–105], at least for some methods. Lee et al. [103] reported four cases of hemispheric dissociation for receptive and expressive language in TLE patients. Using the same semantic decision-making task implemented in many studies from their group (e.g., [10]) they found that IAT and fMRI language lateralization were discordant in three of four cases, though agreement improved when IAT laterality was calculated emphasizing receptive language measures. This finding again highlights the importance of fMRI task selection, as the authors note that their discordant findings may be attributable in part to the lack of sensitivity of this particular task to expressive language. However, these results also demonstrate clinical examples of cases where fMRI alone might not provide sufficient confidence for clinical decision-making. Therefore, a conservative approach would include ESM confirmation of fMRI results.

Special Considerations

In some cases, conducting fMRI prior to more invasive language mapping procedures (e.g., IAT or ESM) can provide important information that significantly alters further evaluation planning. For example, Spreer et al. [106] described the case of a right-handed individual with left frontal onset epilepsy found to have unsuspected right hemisphere language dominance by fMRI (later confirmed by IAT). This finding allowed less invasive intracranial monitoring to be conducted,

Table 11.2 Summary of comparisons of IAT and fMRI language lateralization indices (LIs)

Authors	Sample (age range, years)	IAT language tasks	fMRI language tasks	fMRI LI calculation	Findings
Liegeois et al. 2002 [159]	n = 4 (14–16)	Not reported	Covert generation of nouns to aurally presented verbs	Ratio of the number of significantly activated voxels in each hemisphere using three different statistical thresholds	Some patients showed unambiguous and consistent lateralization at all thresholds, whereas the LI in others decreased in magnitude or even changed as the threshold became less stringent. Concordance with IAT was 100% when all three statistical thresholds were used to determine laterality
Adcock et al. 2003 [77]	n = 19 (15–54)	Speech arrest, naming, spelling, reading, comprehension, and reciting series (e.g., days of the week)	Covert phonemic fluency task	Two LIs, one based on the extent of activation and another based on the magnitude of activity, in volumes of interest	Concordance with IAT was 84% with extent of activation indices and 89% with magnitude of activation index
Deblaere et al. 2004 [85]	n = 17 (9–62)	Reading, naming, and describing scenes	Covert chaining word generation task	Ratio of the number of voxels activated above threshold in ROIs in each hemisphere	Concordance with IAT was 100% with frontal ROIs, 88% with hemispheric ROIs, and 82% with temporal/parietal ROIs
Baciu et al. 2005 [80]	n = 16[a] (mean ≈ 33)	Not reported	Semantic judgment, word stem completion, semantic association, and phonemic association	Ratio of the number of voxels activated above threshold in ROIs in each hemisphere and also using a similar ratio in more specific frontal and temporoparietal areas	Concordance between IAT and fMRI LI ranged from 0 to 83% and varied with task and choice of fMRI LI. Concordance was highest between more liberal LI and semantic association task, but only three subjects were assessed with this LI and task
Benke et al. 2006 [93]	n = 68 (17–60)	Serial speech, naming, comprehension, verbal semantic object decision, reading, and repetition	Semantic decision task	Independent raters defined language dominance (left > right, right > left, or bilateral/equivalent) based on the activation pattern	Concordance with IAT for right TLE patients was 89.3% with frontal ROIs, 78.6% with temporoparietal ROIs, and 75% with combined frontal and temporoparietal ROIs. Concordance with IAT for left TLE patients was 72.5% with frontal ROIs, 62.5% with temporoparietal ROIs, and 62.5% with combined frontal and temporoparietal ROIs
Chlebus et al. 2007 [84]	n = 15 (20–43)	Spontaneous speech, comprehension, reading, naming, and repetition	Covert phonemic fluency task	A variety of LI calculations were compared (e.g., suprathreshold count, t-weighting of voxels)	Concordance between LIs ranged from 33 to 100%, depending upon the ROI used. Correlation between IAT and fMRI LIs ranged from R = 0.64–0.94, depending on LI calculation and ROI used

Lee et al. 2008 [103]	n = 4 (not reported)	Counting, reading, comprehension, naming, and repetition	Semantic decision task	Laterality was calculated for three ROIs (frontal, temporoparietal, and whole hemisphere) as the difference in the number of activated voxels, summed independently for the left and right ROIs, divided by the total number of active voxels in the left and right ROIs	Subjects selected for the study were four from a sample of 269 identified because they had interhemispheric dissociation of language comprehension and production. IAT and fMRI language LI were concordant in 25% of participants but improved to 75% when IAT measures loading on comprehension were used for calculating LI
Szaflarski et al. 2008 [92]	n = 28 (22–53)	Answering four simple yes/no questions and naming four pictures of common objects	Semantic decision and verb generation	Including only voxels with Z scores ≥ 2.58 within an ROI were used in the calculation of laterality, which was defined as the difference in the number of activated voxels, summed independently for the left and right ROIs, divided by the total of active voxels in the left and right ROIs	Correlation between IAT and fMRI LI was r = 0.735 for the semantic decision task and r = 0.652 for the verb generation task
Wellmer et al. 2008 [107]	n = 65 (13–63)	Spontaneous speech, repetition, naming, comprehension, and reading	Semantic decision and verb generation	Ratio of the number of voxels activated above threshold in left and right hemisphere ROIs	Among patients with atypical language dominance according to IAT, fMRI LI ranged from 1 to −1, depending on ROI. In patients where unilateral IAT suggested typical language dominance, fMRI LI ranged from −0.61 to 1, depending on ROI. Although a laterality threshold was not specified a priori, the most conservative threshold would have misclassified 5/22 patients with atypical language dominance
Arora et al. 2009 [78]	n = 40 (14–60)	Spontaneous speech, comprehension, naming, repetition	Sentence comprehension, tone similarity judgment, and verbal fluency	Ratio of the number of significantly activated voxels in left and right hemispheres using a number of quantitative measures of activation and statistical thresholds	IAT and fMRI were concordant in 83.87% patients for the reading task, 83.33% patients for the auditory task, 76.92% patients for the verbal fluency task, and 91.3% patients for the conjunction analysis
Suarez et al. 2008 [91]	n = 14 (23–68)	Spontaneous speech, comprehension, naming, and repetition	Visually presented antonym-generation task with vocalized responses	Threshold-independent LIs were determined by comparing the integrated T score weighted distributions of all the positively correlated voxels between the left and right hemisphere ROIs	Concordance between IAT and threshold-independent laterality for inferior frontal gyrus was 85.7%. Concordance between IAT and threshold-independent laterality for superior marginal gyrus was 92.9%. Both were superior to threshold-dependent LIs

ROI region of interest, *TLE* temporal lobe epilepsy
[a]Subjects did not all complete the same tasks. Mean age reported for different groups based on lesion location

reducing the patient's surgical risk. In cases of dominant hemisphere resection or where language dominance is unclear, intraoperative language mapping is often essential. This caveat is reinforced by recent work by Wellmer et al. [107], who note clinically meaningful intraindividual discrepancies in fMRI LIs calculated from different regions of interest in a group of epilepsy patients found to have atypical language dominance on IAT, as well as fMRI activation patterns in some of these patients which suggested strongly lateralized language functioning, discrepant from IAT results. They conclude that interpretation of fMRI results as typically conducted would be insufficient for language lateralization purposes in such patients. Continued research will allow further refinement of our understanding of the most efficient method of precise fMRI localization of specific language skills. However, the available data suggests that current fMRI paradigms can consistently lateralize language as effectively as the IAT in the majority of cases, and can be used with confidence in place of the IAT in many circumstances (see [108] for Bayesian analysis of the role of fMRI in assessment of language dominance). Many epilepsy surgery centers, including our own, routinely use clinical fMRI to confirm language lateralization in patients with a presumed nondominant (typically right) hemisphere seizure focus, to obviate the need for conducting an IAT. Our clinical team has effectively utilized fMRI word generation tasks to determine language dominance and localization of Broca's area in presurgical epilepsy, tumor, and arteriovenous malformation patients, as well as in patients who cannot undergo the IAT (e.g., due to vascular risk factors). In particular, use of fMRI language paradigms provides a potential alternative for language lateralization in epilepsy patients who would not necessarily be considered for IAT, including adults with medical contraindications and young children, who may be trained to tolerate the fMRI procedure more readily than the IAT, and thus have language laterality assessed without the potential morbidity risks of the IAT.

While studies have noted technical issues that must be considered in the use of fMRI with children [38, 109–112], including tailoring of cognitive paradigms and adjustment of statistical thresholds [85], results from our group and other centers suggest that language can be successfully lateralized using fMRI in pediatric populations. We have routinely achieved successful language lateralization using fMRI word generation paradigms in epilepsy patients age 6 and older, and a few centers have had good success with children as young as 4 years of age (e.g., [21]). Our experience has been that children can effectively perform such fMRI tasks following out-of-scanner preparation, including practicing the fMRI tasks and instruction regarding the importance of remaining motionless, and with minimal in-scanner head restraints (i.e., only foam padding and/or tape across the forehead). With modification of fMRI paradigms as appropriate for level of cognitive functioning, and additional physical assistance in head stabilization, it seems likely that fMRI may come into wider use for lateralization of language in very young children, in whom the IAT is often considered unfeasible or its attendant medical risks too great. Indeed, a series of 35 children and adolescents with frontal or temporal lobe lesions reported by Anderson et al. [113] provides strong support for the utility of fMRI for language lateralization in pediatric patients.

Future Directions

Future directions for fMRI assessment of language skills in presurgical epilepsy patients should include not only consistent lateralization of language dominance, but specific localization of regions subserving the cognitive functions most likely to be negatively affected by surgical resection in the dominant hemisphere [114]. Previous research [115] has demonstrated postoperative decline in naming skills following dominant temporal lobe resection, and other complex language functions such as reading and semantic processing may also be disrupted. Individuals who experience later onset of epilepsy and who have stronger language abilities presurgically have been shown to be at increased risk for postsurgical language deficits following temporal lobe resection in the language-dominant hemisphere (as determined by IAT) [115–118]. Recent work has suggested that fMRI language probes may also prove useful in assessment of risk of postsurgical language deficits. For example, Sabsevitz et al. [119] demonstrated that presurgical activation during an fMRI semantic decision-making task in a group of left TLE patients was significantly related to performance on an out-of-scanner naming task postsurgery. Therefore, while some of the language paradigms used in the studies discussed previously may not provide maximal information regarding overall language lateralization, such tasks may be useful in demonstrating activation of extrafrontal language regions (e.g., temporoparietal association cortex), which may be helpful in assessing the likelihood of postsurgical cognitive impairment and the potential for recovery of function. As TLE patients are those most commonly considered for epilepsy surgery, the importance of delineating temporal lobe language regions as well as memory circuitry becomes evident. In addition, it is important to note that the specific fMRI language task used may not be critical to achieving adequate language lateralization. For example, Grandin et al. [37] found that the number of pixels activated in frontal and temporal language regions did not differ for semantic versus phonemic verbal fluency tasks. Similarly, both tasks lateralized language functioning to the dominant hemisphere, suggesting no particular advantage to one form of verbal fluency task over the other. This information is particularly useful in the study of children, who may not be able to accurately generate words beginning with a particular letter, but who can often generate words to a semantic category such as animals or foods.

Case Examples of fMRI Language Activation

Patients referred to our service for clinical fMRI language mapping complete one or more language paradigms. In our aural word generation paradigm, blocks of nouns are presented alternating with blocks of tones. The patient is instructed to mentally generate as many verbs as possible that go with each noun (e.g., for “frog,” the patient might think “leap,” “croak,” “hop,” etc.). For younger patients or those with cognitive limitations, for whom the noun/verb distinction is less salient, they may be asked simply to generate as many words as possible, without specification of a part of speech. The patient is instructed not to say the words or make any mouth movements. During the control condition (tones) the patient is instructed to simply listen and clear his/her mind. As this task does not involve collection of objective performance data, successful completion of the task is assessed by postscanning debriefing and comparison with performance on similar measures during out-of-scanner neuropsychological testing. Analysis contrasts hemodynamic responses during the two task conditions. The typical pattern of brain activation for this task comprises dominant hemisphere frontal regions, with more posterior temporal lobe activation observed in some patients. Consistent with the literature, cingulate gyrus activation is also often noted.

Examples of left, right, and mixed dominant activation patterns during word generation are shown in Fig. 11.1 (displayed over surface renderings of the patients’ own anatomy). The clinical history of each of these patients is illustrative of cases in which fMRI language mapping can be particularly helpful.

The left hemisphere dominant patient is a 12-year-old, right-handed girl, who began experiencing seizures about 11 months prior to the fMRI scan. Prior brain MRI studies had demonstrated an enhancing lesion in the posterior inferior aspect of the left inferior temporal gyrus, measuring 1.2 × 1 × 2.0 cm, and thought likely to represent a low-grade glioma. Neuropsychological assessment demonstrated intact cognitive abilities, with functioning within normal limits for age across domains. Intraoperative ESM confirmed multiple epileptogenic foci in the temporooccipital region, and pathology was consistent with ganglioglioma (WHO grade I). She underwent gross total lesion resection and has been seizure-free since surgery with no apparent functional deficits. In addition to prominent left inferior frontal activation, in this patient significant left superior

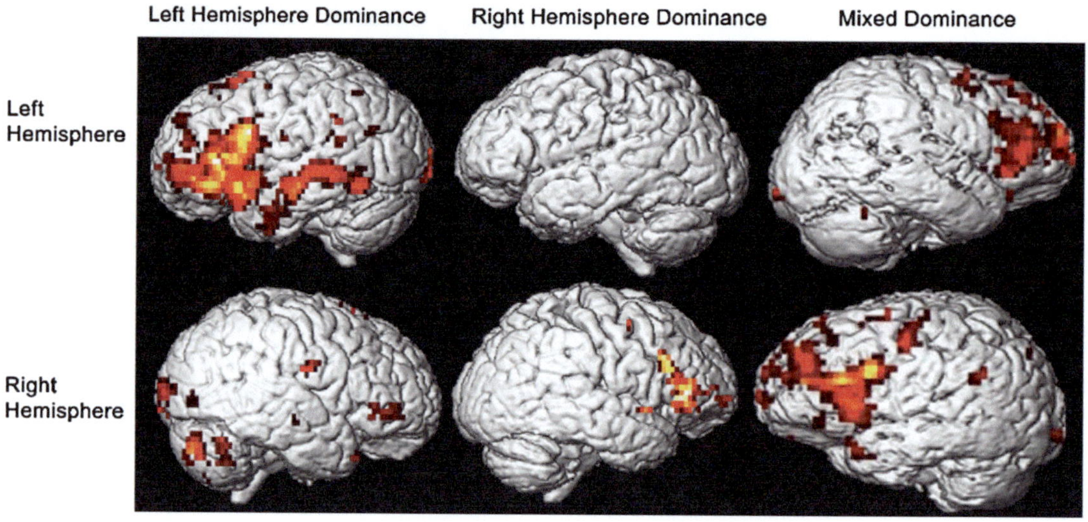

Fig. 11.1 Word generation: fMRI activation maps demonstrating left, right, and mixed language dominance

temporal activation was apparent during word generation, demonstrating good activation of expressive and receptive language regions. Of note, a small cluster of activation can be seen in the inferior frontal lobe of the nondominant hemisphere, in homologous territory. As noted previously, this is not an uncommon finding.

The right hemisphere dominant patient is a 62-year-old, right-handed man, with a history of medication-refractory seizures since age 3. EEG demonstrated right temporal slowing and epileptiform discharges, while brain MRI showed right hippocampal atrophy and T2 prolongation compatible with mesial temporal sclerosis. PET scan showed right temporal hypometabolism. Neuropsychological assessment showed borderline range intellectual ability and impaired verbal memory with variable nonverbal memory. As the patient was right-handed, left hemisphere dominance for language would have been predicted. However, during inpatient video-EEG monitoring pronounced aphasia was apparent during seizures and postictally. As demonstrated on fMRI, this patient was strongly right hemisphere dominant for language, a finding that was later confirmed by IAT. IAT memory testing showed greater right hemisphere impairment. Based on the fMRI and IAT findings of right hemisphere language dominance, the patient underwent a more limited resection than would otherwise have been conducted. Intraoperative ESM confirmed a right temporal seizure focus, and pathology confirmed mesial temporal sclerosis. This patient has also been seizure-free since surgery. For both of these patients clear unilateral hemispheric "dominance" is apparent, in contrast to the case demonstrating mixed dominance. This is a 20-year-old man with mixed handedness (writes predominantly with the left hand, but many other activities are typically conducted with the right), who was diagnosed with a large (Spetzler-Martin grade III–IV) right posterior temporal/inferior parietal arteriovenous malformation. IAT was unsuccessful due to extensive cross-flow. Functional MRI language mapping was therefore conducted prior to embolization of the malformation. While no preoperative neuropsychological data were available, the patient reported a lifelong history of learning and attentional difficulties, including the need for early reading intervention. As can be seen, bilateral frontal activation was apparent. The global peak of activation in the whole brain was observed in the left frontal lobe; however, the presence of such extensive homologous right hemisphere activation argued for mixed dominance for language in this case. This is also of interest in relation to the patient's reported history of learning and attentional problems, given prior research suggesting a relationship between developmental language and reading disorders and abnormal cerebral lateralization of brain regions related to language functioning (for review, see [120]).

fMRI Memory Paradigms and the IAT

While the development of fMRI memory paradigms to replace the IAT has lagged behind that of language paradigms, early data have been encouraging. Functional MRI memory tasks cannot yet serve the critical IAT function of assessing unilateral support of memory functions on an individual basis, as neither hemisphere is anesthetized during stimulus presentation. However, a growing fMRI literature has examined episodic memory encoding and retrieval processes in healthy controls and TLE populations (see Table 11.3 for summary of studies assessing memory functioning in TLE using fMRI and IAT). Research in this area has increased dramatically since the publication of the first edition of this volume, and is encouraging in terms of progress toward the eventual development of paradigms useful for presurgical evaluation on the individual case basis.

Visuospatial/Nonverbal Memory

In TLE patients, Detre et al. [121] used a visual scene encoding fMRI task, previously demonstrated to activate bilateral MTL structures in healthy controls [122], to assess functional asymmetry in comparison with IAT memory lateralization. In controls, comparison of activation during the task condition as compared to a visual control condition demonstrated bilateral posterior temporal and visual association cortex and right frontal activation, with a slight right hemisphere predominance overall in MTL regions of interest. In nine of ten patients, asymmetry ratios were greater than one standard deviation from the control mean; four of ten showed asymmetry ratios greater than two standard deviations away from the control mean. In all patients the direction of hemispheric asymmetry was concordant with IAT memory findings. As two patients demonstrated paradoxically greater fMRI activation and better IAT memory performance ipsilateral to the seizure focus, this pattern was thought not entirely attributable to epilepsy-related structural abnormalities. This finding is clinically significant, as it demonstrates the potential utility of fMRI in demonstrating brain activation patterns that might by extension to the IAT predict memory deficits following temporal lobectomy, and thus inform risk/benefit discussions, or in the extreme case serve as a potential contraindication for surgery.

In subsequent work this group has used the same scene encoding task to explore fMRI predictors of seizure and cognitive outcome following temporal lobectomy. Previous research has demonstrated that postsurgical memory outcome can be predicted by presurgical hippocampal volume [123], severity of hippocampal sclerosis on presurgical structural MRI [124] or pathology of the resected tissue [125, 126], presurgical neuropsychological performance [123, 127, 128], and presurgical IAT memory performance [128–130]. Predictors of seizure outcome following MTL resection have included interictal brain hypometabolism [131, 132] as well as IAT abnormalities [9, 133]. Killgore et al. [134] reported that presurgical fMRI memory lateralization predicted postsurgical seizure status as effectively as IAT in a sample of eight TLE patients (a subset of the sample reported in [121]). Seizure freedom one year postsurgery was associated with presurgical asymmetry of MTL fMRI activation, with higher activation in the nonepileptogenic hemisphere positively correlating with seizure freedom. Comparison of predictive power of fMRI and IAT showed that each method accurately classified seizure outcome for 75% of subjects, but classification improved to 100% when information from fMRI and IAT LIs was combined. In 23 TLE patients, Rabin et al. [135] demonstrated that less activation in the MTL ipsilateral to the seizure focus preoperatively predicted a smaller decline in cognitive performance or improved performance postsurgically. Most recently, Mechanic-Hamilton et al. [136] found that fMRI asymmetry of MTL

Table 11.3 Summary of studies assessing memory performance in TLE using fMRI

Authors	Sample (age range, years)	IAT memory tasks	fMRI memory tasks	Findings
Detre et al. 1998 [121]	Left TLE: $n = 6$ (17–48) Right TLE: $n = 3$ (18–37) Controls: $n = 8$ (18–40)	Free recall and recognition of common objects, low-imagery words, and abstract line drawings	Complex scene encoding	Controls demonstrated generally symmetric MTL activation. Patients showed asymmetric MTL activation, which agreed in all cases with memory asymmetry on IAT
Bellgowan et al. 1998 [142]	Left TLE $n = 14$ (20–57) Right TLE $n = 14$ (28–69)	Not described; IAT memory lateralization data are presented	Semantic and tone decision	Right TLE patients: similar activation in left MTL as previously observed in healthy controls in a separate study Left TLE patients: decreased left MTL activation relative to right TLE patients, but similar whole-brain and left hemisphere activation and task performance
Dupont et al. 2000 [144]	Left TLE: $n = 7$ ((18–53) Controls: $n = 10$ (23–30)	Not described; only IAT data presented are that all patients are left language dominant	Verbal episodic encoding and retrieval	Bilateral parahippocampal gyrus activation during retrieval in both groups, more so in controls, who had stronger task performance Patients also activated left prefrontal regions during encoding and retrieval
Dupont et al. 2001 [145]	Left TLE: $n = 7$ ((18–53) Controls: $n = 10$ (23–31)[a]	Not described; only IAT data presented are that all patients are left language dominant	Verbal retrieval	Relative to the prior scan: Controls: decreased activation in parahippocampal, occipitotemporal, and ventrolateral frontal regions, but new activation in right posterior hippocampus and bilateral parietal cortex Patients: slightly poorer task performance, absent MTL activation, and dramatic decrease in previously noted neocortical fMRI activation
Jokeit et al. 2001 [140]	Left TLE: $n = 16$ (13–55) Right TLE: $n = 14$ (14–54) Controls: $n = 17$ (7–63)	Free recall and recognition of 20 items (e.g., actual and drawn objects, words, and abstract drawings)	Mental navigation and recall	Both groups showed MTL activation, in controls no significant asymmetry was evident Patients: Hemispheric asymmetry in activation lateralized seizure onset in 90% (weaker activation on side of focus); left TLE patients showed correlation between left MTL activation and IAT memory performance using the left hemisphere
Golby et al. 2002 [150]	Left TLE: $n = 6$ (26–33) Right TLE: $n = 3$ (42–54)	Recognition of objects, words, and designs	Encoding and processing of words, faces, scenes, and patterns	fMRI and IAT memory lateralization concordant in 89% of subjects; in each group, greater encoding-related activation was observed in MTL structures contralateral to seizure focus; material specific interaction between side of seizure focus and memory for verbal vs. nonverbal stimuli
Rabin et al. 2004 [135]	Left TLE: $n = 14$ (29–54) Right TLE: $n = 13$ (29–58)	Recognition of objects, words, and designs	Complex visual scene encoding	Asymmetry ratios from the hippocampus, parahippocampus, and fusiform gyrus correlated with memory lateralization by IAT. Asymmetry ratios also correlated with memory outcome, as determined by a change in scene recognition between pre- and postsurgical trials

Szaflarski et al. 2004 [137]	Left TLE: n = 3 (not reported) Right TLE: n = 3 (not reported)	Recognition of objects, words, and line drawings	Complex visual scene encoding	fMRI and IAT laterality indices were concordant in 50% of subjects
Deblaere et al. 2005 [139]	Left TLE: n = 8 (29–54) Right TLE: n = 10 (13–55)	Recognition of words, line drawings, and one abstract item	Line drawing recognition	Regression analysis revealed a significant correlation between fMRI and IAT LIs in the patients with right but not left TLE
Branco et al. 2006 [151]	Left TLE: n = 4 (27–50) Right TLE: n = 1 (34)	Recognition of objects	Encoding of patterns, scenes, and words	Concordance between fMRI and IAT LIs was variable when calculated from suprathreshold voxels only but 100% using weighted LIs
Binder et al. 2003 [143]	Left TLE: n = 56 (mean = 37.4) Right TLE: n = 62 (mean = 40.3)	Recognition of objects	Semantic decision	Preoperative fMRI LIs were better univariate predictors for postoperative memory outcome in patients with left TLE than IAT memory tasks. In a multivariate model IAT did not add predictive power to a model comprised of age, preoperative memory score, onset of epilepsy, and fMRI LI
Mechanic-Hamilton et al. 2009 [136]	Left TLE: n = 21 Right TLE: n = 24 Bilateral TLE: n = 4 (mean ≈ 39)[b]	Not reported	Recognition memory of complex scenes	When compared with IAT laterality, hippocampal structural LIs showed medium-sized correlations without reaching significance, whereas combined hippocampal/parahippocampal/fusiform gyrus LI showed a high correlation

LI laterality index, *MTL* medial temporal lobe, *TLE* temporal lobe epilepsy

[a]Same subjects as Dupont et al. rescanned 24 h after scanning session reported in the previous paper, and asked to recall words learned during the first scanning session

[b]Means are reported for groups scanned at different magnet field strengths

regions relative to healthy controls was found in TLE patients studied on a 3T magnet, though not in those studied at 1.5T. Greater functional asymmetry was observed in patients with a younger age at onset of epilepsy. IAT laterality was also significantly related to MTL fMRI asymmetry across field strengths, though correlations were stronger at 3T. Postoperative memory correlations were strongest in left TLE patients, in whom more intact left MTL structures preoperatively (larger volumetric measurements on structural MRI, more activation on fMRI) was related to greater postoperative decline.

Using a somewhat different scene encoding paradigm Szaflarski et al. [137] studied 19 healthy control subjects and six TLE patients who later underwent temporal lobectomy. Controls demonstrated bilateral MTL activation during scene encoding, while greater lateralization of activation was observed in the TLE group. The degree of concordance between IAT and presurgical fMRI memory lateralization was weak, however, with agreement observed in only 50% of cases, all of whom were seizure-free postsurgery. In two cases with disagreement between IAT and fMRI results, fMRI demonstrated symmetric MTL activation, while IAT demonstrated impaired memory functioning in the epileptogenic hemisphere; both of these subjects had persistent seizures postsurgery (Engel class III). In the remaining case, fMRI lateralized MTL dysfunction to the right hemisphere, while IAT lateralized dysfunction to the left. Comparison of memory performance pre- and postsurgery in the TLE group was not available. Differences in the concordance between IAT and fMRI data in this study and that found in other similar work may be attributable to differences in activation task and/or method of construction and interpretation of LIs; however, these results highlight the caution with which fMRI memory findings must currently be interpreted in terms of predicting postoperative outcomes, given the apparent discrepancies between fMRI and IAT results in this cohort.

In later work, this group examined a larger group of patients, divided by hemispheric seizure onset (most had TLE, though some had extratemporal seizure onset), using the same task [138]. They found that healthy controls and patients with a right hemispheric onset showed a slight left hemisphere lateralization of encoding-related activation. By contrast, patients with left hemispheric seizure onset showed right-lateralized activation. Regardless of side of seizure onset, out-of-scanner verbal memory performance predicted fMRI LI, with better performance correlating with more left-lateralized MTL fMRI activation. Similarly, using a picture encoding and recognition paradigm, Deblaere et al. investigated the concordance of fMRI activation patterns and IAT results in both left and right TLE (LTLE and RTLE) patients relative to controls [139]. This paradigm utilized a novelty detection approach to examine MTL activation, and was found consistently to activate anterior and posterior MTL structures. In both TLE groups, fMRI activation tended to lateralize contralateral to side of seizure focus, consistent with prior studies. Good concordance with IAT results was limited to RTLE patients, however, with no significant correlation found between fMRI and IAT results in LTLE. This finding is somewhat counterintuitive, in that left focus patients would presumably be relying on an intact right MTL, which should be better specialized for visual recognition.

Jokeit et al. [140] utilized fMRI to lateralize declarative memory functioning in a group of 30 TLE patients and 17 healthy control subjects using a mental navigation task involving mental recall and navigation of the subject's hometown, contrasted with a covert counting baseline condition. Both controls and TLE patients (including children, older subjects, and some subjects with lower intellectual functioning) reliably activated MTL structures. Hemispheric asymmetry in MTL activation lateralized seizure onset in 90% of TLE patients, with diminished activation observed on the side of seizure focus. Controls did not demonstrate significant fMRI MTL activation asymmetry. The authors concluded that these activation patterns were specifically related to memory rather than to visuospatial abilities, based on correlations between out-of-scanner neuropsychological testing of memory functions and fMRI MTL activation. Examination of fMRI activation patterns and IAT results demonstrated a significant correlation between number of activated voxels in the left MTL and left hemisphere IAT performance. Unfortunately, too few RTLE subjects were available for the authors to correlate hemispheric asymmetry indices from fMRI and IAT across TLE groups.

Using the same task, Janszky et al. [141] demonstrated a correlation between presurgical fMRI lateralization and postsurgical memory outcome (change in nonverbal memory retention score pre- to postsurgery) in 16 RTLE patients. Relatively reduced MTL activation in the epileptogenic hemisphere (greater activation in the nonepileptic MTL) correlated with better memory outcome. While memory change pre- to postsurgery was not significant at the overall group level, all patients in this sample with greater activation in the MTL ipsilateral to seizure focus or symmetric MTL activation demonstrated decreased memory performance after surgery. These findings provide useful data to support the eventual clinical utility of fMRI in presurgical evaluation of RTLE patients. As already noted, in some epilepsy surgery centers IAT is not routinely performed in RTLE patients, particularly those who are right-handed (presuming left hemisphere language dominance), or who have an apparent right hemisphere lesion on structural MRI. The possibility of using fMRI to predict postsurgical memory outcome in these patients would therefore be a useful clinical tool.

Verbal Memory

Bellgowan et al. [142] were able to discriminate LTLE and RTLE patients based on their fMRI activation patterns on a semantic encoding task. RTLE patients showed predominant left MTL activation, involving the hippocampus, parahippocampal gyrus, and collateral sulcus, whereas those with a left hemisphere seizure focus demonstrated little activation in these regions. This task did not demonstrate bilateral activation of memory structures; neither right nor LTLE patients showed significant right hemisphere activation in MTL regions while completing the task. This is not unexpected, in that semantic tasks do not typically generate right hemisphere activation, and highlights a paradigm potentially useful for preferential activation of the left MTL in presurgical fMRI evaluation of epilepsy patients. The authors hypothesized that the lack of left MTL activation in LTLE patients in spite of relatively intact episodic memory functioning may indicate intra- or interhemispheric reorganization of memory functions in this group, which may be related to factors such as age at seizure onset. Using the same task, these authors investigated factors predictive of postoperative verbal memory decline in a large group of LTLE patients [143]. Their findings were generally consistent with prior neuropsychological and IAT research, and showed that stronger preoperative memory performance, left hemisphere language lateralization on IAT and fMRI, and later age at epilepsy onset all predicted greater verbal memory decline. After including preoperative memory functioning and age at seizure onset in the predictive model, preoperative fMRI accounted for an additional 10% of the variance. Including IAT memory and language asymmetries did not add further predictive power. These authors conclude that preoperative fMRI is therefore useful in predicting patients at high risk for verbal memory declines after surgical treatment for LTLE. Of note is that both of the studies discussed previously [142, 143] utilized the same task as in Binder et al.'s seminal language lateralization paper [10], but focused on its semantic memory properties. This finding has practical clinical significance, as utility of the same task to examine both language and memory functioning as part of presurgical evaluation might offer significant advantages in terms of patient burden and scanner time.

To examine reallocation of verbal memory functions in LTLE, Dupont et al. [144] utilized verbal episodic memory encoding and retrieval tasks in ten healthy control subjects and seven LTLE patients with left hippocampal sclerosis. During fMRI scanning, subjects were asked to encode a supraspan list of 17 words over repeated presentations, then to covertly recall the words. In addition to activation across broader neural networks, both patients and controls demonstrated bilateral parahippocampal gyrus activation (right greater than left) during retrieval, though this effect was more marked in controls. Patients also recruited left prefrontal regions for encoding and retrieval, which were not activated in controls. Given a performance deficit noted in patients relative to controls on postscanner recall testing, Dupont et al. [144] hypothesized that this frontal cortex recruitment reflects ineffective reallocation of memory functions (i.e., cortical dysfunction rather than efficient reorganization) in the patient group, due either to hippocampal dysfunction or epileptogenesis. This group later analyzed differences in brain activation in the same subjects for 24-h delayed retrieval of the verbal material [145]. At the follow-up fMRI session, subjects were asked only to retrieve the words memorized the day before (i.e., the word list was not presented again), and memory was again tested through free recall following the scanner session. For controls, retrieval was similar to prior performance, while patient performance was slightly poorer. Analysis of changes in fMRI brain activation patterns in controls revealed decreases in parahippocampal, occipitotemporal, and ventrolateral frontal activation, and emergence of a new focus of activation in the right posterior hippocampus and bilateral parietal cortex. In the epilepsy patients, no MTL activation was apparent, and activation in neocortical brain regions observed at the previous session was dramatically decreased. These findings were interpreted to support the assertion that MTL structures play a critical role in the neural networks involved in episodic verbal memory, including retrieval of stored information, and that dysfunction of these regions in TLE patients likely underlies the observed memory deficits and alterations in fMRI activation.

Richardson et al. [146] also examined the presumed reorganization of verbal memory functions in a group of 24 LTLE patients with hippocampal sclerosis relative to 12 control subjects. The LTLE group was further subdivided into patients with and without amygdalar sclerosis in addition to hippocampal sclerosis. In the combined patient group, greater activity was observed in the right hippocampus and parahippocampal gyrus during successful verbal encoding relative to the control group. During successfully encoded emotional relative to neutral words, the patient group with left amygdalar and hippocampal sclerosis showed greater right amygdalar activation relative to patients with left hippocampal sclerosis only. In further work, this research team also showed a relationship between hippocampal pathology (hippocampal volume, gray matter density, and sclerosis) and MTL fMRI activation [147]. In 16 LTLE patients, greater left hippocampal volume loss and increased abnormal left hippocampal T2 signal were related to decreased encoding-related fMRI activation in the left hippocampus for neutral words, but increased activation in the right hippocampus. The converse was evident in subjects with less left hippocampal volume loss. A similar shift toward greater right MTL activation was observed related to left amygdalar pathology for encoding of emotional stimuli. Interdependence was found between hippocampal and amygdalar pathology and this putative functional reorganization of encoding-related activation for emotional stimuli, with greater left MTL pathology related to increased right MTL activation. Interaction analyses showed that greater left amygdalar pathology was related to less left hippocampal and greater right hippocampal activation during encoding of emotional stimuli. With greater left hippocampal pathology, diminished left amygdalar activation and increased right amygdalar activation were noted. Taken together, these findings [146, 147] support the argument for reorganization/reallocation of verbal encoding functionality in LTLE to homologous regions in the nonepileptic right MTL, and suggest that such reorganization may become more likely in cases where the left MTL demonstrates more severe pathology.

Richardson et al. then examined the relationship of presurgical fMRI activation to postoperative memory functioning in a subset of 10 of the LTLE patients reported in [146, 147], all of whom were seizure-free postsurgically. Postsurgical memory decline was strongly predicted by a multiple regression model including left hippocampal volume, presurgical verbal memory, and an LI comparing left and right hippocampal fMRI activation during successful encoding of neutral words [123]. Presurgical fMRI assessment of verbal memory encoding was the strongest independent predictor of postoperative memory performance. Consistent with prior work suggesting that greater functional integrity of tissue ipsilateral to seizure focus leads to greater postsurgical cognitive decline, this study found that greater fMRI activation during verbal memory encoding in the left relative to the right hippocampus was correlated with higher degree of postsurgical verbal memory decline. Importantly, the positive predictive value of fMRI data for memory decline was meaningful at the individual level, using standard clinical memory measures as the dependent variable, providing early evidence that fMRI memory probes can show clinical utility.

Further elucidation of alterations in neural networks subserving memory functioning is provided by Köylü et al. who studied 26 LTLE and 24 RTLE patients in addition to 35 control participants [148] using a semantic memory task based on Binder et al. [10]. During verbal semantic memory processing, distinct patterns of fMRI activation were observed. Controls showed bilateral frontotemporal activation, with a left hemisphere predominance. By contrast, LTLE patients showed relatively greater right hemisphere activation, with additional subcortical activation. RTLE patients showed an activation pattern more similar to controls, but with a lower degree of frontal relative to more posterior activation. These findings demonstrate variation in semantic memory processing networks in chronic TLE patients, presumably reflective of alterations in brain function as a result of epilepsy. This demonstration of altered memory networks depending on side of seizure focus highlights an important consideration for interpretation of memory activation patterns in TLE and comparison with IAT results, providing further evidence that side of seizure focus may be a critical factor influencing results. In subsequent work, Köylü et al. demonstrated that preoperative fMRI activation on the same task predicted postoperative memory outcome [149]. Preoperatively their RTLE group showed MTL activation asymmetry favoring the left MTL, whereas the LTLE group showed essentially symmetric MTL activation. Consistent with prior findings, greater preoperative MTL activation ipsilateral to seizure focus correlated with higher preoperative episodic memory performance, while greater MTL activation contralateral to seizure focus was related to higher postoperative memory performance, particularly in LTLE patients.

Multimodality Memory fMRI Paradigms

Golby et al. [150] evaluated hemispheric asymmetry of MTL activation in nine TLE patients during novel stimuli encoding. Subjects were asked to remember four types of stimuli – patterns, faces, scenes, and words – as well as to perform stimulus-related tasks. Performance accuracy was assessed by a recognition paradigm following the encoding phase. In 89% of subjects, fMRI lateralization of memory was concordant with IAT. Overall, RTLE patients demonstrated greater left than right MTL activation across encoding conditions, while the reverse was true for LTLE patients. In addition, group analysis demonstrated an interaction between side of seizure focus and material specificity for memory, such that LTLE patients showed right MTL activation for encoding of verbal material, while RTLE subjects showed left MTL activation for nonverbal information. These data were interpreted to demonstrate functional reorganization of memory circuitry due to TLE. If replicated in larger samples, this approach might provide an fMRI memory paradigm suitable for assessment of memory lateralization in individual patients, and thus possibly lead to eventual replacement of the IAT. Future directions in the study of fMRI memory lateralization and localization in TLE should likewise include assessment of memory across multiple stimulus modalities, to capitalize upon the potential material specificity of hemispheric MTL functioning in memory encoding. Building on their prior study, this research group subsequently assessed the effectiveness of a whole voxel distribution approach to creation of memory LIs [151]. Using three of the four stimuli types used in their prior study (patterns, scenes, and words) they found that LIs calculated using only suprathreshold voxels were more variable than those created from whole weighted statistical distributions (i.e., weighting all voxels with positive T values based on their statistical significance produced more consistent LIs than including only voxels over a specified statistical threshold). Using the latter approach, fMRI memory lateralization was consistent with IAT in all five epilepsy patients assessed.

Prediction of Postsurgical Memory Change

Overall, stronger lateralization of fMRI memory task-related activation has been shown to be related to side of seizure focus (greater activation contralateral to seizure focus), as well as to postsurgical seizure and cognitive outcome (better outcome when presurgical fMRI memory LI favors nonsurgical hemisphere). The finding that fMRI is sensitive to brain dysfunction within the epileptogenic zone indicates potential utility for surgical planning. Two mechanisms for explaining memory changes following temporal lobectomy have been proposed: functional reserve and functional adequacy [152]. The functional reserve model proposes that postoperative memory functioning is dependent on the ability of the nonepileptic MTL to support memory (i.e., greater support of memory in the MTL contralateral to seizure focus presurgically should predict better memory outcome). By contrast, the functional adequacy model hypothesizes that postsurgical memory deficits are related to the extent to which the epileptic MTL supports memory preoperatively (i.e., greater memory support ipsilateral to seizure focus predicts poorer memory outcome). These hypotheses are not mutually exclusive, and the fMRI literature to date appears to offer some support for both theories. Such results are also consistent with previous neuropsychological and pathology findings suggesting that greater presurgical structural and functional integrity of the epileptogenic MTL is related to increased postsurgical functional deficits, and suggest that fMRI probes of memory may eventually achieve the major purpose of IAT memory assessment. While such studies point to the potential utility of fMRI memory activation patterns in predicting postsurgical outcome, they also suggest that at present fMRI and IAT memory data provide complementary information. Demonstration of reliable techniques for evoking MTL activation in TLE patients at the level of the individual may in the future allow fMRI to replace the IAT for memory assessment. Given the evidence for material specificity of hemispheric MTL functioning in memory encoding in TLE, it will be beneficial for future studies to include assessment of memory across multiple stimulus modalities in the same patients. This will allow the development of fMRI paradigms with increased sensitivity to lateralize and localize brain regions critical for memory function, which can then be used to assist in forecasting likely postsurgical outcomes.

Case Examples of fMRI Memory Activation

We have used fMRI probes to elicit activation of memory systems in epilepsy patients before and after resective surgery [153, 154]. Figures 11.2 and 11.3 demonstrate MTL activation using an event-related continuous performance recognition memory task. We patterned this task after the paradigm used by Swick and Knight [155] in their ERP studies of working memory versus delayed recognition, where reaction time and pattern of evoked responses differentiated between patients with focal frontal and hippocampal lesions. This task consists of a list of words or low-verbalizability line drawings [156] with a pseudorandom jittered interstimulus interval of 5–8 s. Each stimulus is presented twice; the second occurrence may be immediately following the first (0–2 intervening stimuli), or may be 9–18 items later in the list. The subject responds by button press to indicate whether a stimulus is being presented for the first or second time. Analysis is performed by dividing items into three event types; first presentations ("new" items, encoding condition), second presentations with a short delay ("working memory" items, up to two stimuli

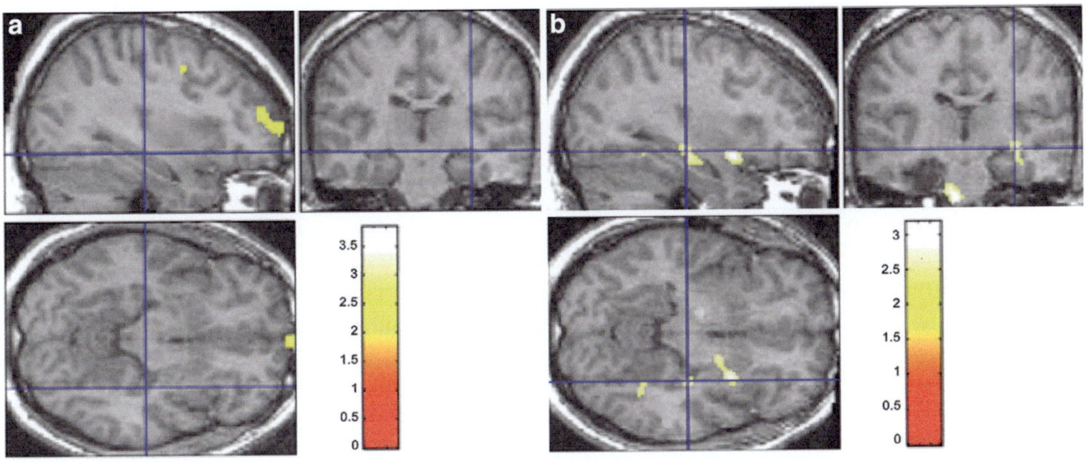

Fig. 11.2 Neurological coordinates. Right hippocampal activation ($p_{\text{crit}} = 0.01$) in a 25-year-old, right-handed male during verbal encoding before (**a**) and after (**b**) left selective amygdalohippocampectomy. Right MTL activation observed after, but not before, surgery in the nonepileptic hippocampus suggests a possible functional release from the irritative seizure focus (see McDonald et al. [153])

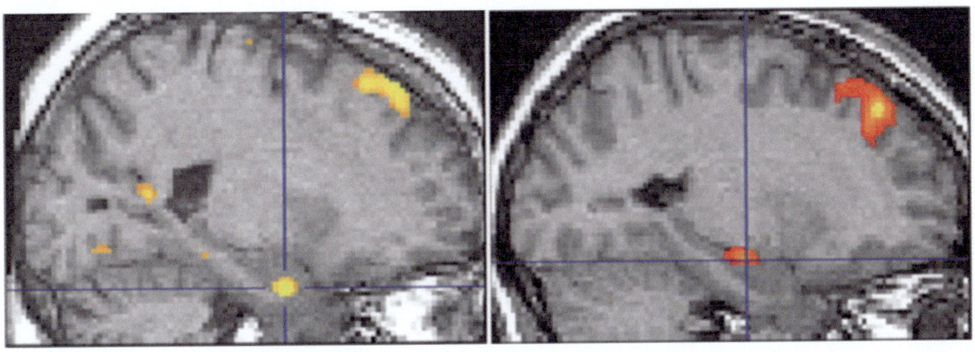

Fig. 11.3 Left medial temporal lobe activation ($p_{\text{crit}} = 0.05$) in two female right temporal lobe resection patients (both right-handed and left-hemisphere dominant for language on IAT), during encoding of novel words showing contralateral memory functioning after surgery (fMRI conducted 2.8 and 4.8 years after surgery, see McDonald et al. [153])

between presentations), and second presentations with a long delay ("long delay items," from 9–18 items between presentations). Contrasts are then made to compare hemodynamic responses between these three types of events. We have observed MTL activation across subjects during encoding on both the verbal and nonverbal (designs) analogs of this task. Functional MRI memory paradigms may prove to be a powerful tool for studying epilepsy-related brain functional reorganization. In Fig. 11.2, we present data from a 25-year-old, right-handed male patient with LTLE, who underwent fMRI pre- and postsurgery. Before surgery no hippocampal activation was evident in the right (nonepileptogenic) hemisphere. After surgery, however, right hippocampal activation was observed during encoding of new words. These findings suggest a possible functional release from the irritative seizure focus following surgery [153]. In Fig. 11.3, data are presented from two right-handed female patients with RTLE who were studied following temporal lobe resection. In both subjects left hippocampal activation was apparent during encoding of new words, demonstrating functional activity in the nonepileptic MTL [153].

We have also utilized a block-design scene encoding paradigm slightly adapted from Detre et al. [121] to examine episodic memory functioning in children and adolescents with TLE and healthy controls [157]. In addition to an encoding phase where analyses compare viewing of novel scenes to viewing a repeated retiled image, we conduct a separate task run with an event-related recognition format, in which participants must distinguish previously seen targets from foils. Data from this task and the verbal analog of the event-related task described previously are presented here for illustration in a group of 11 healthy children aged 8–12 years (Fig. 11.4). Across all three tasks (scene encoding, scene recognition, and detection of novel words), significant bilateral MTL activation is apparent. These findings demonstrate the potential utility of such tasks for examining episodic memory functioning in children, and comparisons between healthy controls and children with TLE are ongoing.

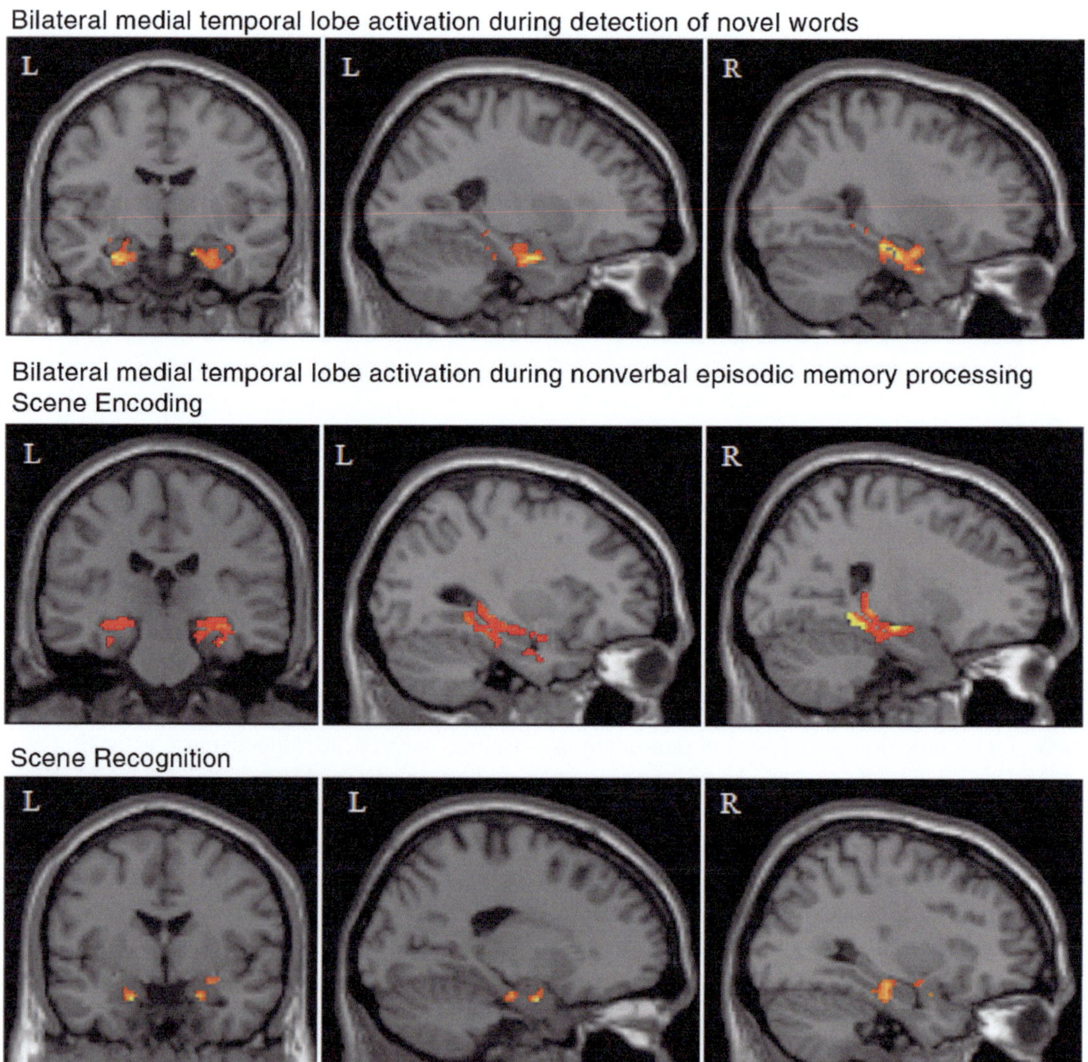

Fig. 11.4 Medial temporal lobe activation during memory processing in 11 healthy children (ages 8–12, see McDonald et al. [157])

Methodological Issues in Creating fMRI Paradigms to Replace the IAT

Technical and Clinical Considerations

Imaging Approach

One critical issue highlighted by review of the current literature in fMRI language and memory paradigms is that of imaging methodology. While some researchers choose only to image specific regions of interest (e.g., scanning only frontal and temporal regions), others conduct whole-brain imaging. Within groups that obtain images of the whole brain some analyze only activation within discrete regions of interest, while others assess alterations in activation patterns throughout the brain. Choices made with regard to which brain regions to image or analyze obviously may have a pivotal effect on statistical power and the results and conclusions that can be drawn regarding the nature and extent of the neural circuits subserving various cognitive functions. For example, those studies that obtain images only of the frontal lobes cannot, by definition, detect functional lateralization or localization of extrafrontal language or memory regions. The choice of imaging plane and slice thickness and positioning (axial, coronal, sagittal, or oblique) may also differentially affect the visualizability of brain regions. The problems of signal dropout and other susceptibility artifacts in memory-related structures (e.g., MTL, frontal poles) also need to be addressed. Continuing improvements in scanning technology will help to diminish the effects of such issues. Conversely, activation in some brain regions that is not specifically task-related may obscure hemispheric lateralization of function. For example, exclusion of midline regions from analyses may improve fMRI language lateralization and its concordance with IAT [78].

The effect of various epileptogenic brain abnormalities (e.g., arteriovenous malformation and related flow disruption, tumor, and cortical dysplasia) on brain anatomy, function, and activation patterns is also of critical importance in evaluation of the effectiveness of fMRI activation tasks in lateralizing and localizing cognitive functions. In particular, patients with structural MRI lesions in the vicinity of brain regions of functional importance have been shown to demonstrate lower LIs and have a greater potential for discordant findings between fMRI and IAT language lateralization [158]. Specific lesion types are more problematic in this respect, including cavernomas, gliomas, mass defects, and severe atrophy.

The statistical significance threshold chosen for a given study can also alter the conclusions drawn from fMRI data in ways that are particularly salient for surgical cases. As noted previously, lowering statistical thresholds for significant activation can lead to increased observed activation, and assist in language lateralization. In some cases, however, lowering the significance threshold can lead to a spurious increase in regionally nonspecific activation, and loss of a significant LI. The need to lower the threshold for significant activation may be greater in younger subjects due to developmental differences in overall levels of observed activation, though this approach could likewise lower the LI due to increased spurious activation or activation in homologous regions in the contralateral hemisphere. Approaches to quantifying language lateralization can be differentially susceptible to changes in significance threshold [80], further highlighting the importance of consideration of this issue with relation to the method being utilized.

In addition, LIs calculated based on a region of interest approach may vary significantly depending on the region analyzed, which can include the whole hemisphere, or regions of frontal and temporal cortex, the boundaries of which are typically defined differently by individual investigators. Liégeois et al. [159] developed a method for direct statistical comparison of task-related activation to ascertain hemispheric language dominance, to circumvent difficulties with the LI approach. Utilizing direct comparison of statistical parametric maps of activation in homotopic voxels of each hemisphere, they eliminated the possible confounding effects of statistical threshold and region of interest boundaries. In a sample of eight adolescents with epilepsy, their results corresponded entirely with results from invasive language lateralization and localization techniques, including IAT and ESM. These findings are clinically meaningful, as this sample included two patients classified as right hemisphere dominant for language, and one classified as having bilateral language representation, in addition to five left hemisphere dominant patients. Therefore, similar methods may have good potential for eliminating current concerns regarding relying on fMRI results to determine language lateralization in place of the IAT. As these authors note, however, review of raw task-induced activation maps remains critical to accurate clinical interpretation of the data generated by the direct statistical comparison method.

Reliability

The question of whether or not fMRI measures of cognition produce reproducible results is also of direct relevance whenever surgical intervention is under consideration. Adcock et al. [77] studied subjects at two time points, about three months apart, using the same fMRI verbal fluency probe. All laterality classifications were in agreement at both points (i.e., laterality categorizations were 100% reliable), with good correlation between LIs between the two studies for all study groups (LTLE, RTLE, and controls). It is important to consider whether laterality conclusions are based on spatial extent of activation (within a whole hemisphere or just a specified region of interest) or magnitude of signal change. The findings from this study suggest that the magnitude of signal change method may be more reproducible. As previously noted, this is in part related to the statistical significance threshold chosen, which dictates the spatial extent of observed activation.

In a sophisticated statistical approach to analyzing the reproducibility of fMRI activation patterns, Fernandez et al. [160] examined the reliability of fMRI lateralization of language functions within and between individual subjects and within and between scanning sessions. They administered a semantic judgment task to 34 epilepsy patients on one occasion and to 12 other patients at two separate scanning sessions on the same day using alternate task forms. Results demonstrated good within-test and test-retest reliability of task-related activation patterns. For test-retest patients, a significant amount of overlap was noted between the first and second evaluations on a voxel-by-voxel basis, with higher significance levels for activation in frontal (e.g., Broca's area, premotor region) than more posterior regions (temporoparietal cortex). This method provided similarly reliable activation patterns for patients with right or mixed hemisphere dominance for language as those with left hemisphere dominance. The authors point out, however, that fMRI may activate some, but not necessarily all, brain regions participating in a given function, and so recommend caution in replacing deactivation procedures (e.g., ESM) entirely for planning surgical resection margins. Furthermore, they note that their data cannot speak to the definition of such surgical margins, as the normalization paradigm required for group statistical analysis introduces spatial distortion of individual activation data.

It should be noted, however, that such spatial normalization is not required for fMRI, and analyses can be performed in native brain space, as is typically done for individual presurgical cases. With regard to setting the surgical margin, the statistical threshold chosen will necessarily affect degree and extent of activation observed. As the overall level of observed fMRI brain activation varies widely between individuals, it is generally not considered appropriate or feasible to set the same a priori threshold for all subjects. Rutten et al. [161] examined fMRI activation patterns in the temporal lobes in nonnormalized scans as compared to ESM. Their study demonstrated a specificity of 61% of subjects, and false-positive activation in 51%, suggesting that fMRI cannot yet be used for direct delineation of the surgical resection margin. Fernandez et al. [160] suggest that one method to alleviate this difficulty would be to create individualized normalization of language regions in relation to brain regions with known, quantifiable relationships between fMRI task stimulation and activation response (e.g., primary visual cortex, where a linear relationship has been demonstrated between changes in neural activity and fMRI signal [162]).

Clinical and Epilepsy-Specific Factors

Future studies examining the potential for fMRI to replace the IAT will also need to address issues related to neurodevelopmental abnormalities in cognition due to factors unique to epilepsy patients. For example, previous research [115, 118, 163, 164] has demonstrated an interaction between factors such as age at seizure onset and age at first risk factor for epilepsy (e.g., febrile convulsions, traumatic brain injury, meningitis, and encephalitis) and cognitive outcomes following temporal lobectomy. As discussed in this chapter, several studies have found that fMRI activation patterns are related to side of seizure onset and risk factors for epilepsy, and can also predict postoperative seizure and cognitive outcome. These findings point to the need for further investigation of the relationship of early risk factors for epilepsy and related abnormalities in neurodevelopment to later brain organization of cognitive functions such as language and memory. Functional MRI may be an ideal tool to study the reorganization suggested by earlier neuropsychological [115, 165] and IAT studies [166].

In pre- [77] and postoperative [167] TLE patients, fMRI studies have demonstrated significant differences between RTLE and LTLE patients and healthy controls in terms of degree of lateralization of language function, with greater bilateral language representation in LTLE patients. This supports prior data suggesting developmental reorganization of language functions in the presence of an epileptic focus in the left hemisphere [27], but also suggests that patients with a left hemisphere seizure focus many show further intra- and interhemispheric reorganization of language functions following surgical resection [167]. Increased understanding of factors that contribute to language lateralization will be important in understanding functional outcomes following neurological insult, not only in epilepsy but in other clinical populations (e.g., brain tumor, traumatic brain injury, etc.). In one study, correlation of fMRI language activation with diffusion tensor imaging (DTI, a structural MRI method for examination of white matter integrity) suggests that white matter abnormalities may be a contributing factor in language reorganization toward the right hemisphere [168]. Atypical dominance and post-surgical language outcome have been associated with earlier age of brain injury and onset of epilepsy [19, 21, 25, 28, 30, 115, 118], while atypical language lateralization has been associated with both weaker [21, 30] and stronger [29] language performance. Further research will be important to clarify the circumstances under which language reorganization improves or impairs functionality.

Functional MRI studies have also demonstrated significant differences in brain connectivity in epilepsy, which should be considered when interpreting presurgical mapping data. In one study, even though language activation maps were generally similar between LTLE patients and controls, resting functional connectivity analysis showed diminished connectivity in patients, perhaps reflective of underlying disruption of the language network [169]. Similarly, Vlooswijk et al. [170] reported on a comparison of 34 epilepsy patients and 20 healthy controls using word generation and reading fMRI tasks. While activation maps were not different between groups, connectivity analyses showed decreased connectivity in patients relative to controls, which related to neuropsychological measures of language function. Other studies have likewise demonstrated alterations in resting and task-related connectivity in TLE relative to healthy individuals [171–175], which show a relationship to measures of white matter integrity [173] and cognitive function [175]. Such disruptions in connectivity have also been examined with relation to postoperative cognitive changes. Wagner et al. [176] found that TLE patients who showed higher task-related coupling between hippocampus and superior temporal gyrus (Brodmann's area 22) preoperatively were more likely to show decreased verbal learning postoperatively. This finding is consistent with prior work indicating that individuals with more intact brain structure and function preoperatively are at greater risk for postsurgical cognitive decline. Other work has also shown alterations in connectivity related to specific epileptic pathology (hippocampal sclerosis) [177], demonstrating potential remote functional effects of localized structural pathology. Hippocampal coupling has been shown to be related to clinical variables in TLE, such that interhippocampal connectivity was positively correlated with age at seizure onset and negatively correlated with disease duration [178]. Such work suggests that differences in brain connectivity are an important consideration when evaluating fMRI maps gained as part of presurgical evaluation, and indicates that patients with focal onset seizures can show disruption in a much broader neural network, which has implications for treatment and assessment of potential postoperative cognitive changes.

Functional MRI studies of cognition in epilepsy have generally not explicitly addressed the potential contribution of antiepileptic drugs (AEDs) to observed activation patterns. AEDs have known or presumed effects on cerebral blood flow and metabolism [179–184], though at present these effects remain unelucidated or poorly understood for many medications. Direct or indirect effects on cortical blood flow may differentially affect the observed BOLD response in epilepsy patients in comparison to healthy, medication-free control subjects. There are differences between AEDs in the nature and extent of influence on neural activity, cortical blood flow, and metabolism, and the role these mechanisms play in the BOLD response requires systematic investigation. This potential confound has not been directly addressed in fMRI studies of epilepsy patients.

Weaker magnitude of fMRI activation has been demonstrated in TLE patients relative to control groups (e.g., [29, 77]). While the reasons for this discrepancy are unclear, factors related to primary CNS dysfunction such as refractory epilepsy and its treatment must be considered, including the potential effects of antiepileptic medications on fMRI brain activation patterns. In one study, patients found to have bilateral language representation on IAT showed weaker fMRI activation than those strongly lateralized to either hemisphere [95]. These observed differences in the strength of activation among epilepsy patients and between patient and control groups also highlight the importance of careful consideration of the statistical significance threshold chosen for analysis of both group and individual fMRI activation maps in this population. Use of lower activation thresholds may be appropriate in patient populations, to detect weaker levels of activation and assist in lateralization of language. On the other hand, use of lower statistical thresholds has been shown in several studies to weaken LIs, and may therefore potentially damage interpretation of laterality categorizations [20, 38, 77]. It may be appropriate to examine a range of thresholds to enhance clinical interpretation. This issue warrants detailed empirical analysis in future studies.

Sex differences in brain language organization also merit consideration when using presurgical IAT results to assess feasibility of surgery or predict postsurgical risk for cognitive deficits [185, 186]. Baxter et al. [187] have utilized fMRI to examine brain activation during a semantic processing task in healthy adult subjects, to assess the applicability of models of intra- versus interhemispheric sex differences in language organization. The results of this study offered some support for both models of language organization; females showed greater bilateral representation of language functions, while males demonstrated more diffuse activation within the left hemisphere. These findings are consistent with previous studies demonstrating sex differences in language lateralization, which may affect predictions regarding cognitive outcome following epilepsy surgery and warrant consideration in presurgical evaluation.

As mentioned previously, it can be difficult to directly compare fMRI and IAT results, as different aspects of language and memory functioning are typically measured in these paradigms. In addition, given the current state of fMRI technology, observed activation patterns may reflect not only activation of regions critical for the function under examination, but also activation of areas related to other functions tapped by a particular fMRI task. For example, some language tasks may reflect brain activation related to attention and planning functions rather than language per se [188]. It may therefore be possible to include some activated areas within the resection margin, to increase the likelihood of obtaining seizure control, without leading to impairment in language and/or memory (though such resection may affect other cognitive functions). Further, brain regions important for a given function may fail to activate during a particular task, suggesting that appropriate caution must be used when interpreting fMRI findings as they relate to surgical intervention. As noted elsewhere in this chapter, task selection is a critically important factor in use of fMRI to localize brain regions specific to a particular cognitive process. Consideration must be given to how well the task paradigm taps the function of interest, and whether control condition(s) adequately address other potentially confounding factors (see prior discussion of auditory versus visual language tasks). In addition, task selection must consider the developmental level and cognitive capacity of the subject population. As already noted, tasks which are particularly complex or require acquired skills such as reading may be inappropriate for use in young children or cognitively impaired patients.

Conclusion: Can We Replace the IAT with fMRI?

The potential for replacement of the IAT with fMRI is quite different for language versus memory. The now extensive language literature indicates that in most cases fMRI can lateralize language as well as IAT and can provide additional information regarding localization of language-critical regions that cannot be obtained with IAT (see Table 11.4 for literature of key significance). For both fMRI and IAT, attempts to lateralize language are nondiagnostic in some cases. In the absence of technical difficulties (for either method) this circumstance is mostly likely in patients with bilateral language representation of

Table 11.4 Summary of key literature

Authors	Article title	Significance
Chelune 1995 [152]	Hippocampal adequacy versus functional reserve: predicting memory functions following temporal lobectomy. Archives of Clinical Neuropsychology 10(5): 413–432	Description of theoretical models of memory functioning in epilepsy (hippocampal adequacy and functional reserve) and their utility for predicting postsurgical outcome
Desmond 1995 [75]	Functional MRI measurement of language lateralization in Wada-tested patients. Brain 118(Pt 6):1411–1419	Seminal early paper demonstrating concordance of fMRI and IAT language lateralization results
Binder et al. 1996 [10]	Determination of language dominance using functional MRI: a comparison with the Wada test. Neurology 46(4): 978–984	Seminal early paper demonstrating concordance of fMRI and IAT language lateralization results
Simkins-Bullock 2000 [13]	Beyond speech lateralization: a review of the variability, reliability, and validity of the intracarotid amobarbital procedure and its nonlanguage uses in epilepsy surgery candidates. Neuropsychology Review 10(1):41–74	Review of clinical uses of the IAT, limitations of IAT-related research, and future directions
Deblaere et al. 2002 [191]	Developing a comprehensive presurgical functional MRI protocol for patients with intractable temporal lobe epilepsy: a pilot study. Neuroradiology 44(8):667–673	Presents an integrated language and memory fMRI exam for potential use in presurgical planning
Woermann et al. 2003 [28]	Language lateralization by Wada test and fMRI in 100 patients with epilepsy. Neurology 61(5):699–701	Largest series to date demonstrating concordance of fMRI and IAT language lateralization results
Gaillard et al. 2007 [21]	Atypical language in lesional and nonlesional complex partial epilepsy. Neurology 69(18):1761–1771	Large series examining fMRI activation patterns on language probes in relation to clinical variables, specifically with regard to language reorganization
Kesavadas et al. 2007 [2]	Real-time functional MR imaging (fMRI) for presurgical evaluation of paediatric epilepsy. Pediatric Radiology 37(10):964–974	Exploration of the potential utility of real-time fMRI for presurgical mapping in epilepsy
Binder et al. 2008 [143]	Use of preoperative functional MRI to predict verbal memory decline after temporal lobe epilepsy surgery. Epilepsia 49(8):1377–1394	Examination of the utility of fMRI activation patterns to predict memory outcomes after epilepsy surgery
Mechanic-Hamilton et al. 2009 [136]	Hippocampal volumetry and functional MRI of memory in temporal lobe epilepsy. Epilepsy & Behavior 16(1): 128–138	Integrated assessment of structural and functional MRI with relation to postsurgical cognitive outcome

language, including those with hemispheric dissociation of receptive and expressive language. As noted previously, a number of epilepsy centers now opt to forego IAT in favor of fMRI in cases where the seizure focus is thought to be in the nondominant hemisphere (typically right hemisphere onset cases), or where memory functioning is less of a concern (i.e., extratemporal seizure onset). Functional MRI does not yet have the proven reliability and validity required to replace current techniques used for setting the surgical margin, including ESM. Data are present, however, indicating that fMRI language activation patterns are predictive of postoperative language outcome, as has previously been shown for IAT. Creation of memory paradigms capable of serving the function of the IAT has proved more challenging. This is in part due to the core difference of the testing methods of fMRI and the IAT (i.e., examination of memory functioning in the context of whole-brain activation versus assessment of each hemisphere while the other is anesthetized). The available literature provides promising data suggesting that fMRI may eventually be able to predict risk of postoperative memory changes, and thus supplant the IAT. However, further investigation is necessary to ascertain the functional utility of these data with regard to surgical planning and outcome, and to extend the applicability to pediatric populations.

Evidence-based standards for the recommendation of new diagnostic tests and treatments have been articulated by relevant professional organizations [189], with the highest (Class I) standard being prospective, randomized controlled clinical trials (RCTs), with masked outcome assessment. Clearly, none of the fMRI research discussed previously meets these stringent standards, but rather falls at the Class IV level (reports of case series). The IAT has likewise never undergone Class I trials, but has become the de facto clinical standard due to its long history and the lack of available alternatives. As with fMRI, a few case studies (e.g., [190]) are available demonstrating reproducibility of IAT results and offering evidence towards reliability and validity. Based on the currently available data it seems unlikely that the field will reach near-term consensus in terms of the acceptability of replacing the IAT with fMRI, particularly for memory. The early results are promising, however, and much more systematic research is needed, including RCTs. A true "gold standard" for language and memory localization will only be ascertained through systematic assessment of postsurgical outcome data in relation to presurgical localization data, a task that has not yet been adequately completed for the IAT or for fMRI.

Overall, it seems likely that optimal fMRI paradigms designed to replace the IAT will include multiple language and memory tasks, to elicit activation of broad neural networks including frontal and temporal language and memory circuitry. Future directions in the development of an fMRI paradigm to replace the IAT may be similar to work recently conducted by Deblaere et al. [191]. In a study unique in its attempt to include fMRI measures for both language and memory functioning, these authors utilized a group of activation paradigms, including complex scene encoding, picture naming, reading, word generation, and semantic decision-making tasks. While this study included only healthy control subjects its findings are promising for future research, as these investigators were able to demonstrate bilateral MTL activation consistent with prior studies [121, 122] during memory encoding, as well as robust language lateralization. While IAT results are obviously not available for comparison, the authors note their intention to utilize this group of fMRI tasks with epilepsy patients, to attempt to determine its feasibility in replicating and eventually replacing the IAT. Furthermore, one criticism of fMRI in attempts to replace the IAT has been the time-consuming and labor-intensive nature of image postprocessing. Functional MRI software analysis packages have grown increasingly sophisticated and amenable to batch data processing, dramatically reducing the time needed for postprocessing, such that in most cases fMRI processing time requirements are comparable to the time requirement for bilateral IAT. Preliminary work using real-time fMRI for language lateralization as well as sensorimotor and visual mapping also suggests that in well-selected cases this level of postprocessing may not be necessary [2, 192], potentially making fMRI more cost-effective and accessible for routine presurgical planning and allowing it to be used more widely.

Future clinical research will continue to demonstrate the value of fMRI as a tool for preoperative assessment of language and memory, as well as other eloquent cortical functions, in various neurosurgical contexts. We expect to see increasing use of fMRI combined with structural imaging and other advanced diagnostic modalities. As an example of the potential of such approaches, Kamada et al. [88] report on a series of 22 patients with lesions adjacent to the arcuate fasciculus in the language-dominant hemisphere. Localization of frontal and temporal language regions was achieved through the use of fMRI and MEG, and this information was utilized in combination with DTI to visualize the arcuate fasciculus. Functional MRI and MEG language lateralization findings were 100% concordant with IAT results. In two patients, the structural and functional neuroimaging data were imported into the surgical navigation system, and ESM confirmed localization of language regions (stimulation of expressive language regions shown by fMRI produced speech arrest, while stimulation of regions near the arcuate fasciculus as shown by DTI produced naming deficits without speech arrest). Further technical advances in field strength, gradient and radiofrequency coils, software, and cognitive paradigms will improve fMRI's sensitivity and specificity. In the not too distant future, accurate results of preoperative fMRI mapping will be registered in the neurosurgeon's computer and microscope and will be routinely used to guide surgery.

Acknowledgments This work was supported in part by members of the Partnership for Pediatric Epilepsy Research, which includes the American Epilepsy Society, the Epilepsy Foundation, the Epilepsy Project, Fight Against Childhood Epilepsy and Seizures (f.a.c.e.s.), and Parents Against Childhood Epilepsy (P.A.C.E.). Aspects of this work were also supported by the Indiana Economic Development Corporation (grant #87884), the National Alliance for Medical Image Computing (NAMIC; NIH grant U54 EB005149), and the Hitchcock Foundation. The authors thank their colleagues in the Surgical Epilepsy Programs at Indiana University Medical Center and Dartmouth-Hitchcock Medical Center for their contributions to the data presented in this chapter.

References

1. Medina LS, Aguirre E, Bernal B, Altman NR. Functional MR imaging versus Wada test for evaluation of language lateralization: cost analysis. Radiology. 2004;230(1):49–54.
2. Kesavadas C, Thomas B, Sujesh S, et al. Real-time functional MR imaging (fMRI) for presurgical evaluation of paediatric epilepsy. Pediatr Radiol. 2007; 37(10):964–74.
3. Wellmer J, Fernandez G, Linke DB, Urbach H, Elger CE, Kurthen M. Unilateral intracarotid amobarbital procedure for language lateralization. Epilepsia. 2005;46(11):1764–72.
4. Loring DW, Meador KJ, Lee GP, King DW. Amobarbital effects and lateralized brain function: The Wada test. New York: Springer-Verlag; 1992.
5. van Emde Boas W, Juhn A. Wada and the Sodium Amytal Test The first (and last?) 50 years. J Hist Neurosci. 1999;8(3):286–92.
6. Gardner WJ. Injection of procaine into the brain to locate speech area in left-handed persons. Arch Neurol Psychiatry. 1941;46:1035–8.
7. Wada J, Rasmussen T. Intracarotid injection of Sodium Amytal for the lateralization of cerebral speech dominance. J Neurosurg. 1960;17:266–82.
8. Milner B, Branch C, Rasmussen T. Study of short-term memory after intracarotid injection of Sodium Amytal. Trans Am Neurol Assoc. 1962;87: 224–6.
9. Sperling MR, Saykin AJ, Glosser G, et al. Predictors of outcome after anterior temporal lobectomy: The intracarotid amobarbital test. Neurology. 1994; 44(12):2325–30.
10. Binder JR, Swanson SJ, Hammeke TA, et al. Determination of language dominance using functional MRI: a comparison with the Wada test. Neurology. 1996;46(4):978–84.
11. Yetkin FZ, Swanson S, Fischer M, et al. Functional MR of frontal lobe activation: comparison with Wada language results. AJNR Am J Neuroradiol. 1998;19(6):1095–8.
12. Rausch R, Risinger M. Intracarotid sodium amobarbital procedure. In: Boulton AA, Baker GB, Hiscock M, editors. Neuropsychology. Clifton, NJ: The Humana Press; 1990. p. 127–46.
13. Simkins-Bullock J. Beyond speech lateralization: a review of the variability, reliability, and validity of the intracarotid amobarbital procedure and its non-language uses in epilepsy surgery candidates. Neuropsychol Rev. 2000;10(1):41–74.
14. Surgery for epilepsy. NIH Consensus Statement Online. Mar 19–21 1990;8(2):1–20.
15. Assessment: Neuropsychological testing of adults. Considerations for neurologists. Report of the Therapeutics and Technology Assessment Subcommittee of the American Academy of Neurology. Neurology. 1996;47(2):592–599.

16. Rausch R. Role of the neuropsychological evaluation and the intracarotid sodium amobarbital procedure in the surgical treatment for epilepsy. Epilepsy Res Suppl. 1992;5:77–86.
17. Tatum IV WO, Benbadis SR, Vale FL. The neurosurgical treatment of epilepsy. Arch Fam Med. 2000; 9(10):1142–7.
18. Carpentier A, Pugh KR, Westerveld M, et al. Functional MRI of language processing: dependence on input modality and temporal lobe epilepsy. Epilepsia. 2001;42(10):1241–54.
19. Devinsky O, Perrine K, Llinas R, Luciano DJ, Dogali M. Anterior temporal language areas in patients with early onset of temporal lobe epilepsy. Ann Neurol. 1993;34(5):727–32.
20. Gaillard WD, Balsamo L, Xu B, et al. Language dominance in partial epilepsy patients identified with an fMRI reading task. Neurology. 2002;59(2): 256–65.
21. Gaillard WD, Berl MM, Moore EN, et al. Atypical language in lesional and nonlesional complex partial epilepsy. Neurology. 2007;69(18):1761–71.
22. Mizrahi EM, Kellaway P, Grossman RG, et al. Anterior temporal lobectomy and medically refractory temporal lobe epilepsy of childhood. Epilepsia. 1990;31(3):302–12.
23. Rasmussen T, Milner B. The role of early left-brain injury in determining lateralization of cerebral speech functions. Ann NY Acad Sci. 1977;299: 355–69.
24. Satz P, Strauss E, Wada J, Orsini DL. Some correlates of intra- and interhemispheric speech organization after left focal brain injury. Neuropsychologia. 1988;26(2):345–50.
25. Springer JA, Binder JR, Hammeke TA, et al. Language dominance in neurologically normal and epilepsy subjects: a functional MRI study. Brain. 1999;122(Pt 11):2033–46.
26. Woods RP, Dodrill CB, Ojemann GA. Brain injury, handedness, and speech lateralization in a series of amobarbital studies. Ann Neurol. 1988;23(5):510–8.
27. Sabbah P, Chassoux F, Leveque C, et al. Functional MR imaging in assessment of language dominance in epileptic patients. Neuroimage. 2003;18(2):460–7.
28. Woermann FG, Jokeit H, Luerding R, et al. Language lateralization by Wada test and fMRI in 100 patients with epilepsy. Neurology. 2003;61(5):699–701.
29. Thivard L, Hombrouck J, du Montcel ST, et al. Productive and perceptive language reorganization in temporal lobe epilepsy. Neuroimage. 2005;24(3): 841–51.
30. Swanson SJ, Binder JR, Possing ET, et al. fMRI language laterality during a semantic task: Age of onset and side of seizure focus effects. J Int Neuropsychol Soc. 2002;8(2):222.
31. Pujol J, Deus J, Losilla JM, Capdevila A. Cerebral lateralization of language in normal left-handed people studied by functional MRI. Neurology. 1999; 52(5):1038–43.
32. Szaflarski JP, Binder JR, Possing ET, McKiernan KA, Ward BD, Hammeke TA. Language lateralization in left-handed and ambidextrous people: fMRI data. Neurology. 2002;59(2):238–44.
33. Knecht S, Drager B, Deppe M, et al. Handedness and hemispheric language dominance in healthy humans. Brain. 2000;123(Pt 12):2512–8.
34. Knecht S, Deppe M, Drager B, et al. Language lateralization in healthy right-handers. Brain. 2000;123(Pt 1):74–81.
35. Binder JR, Rao SM, Hammeke TA, et al. Lateralized human brain language systems demonstrated by task subtraction functional magnetic resonance imaging. Arch Neurol. 1995;52(6):593–601.
36. Gaillard WD, Hertz-Pannier L, Mott SH, Barnett AS, LeBihan D, Theodore WH. Functional anatomy of cognitive development: fMRI of verbal fluency in children and adults. Neurology. 2000;54(1):180–5.
37. Grandin CB, Gaillard WD, Hunter KE, et al. Comparison of phonemic and semantic verbal fluency tasks: An fMRI study. Neuroimage. 1998;7:S133.
38. Hertz-Pannier L, Gaillard WD, Mott SH, et al. Noninvasive assessment of language dominance in children and adolescents with functional MRI: a preliminary study. Neurology. 1997;48(4):1003–12.
39. Beauregard M, Chertkow H, Bub D, Murtha S, Dixon R, Evans A. The neural substrate for concrete, abstract, and emotional word lexica: A positron emission tomography study. J Cogn Neurosci. 1997; 9(4):441–61.
40 Beeman M. Semantic processing in the right hemisphere may contribute to drawing inferences from discourse. Brain Lang. 1993;44(1):80–120.
41. Beeman M, Friedman RB, Grafman J, Perez E, Diamond S, Lindsay MB. Summation priming and coarse coding in the right hemisphere. J Cogn Neurosci. 1994;6(1):26–45.
42. Fletcher PC, Happe F, Frith U, et al. Other minds in the brain: A functional imaging study of "theory of mind" in story comprehension. Cognition. 1995; 57(2):109–28.
43 Gaillard WD, Pugliese M, Grandin CB, et al. Cortical localization of reading in normal children: an fMRI language study. Neurology. 2001;57(1):47–54.
44. Just MA, Carpenter PA, Keller TA, Eddy WF, Thulborn KR. Brain activation modulated by sentence comprehension. Science. 1996;274(5284):114–6.
45. Ross ED, Mesulam MM. Dominant language functions of the right hemisphere? Prosody and emotional gesturing. Arch Neurol. 1979;36(3):144–8.
46. Scoville W, Milner B. Loss of recent memory after bilateral hippocampal lesions. J Neurol Neurosurg Psychiatry. 1957;20:11–21.
47. Loddenkemper T, Morris 3rd HH, Perl 2nd J. Carotid artery dissection after the intracarotid amobarbital test. Neurology. 2002;59(11):1797–8.
48. Morris P. Practical neuroangiography. Baltimore: Williams & Wilkins; 1997.
49. Rausch R, Silfvenius H, Wieser H-G, Dodrill CB, Meador KJ, Jones-Gotman M. Intraarterial amobarbital procedures. In: Engel Jr J, editor. Surgical treatment of the epilepsies. 2nd ed. New York: Raven Press, Ltd.; 1993. p. 341–57.

50. Bookheimer S, Schrader LM, Rausch R, Sankar R, Engel Jr J. Reduced anesthetization during the intracarotid amobarbital (Wada) test in patients taking carbonic anhydrase-inhibiting medications. Epilepsia. 2005;46(2):236–43.
51. Saykin AJ, Sussman NM, Gur RC. Neuropsychological methods in temporal lobectomy: Comparison of traditional batteries and specialized procedures. J Clin Exp Neuropsychol. 1987; 9(1):33–4.
52. Kimura D. Right temporal damage. Arch Neurol. 1963;8:264–71.
53. Green D, Swets J. Signal detection theory and psychophysics. New York: Krieger; 1974.
54. Gerschlager W, Lalouschek W, Lehrner J, Baumgartner C, Lindinger G, Lang W. Language-related hemispheric asymmetry in healthy subjects and patients with temporal lobe epilepsy as studied by event-related brain potentials and intracarotid amobarbital test. Electroencephalogr Clin Neurophysiol. 1998;108(3): 274–82.
55. Epstein CM, Woodard JL, Stringer AY, et al. Repetitive transcranial magnetic stimulation does not replicate the Wada test. Neurology. 2000;55(7): 1025–7.
56. Jennum P, Friberg L, Fuglsang-Frederiksen A, Dam M. Speech localization using repetitive transcranial magnetic stimulation. Neurology. 1994; 44(2):269–73.
57. Pascual-Leone A, Gates JR, Dhuna A. Induction of speech arrest and counting errors with rapid-rate transcranial magnetic stimulation. Neurology. 1991; 41(5):697–702.
58. Bishop DVM, Watt H, Papadatou-Pastou M. An efficient and reliable method for measuring cerebral lateralization during speech with functional transcranial Doppler ultrasound. Neuropsychologia. 2009;47(2): 587–90.
59. Deppe M, Knecht S, Papke K, et al. Assessment of hemispheric language lateralization: a comparison between fMRI and fTCD. J Cereb Blood Flow Metab. 2000;20(2):263–8.
60. Haag A, Moeller N, Knake S, et al. Language lateralization in children using functional transcranial Doppler sonography. Dev Med Child Neurol. 2010;52(4):331–6.
61. Knake S, Haag A, Hamer HM, et al. Language lateralization in patients with temporal lobe epilepsy: a comparison of functional transcranial Doppler sonography and the Wada test. Neuroimage. 2003; 19(3):1228–32.
62. Knecht S, Deppe M, Ebner A, et al. Noninvasive determination of language lateralization by functional transcranial Doppler sonography: a comparison with the Wada test. Stroke. 1998;29(1):82–6.
63. Rihs F, Sturzenegger M, Gutbrod K, Schroth G, Mattle HP. Determination of language dominance: Wada test confirms functional transcranial Doppler sonography. Neurology. 1999;52(8):1591–6.
64. Kamada K, Sawamura Y, Takeuchi F, et al. Expressive and receptive language areas determined by a non-invasive reliable method using functional magnetic resonance imaging and magnetoencephalography. Neurosurgery. 2007;60(2):296–305.
65. Gallagher A, Theriault M, Maclin E, et al. Near-infrared spectroscopy as an alternative to the Wada test for language mapping in children, adults and special populations. Epileptic Disord. 2007;9(3):241–55.
66. Gallagher A, Bastien D, Pelletier I, et al. A noninvasive, presurgical expressive and receptive language investigation in a 9-year-old epileptic boy using near-infrared spectroscopy. Epilepsy Behav. 2008; 12(2):340–6.
67. Watanabe E, Maki A, Kawaguchi F, et al. Non-invasive assessment of language dominance with near-infrared spectroscopic mapping. Neurosci Lett. 1998;256(1):49–52.
68. Akanuma N, Reed LJ, Marsden PK, et al. Hemisphere-specific episodic memory networks in the human brain: a correlation study between intracarotid amobarbital test and [(18)F]FDG-PET. J Cogn Neurosci. 2009;21(3):605–22.
69. Duncan JD, Moss SD, Bandy DJ, et al. Use of positron emission tomography for presurgical localization of eloquent brain areas in children with seizures. Pediatr Neurosurg. 1997;26(3):144–56.
70. Hong SB, Roh SY, Kim SE, Seo DW. Correlation of temporal lobe glucose metabolism with the Wada memory test. Epilepsia. 2000;41(12):1554–9.
71. Hunter KE, Blaxton TA, Bookheimer SY, et al. (15)O water positron emission tomography in language localization: A study comparing positron emission tomography visual and computerized region of interest analysis with the Wada test. Ann Neurol. 1999;45(5):662–5.
72. Kaplan AM, Bandy DJ, Manwaring KH, et al. Functional brain mapping using positron emission tomography scanning in preoperative neurosurgical planning for pediatric brain tumors. J Neurosurg. 1999;91(5):797–803.
73. Pardo JV, Fox PT. Preoperative assessment of the cerebral hemispheric dominance for language with CBF PET. Hum Brain Mapp. 1993;1:57–68.
74. Tatlidil R, Xiong J, Luther S. Presurgical lateralization of seizure focus and language dominant hemisphere with O-15 water PET imaging. Acta Neurol Scand. 2000;102(2):73–80.
75. Desmond JE, Sum JM, Wagner AD, et al. Functional MRI measurement of language lateralization in Wada-tested patients. Brain. 1995;118(Pt 6): 1411–9.
76. Benbadis SR, Binder JR, Swanson SJ, et al. Is speech arrest during wada testing a valid method for determining hemispheric representation of language? Brain Lang. 1998;65(3):441–6.
77. Adcock JE, Wise RG, Oxbury JM, Oxbury SM, Matthews PM. Quantitative fMRI assessment of the differences in lateralization of language-related brain activation in patients with temporal lobe epilepsy. Neuroimage. 2003;18(2):423–38.
78. Arora J, Pugh K, Westerveld M, Spencer S, Spencer DD, Todd Constable R. Language lateralization in

epilepsy patients: fMRI validated with the Wada procedure. Epilepsia. 2009;50(10):2225–41.
79. Baciu M, Kahane P, Minotti L, et al. Functional MRI assessment of the hemispheric predominance for language in epileptic patients using a simple rhyme detection task. Epileptic Disord. 2001; 3(3):117–24.
80. Baciu MV, Watson JM, Maccotta L, et al. Evaluating functional MRI procedures for assessing hemispheric language dominance in neurosurgical patients. Neuroradiology. 2005;47(11):835–44.
81. Bahn MM, Lin W, Silbergeld DL, et al. Localization of language cortices by functional MR imaging compared with intracarotid amobarbital hemispheric sedation. AJR Am J Roentgenol. 1997;169(2): 575–9.
82. Benson RR, FitzGerald DB, LeSueur LL, et al. Language dominance determined by whole brain functional MRI in patients with brain lesions. Neurology. 1999;52(4):798–809.
83. Brockway JP. Two functional magnetic resonance imaging f(MRI) tasks that may replace the gold standard, Wada testing, for language lateralization while giving additional localization information. Brain Cogn. 2000;43(1–3):57–9.
84. Chlebus P, Mikl M, Brazdil M, Pazourkova M, Krupa P, Rektor I. fMRI evaluation of hemispheric language dominance using various methods of laterality index calculation. Exp Brain Res. 2007;179(3): 365–74.
85. Deblaere K, Boon PA, Vandemaele P, et al. MRI language dominance assessment in epilepsy patients at 1.0 T: region of interest analysis and comparison with intracarotid amytal testing. Neuroradiology. 2004;46(6):413–20.
86. Gao X, Jiang C, Lu C, Shen T. Determination of the dominant language hemisphere by functional MRI in patients with temporal lobe epilepsy. Chin Med J. 2001;114(7):711–3.
87. Hirsch J, Ruge MI, Kim KH, et al. An integrated functional magnetic resonance imaging procedure for preoperative mapping of cortical areas associated with tactile, motor, language, and visual functions. Neurosurgery. 2000;47(3):711–21.
88. Kamada K, Todo T, Masutani Y, et al. Visualization of the frontotemporal language fibers by tractography combined with functional magnetic resonance imaging and magnetoencephalography. J Neurosurg. 2007;106(1):90–8.
89. Lehéricy S, Cohen L, Bazin B, et al. Functional MR evaluation of temporal and frontal language dominance compared with the Wada test. Neurology. 2000;54(8):1625–33.
90. Schlosser MJ, Luby M, Spencer DD, Awad IA, McCarthy G. Comparative localization of auditory comprehension by using functional magnetic resonance imaging and cortical stimulation. J Neurosurg. 1999;91(4):626–35.
91. Suarez RO, Whalen S, Nelson AP, et al. Threshold-independent functional MRI determination of language dominance: a validation study against clinical gold standards. Epilepsy Behav. 2009; 16(2):288–97.
92. Szaflarski JP, Holland SK, Jacola LM, Lindsell C, Privitera MD, Szaflarski M. Comprehensive presurgical functional MRI language evaluation in adult patients with epilepsy. Epilepsy Behav. 2008;12(1): 74–83.
93. Benke T, Köylü B, Visani P, et al. Language lateralization in temporal lobe epilepsy: a comparison between fMRI and the Wada Test. Epilepsia. 2006;47(8):1308–19.
94. Gaillard WD, Balsamo L, Xu B, et al. fMRI language task panel improves determination of language dominance. Neurology. 2004;63(8):1403–8.
95. Rutten GJM, Ramsey NF, van Rijen PC, Alpherts WC, van Veelen CWM. fMRI-determined language lateralization in patients with unilateral or mixed language dominance according to the Wada test. Neuroimage. 2002;17(1):447–60.
96. Worthington C, Vincent DJ, Bryant AE, et al. Comparison of functional magnetic resonance imaging for language localization and intracarotid speech Amytal testing in presurgical evaluation for intractable epilepsy: Preliminary results. Stereotact Funct Neurosurg. 1997;69(1–4 Pt 2):197–201.
97. Ramsey NF, Sommer IE, Rutten GJ, Kahn RS. Combined analysis of language tasks in fMRI improves assessment of hemispheric dominance for language functions in individual subjects. Neuroimage. 2001;13(4):719–33.
98. Fitzgerald DB, Cosgrove GR, Ronner S, et al. Location of language in the cortex: A comparison between functional MR imaging and electrocortical stimulation. AJNR Am J Neuroradiol. 1997;18(8): 1529–39.
99. Biega TJ, Levy LM, Bannout F, Gaillard WD, Potolicchio SJ. Bilateral and independent Broca areas confirmed by Wada test and functional magnetic resonance imaging. J Comput Assist Tomogr. 2009;33(4):560–1.
100. Kho KH, Leijten FSS, Rutten G-J, Vermeulen J, Van Rijen P, Ramsey NF. Discrepant findings for Wada test and functional magnetic resonance imaging with regard to language function: use of electrocortical stimulation mapping to confirm results. Case Rep J Neurosurg. 2005;102(1):169–73.
101. Baciu MV, Watson JM, McDermott KB, et al. Functional MRI reveals an interhemispheric dissociation of frontal and temporal language regions in a patient with focal epilepsy. Epilepsy Behav. 2003; 4(6):776–80.
102. Kurthen M, Helmstaedter C, Linke DB, Solymosi L, Elger CE, Schramm J. Interhemispheric dissociation of expressive and receptive language functions in patients with complex-partial seizures: An amobarbital study. Brain Lang. 1992;43(4): 694–712.
103. Lee D, Swanson SJ, Sabsevitz DS, et al. Functional MRI and Wada studies in patients with interhemispheric

dissociation of language functions. Epilepsy Behav. 2008;13(2):350–6.
104. Ries ML, Boop FA, Griebel ML, et al. Functional MRI and Wada determination of language lateralization: a case of crossed dominance. Epilepsia. 2004; 45(1):85–9.
105. Staudt M, Grodd W, Niemann G, Wildgruber D, Erb M, Krageloh-Mann I. Early left periventricular brain lesions induce right hemispheric organization of speech. Neurology. 2001;57(1):122–5.
106. Spreer J, Quiske A, Altenmuller DM, et al. Unsuspected atypical hemispheric dominance for language as determined by fMRI. Epilepsia. 2001; 42(7):957–9.
107. Wellmer J, Weber B, Weis S, et al. Strongly lateralized activation in language fMRI of atypical dominant patients-implications for presurgical work-up. Epilepsy Res. 2008;80(1):67–76.
108. Medina LS, Bernal B, Ruiz J. Role of functional MR in determining language dominance in epilepsy and nonepilepsy populations: a Bayesian analysis. Radiology. 2007;242(1):94–100.
109. Benson RR, Logan WJ, Cosgrove GR, et al. Functional MRI localization of language in a 9-year-old child. Can J Neurol Sci. 1996;23(3):213–9.
110. Bookheimer SY, Dapretto M, Karmarkar U. Functional MRI in children with epilepsy. Dev Neurosci. 1999;21(3–5):191–9.
111. Gaillard WD, Grandin CB, Xu B. Developmental aspects of pediatric fMRI: Considerations for image acquisition, analysis, and interpretation. Neuroimage. 2001;13(2):239–49.
112. Hertz-Pannier L, Chiron C, Vera P, et al. Functional imaging in the work-up of childhood epilepsy. Childs Nerv Syst. 2001;17(4–5):223–8.
113. Anderson DP, Harvey AS, Saling MM, et al. FMRI lateralization of expressive language in children with cerebral lesions. Epilepsia. 2006;47(6):998–1008.
114. Baxendale S. The role of functional MRI in the presurgical investigation of temporal lobe epilepsy patients: a clinical perspective and review. J Clin Exp Neuropsychol. 2002;24(5):664–76.
115. Saykin AJ, Stafiniak P, Robinson LJ, et al. Language before and after temporal lobectomy: specificity of acute changes and relation to early risk factors. Epilepsia. 1995;36(11):1071–7.
116. Hermann BP, Wyler AR, Somes G, Clement L. Dysnomia after left anterior temporal lobectomy without functional mapping: frequency and correlates. Neurosurgery. 1994;35(1):52–6.
117. Hermann BP, Perrine K, Chelune GJ, et al. Visual confrontation naming following left anterior temporal lobectomy: a comparison of surgical approaches. Neuropsychology. 1999;13(1):3–9.
118. Stafiniak P, Saykin AJ, Sperling MR, et al. Acute naming deficits following dominant temporal lobectomy: prediction by age at 1st risk for seizures. Neurology. 1990;40(10):1509–12.
119. Sabsevitz DS, Swanson SJ, Hammeke TA, et al. Use of preoperative functional neuroimaging to predict language deficits from epilepsy surgery. Neurology. 2003;60(11):1788–92.
120. Anderson KC, Brown CP, Tallal P. Developmental language disorders: evidence for a basic processing deficit. Curr Opin Neurol Neurosurg. 1993;6(1): 98–106.
121. Detre JA, Maccotta L, King D, et al. Functional MRI lateralization of memory in temporal lobe epilepsy. Neurology. 1998;50(4):926–32.
122. Stern CE, Corkin S, Gonzalez RG, et al. The hippocampal formation participates in novel picture encoding: Evidence from functional magnetic resonance imaging. Proc Natl Acad Sci USA. 1996;93(16): 8660–5.
123. Richardson MP, Strange BA, Thompson PJ, Baxendale SA, Duncan JS, Dolan RJ. Pre-operative verbal memory fMRI predicts post-operative memory decline after left temporal lobe resection. Brain. 2004;127(Pt 11):2419–26.
124. Trenerry MR, Jack Jr CR, Ivnik RJ, et al. MRI hippocampal volumes and memory function before and after temporal lobectomy. Neurology. 1993;43(9): 1800–5.
125. Hermann BP, Wyler AR, Somes G, Berry 3rd AD, Dohan Jr FC. Pathological status of the mesial temporal lobe predicts memory outcome from left anterior temporal lobectomy. Neurosurgery. 1992;31(4): 652–6.
126. Sass KJ, Westerveld M, Buchanan CP, Spencer SS, Kim JH, Spencer DD. Degree of hippocampal neuron loss determines severity of verbal memory decrease after left anteromesiotemporal lobectomy. Epilepsia. 1994;35(6):1179–86.
127 Helmstaedter C, Elger CE. Cognitive consequences of two-thirds anterior temporal lobectomy on verbal memory in 144 patients: a three-month follow-up study. Epilepsia. 1996; 37(2):171–80.
128. Jokeit H, Ebner A, Holthausen H, et al. Individual prediction of change in delayed recall of prose passages after left-sided anterior temporal lobectomy. Neurology. 1997;49(2):481–7.
129. Bell BD, Davies KG, Haltiner AM, Walters GL. Intracarotid amobarbital procedure and prediction of postoperative memory in patients with left temporal lobe epilepsy and hippocampal sclerosis. Epilepsia. 2000;41(8):992–7.
130. Loring DW, Meador KJ, Lee GP, et al. Wada memory asymmetries predict verbal memory decline after anterior temporal lobectomy. Neurology. 1995; 45(7):1329–33.
131. Manno EM, Sperling MR, Ding X, et al. Predictors of outcome after anterior temporal lobectomy: positron emission tomography. Neurology. 1994;44(12): 2331–6.
132. Weinand ME, Carter LP. Surface cortical cerebral blood flow monitoring and single photon emission computed tomography: prognostic factors for selecting temporal lobectomy candidates. Seizure. 1994; 3(1):55–9.

133. Loring DW, Meador KJ, Lee GP, et al. Wada memory performance predicts seizure outcome following anterior temporal lobectomy. Neurology. 1994; 44(12):2322–4.
134. Killgore WD, Glosser G, Casasanto DJ, French JA, Alsop DC, Detre JA. Functional MRI and the Wada test provide complementary information for predicting post-operative seizure control. Seizure. 1999;8(8):450–5.
135. Rabin ML, Narayan VM, Kimberg DY, et al. Functional MRI predicts post-surgical memory following temporal lobectomy. Brain. 2004;127(Pt 10): 2286–98.
136. Mechanic-Hamilton D, Korczykowski M, Yushkevich PA, et al. Hippocampal volumetry and functional MRI of memory in temporal lobe epilepsy. Epilepsy Behav. 2009;16(1):128–38.
137. Szaflarski JP, Holland SK, Schmithorst VJ, Dunn RS, Privitera MD. High-resolution functional MRI at 3T in healthy and epilepsy subjects: hippocampal activation with picture encoding task. Epilepsy Behav. 2004;5(2):244–52.
138. Vannest J, Szaflarski JP, Privitera MD, Schefft BK, Holland SK. Medial temporal fMRI activation reflects memory lateralization and memory performance in patients with epilepsy. Epilepsy Behav. 2008;12(3):410–8.
139. Deblaere K, Backes WH, Tieleman A, et al. Lateralized anterior mesiotemporal lobe activation: semirandom functional MR imaging encoding paradigm in patients with temporal lobe epilepsy–initial experience. Radiology. 2005;236(3):996–1003.
140. Jokeit H, Okujava M, Woermann FG. Memory fMRI lateralizes temporal lobe epilepsy. Neurology. 2001;57(10):1786–93.
141. Janszky J, Jokeit H, Kontopoulou K, et al. Functional MRI predicts memory performance after right mesiotemporal epilepsy surgery. Epilepsia. 2005;46(2): 244–50.
142. Bellgowan PS, Binder JR, Swanson SJ, et al. Side of seizure focus predicts left medial temporal lobe activation during verbal encoding. Neurology. 1998;51(2):479–84.
143. Binder JR, Sabsevitz DS, Swanson SJ, Hammeke TA, Raghavan M, Mueller WM. Use of preoperative functional MRI to predict verbal memory decline after temporal lobe epilepsy surgery. Epilepsia. 2008;49(8):1377–94.
144. Dupont S, Van de Moortele PF, Samson S, et al. Episodic memory in left temporal lobe epilepsy: a functional MRI study. Brain. 2000;123(Pt 8): 1722–32.
145. Dupont S, Samson Y, Van de Moortele PF, et al. Delayed verbal memory retrieval: a functional MRI study in epileptic patients with structural lesions of the left medial temporal lobe. Neuroimage. 2001;14(5):995–1003.
146. Richardson MP, Strange BA, Duncan JS, Dolan RJ. Preserved verbal memory function in left medial temporal pathology involves reorganisation of function to right medial temporal lobe. Neuroimage. 2003;20 Suppl 1:S112–9.
147. Richardson MP, Strange BA, Dolan RJ. Encoding of emotional memories depends on amygdala and hippocampus and their interactions. Nat Neurosci. 2004;7(3):278–85.
148. Köylü B, Trinka E, Ischebeck A, et al. Neural correlates of verbal semantic memory in patients with temporal lobe epilepsy. Epilepsy Res. 2006; 72(2–3):178–91.
149. Köylü B, Walser G, Ischebeck A, Ortler M, Benke T. Functional imaging of semantic memory predicts postoperative episodic memory functions in chronic temporal lobe epilepsy. Brain Res. 2008;1223: 73–81.
150. Golby AJ, Poldrack RA, Illes J, Chen D, Desmond JE, Gabrieli JDE. Memory lateralization in medial temporal lobe epilepsy assessed by functional MRI. Epilepsia. 2002;43(8):855–63.
151. Branco DM, Suarez RO, Whalen S, et al. Functional MRI of memory in the hippocampus: Laterality indices may be more meaningful if calculated from whole voxel distributions. Neuroimage. 2006;32(2): 592–602.
152. Chelune GJ. Hippocampal adequacy versus functional reserve: predicting memory functions following temporal lobectomy. Arch Clin Neuropsychol. 1995;10(5):413–32.
153. McDonald BC, Saykin AJ, Jobst BC, et al. Brain activation patterns in frontal and temporal memory circuitry following temporal lobe resection for intractable epilepsy: An fMRI study. J Neuropsychiatry Clin Neurosci. 2003;15(2):282.
154. Saykin AJ, Weaver JB, Burr RB, et al. Functional magnetic resonance imaging in the evaluation of epilepsy surgery patients: A memory activation study. Epilepsia. 1994;35:86.
155. Swick D, Knight R. Contributions of prefrontal cortex to recognition memory: Electrophysiological and behavioral evidence. Neuropsychology. 1999;13(2): 155–70.
156. Martin A. Automatic activation of the medial temporal lobe during encoding: Lateralized influences of meaning and novelty. Hippocampus. 1999;9(1): 62–70.
157. McDonald BC, Saykin AJ, West JD, Sullivan JE, 3rd, Detre JA. Medial temporal lobe fMRI activation during episodic memory processing in children. Paper presented at: 37th Annual Meeting of the International Neuropsychological Society 2009; Atlanta, GA.
158. Wellmer J, Weber B, Urbach H, Reul J, Fernandez G, Elger CE. Cerebral lesions can impair fMRI-based language lateralization. Epilepsia. 2009;50(10): 2213–24.
159. Liegeois F, Connelly A, Salmond CH, Gadian DG, Vargha-Khadem F, Baldeweg T. A direct test for lateralization of language activation using fMRI: comparison with invasive assessments in children with epilepsy. Neuroimage. 2002;17(4):1861–7.

160. Fernandez G, Specht K, Weis S, et al. Intrasubject reproducibility of presurgical language lateralization and mapping using fMRI. Neurology. 2003;60(6):969–75.
161. Rutten GJM, Ramsey NF, van Rijen PC, Noordmans HJ, van Veelen CWM. Development of a functional magnetic resonance imaging protocol for intraoperative localization of critical temporoparietal language areas. Ann Neurol. 2002;51(3):350–60.
162. Boynton GM, Engel SA, Glover GH, Heeger DJ. Linear systems analysis of functional magnetic resonance imaging in human V1. J Neurosci. 1996;16(13):4207–21.
163. Saykin AJ, Gur RC, Sussman NM, O'Connor MJ, Gur RE. Memory deficits before and after temporal lobectomy: Effect of laterality and age of onset. Brain Cogn. 1989;9(2):191–200.
164. Saykin AJ, Robinson LJ, Stafiniak P, et al. Neuropsychological changes after anterior temporal lobectomy: Acute effects on memory, language, and music. In: Bennett TL, editor. The neuropsychology of epilepsy. New York: Plenum Press; 1992.
165. Hermann BP, Seidenberg M, Haltiner A, Wyler AR. Relationship of age at onset, chronologic age, and adequacy of preoperative performance to verbal memory change after anterior temporal lobectomy. Epilepsia. 1995;36(2):137–45.
166. Glosser G, Saykin A, Deutsch G, Sperling M, O'Connor M. Patterns of reorganization of memory functions within and between cerebral hemispheres as assessed by the intracarotid amobarbital test. Neuropsychology. 1995;9(4):449–56.
167. Backes WH, Deblaere K, Vonck K, et al. Language activation distributions revealed by fMRI in post-operative epilepsy patients: differences between left- and right-sided resections. Epilepsy Res. 2005;66(1–3):1–12.
168. Briellmann RS, Mitchell LA, Waites AB, et al. Correlation between language organization and diffusion tensor abnormalities in refractory partial epilepsy. Epilepsia. 2003;44(12):1541–5.
169. Waites AB, Briellmann RS, Saling MM, Abbott DF, Jackson GD. Functional connectivity networks are disrupted in left temporal lobe epilepsy. Ann Neurol. 2006;59(2):335–43.
170. Vlooswijk MCG, Jansen JFA, Majoie HJM, et al. Functional connectivity and language impairment in cryptogenic localization-related epilepsy. Neurology. 2010;75(5):395–402.
171. Bettus G, Guedj E, Joyeux F, et al. Decreased basal fMRI functional connectivity in epileptogenic networks and contralateral compensatory mechanisms. Hum Brain Mapp. 2009;30(5):1580–91.
172. Liao W, Zhang Z, Pan Z, et al. Altered functional connectivity and small-world in mesial temporal lobe epilepsy. PLoS ONE. 2010;5(1):e8525.
173. Voets NL, Adcock JE, Stacey R, et al. Functional and structural changes in the memory network associated with left temporal lobe epilepsy. Hum Brain Mapp. 2009;30(12):4070–81.
174. Zhang Z, Lu G, Zhong Y, et al. Impaired perceptual networks in temporal lobe epilepsy revealed by resting fMRI. J Neurol. 2009;256(10):1705–13.
175. Zhang Z, Lu G, Zhong Y, et al. Impaired attention network in temporal lobe epilepsy: a resting FMRI study. Neurosci Lett. 2009;458(3):97–101.
176. Wagner K, Frings L, Halsband U, et al. Hippocampal functional connectivity reflects verbal episodic memory network integrity. Neuroreport. 2007;18(16):1719–23.
177. Frings L, Schulze-Bonhage A, Spreer J, Wagner K. Remote effects of hippocampal damage on default network connectivity in the human brain. J Neurol. 2009;256(12):2021–9.
178. Frings L, Schulze-Bonhage A, Spreer J, Wagner K. Reduced interhemispheric hippocampal BOLD signal coupling related to early epilepsy onset. Seizure. 2009;18(2):153–7.
179. Ketter TA, Kimbrell TA, George MS, et al. Baseline cerebral hypermetabolism associated with carbamazepine response, and hypometabolism with nimodipine response in mood disorders. Biol Psychiatry. 1999;46(10):1364–74.
180. Matheja P, Weckesser M, Debus O, et al. Drug-induced changes in cerebral glucose consumption in bifrontal epilepsy. Epilepsia. 2000;41(5):588–93.
181. Roberts MA, Manshadi FF, Bushnell DL, Hines ME. Neurobehavioural dysfunction following mild traumatic brain injury in childhood: A case report with positive findings on positron emission tomography (PET). Brain Inj. 1995;9(5):427–36.
182. Theodore WH. Antiepileptic drugs and cerebral glucose metabolism. Epilepsia. 1988;29 Suppl 2:S48–55.
183. Theodore WH. Therapeutics: Pharmacologic. In: Mazziotta JC, Toga AW, Frackowiak RSJ, editors. Brain Mapping: The Disorders. San Diego, CA: Academic Press; 2000. p. 599–612.
184. Theodore WH, Bromfield E, Onorati L. The effect of carbamazepine on cerebral glucose metabolism. Ann Neurol. 1989;25(5):516–20.
185. Kimura D. Sex differences in cerebral organization for speech and praxic functions. Can J Psychol. 1983;37(1):19–35.
186. McGlone J. Sex differences in the cerebral organization of verbal functions in patients with unilateral brain lesions. Brain. 1977;100(4):775–93.
187. Baxter LC, Saykin AJ, Flashman LA, et al. Sex differences in semantic language processing: A functional MRI study. Brain Lang. 2003;84(2):264–72.
188. Bookheimer SY, Zeffiro TA, Blaxton T, et al. A direct comparison of PET activation and electrocortical stimulation mapping for language localization. Neurology. 1997;48(4):1056–65.
189. American Academy of Neurology. AAN Clinical Practice Handbook. St. Paul, MN: American Academy of Neurology; 1995–2003.
190. Bramham J, Morris RG. Pre- and postoperative intracarotid Amytal procedure: An assessment of validity. Epilepsy Behav. 2003;4(5):556–63.

191. Deblaere K, Backes WH, Hofman P, et al. Developing a comprehensive presurgical functional MRI protocol for patients with intractable temporal lobe epilepsy: a pilot study. Neuroradiology. 2002;44(8):667–73.

192. Fernandez G, de Greiff A, von Oertzen J, et al. Language mapping in less than 15 minutes: real-time functional MRI during routine clinical investigation. Neuroimage. 2001;14(3):585–94.

fMRI of Human Visual Pathways

12

Edgar A. DeYoe, John L. Ulmer, Wade Mueller, Lotfi Hacein-Bey, Viktor Szeder, Mary Jo Maciejewski, Karen Medler, Danielle Reitsma, and Jedediah Mathis

Introduction

Functional magnetic resonance imaging (fMRI) of the human brain provides images of changes in local blood flow and oxygenation that are evoked by sensory, motor, or cognitive events. Functional MRI has been used since 1991 [1] to identify areas of the brain that respond to visual stimulation and the performance of vision-related tasks. Increasingly, fMRI is accompanied by diffusion tensor imaging (DTI), which provides images of the speed and direction of diffusion of water molecules in the brain. Fortuitously, this allows remarkable differentiation of cerebral white mater and the delineation of a variety of major white matter tracts including vision-related pathways such as the optic radiations. This chapter focuses primarily on fMRI, but DTI data are also discussed where relevant. Together, the two methods provide a wealth of information about the anatomical and functional status of key components of the visual system in individual patients even in the presence of pathology. For example, an imaging-based map of the visual system can be helpful for planning and guiding surgical resection of tumors impacting critical vision-related brain structures. This is especially true when mass effects or previous surgeries have distorted the normal anatomy making it difficult to know where key structures are located and if they are still functional. In difficult cases, identifying the region of "closest approach" of a

E.A. DeYoe, PhD (✉) • D. Reitsma
Department of Radiology, Medical College of Wisconsin, 8701 Watertown Plank Road, Milwaukee, WI 53226, USA
e-mail: deyoe@mcw.edu; dreitsma@mcw.edu

J.L. Ulmer, MD
Medical College of Wisconsin, 8701 Watertown Plank Road, Milwaukee, WI 53226, USA
e-mail: julmer@mcw.edu

W. Mueller, MD
Department of Neurosurgery, Medical College of Wisconsin, 8701 Watertown Plank Road, Milwaukee, WI 53226, USA

L. Hacein-Bey, MD
Radiological Associates of Sacramento Medical Group Inc., 1500 Expo Parkway, Sacramento, CA 95815, USA

V. Szeder, MD, PhD
Division of Stroke, Department of Neurology, Columbia University Medical Center, 630 West 168th Street, New York, NY 10032, USA

M.J. Maciejewski, PhD
Center for Brain Health, University of Texas at Dallas, 2200 W. Mockingbird Lane, Dallas, TX 75235, USA
e-mail: mjm091000@utdallas.edu

K. Medler
Neurolab, Department of Biophysics, Medical College of Wisconsin, 8701 Watertown Plank Road, Milwaukee, WI 53226, USA
e-mail: kmedler@mcw.edu

J. Mathis
Department of Radiology (Neuro Lab), Medical College of Wisconsin, 8701 Watertown Plank Road, Milwaukee, WI 53226, USA

S.H. Faro and F.B. Mohamed (eds.), *Functional BOLD MRI: Principles and Applications*, DOI 10.1007/978-1-4939-1995-6_12,

planned resection to the cortical representation of central vision or to the optic radiations can help to minimize the risk to eloquent neural tissue and thereby avoid significant treatment-induced vision loss while still permitting maximum therapeutic effect.

However, the complexity of MRI technology and the wealth of new information it provides can leave clinicians hard pressed to stay abreast of the latest developments and applications, especially since the field continues to evolve at a brisk pace. The goal of this chapter, then, is to review clinically relevant aspects of fMRI and DTI methods and their use in mapping the visual system to aid diagnosis of vision-related central nervous system (CNS) diseases and to assist treatment planning, delivery, and follow-up. This review does not attempt to review all fMRI- and DTI-related studies of the visual system since the complete literature is quite extensive and covers a wide range of topics that are not always of direct clinical relevance. The authors apologize for the omission of any studies whose relevance may not have been apparent at the time of this writing.

At the outset, it is important to stress that both fMRI and DTI are indirect measures of the underlying neural features of interest: neuronal activation and anatomical connectivity, respectively. For fMRI, a complex sequence of cellular and chemical events link changes in neuronal activity to highly localized changes in blood flow, volume, and oxygenation. In turn, the hemodynamic changes alter local magnetic susceptibility and modify the properties of hydrogen protons that emit the signals detected by the MRI scanner. This neural/hemodynamic cascade is typically referred to as the blood oxygenation-level dependent (BOLD) mechanism and is, as yet, not fully understood [2–4]. It is important to note that the dominant aspect of neuronal activity that drives this mechanism may not necessarily be action potential firing but may include the generation of postsynaptic potentials or other factors [2]. This indirect relationship between fMRI signals and neural activity is particularly important clinically since brain pathologies can interfere with the cascade of hemodynamic events and thereby compromise the fMRI signals. Potentially, this can occur without affecting the neurons themselves. So, a failure to observe an fMRI signal does not always mean that the associated region of brain tissue is nonfunctional and can be resected without consequence. Although cases of such neurovascular uncoupling (NVU) have been documented [3, 5], their incidence in the patient population as a whole is unknown. Similarly, DTI images do not directly show axons. They do show properties of water diffusion that happen to be faster along, rather than across, axonal fiber bundles. Brain pathologies can directly alter the structural properties of fiber fascicles and destroy the anisotropic diffusion that underlies the delineation of axonal tracts. Whether this necessarily compromises axonal conduction is not clear. The important point is that the interpretation of fMRI and DTI images in a clinical context can be complicated by these issues, so awareness of the problem is essential. Accordingly, these and other interpretational issues will be highlighted as part of this review.

The chapter is divided into two sections. The first section reviews basic organizational principles of the human visual system with an emphasis on those properties that may be particularly relevant for clinical applications. Some principles, such as retinotopic organization may be generally familiar, but the ability to map this organization in detail in individual patients and its utility in specific clinical applications may be novel. Other organizational features such as the multiplicity of functionally distinct visual areas have only been revealed comprehensively in humans in recent years. The second section of the chapter focuses on specific clinical applications of visual system mapping with fMRI and presents case studies to highlight such applications. Also, included is a detailed description of methodology aimed at streamlining the clinical workflow and highlighting practical issues that should be considered to obtain high-quality data with clinical patients. The overall goal is to show how it is possible to spend as little as 10 min of fMRI scan time yet obtain information that can be invaluable for diagnosis and treatment of patients with brain tumors, arteriovenous malformations (AVMs), epilepsy, and other pathologies that can impact central visual pathways.

Functional Organization of the Human Visual System

The human visual system is composed of several distinct subsystems including: (1) the geniculostriate system, (2) the retinotectal system, (3) pupillary control systems, (4) the accommodation control system, and (5) eye movement control systems and additional subsystems that exert retinal (light) influence over circadian and endocrine functions. The reader is referred to available texts/reviews concerning the conventional anatomical structure of these various subsystems [6, 7]. Here, we focus on those aspects of human visual system organization that have come to light in recent years through neuroimaging and that may be most relevant for patient diagnosis and treatment of vision-related brain pathologies. Foremost, in this respect is identification and mapping of key cortical areas that, if damaged, could result in loss of critical visual functions thereby compromising a patient's quality of life. Such loss could include blindness within a major portion of the visual field or selective loss of specific visual functions such as face recognition, reading, or the perception of movement or color. With this uniquely clinical orientation in mind, we review those visual system organizational principles that are readily demonstrated and mapped with fMRI in individual patients.

Retinotopic Organization

Since the early 1900s, it has been known that partial damage to the human occipital lobe can produce circumscribed areas of blindness (scotomata) whose topography within the visual field is roughly predictable based on the anatomical pattern of damage [8–11]. Careful analyses of the correlation between the pattern of damage and the resulting scotomata led to the inference that the topographical arrangement of photoreceptors in the retina and, hence, the topography of the visual field is preserved in the subsequent arrangement of anatomical projections to the primary visual cortex. Later, studies of retinotopic organization led to more refined correlations [12–14], which, together with data from animal experiments [15–17], permitted identification of additional retinotopic maps beyond striate cortex. However, it was not until the advent of modern neuroimaging techniques including positron emission tomography (PET) and fMRI that the full complexity of multiple visual areas and their individual retinotopic maps in humans have begun to be appreciated [18–54].

For humans, fMRI-based mapping of the visual field is typically performed using visual stimuli consisting of a slowly expanding, flickering, checkered annulus and a slowly rotating checkered wedge as illustrated at left of Fig. 12.1a. The resulting fMRI maps (Fig. 12.1 – brain maps and Fig. 12.2a, b) are consistent with the earliest analyses of human retinotopy [9, 11]. (Note: Color codes for Figs. 12.1 and 12.2 are different. The center of gaze is blue in Fig. 12.1a but red in Fig. 12.2b.) The representation of the center of gaze (fovea) is typically located at or near the posterior tip of the occipital lobe (red colors in Fig. 12.2b) of each hemisphere with the far peripheral field represented more anteriorly near the junction of the calcarine and parieto-occipital sulci (blue/magenta colors in Fig. 12.2b). However, this cortical representation of the visual field is distorted in that locations increasingly close to the center of gaze subtend a disproportionately larger area of cortex (note large area of red in Fig. 12.2b). For example, the central 5° of the visual field occupies less than 1% of the retinal surface area but encompasses the most posterior 40% of the primary visual cortex, thus reflecting the critical importance of foveal vision [12]. In contrast, the entire monocular field (temporal crescent) from about 55° to the edge of the visible field at 100° covers only about 10% of primary visual cortex at its most anterior extent. This "cortical magnification" of the center of gaze is clinically significant in that large lesions of the posterior visual cortex can cause relatively small-sized deficits in the visual field that can be hard to demonstrate on confrontational neurological testing. Yet, they can cause major impairment of reading and other functions that require high visual acuity. Conversely,

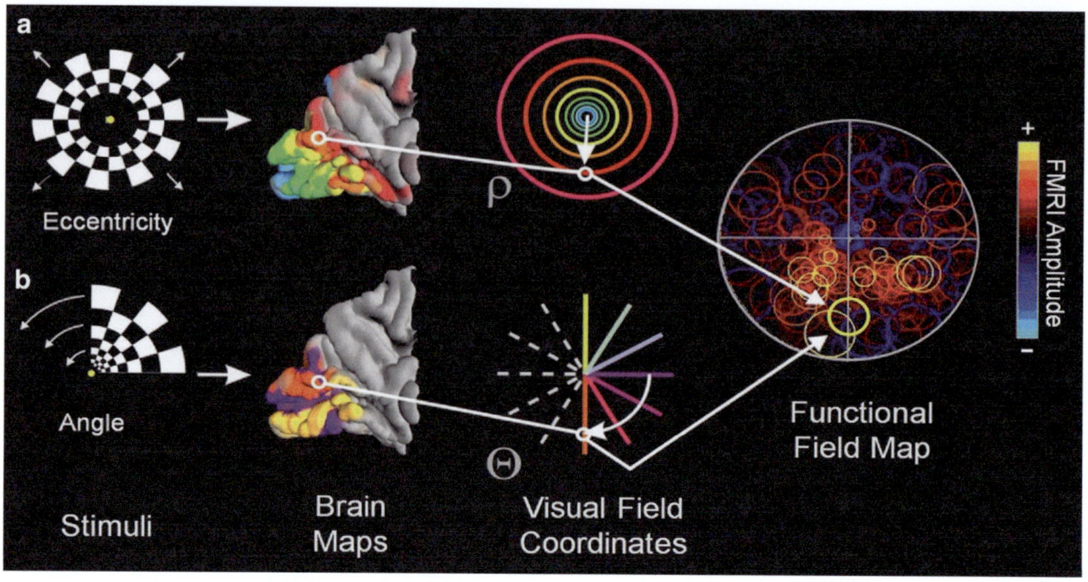

Fig. 12.1 Stimuli for visual field mapping and construction of functional field maps (FFMaps). Retinotopic mapping stimuli consist of an expanding, black-and-white, checkered annulus (**a**) or a rotating wedge (**b**) counterphase flickered at 6 Hz presented in a temporal phase mapping paradigm. A single expansion/rotation sequence takes 32 s and is repeated five times within a 168 s scan run. (The initial 8 s of the scan containing the equilibration transient are discarded.) Outer boundary of stimuli extends to 20° eccentricity. Expanding annuli are not scaled linearly in size and eccentricity but, rather, are scaled nonlinearly so as to activate roughly equal areas of V1 as estimated using the retino-cortical mapping function of Balasubramanian et al. [148]. The subject's task during each mapping sequence is to fix a small dot at the center of the display and press a button when the dot blinks off for 0.125 s varied randomly every 4–8 s. This task helps ensure that the patient attends to the mapping stimulus and maintains gaze at the center of the display. Postprocessing of the resulting fMRI data (see text) yields an estimate of the visual field coordinates (eccentricity [rho], angle [theta]) at which the mapping stimuli activate each voxel most strongly. Using these coordinates, a *circle symbol* can be placed at the corresponding location on a diagram of the patient's view of the stimulus display (*right*). The symbol is colored to show the amplitude of the fMRI response according to the pseudocolor scale at *right*. The size of the symbol represents the error in estimating the preferred stimulus location for that voxel (approximately 70% confidence interval). Symbols for all visually responsive voxels are placed on the diagram to yield a functional field map (FFMap) that allows the physician to determine instantly if the patient's visual cortex is responding to all locations within his/her field of view

lesions of anterior occipital cortex can cause blindness in large portions of the peripheral visual field but may be well-tolerated or even unnoticed unless the patient's activities rely heavily on peripheral vision (e.g., truck driver).

fMRI mapping with a rotating checkered wedge produces a brain map with information that is complementary to that provided by the annular stimulus (Figs. 12.1b and 12.2a. Note that the color codes for Figs. 12.1 and 12.2 are different. The horizontal meridian is purple in Fig. 12.1b but green in Fig. 12.2a). Again consistent with early human studies, the left and right halves of the visual field are represented primarily in the respective contralateral hemispheres [9, 11], though an overlapping portion of the ipsilateral field near the vertical meridian is also found in each hemisphere [55]. However, close inspection of the brain maps reveals, not one, but several representations of the contralateral hemifield in each hemisphere (e.g., brain map of Fig. 12.1b in which three representations of the horizontal meridian are marked in purple). Indeed, multiple maps of the visual hemifield provide de facto evidence for the existence of multiple, distinct visual areas beyond V1. The boundaries between adjacent visual areas are often marked by the representation of either the

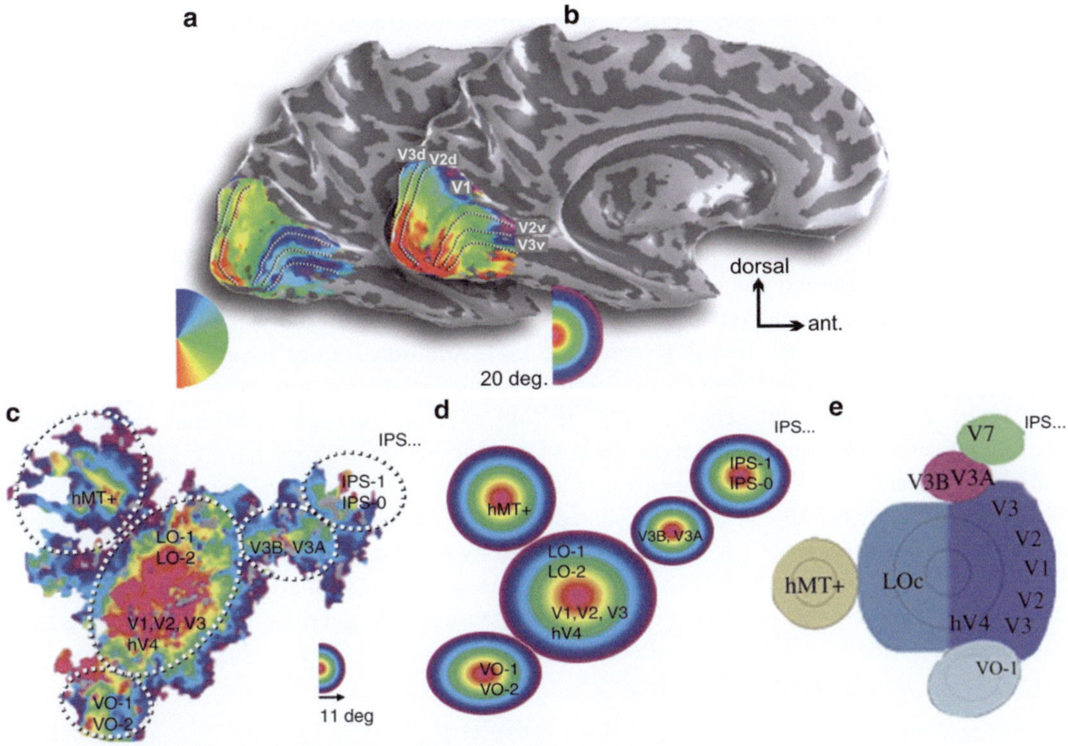

Fig. 12.2 Cortical visual field maps and visual area clusters. Visual field maps in one hemisphere of a single subject measured with expanding ring and rotating wedge stimuli. The color overlay indicates the angle (**a**) or eccentricity (**b**) of the stimulus that produces the most powerful response at each cortical location. The stimuli covered the central 20° radius. For clarity, only responses near the medial occipital cortex are shown. (**c**) Eccentricity measurements spanning 0°–11° are shown on a flattened section of cortex from the left hemisphere of a single subject. *Dotted lines* overlaid on the flattened data illustrate clusters of visual areas that share a common foveal representation (*red/yellow*). Color legend (*inset*) shows the eccentricity that most effectively drives each cortical location. This image is cropped to show only the data within defined visual field maps. (**d**) A schematic diagram of the organization of eccentricity representations in visual cortex is shown. The image shows the visual field map grouped into clusters, as they would appear on flattened cortex. The *concentric colored circles* designate the eccentricity representations of maps within a cluster. Each cluster contains several visual field maps that can be delineated based on the angle maps. (Reproduced with permission from Wandell BA, Dumoulin SO, Brewer AA. Visual field maps in human cortex. Neuron, 2007. 56(2): p. 366–83.) (**e**) A schematic flat map of cluster organization showing some of the constituent areas. Some clusters such as hMT + and LOc each likely contain multiple areas. (Reproduced with permission from Wandell BA, Brewer AA, Dougherty RF. Visual field map clusters in human cortex. Philos Trans R Soc Lond B Biol Sci, 2005. 360(1456): p. 693–707)

vertical or horizontal meridian as indicated by dotted lines in Fig. 12.2. Also note that the superior quadrant of the hemifield is typically represented in ventral occipital cortex (blue colors in Fig. 12.2a), with the inferior field represented dorsally (red/yellow colors in Fig. 12.2a). Thus to a first approximation, the representation of the visual field in medial occipital cortex is "upside down and backwards" within the occipital lobe.

Multiple Visual Areas and Pathways

Recent advances in imaging human visual cortex have made it increasingly evident that the foregoing, classical conception of cortical retinotopic organization and visual area topography is overly simplified. Advanced methods have been used to obtain greater precision and to significantly extend the number of areas that can be mapped in humans [36–40, 42–44, 46–54, 56, 57]. Figure 12.2c, adapted from Wandell et al. [47], illustrates a cortical "flat map" (computationally unfolded cortical surface) showing a more detailed picture of the eccentricity mapping produced by the checkered ring stimulus. Note first that the representation of the center of gaze that in the three-dimensional (3-D) brain is located at the occipital pole (large red patch in Fig. 12.2b, c) is not the only representation of the fovea. Rather, there are additional foveal representations indicated by the white dotted ellipses in Fig. 12.2c and illustrated schematically in Fig. 12.2d. Each foveal representation is believed to mark the center of a cluster of visual areas that are arranged roughly radially around their shared representation of the center of gaze. This organization is outlined schematically in Fig. 12.2d, e. The largest of these clusters surrounds the foveal representation at the occipital pole and consists of visual areas V1, V2 (dorsal and ventral halves), V3 (dorsal and ventral halves), hV4, LO-1, and LO-2 (a.k.a. LO complex). Additional, smaller clusters include (1) visual areas V3B and V3A dorsally, (2) hMT + laterally, (3) VO-1 and VO-2 ventrally extending into the temporal lobe, and (4) a cluster in the intraparietal sulcus (IPS) involving several areas including V7 (a.k.a. IPS-0) and IPS-1. The hMT cluster is very likely to be composed of multiple distinct visual areas [50, 54]. Additional areas have also been proposed within the anterior portion of the IPS [31, 38, 46, 49, 53] and several additional retinotopically organized visual areas have been delineated in ventral occipito-temporal cortex [47, 51].

The more complex picture of cortical eccentricity mapping provided in Fig. 12.2c, d is complemented by a similarly more complex mapping of visual field meridia illustrated in Fig. 12.3 from Swisher et al. [46]. As illustrated in

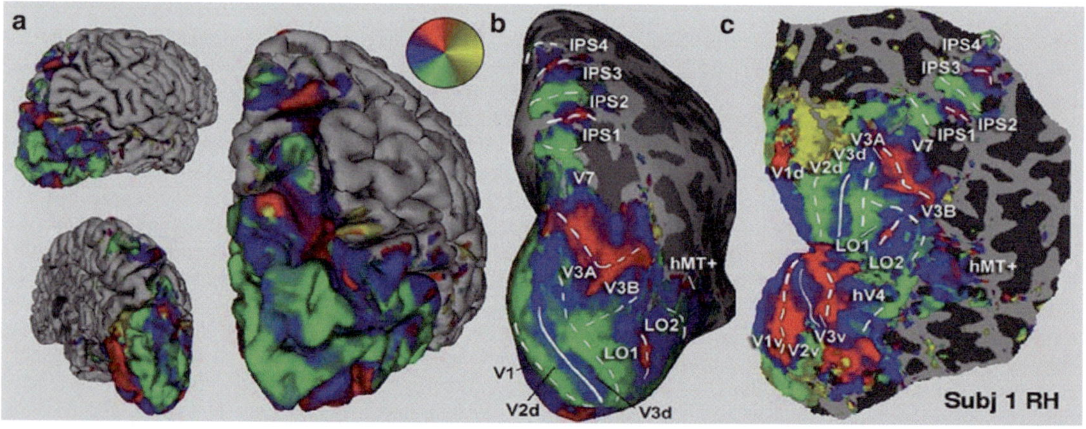

Fig. 12.3 Multiple visual areas mapped throughout occipital and parietal cortex. The angular mapping wedge stimulus reveals visuotopically specific activation throughout a substantial portion of the posterior cerebral cortex. The angular position of the wedge resulting in the greatest significant ($p < 0.05$) response is indicated by the colored overlay (*inset*), with *red* representing the upper visual meridian, *blue* representing the contralateral horizontal meridian, and *green* representing the lower meridian. Potential ipsilateral responses are indicated in *yellow*. The right hemisphere (RH) of a single subject is shown here. (**a**) The reconstructed pial surface is shown from posterior lateral (*top left*), posterior medial (*bottom left*), and posterior (*right*) views. (**b**) Computational inflation of the folded cortical surface reveals visuotopically specific activation within the sulci. Reversals in the represented angular position correspond to areal boundaries in the early visual areas and are shown as overlaid lines. *Dashed lines* indicate reversals at representations of the vertical meridian, whereas *solid lines* indicate reversals at horizontal meridian representations. We find five hemifield maps along the medial bank of the IPS, including area V7 and IPS1–IPS4. (**c**) A flattened representation of the occipital cortex (extending into parietal and temporal regions) showing 14 simultaneously mapped visual regions. (Reproduced with permission from Swisher JD, Halko MA, Merabet LB, McMains SA, Somers DC. Visual topography of human intraparietal sulcus. J Neurosci, 2007. 27(20): p. 5326–37)

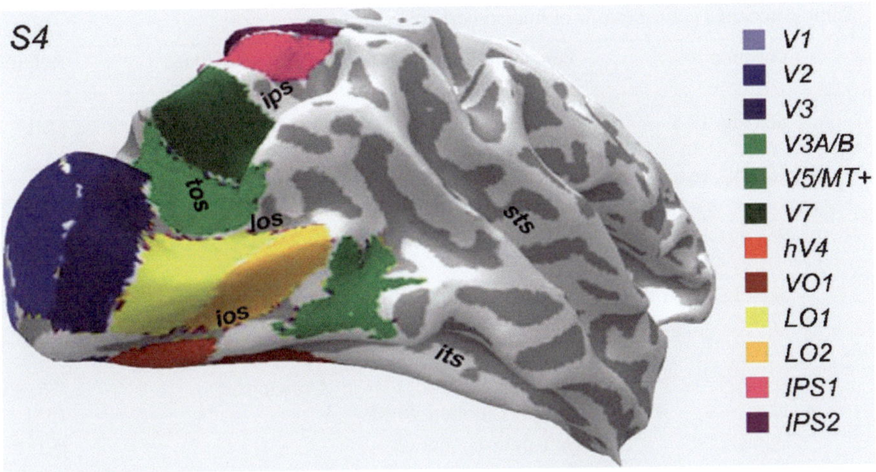

Fig. 12.4 Summary of visual areas on the lateral aspect of the occipital lobe. Locations of LO-1, LO-2, and neighboring visual areas displayed on a partially inflated brain of a representative subject. *los* lateral occipital sulcus, *log* lateral occipital gyrus, *tos* transverse occipital sulcus, *ios* inferior occipital sulcus, *its* inferior temporal sulcus, *sts* superior temporal sulcus, *ips* intraparietal sulcus. Reproduced with permission from Larsson J, Heeger DJ. Two retinotopic visual areas in human lateral occipital cortex. J Neurosci, 2006. 26(51): p. 13128–42

Fig. 12.3b (an "inflated" cortical surface map) and Fig. 12.3c (a cortical "flat map"), fMRI-based mapping of representations of the horizontal meridian (blue) and vertical meridia (red = upper VM, green = lower VM) can be used to identify the boundaries among a host of distinct visual areas, some of which are outlined more clearly in Fig. 12.4 from Larsson and Heeger [42]. It is particularly evident from Figs. 12.3 and 12.4 that distinct visual areas cover the entire occipital lobe and extend well into the parietal and temporal lobes. Careful analysis of such brain maps have revealed several organizational features that are at variance with the classical view of cortical retinotopy. These include upper vertical meridian representations in dorsal occipital cortex associated with areas V3A/B, V7, and within the IPS [31, 38, 46, 49, 53] and lower field representations located ventrally near, or part of, area hV4 and ventromedially within the parahippocampal gyrus [51]. Thus, the classical "upside down and backwards" characterization of cortical retinotopy does not always apply to extrastriate visual areas.

At the time of this writing, the identification and delineation of human visual areas is an ongoing endeavor. Additional distinct visual areas have been proposed, though not necessarily within the scheme of foveal clusters previously described or necessarily congruent with the maps shown in Figs. 12.2–12.4. Some visual areas proposed initially have been subsequently modified or re-named based on new evidence or alternate organizational schemes [58–60].

Functional Specialization

Besides using retinotopy to delineate cortical subdivisions, additional areas have been proposed or further differentiated on the basis of functionally specific fMRI paradigms. As summarized in Table 12.1, such visual areas include the proposed human homolog of the lateral intraparietal area (LIP, a.k.a. IPS1 by some authors) [31, 37, 49], area V6 within the dorsal tip of the parieto-occipital sulcus [43, 52], the fusiform face area (FFA) [61], the visual word form area (WFA) also within the fusiform gyrus [62–64] (but see Price [65]), the parahippocampal place area (PPA) [66] and the biological motion area (BMA) in the posterior superior temporal sulcus [67–69], and the extrastriate body area (EBA) [70, 71]. Also, there has been considerable

Table 12.1 Some perceptual contributions of human cortical visual areas

Cortical area	Location	Perceptual function	Effects of damage	References
Early stages				
V1	See Fig. 12.1	Low-level representation of most visual features	Scotoma	[13]
V2	See Fig. 12.1	Low-level representation of most visual features	Scotoma	[14]
V3d/V3v	See Fig. 12.1	Low-level representation of many visual features	Scotoma?	[14]
V3A/B	See Figs. 12.3 and 12.4	Complex motion, SFM(V3A), stereopsis	?	[28, 151–154]
Dorsal stream				
hMT+/V5	See Figs. 12.3 and 12.4	Object trajectory, complex motion, SFM	Akinetopsia	[25, 86, 153, 155]
V6	Dorsal POS	Self-motion, motion flow	?	[52, 156]
BMA	Posterior STS	Biological motion	Impaired biomotion percept?	[68, 69]
EBA	Posterior ITS	Static body and limbs	?	[70, 157]
V7	See Figs. 12.3 and 12.4	Saccadic eye movements, SFM, stereopsis	?	[153, 154, 158]
IPS1-4/LIP	See Figs. 12.3 and 12.4	Saccadic eye movements, attention control	Neglect	[159–161]
Ventral stream				
hV4	See Figs. 12.3 and 12.4	Form, texture	Impaired texture, form percept	[29, 77, 162–165]
LO-1, -2	See Figs. 12.3 and 12.4	Object form, cue-invariant form, fig./ground segment	Object agnosias	[29]
VO1,2	p. fusiform g., p. collateral s.	Color, form (may overlap with FFA and WFA?)	Achromatopsia, object agnosias	[35, 36, 75, 166]
FFA	p. fusiform g.	Face perception, high level form discrimination	Prosopagnosia	[61, 167]
PPA	Parahippoc. g.	Encode layout of environmental space	Impaired encoding of spatial layout	[168, 169]
WFA	Fusiform g.	Visual recognition of words	Word form agnosia	[62]
Frontal				
FEF	SFS/PCS j.	Eye movements, spatial attention	Impaired eye movements, neglect	[40, 159–161, 170]
DLPFC+	IFS/PCS	Work memory, spatial attention	Neglect	[40, 159–161]

Separation of visual areas into different "streams" is modeled after Felleman and Van Essen [100] and reflects a tendency for areas within each stream to have similarities in response to various types of visual stimuli. This may reflect a tendency for functional and anatomical connections to be stronger within stream, but this has not yet been established conclusively. Cross-connections between visual areas in dorsal versus ventral streams are likely to be abundant as they are in macaque monkeys [100]. Visual area names follow usage in publications cited in last column and in those related to Figs. 12.1–12.4. Note that despite similarities in naming, the homology of human visual areas with macaque monkey areas is typically tentative (though strong for V1, V2, and hMT) and possibly inappropriate (e.g., for V3A [28]).

(continued)

Table 12.1 (continued)

Suggested visual functions reflect inferences from fMRI-based functional studies, effects of lesions, and some inferences from macaque monkeys. Listed perceptual functions for each area are intended to be representative but are not comprehensive. Moreover, most categories of function can be further subdivided and could then further differentiate among areas (e.g., motion processing and form processing). Effects of damage are estimated from selected literature references but often the correspondence between visual or anatomical areas specified in the literature and the visual areas listed in this table is difficult to determine precisely. When a reasonably close correspondence was not apparent, the table entry is marked with a "?". References cited in the table were selected by the authors as being potentially helpful to a clinical readership and do not necessarily reflect publication precedence or the most comprehensive coverage of each topic. *BMA* biological motion area, *DLPFC+* dorsolateral prefrontal cortex, *EBA* extrastriate body area, *FFA* fusiform face area, *hMT+* human visual area MT complex, *hV4* human retinotopically defined visual area V4, *IFS* inferior frontal sulcus, *IPS* intraparietal sulcus, *ITS* inferior temporal sulcus, *LIP* lateral intraparietal visual area, *PCS* precentral sulcus, *POS* parietal occipital sulcus, *PPA* parahippocampal place area, *SFM* structure-from-motion, *SFS* superior frontal sulcus, *WFA* word form area

controversy concerning the identity, location, and function of the human homolog of macaque visual area V4. Though V4 is sometimes referred to as the "color area," it is not clear that it matches the brain area that, when lesioned, produces cerebral achromatopsia [32, 72–77], which may be closer to the VO1,2 complex in ventral occipitotemporal cortex.

Identifying the contributions of different visual areas to perception is not straightforward. For example, it has been known for some time that use of moving visual stimuli of various types can activate a wide range of human visual areas [58, 78–80] in addition to hMT, the human homolog of the monkey "visual motion area" (MT/V5). However, just because a visual area responds to movement does not mean that it necessarily supports, say, the perception of object velocity (speed and direction). Indeed, Serences and Boyton [81] showed that when subjects were asked to report the perceived direction of movement of a stimulus whose motion was actually ambiguous, the direction that subjects reported seeing correlated best with fMRI signals in visual area hMT but not with fMRI responses in other visual areas that were also robustly activated by the same stimuli. Serences and Boynton also point out that inferring perceptual function from the strength of fMRI response alone can be highly misleading. So, why would so many visual areas respond to visual motion stimuli? One key reason is that motion in the retinal image can contribute to a variety of perceptual attributes other than object trajectory [82]. For instance, movement of the observer's head creates relative motion in the retinal image between objects at different distances (motion parallax) that contributes to the perception of depth even when all the objects in the scene (other than the observer) are stationary. In fact, retinal motion information can contribute not only to the perception of object trajectory and depth but to the appreciation of three-dimensional shape, object segmentation (from a stationary or differently moving background), dynamic texture (e.g., riffling on a pond), and the perception of self-motion (via optical flow fields). Even the motions of a few points of light attached to body limb joints can be a potent cue for recognition of body type such as male versus female and emotional states such as happy versus sad [83]. Given the varied uses of retinal image motion, it should not be surprising that many visual areas can be activated by motion, though their contributions to perception are quite varied. The same concept is generally true for other types of retinal image information. With this in mind, Table 12.1 presents a highly simplified listing of some of the most likely perceptual contributions of different human cortical visual areas. It is especially important not to infer from this simplified list that functional specialization of individual visual areas implies that there is an anatomically distinct brain "center" for each visual attribute. In this respect, even lesion data must be considered carefully. Table 12.1 provides an indication of a likely or expected effect of damaging certain visual areas but the scientific evidence for these associations may not be conclusive and, often, a similar deficit may be observed under other lesion conditions (for an informative review see

Girkin and Miller [84]). Though a lesion may produce a highly selective and unique visual deficit, such as akinetopsia [85, 86], it would be invalid to assume that no other visual areas contribute to the processing of visual motion. In general, the neural mechanisms responsible for a particular perceptual function are part of a subnetwork of areas extending from the retina into extrastriate visual cortex. Occurrence of a lesion-induced perceptual deficit thus may reflect a fortuitously vulnerable link in the network as much as it reflects damage to a processing stage at which the lost attribute becomes explicitly represented in the neural activity.

Visual System White Matter Tracts and DTI

Although information concerning the retinotopic organization of cortical visual areas can be important clinically, it is functionally incomplete without an account of the organization of white matter tracts interconnecting the various cortical visual areas and their subcortical inputs (retina, thalamus, and tectum). Prior to the advent of DTI, the differentiation of human white matter tracts in individual patients was limited. Today, DTI-based fiber orientation maps (see Fig. 12.8 later in this chapter) and tractography (Fig. 12.5) have revolutionized surgical planning [87] and deficit interpretation by permitting visualization of a number of important fiber tracts in individual patients [88, 89]. For the human visual system, these include the optic radiations (Fig. 12.5) [90, 91], trans-callosal connections [92], and some cortico-cortical connections among visual areas [93]. However, both the sensitivity and specificity of DTI-based tract identification is typically limited and can be adversely affected by pathologies that alter the properties of water diffusion within the white matter. DTI tractography, which seeks to compute models of white matter fibers from the DTI data, can be compromised by poor quality data and suboptimal methodology [94].

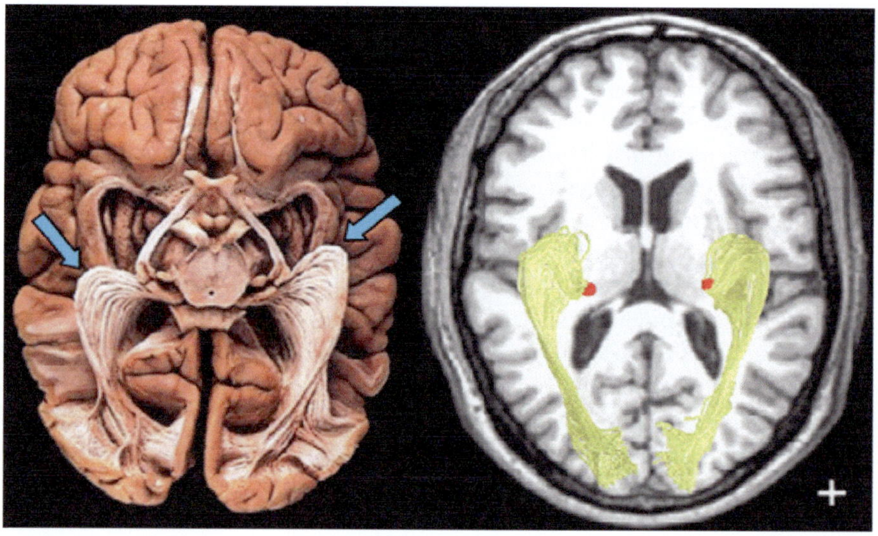

Fig. 12.5 Human optic radiations. (*Left image*) The optic radiation prepared using Klingler's fiber dissection technique in a postmortem brain, as seen from below. The anterior extension of the fibers into the temporal lobe, Meyer's loop, is indicated by the *blue arrows*. (*Right image*) Using diffusion-weighted imaging and fiber tractography, it is possible to identify the optic radiation in living subjects. The fibers are shown against a background of a T1 anatomical image. The fibers connect the lateral geniculate nucleus of the thalamus (*red*) and the calcarine sulcus. Reproduced with permission from Wandell BA, Winawer J. Imaging retinotopic maps in the human brain. Vision Res, 2010 Aug 6. Epub ahead of print

Accurate delineation of fiber tracts can be important for surgical guidance since collateral damage to key white matter structures such as the optic radiations can lead to debilitating scotomata [95]. Moreover, it is conceptually possible to predict the location and extent of surgically induced scotomata from DTI data, but such advanced techniques are not clinically practical at this juncture. So, estimation of the potential effects of optic radiation damage for individual patients is currently limited to inferences based on previous lesion analyses that may or may not be accurate for a given patient. A detailed account of the anatomical connectivity among human cortical visual areas is also not available at the present time. DTI tractography may eventually provide such data but is hampered by issues of accuracy and completeness in the tracing of short cortico-cortical fibers [93]. Another promising approach in this respect is the analysis of "functional connectivity" derived from the pattern of temporal correlations in fMRI signals among different visual areas during "rest" [96] or task-evoked activation [97–99]. For now, however, the detailed anatomical connectivity of cortical visual areas known to exist in monkeys [100] has yet to be elucidated in humans.

Clinical Implications of Visual System Organization

The organizational principles outlined previously have important clinical implications that, if not entirely new, can be expressed at a much greater level of detail than previously possible:

1. Damage to the visual system at any point along the retino-geniculo-striate pathway extending from the retina to visual area V1 and probably to V2 and V3 [14] will generally produce localized visual field blindness (scotoma) that is consistent with the pattern of damage within the retinotopic organization at each level of the hierarchy (but see Merigan [101]).
2. Magnification of the representation of the center of gaze implies that central vision is supported by a particularly large expanse of cortical tissue encompassing much of the occipital pole. Given that the vascular supply of the occipital pole is supported by the middle cerebral artery while medial occipital cortex is supplied from the calcarine artery, selective sparing of the pole can occur and can produce the unique pattern of vision loss referred to as "macular sparing" [13].
3. The existence of multiple functionally distinct visual areas arranged throughout the occipital lobe and nearby portions of the parietal and temporal lobes makes it possible for local lesions to compromise a few or (rarely) even just one visual area. Thus, for higher extrastriate visual areas, damage does not produce blindness but, rather, a selective perceptual loss of one or more visual attributes such as color, movement, complex form (word), or face perception. Detailed retinotopic and functional mapping of human visual cortex provides an increasingly powerful basis for understanding the relationships between local cortical damage and the specific pattern of visual deficits experienced by individual patients [84].
4. The existence of multiple complete maps of the visual field in combination with the existence of multiple functionally distinct visual areas suggests that retinotopically incongruous deficits can occur for different visual attributes. For instance, cortical damage (presumably to medial occipital visual areas while sparing hMT+) may result in incongruous visual field scotomata when behaviorally mapped using static versus moving stimuli [102].
5. Localized lesions of extrastriate visual areas may produce deficits confined to a portion of the visual field that may be difficult or impossible to predict without fMRI visual field mapping. Also note that it is well known from animal experiments that the portion of the visual field to which a neuron is responsive (its receptive field) is smallest in V1 but becomes successively larger for visual areas at successively higher stages of visual processing. This means that mapping the retinotopic organization of these higher areas becomes successively more difficult [48] and, so, it

remains uncertain if all the higher extrastriate areas have complete, regular representations of the visual field – some recent data suggest that they do not [50, 51]. This implies that some visual capacities may not be equally represented throughout the visual field.

6. Modern functional maps of both human and monkey visual cortex indicate that the classically defined cytoarchitectonic boundaries of Brodmann [103] and others [104] often do not correspond with functional boundaries of visual areas defined by electrophysiology and neuroimaging. Though Brodmann's area 17 does correspond closely with visual area V1, Brodmann's area 18 is not necessarily coextensive with area V2 particularly along its anterior border. Moreover, modern imaging techniques can identify more functional subdivisions within the occipital lobe (e.g., Figs. 12.3 and 12.4) than there are areas differentiated by Brodmann. Despite such discrepancies, the Brodmann nomenclature persists in clinical texts and usage, thereby impeding a more detailed and refined dialog concerning the relationships between functionally defined subdivisions of the visual system and the symptomatology of brain-based visual pathologies. Though classical cytoarchitecture may not correlate well with modern functional boundaries, recent advances in defining neurochemical and molecular architecture as well as high-field MRI cytoarchitecture holds great promise for identifying more functionally relevant architectural features that can corroborate fMRI mapping and can provide clues to additional functional distinctions [105–107].

Clinical Applications

Functional MRI-based mapping of the human visual system in current clinical practice is relatively rare, at least compared to mapping of, say, motor and language systems. In part, this may reflect a lower incidence of tumors and other operable pathologies in posterior portions of the brain. However, this also may reflect a lack of awareness of the potential benefits and clinical uses of visual system mapping and the relative ease with which useful fMRI data can be obtained, especially when fMRI is already available. Another impediment has been that fMRI methods that are optimal for clinical use are typically somewhat different than those used for academic research. The goals of clinical fMRI are typically different, such as guidance of surgical resections in individual patients. For such purposes, highly selective fMRI paradigms that isolate unique components of a functional system may be less useful than paradigms that are less selective but permit identification of all or most components of a system. Patients may suffer from disease processes that impair general cognitive abilities, attention, patience, and behavioral performance thereby making complex fMRI tasks unreliable or prohibitively time consuming. Research-oriented fMRI paradigms, then, typically need to be optimized for practical clinical use. So too, the complete imaging workflow typically must be optimized including initial patient assessment, acquisition, data processing, archiving/retrieval, interpretation, treatment guidance, follow-up, and billing. This workflow often involves several physicians (e.g., neurologist, radiologist, and neurosurgeon), nurses, MRI technologists, data processing technicians, and accounting staff. Optimizing and streamlining every aspect of the workflow can help ensure consistent results with minimum impact on physician and patient time.

Due to the unique requirements of clinically oriented functional imaging, the next section reviews the methodology and practical application of fMRI for mapping vision-related brain structures in patients with focal pathologies. (Many of these methods are applicable to the clinical use of fMRI for mapping other functions as well.) This is then followed by a consideration of the use of fMRI and DTI in the context of different types of vision-related brain pathology and the unique issues associated with those pathologies. The emphasis is on relatively focal pathologies such as tumors, AVMs, and infarcts and on treatment procedures such as surgical resection, focal radiation, and brain stimulation that require precise targeting or that may cause localized damage to eloquent tissue as a side effect. Also, it is important to point out that, at the time of this writing, most fMRI (and DTI) paradigms have not been fully validated in clinical trials to establish their reliability as indicators of gray (and white) matter function or to establish their overall impact on clinical outcomes. A number of ongoing studies should help address this problem in the near future.

Methodology

There are a variety of methods and fMRI paradigms that can be used to identify and map various components of the visual system and to distinguish functionally specific subdivisions [25–27, 36, 48, 61, 108]. At present, however, detailed mapping and functional differentiation of single, individual visual areas has not been shown to have a compelling clinical application. Consequently, the following account of the methodology focuses on robust paradigms that can deliver useful data for mapping multiple visual areas in as little as 10 min of MRI scan time and that have been, or are in the process of being, validated for clinical use.

It is important to stress that most fMRI paradigms, including vision mapping, require the patient to perform some sort of behavioral task even if it is simply to rest quietly with minimal head movement. Adequate performance of the behavioral task is as much a determinant of the quality of the fMRI results as any other factor. So, the methodology and workflow that will be outlined in this chapter include features to ensure and verify that the patient performs adequately, or that a failure in this respect is noted and becomes an essential part of the data passed to the attending/consulting physicians.

Visual Field Mapping

fMRI activation of visual cortex can be readily accomplished using a flickering checkerboard pattern, which typically produces robust activation in at least a portion of primary visual cortex and in a number of extrastriate cortical areas [22]. The high black/white contrast and dynamic flickering are both important for strongly activating visual cortex neurons and typically produce strong BOLD activation that rivals or surpasses that obtained in motor cortex with finger tapping. (It should be noted that simply turning the lights on and off in the scanner room may generate detectable activation in the visual cortex but the sensitivity, specificity, repeatability, and "coverage" will be so variable and poorly specified as to be virtually useless for critical clinical applications.) However, the use of an optimized stimulus sequence consisting of an expanding checkered annulus (Fig. 12.1a) combined with a gaze fixation task can improve repeatability and allows differentiation of central versus peripheral visual field representations with no increase in scan time. Stimulus dimensions and timing are described in the caption for Fig. 12.1. Note that this type of stimulus sequence is referred to as a temporal phase mapping design in that each location in the visual field is stimulated at a different time (temporal phase) in the sequence, thereby allowing the spatial preference (best stimulus position) of each voxel to be identified by the timing of its BOLD response. Addition of a second scan using a rotating checkered wedge (Fig. 12.1b) allows differentiation of different angular clock positions within the visual field and permits construction of functional field maps that can provide virtually instant appreciation of the functional status of all portions of the cortical representation of the visual field (Fig. 12.1, right. Explained in more detail later).

There are several advantages of the annulus and wedge stimuli for clinical fMRI. First, this technique is very efficient and provides more information than a simple flashed checkerboard in the same amount of scan time. Together, the ring and wedge scans can be obtained in 10 min, so they can be added to a more extended workup including various types of conventional imaging and additional fMRI scans to map other functional systems. Also note that the size of the annulus and the check patterns of both stimuli are scaled with distance from the center of gaze. This helps compensate for changes in acuity with eccentricity and helps produce a relatively complete mapping of retinotopically organized visual areas throughout occipital cortex (Fig. 12.2a, b). For presurgical mapping, it is important to obtain such a comprehensive mapping since there is a one-to-one relationship between damage to locations in the cortical maps and the pattern of blindness at corresponding locations in the patient's visual field for V1 and probably V2 and V3 [13, 14]. Thus, systematic mapping of all locations in the visual field helps ensure that no visually responsive cortex is missed and allows identification of the representation of central vision (red in Fig. 12.2b), which supports high acuity vision and is critical for reading and other essential functions. Finally, the stimulus sequence includes a fixation marker that dims or disappears for 1/8-s at random times every 4–8 s during the scan sequence. The patient is instructed to watch the fixation point continuously throughout the scan and press a button each time it dims. The dimming of the fixation marker is difficult to detect unless the patient is looking directly at it and so provides ongoing verification that the patient's gaze is directed to the center of the display. Providing such an active task helps the patient attend to the stimulus, which, in turn, enhances the BOLD response and serves to combat sleepiness and distractibility. Though not as fool-proof or precise as eye movement monitoring, the fixation point dimming task is much easier to implement, requires no complex hardware or calibration procedures, and provides verification of behavioral compliance at repeated intervals throughout the entire MRI scan.

The visual stimulation sequence is readily generated using computer graphics and suitable software but can be prerecorded and presented on DVD or videotape if the recording can be started reliably without significant delay. Synchronization of the visual stimulation sequence with the scanner operation is important especially since the previously described paradigm relies on accurate stimulus timing to encode information about each voxel's preferred stimulus location. Best practice is to present the stimuli using a system that uses an electronic trigger pulse produced by the scanner at the beginning of each run to trigger the stimulus presentation hardware/software. Typically, this will provide synchronization accuracy to within the video refresh period of the computer graphics system (typically 16.7 ms for a 60 Hz video projector). However, timing variability up to 1–2 s can be tolerated, thus making it possible to trigger stimulation manually if no other option is available.

Presentation of visual stimuli to patients in the MRI scanner can be accomplished through the use of a video projector or other commercially manufactured system. However, not all systems are optimal for visual field mapping. The most typical limitation is the size of the field of view. In this respect, it is important to note that the important size parameter is the visual angle (expressed in degrees at the eye) and is related to the viewable extent of the stimulus for the patient. A physically small stimulus can subtend a very large visual angle if placed very close to the eye. Obviously, to activate the full expanse of retinotopic visual cortex, it is desirable to have a stimulus that can cover as much of the visual field as possible. As mentioned previously (see section on "Retinotopic Organization"), visual stimulation extending to only 5° eccentricity will activate almost 40% of visual cortex [13], due to cortical magnification of the center of gaze. Commercially available projector systems using back-projection screens placed close to the patient's eyes can produce stimuli that extend to 15–20° of eccentricity and this will typically activate approximately 70% of the V1 retinotopic map [13].

Functionally Specific Tests

Other fMRI-based tests employing more complex visual stimuli can be used to selectively identify specific visual areas involved in the perception of form [29], color [36], motion [52, 80, 109], faces [61], environmental space [66], the human body [70], visual words [63], and visual attention [110]. Such tests have, so far, not been used routinely in clinical practice but may be of use for selected patients. If interested, the reader should consult the references cited previously in the discussion of "Functional Specialization" for details on relevant stimuli and tasks.

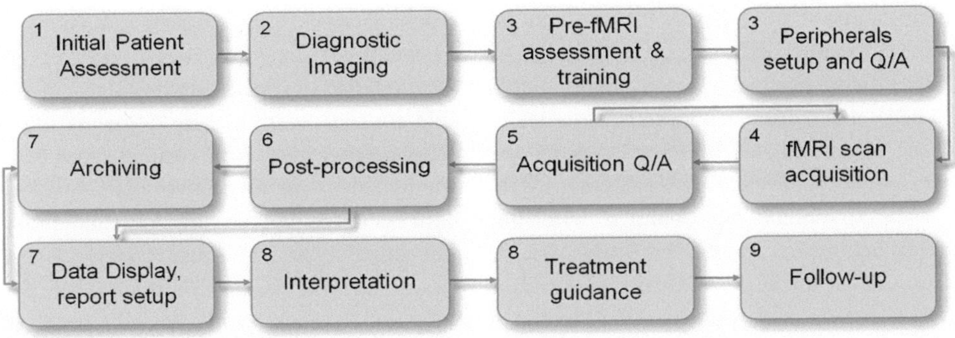

Fig. 12.6 Example of clinical workflow for fMRI mapping of visual cortex. Workflow is representative of current usage but may vary across institutions. Many steps can be automated or performed by professional staff thereby reducing physician time to a minimum. *Numbers in each box* indicate relevant section in text. Note that some steps are discussed in the same text section. *Arrows* indicate workflow sequence, with *backward arrows* indicating steps that may be repeated. Inefficient or inconsistent workflow can significantly impair physician acceptance and utilization, and can impair reliability and repeatability of results

fMRI Workflow (with Details for Visual System Mapping)

Ultimately, the fMRI paradigm and behavioral task are only two of the important components of a complete workflow that should be optimized to achieve accurate, reliable results efficiently with minimum physician involvement. The workflow also should include measures needed to be compliant with the American Medical Association's current procedural terminology (CPT) codes for fMRI [111]. The general features of the workflow described as follows are not unique to vision mapping and have not been standardized across the industry, but do reflect an example of procedures currently in use. Key components of the workflow are outlined in Fig. 12.6. Commercial vendors provide software tools that can aid the setup and routine use of this or a similar workflow [112–114]. Once in place and optimized for a particular institution, a good workflow should help ensure that the imaging data are acquired in the same way with every patient and that all steps needed for quality assurance are performed each time. If a consistent workflow is not established and used daily, the physician is likely to be faced with imaging results whose validity is suspect or that are difficult to interpret with confidence (e.g., This could occur if a patient had nystagmus which was not documented in the imaging session record).

1. *Initial Patient Assessment.* The patient's initial entry into the workflow is typically through conventional methods established at each institution. At some point during the workup, it may become evident that the patient has or may develop a pathology-related vision deficit or that anticipated treatment (e.g., surgery) might damage central visual system components. In such case, ordering fMRI visual system mapping may be indicated either to assist diagnosis or to guide treatment planning and delivery.

Selection of fMRI tests for vision mapping will typically include a general purpose paradigm such as visual field mapping and possibly additional functionally specific tests (faces versus places, word form, or visual movement mapping). One important consideration is whether the patient has difficulty in maintaining stable gaze for a period of 3–4 min (the typical duration of a single fMRI scan). Serious gaze instability can be detected during routine neurological testing and should be noted if present. Functional MRI vision mapping is typically contraindicated if gaze instability is too severe (greater than a few degrees variation – A thumbnail viewed at arm's length is roughly 1° wide).

If fMRI vision mapping is considered, it is important to determine if the patient has any existing vision abnormalities, especially visual field deficits. To reliably screen for existing scotomata, a visual field perimetry test can be obtained (automated Humphrey perimetry or manual Goldmann perimetry, tested monocularly for each eye). It is particularly important to determine if the patient has any monocular or incongruous binocular scotomata. In such case, fMRI vision mapping should be obtained with the patient viewing the test patterns binocularly (as is typical) so that eloquent portions of visual cortex driven by either eye alone are identified as functional. However, there can be a further complication if the patient must view the visual test patterns in the MRI scanner by looking between the bars of a radio-frequency (RF) headcoil. If the bars do not allow each eye a complete view of the entire test pattern, then the BOLD activation patterns in visual cortex can reflect a complex interaction between existing monocular deficits and the portions of the display for each eye that are occluded by the head coil bars. If the patient has intact binocular fields, this is not a problem since all portions of the display are seen by at least one eye. Such difficulties can be circumvented by using either a different RF coil arrangement, a commercially available "binocular" stimulator, or by avoiding fMRI vision mapping for the rare patients for whom this is a problem.

As is appropriate for any fMRI exam, an overall assessment should be made of the patient's alertness, cognitive ability, and behavioral capabilities in order to identify any factors that could compromise the patient's performance of the behavioral task for fMRI. For visual field mapping, the patient must be able to gaze steadily at the fixation marker in the center of the display and press a button when the marker briefly disappears (see section on "Visual Field Mapping"). Also, it is important to determine if the patient suffers from visually induced epilepsy since this can be a risk due to the high contrast, flickering stimuli used for vision mapping. This may not preclude vision mapping but should be discussed with the patient and physician before scheduling a scan session.

2. *Diagnostic Imaging*. fMRI vision mapping is typically ordered as part of a more comprehensive suite of brain imaging, with only a modest increment in imaging time or expense. Other types of convention imaging will likely include T1-weighted anatomy (e.g., spoiled gradient recalled [SPGR]) with or without use of an injectable contrast agent to help delineate tumors and T2-weighted images of various types (e.g., fluid attenuated inversion recovery [FLAIR]) to highlight edema and other pathological factors. These and other types of images (regional cerebral blood volume [rCBV], diffusion or perfusion weighted images, etc.) typically highlight anatomical structure or pathophysiological factors that help identify and localize the pathology to be treated/assessed. It is not uncommon to order an initial imaging screen for diagnosis followed by more specific imaging tests for treatment planning and guidance.

For visual system mapping, conventional anatomical images can permit identification of key structures such as the occipital lobe, calcarine fissure (approximate location of V1), and parieto-occipital sulcus (usual anterior extent of occipital visual areas). Other useful landmarks in this respect are the posterior horns of the lateral ventricles, which at their most posterior extent typically cradle the more medial primary visual cortex within the calcarine fissure. High-resolution anatomical images also can reveal gross physical distortions of visual system structures due to tumor mass effects (e.g., see later Fig. 12.8), congenital malformations (e.g., see later Fig. 12.11), previous surgery (e.g., see later Fig. 12.13) or other CNS damage that can make it difficult or impossible to determine the location and integrity of cortical visual areas and pathways by anatomy alone. In such cases, fMRI and DTI mapping may provide the only method for reliably identifying and localizing key vision-related structures.

3. *Pre-fMRI Assessment and Training. Peripherals Setup and Quality Assurance*. An important part of the workflow involves a series of steps to prepare the patient and equipment for scanning. An essential first step is describing the behavioral task to the patient (e.g., fixation point dimming task) and having them practice it while being observed. This is best accomplished using a system (e.g., laptop computer) that can present the identical stimuli used during scanning and

that can record behavioral responses (e.g., button presses) during the practice session for comparison with response records obtained later during the scan. The patient's ability to perform the task should be carefully assessed and any indication of poor performance, including poor gaze control, should be recorded and passed on to the physician.

MRI scanner operation and quality assurance should be conducted regularly (at least weekly). Besides procedures recommended by the scanner manufacturer, additional procedures to ensure high-quality fMRI should be considered and have been described elsewhere [115, 116]. Though regular Q/A testing of the MRI scanner is desirable to detect serious hardware malfunction, between-subject variability is perhaps the most important factor affecting reliability and reproducibility of fMRI data. Variations among individual scanners, pulse sequences, and field strength also contribute [115, 116].

Testing/calibration of peripheral equipment such as response buttons, video projectors, and sound systems should be performed before each scan in order to document their functionality for later reference by the physician during interpretation. For vision testing, it is particularly important to test, align, "zoom," and focus the video presentation system using a calibration test pattern that extends to the maximum extent of the display screen and contains a focusing pattern such as that illustrated in Fig. 12.7 (Note fine tilted lines within yellow fixation marker to aid focusing). It is recommended that the MRI technician or other staff member conduct an initial adjustment of the display system from within the scanner bore to achieve optimum setup, since patients often have difficulty in conveying problems to the MRI technician. Common mistakes with back-projection systems are using the incorrect screen (typically smaller than optimal) and failing to "zoom" the image to the maximum extent allowed by the screen. The latter typically requires the projector to be placed at a prearranged distance from the screen and the "zoom" control adjusted accordingly. Fixing all components of the projector system in place so they cannot be moved easily is recommended since errors in the size and focus of the stimuli will directly contribute to variability in the fMRI activation patterns. Use of a binocular optical system can avoid some of these issues, but commercially available systems typically have a significantly reduced field of view (leading to incomplete mapping of visual cortex). They also require proper adjustment of focus and eye spacing/centering by the patient to ensure that optical occlusions of the test pattern do not occur if the patient's head position shifts. Such occlusions can block fMRI responses from portions of

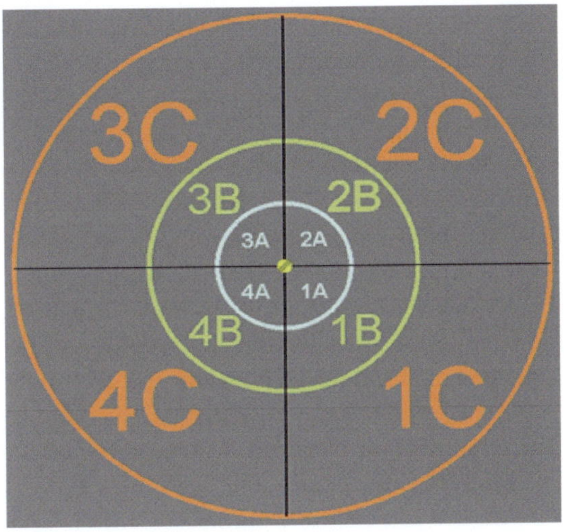

Fig. 12.7 Test pattern for aligning visual stimulus and verifying patient's view. An alignment pattern as illustrated here is used during prescan setup to ensure that the video delivery system is adjusted so that the outer *orange circle* completely fills the display that the patient will view. For a typical back-projection/mirror system, the maximum viewable radius can be 20° of visual angle though as little as 10° can still be useful. Note that the *center yellow* fixation point contains three *thin lines* that can be used to aid focus adjustment. It is recommended that the MR technician verify proper adjustment by viewing the test pattern from within the MRI scanner while having a colleague make final adjustments. Patients often cannot reliably assist detailed adjustment. Once the patient is placed into the scanner, the technician instructs them to stare at the *center dot* and report which number/letter combinations are visible without moving the eyes. They are also asked to report the direction of tilt of the fixation *point lines* (*top to the right*, *left or center*). Any difficulties, omissions, or occlusions should be remedied if possible. Otherwise, it is essential that the problems are described in detail in the session log and passed to the physicians

the test pattern that are not visible, thereby potentially compromising the exam.

Once the patient is placed into the scanner and the video display adjusted, it is important to verify that the entire test pattern is visible and reasonably well focused for him/her. This can be accomplished quickly using the test pattern in Fig. 12.7 by asking the patient which letters/colors they can or cannot see while maintaining gaze on the marker at the center of the display (this test also should be covered in the practice session). Any occlusions or difficulties must be corrected and/or recorded to permit accurate interpretation by the physician.

Finally, just before running the fMRI scan, the technician should briefly repeat a description of the test and the instructions for the behavioral task, preferably using a short written statement that is read verbatim each time to ensure consistency. For patients who are cognitively challenged, sleepy, or distracted, this can be essential since they may readily forget the earlier instructions.

4. *fMRI Scan Acquisition*. Most modern high-field MRI scanners have, or can be equipped to perform, conventional BOLD fMRI, and reliable results usually can be obtained using the pulse sequence provided by the manufacturer. Acceptable visual field mapping can be obtained with both 1.5 and 3.0 Tesla scanners, though the latter can provide superior results and smaller useful voxel size. Use of an 8-channel RF head coil also modestly improves fMRI signals, so is desirable if available. Typical fMRI scan parameters for a General Electric Signa Excite 3T scanner are listed in Table 12.2.

Table 12.2 Example of BOLD fMRI scan parameters for 3T

Parameter/factor	Setting
MRI scanner	General Electric Signa Excite, 3 Tesla
RF head coil	8-Channel birdcage, Model 102859
Pulse sequence	Echo planar, gradient echo EPI
Field of view	24 × 24 cm
Voxel grid	96 × 96
Slice thickness	2.5 mm
Slice number	Maximum allowed by scanner (approx. 25)
Slice orientation	Axial or coronal
Slice position	Whole occipital lobe inclusive of ventral surface + adjacent portions of temporal and parietal lobes
Spacing (skip factor)	0.0
Echo time (TE)	25 ms
Repetition time (TR)	2.0 s
Flip angle	77°
Frequency/phase encode directions	Select after short test scan (see text for details)
NEX	1.0 (actual will be less)
Bandwidth	250 kHz
Scan duration	168 s

Scanner make, model, and head coil configuration are representative of hardware in current use but do not necessarily represent most recent offerings by all scanner vendors. Parameter settings are typical for a 3 Tesla field strength scanner but also may vary somewhat from site to site. Voxel sizes at 1.5 T may need to be larger (e.g., 64 × 64 matrix) to obtain similar data quality. The illustrated parameters with a NEX of 1.0 actually produce a partial K-space scan with a true NEX that is automatically computed by the scanner software

Although 3 Tesla scanners typically yield stronger fMRI signals, this can be accompanied by distortions due to local magnetic susceptibility artifacts. This can be particularly problematic for the occipital lobe and adjacent inferior temporal lobe due to the presence of the midsagittal and transverse vascular sinuses and petrous bone air inclusions [117]. In such case, it can be helpful to select frequency and phase encode directions so as to minimize distortions in or near the occipital pole. This can be accomplished easily by acquiring two very short (10 s) fMRI scans with the frequency and phase encode directions swapped and comparing the resulting images to a T1- or T2-weighted anatomical scan. Additional refinement of shim coil adjustments may also help.

Finally, it is important to note that American Medical Association CPT code requirements for some types of fMRI require the presence of a physician or licensed psychologist during scan acquisition to evaluate patient compliance and performance. This is required under codes 96020 and 70555 for paradigms involving cognitively complex tests, but not for "simple" motor and vision fMRI exams covered by code 70554. Nevertheless in all cases, best practice is to document behavioral compliance/performance objectively to permit valid interpretation by the physician at a later time.

5. *Acquisition Q/A*. Upon completion of each individual fMRI scan, the patient is asked to rate their alertness on a scale of 1–5 and this is recorded. The rating scale is described to the patient in the following manner: 5 indicates completely alert with no drowsiness; 4 indicates generally awake but not always alert, 3 indicates that the patient was not sure if they were awake for the whole scan; 2 indicates that they definitely fell asleep for a short period; and 1 indicates that they were asleep for the majority of the scan. The MRI technician also rates their assessment of the patient's behavior and rates the overall technical quality of the scan acquisition, noting any problems.

During the scan session, it may become clear that the patient is having difficulty in performing the fixation task adequately (by monitoring the online response record) or that imaging time is limited or that fMRI signal quality is poor. In such case, useful data sometimes can be obtained by simply running the checkered annuli with passive fixation while the MRI technician verbally prompts the patient throughout the scan to keep watching the fixation marker in the center of the screen. In such case, the technician should record a description of the problems encountered and any observations concerning patient performance and data quality.

6. *Postprocessing*. Raw fMRI data need to be computationally processed to yield a time series of brain images acquired every repetition time (TR) period during the scan (e.g., 2 s, repetition time). Typically, this time series is further processed to reveal changes in brain activation produced by the visual stimulus/task and to compute various statistical measures that can be used to help identify statistically reliable activation foci. For the visual field mapping stimuli described previously, the data are also processed to identify the stimulus locations (eccentricity and angle) that maximally activate each voxel and to compute functional field maps.

MRI scanner vendors provide software that can produce basic volumetric (slice-oriented) fMRI brain maps but more sophisticated analysis packages that streamline and automate postprocessing and provide helpful tools for clinical use are available from other software vendors [113, 114]. A variety of fMRI analysis packages are also available as "freeware." However, such research-oriented packages are not optimized for routine clinical use and can require considerable effort and dedicated expertise to produce reports in a timely fashion. Typically, in a clinical venue, an "in house" data processing technician will perform the postprocessing, though this can also be performed by commercial vendors as a service on a fee-per-case basis [114].

The following list highlights several of the more common computational steps involved in a typical postprocessing sequence for clinical use.

1. Reconstruction of raw MRI data to produce a time series of 3-D volumes of slice images (typically provided by scanner manufacturer). Ideally yielding DICOM compatible images [118].
2. Combine fMRI images with anatomical and other image data including potential correction for warping and misalignment. This can be critical for accurate spatial localization of BOLD foci and should be checked for each patient.
3. Examination of timecourse data for artifacts, potential rejection thereof, and computation of overall data quality measures. It is helpful to have a checklist of Q/A tests and observations that should be performed on every dataset to assess and document its technical quality.
4. Clustering, region of interest definition (optional).
5. Computation of amplitude/variability metrics and statistical measures such as student's T, Fisher's F, Cross correlation r.
6. Spatial smoothing, normalization [119, 120].
7. Test-specific measures/analyses. For the ring and wedge stimuli described previously, the fMRI time series data must be further analyzed to identify the preferred stimulus location for each voxel. Algorithms for this

analysis are available commercially [121] and through "freeware" such as the "Hilbert Delay" module of AFNI [122, 123].

7. *Display/Report/Archiving*. Once the initial postprocessing has been completed, the postprocessing technician or commercial postprocessing service will prepare the data for physician viewing and generate a technical report summarizing overall data quality and flagging any issues that arose during data acquisition. In this respect, the technical report should include all procedural and Q/A information needed by the physician to perform medical interpretation of the data.

The data are then sent to a software viewing system that may itself perform some of the foregoing postprocessing computations as well as others designed to enhance the display of data for interpretation. Typically, multiple types of conventional MRI, fMRI, DTI, and other imaging data will be combined in the viewer to provide an integrated picture of the patient's condition. Ideally, a virtually unlimited number of data sets can be overlaid and should be co-registered to ensure proper alignment. Viewer settings are then adjusted by the technician and the physician to yield an optimum display for medical interpretation and final medical report generation.

Display packages vary widely in the features they provide and ease of operation. Typical parameters that can be manipulated include selection of data sets to overlay, statistical measures, thresholds for identifying reliable activation foci, degree of smoothing or clustering, pseudocolor scale selection, transparency, and outlining. Since these adjustments are typically customized to help reveal features of interest to the physician, the viewer must provide the ability to record all feature settings and the exact configuration of the images. This ensures that the settings used to make the medical interpretation can be archived as a permanent record and can be recovered at a later time for re-examination if needed. Not all software packages, especially those intended primarily for research, have this capability.

Besides handling image viewing, the software should also permit recording and perusal of other essential information needed to interpret the data. Ideally, all behavioral performance measures, calibration measures, technician evaluations, and comments obtained during patient training and data acquisition should appear in the viewer. Also included should be a complete description of the stimuli/tasks for each fMRI paradigm and the scanner parameter settings (typically included in the DICOM headers of the image data themselves). A good rule of thumb is that all information needed to virtually recreate the imaging session should be available (though not necessarily displayed by default). This information, and especially the behavioral performance data, must be in the final medical report to be compliant with CPT billing requirements.

8. *Interpretation/Treatment Guidance*. Procedures for medical interpretation and diagnosis typically depend on the preferences and practice of physicians at a given institution. Often this may involve a conference among the relevant healthcare professionals including neurologists, radiologists, neurosurgeons, neuro-oncologists, and psychological testing professionals and, if available, may involve interactive use of the display software to explore issues that arise during the conference. At this point in the workflow, it is essential that the technical report contain all relevant information that might be needed by the physicians to assess the imaging procedures, patient performance, technical issues, and quality assurance tests. Obviously, specific expertise in the interpretation of fMRI data and visual system mapping in particular will be needed for accurate interpretation. This includes knowledge of potential artifacts and distortions that could affect the interpretation.

Following medical interpretation and any final adjustment of the imaging displays and report, the viewing software must be capable of exporting the relevant information to other systems such as a picture archiving and communication system (PACS) for long-term storage and to treatment delivery systems such as an intraoperative navigation system. At present, compatibility between image viewing software and all such systems is good but not universal, though efforts are underway to establish standards and thereby enhance portability.

9. *Follow-up.* Depending upon the patient's pathology, prognosis, and treatment, additional follow-up imaging may be required when monitoring tumor progression or re-occurrence, though fMRI is not generally used for this purpose. However, it is not uncommon in cases of tumor recurrence to repeat the complete imaging workflow in order to guide further treatment.

Finally, it is important to point out that there is a need for further validation of fMRI imaging in terms of its ability to accurately reflect the functional status of brain tissue under a wide variety of clinical conditions and its ability to positively affect treatment outcomes. For such purposes, follow-up imaging including fMRI combined with careful outcomes assessment can be invaluable.

Specific Pathologies and Issues

Clinical use of fMRI mapping of vision-related brain structures requires interpretation of the imaging data in terms of the diagnostic/treatment goals and the patient's existing and eventual visual abilities, taking into account potential deficits that may be caused by the treatment procedures themselves. A substantial loss of vision may be acceptable in cases of life threatening illness though, even then, preserving critical foveal vision may be possible. However, when brain tissue is distorted due to tumor mass effects, physical malformation or previous injury/surgery, then identification of eloquent tissue may be difficult or impossible without fMRI mapping. Moreover, individual variation in the size of visual areas and their position relative to sulcal or gyral landmarks can be considerable [34] and avoidance of postoperative deficits may depend on careful surgical resection to within millimeters of key structures [124]. The occurrence of debilitating visual agnosias such as prosopagnosia [125, 126], alexia [127, 128], and akinetopsia [85, 129, 130] are associated with lesions of specific extrastriate visual areas whose locations or functionality are difficult to define for individual patients without functional imaging. It is also becoming apparent that, without fMRI, it may not be possible to fully diagnose/differentiate certain vision pathologies such as attention-related visual neglect versus sensory field loss, and this can have important consequences for surgical planning and outcomes. Finally, if patients learn that techniques are available to maximally preserve vision while still achieving effective treatment, then one must assume that most patients would advocate their use.

The following case studies highlight some of the clinical uses of fMRI-based vision mapping. They were selected from a database of 65 patients who underwent this procedure as part of their pretreatment assessment. Of those tested, 46 yielded high-quality brain maps. These patients suffered from a variety of pathologies including 12 tumors of various types, 3 AVMs, 4 strokes, 19 epilepsy, 2 congenital malformations, and 6 with other types of pathology. Other clinical uses of fMRI and DTI of vision-related brain structures have been published previously [95, 124, 131, 132] and further illustrate the potential advantages of these techniques for particular patients. (Several of these publications report cases that did not use fMRI/DTI but did mention their potential advantage or described situations that the authors felt could be aided by these techniques [133–135]).

Tumor Resection/Radiation

Figure 12.8 illustrates results of a multiparameter imaging study of an adult female with a grade II astrocytoma in the right occipito-parietal cortex. Resection of the tumor and follow-up radiation treatment was indicated, but the proximity to primary visual cortex was a concern. The figure shows a "deck" of five different types of overlaid imaging information represented schematically in the control section at the upper left (only four types of data are visible in the brain image). The bottom layer of the deck is a conventional, T1-weighted SPoiled, GRadient recalled at steady state (SPGR) anatomical image. On top of it, displayed in partial transparency, are DTI data that are color-coded to show the fiber orientation of different white matter pathways. Superimposed on the DTI is a FLuid Attenuated Inversion Recovery (FLAIR) image that has been clipped by intensity thresholding to isolate the tumor bed

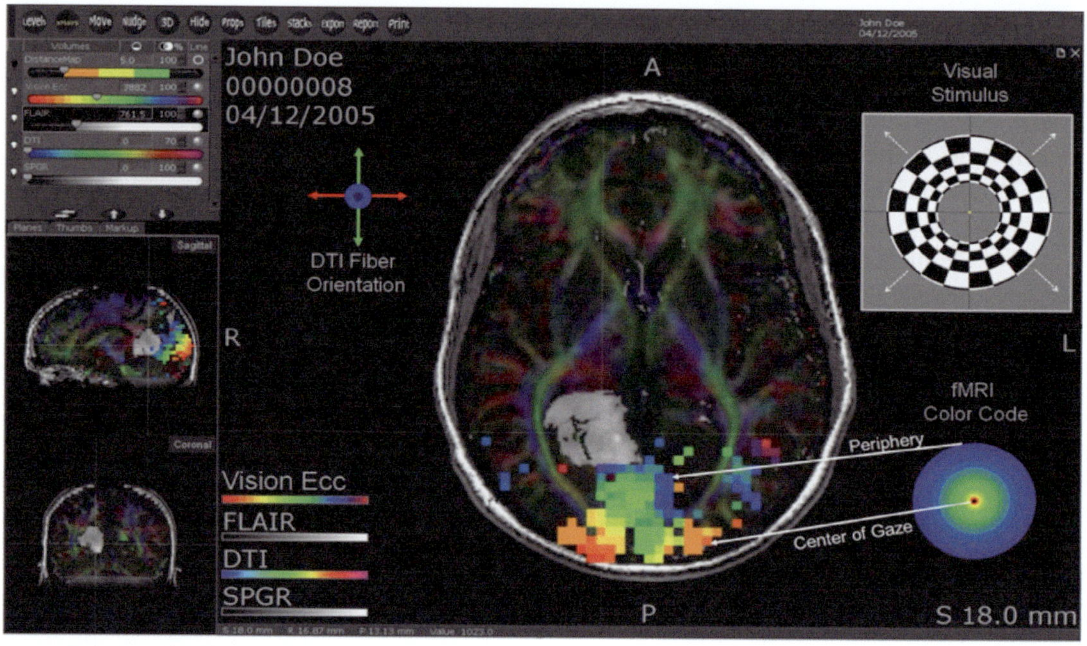

Fig. 12.8 *Case report*. Occipital astrocytoma. Grade II astrocytoma in the right occipital lobe of a 44-year-old female. Eccentricity fMRI map shows proximity of the posterior tumor border to eloquent cortex representing the peripheral visual field (*blue and blue-green voxels*). However, proximity of the optic radiations to lateral tumor border (green fibers in DTI) is of greater concern for surgery-induced vision deficit. *Upper right*: schematic representation of stimulus for fMRI mapping. *Lower right*: fMRI color code indicating mean eccentricity of annulus that maximally activated each colored voxel. Note magnified cortical representation of fovea (*red/orange voxels*). *Upper left*: color code for DTI fiber orientation. *Ecc* eccentricity, *FLAIR* fluid attenuated inversion recovery, *DTI* diffusion tensor imaging, *SPGR* spoiled, gradient recalled

and surrounding edema (light gray). Finally, the small colored squares show the visually evoked, fMRI activation. Here the colors indicate the eccentricity of the stimulus ring (upper right inset) that maximally activated each voxel. This identifies areas supporting critical foveal vision (shown in red-orange) from those representing more peripheral vision (shown in blue-green).

To provide more precise guidance for presurgical planning, a computational routine can be used to compute a "distance map" around the tumor as illustrated in Fig. 12.9. The color coding indicates distances at 5 mm intervals from the tumor margin. Previous research suggests that if the surgeon performs a complete resection out to the margins of the tumor, then any functionally critical structure within a 5–10 mm zone (red, orange shells in Fig. 12.9) is likely to be adversely affected and is at risk for causing a neurological deficit [136, 137]. In this case, the fMRI shows that visually responsive cortex supporting peripheral vision is located within this zone but not critical foveal vision. However, the DTI shows that key white matter tracts including the optic radiations do pass through this zone along the lateral margin of the tumor bed (compare Figs. 12.8 and 12.9). For this patient, loss of some peripheral vision due to gray matter damage might be acceptable, but damage to the optic radiations could cause a severe deficit possibly impairing reading or other essential functions.

Armed with the foregoing detailed information, the surgeon was able to plan a dorsal approach to the tumor and was especially careful along the lateral aspect of the resection. This was facilitated by the use of an ultrasonic aspirator; this particular aspirator (CUSA Excel + by Integra Lifesciences) produces an ultrasonic field to liquefy the tumor tissue and allow it to be easily aspirated. The ultrasonic field has another

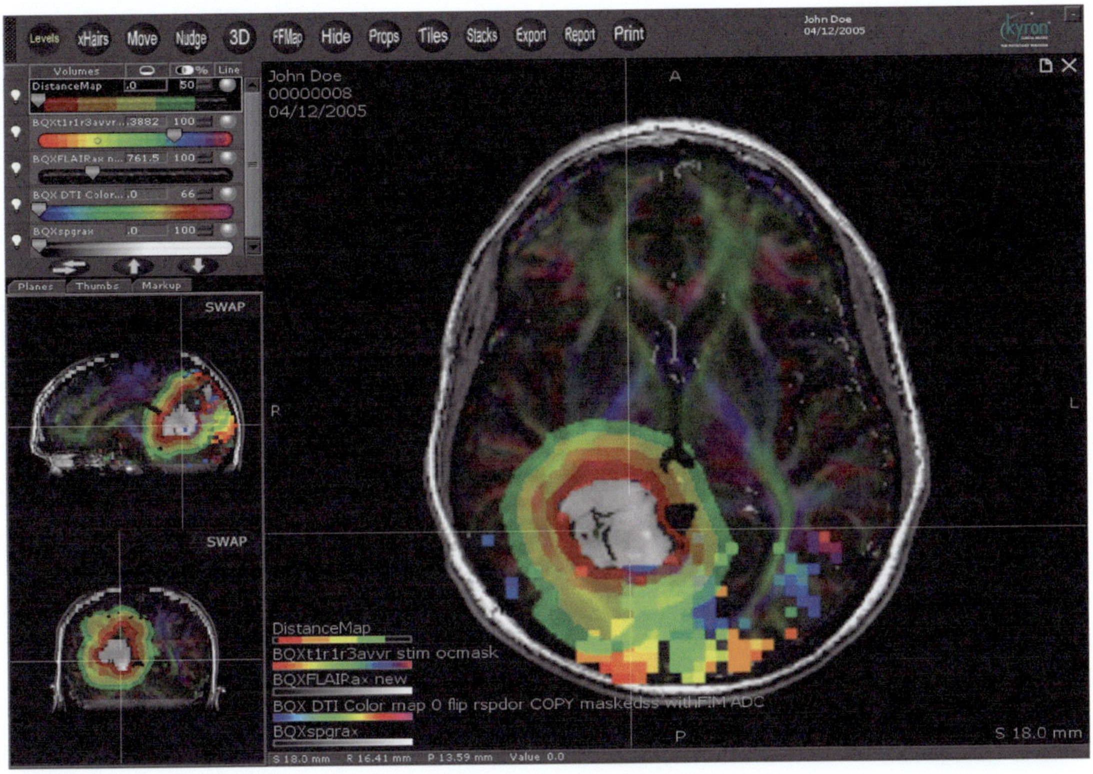

Fig. 12.9 Risk zone surrounding tumor. Same patient as described in Fig. 12.8. Here three-dimensional "shells" have been computed around the tumor and associated edematous tissue. *Color coding* shows shells encompassing distances up to 5 (*red*), 10 (*orange*), 15 (*yellow*), and 20 (*green*) mm from the potential resection margin. Some previous studies suggest that structures within 10 mm of the resection margin have high probability of permanent damage. Note that the three-dimensional shape of the distance shells can be quite complex as shown in the smaller sagittal view at *left*

fortuitous advantage in that it can begin to stimulate/inactivate tissue before it approaches close enough to liquefy it. An alert patient can often detect this stimulation as "seeing stars" or other disruptions of normal vision. The patient's report allows the surgeon to verify the location of a critical structure and advance the resection to the point at which the structure can be reversibly inactivated; thereby removing as much tumor as possible while still preserving visual function.

Epilepsy Treatment

Figure 12.10 illustrates fMRI visual field mapping for a 19-year-old female with extensive congenital malformation of the cerebral hemispheres, corpus callosum, hippocampus, and other structures. She suffered from intractable epilepsy and was a candidate for an extensive left hemisphere resection to remove the epileptic foci found there with EEG recordings. Previous WADA testing showed that language and memory function was right hemisphere dominant. However, it was not clear how much visual and sensorimotor function was present in the left hemisphere and might be at risk from a large resection. Functional MRI-based visual field mapping was performed. The colored voxels indicate that the severely distorted tissue of the left occipital lobe was still visually responsive to the checkered ring stimuli. The color coding indicates that there was a coherent visual field map with a central foveal representation (red voxels). The axial and coronal views at bottom left also showed that both hemispheres were visually responsive. Beyond such gross observations, though, it was virtually impossible to determine by visual examination of the brain activation if there was a complete representation of the visual field. As outlined schematically in Fig. 12.1, the

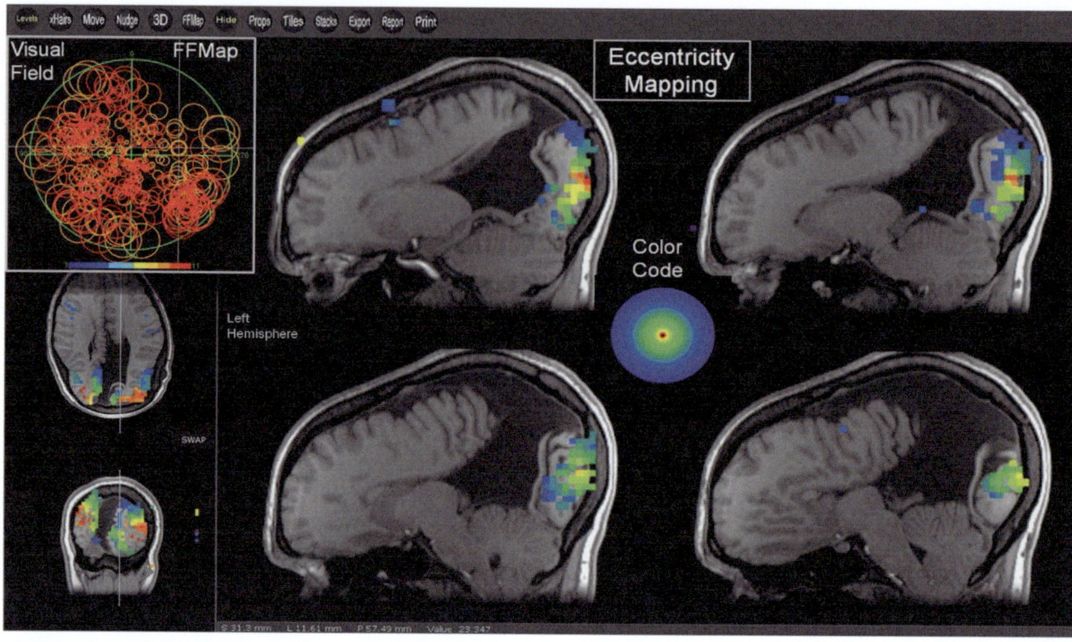

Fig. 12.10 Case report – congenital malformation with epilepsy. FMRI visual field mapping of a 19-year-old female with extensive congenital malformation of the cerebral hemispheres, corpus callosum, hippocampus, and other structures. Vision eccentricity mapping with checkered annuli revealed robust fMRI responses in deformed occipital lobe with preservation of foveal and peripheral topography (note the presence of "rainbow" colors indicating the presence of central and peripheral field representations). Construction of a functional field map (FFMap, *inset upper left*, see text for details) shows that the visual cortex is responsive to virtually all locations within the visual field except a small deficit in the upper right quadrant. (Each *circle* in the FFMap indicates the location of the visual stimuli that best activated a responsive voxel in visual cortex. Together, all the *circle symbols* show instantly what the brain can "see.")

use of both the checkered ring and wedge stimuli permitted construction of a functional field map (FFMap) for this patient (Fig. 12.1 right and Fig. 12.10 upper left). For each visually responsive cortical voxel, the ring and wedge sequences identified the optimal eccentricity [rho] and angle [theta] of the stimuli that produced maximum activation. This information was then used to place a symbol (circle) for each voxel onto a diagram of the patient's visual field. When completed for all visually responsive voxels, the result was a functional field map (Fig. 12.1 right). Each circle in the FFMap corresponds to a single voxel in the brain. The color of the circle indicates the strength of the visual response for that voxel. The size of the circle shows an estimate of the error (70% confidence interval) in determining the location of the stimuli that most strongly activated that voxel. Figuratively speaking, the FFMap depicts what the brain can "see" and allows the clinician to interpret the functional significance of the brain activation at a single glance.

For this patient, the pattern of circles in the FFMap of Fig. 12.10 shows that the brain contains a virtually complete representation of the visual field except, perhaps, for a small portion of the peripheral field in the upper right quadrant where there are relatively few circles (responsive voxels). Thus, despite the severe cerebral malformation, the FFMap revealed that the brain was responsive to visual stimulation throughout almost the entire visual field and, surprisingly, this function appeared to be lateralized normally with the right visual field represented in the left hemisphere (determined by constructing FFMaps separately for each hemisphere, data not shown). This result, combined with the presence of eloquent sensorimotor cortex in the left hemisphere (determined with other fMRI tests) precluded extensive resection of that hemisphere.

In a careful study of 21 patients who underwent surgical removal of epileptic foci involving the occipital lobe, Tandon et al. [135] found that the surgery produced "excellent seizure-free rates" (81%) or an "improvement in seizure control" (19%) and that individually tailored resections could potentially help preserve intact vision. At the time of their study, Tandon et al. did not have access to fMRI. However, they go on to suggest that fMRI vision mapping and DTI would be likely to improve the outcomes even further.

Imaging of the visual system can also be of use for guiding surgical treatment of epileptic patients with medial temporal lobe foci. If the epilepsy is debilitating and unresponsive to pharmacological treatment, the patient may be a candidate for temporal lobectomy to eradicate the offending epileptic focus. In such case, an important consideration is how far posterior to extend the resection. Potentially at risk is the portion of the optic radiation that sweeps into the temporal lobe as it passes from the lateral geniculate nucleus of the thalamus to primary visual cortex in the occipital lobe. Typically referred to as Meyer's loop [138], this portion of the radiation tends to contain fibers representing the upper quadrant of the contralateral visual field. If damaged, it often produces a characteristic "pie in the sky" quadrantanopsia that extends a variable distance into the fovea that is roughly related to the posterior extent of the resection [133]. However, this can be quite variable from patient to patient so that accurate mapping of the optic radiations with DTI and subsequent tractography (computational modeling of the fibers) could provide information about the specific trajectory of the fibers in a given patient, potentially allowing the surgeon to plan the degree of foveal involvement and its likely impact on reading. Though, there are published reports of success using DTI to visualize the radiations [90], care should be exercised since DTI mapping of white matter and particularly tractography can be incomplete. This can be particularly problematic for sharply curving fibers such as those in Myers' loop. Moreover, though DTI can potentially reveal the anatomical trajectory of the radiations, it would be even more informative if the fibers could be labeled according to the visual field location they represent as determined by fMRI mapping of the cortex to which they project (e.g., V1). Currently, such "functional labeling" is not available for routine clinical use, but such advanced capabilities may appear in the not too distant future.

Arteriovenous Malformations

Figure 12.11 illustrates the results of visual field mapping and FFMap construction for a 31-year-old woman who suffered from severe migraine

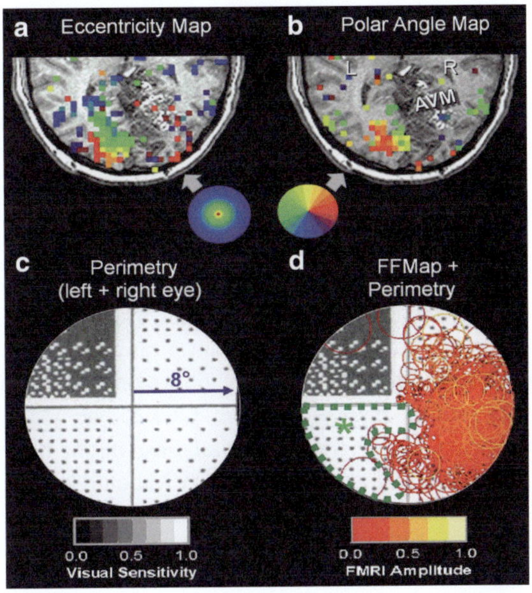

Fig. 12.11 Case report – occipital arteriovenous malformation (AVM) with migraine. A 31-year-old woman suffered from severe migraine headaches due to an AVM of the right occipital lobe. (**a**, **b**) Presurgical vision mapping revealed robust activation of left occipital cortex (left hemisphere is on *left* in this figure) but with only weak, irregular activation in right hemisphere. (**c**) Humphrey perimetry revealed an upper left quadrantanopsia (only central 8° shown). Color scale in (**c**) indicates blindness as *black* with normal visual sensitivity as *white* or lightly stippled. (**d**) Functional field map overlaid on perimetry permits direct comparison of the retinotopic pattern of fMRI responses (*orange circles*) with behavioral perimetry. *Lower left quadrant* indicates a mismatch in that the patient can detect visual stimuli in this quadrant but there are few brain voxels (*circles*) responding to this quadrant. This provides direct evidence for neurovascular uncoupling (NVU) in which the AVM (presumably) has directly impaired the BOLD hemodynamic mechanism responsible for the fMRI response without damaging the associated neurons. Had the NVU not been detected, the physician might have erroneously assumed that the right hemisphere was visually unresponsive

headaches due to an AVM of the right occipital lobe. Surgical removal of the AVM was being considered but the proximity of eloquent visual cortex was a potential contraindication. Routine examination did not reveal any neurological deficits and there were no visual field abnormalities apparent during confrontation testing. However, automated Humphrey perimetry indicated an upper left quadrantanopsia (only the central 8 degrees illustrated in Fig. 12.10c), whereas the FFMap (Fig. 12.11d) indicated that brain responses were confined mainly to the right hemifield. Thus, there appeared to be a clear discrepancy in which the perimetry indicated good visual sensitivity and presumably good brain function in the lower left quadrant, yet there was little fMRI response associated with that region (green dotted outline). This was interpreted as indicative of a zone of pathology-induced uncoupling between the neuronal activity and the vascular response that generates the fMRI signal. Such NVU can be a significant problem for presurgical mapping if such omissions are not detected as they were here. Lack of an fMRI response in the right occipital lobe might have suggested that excision of the AVM could be performed safely. But, in fact this likely would have resulted in a complete left hemianopia and potential reading difficulty.

Diagnosis/Interpretation of Vision Pathologies

Sensory Loss Versus Attentional Neglect. Use of fMRI and DTI to identify key visual system structures for presurgical planning is perhaps the most common clinical application. However, as the use of advanced imaging becomes more common, other unexpected applications can become evident. Figure 12.12 illustrates the case of a 51-year-old woman who suffered from the recurrence of a grade II oligodendroglioma that had been resected 6 years earlier. A follow-up radiotreatment "balloon" had been placed along the parieto-occipital sulcus (white dotted outline of cavity in Fig. 12.12a) and was scheduled for removal with additional resection of the new tumor growth. Visual perimetry for this patient revealed an apparent hemianopsia suggesting sensory blindness in the left visual hemifield (Fig. 12.12d). However, both the fMRI brain map (Fig. 12.12b) and the FFMap for this patient (Fig. 12.12e) revealed ample activation of the apparently blind left hemifield. This indicated that early visual cortex was functionally intact, suggesting that the apparent hemianopsia might not be sensory in nature but, rather, might reflect a higher-order cognitive deficit such as attentional hemi-neglect. This would be consistent with damage to parietal cortex and was later verified with behavioral testing (e.g., line bisection test, target search, and clockface drawing). The potential importance of this insight was subsequently demonstrated upon re-testing after removal of the radiotreatment balloon and the follow-up resection. After surgery, the FFMap showed a loss of activation in the lower left quadrant (Fig. 12.12f) indicating that the surgery had further damaged eloquent sensory cortex. Postoperatively, the patient complained of difficulty reading, which was not apparent preoperatively.

In this case the fMRI, not the perimetry, correctly indicated that visual cortex of the right hemisphere was still functional and potentially at risk from invasive surgery. The postoperative reading deficit raises the possibility (though does not prove) that sensory activity at lower levels of the visual system might contribute to visual functions (e.g., reading) in a manner that may not be obvious to the patient and that may not be apparent in routine behavioral testing. At the very least, this case suggests that visual field deficits apparent on behavioral testing may reflect a combination of both sensory and higher-order cognitive deficits whose relative contributions may be unclear without fMRI mapping.

Agnosias and Extrastriate Visual Areas

Cerebral Achromatopsia. Visual areas VO1,2 can be activated by selective color stimulation and a color discrimination task [77]. These areas appear to be located at or near a ventral occipito-temporal location that when lesioned can cause cerebral achromatopsia [139, 140]. Figure 12.13 illustrates the case of an artist who suffered two strokes during and shortly after cardiac bypass surgery that left him with cerebral dyschromatopsia and

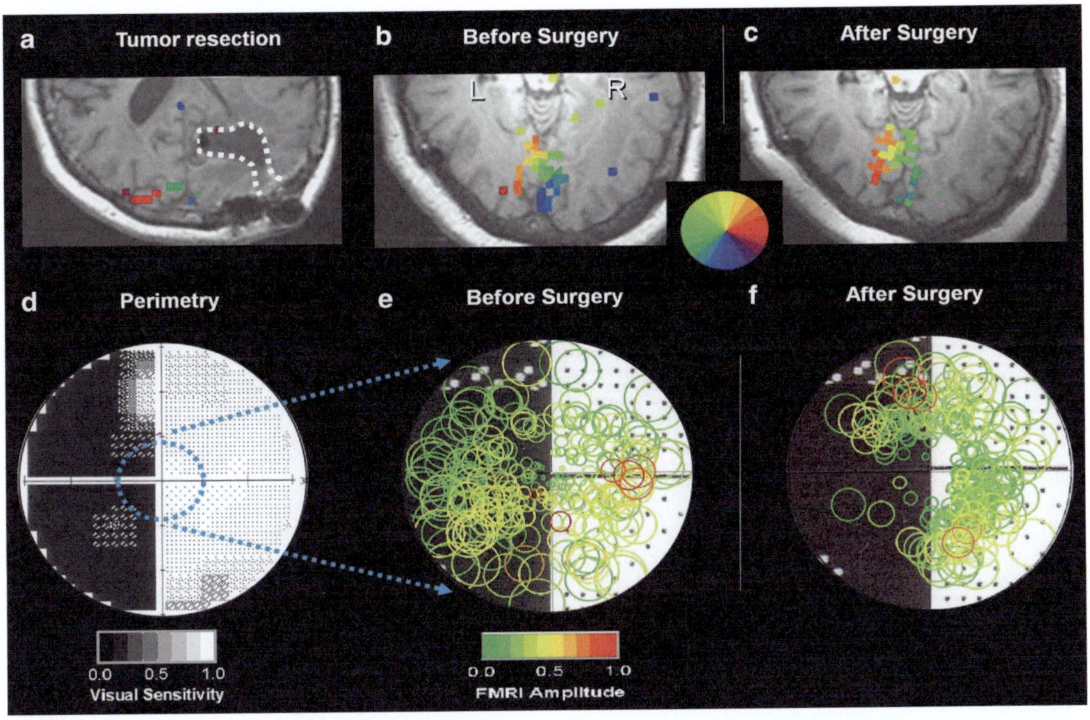

Fig. 12.12 Case report – tumor recurrence with undiagnosed visual neglect. A 51-year-old woman suffered from recurrence of a grade II oligodendroglioma in the *right hemisphere* (right hemisphere displayed here on right). (See text for additional details.) (**a**) Site of previous resection and gliasite balloon implant in occipito-parietal cortex. (**b**) FMRI vision map produced by rotating checkered wedge. Note complete complement of responses at all angular positions within the visual field (rainbow colors). (**c**) Postsurgical fMRI. Note loss of resp-onses for visual field locations marked in *blues/cyan*. (**d**) Humphrey perimetry (30° test field) shows nearly complete left hemianopia. (**e**) Functional field map (*yellow/green circles*) overlaid on perimetry shows that visual cortex is responsive to stimuli presented throughout the visual field even within the supposedly blind hemifield. (Each *circle symbol* indicates the location of the visual stimuli that best stimulated a responsive voxel in visual cortex.) Subsequent behavioral testing showed that apparent hemianopsia was primarily due to visuospatial neglect, not sensory blindness. (**f**) Following surgical removal of the recurrent tumor in the right hemisphere, most of the cortical response to left visual field stimulation is absent. Patient suffered postsurgical reading impairment

"object agnosia" thus effectively ending his career as an artist and his ability to esthetically appreciate his own artwork. (A similar case was reported by Oliver Sacks [141].) Over the 3-year period following the stroke, the patient's ability to perform color discriminations improved to the point that his performance on a standard Farnsworth-Munsell (F-M) color chip sorting test was almost within the normal range. At that time, fMRI responses to an adaptation of the F-M color test revealed responses within a ventral temporal lobe site (Fig. 12.13b) that in healthy controls was activated bilaterally during performance of the same test (Fig. 12.13c, d). It was not possible to determine if the activated site in this patient was responsible for the partial recovery since fMRI data were not acquired immediately following the stroke. Nevertheless, the data are consistent with that possibility and, more importantly, they demonstrate the potential use of fMRI to provide insight into brain mechanisms responsible for long-term recovery of function.

Selective visual agnosias such as those described previously are relatively rare and for many patients may not have a great impact on their overall quality of life. Loss of color vision for most patients might be little more than an annoyance but, for a patient such as the artist described, the effects of selective loss of color vision were devastating. Arguably then, the risks

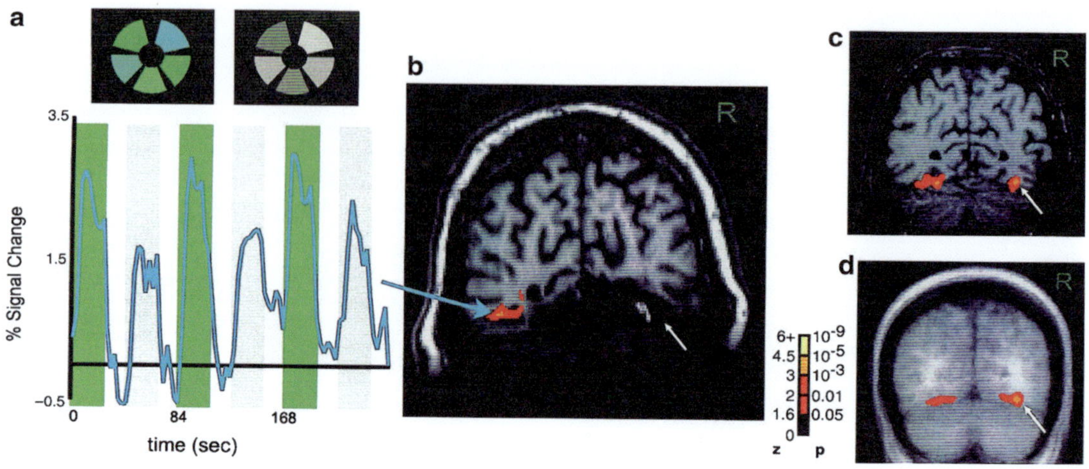

Fig. 12.13 Case report – cerebral achromatopsia patient with color-selective fMRI activation. A 60-year-old male suffered dual strokes during/after coronary artery surgery. (**a**) During fMRI, the patient alternately viewed chromatic and achromatic stimuli (**a**, *top*) interspersed with periods of passive fixation. Average time series (**a**, *blue graph line*) from color-selective voxels in the patient's left ventral cortex illustrates greater MR signal increase during chromatic stimulation (*green bars*) than during achromatic stimulation (*gray bars*). (**b**) Patient's color-selective fMRI response (*orange*) overlaid on coronal section of anatomy. (**c**) Ventral color-selective activity in age-matched control subject. (**d**) Average color-selective activity in 12 young control subjects. Color scale illustrates degree of color-selectivity for (**b**)–(**d**). *White arrows* indicate the location of right ventral color-selective region in normal controls and damaged cortex in KG. Reproduced with permission from [150]

of invasive treatment and the necessity of detailed fMRI mapping should be considered in the context of each individual patient's abilities, vocation, and life style. What is new is that neuroimaging technology can now provide specific information relevant to this issue with relatively little cost and effort.

Stroke

Functional MRI of the visual system has not typically been used in the diagnosis and treatment of stroke patients since there is no established treatment algorithm that could be aided by such information. That said, fMRI-based vision mapping can be performed readily with stroke patients and may be useful for clarifying the cause of stroke-related visual field deficits as described in the previous section on "Sensory Loss versus Attentional Neglect." Such careful diagnosis might prove to be of use in selecting rehabilitation strategies.

Complicating Factors

Neurovascular Uncoupling (NVU). As evident from some of the preceding examples, medical interpretation and use of fMRI and DTI data can be complicated by a variety of factors. Foremost, in this respect is the potential for brain pathology to directly disrupt the BOLD hemodynamic mechanism responsible for fMRI or to disrupt the anisotropic diffusion of water responsible for DTI. In both cases, it appears that it is possible for the imaging signals to be compromised while the underlying neural processes are intact, at least enough to support behavioral functions [142]. As of this writing, however, the incidence rate of BOLD NVU and DTI anisotropy loss is not known. Moreover, their association with particular pathological conditions has not been established, though it seems logical that NVU might be preferentially associated with pathologies involving the vasculature such as AVMs and stroke. In a preliminary analysis of imaging data from patients who received fMRI visual field mapping, three were identified as showing evidence of NVU in a portion of their brain map (DeYoe, personal communication). Figure 12.11 and the associated discussion illustrates one of these cases. Of these three cases, none showed NVU extending throughout an entire hemisphere. One of these patients was re-scanned 5 months later.

The resulting FFMap did not show evidence of NVU. Instead, robust fMRI responses were obtained from the portion of the visual field that had been previously unresponsive. This suggests that the process causing NVU may be reversible, at least in some cases. Besides the method illustrated above for detecting NVU (Fig. 12.11d), other approaches have been tested [143]. Typically, these approaches involve some manipulation or imaging procedure that tests vascular reactivity to a breath-hold [144] or CO_2 challenge [143, 145, 146]. While promising, it is not clear that these tests necessarily detect all causes of NVU. For instance, it is not clear that the BOLD response to a change in neural activity employs the same mechanism as the response to a change in CO_2 level, so it is conceivable that a neurally evoked BOLD response could be blocked even though the vasculature is responsive to a CO_2 challenge. It is also important to point out that a CO_2 challenge or breath-hold may not be an appropriate stressor for patients with cerebral pathology.

Tissue Distortions. A second major complication for use of imaging data in surgical planning/guidance is movement/swelling/distortion of brain tissue after acquisition of the imaging data so that the locations of key features in the imaging data are no longer accurate during surgery. This is a problem even when using an intraoperative navigation system since the brain tissue can move relative to the fiduciary markers used to calibrate and register the navigation system. Though MR imaging during surgery is possible with appropriate scanner hardware, its use has been limited and the imaging procedures are typically disruptive to the ongoing surgical procedures. One helpful approach described previously is to use an ultrasonic aspirator with an alert patient to verify when the resection margin nears a critical eloquent structure such as the optic radiations (pyramidal tracts, etc.). In such case, the presurgical imaging data provide the surgeon with a general orientation to the location of key structures relative to the planned resection, but intraoperative patient reporting is used to provide intrasurgical verification.

Conclusion

Since its inception in the early 1990s, functional MRI has evolved from a novel esoteric technology into a tool used routinely in neuroscience research and increasingly in clinical practice. From the beginning, fMRI has been used to identify visual system pathways [1, 22, 147] and this has advanced to such a degree that today we can routinely map the network of subdivisions whose activity generates the rich and varied experience of vision. Yet, there is a significant gap between the complexity and sophistication of the information that fMRI can provide and our ability to use that information in comparably sophisticated ways to affect the diagnosis and treatment of brain-related vision pathologies. Hopefully advanced knowledge, such as that contained in this chapter, can become the catalyst of future innovation if it is placed into the hands of those at the forefront of daily medical practice.

Acknowledgments and Disclosure This work supported by NIH grants R42CA113186 and R01EB007827. Authors E.A.D. and J.U. are consultants and members of the board of directors of Prism Clinical Imaging Inc.

References

1. Belliveau JW, Kennedy DN, McKinstry RC, Buchbinder BR, Weisskoff RM, Cohen MS, et al. Functional mapping of the human visual cortex by magnetic resonance imaging. Science. 1991;254: 716–9.
2. Logothetis NK, Wandell BA. Interpreting the BOLD signal. Annu Rev Physiol. 2004;66:735–69.
3. Girouard H, Iadecola C. Neurovascular coupling in the normal brain and in hypertension, stroke, and Alzheimer disease. J Appl Physiol. 2006;100(1): 328–35.
4. Logothetis NK. Neurovascular uncoupling: much ado about nothing. Front Neuroener. 2010;2:1–4.
5. Ulmer JL, Hacein-Bey L, Mathews VP, Mueller WM, DeYoe EA, Prost RW, et al. Lesion-induced pseudo-dominance at functional magnetic resonance imaging: implications for preoperative assessments. Neurosurgery. 2004;55(3):569–79. discussion 580–1.
6. Kandel ER, Schwartz JH, Jessell TM, editors. Principles of neural science. 4th ed. New York: McGraw-Hill; 2000. 1414.

7. Mustari MJ, Ono S, Das VE. Signal processing and distribution in cortical-brainstem pathways for smooth pursuit eye movements. Ann NY Acad Sci. 2009;1164:147–54.
8. Inouye T. Die Sehstorungen bei Schussverletzungen der kortikalen Sehsphare. Leipzig, Germany: W Engelmann; 1909.
9. Holmes G, Lister WT. Disturbances of vision from cerebral lesions, with special reference to the cortical representation of the macula. Brain. 1916;39: 34–73.
10. Riddoch G. Dissociation of visual perceptions due to occipital injuries, with especial reference to appreciation of movement. Brain. 1917;40:15–57.
11. Holmes G. Disturbances of vision by cerebral lesions. Br J Ophthalmol. 1918;2:353–84.
12. Horton JC. The central visual pathways. In: Hart WH, editor. Adler's physiology of the eye. St. Louis: Mosby Year book; 1992. p. 728–72.
13. Horton JC, Hoyt WF. The representation of the visual field in human striate cortex. A revision of the classic Holmes map. Arch Ophthalmol. 1991;109: 816–24.
14. Horton JC, Hoyt WF. Quadrantic visual field defects: a hallmark of lesions in extrastriate (V2/V3) cortex. Brain. 1991;114:1703–18.
15. Hubel DH, Wiesel TN. Receptive fields and functional architecture in two nonstriate areas (18 and 19) of the cat. J Neurophysiol. 1965;28:229–89.
16. Allman JM, Kaas JH. A representation of the visual field in the caudal third of the middle temporal gyrus of the owl monkey (*Aotus trivirgatus*). Brain Res. 1971;31:85–105.
17. Allman JM, Kaas JH. Representation of the visual field in striate and adjoining cortex of the owl monkey (*Aotus trivirgatus*). Brain Res. 1971;35:89–106.
18. Fox PT, Miezin FM, Allman JM, Van Essen DC, Raichle ME. Retinotopic organization of human visual cortex mapped with positron-emission tomography. J Neurosci. 1987;7(3):913–22.
19. Corbetta M, Miezin FM, Dobmeyer S, Shulman GL, Petersen SE. Attentional modulation of neural processing of shape, color, and velocity in humans. Science. 1990;248(248):1556–9.
20. Corbetta M, Miezin FM, Dobmeyer S, Shulman GL, Petersen SE. Selective and divided attention during visual discrimination of shape, color, and speed: functional anatomy by positron emission tomography. J Neurosci. 1991;11(8):2383–402.
21. Gulyas B, Roland PE. Cortical fields participating in form and colour discrimination in the human brain. Neuroreport. 1991;2(10):585–8.
22. DeYoe EA, Bandettini P, Neitz J, Miller D, Winans P. Functional magnetic resonance imaging (FMRI) of the human brain. J Neurosci Meth. 1994;54:171–87.
23. Shipp S, Watson JD, Frackowiak RS, Zeki S. Retinotopic maps in human prestriate visual cortex: the demarcation of areas V2 and V3. Neuroimage. 1995;2(2):125–32.
24. Sereno MI, Dale AM, Reppas JB, Kwong KK, Belliveau JW, Brady TJ, et al. Borders of multiple visual areas in humans revealed by functional MRI. Science. 1995;268(268):889–93.
25. Tootell RB, Reppas JB, Kwong KK, Malach R, Born RT, Brady TJ, et al. Functional analysis of human MT and related visual cortical areas using magnetic resonance imaging. J Neurosci. 1995;15(4):3215–30.
26. DeYoe EA, Carman G, Bandettini P, Glickman S, Wieser J, Cox R, et al. Mapping striate and extrastriate visual areas in human cerebral cortex. Proc Natl Acad Sci USA. 1996;93(6):2382–6.
27. Engel SA, Glover GH, Wandell BA. Retinotopic organization in human visual cortex and the spatial precision of functional MRI. Cereb Cortex. 1997; 7:181–92.
28. Tootell RBH, Mendola JD, Hadjikhani NK, Ledden PJ, Liu AK, Reppas JB, et al. Functional analysis of V3A and related areas in human visual cortex. J Neurosci. 1997;17(18):7060–78.
29. Grill-Spector K, Kushnir T, Hendler T, Edelman S, Itzchak Y, Malach R. A sequence of object-processing stages revealed by fMRI in the human occipital lobe. Hum Brain Mapp. 1998;6(4): 316–28.
30. Press WA, Brewer AA, Dougherty RF, Wade AR, Wandell BA. Visual areas and spatial summation in human visual cortex. Vision Res. 2001;41(10–11): 1321–32.
31. Sereno MI, Pitzalis S, Martinez A. Mapping of contralateral space in retinotopic coordinates by a parietal cortical area in humans. Science. 2001; 294(5545):1350–4.
32. Tootell RB, Hadjikhani N. Where is 'dorsal V4' in human visual cortex? Retinotopic, topographic and functional evidence. Cereb Cortex. 2001;11(4): 298–311.
33. Dougherty RF, Koch VM, Brewer AA, Fischer B, Modersitzki J, Wandell BA. Visual field representations and locations of visual areas V1/2/3 in human visual cortex. J Vis. 2003;3(10):586–98.
34. Duncan RO, Boynton GM. Cortical magnification within human primary visual cortex correlates with acuity thresholds. Neuron. 2003;38(4):659–71.
35. Brewer AA, Liu J, Wade AR, Wandell BA. Visual field maps and stimulus selectivity in human ventral occipital cortex. Nat Neurosci. 2005;8(8):1102–9.
36. Liu J, Wandell BA. Specializations for chromatic and temporal signals in human visual cortex. J Neurosci. 2005;25(13):3459–68.
37. Schluppeck D, Glimcher P, Heeger DJ. Topographic organization for delayed saccades in human posterior parietal cortex. J Neurophysiol. 2005;94(2): 1372–84.
38. Silver MA, Ress D, Heeger DJ. Topographic maps of visual spatial attention in human parietal cortex. J Neurophysiol. 2005;94(2):1358–71.
39. Wandell BA, Brewer AA, Dougherty RF. Visual field map clusters in human cortex. Philos Trans R Soc Lond B Biol Sci. 2005;360(1456):693–707.

40. Hagler Jr DJ, Sereno MI. Spatial maps in frontal and prefrontal cortex. Neuroimage. 2006;29(2):567–77.
41. Kastner S, Schneider KA, Wunderlich K. Beyond a relay nucleus: neuroimaging views on the human LGN. Prog Brain Res. 2006;155:125–43.
42. Larsson J, Heeger DJ. Two retinotopic visual areas in human lateral occipital cortex. J Neurosci. 2006;26(51):13128–42.
43. Pitzalis S, Galletti C, Huang RS, Patria F, Committeri G, Galati G, et al. Wide-field retinotopy defines human cortical visual area v6. J Neurosci. 2006; 26(30):7962–73.
44. Hansen KA, Kay KN, Gallant JL. Topographic organization in and near human visual area V4. J Neurosci. 2007;27(44):11896–911.
45. Schira MM, Wade AR, Tyler CW. Two-dimensional mapping of the central and parafoveal visual field to human visual cortex. J Neurophysiol. 2007;97(6): 4284–95.
46. Swisher JD, Halko MA, Merabet LB, McMains SA, Somers DC. Visual topography of human intraparietal sulcus. J Neurosci. 2007;27(20):5326–37.
47. Wandell BA, Dumoulin SO, Brewer AA. Visual field maps in human cortex. Neuron. 2007;56(2):366–83.
48. Dumoulin SO, Wandell BA. Population receptive field estimates in human visual cortex. Neuroimage. 2008;39(2):647–60.
49. Saygin AP, Sereno MI. Retinotopy and attention in human occipital, temporal, parietal, and frontal cortex. Cereb Cortex. 2008;18(9):2158–68.
50. Amano K, Wandell BA, Dumoulin SO. Visual field maps, population receptive field sizes, and visual field coverage in the human MT + complex. J Neurophysiol. 2009;102(5):2704–18.
51. Arcaro MJ, McMains SA, Singer BD, Kastner S. Retinotopic organization of human ventral visual cortex. J Neurosci. 2009;29(34):10638–52.
52. Pitzalis S, Sereno MI, Committeri G, Fattori P, Galati G, Patria F, et al. Human V6: the medial motion area. Cereb Cortex. 2010;20(2):411–24.
53. Silver MA, Kastner S. Topographic maps in human frontal and parietal cortex. Trends Cogn Sci. 2009; 13(11):488–95.
54. Kolster H, Peeters R, Orban GA. The retinotopic organization of the human middle temporal area MT/V5 and its cortical neighbors. J Neurosci. 2010; 30(29):9801–20.
55. Tootell RB, Mendola JD, Hadjikhani NK, Liu AK, Dale AM. The representation of the ipsilateral visual field in human cerebral cortex. Proc Natl Acad Sci USA. 1998;95(3):818–24.
56. Schluppeck D, Curtis CE, Glimcher PW, Heeger DJ. Sustained activity in topographic areas of human posterior parietal cortex during memory-guided saccades. J Neurosci. 2006;26(19):5098–108.
57. Sereno MI, Huang RS. A human parietal face area contains aligned head-centered visual and tactile maps. Nat Neurosci. 2006;9(10):1337–43.
58. Orban GA, Dupont P, De Bruyn B, Vogels R, Vandenberghe R, Mortelmans L. A motion area in human visual cortex. Proc Natl Acad Sci USA. 1995;92(4):993–7.
59. Hadjikhani N, Liu AK, Dale A, Cavanagh P, Tootell RBH. Retinotopy and color sensitivity in human visual cortical area V8. Nat Neurosci. 1998;1: 235–41.
60. Zeki S, Perry RJ, Bartels A. The processing of kinetic contours in the brain. Cereb Cortex. 2003; 13(2):189–202.
61. Kanwisher N, McDermott J, Chun MM. The fusiform face area: a module in human extrastriate cortex specialized for face perception. J Neurosci. 1997;17(11):4302–11.
62. Cohen L, Dehaene S. Specialization within the ventral stream: the case for the visual word form area. Neuroimage. 2004;22(1):466–76.
63. Cohen L, Dehaene S, Naccache L, Lehericy S, Dehaene-Lambertz G, Henaff MA, et al. The visual word form area: spatial and temporal characterization of an initial stage of reading in normal subjects and posterior split-brain patients. Brain. 2000;123 (Pt 2):291–307.
64. Cohen L, Lehericy S, Chochon F, Lemer C, Rivaud S, Dehaene S. Language-specific tuning of visual cortex? Functional properties of the Visual Word Form Area. Brain. 2002;125(Pt 5):1054–69.
65. Price CJ, Devlin JT. The myth of the visual word form area. Neuroimage. 2003;19(3):473–81.
66. Epstein R, Kanwisher N. A cortical representation of the local visual environment. Nature. 1998; 392(6676):598–601.
67. Bonda E, Petrides M, Ostry D, Evans A. Specific involvement of human parietal systems and the amygdala in the perception of biological motion. J Neurosci. 1996;16(11):3737–44.
68. Howard RJ, Brammer M, Wright I, Woodruff PW, Bullmore ET, Zeki S. A direct demonstration of functional specialization within motion-related visual and auditory cortex of the human brain. Curr Biol. 1996;6(8):1015–9.
69. Grossman ED, Blake R. Brain activity evoked by inverted and imagined biological motion. Vision Res. 2001;41(10–11):1475–82.
70. Downing PE, Jiang Y, Shuman M, Kanwisher N. A cortical area selective for visual processing of the human body. Science. 2001;293(5539):2470–3.
71. Astafiev SV, Stanley CM, Shulman GL, Corbetta M. Extrastriate body area in human occipital cortex responds to the performance of motor actions. Nat Neurosci. 2004;7(5):542–8.
72. Lueck CJ, Zeki S, Friston KJ, Deiber MP, Cope P, Cunningham VJ, et al. The colour centre in the cerebral cortex of man. Nature. 1989;340(6232):386–9.
73. Merigan WH. Human V4? Curr Biol. 1993;3(4): 226–9.
74. Heywood CA, Gaffan D, Cowey A. Cerebral achromatopsia in monkeys. Eur J Neurosci. 1995;7: 1064–73.
75. McKeefry DJ, Zeki S. The position and topography of the human colour centre as revealed by functional

magnetic resonance imaging. Brain. 1997;120(Pt 12):2229–42.
76. Zeki S. Improbable areas in the visual brain. Trends Neurosci. 2003;26(1):23–6.
77. Wade A, Augath M, Logothetis N, Wandell B. fMRI measurements of color in macaque and human. J Vis. 2008;8(10):6. 1–19.
78. Dupont P, Orban GA, De Bruyn B, Verbruggen A, Mortelmans L. Many areas in the human brain respond to visual motion. J Neurophysiol. 1994; 72(3):1420–4.
79. Dupont P, De Bruyn B, Vandenberghe R, Rosier AM, Michiels J, Marchal G, et al. The kinetic occipital region in human visual cortex. Cereb Cortex. 1997; 7(3):283–92.
80. Van Oostende S, Sunaert S, Van Hecke P, Marchal G, Orban GA. The kinetic occipital (KO) region in man: an fMRI study. Cereb Cortex. 1997;7(7): 690–701.
81. Serences JT, Boynton GM. The representation of behavioral choice for motion in human visual cortex. J Neurosci. 2007;27(47):12893–9.
82. DeYoe EA, Van Essen DC. Concurrent processing streams in monkey visual cortex. Trends Neurosci. 1988;11(5):219–26.
83. Bio_Motion_Lab. BMLwalker V2.0. 2010. http://www.biomotionlab.ca/Demos/BMLwalker.html.
84. Girkin CA, Miller NR. Central disorders of vision in humans. Surv Ophthalmol. 2001;45(5):379–405.
85. Zihl J, Von Cramon D, Mai N. Selective disturbance of movement vision after bilateral brain damage. Brain. 1983;106:313–40.
86. Zihl J, Von Cramon D, Mai N, Schmid CH. Disturbance of movement vision after bilateral posterior brain damage. Brain. 1991;114:2235–52.
87. Ulmer JL, Salvan CV, Mueller WM, Krouwer HG, Stroe GO, Aralasmak A, et al. The role of diffusion tensor imaging in establishing the proximity of tumor borders to functional brain systems: implications for preoperative risk assessments and postoperative outcomes. Technol Cancer Res Treat. 2004; 3(6):567–76.
88. Wakana S, Jiang H, Nagae-Poetscher LM, van Zijl PC, Mori S. Fiber tract-based atlas of human white matter anatomy. Radiology. 2004;230(1):77–87.
89. Jellison BJ, Field AS, Medow J, Lazar M, Salamat MS, Alexander AL. Diffusion tensor imaging of cerebral white matter: a pictorial review of physics, fiber tract anatomy, and tumor imaging patterns. AJNR Am J Neuroradiol. 2004;25(3):356–69.
90. Sherbondy AJ, Dougherty RF, Napel S, Wandell BA. Identifying the human optic radiation using diffusion imaging and fiber tractography. J Vis. 2008;8(10):12. 1–11.
91. Toosy AT, Ciccarelli O, Parker GJ, Wheeler-Kingshott CA, Miller DH, Thompson AJ. Characterizing function-structure relationships in the human visual system with functional MRI and diffusion tensor imaging. Neuroimage. 2004;21(4): 1452–63.
92. Dougherty RF, Ben-Shachar M, Bammer R, Brewer AA, Wandell BA. Functional organization of human occipital-callosal fiber tracts. Proc Natl Acad Sci USA. 2005;102(20):7350–5.
93. Kim M, Ducros M, Carlson T, Ronen I, He S, Ugurbil K, et al. Anatomical correlates of the functional organization in the human occipitotemporal cortex. Magn Reson Imaging. 2006;24(5):583–90.
94. Sherbondy AJ, Dougherty RF, Ananthanarayanan R, Modha DS, Wandell BA. Think global, act local; projectome estimation with BlueMatter. Med Image Comput Comput Assist Interv. 2009;12(Pt 1): 861–8.
95. Shinoura N, Suzuki Y, Yamada R, Tabei Y, Saito K, Yagi K. Relationships between brain tumor and optic tract or calcarine fissure are involved in visual field deficits after surgery for brain tumor. Acta Neurochir (Wien). 2010;152(4):637–42.
96. Biswal BB, Mennes M, Zuo XN, Gohel S, Kelly C, Smith SM, et al. Toward discovery science of human brain function. Proc Natl Acad Sci USA. 2010;107(10):4734–9.
97. McIntosh AR, Grady CL, Ungerleider LG, Haxby JV, Rapoport SI, Horwitz B. Network analysis of cortical visual pathways mapped with PET. J Neurosci. 1994;14(2):655–66.
98. Marreiros AC, Kiebel SJ, Friston KJ. Dynamic causal modelling for fMRI: a two-state model. Neuroimage. 2008;39(1):269–78.
99. Bianciardi M, Fukunaga M, van Gelderen P, Horovitz SG, de Zwart JA, Duyn JH. Modulation of spontaneous fMRI activity in human visual cortex by behavioral state. Neuroimage. 2009;45(1):160–8.
100. Felleman DJ, Van Essen DC. Distributed hierarchical processing in the primate cerebral cortex. Cereb Cortex. 1991;1:1–47.
101. Merigan WH, Nealey TA, Maunsell JH. Visual effects of lesions of cortical area V2 in macaques. J Neurosci. 1993;13(7):3180–91.
102. Zeki S, Ffytche DH. The Riddoch syndrome: insights into the neurobiology of conscious vision. Brain. 1998;121(Pt 1):25–45.
103. Brodmann K. Vergleichende Lokalisationslehre der Grosshirinde in ihren Prinzipien dargestellt auf Grund des Zellenbaues. Leipzig: J.A. Barth; 1909.
104. von Economo C, Koskinas GN. Atlas of cytoarchitectonics of the adult human cerebral cortex: first English edition. In: Triarhou LC, editors. Basel: Karger; 2008.
105. Schleicher A, Morosan P, Amunts K, Zilles K. Quantitative architectural analysis: a new approach to cortical mapping. J Autism Dev Disord. 2009;39(11):1568–81.
106. Zilles K, Amunts K. Receptor mapping: architecture of the human cerebral cortex. Curr Opin Neurol. 2009;22(4):331–9.
107. de Sousa AA, Sherwood CC, Schleicher A, Amunts K, MacLeod CE, Hof PR, et al. Comparative cytoarchitectural analyses of striate and extrastriate areas in hominoids. Cereb Cortex. 2010;20(4):966–81.

108. Buracas GT, Boynton GM. Efficient design of event-related fMRI experiments using M-sequences. Neuroimage. 2002;16(3 Pt 1):801–13.
109. Seiffert AE, Somers DC, Dale AM, Tootell RB. Functional MRI studies of human visual motion perception: texture, luminance, attention and after-effects. Cereb Cortex. 2003;13(4):340–9.
110. Brefczynski J, Datta R, Lewis JW, DeYoe EA. The topography of visuospatial attention as revealed by a novel visual field mapping technique. J Cogn Neurosci. 2009;21(7):1447–60.
111. American Medical Association. Coding billing insurance: CPT. 2010. http://www.ama-assn.org/ama/pub/physician-resources/solutions-managing-your-practice/coding-billing-insurance/cpt.shtml.
112. Invivo. Invivo. 2010. http://www.invivocorp.com/.
113. NordicNeuroLab. NordicNeuroLab. 2010. http://www.nordicneurolab.com/.
114. Prism Clinical Imaging. Prism clinical imaging Inc. 2010. http://www.prismclinical.com/index.html.
115. Greve DN, Mueller BA, Liu T, Turner JA, Voyvodic J, Yetter E, Diaz M, McCarthy G, Wallace S, Roach BJ, Ford JM, Mathalon DH, Calhoun VD, Wible CG, Brown GG, Potkin SG, Glover G. A novel method for quantifying scanner instability in fMRI. Magn Reson Med. 2011;65(4):1053–61.
116. Brown GG, Mathalon DH, Stern H, Ford J, Mueller B, Greve DN, McCarthy G, Voyvodic J, Glover G, Diaz M, Yetter E, Ozyurt IB, Jorgensen KW, Wible CG, Turner JA, Thompson WK, Potkin SG. Multisite reliability of cognitive BOLD data. Neuroimage. 2011;54(3):2163–75.
117. Ojemann JG, Akbudak E, Snyder AZ, McKinstry RC, Raichle ME, Conturo TE. Anatomic localization and quantitative analysis of gradient refocused echo-planar fMRI susceptibility artifacts. Neuroimage. 1997;6(3):156–67.
118. National Electrical Manufacturers Association. DICOM. 2010. http://medical.nema.org/dicom/geninfo/Brochure.pdf.
119. Voyvodic JT. Activation mapping as a percentage of local excitation: fMRI stability within scans, between scans and across field strengths. Magn Reson Imaging. 2006;24(9):1249–61.
120. Voyvodic JT, Petrella JR, Friedman AH. fMRI activation mapping as a percentage of local excitation: consistent presurgical motor maps without threshold adjustment. J Magn Reson Imaging. 2009;29(4):751–9.
121. Prism Clinical Imaging. Prism process. Elm Grove, WI: Prism Clinical Imaging; 2010.
122. Saad ZS, Ropella KM, Cox RW, DeYoe EA. Analysis and use of FMRI response delays. Hum Brain Mapp. 2001;13(2):74–93.
123. Cox DD, Savoy RL. Functional magnetic resonance imaging (fMRI) "brain reading": detecting and classifying distributed patterns of fMRI activity in human visual cortex. Neuroimage. 2003;19(2 Pt 1):261–70.
124. Coenen VA, Krings T, Weidemann J, Spangenberg P, Gilsbach JM, Rohde V. Diffusion weighted imaging combined with intraoperative 3D-ultrasound and fMRI for the resection of an optic radiation cavernoma. Zentralbl Neurochir. 2003;64(3):133–7.
125. Damasio AR, Damasio H, Van Hoeson GW. Prosopagnosia: anatomical basis and behavioral mechanisms. Neurology. 1982;32:331–41.
126. Andreasen NC, O'Leary DS, Arndt S, Cizadlo T, Hurtig R, Rezai K, et al. Neural substrates of facial recognition. J Neuropsychiatry Clin Neurosci. 1996;8(2):139–46.
127. Warrington EK, Shallice T. Word-form dyslexia. Brain. 1980;103(1):99–112.
128. Feinberg TE, Schindler RJ, Ochoa E, Kwan PC, Farah MJ. Associative visual agnosia and alexia without prosopagnosia. Cortex. 1994;30(3):395–411.
129. Zeki S. Cerebral akinetopsia (visual motion blindness). Brain. 1991;114:811–24.
130. Rizzo M, Mawrot M, Zihl J. Motion and shape perception in cerebral akinetopsia. Brain. 1995;118:1105–27.
131. Bernal B, Altman N. Visual functional magnetic resonance imaging in patients with Sturge-Weber syndrome. Pediatr Neurol. 2004;31(1):9–15.
132. Pantelis E, Papadakis N, Verigos K, Stathochristopoulou I, Antypas C, Lekas L, et al. Integration of functional MRI and white matter tractography in stereotactic radiosurgery clinical practice. Int J Radiat Oncol Biol Phys. 2010;78(1):257–67.
133. Barton JJ, Hefter R, Chang B, Schomer D, Drislane F. The field defects of anterior temporal lobectomy: a quantitative reassessment of Meyer's loop. Brain. 2005;128(Pt 9):2123–33.
134. Bartolomeo P, Thiebaut de Schotten M, Duffau H. Mapping of visuospatial functions during brain surgery: a new tool to prevent unilateral spatial neglect. Neurosurgery. 2007;61(6):E1340.
135. Tandon N, Alexopoulos AV, Warbel A, Najm IM, Bingaman WE. Occipital epilepsy: spatial categorization and surgical management. J Neurosurg. 2009;110(2):306–18.
136. Haberg A, Kvistad KA, Unsgard G, Haraldseth O. Preoperative blood oxygen level-dependent functional magnetic resonance imaging in patients with primary brain tumors: clinical application and outcome. Neurosurgery. 2004;54(4):902–15.
137. Krishnan R, Raabe A, Hattingen E, Szelenyi A, Yahya H, Hermann E, et al. Functional magnetic resonance imaging-integrated neuronavigation: correlation between lesion-to-motor cortex distance and outcome. Neurosurgery. 2004;55(4):904–14. discussion 914–5.
138. Meyer A. The connections of the occipital lobes and the present status of the cerebral visual affections. Trans Assoc Am Physicians. 1907;22:7–15.
139. Zeki S. A century of cerebral achromatopsia. Brain. 1990;113:1721–77.

140. Heywood CA, Cowey A, Newcombe F. On the role of parvocellular (P) and magnocellular (M) pathways in cerebral achromatopsia. Brain. 1994;117(Pt 2):245–54.
141. Sacks O. An anthropologist on mars. New York: Alfred A. Knopf; 1995.
142. Burke M, Buhrle C. BOLD response during uncoupling of neuronal activity and CBF. Neuroimage. 2006;32(1):1–8.
143. van der Zande FH, Hofman PA, Backes WH. Mapping hypercapnia-induced cerebrovascular reactivity using BOLD MRI. Neuroradiology. 2005; 47(2):114–20.
144. Hsu YY, Kuan WC, Lim KE, Liu HL. Breathhold-regulated blood oxygenation level-dependent (BOLD) MRI of human brain at 3 tesla. J Magn Reson Imaging. 2010;31(1):78–84.
145. Riecker A, Grodd W, Klose U, Schulz JB, Groschel K, Erb M, et al. Relation between regional functional MRI activation and vascular reactivity to carbon dioxide during normal aging. J Cereb Blood Flow Metab. 2003;23(5):565–73.
146. Rauscher A, Sedlacik J, Barth M, Haacke EM, Reichenbach JR. Nonnvasive assessment of vascular architecture and function during modulated blood oxygenation using susceptibility weighted magnetic resonance imaging. Magn Reson Med. 2005;54(1): 87–95.
147. Kwong KK, Belliveau JW, Chesler DA, Goldberg IE, Weisskoff RM, Poncelet BP, et al. Dynamic magnetic resonance imaging of human brain activity during primary sensory stimulation. Proc Natl Acad Sci USA. 1992;89(12):5675–79.
148. Balasubramanian M, Polimeni J, Schwartz EL. The V1–V2-V3 complex: quasiconformal dipole maps in primate striate and extra-striate cortex. Neural Netw. 2002;15(10):1157–63.
149. Wandell BA, Winawer J, Imaging retinotopic maps in the human brain. Vision Res. 2010. Epub ahead of print.
150. Beauchamp MS, Haxby JV, Rosen AC, DeYoe EA. A functional MRI case study of acquired cerebral dyschromatopsia. Neuropsychologia. 2000; 38(8):1170–9.
151. Smith AT, Greenlee MW, Singh KD, Kraemer FM, Hennig J. The processing of first- and second-order motion in human visual cortex assessed by functional magnetic resonance imaging (fMRI). J Neurosci. 1998;18(10):3816–30.
152. Greenlee MW, Smith AT. Detection and discrimination of first- and second-order motion in patients with unilateral brain damage. J Neurosci. 1997; 17(2):804–18.
153. Brouwer GJ, van Ee R. Visual cortex allows prediction of perceptual states during ambiguous structure-from-motion. J Neurosci. 2007;27(5):1015–23.
154. Tsao DY, Vanduffel W, Sasaki Y, Fize D, Knutsen TA, Mandeville JB, et al. Stereopsis activates V3A and caudal intraparietal areas in macaques and humans. Neuron. 2003;39(3):555–68.
155. Watson JDG, Myers R, Frackowiak RSJ, Hajnal JV, Woods RP, Mazziotta JC, et al. Area V5 of the human brain: evidence from a combined study using positron emission tomography and magnetic resonance imaging. Cereb Cortex. 1993;3:79–94.
156. Rosa MG, Tweedale R. The dorsomedial visual areas in New World and Old World monkeys: homology and function. Eur J Neurosci. 2001;13(3):421–7.
157. Peelen MV, Wiggett AJ, Downing PE. Patterns of fMRI activity dissociate overlapping functional brain areas that respond to biological motion. Neuron. 2006;49(6):815–22.
158. Tootell RBH, Hadjikhani N, Hall EK, Marrett S, Vanduffel W, Vaughan JT, et al. The retinotopy of spatial attention. Neuron. 1998;21:1409–22.
159. Corbetta M, Kincade MJ, Lewis C, Snyder AZ, Sapir A. Neural basis and recovery of spatial attention deficits in spatial neglect. Nat Neurosci. 2005; 8(11):1603–10.
160. Corbetta M, Patel G, Shulman GL. The reorienting system of the human brain: from environment to theory of mind. Neuron. 2008;58(3):306–24.
161. Mesulam MM. Spatial attention and neglect: parietal, frontal and cingulate contributions to the mental representation and attentional targeting of salient extrapersonal events. Philos Trans R Soc Lond B Biol Sci. 1999;354(1387):1325–46.
162. Merigan W, Freeman A, Meyers SP. Parallel processing streams in human visual cortex. Neuroreport. 1997;8(18):3985–91.
163. Merigan WH, Pham HA. V4 lesions in macaques affect both single- and multiple-viewpoint shape discriminations. Vis Neurosci. 1998;15(2):359–67.
164. Merigan WH. Cortical area V4 is critical for certain texture discriminations, but this effect is not dependent on attention. Vis Neurosci. 2000;17(6):949–58.
165. Kastner S, De Weerd P, Ungerleider LG. Texture segregation in the human visual cortex: a functional MRI study. J Neurophysiol. 2000;83(4):2453–7.
166. Beauchamp MS, Haxby JV, Jennings JE, DeYoe EA. An fMRI version of the Farnsworth-Munsell 100-Hue test reveals multiple color-selective areas in human ventral occipitotemporal cortex. Cereb Cortex. 1999;9(3):257–63.
167. Steeves JK, Culham JC, Duchaine BC, Pratesi CC, Valyear KF, Schindler I, et al. The fusiform face area is not sufficient for face recognition: evidence from a patient with dense prosopagnosia and no occipital face area. Neuropsychologia. 2006;44(4):594–609.
168. Epstein R, Harris A, Stanley D, Kanwisher N. The parahippocampal place area: recognition, navigation, or encoding? Neuron. 1999;23(1):115–25.
169. Epstein R, DeYoe EA, Press DZ, Rosen AC, Kanwisher N. Neuropsychological evidence for a topographical learning mechanism in parahippocampal cortex. Cogn Neuropsychol. 2001;18(6): 481–508.
170. Paus T. Location and function of the human frontal eye-field: a selective review. Neuropsychologia. 1996;34(6):475–83.

Brain Mapping for Neurosurgery and Cognitive Neuroscience

13

Joy Hirsch

Introduction

The Unity Principle: Cortical Processes Are Linked to Mental Events; Lesion Studies to Neuroimaging

One of the primary goals of neural science is to understand the biological underpinnings of cognition. This goal is based on the assumption that cognitive events emerge from brain events and that behavior can be explained in terms of neural processes. Francis Crick referred to this as "the Astonishing Hypothesis" [1]. According to this view, the biological principles that underlie cognition link the structure and function of the brain.

> "The Astonishing Hypothesis is that 'You,' your joys and your sorrows, your memories and your ambitions, your sense of personal identity and free will, are in fact no more than the behavior of a vast assembly of nerve cells and their associated molecules."
> Francis Crick, 1994, The Astonishing Hypothesis, p. 3

The emergence of functional magnetic resonance imaging (fMRI) has transformed this "hypothesis" into a common assumption. Using neuroimaging methods, it is possible to observe active cortical areas associated with cognitive processes in healthy human volunteers. This capability has stimulated a renewed focus on the physiological bases of mental events. In particular, the implementation of noninvasive, functional imaging techniques such as fMRI offers an unprecedented view of the complexities of the intact working human brain, including local neural circuits (cortical columns), regions, and large-scale systems of interconnected regions. Functional imaging provides a unique view of the cortical activation patterns associated with specific functional processes such as seeing, hearing, feeling, moving, talking, and thinking. Thus, the potential to realize a neural basis for cognition has emerged with the development of neuroimaging.

Conventional definitions of cognition do not directly address the biological components of mental events. For example, *Dorland's Illustrated Medical Dictionary* defines cognition as "operations of the mind by which we become aware of objects of thought or perception; it includes all aspects of perceiving, thinking and remembering." [2] *The American Heritage Dictionary* offers a similar definition for cognition as "the mental process of knowing, including aspects such as awareness, perception, reasoning and judgment, and that which comes to be known, as through perception, reasoning, or intuition, and knowledge." [3]. However, in his seminal book, *Cognitive Psychology*, Ulrich Neisser defined cognition as "all processes by which the sensory

J. Hirsch, PhD (✉)
Departments of Radiology, Neuroscience, and Psychology, Columbia University Medical Center, 710 W 168th St, B-41, 108, New York, NY 10032, USA
e-mail: joyhirsch@yahoo.com

S.H. Faro and F.B. Mohamed (eds.), *Functional BOLD MRI: Principles and Applications*,
DOI 10.1007/978-1-4939-1995-6_13, © Springer Science+Business Media New York 2015

input is transformed, reduced, elaborated, stored, recovered, and used" [4]. This definition could be interpreted to encompass biological processes, although none were specifically proposed by Neisser.

Medical reports of associations between specific brain injuries and functional deficits provided the initial basis for the assumed linkage between specific brain areas and behavior. As early as 1841, Broca reported language production deficits in patients with specific damage to the left frontal lobe, and in 1874, Wernicke reported deficits in language comprehension and expression in patients following specific damage to the left temporal lobe. Since then, Broca's and Wernicke's areas have become established as regions of cortex associated with aspects of speech production and comprehension, respectively. Around the same time, Harlow reported profound personality changes following an unfortunate frontal lobe injury in his now well-known patient, Phineas Gage [5]. Nearly a century later, Penfield pioneered the experimental technique of direct cortical stimulation during neurosurgical procedures. His observations confirmed the functional specializations of the speech-related areas and demonstrated topographical maps associated with sensory and motor functions [6]. Along with the documented associations between lesions and specific functions, Penfield's reports of cortical stimulations that elicited memories, tastes, and other mental events supported the profound link between brain structure and cognitive function widely accepted within the mainstream of clinical neurology and neurosurgery. For example, it had been noted that severing a segment of the optic nerve always resulted in visual field loss (Fig. 13.1), and similarly, severing a primary motor projection always resulted in a contralateral plegia.

One of the key principles that links brain function and mental events is the relationship between neural activity and blood flow. In 1881, Angelo Mosso, a physiologist, studied a patient who had survived an injury to the skull. Due to the nature of the injury, it was possible to observe blood flow-related pulsations to the left frontal lobe that occurred during certain cognitive events. Mosso concluded that blood flow within the brain was coupled to mental events. Roy and Sherrington [7] subsequently proposed a specific mechanism to couple blood flow and neural activity based on direct measurements on dogs. More recently, using H215O as a tracer of blood flow in the human brain, Raichle et al. [8] confirmed this fundamental relationship between blood flow and local neural activity. This seminal physiology work provided the basis for positron emission tomographic (PET) imaging of active cortical tissue during the execution of a task. The technique was demonstrated by Fox and Raichle [9] with a simple sensory and motor activation paradigm, where hemodynamic variations (as indicated by a radioactive tracer of water molecules) were observed within the pre- and postcentral gyri.

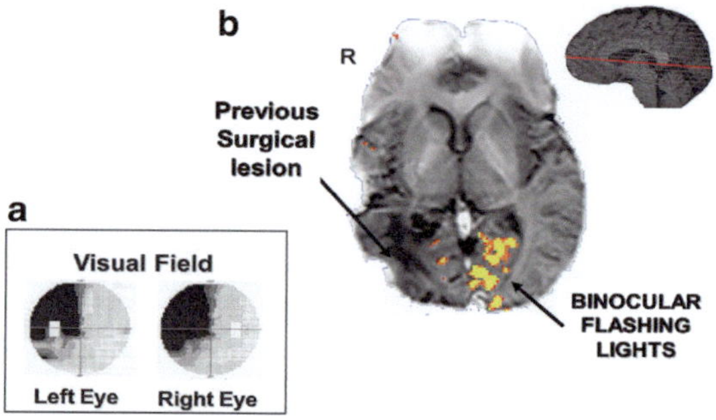

Fig. 13.1 Static visual fields indicate a homonymous quadrantic field defect in the left superior quadrant that is associated with damage to the visual projection fibers within the right occipital lobe following resection of a lesion within the right hemisphere occipital region. Functional magnetic resonance imaging activation during binocular viewing of flashing lights (8 Hz) demonstrates unilateral cortical responses (left hemisphere only), reflecting the loss of visual responses in this topographically mapped area of the visual field

Typically, PET activation studies depend upon subtractive comparisons of images acquired during a task and images acquired during a rest or control condition. The logic of this technique is that the difference in image represents the neural activity present in the task condition and not in the control; for example, activity associated with viewing a flashing checkerboard minus activity associated with viewing a fixation dot presumably reveals the effect of the flashing checkerboard on specialized neural structures. Unfortunately, the PET camera does not provide a detailed image of brain structure; therefore, computational techniques to register the locations of the gamma ray events to brain anatomy obtained by other higher resolution techniques such as magnetic resonance imaging (MRI) were developed. These procedures also include algorithms to register the anatomical and PET images of multiple subjects based on a standard human brain atlas. When all subject brains are registered to the same atlas, the difference in images of multiple subjects can be averaged to obtain conserved and generalizable results.

These advances in PET techniques enabled the first neuroimaging study of cognitive processes relating to language [10]. The study differentiated cortical patterns of activation associated with four separate word tasks: passively viewing words, listening to words, speaking words, and generating words. These early PET studies firmly established the proof of principle that activity associated with cognitive events was observable in the living human brain via hemodynamic variations within locally active neural areas. However, due to risks associated with injections of radioactive tracers, limitations to the number of times a subject can be studied, the relatively coarse resolution, and the relatively few PET facilities available for research, the imaging of cortical activity associated with cognitive processes has advanced most rapidly using a newer, noninvasive, higher resolution, and more available technique: fMRI.

Development of MRI to Visualize Living Brain Structure

Since the invention of the microscope in 1664, imaging technology has guided the mainstream of basic research in biology by revealing structures not visible to the naked eye, including the cell, organelles, molecules, and even atoms. Despite its electronic and computational developments, the microscope is not suited for the imaging of living structures occluded beneath surface tissues such as skin, muscle, and bone. This occlusion problem was solved with the development of MRI, where internal structures within the living body can be resolved at submillimeter scales.

The development of MRI incorporated a long chain of discoveries, beginning with the discovery of molecular beam magnetic resonance in 1936 by Isidor Rabi at Columbia University. Shortly thereafter, in 1945, Edward Purcell and Felix Bloch independently discovered nuclear magnetic resonance (NMR) in condensed matter, followed by Erwin Hahn's observations of nuclear magnetic relaxation and the discovery of spin echo in 1949. A pinnacle event in the development of MRI was made in 1971 by Raymond Damadian who discovered that biological tissues have different relaxation rates. A year later, the first magnetic resonance image of a tube phantom was produced by Paul Lauterbur using a magnetic gradient to produce spatial resolution of the image. The first MRI of a human body part (a finger) was published in 1976 by Peter Mansfield and colleagues. Mansfield and colleagues also developed a key enhancement of a high-speed imaging sequence, echo-planar imaging (EPI), which enabled three-dimensional (3D) acquisitions of body organs (such as the brain) within seconds. A year later, Damadian produced the first magnetic resonance image of a human whole body (cross-sectional chest) and in 1980 produced the first human whole body commercial MRI scanner.

The Development of fMRI to Visualize Living Brain Function

Recent advances in MRI have extended imaging of brain structures to include the identification of active neural tissue in the cortex. The chain of discoveries that led to the generation of MR images of the working brain include Michael Faraday's discovery in 1845 that dried blood has magnetic properties, and Linus Pauling's discovery in 1936 that the magnetic properties of hemoglobin change with the state of oxygenation.

The BOLD Response

These discoveries lay dormant with respect to functional neuroimaging until after the development of high-speed MRI of brain structure and PET imaging of active neural tissue based on the coupling of blood flow. The fundamental breakthrough discovery of the blood oxygen level-dependent (BOLD) signal in 1990 by Seiji Ogawa and colleagues followed the observation that the MR signal originating from the occipital lobe (the area of the brain specialized for visual processing) in rats had a higher contrast when the room lights were on than when the lights were off. Ogawa reasoned that the increased magnetic resonance signal was related to changes in oxygenated hemoglobin (HGB) resulting from blood flow coupled to neural activity [11].

The BOLD signal	
Physiology	Physics
Neural activation is associated with an increase in blood flow O_2 extraction is relatively unchanged.	Deoxy-HGB is paramagnetic and distorts the local magnetic field, causing signal loss.
Result: Reduction in the proportion of deoxy-HGB in the local vasculature.	*Result*: Less distortion of the magnetic field results in local signal increase.

Within a short time, Belliveau and colleagues replicated Ogawa's visual stimulation studies in humans using echo-planar MRI, demonstrating the potential to reveal not only brain structure, but also brain function using MRI. This technique, which exploited the fundamental link between the MR signal, blood flow, and neural events, was referred to as fMRI (see review by John Gore [12] for a more detailed description of these relationships). Figure 13.2 illustrates a BOLD signal (right) originating from the right hemisphere (R) region of postcentral gyrus (indicated by the arrow and yellow cluster) in response to touch of the left hand. The active region is contralateral to the stimulation and well established as an area functionally specialized for tactile sensation.

The "Real Estate" Principle: Functional Specialization from "Bottom–up" and "Top–down"

One of the central principles that drives clinical applications that link cortical structure and function behavior is that specific brain areas are involved in specific aspects of behavior such as action, perception, cognition, affect, and consciousness. We refer to this as the "Real Estate" principle.

In the case of the well-studied visual system, multiple distinct visual cortical areas are organized into well-defined processing pathways. Visual signals from the retina are transmitted to the lateral geniculate nucleus of the thalamus, and then to primary visual cortex where visual information fans out to the extrastriate visual cortical areas. The extrastriate visual areas serve many different aspects of visual perception and visually guided behavior. Among the dimensions suggested for independent visual analysis are brightness, texture, color, depth, movement, shape, face recognition, and object recognition. While specializations for these functions are active topics for investigation, Fig. 13.3 illustrates the well-known specialization of primary visual cortex for primitive stimuli such as on–off full-field stimulation. Similar specializations exist for language, sensory, motor, and auditory systems, and provide the focus for recent developments in cortical function mapping that protect these systems during invasive neurosurgical procedures.

Identification and Preservation of Cortical Areas Specialized for Essential Tasks

Functional maps for individual subjects aim to identify functional specializations specific to that particular subject. In the case of functional mapping prior to a surgical procedure, the goal is to identify regions of the individual patient's brain that are employed for functions (such as motor

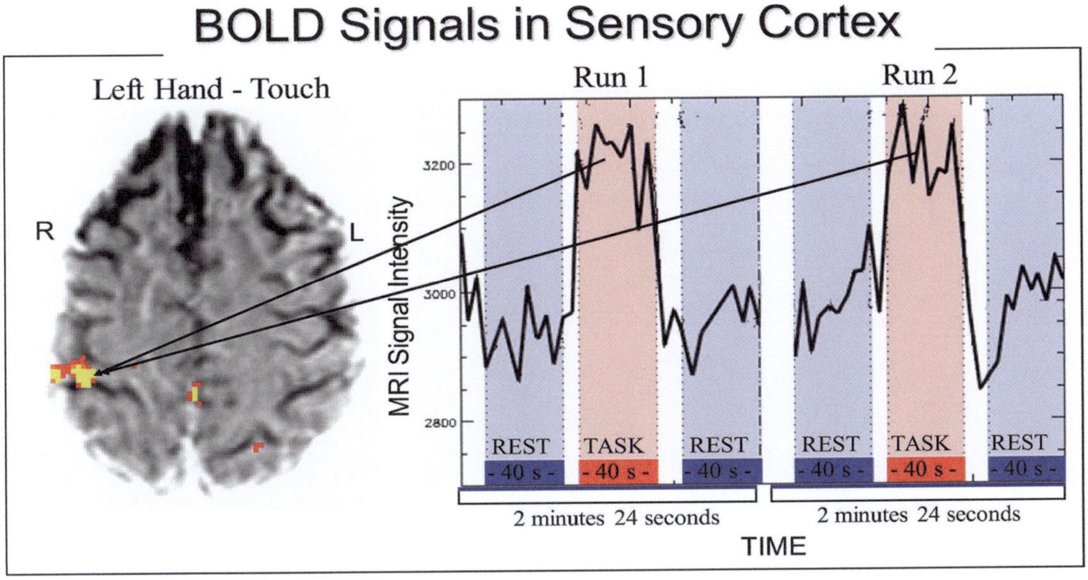

Fig. 13.2 Blood oxygen level-dependent (BOLD) signals associated with tactile stimulation of the left hand. Signals illustrate the changes in MR susceptibility observed in response to passive tactile stimulation of the left hand for a single voxel (1.5 × 1.5 × 4.5 mm) without the benefit of smoothing or "pre-processing." Signals are acquired on two separate short runs. Each run lasted 2 min 24 s, during which 36 images were acquired, including ten images for each of three epochs: initial resting baseline (*purple bar*), task (left-hand touch) (*pink bar*), and final resting baseline (*purple bar*). All voxels in the brain for which the statistical criteria were met (the average amplitude of the signal during the activity epoch was statistically different from the baseline signal) are indicated by either a *yellow or a red* color superimposed on the T2*-weighted image at the voxel address and signify decreasing levels of statistical confidence. *Arrows* point to the source voxel, which is centered within a cluster of similar (*yellow*) voxels and located in the right (R) hemisphere of the brain along the postcentral gyrus. Reprinted with permission from Hirsch J, Ruge MI, Kim KHS, et al. An integrated fMRI procedure for preoperative mapping of cortical areas associated with tactile, motor, language, and visual functions. Neurosurgery 2000;47(3):711–22. Copyright © 2000 Lippincott Williams & Wilkins

movements, tactile sensation, language functions, vision, and audition) that might be at risk because of the location of the surgical procedures. The presence of a space-occupying lesion or long-term seizure-genic conditions can modify or shift functional foci, and normal assumptions do not necessarily apply. In these cases, functional images are acquired at the highest possible resolution and integrated into the appropriate treatment plan. Ideally, individual effects are studied by comparisons that occur before and after a therapeutic intervention where functional changes would be expected.

The preservation of function during a resection or other new surgical procedure is an essential goal of neurosurgery, and various intraoperative and preoperative brain mapping techniques are currently employed for this purpose. These techniques aim to identify cortical areas involved in sensory, motor, and language functions and have become standard practice. They include intraoperative electrophysiology with motor and language mapping, preoperative Wada tests, and visual field examinations. However, the added risk, time, and expense of multiple mapping procedures favor a single, noninvasive, preoperative procedure that could prove effective for mapping these functions. Functional MRI has emerged as such a technique. Functional MRI maps of sensory and motor functions, either alone or in combination with other neuronavigation techniques [13–15], have been shown effective in directing brain tumor resection procedures away from cortical regions with residual function [13, 16–22].

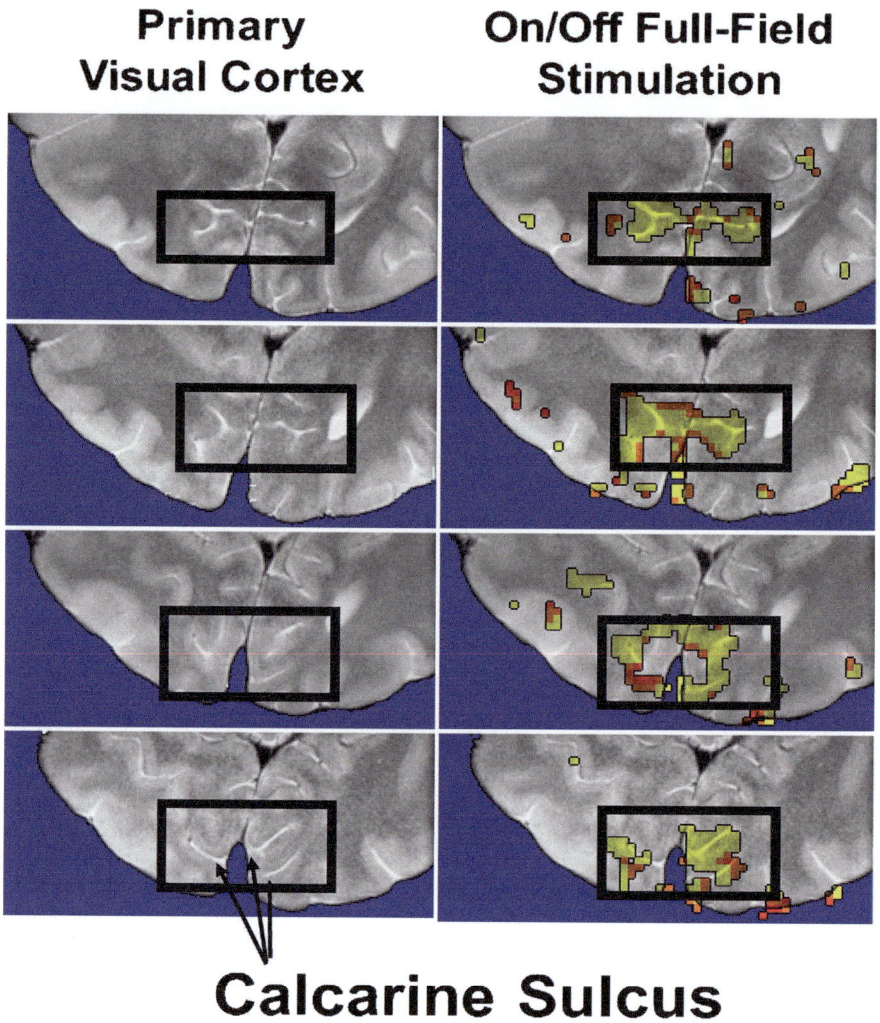

Fig. 13.3 *Boxed* areas surround the anatomical calcarine sulcus in contiguous 3-mm-thick axial slices (*left column*). The *right column* illustrates cortical activity (fMRI) observed during viewing of full-field 8-Hz on–off stimulation. The proximity of the activity patterns and the calcarine sulcus (primary visual cortex) is consistent with the known of functional specificity for this region

Standard of Care and CPT Codes

A series of evaluation/procedural codes were approved to the American Medical Association (AMA) CPT Editorial Panel for use in billing for these procedures by physicians or licensed clinical psychologists. As of January 2007, three CPT codes were approved for use in billing for services provided during an fMRI procedure, grouped as follows:

70554: MRI, brain, fMRI; including test selection and administration of repetitive body part movement and/or visual stimulation, not requiring physician or psychologist administration (do not report 70554 when 96020 is performed).

And

70555: MRI, brain, fMRI; requiring physician or psychologist administration. This code is intended to be reported with 96020: neurofunctional testing selection and administration during noninvasive imaging functional brain mapping, with test administered entirely by a physician or psychologist, with review of test results and report [23].

These codes and their intended applications are described below.

Code 70554

This code is to be used by the physician acquiring the images of the brain and interpreting the locations of activations when the neurofunctional tests to be administered are limited to repetitive body part movement and/or simple visual stimulation. These simple motor and visual tasks can be administered by a radiologic technician under the supervision of the physician in charge of the procedure. If the indication for fMRI procedure is the treatment of a brain lesion and for locating it, then in these cases, it requires only an assessment of simple perceptual and/or sensorimotor functions. This procedure may then be appropriate in the judgment of the referring physician.

The preservice work of the physician typically includes reviewing the patient's clinical history and prior imaging studies, and preliminary planning of the neurofunctional tasks to be performed. The typical intraservice work consists of a limited examination to determine if the patient can perform the tasks. The patient is then placed in the scanner, simple motor and/or visual testing is administered by radiologic technician or physicist during scanning and data acquisition, image data are analyzed, and coregistered fMRI images are interpreted by the physician. Postservice work includes report generation and communication to the neurosurgeon.

Codes 70555 and 96020

In the fMRI studies requiring mapping of neurologic/cognitive functions (e.g., language, memory, cognition, higher order movements, and perception) beyond simple motor a sensory assessment, both the 70555 and 96020 are reported together. Either the referring physician or the physician supervising fMRI procedure determines that mapping of brain functions in these patients will require more extensive neurofunctional testing than those covered by 70554. The choice to map cognitive functions will be determined in part by the patient status, age, presence of neurologic deficit, specific cognitive expertise, location of the lesion, and/or lesions in brain regions known to affect cognition, language, or other higher order operations.

Faro 2007, ACR Standards and Guidelines for fMRI [24]

Hart, 2007, Clinical functional magnetic resonance imaging, p. 142 [23]

http://www.ASFNR.org for more information

Tasks for fMRI and Mapping of Essential Functions

Tasks employed for functional mapping of sensory and motor-sensitive regions have generally been developed by separate research groups in the service of neurosurgical planning. As a consequence, many task variants have been employed. For example, motor tasks are sometimes accomplished by single finger–thumb tapping [19], and in other cases by multiple finger–thumb tapping [17, 25, 26]. Other approaches include self-paced clenching and spreading of the hand [22, 27–29], or sponge squeezing [18, 20]. Tactile stimulation has included palm brushing [18], compressed air puffs to the hand [20], and scratching the ventral surface of the hand [19]. Similarly, functional mapping of language areas has also been accomplished by a range of tasks and procedures including object naming and verb generation [30], production of the names of animals starting with a given letter [17], word generation in alphabetical order [31], or auditory noun presentations with a required category response [32]. It is not known, however, how these various tasks compare with respect to sensitivity or targeted regions of interest. Assessment of cortical activity associated with visual stimulation has been accomplished with intermittent binocular photic stimulation [17, 26, 33], and with various projected pattern stimuli [34]. The length of the activity period and the number of epochs in a run are also nonstandard. Additional variation is introduced to the literature by different levels of statistical stringency and multiple data-processing procedures. Although all of these tasks for sensory, motor, language, and visual functions may be individually effective, an integrated and standardized battery of tasks could optimize application for neurosurgical planning.

Within a cohesive task battery, it is desirable to maximize reliability by using multiple tasks to target related functions. One such battery of fMRI tasks targets cortical regions associated with tactile, motor, language, and visual-sensitive cortical areas [35]. The task battery targets functions selective for regions frequently considered most critical for surgical decisions. All functions are repeated using both active (volitional) and passive (receptive) modes to assure that it is applicable to patients with a range of symptoms and performance capabilities. Any subset of these tasks may be selected for specific clinical objectives while retaining the advantages of the standardized procedures with validations based on responses of both healthy volunteers and patients.

fMRI Task Battery for Cortical Mapping of Sensory, Motor, Language and Vision-Related Areas

1.	SENSORY Touch/hand	+	VISION Reversing Checkerboard
2.	MOTOR Finger/Thumb tapping	+	VISION Reversing Checkerboard
3.	LANGUAGE/active Picture Naming	+	VISION Pictures
4.	LANGUAGE/passive Listening to Words	+	AUDITION Spoken words

Fig. 13.4 A summary of the functions mapped by the four conditions in the fMRI task battery. Reprinted with permission from Hirsch J, Ruge MI, Kim KHS, et al. An integrated fMRI procedure for preoperative mapping of cortical areas associated with tactile, motor, language, and visual functions. Neurosurgery 2000;47(3):711–22. Copyright © 2000 Lippincott Williams & Wilkins

An Example of a Multifunction Task Battery

The specific tasks selected for this task battery are intended to be nearly universally applicable and employ common stimuli and procedures [36]. The tasks consist of four separate procedures (Fig. 13.4) including the following:

1. Passive tactile stimulation of a hand (either the dominant hand or the hand relevant to the hemisphere of surgical interest) with a mildly abrasive plastic surface that is gently rubbed on the palm and fingers. Simultaneously, the patient views a reversing checkerboard pattern (8 Hz). This visual stimulation also aids in head stabilization of the patient.
2. Active hand movement (finger–thumb tapping) using either the same hand, as in the passive tactile stimulation, or both hands during a repeat of the simultaneous visual stimulation (reversing checkerboard).
3. Picture naming by internal (silent) speech in response to visually displayed, black-and-white, line drawings [37] presented at 4-s intervals. These drawings are selected from an appropriate range of the Boston Naming test.
4. Listening to recordings of spoken words (names of objects) presented through headphones designed to reduce scanner noise. A visual fixation cross helps prevent head movement.

The aims of these four task conditions include the following:

1. Localization of sensory and motor cortices, and by inference, location of the central sulcus.
2. Localization of language-related activity, and by inference, the locations of Broca's and Wernicke's areas and the dominant hemisphere for speech.
3. Localization of primary and secondary visual and auditory areas.

Each of the targeted functions and structures associated with each task is illustrated in Fig. 13.5 for a healthy volunteer. The sensory and motor tasks target post- and precentral gyrus (GPoC and GPrC), respectively, and are illustrated in the left panels. These figures also illustrate the expected

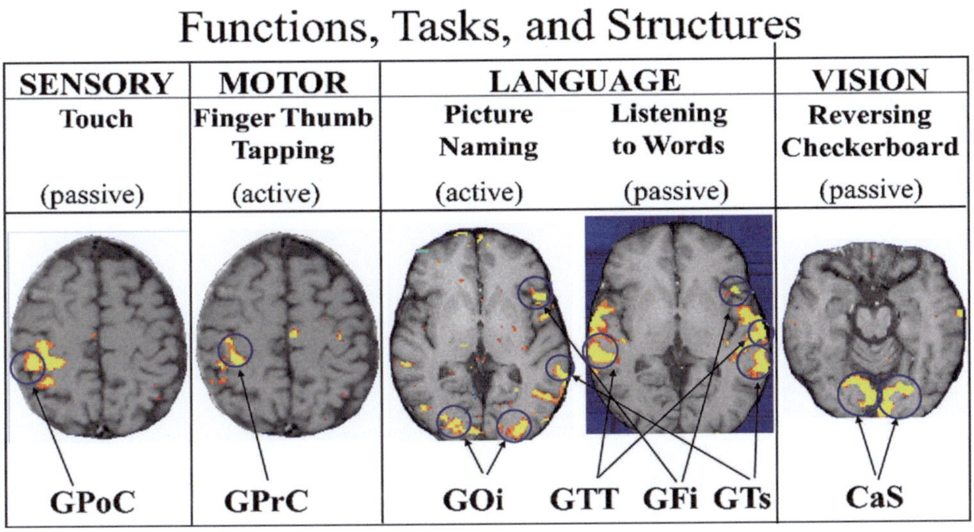

Fig. 13.5 Selected slices for a healthy brain illustrate targeted (*circled*) structures each of the functions and tasks: sensory, passive touch of the hand (*left*) using a rough plastic surface targets the postcentral gyrus (GPoC); motor, active finger–thumb tapping targets the precentral gyrus (GPrC); language, picture naming (expressive), and listening to spoken words (receptive) target the inferior frontal gyrus (GFi; Broca's area) and the superior temporal gyrus (GTs; Wernicke's area) on the dominant hemisphere; and vision, viewing of the reversing checkerboard and picture naming target the calcarine sulcus (CaS) and the inferior occipital gyrus (GOi). Primary auditory activity expected to be associated with the listening task also is observed bilaterally in the transverse temporal gyrus (GTT), middle panel. Reprinted with permission from Hirsch J, Ruge MI, Kim KHS, et al. An integrated fMRI procedure for preoperative mapping of cortical areas associated with tactile, motor, language, and visual functions. Neurosurgery 2000;47(3):711–22. Copyright © 2000 Lippincott Williams & Wilkins

overlap along the pre- and postcentral gyrus between activity associated with sensory and motor stimulation. The language tasks target putative Broca's and Wernicke's areas that are found within inferior frontal gurus (GFi) and superior temporal gyrus (GTs), respectively, on the dominant hemisphere for language (middle panels of Fig. 13.5). Both areas are redundantly targeted by expressive (active) and receptive (passive) language tasks, and by both visual and auditory modalities. Visual and auditory systems also are revealed by the activity in inferior occipital gyrus (GOi) and the transverse temporal gyrus (GTT), respectively, left and right language panels. Vision-related activity elicited by the reversing black-and-white checkerboard stimulations also targets primary visual cortex found along the calcarine sulcus (CaS), illustrated in the far-right panel of Fig. 13.5. Given the high levels of statistical confidence (p values from ≤ 0.0001 to ≤ 0.0005), it can be assumed that activity not circled also represents true physiological activations that are task related and distributed outside the targeted regions of interest.

Healthy Volunteers and Patients

Development of this test battery was based upon a total of 63 healthy volunteers (24 females and 39 males) who participated in the evaluation of the specific set of tasks targeted to identify brain regions most likely to be surgical regions of interest for (1) primary brain tumor, (2) brain metastasis, (3) seizure disorder, or (4) cerebral vascular malformation. A total of 125 patients also participated. These patients were surgical candidates and presented with surgical regions of interest that included sensorimotor (n = 63), language (n = 56), or visual (n = 6) functions.

Sensitivity of Task Battery: Healthy Volunteers

Each task was associated with the targeted region of interest, and the percentage of cases showing activity in those regions (sensitivity) was determined [Table 13.1 (A)]. This task battery provides two opportunities to observe the targeted region; for example, whereas the GTs was

Table 13.1 Evaluation of task sensitivity

		A. Healthy subjects				B. Surgical patients			
		Targeted regions of interest				Surgical regions of interest			
Task	Structure	Central sulcus (n = 30)	Broca's area (n = 45)	Wernicke's area (n = 45)	Visual cortex (n = 15)	Central sulcus (n = 63)	Broca's area (n = 22)	Wernicke's area (n = 34)	Visual cortex (n = 6)
Touch	GPoC	100%				94%			
Finger–thumb	GPrC	100%				89%			
Tapping									
Picture	GFi		90%				72%		
Naming	GTs			73%				65%	
Listening to	GFi		93%				54%		
Spoken words	GTs			100%				88%	
Checkerboard	CaS				100%				100%
Pictures	GOi				100%				100%
Composite sensitivity		100%	93%	100%	100%	97%	77%	91%	100%
(Logical OR)									

activated in only 73% of cases during picture naming, it was activated in 100% of healthy volunteers during listening to spoken words [Table 13.1 (A), column 5]. Overall, the sensitivity of the entire battery to identify language-related cortex in the GTs is 100% for the population of healthy volunteers, as indicated on the bottom row: composite sensitivity. Specifically, the composite sensitivity is the result of a logical operating room (OR) decision rule based on two tasks that target a specific region. Central sulcus and visual cortex were identified in 100% of cases and Broca's area in 93%.

Sensitivity of Task Battery: Surgical Population

Following task-sensitivity determinations for healthy volunteers, similar determinations were made for surgical candidates with pathology in the specified cortical regions of interest. This enabled assessment of the fMRI task within the affected pathological cohort. These subgroups served as the basis for evaluation of the respective tasks, although all patients completed all tasks in the battery, regardless of the region of surgical interest. Table 13.1 (B) reports the task sensitivity within each surgical group, thus indicating the sensitivity in the presence of pathology. The tactile stimulation revealed activity in the postcentral gyrus in 94% of patients with lesions in or close to the motor strip, whereas the finger–thumb tapping task predominantly demonstrated function in the area of the precentral gyrus in 89%. Of the two patients for whom the central sulcus was not identified, one was characterized by excessive (not correctable) head movement and marginal compliance. Neurological deficits were the most likely contributing factor in the second case. Overall, the location of central sulcus, as indicated by either its posterior or anterior margins, was obtained in 97% of the cases with pathology in this region and is indicated as the composite sensitivity (bottom row). This boost in sensitivity is achieved by exploiting the two approaches to locate central sulcus and the employment of a logical OR combination decision rule between the two tasks.

With the combined performances of the picture-naming task, as well as the passive listening task, the fMRI signal was observed in Wernicke's area in 31 of 34 (91%) patients with pathology in GTs and Broca's area in 17 of the 22 patients (77%) with pathology in inferior frontal gyrus. Explanations for the three unsuccessful Wernicke's area patients included movement artifact ($n = 1$) and probable lack of compliance ($n = 2$). Explanations for the five unsuccessful Broca's area patients included neurological deficits ($n = 3$), probable marginal compliance ($n = 1$), and head-movement artifact that was not correctable ($n = 1$), although a false-negative finding cannot be ruled out. The fMRI signal was observed in the visual cortex (CaS and GOi) in all six patients with lesions in these cortical areas.

Comparison of Task Sensitivity for Patients and Healthy Volunteers

Although the sensory and motor probes of GPoC and GPrC were each 100% effective in healthy volunteers, they were individually 94 and 89% effective in patients with tumors in those regions. These observations include patients with severe symptoms such as hemiparesis and loss of sensory function. However, by combining the two tasks with the Either/Or decision rule, the central sulcus was identified in 97% of cases. By combining the hit rates of the picture-naming and the listening to spoken words tasks for the healthy volunteers, the targeted Broca's (GFi) and Wernicke's (GTs) areas were activated in 93 and 100% of cases, respectively. Correspondingly, for the surgical cases, these areas were activated in 77 and 91% of the cases, respectively.

The reduction in patient sensitivity for the language areas presumably reflects tumor-related receptive and expressive aphasias, as well as related cognitive losses. The visual functions within CaS and GOi were 100% effective in both healthy subjects and also for surgical patients where the unaffected hemisphere provided the comparison. Accuracy of the fMRI observations also can be assessed in all surgical patients for whom multiple procedures were included in the treatment plan by comparison of the fMRI maps with conventional techniques such as intraoperative mapping, Wada, and visual fields testing methods. This method of comparison serves to establish the concordance of the fMRI technique with other accepted techniques.

Accuracy of Task Battery: Comparison with Intraoperative Electrophysiology

Both fMRI preoperative maps and intraoperative electrophysiology were performed in 16 cases. Intraoperative recording of somatosensory evoked potentials (SSEPs) were performed to localize the central sulcus [37], and successful recordings were obtained in 15 cases. Direct cortical stimulation was performed in 11 of these cases with successful stimulations in nine. The areas of electrophysiological response were referenced to axial images with the use of an intraoperative frameless-based stereotactic navigation device and compared to the preoperative fMRI images. Due to the differences in the orientations of the acquired slices, however, precise measurements of the localizations of the two techniques were not possible. In each case, the surgeon judged the correspondence as consistent (see case example).

The fMRI maps revealed precentral gyrus activity in 16 of 16 (100%) cases and postcentral gyrus in 13 of 16 (81%) cases. However, the combined maps revealed the location of the central sulcus in all cases. When both methods (fMRI and electrophysiology) reported the central sulcus, the locations concurred in 100% of the cases for the SSEPs (15 of 15) and 100% for the direct cortical stimulation (9 of 9), as determined within the spatial accuracy of both methods, and in accord with previous findings of other investigators [20, 38, 39].

Comparison of fMRI, Wada, and Intraoperative Language Mapping

Hemispheric language dominance as predicted by the fMRI language-related maps was compared to preoperative Wada procedures [40] in 13 cases. The dominant hemisphere for language as determined by Wada testing was consistent with fMRI results in all 13 cases (double-blind study), and is consistent with findings of previous investigations [32]. In a subsequent cohort of five patients, this integrated battery of tasks was applied prior to intraoperative language mapping, with consistent findings between the two methods [41].

Comparison of fMRI and Visual Fields

Homonymous visual field defects were compared with fMRI response patterns in primary visual cortex in six cases (illustrated in Fig. 13.1). Visual fields determined by formal static perimetry indicated hemianopic or quadrantanoptic field deficits consistent with known disruptions of visual projection pathways and were consistent with the fMRI cortical maps when compared with activity within the unaffected hemisphere. That is, gross absences of hemispheric symmetry along the calcarine sulcus in regions expected to correspond to the visual field were taken as demonstrations of field and fMRI consistency.

Case Example 13.1 Motor and Language Mapping

In this case, a 43-year-old, right-handed man presented with mild headaches and brief episodes of receptive language disturbance, as well as occasional word-finding difficulties. Preoperative neuropsychological evaluation revealed no language deficits. MRI revealed a rounded, partially hemorrhagic lesion, 4.5 cm in diameter located in the left posterior temporal lobe. To optimize a therapeutic plan, functional maps were obtained using the multifunction task battery (results are

(continued)

Case Example 13.1 (continued)

Summary of fMRI Task Battery (Illustrative Case)

FUNCTION	TASK	AREA	fMRI
Motor	Finger-Thumb Tapping	GPrC	
Sensory	Touch	GPoC	
Broca's Area	Picture Naming	GFi	
Wernicke's Area	Listening to Spoken Words	GTs	
Visual Cortex	Reversing Checkerboard	CaS	

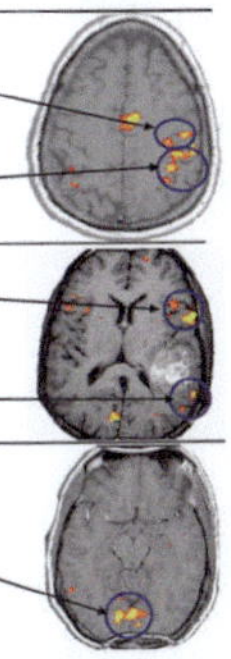

Fig. 13.6 Selected slices (*right*) illustrate cortical responses associated with each of the tasks and the targeted regions of interest for case example 1. Sensory and motor tasks elicited activity within pre- and postcentral gyri and predicted the location of the central sulcus on multiple contiguous slices. The slice illustrated in the *right top row* shows a relatively inferior representation. The two language tasks – picture naming and listening to spoken words – elicited activity in the left hemisphere within the inferior frontal gyrus (GFi) and the superior temporal gyrus (GTs; *arrows*). In this case, the specific locations of the activity within the GFi and GTs were replicated on both tasks and the overlapping regions were taken as the best predictor of Broca's and Wernicke's areas, respectively. Finally, the reversing checkerboard (*bottom row*) indicated primary visual cortex, as illustrated by the activity labeled calcarine sulcus (CaS). Similar to the language-related regions, these regions were replicated across the multiple visual tasks and served to increase confidence in these results. Reprinted with permission from Hirsch J, Ruge MI, Kim KHS, et al. An integrated fMRI procedure for preoperative mapping of cortical areas associated with tactile, motor, language, and visual functions. Neurosurgery 2000;47(3):711–22. Copyright © 2000 Lippincott Williams & Wilkins

summarized in Fig. 13.6). The central sulcus was identified clearly by the sensory and motor tasks (top rows). The language tasks revealed language-related activity on the left hemisphere adjacent to both the posterior margins and the anterior margins of the mass (GTs and GFi; middle rows). The visual stimulation was reliably associated with signals within and along the primary visual areas (CaS). Due to the proximity of the language-related activity to the tumor, an awake craniotomy with electrophysiological mapping of motor and language functions was performed.

Integrative Mapping of Sensory and Motor Functions

Recording of SSEPs indicated the location of the central sulcus (Fig. 13.7, left columns), which was confirmed by direct cortical stimulation of precentral gyrus (middle columns). Comparison with the location of central sulcus by fMRI (right column) indicates good agreement with both techniques, as illustrated by the arrows.

Interoperative Mapping of Language Functions

Direct cortical stimulation of the left inferior frontal gyrus with the Ojemann Bipolar stimulator disrupted the patient's ability to count, and a similar stimulation of the GTs produced language disturbances, including literal paraphasic errors and word-finding difficulties, respectively (Fig. 13.8). Sites of observable responses were tagged with

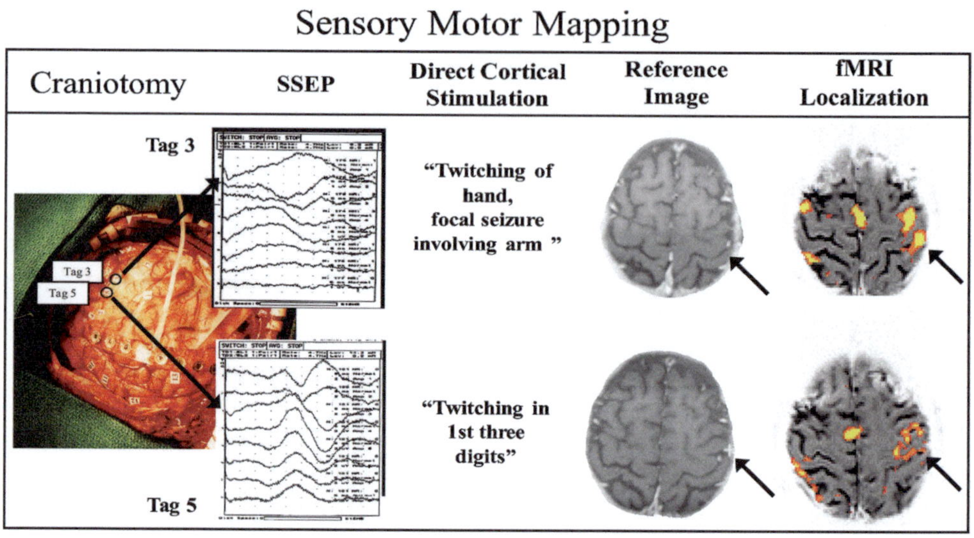

Fig. 13.7 Needle-recording electrodes were placed at Erb's Point and stimulating electrodes were placed over the left or right median nerve at the wrist. Following craniotomy and exposure of cortex, subdural strip electrodes were placed in the operative field. The median nerve was stimulated to elicit epicortical responses measured with the electrodes. A consistent phase reversal between electrode sites (tags 3 and 5, column 2) was taken as the physiological identification of sensorimotor cortex, and therefore, the central sulcus (indicated by *arrows* on the reference images in column 4). These recordings of somatosensory evoked potentials (SSEPs) were made with an eight-Channel Viking IV7 and standard filter settings (30 Hz to 3 kHz). Direct cortical stimulation of the exposed cortex directed by the SSEP results was performed using the Ojemann bipolar stimulator (1 s trains of 1 ms pulses at 60 Hz) varied from 2 milliamperes (mA) to 18 mA, peak to peak, resulting in hand twitching and a focal seizure of the right arm (*top row*) and twitching of the first three digits of the hand (*bottom row*). Using a frameless-based intraoperative navigation system (BrainLAB GmbH, Munich, Germany), the tagged locations were referenced to anatomical axial MR images localized using a viewing wand and subsequently compared with areas of activation on corresponding fMRI images, as illustrated by comparison of the images in columns 4 and 5 (*arrows*). The T2* images (*right column*) and the conventional T1 images (reference image) were not acquired at exactly corresponding plane orientations, accounting for the variation in the two structural images and limiting the precision with which the electrophysiological and fMRI locations can be compared. Reprinted with permission from Hirsch J, Ruge MI, Kim KHS, et al. An integrated fMRI procedure for preoperative mapping of cortical areas associated with tactile, motor, language, and visual functions. Neurosurgery 2000;47(3):711–22. Copyright © 2000 Lippincott Williams & Wilkins

numbers, photographically documented, and cross referenced to the fMRI, as illustrated by arrows.

Postsurgical Status

A total resection was achieved that spared these functional regions. The pathology was consistent with an ependymoma. Immediately postsurgery, no impairments in language function were detected. However, the postoperative recovery of the patient was complicated by a temporary mixed aphasia and seizures. Subsequently, within 10 days, the patient's condition was substantially improved, and no further adjuvant treatment was planned. A 6-month postsurgical fMRI scan was consistent with previous findings, and neuropsychological evaluation revealed residual, mild word-finding difficulties and occasional literal paraphasic errors.

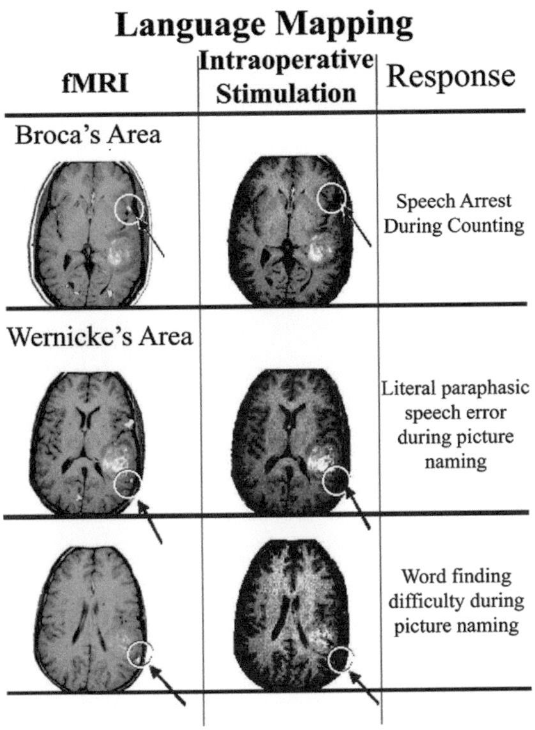

Fig. 13.8 After craniotomy and recording of SSEPs, the patient was awakened and asked to count forward and backward while the cortex in putative Broca's area was stimulated. Subsequently, the picture-naming paradigm used in the fMRI battery of tasks was administered and stimulation at the site where fMRI maps indicated the location of Broca's area resulted in speech disruption (*top row*). Stimulation was systematically repeated and extended to temporal lobe cortex, and sites of activation revealed by the fMRI maps were specifically targeted as indicated by the *circles* in the *middle* and *bottom column*. These stimulations resulted in paraphasic speech errors and word-finding difficulties as indicated, consistent with disruption of Wernicke's area-related functions that occurred in the two separate locations as indicated. The corresponding preoperative fMRI maps shown on the *left* column confirm the correspondence of cortical areas (*circles* and *arrows*). Reprinted with permission from Hirsch J, Ruge MI, Kim KHS, et al. An integrated fMRI procedure for preoperative mapping of cortical areas associated with tactile, motor, language, and visual functions. Neurosurgery 2000;47(3):711–22. Copyright © 2000 Lippincott Williams & Wilkins

Case Example 13.2 Language Mapping – Late Bilingual Patient

In this case, the patient was a native of Italy who emigrated to the USA as a young adult and then learned English. When she was 44 years old, she began to experience episodes of word-finding difficulty in both Italian and English, as well as slowed speech production. An MRI obtained during a medical evaluation revealed a large tumor in the left inferior posterior frontal region of her brain expected to be associated with speech production (Fig. 13.9a). In order to determine the location of her language areas relative to her tumor, an fMRI was acquired using the task battery previously described for each language, which revealed (1) separate locations for her native (Italian) and second language (English) and (2) that both languages were displaced from the expected locations by the tumor. These displacements were confirmed during surgery and the tumor was resected without damage to either language function. Approximately 2 years later, she remains tumor free, with excellent English and Italian language function. A follow-up fMRI scan indicated the language areas associated with each language have shifted back to the expected locations within the brain (Fig. 13.9b). The separation of the locations active during the native language and the second language within Broca's area is consistent with previous findings of separation between L1- and L2-sensitive areas, when L2 was acquired during adulthood [42].

(continued)

Case Example 13.2 (continued)

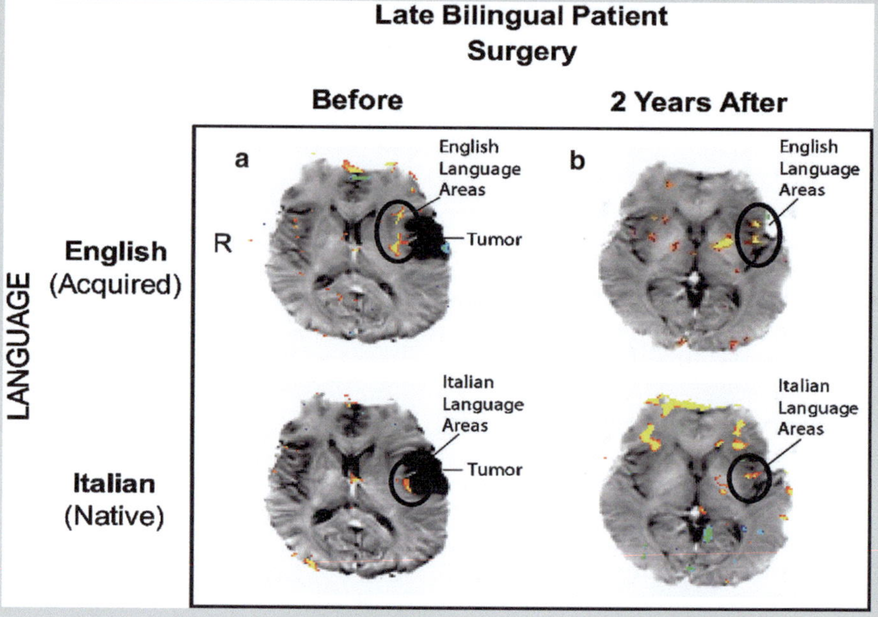

Fig. 13.9 Language mapping of a late bilingual patient. Object naming was performed in the native language (Italian), and also in the acquired language (English). Typical of late bilingual individuals, the languages occupied distinct regions of Broca's area (**a**). These distinct regions were preserved following surgery and are consistent with her clinical outcome of no deficits in either language (**b**)

Case Example 13.3 Language Mapping – Early Bilingual Patient

A 23-year-old, right-handed bilingual woman who works as a waitress in her father's Italian restaurant was seen on an emergency basis following the sudden onset of supplementary motor seizures. An MRI revealed the presence of a left posterior frontal cystic lesion suggestive of cystic astrocytoma. Although the patient was born and educated in the USA, she was raised in a household that spoke Italian and became bilingual during her early language development. fMRI of her language areas for both languages revealed overlapping clusters in putative Broca's area (left inferior frontal gyrus) as illustrated in Fig. 13.10a, which was not changed following surgery (Fig. 13.10b), consistent with the absence of postsurgical morbidity.

(continued)

Case Example 13.3 (continued)

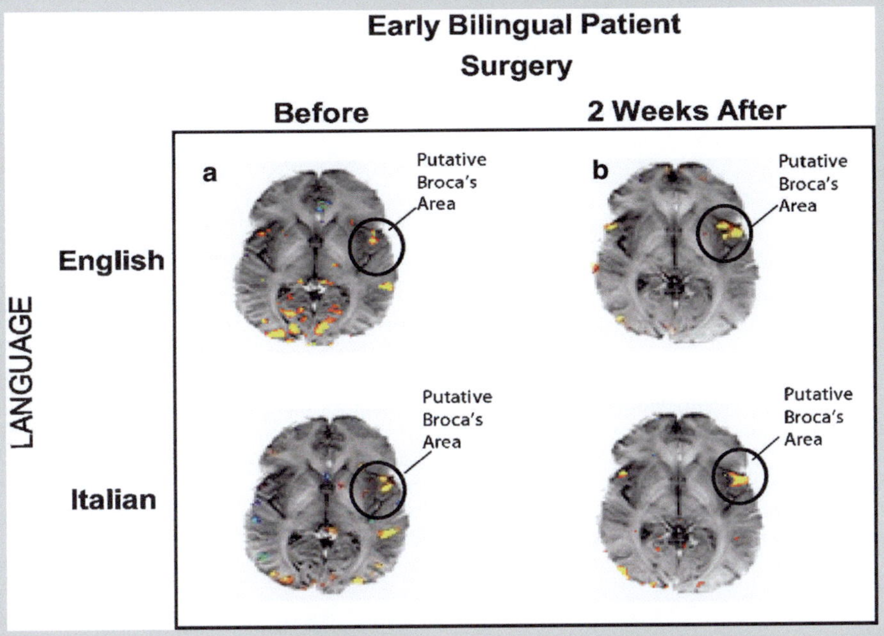

Fig. 13.10 Language mapping of an early bilingual patient. Object naming, as for the late bilingual patient (Fig. 13.9), was performed in both languages, Italian and English. Typical of early bilingual individuals, the activity clusters associated with both languages were largely overlapping within Broca's area (**a**). This single language area was preserved following resection (**b**), consistent with the absence of postsurgical morbidity

Individual variations in language maps that depend upon language experience is confirmed by previous reports that compared activity patterns in Broca's area for L1 and L2 for early and late bilinguals (Fig. 13.11).

Cases 13.2 and 13.3 illustrate earlier findings that document different cortical organization with respect to early and late acquisition of a second language. Kim and colleagues [42] showed that the average centroid separation in putative Broca's area during L1 and L2 production in late bilingual subjects was approximately 7 mm, whereas in early bilingual subjects, the language activations were indistinguishable (Fig. 13.11).

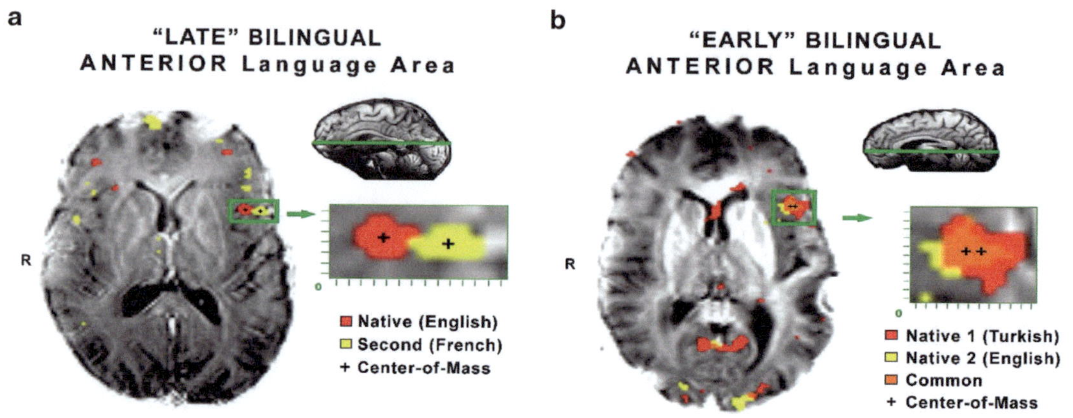

Fig. 13.11 Examples of main findings based on two samples of healthy volunteers who were either late (**a**) or early (**b**) bilinguals. Cluster centroids and variances (spreads) were determined for activity associated with each language. A significant separation between centroids of activity was found for late bilingual subjects and not for the early bilingual subjects in Broca's area. No differences were observed within Wernicke's area. Reprinted with permission from Kim KHS, Relkin NR, Lee K-M, Hirsch J. Distinct cortical areas associated with native and second languages. Nature 1997;388:171–4

Case Example 13.4 Motor Mapping

An 11-year-old female with a completely unremarkable medical history presented following the occurrence of a grand mal seizure. Imaging revealed a large mass along the lateral margin of right central sulcus (Fig. 13.12a). Due to the risk to sensory and motor functions, a surgical resection was recommended, and recommended treatment consisted of seizure management. Seeking a second opinion, parents sought a medical center with fMRI mapping capability; the functional map revealed that the tumor had displaced eloquent sensory- and motor-sensitive cortex medially and posteriorly from the expected positions (Fig. 13.12b). Based on this information, an anterior surgical route resulted in a complete and total resection of a ganglioglioma without functional deficit. Six months postsurgery, she returned for a follow-up map that revealed the expected functional pattern (Fig. 13.12c). She had returned to her normal activities, including soccer, dance, and rock climbing.

(continued)

Case Example 13.4 (continued)

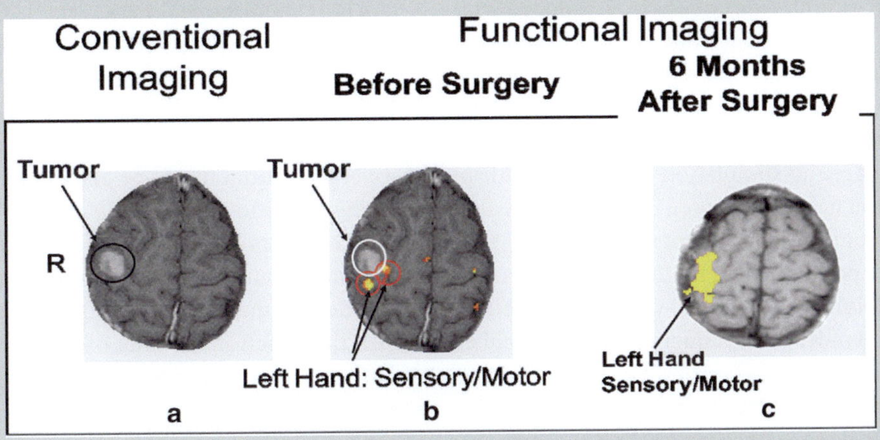

Fig. 13.12 (**a**) Conventional T1 image reveals right hemisphere mass located on the margins of the central sulcus. (**b**) Functional map of tactile and finger–thumb tapping suggests displacement of eloquent cortex. (**c**) Six months after surgery, the patient is disease free, without deficits consistent with the sensory and motor activity revealed by fMRI

A novel feature of this battery of integrated fMRI tasks is the redundancy in the measurements; for example, language-sensitive regions are mapped by both active (expressive) and passive (receptive) tasks, as are the regions sensitive to motor (active tapping) and sensory (passive touching) tasks. Visual areas also are assessed by passive viewing of the reversing checkerboard stimulus (no response required) and active viewing of pictures during a naming task in which a response was required. Advantages to employing more than one task associated with a particular function to isolate eloquent cortical areas include improved confidence when replications are observed, and improved sensitivity when the activity is observed during either an active or a passive performance. This feature translates into a greater likelihood of a successful map for patients with neurologic deficits. Together, the task sensitivity and accuracy observed for these fMRI maps suggests that this multifunction task battery yields a reliable estimate of the locations of critical functions potentially at risk during brain surgery, and thus extends the potential of a single preoperative fMRI brain mapping procedure to facilitate optimal outcomes for neurosurgery.

Based on our experience with this fMRI task battery, the images serve both pre- and intraoperative objectives. On the preoperative side, the fMRI maps have contributed to our estimates of the risk–benefit ratio and to the decision whether or not to offer surgery to the patient, although these decisions are based on the entire medical situation taken together, and not on any single factor. Communication between the surgeon and the patient is also facilitated by images that summarize the relevant structure and function issues. On the intraoperative side, as illustrated previously, the fMRI results have also served to direct the intraoperative electrophysiology, and thereby have contributed to the efficiency of the intraoperative procedures. However, it has been observed that the information offered by the preoperative fMRI map is often more distributed than that of the intraoperative map, and the question of which active regions are essential to the function is not directly addressed by fMRI [43]. A false-positive interpretation is, therefore, possible based on these associated patterns of activity, whereas a false-negative finding is also possible due to sensitivity, compliance, and imaging artifacts. The likelihood of both types of errors is reduced with repetitions and checks for internal consistency, as suggested by this integrated task battery. However, advances to resolve these issues may depend upon additional techniques, such as transcranial magnetic stimulation (TMS), to confirm the essential nature of an area identified by fMRI.

Many future enhancements of this initial task battery are possible using methods that determine task sensitivity and clinical validity, as well as improve confidence by reducing the risk of either false-positive or false-negative findings. The battery could be extended to include memory functions, high-level cognitive tasks, and perhaps even emotion and affect, and continued development could improve the tasks to target the sensory/motor and language areas. Techniques employed for the development of this integrated battery of functions could serve as a basis to develop other similar probes, and thus extend the potential role of fMRI in neurosurgical planning to encompass more precision and diversity in structure and function relationships.

Functional MRI During Loss of Consciousness: A "Voice" for Unresponsive Patients

Applications of functional neuroimaging now extend beyond mapping the primary stages of perception, language, and motor systems to characterize cortical function in patients with disorders of consciousness (DOC) [44]. At first pass, this objective appears paradoxical because conventional investigations of cognitive processes require patient cooperation with a task. For example, to map the location of language-sensitive cortex, a language-related task is performed according to a temporal sequence that alternates the task with rest (no-task) periods. However, another strategy employs the use of *passive stimulations* of patients who are not conscious. Comparisons between patients with altered states of consciousness due to sedation or brain injury and healthy subjects may be employed to map eloquent cortex and to infer readiness and potential to sustain awareness.

As if a "mindscope," fMRI enables a view of occluded neural processes to inform medical practitioners about the health of the neurocircuitry mediating cognitive processes. An underlying point of view is that assessment of recovery potential might be enhanced by neuroimaging techniques that reveal the status of residual systems specialized for essential cognitive and volitional tasks for each patient. Thus, development of imaging techniques that assess the functional status of individual unresponsive patients is a primary goal for current investigations.

The structural integrity of injured brains is often compromised depending on the specific traumatic event, and, therefore, images cannot be grouped across patients as is standard practice for investigations of cognitive systems in healthy volunteers. Thus technical adaptations associated with individual patient assessments where there is "zero tolerance for error," as for neurosurgical planning, and confidence in the results must meet the highest standards of care, can be applied to assessments of cognitive capacity in patients with DOC. Adaptations that have been developed for the purpose of personalized planning for neurosurgical procedures by mapping the locations of essential functional systems such as language, perception, and sensory/motor for each individual patient give rise to assessment techniques useful for assessments of neurocognitive health in patients who are unresponsive.

"Zero Tolerance" for Error

In contrast to population-based studies where error bars are considered to be variations largely due to individual differences, clinical tests focus on the individual for diagnosis, treatment, and follow-up. Thus, the burden for accuracy for the "n of one" case is 100% and dictates methodological adaptations to meet this standard. These adaptations include an extraordinary standard for high image quality as well as clarity, accuracy, and precision for interpretation.

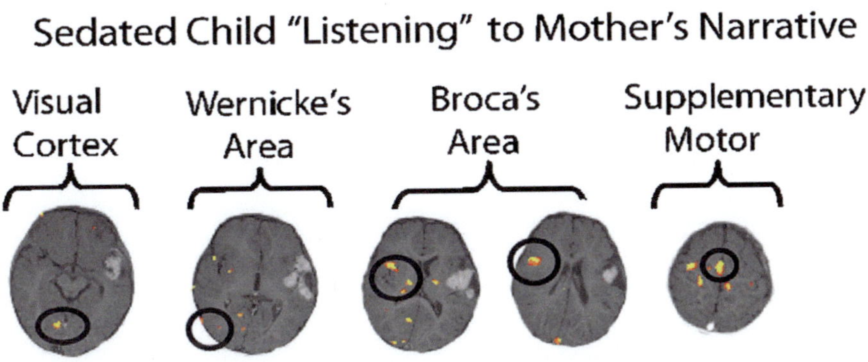

Fig. 13.13 Functional imaging during sedation. Fourteen continuous 4.5-mm slices covering the whole brain of a 15-month-old female with an aggressive tumor (PNET) in the left hemisphere (hyperintense region, slices 1–8 where slice 1, located in the *upper left* of the figure is the most ventral). In-plane resolution was 1.5 × 1.5 mm, and the double-pass paradigm and analysis (see text) were employed. The patient was sedated with propofol and maintained at the lightest level that prevented movement of the head. A recorded passage of the mother talking to the patient was played through earphones worn by the patient while scanning. The *circles* indicate putative Wernicke's area, Broca's area, and supplementary motor area, consistent with the expected language network in preparation for the emerging language function

The "Zero Tolerance for Error" standard is further complicated by the special circumstances of many patients. Some key factors include functional deficits that challenge execution of the task, high levels of anxiety leading to claustrophobia, inability to remember or perform instructions, excessive head movements, probability of a seizure or other sudden event that interrupts a scan, the effects of therapeutic drugs, and susceptibility artifacts often resulting from a previous surgical bed, implant, or a vascular abnormality. The methodological adaptations developed to accommodate neurosurgical applications are discussed earlier in this chapter and include standardized paradigms and tasks that map most relevant functions and employ short imaging runs, high-resolution grids, and least number of assumptions for data analysis. All of these adaptations are relevant to the even more challenging task of imaging unresponsive patients with DOC where passive (rather than volitional) responses are required.

Functional Mapping During Sedation

Following the development of the basic standard battery of tasks for neurosurgical planning, we were challenged by the need to provide similar maps for patients who were sedated during the imaging procedure. The population for which this was generally necessary included children under 6 years old. In the face of specific medical needs, the passive tasks (listening, tactile, and visual photic stimulation) were adapted for use under sedation with propofal [45]. One of the adaptations was the use of a familiar speaker for the passive listening, and meaningful narratives were recorded for the purpose of the functional maps. As illustrated for the case of a 15-month-old sedated female (Fig. 13.13), this technique yields a system of regions consistent with known language-related areas. In the case of this patient, the language dominant hemisphere was on the right side, which is consistent with the absence of morbidity following a complete and total resection on the left hemisphere. These studies confirm that "consciousness" is not a prerequisite to confirming the presence of an active language-related system in the cortex.

The discovery that the neural correlates for language processes could be engaged during sedation raised the possibility that unresponsive patients due to a disorder of consciousness could be similarly aroused. The first example of FMRI in patients with DOC is illustrated as follows.

Functional Mapping of Minimally Conscious Patients

An Illustrative Case

A 33-year-old, right-handed male without prior history of neurological disorders suffered severe head trauma secondary to a blow to the right frontal region with a blunt object leading to bilateral subdural hematoma and brainstem compression injury [46]. Bedside examinations were consistent with the diagnosis of MCS [47], and the functional imaging study was performed 24 months after the injury. Neurological examination at the time of the study revealed oculocephalic responses with intact visual tracking and saccades to both stimuli and to commands, marked increased motor tone bilaterally, and frontal release signs. The highest level behavior observed in this patient was his ability to inconsistently follow complex commands including go, no-go, countermanding tasks, and occasional verbalization. Right frontal lobe encephalomalacia and paramedian thalamic infarction were present on the structural MRI and on the functional (T2*) scans. Resting fluorodeoxyglucose PET demonstrated 40.6% of normal regional cerebral metabolic rate.

Imaging methods were as described previously for neurosurgical patients, and employed passive auditory stimulation by presenting a prerecorded narrative of a family member recalling past experiences that she had shared with the patient. The narrative was also presented as reversed speech including the same content but without linguistic meaning. Passive tactile stimulation was also employed. Single epoch runs each lasting 2 min 24 s and the double-pass short-block paradigm were employed. Single-voxel confidence levels were set at $p \leq 0.0001$ corrected for false positives (Fig. 13.2). Voxel size was 1.5 × 1.5 × 4.5 mm and 21 continuous slices covered the whole brain. The scanner was a 1.5-T GE equipped for EPI with a standard fMRI sequence (TR = 4,000, TE = 60, flip angle = 60).

Figure 13.14 shows the results of activity associated with the forward speech excluding areas associated with the backward speech in order to evaluate the hypothesis that the patient

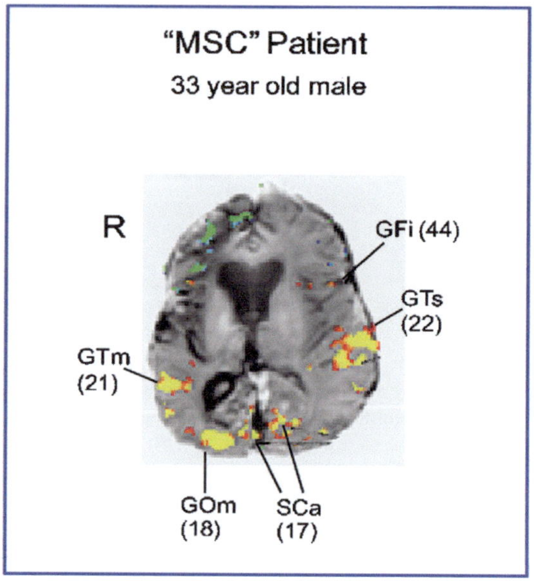

Fig. 13.14 Functional imaging of cognitive processes in minimally conscious states. Neuroimaging While Listening to Narratives presented as normal speech (Forward) excluding responses elicited when the same speech was presented in reversed time (AND/NOT Backward). Note the structural abnormalities in the anterior right hemisphere secondary to the injury. Activity in left inferior frontal gyrus (GFi), Brodmann's area (BA) 44, putative Broca's area; left hemisphere temporal gyrus (GT's), BA 22, putative Wernicke's area; and middle temporal gyrus (GTm), BA21, bilaterally, putative auditory-cortex as expected for language tasks is observed. Additionally, the MCS subject shows activity in the extrastriate visual cortex (middle occipital gyrus, GOm, BA18), and in primary visual cortex (calcarine sulcus, SCa, BA17). The levels of statistical stringency and analysis procedures were identical for the patient and a comparison healthy volunteer, suggesting that the responses elicited by the patient were (1) more robust as they activated a large volume of cortex (larger number of significant voxels) and (2) more distributed as the global pattern of activity included visual system responses. This was unexpected since there was no visual stimulation (only auditory), and the patient had his eyes closed. We cannot rule out the possibility that this patient was "visualizing" some representation of the narrative that was personalized for him

was responsive to the "meaning" of the narrative not just the sound. Most notable is the similarity between the patient and both the group and healthy individuals who performed the same task. In particular, activity observed in the left temporal gyres (GTs) and left inferior frontal gyres (GFi) are consistent with Wernicke's and

Broca's areas, respectively. Of notable interest is the additional activity in the occipital region (calcarine sulcus [CaS] and middle occipital gyres [GOm]) of the patient suggestive of mental imagery and/or top–down information processing in response to the narrative.

The neural activity associated with this stimulation, and the forward–backward narrative comparison are not only remarkably robust for the patient, but are also basically indistinguishable from the normals.

These findings and similar cases [48] raise a number of complex questions including "Does this patient have an inner cognitive life that is not reflected by his bedside responses?" If so, what can we do about it? Are any of these findings evidence for "neural preparedness" for emergence? What ethical issues do these findings suggest? [49] What investigations need to be done to lead us to informed and aggressive therapies? Can neuroimaging contribute to assessments that will guide and inform therapies for individual patients? Recent investigations suggest that imaging paradigms established to investigate the neural underpinnings of cognition in normals also provide foundations for emerging investigations of the neural underpinnings of consciousness. Both bring neural science closer to the goal of understanding the biological underpinnings of the mind, and perhaps closer to the goal of treating patients with DOC.

Objective Assessment of Patient States During a Disorder of Consciousness Based on the Extent of the Network Engaged by a Command to Name Objects

The aforementioned studies document that even during states where consciousness is lost, evidence of cognitive engagement is obtainable using fMRI. More recent advances suggest that the integrity of the long-range networks elicited by an instruction to name pictures can inform the neurophysiology. Patients with DOC can be stratified by completeness of the neural system engaged by the task [50]. Suggesting that activity of the language network may serve as a proxy for behavioral evidence of awareness. Command-following paradigms that employ fMRI rather than overt motor responses to assess cognitive capacity in DOC patients have emerged as an important clinical advance.

Awareness of self or environment is considered a prerequisite for conscious processing and it is conventionally assessed by overt motor responses. Subjects in the minimally conscious state (MCS) show fluctuations in awareness and clear, but inconsistent, minimal behavioral signs of conscious awareness [47]. In contrast, subjects in the vegetative state (VS) are awake but not aware, and do not show behavioral response to environmental stimuli, indicating lack of conscious processing [51]. Subjects in the locked-in syndrome (LIS) show very limited signs of awareness due to profound sensory and motor deficits but have preserved self-awareness and normal or near-normal cognitive capacities [52]. Impairments of the sensory and motor systems in these patient populations render conventional bedside diagnosis inadequate and it is thought to have contributed to high rates of misdiagnosis of LIS, MCS, and VS patients [53, 54], as well as underestimation of cognitive capacity. It has become evident that assessment of these patients' cognitive abilities requires diagnostic tools that do not rely exclusively on overt motor responses. Recent studies using passive tasks [46, 54], imagery tasks [55, 56], and covert tasks [54–56] have suggested that a larger number of patients with DOC than previously suspected may retain awareness of self or environment undetected by conventional behavioral response methods. Thus, improved assessments of awareness and cognitive abilities that do not depend upon motor responses provide a significance advance for the assessment, treatment, and care of patients with DOC [57–59].

Internal picture naming was employed to assess conscious awareness in patients who fail to demonstrate clearly discernible evidence of awareness on bedside examination. Areas related to visual processing, language, and executive regions would be expected to be activated in a task-contingent manner and be most and least prominent in LIS and VS, respectively. In particular, this task is known to elicit activity in Broca's and Wernicke's areas and medial frontal gyrus [35, 36].

The Coma Recovery Scale-Revised (CRS-R) [60] consists of 23 items organized in six subscales that address arousal, auditory, visual, motor, oromotor/verbal, and communication systems. Each subscale is organized hierarchaly, with lower items representing reflexive activity and higher items representing cognition-based behaviors.

Findings demonstrate variations in the underlying brain activity of the MCS patients for the command-following task that generally correspond to the CRS-R. The comparison of the naming network observed in healthy volunteers with DOC patients allows a functional differentiation of patients into three groups: (1) complete network: patients with activation of all brain areas observed in healthy volunteers; (2) partial network: patients with activation of some brain areas observed in healthy volunteers; and (3) absent network: patients with no activation of any brain areas observed in healthy volunteers. These neural categories are related to behavioral measures of status. As expected, patient with high CRS-R scores, including LIS1, EMCS1, MCS, and MCS2, showed patterns of activity similar to those of control subjects elicited by Boston Naming task (complete network group). Conversely, patients with low CRS-R scores (i.e., VS1) show a very unresponsive brain as expected for this population (absent network group). Remarkably, patients in the partial network group are characterized by lack of activation in the medial frontal gyrus and lower CRS-R scores, i.e., MCS3 to MCS5 (Fig. 13.15).

To our knowledge, this is the first fMRI study to employ covert picture naming (internal speech) as a command-following task in a series of patients with a range of DOC and behavioral profiles [50]. Picture naming is considered a complex process that requires access to various representations of the object, including stored knowledge about the structural description (physical properties of the object), semantic (functional and associative properties), and phonological (name) representations of the object [60–63]. Boston Naming is thought to recruit stimulus-driven (bottom–up) [64] and purpose-driven (top–down) [62] brain circuits: visual input processing areas, language areas, short-term memory regions, motor areas, and executive regions. The initial step of the Boston Naming task is the processing of the visual stimuli. Therefore, the presence of visual cortex activation is taken as a prerequisite for successful performance of the task. All the patients reported showed early visual processing as it was used as an inclusion criteria. It has been shown that picture processing during naming tasks is not

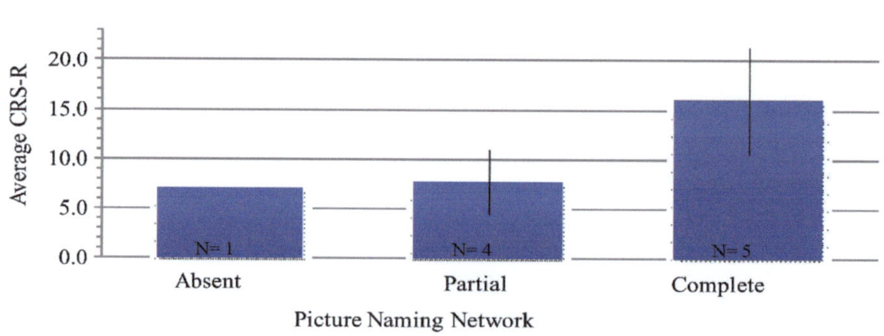

Fig. 13.15 Relationship between CRS-R scores and preservation of the picture-naming network. DOC patients are grouped according to preservation of the naming network previously observed in healthy volunteers: (1) complete network: patients with activation of all brain areas observed in healthy volunteers (LGTs, LGFi(v), LGFi(d), and Pre-SMA); (2) partial network: patients with activation of some brain areas observed in healthy volunteers; and (3) absent network: patients with no activation of any brain areas observed in healthy volunteers. The *bars* show the average CRS-R score for each group with the corresponding standard deviation

automated but rather an effortful process that involves controlled attentional resources [65]. Object recognition involves top–down modulation of early visual cortex by regions on the occipitotemporal associated with semantic knowledge of the object [65, 66]. Previous studies highlight the importance of traditional language areas in object naming. For example, the left BA22 of the GTs, also referred to as Wernicke's area, has been associated to semantic knowledge [67, 68] and to phonological code retrieval [69], the left ventral region of the inferior frontal gyrus, Broca's area (BA 44/45), has been linked to phonological processing [70], phonetic sequencing [71], selection of competing semantic representations [72], and dorsal Broca's area (BA 44/6) associated to executive processes to select a lexical representation and processes related to motor programming and planning of articulation [72–75]. Overt picture naming has a very similar activity pattern relative to covert picture naming [72], although the degree of activation might be higher in inferior frontal regions during overt naming in comparison to covert naming [77]. Although emphasis has been commonly placed in the linguistic aspects of picture naming, it was used as a command-following task in this application and expected to engage regions associated in volitional control. Previous imaging reports have associated midline regions (pre-supplementary motor area [pre-SMA]) with volitional aspects of cognition and actions [76]. Boly et al. [78] found pre-SMA activation on all subjects performing four different imagery tasks in comparison to rest and interpreted the activation as reflecting cognitive control or the intention to perform the task. A recent study also found medial frontal cortex activation in healthy controls and one MCS patient when subjects counted a target word in comparison to listening to the words [58].

Activity in the GTs BA 22 (including Wernicke's area), inferior frontal gyrus BA44/45 (including Broca's area), and medial frontal gyrus (pre-SMA, BA 6/8) is typically reported during covert picture naming [35, 36]. Similar patterns of activity have also been found to include parietal regions [61, 62, 75]. Observation of this expected functional specificity for the picture-naming task can thus be considered as evidence for awareness in these patients, suggesting that conscious, volitional execution of the task may depend on the engagement of visual, temporal, and inferior frontal regions engaged by visual stimuli and linked to activity in the frontal regions to execute cognitive control of the task. This interpretation is in accord with the view that consciousness is characterized by simultaneous activation of multiple brain areas to form a single long-distance network [79]. The comparison of patients' naming networks with that of healthy volunteers allows a classification of patients into three categories: patients who retain all components of the reference network (complete network), patients who engage only some of those brain regions (partial network), and patients who show no activation of any of those components (absent network). For the MCS cohort, activation of neural networks associated with language is counter-posed against the lack of consistent verbal expression in these patients. The finding of unresponsiveness at the behavioral level accompanied by extensive preservation of cognitive networks raises challenges to our ability to identify VS by behavioral assessment alone in some patients, as recently shown by Owen et al. [48] using motor imagery.

The functional capacity of these systems can be influenced by anxiety and fluctuations in arousal and awareness. In addition to these caveats, fMRI data acquisition allows for very limited motion; and interpretation of imaging data can be challenged in the presence of structural abnormalities or temporal mismatch between presentation of the target stimulus and the patient's response.

Summarizing, this work provides a framework to identify patients in various levels or states of consciousness that retain neural circuits capable of supporting high-level volitional processes not discerned through conventional behavioral assessment alone. Information provided by fMRI has not yet been sufficiently vetted to justify changing the behavior-based diagnosis in most cases. However, these findings indicate a clear need to consider the capacity for covert cognitive processing in addition to the overt behaviors when conducting diagnostic assessment, particularly in patients with ambiguous findings or significant sensory and motor impairments. Determining where patients lie on the spectrum of consciousness is key to optimal clinical management, application of available therapies, and maximization of quality of life for this population. These new findings indicate that neuroimaging studies provide novel information that may aid in differential diagnosis, identifying patients in DOC with substantially preserved neural circuits that may serve as a marker for retention of high-level cognitive capacities not apparent on bedside examination.

Determination of the Anatomy and Topography of Cortical Areas Specialized for Cognitive Tasks

In contrast to language, sensory/motor, and visual systems, our current understanding of the mechanisms of higher functions is not so closely linked to a specified neurophysiological substrate. This is due, in part, to the fact that many aspects of cognition are dynamic processes that involve many working parts, and often cannot be studied in animals. The emergence of neuroimaging provides a new opportunity to test hypotheses and map the underlying mechanisms of cognition in healthy individuals without reliance on lesions or disease processes. However, these investigations remain in their early stages. Determinations of the anatomy and topography of cortical areas specialized for cognitive tasks can contribute to models that integrate multiple functionally specialized areas. These objectives will be discussed later in the context of specific functions, including attention, working memory, executive processes, and consciousness, with an emphasis on the unifying notion that the neurobiological pathways are multiregional with complex covariations. Clinical applications for these maps are currently under development in specialties such as psychiatry, neurology, rehabilitation, and even nonmedical specialties such as neuroeconomics and neurolaw.

> "While there has been general agreement that operations performed by the sensory and motor systems are localized, there has been much more dispute about higher-level cognitive processes. It is still undetermined whether higher-level processes have defined locations, and if so, where these locations would be." Posner and Raichle, *Images of Mind*, 1994, p. 16 [80]

As previously discussed, the functional neuroanatomy of cognitive processes is revealed by comparing the BOLD response elicited by various experimental and control tasks and is typically characterized by a voxel-by-voxel statistical comparison of the signal amplitude during the activity epoch, with the average signal amplitude during a baseline resting or control epoch. The basic assumption is that neuronal activity is increased in a functionally specialized area during the execution of a task that employs that specialization. Locations of active areas, cluster sizes, and dynamic properties of the signal such as covariation can be compared across cognitive conditions. Tasks are designed to either include or exclude the cognitive component of interest and the signals elicited from these tasks are compared.

Conservation of Effects Versus Individual Differences: Generalizing the Results

Investigations of the neural basis for cognitive processes are aimed toward findings generalizable to the population at large. Neuroimaging studies on single subjects can be assumed to include effects that are conserved across all subjects (generalizable), and effects that are specific to that individual subject [81]. Results that are present in all or most cases given a sufficiently large sample size can be assumed to reflect a fundamental specialization characteristic of the population, whereas intermittently present results can be assumed to represent other less-conserved (individual) processes. A theoretical basis for inferences to a population based on functional imaging data is currently under development. Based on models using a two-tailed test of significance at a criterion level of $p \leq 0.05$ and a power of 80%, Desmond and Glover [82] suggested that analyses of covariation and connectivity may require sample sizes up to 20 or more subjects.

Inferences to a population based on imaging data generally require registration of individual brains and a standard stereotactic coordinate system. Although registration procedures are an area of active development, the conventional method (originally developed for PET studies) employs the Co-Planar Stereotaxic Atlas of the Human Brain [83]. Acquired brain images are registered to that atlas by reference to the anterior–posterior commissure line and active areas are labeled accordingly and assigned an address in x, y, z stereotactic coordinates. One popular tool for accomplishing this objective is available in Statistical Parametric Mapping (SPM) [84], a software package developed for processing neuroimaging data. Other representations of brain structure and functions include flat maps and inflated brains.

Method of Cognitive Subtraction

The cognitive subtraction paradigm requires two tasks: an experimental task that engages the cognitive component of interest, and a baseline or control task that engages all of the processes included in the cognitive task except for the cognitive component of interest. The neural correlates of the cognitive task of interest are presumed to be revealed by a subtraction of the baseline activity from the activity observed during the experimental task. Examples of the cognitive subtraction design are found in the early PET studies, where, for example, the effect of viewing a fixation dot was subtracted from the effect of viewing a flashing checkerboard to reveal the neural effect of the checkerboard alone. Although the subtractive approach was employed successfully in those early studies, it is limited by the difficulty of selecting tasks that differ only with respect to the cognition of interest. If differences between the experimental task and the comparison baseline task are due to a combinatorial effect not present with either task alone, then the conclusion could be misguided. These assumptions often are referred to as the assumptions of linear additivity or pure insertion, and depend upon the partitioning of complex cognitive tasks into independent subcomponent processes.

Method of Cognitive Conjunction

In contrast to the identification of differences between the elicited activity of two cognitive tasks by subtraction, a conjunction analysis reveals the activity common to multiple tasks. For example, in an investigation to identify the neural substrate specialized for object naming, the same task can be performed using multiple sensory systems – that is, objects that are seen, heard, and felt are named during an imaging study. The conjunction of neural activity present in all three naming tasks is assumed to represent the neural activity associated with naming alone, and the processes associated with the sensory-related activity are assumed to be excluded by virtue of the fact that such activity is not common to all tasks (as illustrated in Fig. 13.16).

Some of the same assumptions for the subtractive approach previously described apply. First, it is assumed that the cognitive processes engaged by each task are performed similarly across the sensory modalities. However, there is considerable evidence for intermingling of modality-specific and domain-general mechanisms in some tasks.

For example, mental imagery tasks may draw upon modality-specific subsystems, which would not be observed by this method. Thus, the conjunctive method applied to cross-modal studies identifies a subset of domain-general processes, but may fail to recognize all components critical to task performance.

On the contrary, the conjunctive approach, applied to within-modal studies, can serve to enhance confidence in a result by isolating activity that is repeated on multiple runs of the same task. This strategy is based on the assumption that signals originating from noise sources are distinguished from signals originating from real events by the probability of a repeat occurrence at

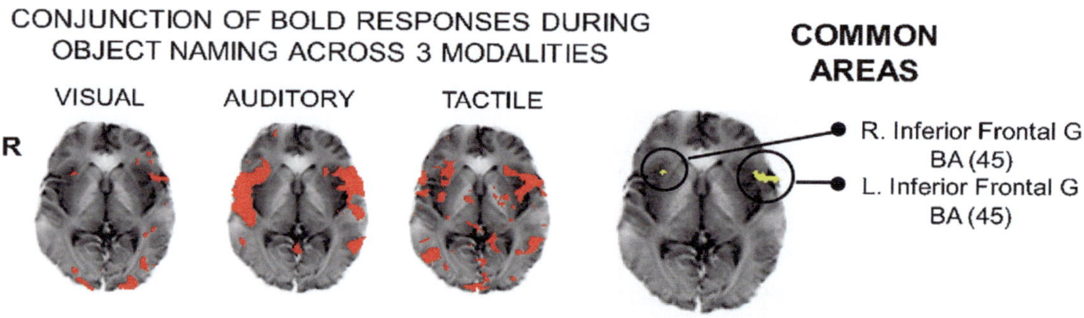

Fig. 13.16 Conjunction of BOLD responses during object naming across three sensory modalities. Voxels active during visual stimulation (*left*), auditory stimulation (*middle*), and tactile stimulation (*right*) are indicated in orange for one slice of brain. The conjunction image (*yellow*) illustrates the supramodal activity common to all three modalities of stimulation following a Boolean AND operation. This activity occurs in left and right inferior frontal gyrus (BA 45) and is taken to represent the aspects of object naming not primarily associated with a specific sensory modality for this single subject. Reprinted with permission from Hirsch J, Rodriguez-Moreno D, Kim KHS. Interconnected large-scale systems for three fundamental cognitive tasks revealed by functional MRI. J Cogn Neurosci. 2001;13(3):1–16. MIT Press Journals

the same location. Voxels that are reliably activated on multiple separate occasions result in a low false-positive rate that can be empirically determined based on images acquired either during resting states or on images acquired on a spherical container of copper sulfate solution that simulates brain (phantom). For this reason, conjunctions often are employed in clinical and neurosurgical applications to enhance confidence in a result by isolating the activity that is elicited on multiple runs of the same task [36, 41, 42]. However, because repeated stimuli do not usually elicit as robust a response as novel stimuli, all repetitions of a task are optimally performed using equal but different stimuli. Thus, in the case of an object-naming task, all objects would be novel but equated for variables such as familiarity and difficulty during the multiple runs in order to be optimized for the within-modal conjunction approach.

Integration of Functionally Specialized Areas Associated with Cognitive Tasks: The Network Approach

Although functional differentiation of single brain areas is a well-established principle of cortical organization, recent approaches to human cognition have focused on the integration of groups of specialized areas into long-range units that may collectively serve as the comprehensive neural substrate for specific cognitive tasks. An early empirical foundation for this emerging view is found in the work of Mishkin and Ungerleider [85], who described ventral and dorsal pathway segmentation during visual tasks that required either object identification or object localization, respectively. More recently, direct interactions between brain regions that participate in specific functions have been proposed as evidence for this systems model; for example, covariations between BOLD responses in separate cortical areas during complex attention tasks have been examined using a statistical approach called structural equation modeling, which can determine whether the covariances between areas are due to direct or indirect interactions [86]. This analysis technique identifies the groups of areas associated with a task, and also characterizes changes in regional activity and interactions between regions over time. Other approaches to identify function-specific long-range systems associated with language and attention processes are illustrated later in this chapter.

> "A central feature in the organization of the large-scale network is the absence of one-to-one correspondences among anatomical sites, neural computations and complex behaviors. According to this organization, an individual cognitive or behavioral domain is subserved by several interconnected

macroscopic sites, each of which subserves multiple computations, leading to a distributed and interactive but also coarse and degenerate (one-to-many and many-to-one) mapping of anatomical substrate onto neural computation and computation onto behavior." M. Marsel Mesulam, 1998 [87]

Functional Neuroanatomy of Language Processes: A Large-Scale Network

Models of the neural correlates for elementary language processes often include left hemisphere regions involved in a variety of language functions, including Broca's and Wernicke's areas, and are generally consistent with a network model. To demonstrate this network, an object-naming task using auditory, visual, and tactile stimuli can be employed. A cross-modality conjunction technique (above) isolates effects not dependent upon sensory processes. Results are consistent with the view that the task of naming objects elicits activity from a set of areas within a neurocognitive system specialized for language-related functions (Fig. 13.17). The colored circles on the glass brain represent average locations of activity centroids on the standard atlas brain (*x*, *y*, *z* coordinates) as indicated on the table in Fig. 13.17. There are five regions in this neurocognitive system (all located within the left hemisphere), including putative Broca's area (inferior frontal gyrus, BA 44 and 45), putative Wernicke's area (GTs, BA 22), and medial frontal gyrus (BA 6). Thus, these results are consistent with the view that the functional specialization for this elementary language task involves a system of language-related areas rather than a single area.

OBJECT NAMING NETWORK

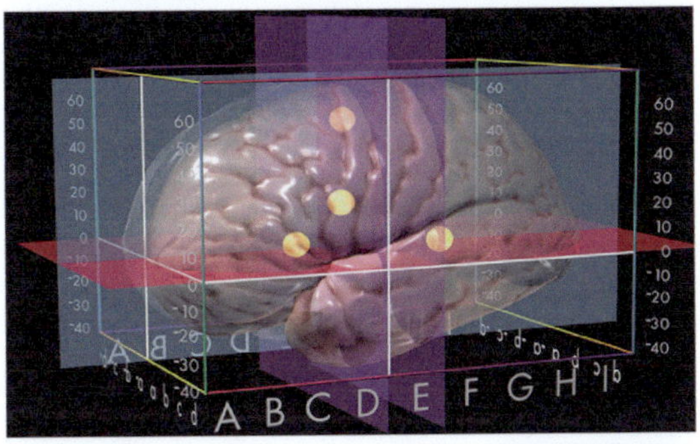

Anatomical Region	Area	Center of mass x	y	z
Medial Frontal Gyrus (GFd)	6	9	-6	53
Superior Temporal Gyrus (GTs)	22	57	-26	9
Inferior Frontal Gyrus (Gfi)	44	49	10	25
Inferior Frontal Gyrus (Gfi)	45	40	25	8

Fig. 13.17 A fixed large-scale network for object naming. The network of areas that subserve object naming as determined by conjunction across three sensory modalities consists of medial frontal gyrus (GFd, BA 6), superior temporal gyrus (GTs, BA 22; putative Wernicke's area), and inferior frontal gyrus (Gfi, BA 44,45; putative Broca's area) in the left hemisphere. These areas are portrayed as *colored circles* in a 3D glass brain based upon the Talairach and Tournoux Human Brain Atlas45 and stereotactic coordinate system. The table appearing below contains the average group coordinates (*x*, *y*, *z*) of the included regions. Reprinted with permission from Hirsch J, Rodriguez-Moreno D, Kim KHS. Interconnected large-scale systems for three fundamental cognitive tasks revealed by functional MRI. J Cogn Neurosci. 2001;13(3):1–16. MIT Press Journals.

Functional Neuroanatomy of Attention Processes: A Large-Scale Network

Like language, the ability to direct attention is involved in a range of cognitive tasks. Functional imaging studies by Mesulam [87] and others suggest that spatial attention is mediated by a large-scale distributed network of interconnected cortical areas within the posterior parietal cortex, the region of frontal eye fields, and the cingulate cortex. Kim and colleagues [88] used a conjunction analysis to compare activity associated with two different types of visuospatial attention shifts: one based on spatial priming and the other based on cues that directed spatial expectancy to test the hypothesis of a fixed area network for both tasks. The activation foci observed for the two tasks were nearly overlapping, indicating that both were subserved by a common network of cortical and subcortical areas. The main findings of this study were consistent with a model of spatial attention that is associated with a fixed large-scale distributed network specialized to coordinate multiple aspects of attention. Alternative hypotheses that predict that task variations are associated with an increase in the number of involved areas can be rejected. However,

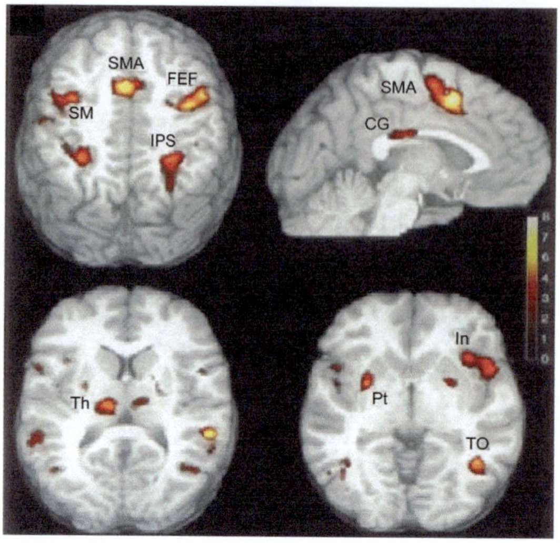

Fig. 13.18 A fixed large-scale network for spatial attention. The network of areas that subserve visuospatial attention shifts consists of supplementary motor area – anterior cingulate cortex (SMA, BA 6), frontal eye fields (FEF, BA 6), and the banks of the intraparietal sulcus (IPS, BA 7,40). This network was determined by a conjunction analysis of activation related to visuospatial attention tasks based on two different types of information, spatial priming and spatial expectancy. Although the same areas are involved in both tasks, a rightward bias in the intraparietal sulcus (IPS) was observed for the spatial priming task and suggests that, within this network, task-related variations are present. Reprinted with permission from NeuroImage Vol. 9. Kim Y-H, Gitelman Dr, Nobre AG, Parrish TB, LaBar KS, Mesulam M-M. The large-scale neural network for spatial attention displays multifunctional overlap but differential asymmetry, 269–277. Copyright © 1999, Elsevier. (Neurologic coordinates)

an observed rightward bias for the spatial priming task suggested that activation within the system showed variations specific to the attributes of the attentional task (Fig. 13.18).

Tests of Cognitive Theory Based on Mapping of Neural Correlates

Advances in our understanding of the biological components of cognition are dependent upon the development of functional tasks that reveal specific cognitive processes; therefore, tasks are selected to target some aspect of cognition that can be varied so that the specific processing requirements are increased or decreased. Current neuroimaging investigations of language, attention, memory, executive processes, and even consciousness generate hypotheses based on theoretical frameworks and behavioral models and develop stimulation paradigms that cause the subject to engage the targeted functions. This section presents a selection of models, hypotheses, cognitive functions, and tasks that have been investigated by neuroimaging techniques.

Although more in-depth coverage of many of these topics is presented elsewhere, the objective here is to illustrate the advantages of neuroimaging for understanding the biological components of various cognitive processes rather than to provide a comprehensive survey of each of these cognitive processes.

Functional Neuroanatomy of Working Memory: A Fixed- or Variable-Area Network

Mechanisms for cognitive functions such as reasoning, problem solving, and language are critically dependent upon working memory processes that briefly maintain a limited amount of information in a mental scratch pad for ongoing processing. To test the hypothesis that a working memory system is subserved by a fixed number of brain areas, Smith and Jonides [89] employed a memory task (N-Back) that varied cognitive load. The logic of the experiment follows: If the hypothesis of a fixed number of regions was supported, then increasing the difficulty of the task, and thereby the cognitive load, would increase the amount of activity in each of the component areas. However, if the hypothesis of a variable area network was supported, then increasing the difficulty of the task would activate additional areas.

The *N*-Back Task and a Test of a Cognitive Theory

The *N*-Back task, illustrated in Fig. 13.19, was developed as a cognitive tool to vary memory task difficulty (load). The subject views a series of letters separated by fixation points. In the 0-Back condition, the subject responds whenever one of the presented letters matches a standard

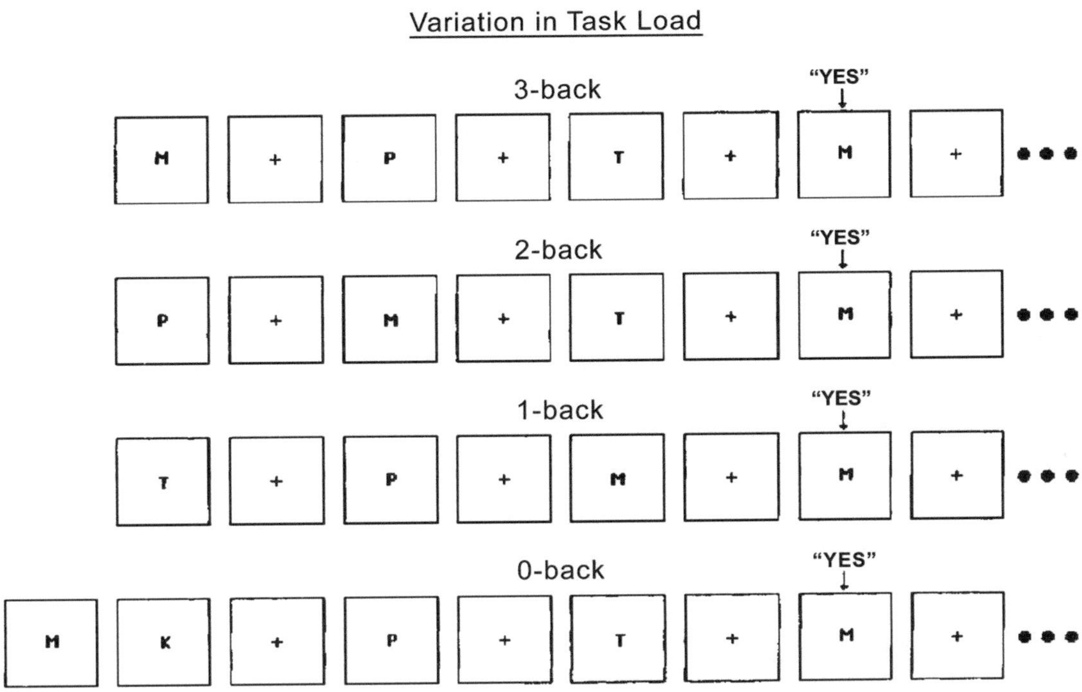

Fig. 13.19 Variation in working memory load based on the *N*-Back task. The *N*-Back task engages working memory by requiring the subject to remember a previous event and respond if a present stimulus (target) is identical to that previously presented stimulus. Task load can be increased by increasing the distance between the target and its match, e.g., 0-, 1-, 2-, and 3-Back. Reprinted with permission from Cognitive Psychology, Vol. 33, Smith EE, Jonides J. Working memory: a view from neuroimaging, 5–42. Copyright © 1997, Elsevier

presented at the beginning of the run. In the 1-Back condition, the subject responds when there is a match to the preceding letter. In the 2-Back condition, the subject responds when there is a match to the letter 2-Back in the series, and similarly for the 3-Back condition.

Results of this study showed a clear increase in the volume of activity, with the increase in difficulty (load) of the task (Fig. 13.20). However, the specific regions involved did not vary with increases in load supporting the "fixed number of areas" hypothesis for a working memory system.

Functional Neuroanatomy of Selective Attention: A Neurological Model of Cognitive Interference

The ability to filter task-related stimuli to guide responses is referred to as selective attention. An experimental task that requires the subject to attend to certain stimulus characteristics while ignoring others that elicit a competing response engages a system of selective attention. The Stroop task is a classical cognitive task first developed for use in behavioral studies of cognitive interference and is an ideal task for functional imaging studies that seek to identify the neural substrate associated with selective attention mechanisms.

The Stroop Task

In the classical Stroop task, a subject views a series of words in different colored inks. Each word is the name of a color. The subject is instructed to produce the color of the ink. In the incongruent case, the word and the ink color of the written word are different, resulting in longer reaction times than in the congruent case where the word and ink color match. For example, if the ink color was blue but the word was red (incongruent), the reaction time to report "blue" (the

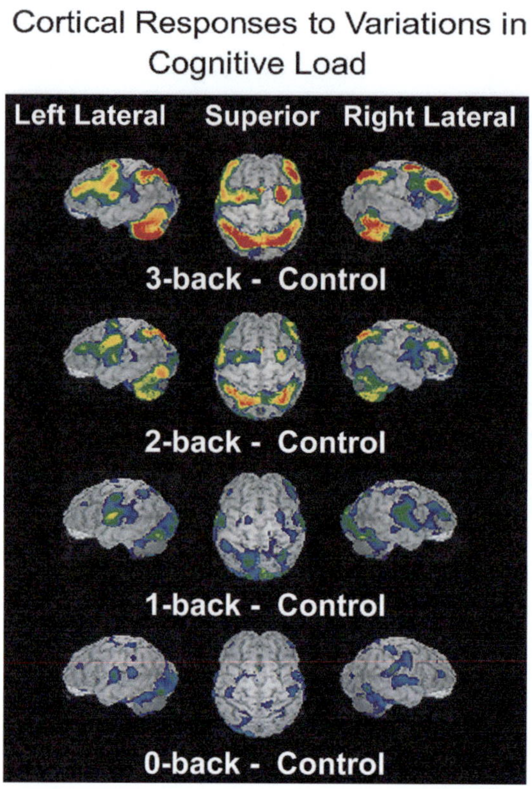

Fig. 13.20 Cortical responses during the *N*-Back task. Left and right lateral, as well as a superior, views of the average PET images are shown. All images are difference images that reflect the subtraction of a control condition in which subjects responded to every stimulus. The different colors reflect the significance of the activation, with *red areas* being most significant. Robust responses for the 3-Back condition relative to 0-, 1-, and 2-Back conditions are taken as evidence of increased neural activity associated with increased memory load. Reprinted with permission from Cognitive Psychology, Vol. 33, Smith EE, Jonides J. Working memory: a view from neuroimaging, 5–42. Copyright © 1997, Elsevier

ink color) would be longer than when the word and the ink color were both blue (congruent) (Fig. 13.20).

Cognitive models that account for results obtained by the Stroop task propose that subjects must inhibit the automatic reading response and selectively attend to the color of the letters in order to perform the color-naming task successfully. A neuroimaging study designed to probe the neural basis for this type of cognitive interference, that is, the mechanisms of selective attention [90], compared BOLD responses to congruent and incongruent conditions in an event-related neuroimaging study (see following section on event-related paradigms). The results are shown in Fig. 13.21 for incongruent and congruent conditions, respectively. The incongruent condition is associated with robust distributed responses as compared to the congruent condition, suggesting that a distributed large-scale neural network is employed during selective attention. The results also suggest a possible correspondence between the selective attention mechanisms engaged in this study and visuospatial attention mechanisms (Fig. 13.22).

Functional Neuroanatomy of Executive Processes: Separate or Combined Systems

Current models of cognition often include undefined mechanisms (frequently referred to as a black box) to account for executive processes such as the allocation of attentional resources among competing tasks. Functional neuroimaging techniques and experimental paradigms, such as the dual performance task and the Go/No-Go task, have been developed to observe the neural correlates of these executive functions and attempt to define the black box in neurophysiological terms.

D'Esposito et al. [91] introduced an fMRI task paradigm that required subjects to perform two tasks simultaneously, referred to as a dual performance task. Comparison of the BOLD responses elicited during each task alone and both tasks together enabled tests of hypotheses about the neural system involved in the execution of competing tasks. Specifically, the hypothesis of a modular executive system predicts the recruitment of additional regions during the dual-task condition, whereas the fixed-areas hypothesis predicts an increase in volume of the areas activated by a single task. Adcock et al. [92] employed this paradigm with paired combinations of spatial rotation tasks (visual), semantic categorization tasks (auditory), and facial identification tasks (visual). Results indicated that the activated areas varied with the sensory modality of component

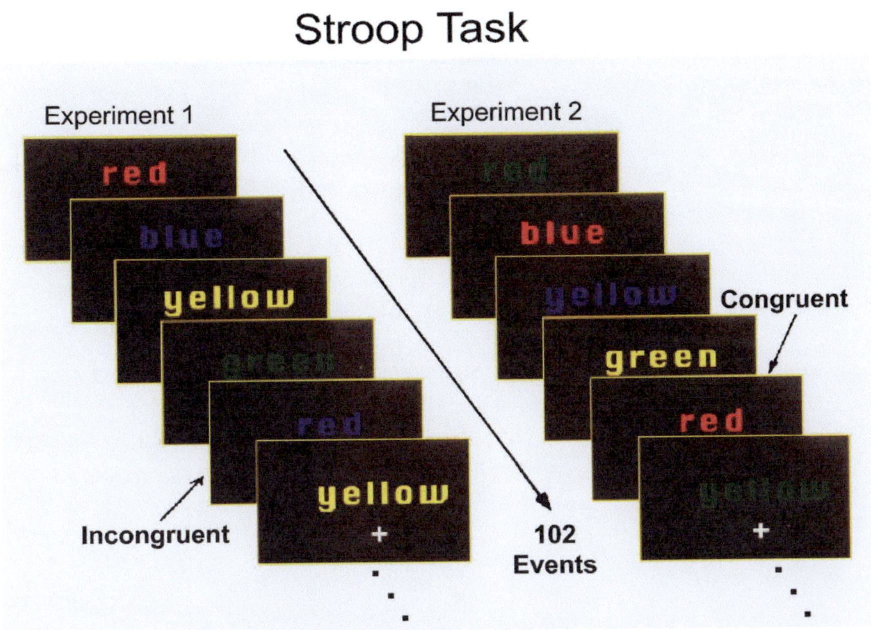

Fig. 13.21 The classical Stroop color word interference task. In congruent cases, the color of the ink matches the color of the word. In incongruent cases, the color of the ink is different from the color of the word. The words are presented sequentially to subjects who respond by indicating the color of the ink for each word. Reprinted with permission from Leung H-C, Skudlarski P, Gatenby JC, Peterson BS, Gore JC. An event-related functional MRI study of the Stroop color word interference task. Cereb Cortex. 2000;10:552–60. Oxford University Press

tasks as expected based on these domain-specific functional specializations. However, all of the areas activated during the dual-task performance were also activated during the component tasks; that is, there was no evidence for a separate executive system. Increases in activity within a given area during the dual task are related to the additional load of the second task. These results can be interpreted as generally consistent with the hypothesis that these executive processes may be implemented by interactions between anatomically and functionally distinct systems engaged in the performances of component tasks rather than by a specific area or areas dedicated to a modular and separable executive system.

The Go/No-Go Task

Another classical executive function is the ability to inhibit a prepotent or habitual response that has been studied psychophysically using a Go/No-Go task paradigm. Neuroimaging investigations of the neural correlates of response inhibition have employed a version of the task to investigate the neural correlates of response inhibition in children and adults [93]. The hypothesis was that the ability to inhibit a response successfully varies with maturity. This variation could be neurally represented as either the recruitment of different areas in children versus adults or variations in the volumes within a fixed set of areas. During the Go/No–Go task, the subject views a series of letters presented sequentially and presses a button on each successive presentation except when the letter is an X. On the X trials, the subject must inhibit the response.

The BOLD responses for children (ages 7–12 years) and adults were compared within five selected areas of the prefrontal cortex using an event-related paradigm and an analysis of variance (ANOVA) where subject age and the task conditions (Go vs. No-Go) were taken as factors. The areas demonstrating significant activity

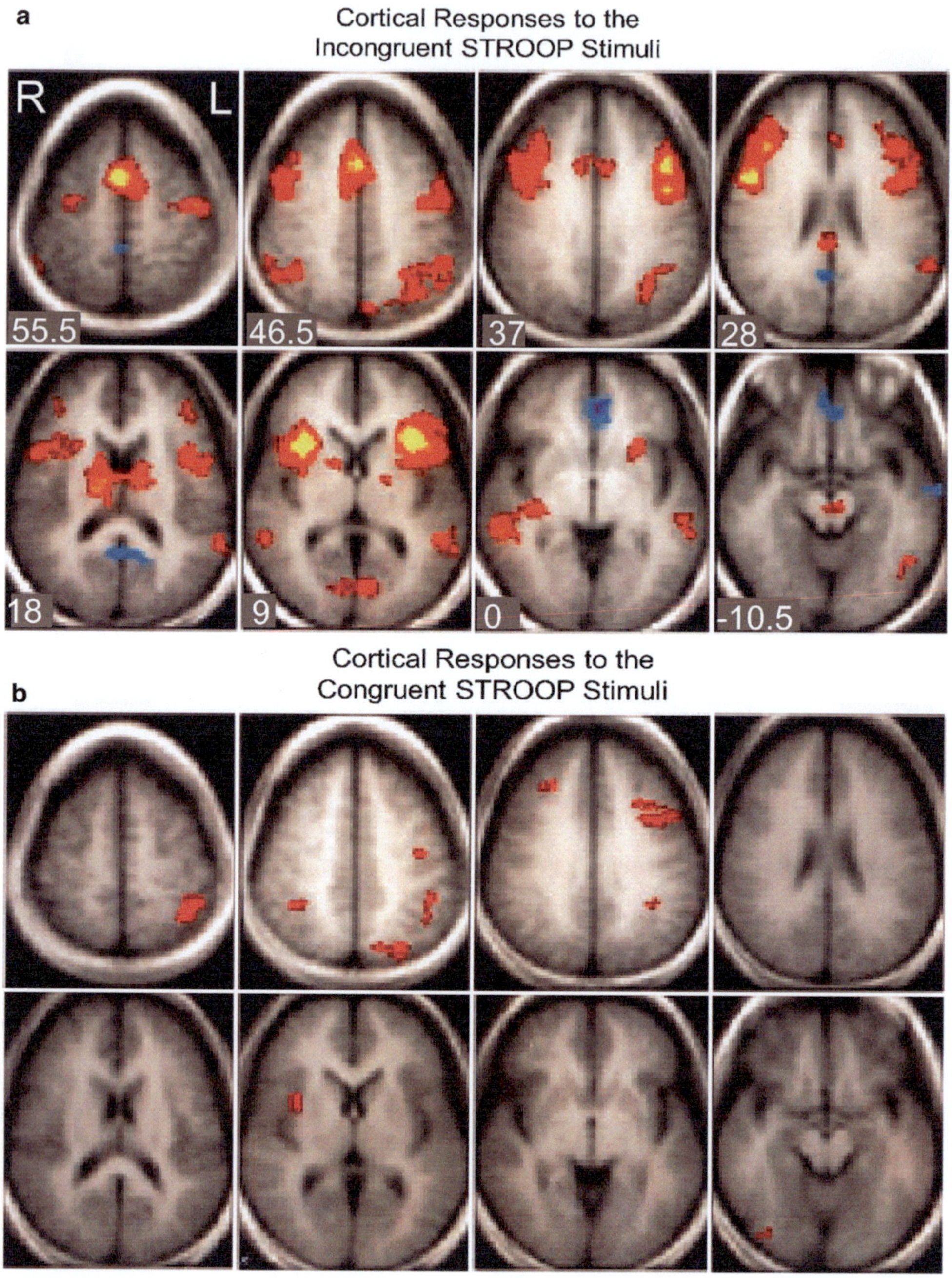

Fig. 13.22 Activation related to the classical Stroop task versus the inverse Stroop task. Images represent composite maps of 13 subjects performing the Stroop task. In Experiment 1, the classical Stroop task was employed, that is, incongruent words appear infrequently whereas congruent words appear frequently (**a**). In Experiment 2 (**b**), an inverse Stroop task was employed; that is, congruent words are infrequent events and incongruent words appear frequently. The robust response for the incongruent condition (**a**) relative to the congruent condition (**b**) is taken as evidence of a neural basis for response inhibition. Reprinted with permission from Leung H-C, Skudlarski P, Gatenby JC, Peterson BS, Gore JC. An event-related functional MRI study of the Stroop color word interference task. Cereb Cortex 2000;10:552–560. Oxford University Press

related to the No-Go task include anterior cingulate and four frontal gyri, including inferior, middle, orbital, and superior. The areas involved in the response inhibition function did not vary between adults and children. However, during No-Go trials, the amount of activity was higher in children, particularly in the dorsal and lateral prefrontal sites.

This observation is consistent with the hypothesis of a distributed system for response inhibition and further suggests that the elements include anterior cingulate and four frontal gyri, including inferior, middle, orbital, and superior. The areas involved in the response inhibition function did not vary between adults and children. However, during No-Go trials, the amount of activity was higher in children, particularly in the dorsal and lateral prefrontal sites.

Integration of Temporal and Spatial Information to Map Executive Processes

A common theme in the aforementioned neuroimaging studies of cognitive functions is the identification of the underlying cortical networks associated with each function and the question of fixed versus variable areas for related functions. In the case of the language, attention, memory, and cognitive control systems illustrated previously, the results suggest that a fixed number of areas (rather than the recruitment of new areas) are modulated with increased load. This is an active area of research, and new evidence from studies using techniques such as electrophysiological recordings, developing connectivity analyses, and tractography to probe within-system effects may be required to elucidate the modulation of processes both within and across these systems.

Integration of ERP and fMRI

New investigations that focus on within-system processes and the modulation of a specialized system consisting of a fixed set of distributed areas require probes of the computations performed within neural systems. A new class of multi-technique experiments are currently being developed that elucidate the spatial localization of active regions (fMRI), and the temporal covariations between these cortical or subcortical regions, as reflected in event-related potentials (ERP). These techniques may be employed either simultaneously or sequentially and require an adaptation of the blocked fMRI experiments (event-related fMRI) and a task specialized for both fMRI and electrophysiological approaches.

Event-Related fMRI

As in conventional event-related electrophysiology, individual trials (events) are presented separately (rather than in a continuous block), and the signal is selectively averaged across like trials. This acquisition scheme is illustrated in Fig. 13.23, where both block and event-related schemes are shown [94]. Event-related fMRI offers an additional class of task designs that expand and elaborate investigations of cognitive processes. Given that the BOLD response tracks neuronal activity with hemodynamic delays on the order of about 2–4 s, it is possible to identify the activity associated with each successive trial reliably.

There are several advantages to event-related fMRI:

1. By detecting signals that are linked to individual trial events rather than to blocks, the observations can parallel other behavioral and evoked response potential studies that are also linked to individual events. Thus, the added value of precise temporal data from other integrated methods in combination with the high-resolution data of fMRI extends the range of questions that can be addressed.
2. An event-related approach is particularly useful when subject response is a factor, as in the case where it is necessary to separate trials in which there was a correct response from trials in which the response was not correct, or trials where the stimulus was novel from trials where the stimulus was repeated, or to isolate the acquisitions associated with bistable

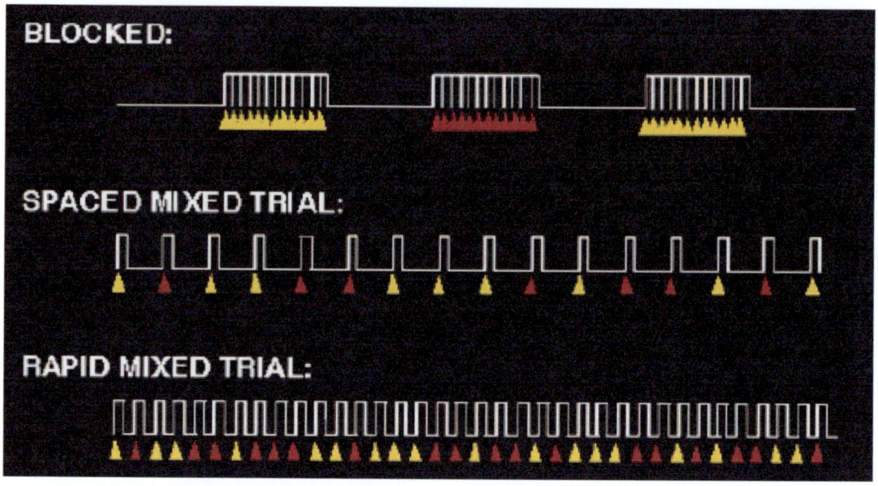

Fig. 13.23 Blocked versus event-related fMRI paradigms. Schematic diagrams illustrate the difference between two forms of imaging paradigms: blocked trials and event-related trials. Each schematic shows two trial types indicated by either *yellow or red arrows*. In blocked trial paradigms (labeled Blocked), the trial types are clustered together in succession so that the same trial type or condition occurs for an extended period of time. Event-related trials, by contrast, intermix different trial types either by spacing them widely apart to allow the hemodynamic response from one trial to decay before the next trial occurs (labeled Spaced Mixed Trial), or by presenting them rapidly (labeled Rapid Mixed Trial). Reprinted with permission from Dale AM, Buckner RL. Selective averaging of rapidly presented individual trials using fMRI. Hum Brain Mapp. 1997;5:329–40. Copyright © 1997 Wiley-Liss, Inc., a subsidiary of John Wiley & Sons, Inc

perspectives of ambiguous figures as reported by the subject during the experiment. Thus, the event-related approach allows trials to be categorized post hoc on the basis of the subject's behavior.

3. Some events cannot be presented in a blocked design, as in cases involving a surprise element or the occurrence of an oddball stimulus that is distinguished from the expected context. In those cases, an event-related approach is required.

The Oddball Task

Cortical mechanisms specialized for novelty oddball detection compare incoming information with relevant memories to register a novel event. Opitz et al. [95] reported the spatial and temporal properties of cortical mechanisms involved in the detection of novel tones by combining evoked response potential and fMRI measures. The evoked response potential methods lack precision with respect to the spatial source of the signal as detected by scalp electrodes because these sources must be inferred from 2D scalp topography and using dipole fitting algorithms. Temporal resolution of signals, however, is within milliseconds. By combining evoked response potential and fMRI, both temporal and spatial properties of the cortical responses corresponding to novelty can be investigated. Although registration of these separate data domains remains a challenge, results of the Opitz study relate specific evoked response potential responses to bilateral GTs and right prefrontal cortex, suggesting coordinated activity between areas previously associated with novelty using event-related fMRI techniques.

A similar evoked response potential and fMRI experiment by Kruggel et al. [96] employed a visual oddball task using illusory contours that deviated from the prevailing visual stimuli (no illusory contours). Results replicated previous fMRI findings, indicating the activation of extrastriate visual cortex in the appreciation of the illusory contours (perceived between the corner elements of Kanizsa squares) and the lack of this activation during viewing of stimuli in which the corner elements were rotated out of alignment. Additionally, the evoked response potential results confirmed a sequential activation of striate to extra striate visual cortex consistent with hierarchal models of visual processing. Thus, integration of approaches that optimize both spatial and temporal information relating to neural mechanisms and both perceptual and cognitive processes offers new directions and precision to probe the neural basis of mental events.

The Functional Neuroanatomy of Very High-Level Cognitive Processes

Guided by the Astonishing Hypothesis of Francis Crick [1], it is assumed that the biological components of even very high-level cognitive processes, such as decision making, moral judgments, altruism, and fairness, are observable. As in the neuroimaging of related cognitive processes, including language, attention, working memory, and executive control, an investigation of consciousness is also rigorously investigated.

Dehaene and Naccache [79] have developed one theoretical framework for the investigation of consciousness that consists of a global neuronal workspace. This framework postulates that "at any given time, many modular cerebral networks are active in parallel and process information in an unconscious manner." As information becomes conscious, however, the neural population that represents the information is mobilized by top–down attentional amplification into a state of coherent activity that involves many neurons distributed throughout the brain. The long-distance connectivity of these workspace neurons can, when they are active for a minimal duration, make the information available to a variety of processes, including perceptual categorization, long-term memorization, evaluation, and intentional action. According to this theoretical framework, the global availability of information throughout the workspace is what is subjectively experienced as a conscious state.

> "The fact that consciousness is a private, first-person phenomenon makes it more difficult to study than other cognitive phenomena that, although being equally private, also have characteristic behavioral signatures. Nonetheless, by combining cognitive and neurobiological methods, it is possible to approach consciousness, to describe its cognitive nature, its behavioral correlates, its possible evolutionary origin and functional role; last but not least, it is possible to investigate its neuroanatomical and neurophysiological underpinnings."
> Antonio R. Damasio, 1998 [97]

A major obstacle to applying neuroimaging techniques to the investigation of consciousness is the inability to establish a task that varies the state of consciousness; that is, consciousness is not started and stopped in synchrony with a particular task, as is assumed in many cognitive tasks. The global workspace hypothesis suggests a distributed neural system or workspace with long-distance connectivity that interconnects multiple specialized brain areas in a coordinated, although variable, manner [98]. This framework challenges current neuroimaging paradigms based on conventional experimental paradigms and views of functional specialization.

One approach to circumvent this obstacle is based on the specific hypothesis that conscious humans are engaged continuously during resting states in "adaptive cognitive processes that involve semantic knowledge retrieval, representation in awareness and directed manipulation of represented knowledge for organization, problem solving and planning." Thus, comparison of resting activation and task activations during a neuroimaging study might reveal neural processes associated with consciousness. Binder and colleagues [99] used fMRI to measure brain activity during rest and during several contrasting activation paradigms, including a perceptual task (tone monitoring) designed to interfere with ongoing thought processes and a semantic retrieval task (noun categorization) designed to engage ongoing thought processes similar to those hypothesized to occur during rest. Higher signal values were observed during the resting state than during the tone-monitoring task in a network of left hemisphere cortical regions. These areas were equally active during the semantic task.

This finding is consistent with the hypothesis that perceptual tasks interrupt specific ongoing processes during rest that are associated with many of the same brain areas engaged during semantic retrieval. Thus, neuroimaging observations suggest that ongoing processing during a conscious resting state involves an underlying neural substrate similar to that employed in cognitive tasks such as semantic processing.

Another paradigm that employs masked (too brief for cognitive awareness) presentations of emotional facial expressions has been found to modulate BOLD and PET-related hemodynamic responses originating in the amygdala [100, 101]. In these studies, the amygdala was involved in (1) nonconscious responses that reflected the emotional valence of stimuli and (2) was spatially differentiated depending upon level of awareness. Both findings confirm a neural substrate that is active and responsive without awareness.

Conclusion

The resting-state and masking paradigms, as well as other ongoing neuroimaging investigations of related aspects of consciousness, including perceptual awareness, awareness during varying levels of anesthesia, and awareness in patients in vegetative and MCSs, can be expected to contribute to an emerging understanding of the neural basis of consciousness and the neural basis for related events that occur without awareness. Imaging paradigms that are established to investigate the neural underpinnings of cognition also provide foundations for emerging investigations of the neural underpinnings of consciousness and bring neural science closer to the goal of understanding the biological underpinnings of the mind (see Table 13.2 for summaries of key brain mapping studies).

Table 13.2 Summary of key brain mapping studies

Title	Authors	Year	fMRI paradigm(s)	Summary
The JFK coma recovery scale revised: measurement characteristics and diagnostic utility	Giacino JT, Kalmar K, Whyte J	2004	Behavioral measures.	Defines the current behavioral paradigms to distinguish between minimally conscious and vegetative states.
fMRI reveals large-scale network activation in minimally conscious patients	Schiff ND, Rodriguez Moreno D, Kamal A, et al.	2005	Passive auditory stimulation using personalized narratives.	This is the first study to document that minimally conscious patients can engage neural circuitry associated with cognitive function.
Detecting awareness in the vegetative state	Owen AM, Coleman MR, Boly M, Davis MH, Laureys S, Pickard JD	2006	Passive stimulation and command following (motor and memory).	A case report that documents command following in a vegetative patient using fMRI documenting the need for neuralimaging as an assessment tool for awareness.
Clinical functional magnetic resonance imaging	Hart J, Rao SM, Nuwer M	2007	Block design for single patient assessments.	CPT codes for billing of MRI procedures that map active cortex engaged during specific tasks including language, sensory, motor, and perceptual functions.
A network approach to assess cognition in disorders of consciousness	Rodriguez Moreno D, Schiff ND, Giacino J, Kalmar K, Hirsch J	2010	Passive stimulation and command following (language).	Patients who are unresponsive may be able to communicate awareness, or emerging signs of awareness, using fMRI. The extent to which a canonical language network is engaged can be related to the bedside coma recovery scale.

Acknowledgments The first edition of this chapter was written in collaboration with Sarah Callahan, who was a psycholinguistic student in my laboratory. She not only researched and provided essential original sources, but also was a partner in the development of the ideas and conceptual organization. Without her critical contributions, this chapter would not have emerged in print. Recent editions were done with the assistance of Melissa Sy, a research assistant in my laboratory at Columbia University.

References

1. Crick F. The astonishing hypothesis: the scientific search for the soul. New York: Charles Scribner's Sons; 1994.
2. Dorland's Illustrated Medical Dictionary. 27th ed. Philadelphia, PA: W.B. Saunders Co. (Harcourt Brace Jovanovich Inc.); 1988.
3. The American Heritage Dictionary of the English Language. 4th ed. Boston, MA: Houghton Mifflin Co.; 2000.
4. Neisser U. Cognitive psychology. New York: Appleton; 1967.
5. Damasio H, Grabowski T, Frank R, Galaburda AM, Damasio AR. The return of Phineas Gage: clues about the brain from the skull of a famous patient. Science. 1994;264:1102–5.
6. Penfield W. The mystery of the mind. Princeton, NJ: Princeton University Press; 1975.
7. Roy, CS, Sherrington, CS. On the regulation of the blood supply of the brain. J. Physiol. 1890;11(1): 85–158.
8. Raichle ME, Martin WRW, Herscovitch P, Mintun MA, Markham J. Brain blood flow measured with intravenous H215O. II. Implementation and validation. J Nucl Med. 1983;24:790–8.
9. Fox PT, Raichle ME. Stimulus rate dependence of regional cerebral blood flow in human striate cortex demonstrated by positron emission tomography. J Neurophysiol. 1984;51:1109–20.
10. Peterson SE, Fox PT, Posner MI, Mintun M, Raichle ME. Postiron emission tomographic studies of the processing of single words. J Cogn Neurosci. 1989; 1(2):153–70.
11. Ogawa S, Lee T-M, Nayak AS, Glynn P. Oxygenation-sensitive contrast in magnetic resonance image of rodent brain at high magnetic fields. Magn Reson Med. 1990;14:68–78.
12. Gore JC. Principles and practice of functional MRI of the human brain. J Clin Invest. 2003;112:4–9.
13. George JS, Aine CJ, Mosher JC, Schmidt MD, et al. Mapping function in the human brain with magneto encephalography, anatomical magnetic resonance imaging, and functional magnetic resonance imaging. J Clin Neurophysiol. 1995;12:406–29.
14. Nimsky C, Ganslandt O, Kober H, Moller M, Ulmer S, Tomandl B, et al. Integration of functional magnetic resonance imaging supported by agnetoencephalography in functional neuronavigation. Neurosurgery. 1999;44(6):1249–55.
15. Stapleton SR, Kiriakopoulos E, Mikulis D, Drake LM, Hoffman HJ, Humphreys R, et al. Combined utility of functional MRI, cortical mapping, and frameless stereotaxy in the resection of lesions in eloquent areas of brain in children. Pediatr Neurosurg. 1997;26:68–82.
16. Atlas SW, Howard RS, Maldjian J, Alsop D, Detre JA, Listerud J, et al. Functional magnetic resonance imaging of regional brain activity in patients with intracerebral gliomas: findings and implications for clinical management. Neurosurgery. 1996;38(2): 329–38.
17. Latchaw RE, Xiaoping HU, Ugurbil K, Hall WA, Madison MT, Heros RC. Functional magnetic resonance imaging as a management tool for cerebral arteriovenous malformations. Neurosurgery. 1995; 37(4):619–25.
18. Lee CC, Jack Jr CR, Riederer SJ. Mapping of the central sulcus with functional MR: active versus passive activation tasks. Neuroradiology. 1998;19: 847–52.
19. Mueller WM, Yetkin FZ, Hammeke TA, Morris III GL, Swanson SJ, Reichert K, et al. Functional magnetic resonance imaging mapping of the motor cortex in patients with cerebral tumors. Neurosurgery. 1996;39(3):515–21.
20. Puce A, Constable T, Luby ML, Eng M, McCarthy G, Nobre AC, et al. Functional magnetic resonance imaging of sensory and motor cortex: comparison with electrophysiological localization. J Neurosurg. 1995;83:262–70.
21. Schulder M, Maldijian JA, Liu WC, Holodny AI, Kalnin AT, Mun IK, et al. Functional image-guided surgery of intracranial tumors located in or near the sensorimotor cortex. Neurosurgery. 1998;89:412–8.
22. Yousry TA, Schmid UD, Jassoy AG, Schmidt D, Eisener WE, Reulen HJ, et al. Topography of the cortical motor hand area: prospective study with functional MR imaging and direct motor mapping at surgery. Radiology. 1995;195:23–9.
23. Hart J, Rao SM, Nuwer M. Clinical functional magnetic resonance imaging. Cogn Behav Neurol. 2007;20(3):141–4.
24. Faro SH, Mukherji SK, Dolinskas CA, et al. ACR guidelines and standards committee ACR–ASNR practice guideline for the performance of functional magnetic resonance imaging of the brain (fMRI). 2007 (Resolution 3). http://www.acr.org/guidelines
25. Debus J, Essig M, Schad LR, Wenz F, Baudendistel K, Knopp MV, et al. Functional magnetic imaging in a stereotactic setup. Magn Reson Imaging. 1996; 14(9):1007–12.
26. Fried I, Nenov VI, Ojemann SG, Woods RP. Functional MR and PET imaging of rolandic and visual cortices for neurosurgical planning. J Neurosurg. 1995; 83:854–61.

27. Chapman PH, Buchbinder BR, Cosgrove GR, Jiang HJ. Functional magnetic resonance imaging for cortical mapping in pediatric neurosurgery. Pediatr Neurosurg. 1995;23:122–6.
28. Fandino J, Kollias S, Wieser G, Valavanis A, Yonekawa Y. Intraoperative validation of functional magnetic resonance imaging and cortical reorganization patters in patients with brain tumors involving the primary motor cortex. J Neurosurg. 1999;91: 238–50.
29. Pujol J, Conesa G, Deus J, Lopez-Obarrio L, Isamat F, Capdevila A. Clinical application of functional magnetic resonance imaging in presurgical identification of the central sulcus. J Neurosurg. 1998;88: 863–9.
30. Herholz K, Reulen H, von Stockhausen H, Thiel A, Ilmberger J, Kessler J, et al. Preoperative activation and intraoperative stimulation of language-related areas in patients with glioma. Neurosurgery. 1997;41(6):1253–62.
31. Hinke RM, Hu X, Stillman AE, Kim SG, Merkle H, Salmi R, et al. Functional magnetic resonance imaging of Broca's area during internal speech. Neuroreport. 1993;4:675–8.
32. Binder JR, Frost JA, Hammeke TA, Bellgowan PSF, Rao SM, Cox RW. Conceptual processing during the conscious resting state: a functional MRI study. J Cogn Neurosci. 1999;11(1):80–93.
33. Kollias SS, Landau K, Khan N, Golay X, Bernays R, Yonekawa Y, et al. Functional evaluation using magnetic resonance imaging of the visual cortex in patients with retrochiasmatic lesions. Neurosurgery. 1998;89:780–90.
34. Tootell RB, Reppas JB, Kwong KK, Malach R, Born RT, Brady TJ, et al. Functional analysis of human MT and related visual cortical areas using magnetic resonance imaging. J Neurosci. 1995;15: 3215–30.
35. Hirsch J, Rodriguez-Moreno D, Kim KHS. Interconnected large-scale systems for three fundamental cognitive tasks revealed by functional MRI. J Cogn Neurosci. 2001;13(3):1–16.
36. Hirsch J, Ruge MI, Kim KHS, Correa DD, Victor JD, Relkin NR, et al. An integrated fMRI procedure for preoperative mapping of cortical areas associated with tactile, motor, language, and visual functions. Neurosurgery. 2000;47(3):711–22.
37. Kaplan EF, Goodglass H, Weintraub S. The Boston naming test. 2nd ed. Philadelphia, PA: Lea & Febiger; 1983.
38. Cedzich C, Taniguchi M, Schafer S, Schramm J. Somatosensory evoked potential phase reversal and direct motor cortex stimulation during surgery in and around the central region. Neurosurgery. 1996; 38:962–70.
39. Puce A. Comparative assessment of sensorimotor function using functional magnetic resonance imaging and electrophysiological methods. J Clin Neurophysiol. 1995;12:450–9.
40. Wada J, Rasmussen T. Intracarotid injection of sodium amytal for the lateralization of cerebral speech dominance. J Neurosurg. 1960;17:266–82.
41. Ruge MI, Victor JD, Hosain S, Correa DD, Relkin NR, Tabar V, et al. Concordance between functional magnetic resonance imaging and intraoperative language mapping. J Stereotact Funct Neurosurg. 1999; 72:95–102.
42. Kim KHS, Relkin NR, Lee K-M, Hirsch J. Distinct cortical areas associated with native and second languages. Nature. 1997;388:171–4.
43. Ojemann G, Ojemann J, Lettich E, Berger M. Cortical language localization in left, dominant hemisphere. J Neurosurg. 1989;71:316–26.
44. Hirsch J. Functional neuroimaging during altered states of consciousness: how and what do we measure? In the boundaries of consciousness: neurobiology and neuropathology (Steven Laureys, editor) progress in brain research, vol. 150. Amsterdam: Elsevier; 2005. p. 25–44.
45. Souweidane MM, Kim KHS, McDowall R, Ruge MI, Lis E, Krol G, et al. Brain mapping in sedated infants and young children with passive-functional magnetic resonance imaging. Pediatr Neurosurg. 1999;30:86–91.
46. Schiff ND, Rodriguez Moreno D, Kamal A, et al. fMRI reveals large-scale network activation in minimally conscious patients. Neurology. 2005;64: 514–23.
47. Giacino JT, Ashwal S, Childs N, et al. The minimally conscious state: definition and diagnostic criteria. Neurology. 2002;58:349–53.
48. Owen AM, Coleman MR, Boly M, Davis MH, Laureys S, Pickard JD. Detecting awareness in the vegetative state. Science. 2006;313:1402.
49. Fins JJ. Constructing an ethical stereotaxy for severe brain injury: balancing risks, benefits and access. Nat Rev Neurosci. 2003;4:323–7.
50. Rodriguez Moreno D, Schiff ND, Giacino J, Kalmar K, Hirsch J. A network approach to assessing cognition in disorders of consciousness. Neurology. 2010;75(21):1871–8.
51. The Multi-Society Task Force on PVS. Medical aspects of the persistent vegetative state (1). N Engl J Med. 1994;330:1499–508.
52. Haig AJ, Katz RT, Sahgal V. Mortality and complications of the locked-in syndrome. Arch Phys Med Rehabil. 1987;68:24–7.
53. Childs NL, Mercer WN, Childs HW. Accuracy of diagnosis of persistent vegetative state. Neurology. 1993;43:1465–7.
54. Andrews K, Murphy L, Munday R, Littlewood C. Misdiagnosis of the vegetative state: retrospective study in a rehabilitation unit. BMJ. 1996;313:13–6.
55. Boly M, Coleman MR, Davis MH, Hampshire A, et al. When thoughts become actions: an fMRI paradigm to study volitional brain activity in non-communicative brain injured patients. Neuroimage. 2007;36:979–92.

56. Monti MM, Vanhaudenhuyse A, Coleman MR, Boly M, et al. Willful modulation of brain activity in disorders of consciousness. N Engl J Med. Epub 3 Feb 2010.
57. Bekinschtein TA, Coleman MR, Niklison III J, Pickard JD, Manes FF. Can electromyography objectively detect voluntary movement in disorders of consciousness? J Neurol Neurosurg Psychiatry. 2008;79(7):826–8.
58. Schnakers C, Perrin F, Schabus M, et al. Voluntary brain processing in disorders of consciousness. Neurology. 2008;71(20):1614–20.
59. Monti MM, Coleman MR, Owen AM. Executive functions in the absence of behavior: functional imaging of the minimally conscious state. Prog Brain Res. 2009;177:249–60.
60. Giacino JT, Kalmar K, Whyte J. The JFK coma recovery scale revised: measurement characteristics and diagnostic utility. Arch Phys Med Rehabil. 2004;85:2020–9.
61. Price CJ, Devlin JT, Moore CJ, Morton C, Laird AR. Meta-analyses of object naming: effect of baseline. Hum Brain Mapp. 2005;25:70–82.
62. Liljestrom M, Takianinen A, Parviainen T, et al. Perceiving and naming actions and objects. Neuroimage. 2008;41(3):1132–41.
63. Friederici AD, Ruschemeyer SA, Hahne A, Fiebach CJ. The role of left inferior frontal and superior temporal cortex in sentence comprehension: localizing syntactic and semantic processes. Cereb Cortex. 2003;13:170–7.
64. Grossberg S. How does the cerebral cortex work? Development, learning, attention, and 3-D vision by laminar circuits of visual cortex. Behav Cogn Neurosci Rev. 2003;2(1):47–76.
65. Greenham SL, Stelmack RM, Campbell KB. Effects of attention and semantic relation on event-related potentials in a picture-word naming task. Biol Psychol. 2000;50:79–104.
66. Humphreys GW, Riddoch MJ, Price J. Top-down processes in object identification: evidence from experimental psychology, neuropsychology and functional neuroanatomy. Philos Trans R Soc Lond B. 1997;352:1275–82.
67. Booth JR, Burman DD, Meyer JR, Gitelman DR, Parrish TB, Mesulam MM. Functional anatomy of intra- and cross-modal lexical tasks. Neuroimage. 2002;16:7–22.
68. Okada K, Hickik G. Left posterior auditory-related cortices participate both in speech perception and speech production: neural overlap revealed by fMRI. Brain Lang. 2006;98:112–7.
69. Indefrey P, Levelt WJ. The spatial and temporal signatures of word production components. Cognition. 2004;92:101–44.
70. Burton MW. Understanding the role of the prefrontal cortex in phonological processing. Clin Linguist Phon. 2009;23(3):180–95.
71. Damasio H, Tranel D, Grabowski T, Adolphs R, Damasio A. Neural systems behind word and concept retrieval. Cognition. 2004;92:179–229.
72. Kan IP, Thompson-Schill SL. Effect of name agreement on prefrontal activity during overt and covert picture naming. Cogn Affect Behav Neurosci. 2004;4(1):43–57.
73. Blank SC, Scott SK, Murphy K, Warburton E, Wise RJ. Speech production: Wernicke, Broca and beyond. Brain. 2002;125(8):1829–38.
74. Coleman MR, Rodd JM, Davis MH, et al. Do vegetative patients retain aspects of language comprehension? Evidence from fMRI. Brain. 2007;130:2494–507.
75. DeLeon J, Gottesman RF, Kleinman JT, et al. Neural regions essential for distinct cognitive processes underlying picture naming. Brain. 2007;130:1408–22.
76. Passigngham RE. The frontal lobes and voluntary action. Oxford: Oxford University Press; 1995.
77. Basho S, Palmer ED, Rubio MA, Wulfeck B, Muller RA. Effects of generation mode in fMRI adaptation of semantic fluency: pace production and overt speech. Neuropsychologia. 2007;45(8):1697–706.
78. Boly M, Coleman MR, Davis MH, et al. When thoughts become action: an fMRI paradigm to study volitional brain activity in non-communicative brain injured patients. Neuroimage. 2007;36:979–92.
79. Dehaene S, Naccache L. Towards a cognitive neuroscience of consciousness: basic evidence and a work-space framework. Cognition. 2001;79:1–37.
80. Posner MJ, Raichle ME. Images of mind. New York: Scientific American Library; 1994. p. 16.
81. Friston KJ, Holmes AP, Price CJ, Büchel C, Worsley KJ. Multisubject fMRI studies and conjunction analysis. Neuroimage. 1999;10:385–96.
82. Desmond JE, Glover GH. Estimating sample size in functional MRI (fMRI) neuroimaging studies: statistical power analyses. J Neurosci Methods. 2002;118: 115–28.
83. Talairach J, Tournoux P. Co-planar stereotaxic atlas of the human brain. New York: Thieme; 1988.
84. Friston KJ et al. Statistical parametric maps in functional imaging: a general linear approach. Hum Brain Mapp. 1995;2:189.
85. Mishkin M, Ungerleider LG. Contribution of striate inputs to the visuospatial functions of parieto-preoccipital cortex in monkeys. Behav Brain Res. 1982;6(1):57–77.
86. Buchel C, Friston KJ. Modulation of connectivity in visual pathways by attention: Cortical interactions evaluated with structural equation modeling and fMRI. Cereb Cortex. 1997;7(8):768–78.
87. Mesulam M-M. From sensation to cognition. Brain. 1998;121:1013–52.
88. Kim Y-H, Gitelman DR, Nobre AC, Parrish TB, LaBar KS, Mesulam M-M. The large-scale neural network for spatial attention displays multifunctional overlap but differential asymmetry. Neuroimage. 1999;9:269–77.
89. Smith EE, Jonides J. Working memory: a view from neuroimaging. Cogn Psychol. 1997;33:5–42.
90. Leung H-C, Skudlarski P, Gatenby JC, Peterson BS, Gore JC. An event-related functional MRI study of the Stroop color word interference task. Cereb Cortex. 2000;10:552–60.

91. D'Esposito M, Detre JA, Alsop DC, Shin RK, Atlas S, Grossman M. The neural basis of the central executive system of working memory. Nature. 1995;378:279–81.
92. Adcock RA, Constable RT, Gore JC, Goldman-Rakic PS. Functional neuroanatomy of executive processes involved in dual-task performance. Proc Natl Acad Sci U S A. 2000;97(7):3567–72.
93. Casey BJ, Trainor RJ, Orendi JL, Schubert AB, Nystrom LE, Giedd JN, et al. A developmental functional MRI study of prefrontal activation during performance of a Go-No-Go task. J Cogn Neurosci. 1997;9(6):835–47.
94. Rosen BR, Buckner RL, Dale AM. Event-related functional MRI: past, present, and future. Proc Natl Acad Sci U S A. 1998;95:773–80.
95. Opitz B, Mecklinger A, Friederici AD, von Cramon DY. The functional neuroanatomy of novelty processing: integrating ERP and fMRI results. Cereb Cortex. 1999;9(4):379–91.
96. Kruggel F, Herrmann CS, Wiggins CJ, von Cramon DY. Hemodynamic and electroencephalographic responses to illusory figures: recording of the evoked potentials during functional MRI. Neuroimage. 2001;14:1327–36.
97. Damasio AR. Investigating the biology of consciousness. Philos Trans R Soc Lond B Biol Sci. 1998;353:1879–82.
98. Dehaene S, Kerszberg M, Changeux JP. A neuronal model of a global workspace in effortful cognitive tasks. Proc Natl Acad Sci U S A. 1998;95(24):14529–34.
99. Binder JR, Price CJ. Functional imaging of language. In: Cabeza R, Kingstone A, editors. Handbook of functional neuroimaging of cognition. Cambridge, MA: MIT Press; 2001. p. 187–251.
100. Whalen PJ, Rauch SL, Etcoff NL, McInerney SC, Lee MB, Jenike MA. Masked presentations of emotional facial expressions modulate amygdala activity without explicit knowledge. J Cogn Neurosci. 1998;18(1):411–8.
101. Morris JS, Ohman A, Dolan RJ. Conscious and unconscious emotional learning in the human amygdala. Nature. 1998;393:467–70.

14 Pediatric Applications of fMRI

Nolan R. Altman and Byron Bernal

Introduction

Functional magnetic resonance imaging (fMRI) has become an important pillar in the evaluation of children's brain function. The technique has made it possible to map almost any brain function, from hearing to language, from memory to learning, and from normal executive functions to some other unique human functions not previously studied with imaging procedures.

One measure of the interest that functional magnetic resonance imaging (fMRI) has produced in the pediatric clinical and research community is the number of articles published. A search on PubMed utilizing the word "fMRI" limited to ages between 0 and 18 years, resulted in 1,584 articles (accessed September 24, 2009). Part of the success of fMRI is due to the fact that, for the first time, there is a functional study with the definition, beauty, versatility, and easiness already achieved by anatomic exams.

Although fMRI has been utilized in the study of normal subjects and an extensive number of pediatric abnormal conditions, its most useful application to date is in preoperatory cortical mapping. Functional MRI has become a cost-effective study [1] that can replace more invasive procedures in children, such as the intracarotid amobarbital test (Wada test). As acknowledgment of these facts, fMRI has received CPT billing codes to be utilized within these parameters.

Numerous pediatric conditions have been studied with fMRI including autism, dyslexia, speech delay, attention deficit hyperactive disorder (ADHD), schizophrenia, stuttering, and many other neurologic and psychiatric conditions. These disorders have challenged medicine since no chemical, genetic, or anatomic markers have been described regardless of the severity of the problem. Functional MRI findings have been described in all of them, but their impact is still a matter of research.

Most recently, important advances have appeared in the development of fMRI techniques based on the detection of slow spontaneous brain activations by means of independent component analysis (ICA). Similarly, a great many publications are now exploring the role of fMRI in pharmacology. Functional MRI shows brain changes associated with neuropharmaceuticals, vasoactive drugs, and toxins, among others. Thus, the field of fMRI is continuously expanding, making visible a constellation of previously mysterious mental processes, revealing their nature, and opening avenues for understanding, cure, or control.

N.R. Altman, MD
Department of Radiology, Miami Children's Hospital, 3100 SW 62nd Avenue, Miami, FL 33155, USA
e-mail: nolan.altman@mch.com

B. Bernal, MD, CCTI (✉)
Department of Radiology, Miami Children's Hospital, 10529 SW 103rd Avenue, Miami, FL 33176, USA
e-mail: byron.bernal@mch.com

S.H. Faro and F.B. Mohamed (eds.), *Functional BOLD MRI: Principles and Applications*,
DOI 10.1007/978-1-4939-1995-6_14,

Uniqueness of fMRI in Children

Functional MRI in children has some important differences when compared with adults. These differences are not limited to anatomy and include vascularity, metabolism, comprehension, and educational level – variables that change with age. Children undergo many changes in the first few years of life. The brain increases in volume in the first 5 years to 95% of the adult size [2–4]. Myelination is almost completed by the end of the second year [2, 3]. The brain synapse number peaks around 8 months of age and is followed by selective synaptic regression in which sprouts are pruned until the age of 16 [4]. Neurons suffer drastic apoptosis from birth. By the ripe old age of 19 months, neurons are reduced to less than one-third of that with which we are born [5]. These dynamic structural changes result in higher metabolism in the younger brain, which peaks at 3–4 years, and reaches adult levels by the end of the second decade [6]. This is the reason that blood volume is higher and the vascular response is greater in children. Children activate 60–400% more voxels than adults using standard fMR post-processing techniques [7–9]. This difference is due to the increased metabolism, resulting in better signal-to-noise ratio of the activated voxels [7, 10, 11]. The increase of activation takes place without changes of onset time, rise, and peak amplitude of the hemodynamic response [9]. Children, however, are similar to adults in the variance of the MR signal [10]. These neurobiological facts influence brain activation in children. For example, language tasks in children have more intensity, extent, and bilateral activation [8].

The aforementioned functional changes may partially explain age-related differences. Structural changes may also play an important role. Intra-subject comparisons across time reveal these maturational changes. Myelination of the human brain proceeds from inferior to superior, posterior to anterior, central loci to lobar poles, and proximal to distal pathways [12]. The frontal lobes mature in the last stages of myelination (after 5 years), which may explain the finding of hypofrontality in children and adolescents [13]. The right frontal lobe seems to mature before the left [13, 14]. Fronto-striatal areas show a progressive increased activation related to age [18]. Synapse accretion and pruning proceeds at different rates from region to region. It peaks at 8 months in the visual cortex, and at 4 years in auditory and frontal cortices [15]. Although pruning peaks at these ages, adult patterns may be acquired at earlier ages. For example, the auditory cortex has an adult pattern in the infant. The frontal lobes will acquire an adult pattern by the third or fourth month of life [15]. In contrast, the visual cortex shows a different pattern of activation in children between 7 weeks and 5–7 years that has been claimed to be related to maturational milestones. Cognitive and fine motor functions that develop over long periods of time, such as language, are also associated with an increase of activation over time [16, 17]. In infants and small children, sedation is often required and the medications may have a direct effect on cerebral blood flow (CBF) and cortical metabolism.

fMR Technical Challenges in Children

Study Design

Study design in children is critical. The blood-oxygen-level-dependent (BOLD) response of target areas (areas of activation) can be affected by endogenous factors such as the subject's education and skillfulness. In general, activation is lower when the task is too easy or too difficult [18, 19]. The degree of difficulty may be manifested by an increase in regional blood flow as seen in motor [20], sensory [21], and cognitive tasks. However, too difficult task may produce poor activation [22].

Increased difficulty and practice alter the magnitude of signal and pattern of activation. For example, a subject who activates the left inferior frontal gyrus in a verb generation task may show a change of the activation toward the anterior aspect of the insula, if the same task is practiced [23]. This variability of brain activation has implications on study design, application, and interpretation when performing fMR in children. The more complicated the study, the more likely it will obtain spurious activation. Therefore, in clinical cases, it is best to keep the tasks as simple as possible, since children may get confused when complexities are added to the paradigms. Attempts to control too many variables may subtract out activation in brain regions critical for a target function [24].

There may be a trade-off between varying the task to match the patient performance and keeping the task simple. For clinical purposes, we prefer to keep the task constant and look at areas of activation as related to time, development, anatomic abnormality, or reorganization. Degree of task difficulty must be considered with different ages or, more importantly, ability. We have taken a practical approach using two or three paradigms with different degrees of difficulty depending on the child's ability. Passive paradigms allow the most consistency and are included when feasible.

Sedation

Many fMRI studies in the pediatric population need to be conducted under sedation, particularly in children younger than 6 years or otherwise affected by cognitive or behavioral conditions. Sedation has been utilized in many pediatric fMR studies with success (e.g., [25–34]). Pentobarbital, propofol, and chloral hydrate are the most commonly utilized sedatives. The typical paradigms are presentation of light, sounds, human voice, rubbing of the skin, or passive movement of the hand or foot. Light is delivered through the closed eyes most frequently by goggles directly placed over the eyelids. Sounds vary from tones to mother's voice.

Sedation of Choice

There is a paucity of studies comparing the outcome of fMRI exams with different drugs, in children. Propofol and midazolan have been compared in a study of auditory fMRI in 14 children between 3 and 7 years. Brain activation with propofol was localized in the primary auditory area resembling the activation seen in adults. Midazolam produced more scattered and delayed activation [35].

The authors have empirically tested several sedative schemes utilizing different drugs alone and combined. The best results were obtained with propofol alone, followed by amobarbital. Chloral hydrate is also a good choice in small children.

The dosage of medication seems to be critical to obtain good activation. Sevofluorane, if necessary, may be used at three different levels (0.5, 0.75, and 1.0) of minimum alveolar concentration (MAC) of the gas. The best activation is seen at 0.75 MAC [36]. Based on our experience, doses of propofol above 120 μg/kg per minute usually result in failure of brain activation. We have had our best results with single drug protocols and performing the fMR exam at the start of the imaging session when less sedation is on board.

Motion

Patient motion is a significant challenge in the fMR examination of children. The imaging usually takes several minutes per task and the post-processing methods used require minimal motion for accurate results. Small children have significant difficulty remaining still in the MR magnet [37]. A recent study conducted in 323 healthy children between 5 and 18 years found that boys have a tendency to move more than girls, particularly when comparing the younger groups [38]. Remaining motionless is a demanding pro-active function, requiring working memory to store the command, frontal inhibition, and the ability to monitor small body movements. The bore of the magnet is a confining space and may be frightening to children. To determine if the child will successfully cooperate for the exam may be best done by the child undergoing a simple test before the exam is performed. This is accomplished by the use of a simulator, which consists of a mockup of the magnet using an MR table, head coil, magnet housing, and any hardware specific to the task such as earphones, video screen, or finger buttons. Taped scanner noise can also be added.

Electronic devices that track head movement can be coupled to video-projectors setting up a feedback in which head movement beyond a given threshold turns off the video display. The child learns how to control head movement as the tolerance for the feedback is narrowed [39]. Use of these techniques may improve the likelihood of successful exams, although its use is limited [25].

Immobilization aids may be used such as bite bars, external cushions, and tape. The bite bar is uncomfortable and not well tolerated by children. These techniques are not widely used as success is limited.

We pack the head holder with cushions surrounding the head and support with cloth medical tape between the borders of the head holder and forehead. This results in a somatosensory feedback of the forehead skin producing easy detection by the child of head motion. Neonates and sleep-deprived children may be examined sleeping; however, this technique is limited. Sedation may be required with concomitant use of passive paradigms.

Based on our pediatric radiology experience of more than 1,000 fMR paradigms applied in children, we feel that children younger than 5 years usually cannot perform the exam without sedation. Children between 5 and 7 years of age with appropriate training may be successful in completing a short study of 5–10 min and those between 7 and 9 years may tolerate a longer exam. Children older than 9 years usually will cooperate to allow four to six paradigms plus the anatomical sequences required for coregistration. Girls tend to stay still longer than boys. As with all exams there are some children who despite careful instructions and preparation can still not perform the study, particularly if they are mentally challenged.

A recent study has investigated the success rate of fMRI in normal children and patients with three different common conditions: epilepsy, ADHD, and autism spectrum disorder. A study was judged as successful if it yields interpretable results and can be pooled with other studies. Successful fMRI exams were obtained in 87% of normal controls, 80% of epilepsy patients, and 77% of ADHD patients off methylphenidate and in 81% of ADHD patients on methylphenidate [40]. This failure rate should be taken into consideration when research and clinical studies are planned. Research subjects between 4 and 6 years may require 20–40% additional participants and studies with 10- to 18-year-olds may require 10–15% additional participants [40].

Motion Correction (Image Post-processing)

Sedated cases, and those patients with motion less than 20% of the inplane voxel diameter, do not require motion correction. For an FOV of 240 mm and a matrix size of 64 × 64, the transverse inplane diameter is 3.75 mm. Hence, motion less than 0.75 mm does not need to be corrected. Post-processing motion correction tools and surface algorithms may correct for patient motion not task correlated. When there is movement associated with the task (Fig. 14.1), the correction is very difficult to perform and most of these algorithms fail. Inclusion of motion parameters in the statistical post-processing often results in a decrease of the overall level of activation, although an increase may be observed when motion is random not correlated with the task [37]. Moreover, spurious activation has been demonstrated when motion correction is applied to motionless phantoms [41]. One should be cautious when rejecting or accepting abnormal brain activation that varies after motion correction.

Spatial Normalization

The most popular atlases for spatial normalization of fMRI studies are based on adult brains. These are the Talairach and Tournoux [42] atlas, and the Montreal Neurological Institute (MNI) template based in 152 young adult brains. However, it has been shown that brains of children from age 7 may be compared with the adult brain utilizing the same atlases [43]. Due to the intrinsic variability of the maturing brain, pediatric fMRI research would require numerous sets of templates to perform group comparisons with other child groups. Change in shape and distortion due to pathology may prevent good coregistration.

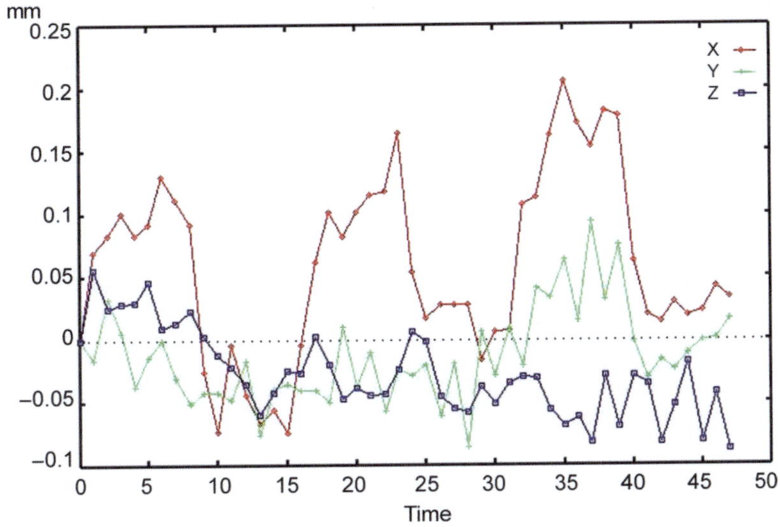

Fig. 14.1 Phasic movement of the head related to a motor task. Graph of patient head motion in the three orthogonal axes: *x* (*red*), *y* (*green*), and *z* (*blue*). *Y*-axis scale is in millimeter, *X*-axis: time-points (TP). Patient is performing a tapping task with the right hand. The paradigm consists of 48 TP (TP 0 is the first), starting in OFF and switching every 8 time-points. The graph shows weak phasic movement, less than 0.2 mm in the *x*-axis (*red*). Changes are seen at 8, 16, 24, 32, and 40 time-points, correlating the paradigm frequency. This produces spurious activation and ring-shaped artifacts on the fMR images, which are difficult to correct with post-processing

This may not be as critical in research as in the clinical arena. The authors always perform manual coregistration in clinical cases. Comparison may be performed on the basis of anatomical landmarks; however, many investigators prefer to use stereotactic three-dimensional templates.

Statistical Analysis

Although the standard methods of statistical analysis utilized in adult fMR are also useful in children, some peculiar facts should be considered in children. The most popular statistical methods applied to the data analysis are correlation coefficient and general linear model. Correlation coefficient analysis looks at variation of the time-course intensities in relation to a predefined function. The general linear model technique looks at the variation of the BOLD signal at each voxel compared with the baseline and usually includes the modeling of the hemodynamic response function (HRF).

Little is currently known of the differences of the hemodynamic response in sick infants and children when compared with adults. Longer peak times of the hemodynamic response have been found in children and infants with epilepsy [44]. The shape of the BOLD time course is also different in children [45], but the practical effects of this difference in fMRI processing is not clear. In addition, variability of subject performance is a significant challenge that is difficult to incorporate into these models.

In group analysis, comparison of activation of different age groups is difficult. The number of voxels activated over a given threshold of different age groups is not a reliable measure of response magnitude [46]. A more valid approach may be magnitude measurements of actual change in signal intensity as percent change from baseline. Another alternative is to have a primary cortex activation as an internal reference (e.g., the occipital activation elicited by flashing lights) compared with the activation of cognitive tasks. At least, with this baseline, the neuroscientist may have an insight of how "good an activator" the subject is.

Thresholding

In keeping with thresholding, there is a trade-off between sensitivity and specificity, that is, between false positives and false negatives. Typically, thresholds are set high in research to avoid false-positive activation. There are no established guidelines on thresholds for post-processing analysis except what is regarded by statisticians as appropriate. However, significant areas of true activation may go undetected [47], an aspect of crucial significance in clinical settings. For practical and clinical purposes, when no activation is seen utilizing the standard higher thresholds, the authors advise to check for activation at softer thresholds and to perform a reexamination of the raw Z-score map looking for activation that cannot be explained as random. Activation seen in canonical regions, as dictated by clinical experience, is then evaluated on a case-by-case basis. This technique has been utilized by different authors investigating language function in adults and children with epilepsy (e.g., [48–50]). Studies may show significant areas of activation not demonstrated by conventional statistical methods. These areas can be mined by a practical empirical approach. This requires three criteria: clusterized activation, cannonical activation, and Gaussian distribution. Clusters are typical of neighbor-correlated activation prompting for cortical functional modules (i.e., Brodmann's areas). Activations located in canonical areas, which are areas matching activation maps established in normal children, may be considered not spurious particularly if they are expected to be activated by the applied paradigm. Gaussian distribution of signal intensities stands for an organized array of the intensities with higher signal values of activation located toward the center of the cluster, a feature not expected to happen at random. These cases are not frequent, but they will require a nonstandard low thresholding to produce a clean map of activation (Fig. 14.2).

Applications

Currently, the primary application of pediatric fMRI is in surgical planning. Within this application, an important number of clinical fMRI studies are used to lateralize and localize critical areas of language and motor function related to the dominant hand. Other pediatric applications have also been increasing. A great many publications on fMRI in children has looked at pediatric conditions including autism, epilepsy, ADHD, dyslexia, and others. We will review and address the key publications on these topics.

Cortical Functional Mapping for Surgical Planning

The localization of language and the motor area of the dominant hand are of key importance for neurosurgical planning. Auditory, visual, memory, and other cognitive mapping are currently performed in different clinical and research settings, although without the practical importance of the localization of eloquent and motor cortex in presurgical cases.

Language Mapping

Language Mapping of Noncooperative Patients

Early stages of language have been assessed with functional MRI using passive paradigms in sedated infants and children or under natural sleep. Left lateralization of language areas may be obtained by listening to the mother's voice [29]. Infants as early as 3 months have been found to activate similar areas activated by canonical language tasks in adults. They lateralize to the left superior temporal and angular gyri [51]. The activation remains similar regardless if the patient is awake or sedated (same authors). Similar results were reported in a patient [52] and have been also observed by us in a large number of clinical cases who ultimately underwent epilepsy surgery. We have described utilizing a paradigm that allows

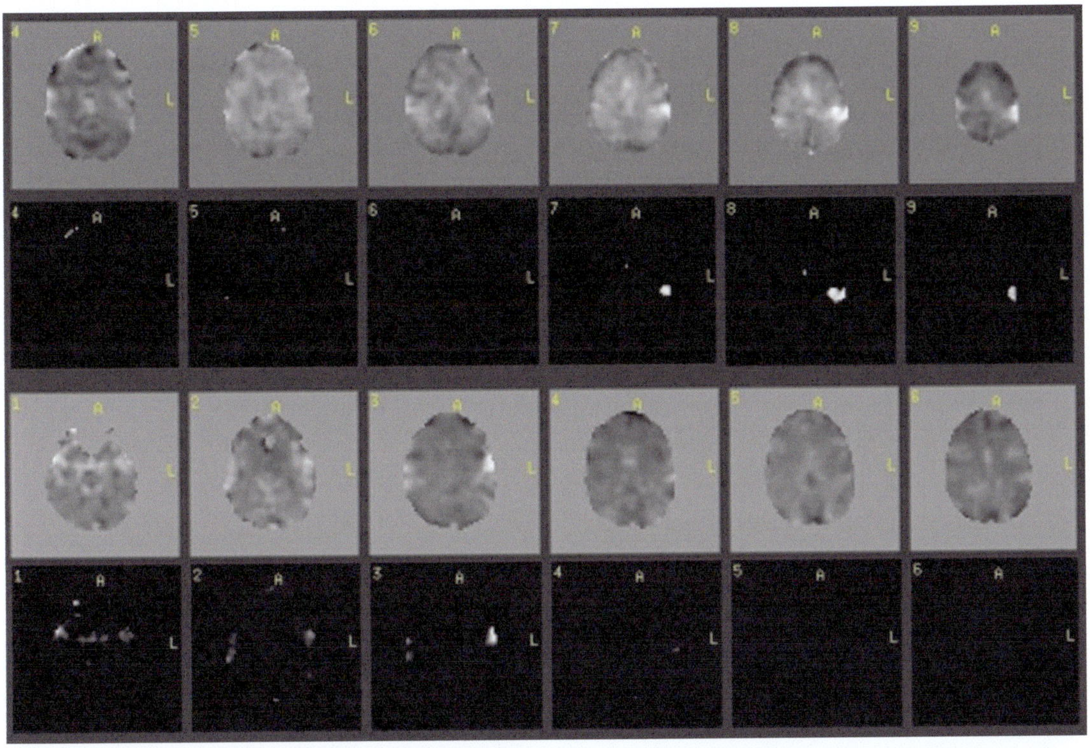

Fig. 14.2 Activation detection using raw Z-score maps for motor and listening to a story tasks. *Gray images* are the composite EPI images with raw Z-score statistical activation far below maximum Z value of 2.33 ($p < 0.05$), which would not survive any "acceptable" statistical analysis. Well-defined clusters of activation from tasks, *upper rows* are for motor tasks, *lower rows* for listening to a story, are seen in the expected areas without any other areas demonstrating activation. The *black rows* demonstrate only positive values, which can be superimposed on the anatomic images

the mother to speak with intonation, which involves prosody, a well-known right hemisphere function, lateralization appearing more toward the right hemisphere in sedated children less than 3 years (Fig. 14.3a). After 4 years, children tend to lateralize to the left temporal lobe (Fig. 14.3b). Strikingly, this passive receptive paradigm may also activate Broca's area in a few cases.

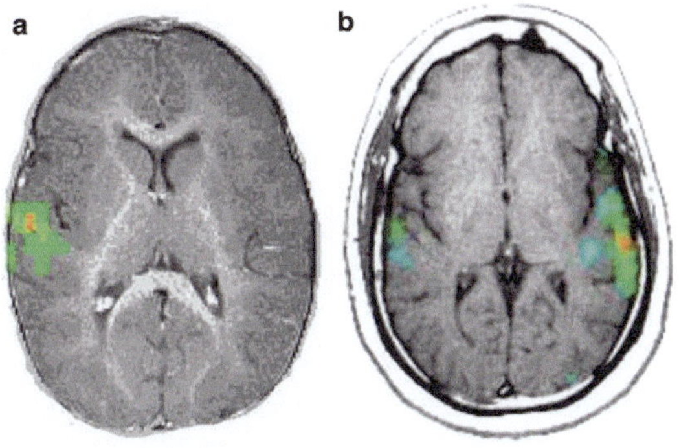

Fig. 14.3 Functional MRI of changing language lateralization with aging of the child. (**a**) Sedated 2-year-old infant with right lateralization of language. (**b**) Nonsedated 11-year-old with left lateralization of language

Language Mapping of Cooperative Children

Mapping of expressive and receptive language in cooperative awake preschoolers and older children has been performed by many authors. Language is best mapped with the use of multiple task paradigms to evaluate expressive and receptive functions.

Expressive tasks demonstrate inferior and middle frontal gyrus activation. Tasks consist of: phonological fluency, thinking of words that start with specified letters [49, 53, 54]; semantic fluency, thinking of specific groups of items such

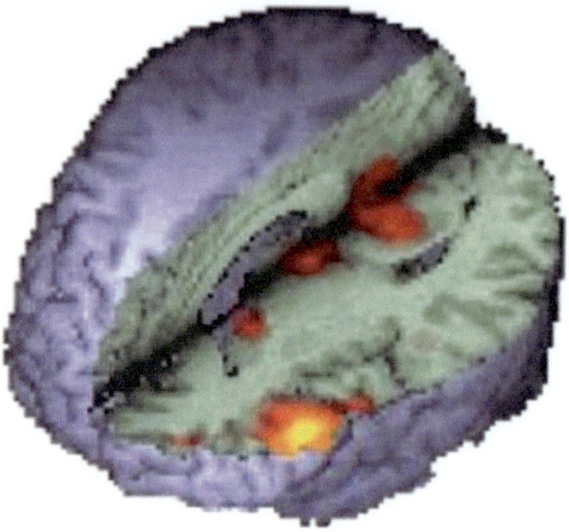

Fig. 14.4 Three-dimensional (3-D) MR with coregistration of language mapped by semantic fluency task. The *yellow* cluster corresponds to the highest intensities located in Broca's area (left inferior frontal gyrus). Activation of left caudate nucleus, thalamus, and occipital cortex are also seen. The 3-D representation can aid the neurosurgeon in the localization of deeper areas related to cognitive task

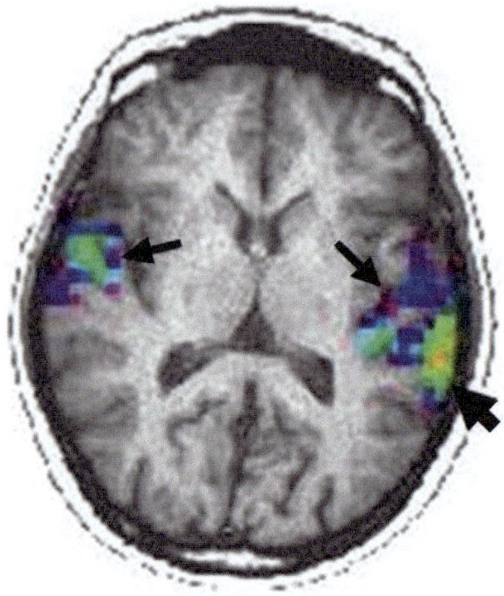

Fig. 14.5 Typical brain activation with a passive listening-to-a-story task. Axial view at the level of the Heschl's gyrus. The left hemisphere appears on the right side (radiological convention). Color-coded fMRI signal intensities vary from *yellow* (*highest*) to *blue* (*lowest*). In addition to the activation of the primary auditory areas (Heschl's gyrus, *bilateral short arrows*), there is another cluster with higher intensity located in the left hemisphere (*short arrow*). This cluster corresponds to the secondary auditory cortex or Wernicke's area

as clothes, animals, toys, etc. (Fig. 14.4) [49, 54]; silent spelling [59, 60]; verb generation [8, 55–59]; and reading [8, 56, 60].

Receptive language paradigms include listening to a story [61–63], auditory comprehension [55, 64, 65], naming objects presented visually [66, 67], and reading. Areas of activation include the posterior third of the superior and middle temporal gyrus, the supramarginal gyrus, the fusiform gyrus, and angular gyrus. Expressive paradigms may produce activation of receptive areas and vice versa. The verb generation task most frequently activates Broca's and Wernicke's areas.

Listening to a story is an important task in the evaluation of language in children. This task is so familiar to children that it is readily accepted, particularly when the story is narrated by a parent, even in the unusual and uncomfortable environment of the MR scanner. The passive nature of the task lends itself to the evaluation of the sedated or sleeping child. Initially, early investigators [68] did not find lateralization on this passive task comparing number of voxels activated on each side. However, more recent studies indicate lateralization to the left supramarginal and angular gyri in both sexes [63, 69] with listening to a story. Primary and secondary auditory activation with lateralization in Wernicke's region has been consistently found with fMR and has proven to be a good indicator of receptive language representation (Fig. 14.5).

Combining two or more tasks has been proposed to increase the certainty of language lateralization with fMRI. A study of Gaillard and colleges [70] evaluated nine normal right-handed children, 7–13 years, utilizing two tasks. These consisted of reading Aesop's Fables and a "Read Response Naming" task that consists of the subject naming an object described by a sentence; i.e., "*What is a purring house pet?*" These tasks predominantly activated the left middle temporal gyrus, left middle frontal gyrus, and inferior occipital cortex including fusiform and lingual gyrus. Reading the fable activates the left inferior frontal gyrus as well and produces more activation of the left superior temporal gyrus. Strikingly, the primary auditory area was also left dominant in all subjects when low thresholds were utilized [70]. Passive listening tasks do not differ significantly from other listening tasks involving active responses from the subjects [63]. They also seem to produce similar activation during awake or natural sleep conditions [52].

Despite the experience accumulated with language mapping in adults and children, it is important to stress that in those cases where results are divergent or activation is highly atypical or absent it would seem prudent to repeat the study to confirm the results. Alternatively, these patients may be assessed with intraoperative cortical electrical stimulation or Wada tests, if there are important surgical planning issues.

Anatomical or functional lesions may produce language variability in cortical localization in adults [71, 72], but atypical language localization is more frequent in epilepsy patients with early established cerebral lesions [73]. Essential centers of speech and motor function may be altered in patients with tumors, vascular malformations, cortical dysgenesis, and epilepsy [74–76]. These functions may be transferred to the contralateral hemisphere, ipsilateral neighboring areas, or scattered in one or both hemispheres. Appropriate tailoring of elective surgery deems that the neurosurgeon should have knowledge of at least the lateralization of language.

fMRI Versus Wada or Electrocortical Stimulation in Children

Formerly language lateralization was determined either by the Wada test or intracortical stimulation. The Wada test is performed assessing the cognitive deficit produced by the injection of amobarbital into an internal carotid artery. Electrocortical stimulation requires the placement of electrodes on the cerebral cortex. This is done either as an initial separate procedure with surgical placement of subdural grids and electrodes or during the definitive surgical resection.

The effect of the amobarbital injection of the Wada test is usually too frightening for small children and even adolescents, since they have to experience a temporary hemiplegia and aphasia. The procedure is invasive, expensive, and nonlocalizing. Equivocal results may occur, if the child is oversedated and cannot respond, and some patients may show speech arrest after injection of the nondominant hemisphere [77]. The cortico-electrical stimulation requires the child to be awake during surgery, if language is to be determined. In addition, only one hemisphere can be evaluated. These limitations suggest that Wada or cortical stimulation may not be the gold standard for language localization in children.

Functional MRI can noninvasively determine the lateralization and localization of language centers. The procedure is safe, cost-effective [1], and replicable. Several studies conducted in adults and children have compared language mapping with fMRI to Wada tests and electrocortical mapping (Table 14.1). Most of these studies have been done utilizing a quantitative approach based on lateralization indexes of both tests. The vast majority of the studies describe a positive correlation ranging between 0.88 and 0.96 (e.g., [48, 61, 78–82]). However, a few conflicting results have been reported in patients with left temporal epilepsy (<0.75) [83]. Anecdotic cases in which fMRI and Wada test have been compared with electrocortical stimulation have shown fMRI to be more reliable [84]. Similar failures of the Wada test have been demonstrated for motor hemispheric localization, verified with motor- and sensory-evoked potentials [85]. Electrocortical stimulation has also been compared with fMRI in adults, confirming the fMRI findings with rare exceptions [86, 87]. Possible discrepancies may be due to failure of the cortico-electrical stimulation to account for interhemispheric dissociation of receptive and expressive areas.

BOLD responses for language tasks are transitory and severely diminished in the postictal temporal lobe (Fig. 14.6) [88]. The timing of the exam in seizure patients is critical. The exam should be performed preferably before the patient is taken off antiseizure medication or at least 24 h following a seizure. Main contributory studies in pediatric fMRI and language have been summarized in Table 14.1.

Motor Mapping

In general, there is no differences in the brain activation elicited with motor tasks when comparing adults and children [89] (Table 14.2).

Table 14.1 Selected fMRI research of language mapping

Authors	Subjects	fMRI paradigm	Main findings
Hertz-Pannier et al. (1997)	Right-handed children with partial epilepsy	Word generation task (phonological or semantic fluency tasks)	Complete concordance with intra-arterial amobarbital test or intraoperative electrocortical stimulation
Gaillard et al. (2000)	Normal children and adults	Covert word generation task	Children and adults activate similar areas. Children activate 60% greater extent than adults
Lehericy et al. (2000)	Patients with temporal lobe epilepsy	Listening to a story Semantic fluency and sentence repetition	Good concordance with intracarotid amobarbital test findings, better for the frontal lobe
Gaillard et al. (2001)	Right-handed children	Listening to a story, read response naming	Typical auditory/language activation observed with these paradigms. Increased yield combining paradigms
Holland et al. (2001)	Children between 7 and 18 years	Verb generation	The degree of left lateralization increased with age
Dehaene-Lambert et al. (2002)	Non-sedated 2- to 3-month-old infants	Highly intonated female voice reading a history	Left lateralized superior temporal and angular activation
Jayakar et al. (2002)	Right-handed child	Listening to a story, fluency tasks	BOLD responses for language tasks are transitory and severely diminished in the postictal temporal lobe
Ahmad et al. (2003)	Right-handed children	Listening to a story	Auditory language processing is localized and lateralized by age 5

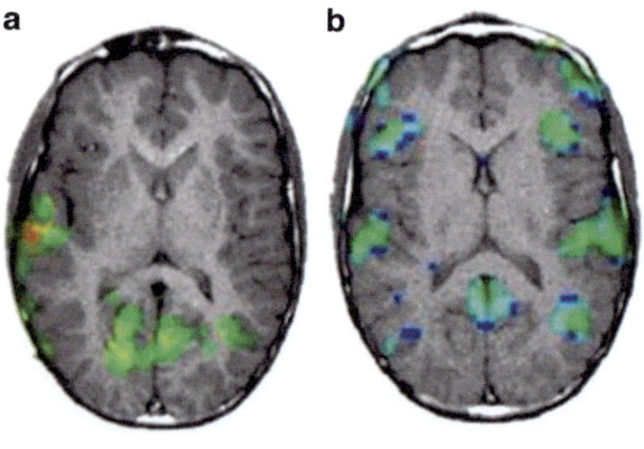

Fig. 14.6 Postictal versus interictal fMR. Functional MRI of a right-handed patient performing a listening to a story task postictal (**a**) and interictal (**b**). The postictal image, obtained a few hours following the seizure, shows right temporal lobe dominance. The same procedure, performed seizure free for 24 h several days later (interictal), revealed bilateral frontal and temporal lobe activation with left-sided dominance

Evaluation of motor and sensory function in the sedated infant and child has met with limited success. In the study of Soweidane and coworkers [29], sensorimotor areas were activated using passive tactile stimulus by rubbing the hands. However, this finding has not been replicated. We have obtained sensorimotor activation in up to 50% of sedated cases with passive repetitive maximal extension of the hand and fingers. Caution must be maintained to not provoke motion artifact. Activation of the central cortex has been obtained in adults with electrical stimulation of the median nerve by several authors (e.g., [73, 90, 91]). This technique holds promise for mapping the sensorimotor areas of children under sedation.

Motor mapping in the young sedated infant is possible in some cases utilizing a modified version of the "nonnutritive high-amplitude sucking procedure." This procedure is originally performed by presenting a verbal stimulus (e.g., the syllable/pa/) to an infant with a pacifier in its mouth. This results in a high frequency of strong sucking. Repeated presentation of the stimulus results in a gradual decrease in the intensity of sucking. When such habituation occurs, a new speech stimulus is presented to reinitiate the

Table 14.2 Selected fMRI research of motor and sensory mapping

Authors	Subjects	fMRI paradigm	Main findings
Souweidane et al. (1999)	Sedated infants and children	Rubbing the hands	Sensory-motor activation
Hirsch et al. (2000)	Adolescents and adults	Rubbing the palm and fingers	Central sulcus identified in 97% of cases
Hartnick et al. (2001)	Children and adults	Swallowing	Bilateral activation of pre- and postcentral gyrus, insula, inferior frontal gyrus, and superior temporal gyrus
Vandermeeren et al. (2002)	A child with schizencephaly	Tapping fingers	Paretic hand showed ipsilateral activation
Kang et al. (2003)	Children vs. adults	Pressing buttons in response to a visual stimulus	No differences in the brain activation elicited with motor tasks when comparing adults and children

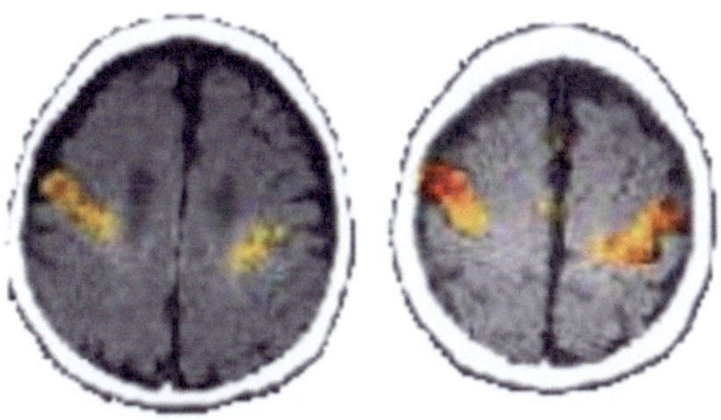

Fig. 14.7 Motor activation of the oral facial cortex associated with sucking reflex in a sedated 2-month-old. There is bilateral activation of the precentral gyri in the oral-facial region. This is related with the habituation-dishabituation of high-amplitude sucking in response to linguistic stimuli

sucking. This paradigm has shown that newborns and infants are able to perform phonemic discrimination [92] and extract differences between allophonic words such as *nitrate* and *night rate* [93]. The task with fMRI consists of placing the child in the magnet with a pacifier and delivering mothers voice through headphones during ON epochs to elicit the sucking response. During the OFF epoch her voice is halted. Motor activation can be obtained using this paradigm in a sedated infant (Fig. 14.7). The areas activated are bilateral, located on the homunculus caudal to the hand area representing the mouth and tongue region.

Motor Mapping of Cooperative Patients

The vast majority of the motor mapping in cooperative children has been focused, given its importance, on the hand. Two tasks are standard: finger tapping (e.g., [94–97]) or squeezing a foam pad (e.g., [16, 98]). Other tasks that may be used consist of flexing and extending the fingers (hand clenching) repetitively [54, 99, 100]. Typical activation is obtained in the contralateral areas of the precentral gyrus in the "hand knob" (Fig. 14.8). Additional regions may also be activated such as the bilateral supplemental motor areas (SMA), ipsilateral cerebellum, and basal ganglia. There usually is sensory cortex activation due to propioceptive and tactile input. Activation is usually isolated to the contralateral hemisphere but frequently some activation is seen in the ipsilateral hemisphere. The non-dominant hand is more frequently associated with bilateral activation (Fig. 14.8). Finger tapping tasks promote more activation than hand squeezing tasks. Young children and hemiparetic patients, however, appear to better understand and perform the squeezing task. Adult patients with hemiparesis have decreased activation in primary motor areas with significant increase of activation in secondary motor areas including contralateral or ipsilateral SMA and basal ganglia [101].

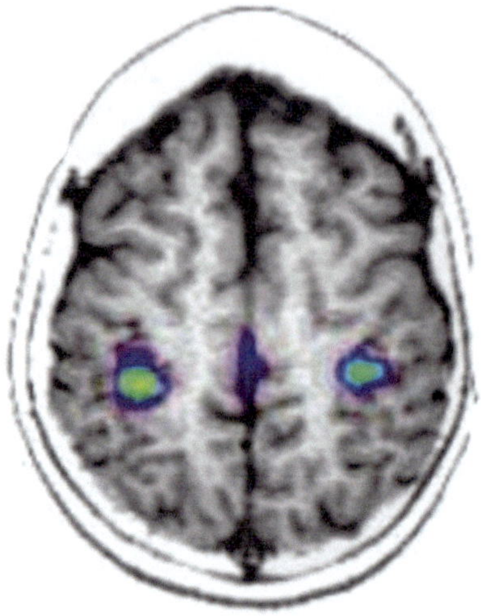

Fig. 14.8 Finger-tapping task activation map of the left hand in a right-handed patient. There is bilateral motor cortex activation with slight right-sided dominance

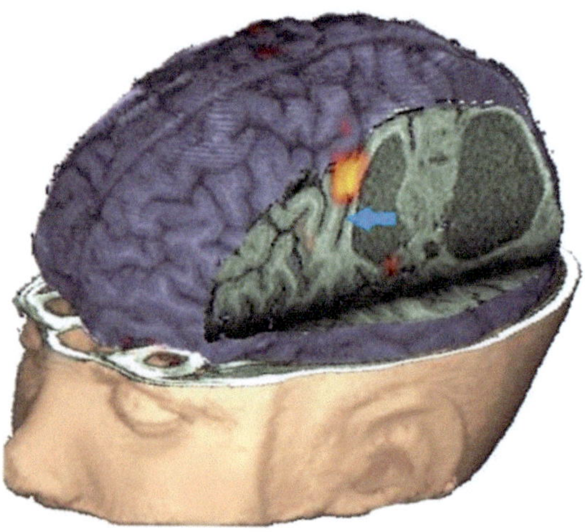

Fig. 14.9 Right finger-tapping task in patient with large tumor. A 3-D fMR that demonstrates a large left parietal ganglioglioma. The left motor cortex is located by the central sulcus (*blue arrow*). This is displaced rostrally by the tumor. Small activation is also seen of the right motor cortex

Patients of different ages, including adolescents, with tumors or dysgenesis may show displacement of the motor cortex (Fig. 14.9). In addition to displacement, activation may be reduced, scattered or transferred to the contralateral hemisphere [101–103]. Children with congenital malformations such as schizencephaly performing a finger-tapping task demonstrate increased, dispersed, and wider areas of activation in the unaffected hemisphere [104]. Extreme examples of reorganization are encountered in severe cases of hemimegalencephaly where both hands may show activation in the normal hemisphere [104, 105].

Motor mapping of the face may be obtained by pronouncing the syllables bah/dah/gah alternatively throughout the ON periods. The combination of these syllables alternates lips, tongue, and pharynx movements. The subject should be instructed to do it as softly as possible, as if he/she were whispering it. Motor mapping of the foot may be elicited by flexing and extending the toes. A cushion placed below the knees may help to prevent concomitant motion of the head. Swallowing studies in children have demonstrated activation in pre- and postcentral gyrus, superior motor cortex, insula, inferior frontal cortex, Heschl's gyrus, lenticular nucleus, and nucleus ambiguous [106]. The significance of these findings may aid in the development of novel rehabilitative strategies in compromised patients.

The concordance of motor fMRI and intraoperative electrophysiology utilizing somatosensory evoked potential and direct cortical stimulation is excellent [107–109].

Sensory Mapping

Pure sensory fMRI studies are scanty in adults and children. Most of the motor and sensory paradigms activate both brain areas since they are functionally intermingled. Activation has been obtained using tactile stimulation of the hand by rubbing the patient's palm and fingers with a mildly abrasive surface [94]. Cortical activation has been described on fMR exams by brief innocuous electrical stimuli applied to the fingers in adults [110]. This technique shows promise to use as a passive technique in children who are sedated or comatose. No studies in children have been reported using this method.

Visual Mapping

Noncooperative Patients

Sedated children show a negative BOLD response in the rostral aspect of the calcarine fissure when stimulated with flashing lights [27, 33]. This response is not well understood. The effect of the sedative medication may or may not play a marginal role, since negative BOLD response has been reported not only in sedated children but also on exams performed during natural sleep. BOLD response immaturity also has been implicated, but some adults present this type of activation [111]. Measurements of blood flow done in children performing the visual task with near-infrared spectroscopy shows that deoxyhemoglobin and oxyhemoglobin increase with photic stimulation [112], suggesting local blood flow increase. Opposing results, however, were reported in a PET study that demonstrated regional cerebral-blood-flow decrease in the visual area in control subjects under sleep [111]. The same subjects have had a BOLD signal decrease during visual stimulation in the anterior visual cortex. Similar results were also obtained utilizing arterial spin labeling (ASL) MRI. ASL has demonstrated that photic stimulation of sedated children (or under natural sleep) reduces the rCBF of the occipital cortex [113]. Taken together, these studies suggest that the lack of signal is due to a true deactivation of the occipital cortex, a sort of active inhibition, and not from overextraction of oxygen due to immature uncoupling of the stimulus-BOLD response, or as the consequence of redundant synaptic connections in the immature visual system activating a larger neuronal population as it was suggested previously [114]. The nonconcordant results of the study with near-infrared spectroscopy probably could be explained by the limitation to detect changes occurring in the deep sulci as the activation is seen in the rostral aspect of the visual cortex.

It is still unclear the role of other complex mechanisms involved in the visual function. There are retinal ganglion cells and neurons of the striatal system that respond to "black" or absence of light. These cells outnumber the white-reacting cells. They are more sensitive and have a fairly more rostral distribution in area V1, at least in monkeys [115]. Photic stimulation with diffuse red light selectively suppresses the magnocellular visual system in monkeys [116] and humans [117]. This system is tightly related to the "black" system mentioned previously. Light stimulation in sedated or sleeping patients is given through the closed eyes. The blood of the eyelids produces a red-shift in the color delivered to the retina and diffuses the light.

Other factors seem to have been overlooked. Astrocytes can regulate vascular tone by modifying the cytosolic calcium. Thus, they play a role in the functional hyperemia related to neuronal activation [118]. All of these factors may play a significant role in the activation/deactivation pattern observed in children with visual fMRI under sedation. However, as of yet, there is not a model strong enough to explain all the findings. Indeed, no statistical differences in the fMRI responses of sedated and non-sedated infants were documented by Martin et al. [28]; sedated adults usually show positive BOLD responses during visual stimulation [27]; and Altman and Bernal [33] demonstrated both positive and negative BOLD responses in the visual cortex in sedated children.

Functional dominance of the visual cortex may be derived from fMR exams. Contralateral eye dominance is observed in adults and children manifested as greater activation of the anterior striate cortex where the calcarine sulcus merges with the parieto-occipital sulcus [119]. This finding may provide a test in infants and children who cannot cooperate to perform formal visual field testing. Clinical evaluation of visual fields in infants and children is difficult and limited. Formal testing is not usually done. Functional MR evaluation of the visual cortex in premature infants is underway. One study conducted in 28 sedated 18-month-old infants with and without periventricular leukomalacia (PVL) revealed no correlation between functional activation and the presence of the white matter abnormality [120]. Strikingly, those infants with higher amounts of PVL tended to have larger regions of activation.

Amblyopic eyes show reduced calcarine activation compared with the contralateral normal

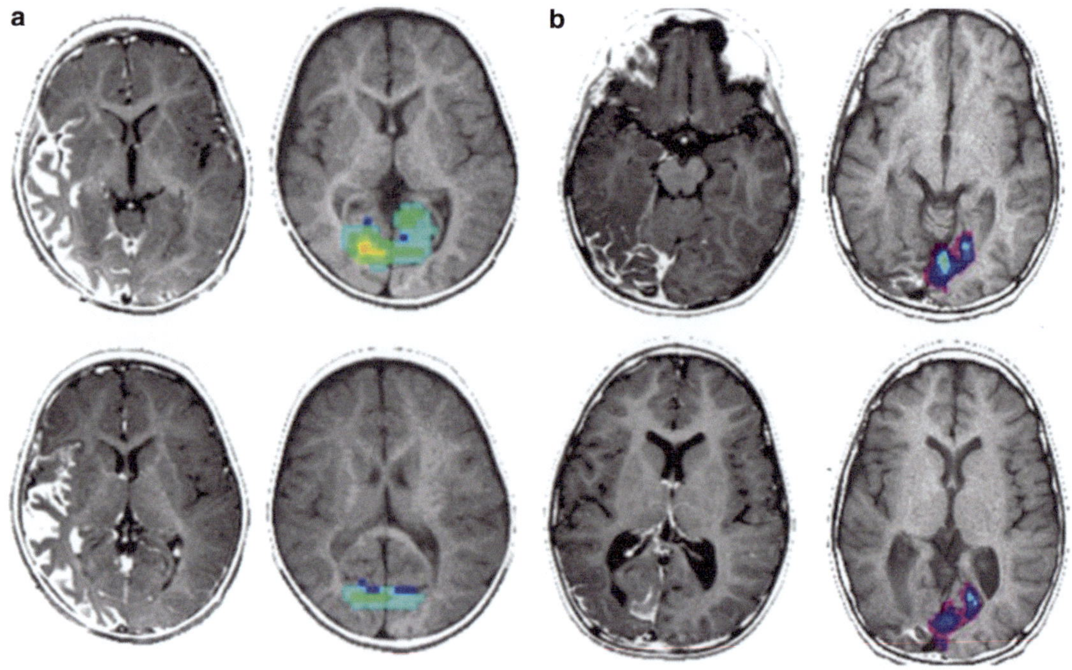

Fig. 14.10 Visual fMRI in Sturge-Weber patient. (**a**) Sedated 6-month child with large malformation and fMR that shows symmetrical activation of the visual cortex. (**b**) Sleeping 12-year-old child with small malformation that shows absent activation of the involved right hemisphere

eye [121]. Differentiation between anisometric and strabismic amblyopic eyes have been described [122]. Functional MRI also has been shown to be useful in objectively documenting residual visual function in children with severe visual loss [123]. Unilateral damage of the optic radiations produces strong asymmetrical activation [124]. We have used fMRI to identify visual cortex functionality in patients with Sturge-Weber syndrome prior to hemispherectomy [125]. The activation does not appear related to the size of the vascular malformation. An fMR performed with sedation on a 6-month-old Sturge-Weber patient with a large vascular lesion shows bilateral symmetrical activation of the anterior visual cortex (Fig. 14.10a). An additional Sturge-Weber patient with a much smaller vascular lesion, who was scanned sleeping, shows absent activation of the involved hemisphere (Fig. 14.10b). The lack of activation appears due to dysfunction of the cortex and not due to the vascular malformation. The most relevant studies on visual mapping in children have been summarized in Table 14.3.

Auditory Mapping

Non-cooperative Patients

Primary auditory function is crucial to the normal development of language [126–128]. Mapping of the primary auditory areas have been performed utilizing passive auditory paradigms in sedated children [29, 33]. Although negative BOLD responses have been found with auditory stimulation in non-sedated newborns [128], older children under sedation show normal positive BOLD activation in 70% of cases in the auditory temporal lobes. Children older than 18 months of age may show frontal lobe activation as well (Fig. 14.11) [33]. In some cases, the temporal activation encompasses the secondary auditory cortex extending backwards to the angular gyrus or the inferior parietal lobule, in an asymmetrical manner. This asymmetrical extension toward secondary auditory areas in preverbal infants is remarkable, although, possibly explained by the fact that cognition-development appears based on a biological hard-wire preprogramming of the newborn [129]. We have found lateralization

Table 14.3 Selected fMRI research of visual mapping

Authors	Subjects	fMRI paradigm	Main findings
Born et al. (1999)	Infants and children under natural sleep	Flashing lights	Negative BOLD response in the occipital cortex
Born et al. (2000)	Sedated infants and young children, with posterior brain lesions	Stroboscopic lights	Unilateral damage of the optic radiations is associated with strong asymmetrical activation
Altman and Bernal (2001)	Children and infants under sedation	Flashing lights	Negative BOLD response in the rostral aspect of the calcarine fissure
Sie et al. (2001)	Infants with periventricular leukomalacia	Flashing lights	No correlation between functional activation and the presence of periventricular leukomalacia lesions
Born et al. (2002)	Sedated children	Flashing lights Arterial spin-labeling MRI	Decreased cerebral blood flow in primary visual cortex
Bernal and Altman (2004)	Children with Sturge-Weber syndrome	Flashing lights	Visual activation is not related to the size of the vascular malformation

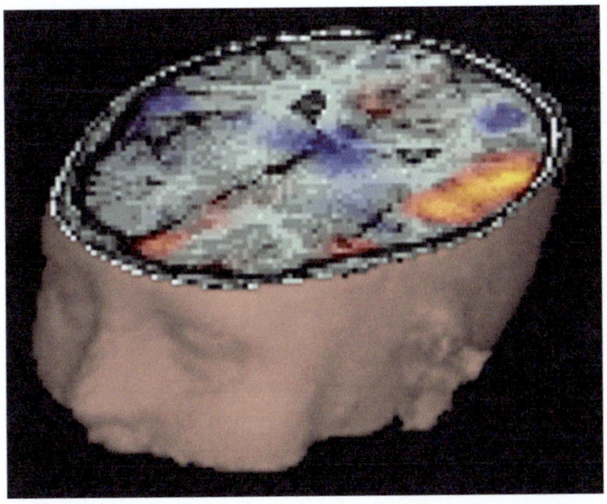

Fig. 14.11 Auditory fMRI under sedation, with 3-D rendering. Axial cut at the level of the superior temporal gyrus. Mesial frontal activation of the left hemisphere is seen along with language areas. *Blue bubbles* correspond to areas of deactivation

trends supporting this assumption in the vast majority of the studies using sedation.

FMR may provide an important tool for assessing language development and organization in infants and children. This has important implications for early diagnosis, intervention, and treatment of children with language delays. The medical delay in diagnosis is often directly related to the degree of language delay in these children who benefit most with the treatment of these disorders. Human hearing has been shown to begin at 27 weeks of gestation [130]. There are studies showing auditory activation in the fetal human brain [131–134]. In term neonates, auditory activation is obtained in 70% of cases utilizing a frequency-modulated pure tone centered at 1.3 kHz at a rate of 7 Hz [128].

Functional MRI may be utilized as a prognostic indicator for the outcome of cochlear implantation in infants. In a recent study, fMRI was utilized to assess residual and post-cochlear implantation function in the primary auditory cortex in sedated hearing-impaired toddlers. The improvement in hearing threshold after cochlear implantation correlated strongly with the amount of activation in the auditory cortex detected before cochlear implantation [135]. The most relevant studies of pediatric auditory fMRI have been summarized in Table 14.4.

Memory Mapping

The majority of fMRI studies of memory are related to working memory (WM) (Table 14.5). As in adults, children exhibit similar hemispheric asymmetry in activation, greater on the right for spatial WM and on the left for verbal WM [136]. Nelson and coworkers [137] have shown that

Table 14.4 Selected fMRI research of auditory mapping

Authors	Subjects	fMRI paradigm	Main findings
Hykin et al. (1999)	Fetuses	Mother speech	Activation of temporal lobes
Souweidane et al. (1999)	Sedated children	Mother or father's voice	Multiple areas of activation including primary and secondary auditory areas
Altman and Bernal (2001)	Sedated children	Mother's voice	Primary auditory cortex, predominantly in the left hemisphere in 70% of cases Some with activation in the secondary auditory area
Anderson et al. (2001)	Non-sedated neonates	Pure tone of 1.300 Hz	Signal decrease in temporal regions
Patel et al. (2007)	Awake and sedated hearing impaired children	Random sequence of tones	Hearing improvement after cochlear implantation correlated strongly with activation in the auditory area as detected by pre-op fMRI

Table 14.5 Selected fMRI research of memory

Authors	Subjects	fMRI paradigm	Main findings
Casey et al. (1995)	Pre-pubertal children	Nonspatial working memory	Activation similar to previously described in adults – inferior and middle frontal gyri (L > R)
Nelson et al. (2000)	Children	*N*-back visual-spatial working memory task	Dorsal prefrontal, posterior parietal and anterior cingulate cortex activation (as in adults)
Jokeit et al. (2001)	Children, adolescents, and adults	Spatial memory-based navigational task	90% of patients with temporal lobe epilepsy show dominant mesial temporal activation contralateral to the seizure focus
O'Hare et al. (2008)	Children, adolescents, and adults	Verbal working memory task with three load levels	Children recruit only left ventral prefrontal cortex in response to increasing load, while adolescents and adults also enlist the frontal, parietal, and cerebellar regions
Geier et al. (2009)	Children, adolescents, and adults	Visual spatial working memory	Children and adolescents have more extensive distributed activation than adults
Libertus et al. (2009)	Children and adults	Domain-specific working memory tasks (digits, letters, and faces)	Adults, but not children, show category-specific activation. Face activates the fusiform gyrus with no developmental differences. Letter-based working memory task may predict children's spelling performance
Thomason et al. (2009)	Children and adults	Verbal and spatial working memory	Children and adults exhibit similar task-specific asymmetry – greater on the right for spatial and on the left for verbal working memory

spatial working memory tasks applied in children between 8 and 11 years elicit fMR activation in several cortical areas, including the dorsal aspects of the prefrontal cortex and in the posterior parietal and anterior cingulate gyrus. Similar results were found previously by Casey et al. in 1995 [10], utilizing a nonspatial task. They also found an increase of signal intensity in children ages 9–11 in the bilateral inferior and middle frontal gyri with dominance on the left. It has been described that brain activation of children and adolescents performing a visual spatial working memory task is more extensively distributed when compared with adults [138].

Adults, but not children, have shown category-specific activation related to working memory tasks based on digits (intraparietal sulcus) or letters (left occipitotemporal areas), while working memory tasks based on faces activate the fusiform gyrus with no developmental differences [139]. The same authors found that brain activity in letter-responsive areas predicts children's spelling performance.

On working memory tasks, children recruit only left ventral prefrontal cortex in response to increasing load, while adolescents and adults also enlist the frontal, parietal, and cerebellar regions [140]. Similar results are reported in another study, where children failed to exhibit the same degree of increasing activation across working memory loads when compared with adults who showed this change in multiple frontal and parietal cortical regions [136].

Functional MRI evaluation of long-term memory has potential clinical applications in the work-up of temporal lobe epilepsy. Although a long-term memory paradigm has not been presented yet, there are some paradigms tested in adults capable to activate the same structures that are felt to be involved in this process, namely the mesial temporal lobes. Differences of activation in the mesial aspect of the temporal lobes elicited by mental navigation and visuo-discriminatory tasks [141] give clues of long-term memory lateralization. Asymmetry of lateralization of the parahippocampal activation in navigational/discriminatory tasks correlates with the opposite hemisphere temporal lobe seizure onset in 90% of adult and child patients with symptomatic temporal lobe epilepsy [142]. These types of tasks have been tried in our service with good results (Fig. 14.12).

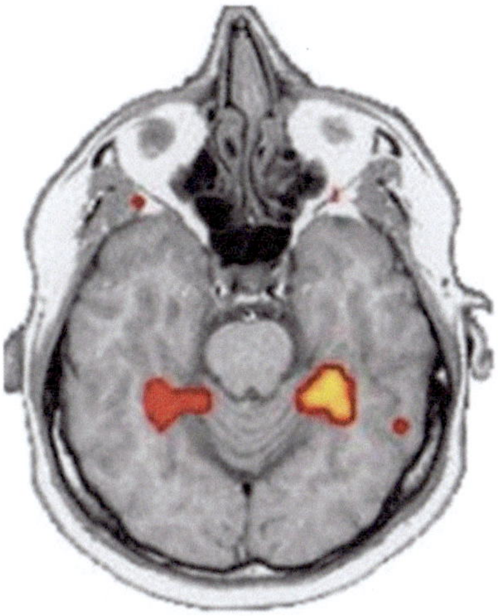

Fig. 14.12 Functional MRI of the memory circuitry. Axial cut at the level of the parahippocampus. The subject was performing a navigational task. Along with visual activation (data not shown), there was activation of the parahippocampal gyri with clear left hemisphere dominance. In this example, a better outcome for memory would be expected for a right-sided temporal resection

Complex Cognitive Functions

Complex cognitive functions including attention, inhibition, theory of mind, and face recognition also have been investigated with fMRI, but mostly in young adults. Studies limited to children are still scanty (Table 14.6). Spatial selective attention and response inhibition tasks show some differences between adults and children. Children show greater activation than adults in the anterior cingulate and thalamus in the selective attention task. Children also show greater activation than adults in the middle and posterior cingulate, medial frontal gyrus, medial aspects of bilateral superior frontal gyrus, thalamus, hippocampo-amygdaloid region, and the caudate nucleus on the left in response inhibition tasks [143].

Children show reduced brain activation in the right frontal-mesial regions during alerting, and in the right temporo-parietal junction during

Table 14.6 Selected fMRI research on complex cognitive functional mapping

Authors	Subjects	fMRI paradigm	Main findings
Booth et al. (2003)	Children and adults	Go-no-go task. Visual attention (searching a target shape)	Children show greater activation than adults in subcortical and striatal cortical areas
Konrad et al. (2005)	Children and adults	Attention nonverbal task (detecting an arrow direction amidst flanker arrows)	Children show reduced brain activation in the right frontal-mesial regions during alerting, and in the right temporo-parietal junction during reorienting of attention, when compared with adults
Lawrence et al. (2009)	Preterm-born adults and normal adults	Go-no-go task	Reduced activation of inhibitory-control areas in preterm group

reorienting of attention, when compared with adults [144]. In contrast, children show more brain activation in the superior frontal gyrus during reorienting and the superior temporal gyrus during executive control of attention [144]. These findings suggest a transition from functional immature systems to adult networks in attention.

Children and adolescents born before 33 weeks of gestation show differences in brain activation when compared with normal term-born controls in brain activation related to motor inhibition and attention tasks. During motor response inhibition, preterm-born subjects show increased activation in the medial and right lateral posterior brain regions, including middle temporal/occipital gyrus, posterior cingulate gyrus, and precuneus. During a task demanding spatial attention, preterm-born young adults showed diminished brain activation in the fronto-parietal areas and the cerebellum, a network involved in mediating attention [145]. These patterns may reflect a developmental delay secondary to preterm birth.

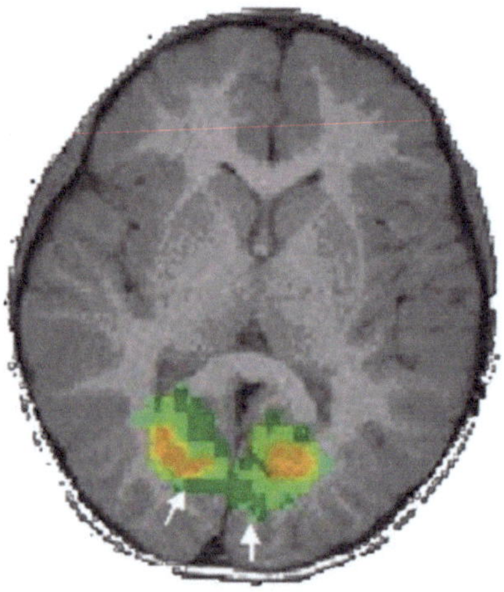

Fig. 14.13 Visual activation. Axial fMR images of a sedated child that demonstrates negative BOLD activation along the anterior calcarine cortex (*white arrows*)

fMRI in Specific Pediatric Conditions

Development

Functional MR provides a window to view developmental changes in morphogenesis, myelination, synaptogenesis, and neurotransmitter receptor density, not only in normal but also in pathologic cases. These may be associated with specific structural, metabolic, and congenital conditions.

There appears to be an age-related visual pattern activation. The expected positive BOLD response is seen in the occipital cortex of infants less than 4–7 weeks that are sleeping or sedated [32, 124]. Children more than 2 months show a negative BOLD response to the presentation of light. This occurs along the anterior aspect of the calcarine fissure (Fig. 14.13). In some cases, there may be concomitantly positive and negative voxels of activation in the visual cortex [33].

Children less than 15 years show less activation of the bilateral sensorimotor cortex, parietal areas, the supplementary motor area, and the cerebellum, in a simple motor task, compared with adults [16]. After the age of 10, there is a shift of the cortical allocation for categorical working memory from the dorsal visual and premotor/cerebellar networks to the ventral prefrontal and inferior temporal networks seen in adults [146]. Functional MRI of cognitive inhibition (e.g., self-regulatory control) has shown that the magnitude of fMRI signal change increases with age in the right inferior frontal gyrus and right lenticular nucleus. Activation of the frontal areas correlated with better response inhibition [147]. Similar results have been published with motor inhibition tasks [148]. Functional MRI of studies in children exposed to a task consisting of positive and negative feedback has revealed that the lateral orbitofrontal cortex reaches an adult-like activation by age 9, whereas parietal cortex reaches its adult-like response by age 15. The dorsolateral prefrontal cortex and anterior cingulate gyrus still develop after age 15 [149]. Dissociation for positive versus negative feedback and age has been described [150] – dorsolateral prefrontal cortex and superior parietal cortex more active after negative feedback for adults, and positive feedback for children under 9 years. Neuromaturational changes associated with visuospatial relational reasoning have been described as a shift from widespread fronto-cingulate-striatal pattern in childhood to predominant parieto-frontal activation pattern in late adolescence [151]. Children also show more widespread activation when compared with adults in working memory tasks [138].

Epilepsy

Functional MRI has been utilized as a tool for seizure localization. Anecdotic cases have been described of patients having an accidental subtle seizure, while an fMRI is performed. Cortical activation triggered by seizures provokes the BOLD response. This may be localized with fMR, if the seizure is captured in the MR scanner and does not produce head movement. Jackson and coworkers [152] performed an ictal fMRI in a 4-year-old boy with frequent partial motor seizures, revealing the epileptic focus. The paradigm consisted of contrasting periods of clinical seizures to baseline images acquired during a 10-min sequence. Another incidental ictal activity was mapped with fMRI in a 16-year-old boy performing different tasks for presurgical mapping of a dysplastic lesion [153]. Four cases with eyelid myoclonias and absence show BOLD responses localized to the thalamus, mesial frontal cortex, middle parietal lobe, temporal lobe, insula, and cerebellum [154]. Another case with hypothalamic hamartoma and gelastic seizures showed activation of the hamartoma, as well as the left hypothalamus, hippocampus, parietal-occipital area, cingulate gyrus, and dorsal-lateral frontal area [155]. Subclinical ictal activity has also been detected in adults with fMRI and confirmed with invasive monitoring in adolescent patients with frequent partial motor seizures [156].

In reflexogenic epilepsy, a specific stimulus triggers the seizures. Usually, the stimulus is reading or listening to music. Several cases have been reported utilizing the known triggering stimulus during an fMRI session. Obviously the provoked seizure needs to be of sensory or partial complex type, since the movement of motor seizures precludes imaging and post-processing.

Many studies have reported BOLD responses associated with interictal discharges, by triggering fMRI acquisition with discharges observed in an fMR with compatible electroencephalogram (EEG) obtained during the fMRI acquisition (e.g., [157–160]). This technique may demonstrate the epileptogenic focus in up to 60% of cases. Epileptogenic areas of the frontal, occipital, and parietal lobes were reliably detected. Areas close to the sinuses that create a profound paramagnetic effect on the images are not well served with this technique. This unfortunately occurs in the mesial temporal region, which is the most frequent epileptogenic region. A different approach may allow functional MR to localize the seizure origin in cases of occipital lobe epilepsy using a visual paradigm [161]. A summary of the most relevant studies of pediatric fMRI in epilepsy is presented in Table 14.7.

Table 14.7 Selected fMRI research in epilepsy

Authors	Subjects	fMRI paradigm	Main findings
Jackson et al. (1994)	One 4-year-old boy	ON: clinical seizures OFF: baseline (10 min observation)	Specific activation within the left hemisphere with each of five consecutive clinical seizures
Seeck et al. (1998)	One adolescent with frequent interictal frontal discharges	EEG-triggered fMRI (Event-related type)	Multiple areas of BOLD response of the left frontal lobe, where EEG source localization confirmed the focus
Schwartz et al. (1998)	One 16-year-old female	Incidental 20-s sensorymotor seizure used as ON epoch	Demonstration of the inherent epileptogenicity of a dysplastic cortex
Masuoka et al. (1999)	Children and adolescents with occipital lobe epilepsy	ON: Alternating checkerboard patterns OFF: Blank screen	Asymmetric activation pattern in six of ten patients. The side with less activation was concordant with laterality of seizure onset
Lazeyras et al. (2000)	Adolescents and adults with partial epilepsy	EEG-triggered fMRI	Activation of epileptogenic area. Areas confirmed in five of six subjects with intra-cranial recordings (ECoG)
Leal et al. (2006)	Children with occipital lobe epilepsy	ON: Periods of spikes in simultaneous EEG/fMRI recordings	The BOLD activation and the EEG were concordant to the same lobe, but with little spatial overlap between them. BOLD localization found more consistent with the ictal clinical manifestations
Liu et al. (2008)	Children	ON: Eyelid myoclonias and absences OFF: Baseline	Activation of the thalamus, mesial frontal cortex, middle parietal lobe, temporal lobe, insula, and cerebellum associated with the abnormal movements
Leal et al. (2009)	One child with gelastic seizures	ON: several gelastic episodes OFF: Baseline as per simultaneous EEG	Activation of the hamartoma, left hypothalamus, hippocampus, dorsolateral frontoparietal, and cingulate gyrus

Autism

The vast majority of the fMR studies in autism are limited to patients cooperative enough to hold still and follow commands. These are usually young adult patients of the *high-functioning Autism* subtype. In general, patients with autism show abnormal variability and scatter of functional maps in visuomotor tasks [162]. A distinctive feature of autism resides in the lack of social communication and inability to put oneself in someone else's shoes (theory of mind). A number of studies have attempted to map those functions.

The fusiform gyrus is involved in the perception of human faces. Functional MRI studies in adults have shown that the fusiform gyrus shows hypoactivity when faces are presented to autistic patients [163]. Other structures such as the amygdala, temporal pole, medial prefrontal cortex, inferolateral frontal cortex, and superior temporal sulci may play a secondary role [164]. Autistic patients demonstrate activation of the fusiform gyrus perceiving non-human stimulus such as cartoons but not with faces [165]. Autistic adult patients do not show significant changes in the fusiform gyrus activation after cognitive

Table 14.8 Selected fMRI research in autism

Authors	Subjects	fMRI paradigm	Main findings
Muller et al. (2001)	Autistic and normal adolescents and young adults	Visually paced finger movements vs. visual stimulation in the absence of motor response	Activation less pronounced in the autism group (when compared with controls) of contralateral perirolandic cortex, basal ganglia, thalamus, bilateral supplementary motor area, and ipsilateral cerebellum
Takeuchi et al. (2004)	Children and adolescents with autism vs. controls	Language task requiring understanding another's mental state	Activation of bilateral prefrontal areas and occipito-temporal regions. Autistic patients demonstrated more activation of the right frontal lobe than controls
Grelotti et al. (2005)	One child with autism	Face/object/cartoon discrimination task	The amygdala and the fusiform gyrus were activated with cartoons but not with faces
Dapretto et al. (2006)	High functioning autism children	Imitating and observing emotional expressions	Children with autism showed no mirror neuron activity in the inferior frontal
Gomot et al. (2006)	Autistic children between 10 and 15 years of age	Passive detection of deviant and complex novel sounds	Children with autism showed reduced activation of the left anterior cingulate cortex with both tasks, and bilateral temporoparietal region and right inferior and middle frontal areas during novelty detection

intervention with computer-based programs intended to teach facial affect identification [166]. However, they do show greater activation in the superior parietal lobule that correlates with improvement on behavioral scores.

Language is a major problem in autistic patients. Very few studies of language function have been conducted as of yet. In one study, autistic patients demonstrated right-hemisphere dominance for language when compared with normal controls [167].

Autistic children have a noticeable resistance to change. This resistance to change seems to be rooted in atypical processing of unexpected stimuli. Brain activity associated with a passive detection of frequency-deviant and complex novel sounds has shown differences between autistic children and age-matched controls. Children with autism showed reduced activation of the left anterior cingulate cortex with both tasks, and bilateral temporoparietal region and right inferior and middle frontal areas during novelty detection [168].

Motor activation appears generally less pronounced in autism patients [169]. Mirror neuron abnormalities have also been found in autism with fMRI. Children with autism show no mirror neuron activity in the inferior frontal gyrus (pars opercularis) when compared with normal controls. Activity in the pars opercularis is inversely related to social domain symptoms [170]. Interestingly, fMRI has found differences in brain activation of parents of autistic children when compared with normal controls performing tasks of visual search and emotional recognition [171]. A summary of relevant fMR studies in autistic children is presented in Table 14.8.

ADHD

Attention deficit hyperactivity disorder (ADHD) lacks clear anatomical markers [172]. Difficulty with compliance in ADHD patients is expected. However, with the use of the proper paradigms, fMR has been proven to be feasible in children

Table 14.9 Selected fMRI research in ADHD

Authors	Subjects	fMRI paradigm	Main findings
Durston et al. (2003)	Children with ADHD vs. controls	Parametric go/no-go task	Normal children activate bilateral fronto-striatal network ADHD children show widespread dorsolateral and parietal-occipital activation Children with ADHD present easier interference with conflicting trials (even with a single go trial)
Rubia et al. (2005)	Medication-naïve adolescents with ADHD and healthy volunteers	Response inhibition tasks	Medication-naive adolescents with ADHD show reduced brain activation in the right inferior prefrontal cortex during motor inhibition, and in the precuneus and posterior cingulate gyrus during inhibition failure
Vaidya et al. (2005)	Children with combined type of ADHD vs. controls	Visual interference task (flanker task)	ADHD subjects: reduced activation of the frontal-striatal-temporal-parietal network Distinct localization: Normal volunteers: frontal-striatal. ADHD children right superior temporal
Bernal and Altman (2009)	Normal children	Go/no-go task; Color Stroop task	Normal activation to inhibition tasks involves the middle frontal gyri, anterior cingulate gyrus, superior parietal lobules, and inferior parietal lobules
Solanto et al. (2009)	Children with ADHD (inattentive vs. combined forms)	Go/no-go task	No significant group differences in task performance. Activation was seen in the right inferior frontal gyrus, right superior temporal lobe, and left inferior parietal lobe during inhibitory control. Activation was greater in the inattentive than in the combined group, except the medial occipital lobe activation that was greater in the combined group
Rubia et al. (2009)	Medication-naive children with ADHD. Normal controls	Selective attention with rewarded performance Task presented twice, single methylphenidate dose or placebo, randomized double blinded design	Methylphenidate enhances the activation of fronto-striato-cerebellar and parietotemporal regions, and normalizes the enhanced orbitofrontal activation in children with ADHD in response to reward

with ADHD (Table 14.9). These tasks include sustained visual vigilance or sustained attention [173, 174], inhibition of motor response ("go-no-go paradigms," stop or delayed response) [173, 175–178], and Stroop and Stroop-like tasks (Fig. 14.14) [179, 180].

Children with ADHD have a characteristic impairment of inhibition. Normal activation to inhibition tasks involves the middle frontal gyri, anterior cingulate gyrus, the superior parietal lobules (predominantly on the left), and the inferior parietal lobules [181]. Adult ADHD patients

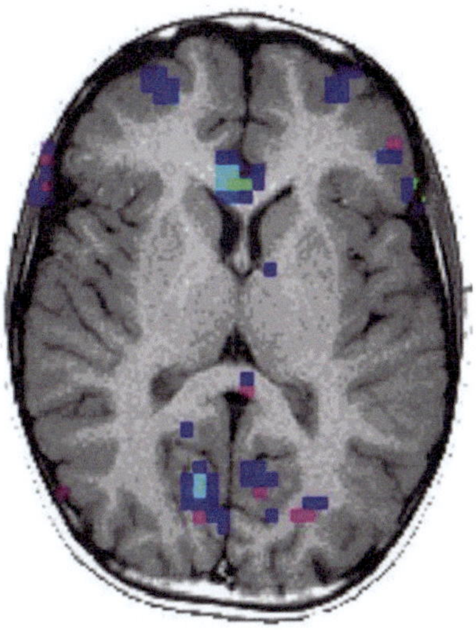

Fig. 14.14 Functional MR of normal child performing a Stroop task. Activation in the anterior cingulate gyrus and bilateral middle frontal gyrus is associated with inhibition tasks. The bilateral calcarine cortex is related to the visual demands of the task

show less activation of the anterior cingulate gyrus on Stroop paradigms than normal patients [179, 182]. Motor inhibition tasks in ADHD cases do not activate frontostriatal regions in the same manner as normally developing children, but rather rely on a more diffuse network of regions, including more posterior and dorsolateral prefrontal regions [175]. Children with ADHD present easier interference with conflicting trials (even with a single go trial) in motor tasks when compared with normal children [175]. More recent studies have shown a dissociation of the activation abnormalities with respect to the inhibition tasks. During motor response inhibition, medication-naive adolescents with ADHD show reduced brain activation in the right inferior prefrontal cortex [177].

Children with hyperactive predominant ADHD activate more right inferior frontal gyrus, right superior temporal lobe, and left inferior parietal lobe during inhibitory control than patients with the combined form [183]. These results are consistent also with the reported dissociation of brain activation related to motor and cognitive inhibitory control in normal children [184] and children with ADHD [180].

Functional MRI results have demonstrated image correlates to clinical findings in ADHD. Methylphenidate enhances the activation of fronto-striato-cerebellar and parietotemporal regions and normalizes the enhanced orbitofrontal activation in children with ADHD in response to reward [185].

Dyslexia

Numerous studies have been performed comparing dyslexic to normal children looking at patterns of activation of reading paradigms (Table 14.10). Dyslexic children have less activation in the left temporal-parietal cortex [186, 187]. Children with dyslexia show reduced activation in the left middle and inferior frontal gyri, right superior frontal gyrus, left middle and inferior temporal gyri, and bilateral superior parietal regions when performing phonological and morphological tasks, when compared with normal controls [188, 189]. However, it has been reported significant hyperactivation in the left inferior frontal gyrus associated with tasks of reading nonwords or performing phonological transformations [53]. A deficit in processing rapid acoustic stimuli in children with dyslexia has been demonstrated utilizing fMRI. Normal children performing a reading task show higher prefrontal activation for rapid versus slow phonological transitions in the left prefrontal cortex. Children with developmental dyslexia do not show any differential response in these regions. [190]. Verb generation tasks produce bilateral posterior cerebellar activations (along with the canonical left frontal and parietal activations) in normal children. Patients with developmental dyslexia show widespread and diffuse activations in the cerebral and cerebellar level [191].

Brain Plasticity

Brain plasticity refers to the nervous system's ability to organize change on the basis of development, experience, and lesions acquired during one's lifespan. This phenomenon has different

Table 14.10 Selected fMRI research in dyslexia

Authors	Subjects	fMRI paradigm	Main findings
Georgieva et al. (1999)	Normal and dyslexic children	Several tasks of reading from letters to words	Dyslexic patients show increased activation of the left inferior frontal gyrus, in nonwords and phonological transformation tasks when compared to normals
Temple et al. (2001)	Normal and dyslexic children	Phonological and orthographic tasks of rhyming and matching visually presented letter pairs	Dyslexic children have less activation in left temporal-parietal cortex
Backes et al. (2002)	Normal and dyslexic children	Visuospatial, orthographic, phonologic, and semantic processing	Dyslexic children predominantly show activation in the right prefrontal cortex on orthographic processing. Normal readers show activation of left prefrontal cortex
Aylward et al. (2003)	Normal and dyslexic children	Decoding phonemes and morphemes, pre- and postreading training intervention	Dyslexic children show reduced activation in the left middle and inferior frontal gyri, right superior frontal gyrus, left middle and inferior temporal gyri, and bilateral superior parietal regions when performing phonological tasks, when compared with normal controls Training improves scores and brain activation
Gaab et al. (2007)	Normal and dyslexic children	Listening to nonlinguistic acoustic stimuli, with either rapid or slow transitions	Children with dyslexia did not show any differential response in the left frontal areas, to rapid versus slow transitions as was found in normal controls. Training improved reading and brain activation
Baillieux et al. (2009)	Normal and dyslexic children	Noun-to-verb association paradigm	Patients with dyslexia show widespread and diffuse activation in the cerebrum and the cerebellum compared with focal well-defined activation seen in normals

levels of expression that involves the synaptic population and the complexities of neural network reorganization observed with cognition recovery. The study of neural organization is of crucial importance in the understanding of normal brain development and in neurological recovery following brain injury. Brain plasticity associated with development and learning is known as natural plasticity. These changes have been identified as changing patterns seen by fMR in the developing brain. Brain plasticity associated with brain injury is known as postlesional brain plasticity. Postlesional brain plasticity depends on the ability of neurons to connect with those neurons whose function has been halted or to invade networks adjacent to the damaged regions competing with them [192]. These changes occur by axonal regeneration and reactional synaptogenesis guided by gradients of trophic substances released by the postsynaptic cells.

The greater plasticity observed in children may be explained by the greater ability of collaterals to utilize connectional redundancy allowing ectopic pathways to be settled. Infants less than 6 years may recover language deficits after

Table 14.11 Selected fMRI research of brain plasticity

Authors	Subjects	fMRI paradigm	Main findings
Staudt et al. (2001)	Young adults with pre- and perinatal left periventricular lesions	Phonological fluency task	Deep motor tract involvement of the left hemisphere correlates with right-hemisphere activation
Hertz-Pannier et al. (2002)	A boy with left-sided Rasmussen's syndrome scanned at age 6 and 10	Covert semantic fluency task (first fMRI). Word generation and story listening (second fMRI)	First fMRI: left lateralization After hemispherectomy and profound subsequent aphasia the patient showed partial recovery of language. Second fMRI: right activation of language areas
Liegeois et al. (2004)	Children and adolescents with intractable partial seizures and early acquired focal lesions of the left hemisphere	Covert verb generation task	50% of cases showed bilateral or right language lateralization. Lesions in or near Broca's area were mostly associated with perilesional activation. Paradoxically, lesions remote from the canonical language areas were associated with bilateral or right-sided activation
Anderson et al. (2006)	Children with epilepsy and frontal or temporal lesions	Covert word generation task	Involvement of the left inferior or middle frontal gyri increased the likelihood of atypical language lateralization
Jacola et al. (2006)	Children with perinatal infarctions of the left hemisphere vs. controls	Verb generation task and story listening	Patients showed activation either bilaterally or in the right hemisphere during both tasks when compared with controls who showed bilateral or left language areas activation
Hadac et al. (2007)	Children with pre- and postnatal eoileptogenic lesions of the left hemisphere	Verbal fluency task	Reorganization was strongly influenced by age of onset and duration of epilepsy
Guzzetta et al. (2008)	Children with perinatal stroke of the left hemisphere, with right hemiplegia	Covert phonological task	80% of patients showed right hemisphere Broca's activation

hemispherectomy. However, prenatal brain injury concurrent with the neuronal proliferation, organization, and differentiation stages are the cause of the most diffuse and unrecoverable deficits of children [193]. Factors such as the size of the lesion, localization, contralateral tissue integrity, epilepsy, drugs, medications, and external stimulation may influence neural plasticity and recovery. Prior to fMRI, very few studies on postlesional plasticity were done in infants and children. Previous functional studies on evoked potentials [194], magnetoencephalography [195, 196], transcranial magnetic stimulation [197, 198], and positron emission tomography (PET) [199–201] have shown variability of localization, diffuse distribution of activation, and frequent involvement of the hemisphere contralateral to the lesion. However, the burden or the risk involved in PET studies has made it difficult to compare these results with normal children.

Functional MRI in children has confirmed these findings and brought new perspectives to the study of postlesional brain plasticity (Table 14.11). Infants and adolescents with low-grade tumors in the rolandic region without motor deficits show significant recruitment of the hemisphere ipsilateral to the hand doing a tapping task. In addition, scattered activation

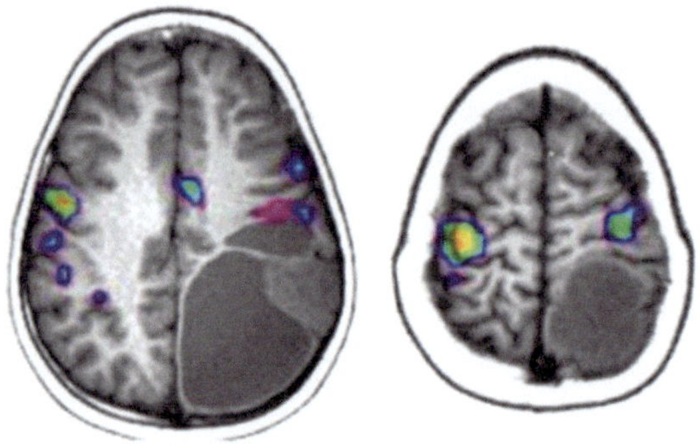

Fig. 14.15 Functional MR demonstrating motor cortex plasticity in a child with large brain tumor. Axial fMR images of a right-handed child performing a right-hand finger tapping task. There is asymmetric bilateral motor cortex activation greater on the right. Bilateral scattered areas of activation and contralateral SMA activation are seen suggesting reorganization of function in this child with a slowly growing tumor

indicating reorganization may appear in the contralateral hemisphere (Fig. 14.15) [202]. In such cases, surgical resection is not followed by significant motor deficit. Functional MRI studies in children with other types of lesions of the left hemisphere including encephaloclastic lesions, severe and precocious epilepsy, or dysplasias may show right hemisphere transference [57, 62, 203–207]. Similarly, fMRI has shown that early left periventricular lesions also induce right hemisphere transference of language [208]. Late brain plasticity for language has been demonstrated with fMRI in a patient who suffered from Rasmussen's encephalitis after normal language acquisition at the age of 5. Left hemispherectomy was performed at age 9. Pre- and postoperative fMRI were obtained. After profound aphasia, the patient recovered receptive language but very limited expressive skills. Presurgical fMRI revealed left lateralization. Postoperative fMRI performed at age 10 showed a shift of activation for both receptive and expressive language tasks to the right. These areas mirrored those previously found in the left hemisphere [203].

Dysinhibition and functional enlargement of the motor cortex associated with the removed limb in patients amputated during childhood have been demonstrated with transcranial magnetic stimulation and confirmed by fMRI [209]. These patients also show ipsilateral functional reorganization.

Brain plasticity has been described in three young adults with brachial plexus injury who underwent nerve transfer surgery. In all cases, the authors found that the areas activated by flexing the elbow on the operated side was symmetrical to the fMR activation of the motor cortex elicited by flexing the other elbow [210]. The fMRI was done 4–12 months after surgery and was confirmed with magnetoencephalography.

Other fMRI Studies in Specific Pediatric Conditions

Fragile X syndrome is a relatively common genetic cause of developmental and learning problems [211]. MRI is usually normal, although atrophy of the brainstem and cerebellum has been described [212]. A reduced gray matter to white matter ratio has also been noted [213]. Functional MRI performed on 14 age-matched girls with fragile X, using a counting Stroop task, showed more extensive activation in the anterior prefrontal cortex, reduced activation in the left orbitofrontal gyrus, and lack of activation in the parietal cortex when compared with normal children [214].

Children with Tourette's syndrome have been studied by presentation of a complex inhibition paradigm involving tactile stimulus demonstrating an inhibitory deficit of the startling coupling response [215]. Similarly, Tourette's patients show abnormal activation of circuitry involved in cognitive self-control when compared with normal children [216]. It has been described that the tic severity is associated with the activation of dopaminergic nuclei (substantia nigra/ventral tegmental area) and cortical, striatal, thalamic, and subthalamic regions [217]. Tourette's syndrome patients also have a significantly greater activation of motor areas on tapping-finger tasks [218].

New Trends in Pediatric fMRI

Functional MRI has evolved rapidly. There are many new developments in the technique that impact the way the procedure is done, the manner in which the activation is obtained, and how the images are analyzed. The most promising of these are pharmacology-fMRI and resting-state fMRI.

Pharmacology-fMRI (ph-fMRI) in Children

Functional MRI has shown a strong intra-subject reproducibility with low variance over time. This allows for observing changes in patterns of brain activation after the administration of a given pharmaceutical or biological active substance. The BOLD response is effected by vasodilators; vasoconstrictors; metabolic rate; oxy/deoxyhemoglobin changes; neurotransmitter agonists, antagonists, blockers or modulators, and many other circumstances.

Pharmacology-fMRI has demonstrated very promising results in several areas. Patients with ADHD (off medication) show hypoactivation of prefrontal lateral areas and in striatal subcortical structures in motor inhibition tasks. When these patients are evaluated with fMR after administration of methylphenidate, they show improved response inhibition [176] as seen by increasing frontal activation to an extent similar to healthy controls. The pharmaceutical increases striatal activation only in ADHD children and not in healthy controls where the effect is the opposite, as it appears clinically. There also appears to be a different response to the medication in adults and children with ADHD. In adults, compared with children, there is no increase of prefrontal activation, and it is only confined to the subcortical striatum [219].

Children with growth hormone deficiency, who have memory problems, have been scanned with fMRI pre- and post-growth hormone administration. The interval between the exams was 6 months on average. The replacement of the hormone produced better memory performance and correlated with a reduction of the activation of the basal and lateral aspect of the frontal lobes, which was felt a product of effort [220].

Children with mood dysregulation, but not bipolar disorder, show a decrease in the activation of the prefrontal brain areas, which correlates with the degree of decrease in depressive symptom severity after the administration of divalproex for 12 weeks [221].

A combined study of ph-fMRI and default resting-state fMRI in adolescents has shown that stimulant medication significantly improves the suppression of the default-mode activity in the ventral anterior cingulate cortex in the ADHD group while performing a Stroop task. When off medication, this group was unable to suppress default-mode activity to the same degree as healthy controls. More interestingly, the degree of prefrontal activation, when off medication, was able to predict the reduction in the ADHD symptoms when on medication [222].

Resting-State fMRI in Children

Usually, fMRI interrogates the areas of the brain responding to a given stimulus. This stimulus is presented discontinuously either in a block-designed or event-related manner. Mathematical procedures analyze the variance of the data in relationship to the timing of the stimulus. These standard analyses require prior assumptions about the time course of the measured signal. However, there are techniques that can mine the data looking for spatial and temporal correlations independent of the timeline of the stimuli. One of these techniques is called independent component analysis or ICA [223]. ICA, "extracts" independent patterns of spatial or temporal correlated activations within the entire data set. A subject listening to music, for example, will have in addition to the activation located in the superior temporal gyrus, several other components not associated (hence, independent) with the stimulus frequency of presentation. Moreover, these independent components remain even if the same analysis is done without a task being presented during the sequence. These spontaneous

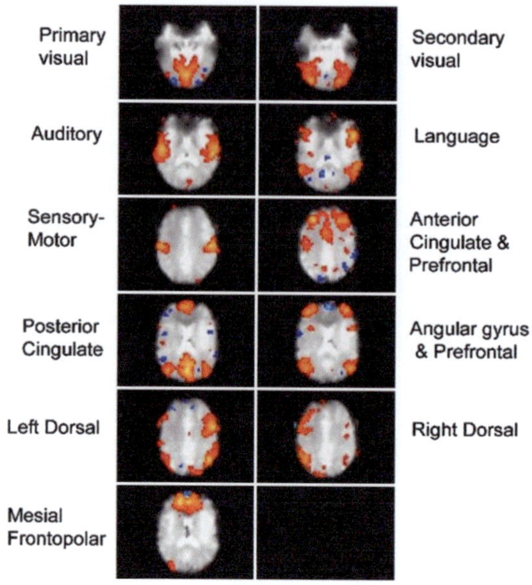

Fig. 14.16 Resting-state fMRI. Normal components observed in a 17-year-old boy. The components were extracted by visual inspection. All of them show cortical localization and fast Fourier frequency below 0.05 Hz (criteria for selection). Notice the bilateral and rather symmetrical distribution for all of them but three – the fronto-parietal dorsal components (*second row from bottom to top*) and the component interpreted as language circuitry (*second row from top to bottom, right figure*)

components have a very low frequency (<0.08 Hz), and they reflect an intrinsic connectivity network, due to their temporal correlation.

Seven to nine components have been described in adults [224]. We have demonstrated at least 11 different normal components in children (Fig. 14.16). In newborn babies under natural sleep, five components have been described [225], including parietal, temporal, and prefrontal cortices and bilateral basal ganglia. Resting-state independent components are present under natural sleep, sedation, and even under anesthesia [226–228].

An interesting feature of the resting-state network is that its medial structures – including the prefrontal cortex, rostral anterior cingulate gyrus, posterior cingulate gyrus, and precuneus–deactivates during cognitively demanding tasks [229], but not during sensory tasks [230]. This suppression of activity is observed as "deactivation," which is thought to be indicative of an interruption of mental activity that persists during rest. Children over 13 years show the same pattern of deactivation than adults [231]. In adults, some other neocortical areas of the resting-state mode activate in an anti-correlated fashion with the medial structures [232].

Resting-state fMRI has been utilized in pediatric conditions. Contrasted to healthy controls, patients with ADHD exhibit significant resting-state temporal coactivation with the dorsal aspect of the anterior cingulate gyrus (bilaterally) with bilateral thalamus, bilateral cerebellum, bilateral insula, and the pons [233]. The low-frequency spontaneous fluctuations that characterize resting-state show less amplitude in ADHD children contrasted to normal volunteers [234]. Boys with ADHD showed decreased regional homogeneity in the frontal-striatal-cerebellar circuits, but increased regional homogeneity mainly in the occipital cortex [235]. Psychostimulants in children with ADHD improves the deactivation of the default mode related to demanding tasks as is seen in the normal age-matched controls [236].

There is a procedure derived from the resting-state fMRI sequence in which the connectivity of a given region of interest (ROI) is explored by looking into the commonality of activation with remote cortical areas. In these types of studies, the signal profile, throughout the entire number of time-points of the ROI, is chosen as the convolved function to detect correlated areas. With this technique, it has been found that children evolve from a localized to a distributed connectivity [237], and it is larger in sensory-motor areas than visual areas before the age of 2[238]. ADHD patients show abnormal functional connectivity between the putamen and the cortical-striatal-thalamic circuits [239].

Adults with high functioning autism fail to demonstrate default-network deactivation that normally appears associated with cognitive load [240]. They also show a weaker connectivity between the posterior cingulate gyrus and superior frontal gyrus, but stronger connectivity between the posterior cingulate and both the right temporal lobe and right parahippocampal gyrus [241].

Table 14.12 Selected fMRI articles on resting-state fMRI research

Authors	Subjects	fMRI condition/processing	Main findings
Kiviniemi et al. (2000)	Children under general anesthesia with thiopental	Independent component analysis	Thiopental increases magnitude and decreases frequency of the spontaneous slow fluctuations of the BOLD signal associated with resting-state
Kiviniemi et al. (2003)	Children under general anesthesia	Taskless fMR. Independent component analysis	Components were found in all primary sensory areas, with a frequency spectra power of 0.03 Hz
Tian et al. (2006)	Adolescents with ADHD and normal controls	Resting-state. Anterior Cingulate Gyrus outlined to serve as ROI to explore functional connectivity	ADHD patients exhibit more significant connectivity with the anterior cingulate gyrus, bilateral thalamus, bilateral cerebellum, bilateral insula, and bilateral brainstem when compared with normal controls
Zang et al. (2007)	Boys with ADHD and controls	Analysis of amplitude of spontaneous low frequency fluctuations	Decreased connectivity in the right inferior frontal cortex, left sensorimotor cortex, and bilateral cerebellum and the vermis
Cao et al. (2007)	Children with ADHD (two subtypes) and normal controls	Regional homogeneity	Decreased regional homogeneity in the frontal-striatal-cerebellar circuits. Increased regional homogeneity in the occipital cortex
Fair et al. (2009)	Children and young adults	ROI-based functional connectivity	Connectivity evolves from "segregated-type" where correlation strength is mainly seen between regions close in anatomical space, to "integration," where an increased correlation strength is seen among regions distant in space
Fransson et al. (2009)	Full-term born unsedated infants	Natural sleep/independent component analysis	Five components found: parietal, frontal, temporal, prefrontal, and basal ganglia
Vuontela et al. (2009)	Children	Working memory tasks/ resting-state fMR	Children exhibited similar pattern of cortical deactivation reported in adults during cognitive task performance compared with a resting-state

There is a direct correlation between social functioning in autistic patients and connectivity between the posterior cingulate cortex and the superior frontal gyrus [241].

Critical functional networks have been identified from resting-state fMRI data in adult patients with brain tumors [242] providing valuable presurgical information. This approach may be useful in child patients who cannot cooperate with the traditional task-based fMRI. A summary of the most relevant studies on pediatric-resting-state fMRI is presented in Table 14.12.

Conclusion

Functional MRI has begun to show considerable clinical benefits in the understanding of crucial aspects of cognitive development in both normal and impaired children. Presurgical mapping is an alternative to more invasive and costly procedures. Functional MRI is utilized in close to 70% of children's hospitals who work-up of patients with intractable epilepsy. Pharmacology fMRI may become a standard for the evaluation of neuropharmaceutical compounds in the diagnosis and treatment of ADHD and, perhaps, autism. Treatment will be better tailored and monitored. Resting-state fMRI will grow significantly in the years to come. Several articles are suggesting its importance to reveal clinical biomarkers in different functional conditions. Conditions such as ADHD, autism, dyslexia, and psychiatric disorders will be better diagnosed and understood. The clinical contribution of fMRI in the understanding of physiologic processes of the brain will be as significant as MRI was in the understanding of anatomic abnormalities.

References

1. Medina LS, Aguirre E, Bernal B, Altman NR. Functional MR imaging versus Wada test for evaluation of language lateralization: cost analysis. Radiology. 2004;230(1):49–54.
2. Barkovich AJ, Kjos BO, Jackson Jr DE, Norman D. Normal maturation of the neonatal and infant brain: MR imaging at 1.5 T. Radiology. 1988;166(1 Pt 1):173–80.
3. Staudt M, Krageloh-Mann I, Grodd W. Normal myelination in childhood brains using MRI – a meta analysis. Rofo. 2000;172(10):802–11.
4. Huttenlocher PR. Synaptic density in human frontal cortex – developmental changes and effects of aging. Brain Res. 1979;163(2):195–205.
5. Huttenlocher PR. Morphometric study of human cerebral cortex development. Neuropsychologia. 1990;28(6):517–27.
6. Chugani HT, Phelps ME, Mazziotta JC. Positron emission tomography study of human brain functional development. Ann Neurol. 1987;22(4): 487–97.
7. D'Esposito M, Zarahn E, Aguirre GK, Rypma B. The effect of normal aging on the coupling of neural activity to the bold hemodynamic response. Neuroimage. 1999;10(1):6–14.
8. Gaillard WD, Hertz-Pannier L, Mott SH, Barnett AS, LeBihan D, Theodore WH. Functional anatomy of cognitive development: fMRI of verbal fluency in children and adults. Neurology. 2000;54(1):180–5.
9. Huettel SA, Singerman JD, McCarthy G. The effects of aging upon the hemodynamic response measured by functional MRI. Neuroimage. 2001;13(1): 161–75.
10. Casey BJ, Cohen JD, Jezzard P, et al. Activation of prefrontal cortex in children during a nonspatial working memory task with functional MRI. Neuroimage. 1995;2(3):221–9.
11. Zarahn E, Aguirre GK, D'Esposito M. Temporal isolation of the neural correlates of spatial mnemonic processing with fMRI. Brain Res Cogn Brain Res. 1999;7(3):255–68.
12. Volpe JJ. Neurology of the newborn. 5th ed. Philadelphia, PA: WB Saunders/Elsevier; 2008; 97–8.
13. Rubia K, Overmeyer S, Taylor E, et al. Functional frontalisation with age: mapping neurodevelopmental trajectories with fMRI. Neurosci Biobehav Rev. 2000;24(1):13–9.
14. Klingberg T, Vaidya CJ, Gabrieli JD, Moseley ME, Hedehus M. Myelination and organization of the frontal white matter in children: a diffusion tensor MRI study. Neuroreport. 1999;10(13):2817–21.
15. Huttenlocher PR, Dabholkar AS. Regional differences in synaptogenesis in human cerebral cortex. J Comp Neurol. 1997;387(2):167–78.
16. Mall V, Linder M, Herpers M, et al. Recruitment of the sensorimotor cortex – a developmental FMRI study. Neuropediatrics. 2005;36(6):373–9.
17. Rotte M. Age-related differences in the areas of Broca and Wernicke using functional magnetic resonance imaging. Age Ageing. 2005;34(6):609–13.
18. Bookheimer SY. Functional MRI applications in clinical epilepsy. Neuroimage. 1996;4(3 Pt 3): S139–46.
19. Nagel BJ, Barlett VC, Schweinsburg AD, Tapert SF. Neuropsychological predictors of BOLD response during a spatial working memory task in adolescents: what can performance tell us about fMRI response patterns? J Clin Exp Neuropsychol. 2005;27(7):823–39.
20. Kastrup A, Krüger G, Neumann-Haefelin T, Glover GH, Moseley ME. Changes of cerebral blood flow, oxygenation, and oxidative metabolism during graded motor activation. Neuroimage. 2002;15(1): 74–82.
21. Price C, Wise R, Ramsay S, et al. Regional response differences within the human auditory cortex when listening to words. Neurosci Lett. 1992;146(2):179.
22. Bookheimer S. Functional MRI of the hippocampus during short term memory tasks: parametric responses to task difficulty and stimulus novelty. Neuroimage. 1996;3(3):531.

23. Raichle ME, Fiez JA, Videen TO, et al. Practice-related changes in human brain functional anatomy during nonmotor learning. Cereb Cortex. 1994;4(1):8–26.
24. Bookheimer SY, Dapretto M, Karmarkar U. Functional MRI in children with epilepsy. Dev Neurosci. 1999;21(3–5):191–9.
25. Rosenberg DR, Sweeney JA, Gillen JS, et al. Magnetic resonance imaging of children without sedation: preparation with simulation. J Amer Acad Child Adolesc Psychiatry. 1997;36(6):853.
26. Yamada H, Sadato N, Konishi Y, et al. A rapid brain metabolic change in infants detected by fMRI. Neuroreport. 1997;8(17):3775–8.
27. Born P, Leth H, Miranda MJ, et al. Visual activation in infants and young children studied by functional magnetic resonance imaging. Pediatr Res. 1998; 44(4):578–83.
28. Martin E, Joeri P, Loenneker T, et al. Visual processing in infants and children studied using functional MRI. Pediatr Res. 1999;46(2):135–40.
29. Souweidane MM, Kim KH, McDowall R, et al. Brain mapping in sedated infants and young children with passive-functional magnetic resonance imaging. Pediatr Neurosurg. 1999;30(2):86–92.
30. Born AP, Miranda MJ, Rostrup E, et al. Functional magnetic resonance imaging of the normal and abnormal visual system in early life. Neuropediatrics. 2000;31(1):24–32.
31. Morita T, Kochiyama T, Yamada H, et al. Difference in the metabolic response to photic stimulation of the lateral geniculate nucleus and the primary visual cortex of infants: a fMRI study. Neurosci Res. 2000;38(1):63–70.
32. Yamada H, Sadato N, Konishi Y, et al. A milestone for normal development of the infantile brain detected by functional MRI. Neurology. 2000;55(2): 218–23.
33. Altman NR, Bernal B. Brain activation in sedated children: auditory and visual functional MR imaging. Radiology. 2001;221(1):56–63.
34. Carmody DP, Moreno R, Mars AE, Seshadri K, Lambert GH, Lewis M. Brief report: brain activation to social words in a sedated child with autism. J Autism Dev Disord. 2007;37(7):1381–5.
35. Gemma M, de Vitis A, Baldoli C, et al. Functional magnetic resonance imaging (fMRI) in children sedated with propofol or midazolam. J Neurosurg Anesthesiol. 2009;21(3):253–8.
36. Marcar VL, Schwarz U, Martin E, Loenneker T. How depth of anesthesia influences the blood oxygenation level-dependent signal from the visual cortex of children. AJNR Am J Neuroradiol. 2006;27(4): 799–805.
37. Poldrack RA, Pare-Blagoev EJ, Grant PE. Pediatric functional magnetic resonance imaging: progress and challenges. Top Magn Reson Imaging. 2002; 13(1):61–70.
38. Yuan W, Altaye M, Ret J, et al. Quantification of head motion in children during various fMRI language tasks. Hum Brain Mapp. 2009;30(5):1481–9.
39. Slifer KJ, Cataldo MF, Cataldo MD, Llorente AM, Gerson AC. Behavior analysis of motion control for pediatric neuroimaging. J Appl Behav Anal. 1993;26:469–70.
40. Yerys BE, Jankowski KF, Shook D, et al. The fMRI success rate of children and adolescents: typical development, epilepsy, attention deficit/hyperactivity disorder, and autism spectrum disorders. Hum Brain Mapp. 2009;30(10):3426–35.
41. Freire L, Mangin JF. Motion correction algorithms may create spurious brain activations in the absence of subject motion. Neuroimage. 2001;14(3): 709–22.
42. Talairach J, Tournoux P. Co-planar stereotaxic atlas of the human brain: 3-dimensional proportional system: an approach to cerebral imaging. Thieme. 1988.
43. Burgund ED, Kang HC, Kelly JE, et al. The feasibility of a common stereotactic space for children and adults in fMRI studies of development. Neuroimage. 2002;17(1):184–200.
44. Jacobs J, Hawco C, Kobayashi E, et al. Variability of the hemodynamic response as a function of age and frequency of epileptic discharge in children with epilepsy. Neuroimage. 2008;40(2):601–14.
45. Richter W, Richter M. The shape of the fMRI BOLD response in children and adults changes systematically with age. Neuroimage. 2003;20(2):1122–31.
46. Cohen MS, DuBois RM. Stability, repeatability, and the expression of signal magnitude in functional magnetic resonance imaging. J Magn Reson Imaging. 1999;10(1):33–40.
47. Gaillard WD, Grandin CB, Xu B. Developmental aspects of pediatric fMRI: considerations for image acquisition, analysis, and interpretation. Neuroimage. 2001;13(2):239–49.
48. Binder JR, Swanson SJ, Hammeke TA, et al. Determination of language dominance using functional MRI: a comparison with the Wada test. Neurology. 1996;46(4):978–84.
49. Hertz-Pannier L, Gaillard WD, Mott SH, et al. Noninvasive assessment of language dominance in children and adolescents with functional MRI: a preliminary study. Neurology. 1997;48(4):1003.
50. Stapleton SR, Kiriakopoulos E, Mikulis D, et al. Combined utility of functional MRI, cortical mapping, and frameless stereotaxy in the resection of lesions in eloquent areas of brain in children. Pediatr Neurosurg. 1997;26(2):68–82.
51. Dehaene-Lambertz G, Dehaene S, Hertz-Pannier L. Functional neuroimaging of speech perception in infants. Science. 2002;298(5600):2013–5.
52. Wilke M, Holland SK, Ball Jr WS. Language processing during natural sleep in a 6-year-old boy, as assessed with functional MR imaging. AJNR Am J Neuroradiol. 2003;24(1):42–4.
53. Georgiewa P, Rzanny R, Hopf JM, et al. fMRI during word processing in dyslexic and normal reading children. Neuroreport. 1999;10(16):3459–65.
54. Cravo I, Palma T, Conceição C, Evangelista P. Preoperative applications of cortical mapping with

functional magnetic resonance. Acta Méd Port. 2001;14(1):21–5.

55. Booth JR, Macwhinney B, Thulborn KR, Sacco K, Voyvodic J, Feldman HM. Functional organization of activation patterns in children: whole brain fMRI imaging during three different cognitive tasks. Prog Neuropsychopharmacol Biol Psychiatry. 1999;23(4):669–82.
56. Holland SK, Plante E, Weber Byars A, Strawsburg RH, Schmithorst VJ, Ball Jr WS. Normal fMRI brain activation patterns in children performing a verb generation task. Neuroimage. 2001;14(4): 837–43.
57. Liégeois F, Connelly A, Cross JH, et al. Language reorganization in children with early-onset lesions of the left hemisphere: an fMRI study. Brain. 2004; 127(Pt 6):1229–36.
58. Schapiro MB, Schmithorst VJ, Wilke M, Byars AW, Strawsburg RH, Holland SK. BOLD fMRI signal increases with age in selected brain regions in children. Neuroreport. 2004;15(17):2575–8.
59. Szaflarski JP, Holland SK, Schmithorst VJ, Byars AW. fMRI study of language lateralization in children and adults. Hum Brain Mapp. 2006;27(3): 202–12.
60. Gaillard WD, Balsamo L, Xu B, et al. fMRI language task panel improves determination of language dominance. Neurology. 2004;63(8):1403–8.
61. Lehéricy S, Cohen L, Bazin B, et al. Functional MR evaluation of temporal and frontal language dominance compared with the Wada test. Neurology. 2000;54(8):1625–33.
62. Jacola LM, Schapiro MB, Schmithorst VJ, et al. Functional magnetic resonance imaging reveals atypical language organization in children following perinatal left middle cerebral artery stroke. Neuropediatrics. 2006;37(1):46–52.
63. Vannest JJ, Karunanayaka PR, Altaye M, et al. Comparison of fMRI data from passive listening and active-response story processing tasks in children. J Magn Reson Imaging. 2009;29(4):971–6.
64. Ahmad Z, Balsamo LM, Sachs BC, Xu B, Gaillard WD. Auditory comprehension of language in young children: neural networks identified with fMRI. Neurology. 2003;60(10):1598–605.
65. Gaillard WD, Berl MM, Moore EN, et al. Atypical language in lesional and nonlesional complex partial epilepsy. Neurology. 2007;69(18):1761–71.
66. Rutten GJ, van Rijen PC, van Veelen CW, Ramsey NF. Language area localization with three-dimensional functional magnetic resonance imaging matches intrasulcal electrostimulation in Broca's area. Ann Neurol. 1999;46(3):405–8.
67. Turkeltaub PE, Flowers DL, Lyon LG, Eden GF. Development of ventral stream representations for single letters. Ann NY Acad Sci. 2008;1145: 13–29.
68. Ulualp SO, Biswal BB, Yetkin FZ, Kidder TM. Functional magnetic resonance imaging of auditory cortex in children. Laryngoscope. 1998;108(12): 1782–6.
69. Kansaku K, Yamaura A, Kitazawa S. Sex differences in lateralization revealed in the posterior language areas. Cereb Cortex. 2000;10(9):866–72.
70. Gaillard WD, Pugliese M, Grandin CB, et al. Cortical localization of reading in normal children: an fMRI language study. Neurology. 2001;57(1): 47–54.
71. Ojemann GA. Cortical organization of language. J Neurosci. 1991;11(8):2281–7.
72. Sanai N, Mirzadeh Z, Berger MS. Functional outcome after language mapping for glioma resection. N Engl J Med. 2008;358(1):18–27.
73. Boakye M, Huckins SC, Szeverenyi NM, Taskey BI, Hodge Jr CJ. Functional magnetic resonance imaging of somatosensory cortex activity produced by electrical stimulation of the median nerve or tactile stimulation of the index finger. J Neurosurg. 2000; 93(5):774–83.
74. Chapman SB, McKinnon L. Discussion of developmental plasticity: factors affecting cognitive outcome after pediatric traumatic brain injury. J Commun Disord. 2000;33(4):333–44.
75. Jacobs KM, Graber KD, Kharazia VN, Parada I, Prince DA. Postlesional epilepsy: the ultimate brain plasticity. Epilepsia. 2000;41 Suppl 6:S153–61.
76. Schwartzkroin PA. Mechanisms of brain plasticity: from normal brain function to pathology. Int Rev Neurobiol. 2001;45:1–15.
77. Benbadis SR, Binder JR, Swanson SJ, et al. Is speech arrest during wada testing a valid method for determining hemispheric representation of language? Brain Lang. 1998;65(3):441–6.
78. Yetkin FZ, Swanson S, Fischer M, et al. Functional MR of frontal lobe activation: comparison with Wada language results. AJNR Am J Neuroradiol. 1998;19(6):1095–8.
79. Spreer J, Arnold S, Quiske A, et al. Determination of hemisphere dominance for language: comparison of frontal and temporal fMRI activation with intracarotid amytal testing. Neuroradiology. 2002;44(6): 467–74.
80. Woermann FG, Jokeit H, Luerding R, et al. Language lateralization by Wada test and fMRI in 100 patients with epilepsy. Neurology. 2003;61(5): 699–701.
81. Baciu MV, Watson JM, Maccotta L, et al. Evaluating functional MRI procedures for assessing hemispheric language dominance in neurosurgical patients. Neuroradiology. 2005;47(11):835–44.
82. Arora J, Pugh K, Westerveld M, Spencer S, Spencer DD, Todd Constable R. Language lateralization in epilepsy patients: fMRI validated with the Wada procedure. Epilepsia. 2009;50:2225–41.
83. Benke T, Köylü B, Visani P, et al. Language lateralization in temporal lobe epilepsy: a comparison between fMRI and the Wada Test. Epilepsia. 2006; 47(8):1308–19.

84. Kho KH, Leijten FS, Rutten GJ, Vermeulen J, Van Rijen P, Ramsey NF. Discrepant findings for Wada test and functional magnetic resonance imaging with regard to language function: use of electrocortical stimulation mapping to confirm results. Case report. J Neurosurg. 2005;102(1):169–73.
85. Lanzenberger R, Wiest G, Geissler A, et al. FMRI reveals functional cortex in a case of inconclusive Wada testing. Clin Neurol Neurosurg. 2005;107(2): 147–51.
86. Ruge MI, Victor J, Hosain S, et al. Concordance between functional magnetic resonance imaging and intraoperative language mapping. Stereotact Funct Neurosurg. 1999;72(2–4):95–102.
87. Schlosser MJ, Luby M, Spencer DD, Awad IA, McCarthy G. Comparative localization of auditory comprehension by using functional magnetic resonance imaging and cortical stimulation. J Neurosurg. 1999;91(4):626–35.
88. Jayakar P, Bernal B, Santiago Medina L, Altman N. False lateralization of language cortex on functional MRI after a cluster of focal seizures. Neurology. 2002;58(3):490–2.
89. Kang HC, Burgund ED, Lugar HM, Petersen SE, Schlaggar BL. Comparison of functional activation foci in children and adults using a common stereotactic space. Neuroimage. 2003;19(1):16–28.
90. Ferretti A, Del Gratta C, Babiloni C, et al. Functional topography of the secondary somatosensory cortex for nonpainful and painful stimulation of median and tibial nerve: an fMRI study. Neuroimage. 2004;23(3):1217–25.
91. Manganotti P, Formaggio E, Storti SF, et al. Steady-state activation in somatosensory cortex after changes in stimulus rate during median nerve stimulation. Magn Reson Imaging. 2009;27:1175–86.
92. Eilers RE, Minifie FD. Fricative discrimination in early infancy. J Speech Hear Res. 1975;18(1): 158–67.
93. Hohne EA, Jusczyk PW. Two-month-old infants' sensitivity to allophonic differences. Percept Psychophys. 1994;56(6):613–23.
94. Hirsch J, Ruge MI, Kim KH, et al. An integrated functional magnetic resonance imaging procedure for preoperative mapping of cortical areas associated with tactile, motor, language, and visual functions. Neurosurgery. 2000;47(3):711–21. discussion 721–2.
95. Rivkin MJ, Vajapeyam S, Hutton C, et al. A functional magnetic resonance imaging study of paced finger tapping in children. Pediatr Neurol. 2003; 28(2):89–95.
96. Ullen F, Forssberg H, Ehrsson HH. Neural networks for the coordination of the hands in time. J Neurophysiol. 2003;89(2):1126–35.
97. Mostofsky SH, Rimrodt SL, Schafer JG, et al. Atypical motor and sensory cortex activation in attention-deficit/hyperactivity disorder: a functional magnetic resonance imaging study of simple sequential finger tapping. Biol Psychiatry. 2006;59(1): 48–56.
98. Lee CC, Jack Jr CR, Riederer SJ. Mapping of the central sulcus with functional MR: active versus passive activation tasks. AJNR Am J Neuroradiol. 1998;19(5):847–52.
99. Roux FE, Ibarrola D, Lazorthes Y, Berry I. Chronic motor cortex stimulation for phantom limb pain: a functional magnetic resonance imaging study: technical case report. Neurosurgery. 2001;48(3):681–7. discussion 687–8.
100. Hoeller M, Krings T, Reinges MH, Hans FJ, Gilsbach JM, Thron A. Movement artefacts and MR BOLD signal increase during different paradigms for mapping the sensorimotor cortex. Acta Neurochir (Wien). 2002;144(3):279–84. discussion 284.
101. Krings T, Töpper R, Willmes K, Reinges MH, Gilsbach JM, Thron A. Activation in primary and secondary motor areas in patients with CNS neoplasms and weakness. Neurology. 2002;58(3): 381–90.
102. Fandino J, Kollias SS, Wieser HG, Valavanis A, Yonekawa Y. Intraoperative validation of functional magnetic resonance imaging and cortical reorganization patterns in patients with brain tumors involving the primary motor cortex. J Neurosurg. 1999;91(2):238–50.
103. Carpentier AC, Constable RT, Schlosser MJ, et al. Patterns of functional magnetic resonance imaging activation in association with structural lesions in the rolandic region: a classification system. J Neurosurg. 2001;94(6):946–54.
104. Vandermeeren Y, De Volder A, Bastings E, et al. Functional relevance of abnormal fMRI activation pattern after unilateral schizencephaly. Neuroreport. 2002;13(14):1821–4.
105. Staudt M, Pieper T, Grodd W, Winkler P, Holthausen H, Krägeloh-Mann I. Functional MRI in a 6-year-old boy with unilateral cortical malformation: concordant representation of both hands in the unaffected hemisphere. Neuropediatrics. 2001;32(3):159–61.
106. Hartnick CJ, Rudolph C, Willging JP, Holland SK. Functional magnetic resonance imaging of the pediatric swallow: imaging the cortex and the brainstem. Laryngoscope. 2001;111(7):1183–91.
107. Puce A. Comparative assessment of sensorimotor function using functional magnetic resonance imaging and electrophysiological methods. J Clin Neurophysiol. 1995;12(5):450–9.
108. Puce A, Constable RT, Luby ML, et al. Functional magnetic resonance imaging of sensory and motor cortex: comparison with electrophysiological localization. J Neurosurg. 1995;83(2):262–70.
109. Yousry T, Schmid UD, Schmidt D, et al. The motor hand area. Noninvasive detection with functional MRI and surgical validation with cortical stimulation. Radiologe. 1995;35(4):252–5.
110. Deuchert M, Ruben J, Schwiemann J, et al. Event-related fMRI of the somatosensory system using

electrical finger stimulation. Neuroreport. 2002; 13(3):365–9.
111. Born AP, Law I, Lund TE, et al. Cortical deactivation induced by visual stimulation in human slow-wave sleep. Neuroimage. 2002;17(3):1325–35.
112. Meek JH, Firbank M, Elwell CE, Atkinson J, Braddick O, Wyatt JS. Regional hemodynamic responses to visual stimulation in awake infants. Pediatr Res. 1998;43(6):840–3.
113. Born AP, Rostrup E, Miranda MJ, Larsson HB, Lou HC. Visual cortex reactivity in sedated children examined with perfusion MRI (FAIR). Magn Reson Imaging. 2002;20(2):199–205.
114. Marcar VL, Strässle AE, Loenneker T, Schwarz U, Martin E. The influence of cortical maturation on the BOLD response: an fMRI study of visual cortex in children. Pediatr Res. 2004;56(6):967–74.
115. Yeh CI, Xing D, Shapley RM. "Black" responses dominate macaque primary visual cortex v1. J Neurosci. 2009;29(38):11753–60.
116. Wiesel TN, Hubel DH. Spatial and chromatic interactions in the lateral geniculate body of the rhesus monkey. J Neurophysiol. 1966;29(6):1115–56.
117. Bedwell JS, Miller LS, Brown JM, Yanasak NE. Schizophrenia and red light: fMRI evidence for a novel biobehavioral marker. Int J Neurosci. 2006;116(8):881–94.
118. Wang X, Takano T, Nedergaard M. Astrocytic calcium signaling: mechanism and implications for functional brain imaging. Methods Mol Biol. 2009;489:93–109.
119. Miki A, Liu GT, Fletcher DW, Hunter JV, Haselgrove JC. Ocular dominance in anterior visual cortex in a child demonstrated by the use of fMRI. Pediatr Neurol. 2001;24(3):232–4.
120. Sie LTL, Rombouts SA, Valk IJ, Hart AA, Scheltens P, van der Knaap MS. Functional MRI of visual cortex in sedated 18 month-old infants with or without periventricular leukomalacia. Dev Med Child Neurol. 2001;43(7):486–90.
121. Liu GT, Miki A, Francis E, et al. Eye dominance in visual cortex in amblyopia using functional magnetic resonance imaging. J AAPOS. 2004;8(2): 184–6.
122. Choi MY, Lee KM, Hwang JM, et al. Comparison between anisometropic and strabismic amblyopia using functional magnetic resonance imaging. Br J Ophthalmol. 2001;85(9):1052–6.
123. Miki A, Nakajima T, Hasebe H, Abe H. Functional magnetic resonance imaging of visual function in postpapilledema optic atrophy. J Neuroophthalmol. 1997;17(4):223–5.
124. Born AP, Miranda MJ, Rostrup E, et al. Functional magnetic resonance imaging of the normal and abnormal visual system in early life. Neuropediatrics. 2000;31(1):24–32.
125. Bernal B, Altman N. Visual functional magnetic resonance imaging in patients with Sturge-Weber syndrome. Pediatr Neurol. 2004;31(1):9–15.
126. Sininger YS, Doyle KJ, Moore JK. The case for early identification of hearing loss in children. Auditory system development, experimental auditory deprivation, and development of speech perception and hearing. Pediatr Clin North Am. 1999;46(1):1–14.
127. Paradise JL, Dollaghan CA, Campbell TF, et al. Language, speech sound production, and cognition in three-year-old children in relation to otitis media in their first three years of life. Pediatrics. 2000;105(5):1119–30.
128. Anderson AW, Marois R, Colson ER, et al. Neonatal auditory activation detected by functional magnetic resonance imaging. Magn Reson Imaging. 2001; 19(1):1–5.
129. Spreen O, Risser A, Edgell D. Developmental neuropsychology. USA: Oxford University Press; 1995.
130. Johansson B, Wedenberg E, Westin B. Measurement of tone response by the human foetus. A preliminary report. Acta Otolaryngol. 1964;57:188–92.
131. Hykin J, Moore R, Duncan K, et al. Fetal brain activity demonstrated by functional magnetic resonance imaging. Lancet. 1999;354(9179):645–6.
132. Moore RJ, Vadeyar S, Fulford J, et al. Antenatal determination of fetal brain activity in response to an acoustic stimulus using functional magnetic resonance imaging. Hum Brain Mapp. 2001;12(2):94–9.
133. Fulford J, Vadeyar SH, Dodampahala SH, et al. Fetal brain activity and hemodynamic response to a vibroacoustic stimulus. Hum Brain Mapp. 2004;22(2): 116–21.
134. Jardri R, Pins D, Thomas P. A case of fMRI-guided rTMS treatment of coenesthetic hallucinations. Am J Psychiatry. 2008;165(11):1490–1.
135. Patel AM, Cahill LD, Ret J, Schmithorst V, Choo D, Holland S. Functional magnetic resonance imaging of hearing-impaired children under sedation before cochlear implantation. Arch Otolaryngol Head Neck Surg. 2007;133(7):677–83.
136. Thomason ME, Race E, Burrows B, Whitfield-Gabrieli S, Glover GH, Gabrieli JD. Development of spatial and verbal working memory capacity in the human brain. J Cogn Neurosci. 2009;21(2): 316–32.
137. Nelson CA, Monk CS, Lin J, Carver LJ, Thomas KM, Truwit CL. Functional neuroanatomy of spatial working memory in children. Dev Psychol. 2000; 36(1):109–16.
138. Geier CF, Garver K, Terwilliger R, Luna B. Development of working memory maintenance. J Neurophysiol. 2009;101(1):84–99.
139. Libertus ME, Brannon EM, Pelphrey KA. Developmental changes in category-specific brain responses to numbers and letters in a working memory task. Neuroimage. 2009;44(4):1404–14.
140. O'Hare ED, Lu LH, Houston SM, Bookheimer SY, Sowell ER. Neurodevelopmental changes in verbal working memory load-dependency: an fMRI investigation. Neuroimage. 2008;42(4):1678–85.

141. Golby AJ, Poldrack RA, Illes J, Chen D, Desmond JE, Gabrieli JD. Memory lateralization in medial temporal lobe epilepsy assessed by functional MRI. Epilepsia. 2002;43(8):855–63.
142. Jokeit H, Okujava M, Woermann FG. Memory fMRI lateralizes temporal lobe epilepsy. Neurology. 2001;57(10):1786–93.
143. Booth JR, Burman DD, Meyer JR, et al. Neural development of selective attention and response inhibition. Neuroimage. 2003;20(2):737–51.
144. Konrad K, Neufang S, Thiel CM, et al. Development of attentional networks: an fMRI study with children and adults. Neuroimage. 2005;28(2):429–39.
145. Lawrence EJ, Rubia K, Murray RM, et al. The neural basis of response inhibition and attention allocation as mediated by gestational age. Hum Brain Mapp. 2009;30(3):1038–50.
146. Ciesielski KT, Lesnik PG, Savoy RL, Grant EP, Ahlfors SP. Developmental neural networks in children performing a categorical N-back task. Neuroimage. 2006;33(3):980–90.
147. Marsh R, Zhu H, Schultz RT, et al. A developmental fMRI study of self-regulatory control. Hum Brain Mapp. 2006;27(11):848–63.
148. Rubia K, Smith AB, Taylor E, Brammer M. Linear age-correlated functional development of right inferior fronto-striato-cerebellar networks during response inhibition and anterior cingulate during error-related processes. Hum Brain Mapp. 2007; 28(11):1163–77.
149. Crone EA, Zanolie K, Van Leijenhorst L, Westenberg PM, Rombouts SA. Neural mechanisms supporting flexible performance adjustment during development. Cogn Affect Behav Neurosci. 2008;8(2): 165–77.
150. van Duijvenvoorde AC, Zanolie K, Rombouts SA, Raijmakers ME, Crone EA. Evaluating the negative or valuing the positive? Neural mechanisms supporting feedback-based learning across development. J Neurosci. 2008;28(38):9495–503.
151. Eslinger PJ, Blair C, Wang J, et al. Developmental shifts in fMRI activations during visuospatial relational reasoning. Brain Cogn. 2009;69(1):1–10.
152. Jackson GD, Connelly A, Cross JH, Gordon I, Gadian DG. Functional magnetic resonance imaging of focal seizures. Neurology. 1994;44(5):850–6.
153. Schwartz TH, Resor Jr SR, De La Paz R, Goodman RR. Functional magnetic resonance imaging localization of ictal onset to a dysplastic cleft with simultaneous sensorimotor mapping: intraoperative electrophysiological confirmation and postoperative follow-up: technical note. Neurosurgery. 1998;43(3):639–44. discussion 644–5.
154. Liu Y, Yang T, Liao W, et al. EEG-fMRI study of the ictal and interictal epileptic activity in patients with eyelid myoclonia with absences. Epilepsia. 2008;49(12):2078–86.
155. Leal AJ, Monteiro JP, Secca MF, Jordão C. Functional brain mapping of ictal activity in gelastic epilepsy associated with hypothalamic hamartoma: a case report. Epilepsia. 2009;50(6):1624–31.
156. Detre JA, Sirven JI, Alsop DC, O'Connor MJ, French JA. Localization of subclinical ictal activity by functional magnetic resonance imaging: correlation with invasive monitoring. Ann Neurol. 1995; 38(4):618–24.
157. Seeck M, Lazeyras F, Michel CM, et al. Non-invasive epileptic focus localization using EEG-triggered functional MRI and electromagnetic tomography. Electroencephalogr Clin Neurophysiol. 1998;106(6):508–12.
158. Krakow K, Woermann FG, Symms MR, et al. EEG-triggered functional MRI of interictal epileptiform activity in patients with partial seizures. Brain. 1999;122(Pt 9):1679–88.
159. Lazeyras F, Blanke O, Perrig S, et al. EEG-triggered functional MRI in patients with pharmacoresistant epilepsy. J Magn Reson Imaging. 2000;12(1): 177–85.
160. Leal A, Dias A, Vieira JP, Secca M, Jordão C. The BOLD effect of interictal spike activity in childhood occipital lobe epilepsy. Epilepsia. 2006;47(9): 1536–42.
161. Masuoka LK, Anderson AW, Gore JC, McCarthy G, Spencer DD, Novotny EJ. Functional magnetic resonance imaging identifies abnormal visual cortical function in patients with occipital lobe epilepsy. Epilepsia. 1999;40(9):1248–53.
162. Müller RA, Kleinhans N, Kemmotsu N, Pierce K, Courchesne E. Abnormal variability and distribution of functional maps in autism: an FMRI study of visuomotor learning. Am J Psychiatry. 2003;160(10): 1847–62.
163. Schultz RT, Gauthier I, Klin A, et al. Abnormal ventral temporal cortical activity during face discrimination among individuals with autism and Asperger syndrome. Arch Gen Psychiatry. 2000;57(4): 331–40.
164. Schultz RT, Grelotti DJ, Klin A, et al. The role of the fusiform face area in social cognition: implications for the pathobiology of autism. Philos Trans R Soc Lond B Biol Sci. 2003;358(1430):415–27.
165. Grelotti DJ, Klin AJ, Gauthier I, et al. fMRI activation of the fusiform gyrus and amygdala to cartoon characters but not to faces in a boy with autism. Neuropsychologia. 2005;43(3):373–85.
166. Bölte S, Hubl D, Feineis-Matthews S, Prvulovic D, Dierks T, Poustka F. Facial affect recognition training in autism: can we animate the fusiform gyrus? Behav Neurosci. 2006;120(1):211–6.
167. Takeuchi M, Harada M, Matsuzaki K, Nishitani H, Mori K. Difference of signal change by a language task on autistic patients using functional MRI. J Med Invest. 2004;51(1–2):59–62.
168. Gomot M, Bernard FA, Davis MH, et al. Change detection in children with autism: an auditory event-related fMRI study. Neuroimage. 2006;29(2): 475–84.

169. Müller RA, Pierce K, Ambrose JB, Allen G, Courchesne E. Atypical patterns of cerebral motor activation in autism: a functional magnetic resonance study. Biol Psychiatry. 2001;49(8):665–76.
170. Dapretto M, Davies MS, Pfeifer JH, et al. Understanding emotions in others: mirror neuron dysfunction in children with autism spectrum disorders. Nat Neurosci. 2006;9(1):28–30.
171. Baron-Cohen S, Ring H, Chitnis X, et al. fMRI of parents of children with Asperger Syndrome: a pilot study. Brain Cogn. 2006;61(1):122–30.
172. Baumeister AA, Hawkins MF. Incoherence of neuroimaging studies of attention deficit/hyperactivity disorder. Clin Neuropharmacol. 2001;24(1):2–10.
173. Sunshine JL, Lewin JS, Wu DH, et al. Functional MR to localize sustained visual attention activation in patients with attention deficit hyperactivity disorder: a pilot study. AJNR Am J Neuroradiol. 1997;18(4):633–7.
174. Booth JR, Burman DD, Meyer JR, et al. Larger deficits in brain networks for response inhibition than for visual selective attention in attention deficit hyperactivity disorder (ADHD). J Child Psychol Psychiatry. 2005;46(1):94–111.
175. Durston S, Tottenham NT, Thomas KM, et al. Differential patterns of striatal activation in young children with and without ADHD. Biol Psychiatry. 2003;53(10):871–8.
176. Vaidya CJ, Austin G, Kirkorian G, et al. Selective effects of methylphenidate in attention deficit hyperactivity disorder: a functional magnetic resonance study. Proc Natl Acad Sci USA. 1998;95(24):14494–9.
177. Rubia K, Smith AB, Brammer MJ, Toone B, Taylor E. Abnormal brain activation during inhibition and error detection in medication-naive adolescents with ADHD. Am J Psychiatry. 2005;162(6):1067–75.
178. Rodriguez PD, Baylis GC. Activation of brain attention systems in individuals with symptoms of ADHD. Behav Neurol. 2007;18(2):115–30.
179. Bush G, Frazier JA, Rauch SL, et al. Anterior cingulate cortex dysfunction in attention-deficit/hyperactivity disorder revealed by fMRI and the Counting Stroop. Biol Psychiatry. 1999;45(12):1542–52.
180. Vaidya CJ, Bunge SA, Dudukovic NM, Zalecki CA, Elliott GR, Gabrieli JD. Altered neural substrates of cognitive control in childhood ADHD: evidence from functional magnetic resonance imaging. Am J Psychiatry. 2005;162(9):1605–13.
181. Bernal B, Altman N. Neural networks of motor and cognitive inhibition are dissociated between brain hemispheres: an fMRI study. Int J Neurosci. 2009;119(10):1848–80.
182. Peterson BS, Skudlarski P, Gatenby JC, Zhang H, Anderson AW, Gore JC. An fMRI study of Stroop word-color interference: evidence for cingulate subregions subserving multiple distributed attentional systems. Biol Psychiatry. 1999;45(10):1237–58.
183. Solanto MV, Schulz KP, Fan J, Tang CY, Newcorn JH. Event-related FMRI of inhibitory control in the predominantly inattentive and combined subtypes of ADHD. J Neuroimaging. 2009;19(3):205–12.
184. Bernal B, Altman N. Neural networks of motor and cognitive inhibition are dissociated between brain hemispheres: an fMRI study. Int J Neurosci. 2009;119(10):1848–80.
185. Rubia K, Halari R, Cubillo A, Mohammad AM, Brammer M, Taylor E. Methylphenidate normalises activation and functional connectivity deficits in attention and motivation networks in medication-naive children with ADHD during a rewarded continuous performance task. Neuropharmacology. 2009;57(7–8):640–52.
186. Temple E, Poldrack RA, Salidis J, et al. Disrupted neural responses to phonological and orthographic processing in dyslexic children: an fMRI study. Neuroreport. 2001;12(2):299–307.
187. Backes W, Vuurman E, Wennekes R, et al. Atypical brain activation of reading processes in children with developmental dyslexia. J Child Neurol. 2002;17(12):867–71.
188. Aylward EH, Richards TL, Berninger VW, et al. Instructional treatment associated with changes in brain activation in children with dyslexia. Neurology. 2003;61(2):212–9.
189 Cao F, Bitan T, Chou TL, Burman DD, Booth JR. Deficient orthographic and phonological representations in children with dyslexia revealed by brain activation patterns. J Child Psychol Psychiatry. 2006;47(10):1041–50.
190. Gaab N, Gabrieli JD, Deutsch GK, Tallal P, Temple E. Neural correlates of rapid auditory processing are disrupted in children with developmental dyslexia and ameliorated with training: an fMRI study. Restor Neurol Neurosci. 2007;25(3–4):295–310.
191. Baillieux H, Vandervliet EJ, Manto M, Parizel PM, De Deyn PP, Mariën P. Developmental dyslexia and widespread activation across the cerebellar hemispheres. Brain Lang. 2009;108(2):122–32.
192. Schneider G. Early lesions and abnormal neuronal connections. Trends Neurosci. 1981;4(18):192.
193. Hebb D. The effect of early and late brain injury upon test scores, and the nature of normal adult intelligence. Proc Am Philos Soc. 1942;85:275–92.
194. Mills DL, Coffey-Corina SA, Neville HJ. Variability in cerebral organization during primary language acquisition. In: Dawson G, Fischer KW, editors. Human behavior and the developing brain. New York: The Guilford Press; 1994. p. 427–55.
195. Papanicolaou AC, Simos PG, Breier JI, et al. Brain plasticity for sensory and linguistic functions: a functional imaging study using magnetoencephalography with children and young adults. J Child Neurol. 2001;16(4):241–52.
196. Lewine JD, Astur RS, Davis LE, Knight JE, Maclin EL, Orrison Jr WW. Cortical organization in adulthood is modified by neonatal infarct: a case study. Radiology. 1994;190(1):93–6.
197. Carr LJ, Harrison LM, Evans AL, Stephens JA. Patterns of central motor reorganization in

hemiplegic cerebral palsy. Brain. 1993;116(Pt 5): 1223–47.

198. Benecke R, Meyer BU. Magnetic stimulation of corticonuclear systems and of cranial nerves in man: physiological basis and clinical application. Electroencephalogr Clin Neurophysiol Suppl. 1991;43:333–43.

199. Müller RA, Rothermel RD, Behen ME, et al. Brain organization of language after early unilateral lesion: a PET study. Brain Lang. 1998;62(3):422–51.

200. Müller RA, Rothermel RD, Behen ME, Muzik O, Mangner TJ, Chugani HT. Differential patterns of language and motor reorganization following early left hemisphere lesion: a PET study. Arch Neurol. 1998;55(8):1113–9.

201. Müller RA, Rothermel RD, Behen ME, Muzik O, Chakraborty PK, Chugani HT. Language organization in patients with early and lateleft-hemisphere lesion: a PET study. Neuropsychologia. 1999; 37(5):545–57.

202. Hertz-Pannier L. Brain plasticity during development: physiological bases and functional MRI approach. J Neuroradiol. 1999;26(1 Suppl):S66–74.

203. Hertz-Pannier L, Chiron C, Jambaqué I, et al. Late plasticity for language in a child's non-dominant hemisphere: a pre-and post-surgery fMRI study. Brain. 2002;125(2):361.

204. Staudt M, Grodd W, Gerloff C, Erb M, Stitz J, Krägeloh-Mann I. Two types of ipsilateral reorganization in congenital hemiparesis: a TMS and fMRI study. Brain. 2002;125(Pt 10):2222–37.

205. Anderson DP, Harvey AS, Saling MM, et al. FMRI lateralization of expressive language in children with cerebral lesions. Epilepsia. 2006;47(6):998–1008.

206. Hadac J, Brozová K, Tintera J, Krsek P. Language lateralization in children with pre- and postnatal epileptogenic lesions of the left hemisphere: an fMRI study. Epileptic Disord. 2007;9 Suppl 1:S19–27.

207 Guzzetta A, Pecini C, Biagi L, et al. Language organisation in left perinatal stroke. Neuropediatrics. 2008;39(3):157–63.

208. Staudt M, Grodd W, Niemann G, Wildgruber D, Erb M, Krägeloh-Mann I. Early left periventricular brain lesions induce right hemispheric organization of speech. Neurology. 2001;57(1):122–5.

209. Hamzei F, Liepert J, Dettmers C, Adler T, Kiebel S, Rijntjes M, et al. Structural and functional cortical abnormalities after upper limb amputation during childhood. Neuroreport. 2001;12(5):957–62.

210. Iwase Y, Mashiko T, Ochiai N, Kurosawa H. Postoperative changes on functional mapping of the motor cortex in patients with brachial plexus injury: comparative study of magnetoencephalography and functional magnetic resonance imaging. J Orthop Sci. 2001;6(5):397–402.

211. Crawford D, Acuna J, Sherman S. FMRI and fragile X syndrome: human genome epidemiology. Review. Genet Med. 2001;3:359–71.

212. Guerreiro MM, Camargo EE, Kato M, et al. Fragile X syndrome. Clinical, electroencephalographic and neuroimaging characteristics. Arq Neuropsiquiatr. 1998;56(1):18–23.

213. Eliez S, Blasey CM, Freund LS, Hastie T, Reiss AL. Brain anatomy, gender and IQ in children and adolescents with fragile X syndrome. Brain. 2001;124(Pt 8):1610–8.

214. Tamm L, Menon V, Johnston CK, Hessl DR, Reiss AL. fMRI study of cognitive interference processing in females with fragile X syndrome. J Cogn Neurosci. 2002;14(2):160–71.

215. Swerdlow NR, Karban B, Ploum Y, Sharp R, Geyer MA, Eastvold A. Tactile prepuff inhibition of startle in children with Tourette's syndrome: in search of an "fMRI-friendly" startle paradigm. Biol Psychiatry. 2001;50(8):578–85.

216. Marsh R, Zhu H, Wang Z, Skudlarski P, Peterson BS. A developmental fMRI study of self-regulatory control in Tourette's syndrome. Am J Psychiatry. 2007;164(6):955–66.

217. Baym CL, Corbett BA, Wright SB, Bunge SA. Neural correlates of tic severity and cognitive control in children with Tourette syndrome. Brain. 2008;131(Pt 1):165–79.

218. Biswal B, Ulmer JL, Krippendorf RL, et al. Abnormal cerebral activation associated with a motor task in Tourette syndrome. AJNR Am J Neuroradiol. 1998;19(8):1509–12.

219. Epstein JN, Casey BJ, Tonev ST, et al. ADHD- and medication-related brain activation effects in concordantly affected parent-child dyads with ADHD. J Child Psychol Psychiatry. 2007;48(9):899–913.

220. Arwert LI, Veltman DJ, Deijen JB, van Dam PS, Drent ML. Effects of growth hormone substitution therapy on cognitive functioning in growth hormone deficient patients: a functional MRI study. Neuroendocrinology. 2006;83(1):12–9.

221. Chang K, Karchemskiy A, Kelley R, et al. Effect of divalproex on brain morphometry, chemistry, and function in youth at high-risk for bipolar disorder: a pilot study. J Child Adolesc Psychopharmacol. 2009;19(1):51–9.

222. Peterson BS, Potenza MN, Wang Z, et al. An FMRI study of the effects of psychostimulants on default-mode processing during Stroop task performance in youths with ADHD. Am J Psychiatry. 2009; 166(11):1286–94.

223. McKeown MJ, Makeig S, Brown GG, et al. Analysis of fMRI data by blind separation into independent spatial components. Hum Brain Mapp. 1998;6(3): 160–88.

224. Beckmann CF, DeLuca M, Devlin JT, Smith SM. Investigations into resting-state connectivity using independent component analysis. Philos Trans R Soc Lond B Biol Sci. 2005;360(1457):1001–13.

225. Fransson P, Skiöld B, Engström M, et al. Spontaneous brain activity in the newborn brain during natural sleep – an fMRI study in infants born at full term. Pediatr Res. 2009;66:301–5.

226. Redcay E, Kennedy D, Courchesne E. fMRI during natural sleep as a method to study brain function

during early childhood. Neuroimage. 2007;38(4): 696–707.
227. Kiviniemi V, Jauhiainen J, Tervonen O, et al. Slow vasomotor fluctuation in fMRI of anesthetized child brain. Magn Reson Med. 2000;44(3):373–8.
228. Kiviniemi V, Kantola JH, Jauhiainen J, Hyvärinen A, Tervonen O. Independent component analysis of nondeterministic fMRI signal sources. Neuroimage. 2003;19(2 Pt 1):253–60.
229. Harrison BJ, Pujol J, López-Solà M, et al. Consistency and functional specialization in the default mode brain network. Proc Natl Acad Sci USA. 2008;105(28):9781–6.
230. Greicius MD, Krasnow B, Reiss AL, Menon V. Functional connectivity in the resting brain: a network analysis of the default mode hypothesis. Proc Natl Acad Sci USA. 2003;100(1):253.
231. Vuontela V, Steenari MR, Aronen ET, Korvenoja A, Aronen HJ, Carlson S. Brain activation and deactivation during location and color working memory tasks in 11–13-year-old children. Brain Cogn. 2009;69(1):56–64.
232. Fox MD, Zhang D, Snyder AZ, Raichle ME. The global signal and observed anticorrelated resting state brain networks. J Neurophysiol. 2009; 101(6):3270–83.
233. Tian L, Jiang T, Wang Y, et al. Altered resting-state functional connectivity patterns of anterior cingulate cortex in adolescents with attention deficit hyperactivity disorder. Neurosci Lett. 2006;400(1–2): 39–43.
234. Zang YF, He Y, Zhu CZ, et al. Altered baseline brain activity in children with ADHD revealed by resting-state functional MRI. Brain Dev. 2007;29(2):83–91.
235. Cao Q, Zang Y, Sun L, Sui M, Long X, Zou Q, et al. Abnormal neural activity in children with attention deficit hyperactivity disorder: a resting-state functional magnetic resonance imaging study. Neuroreport. 2006;17(10):1033–6.
236. Peterson BS, Potenza MN, Wang Z, et al. An fMRI study of the effects of psychostimulants on default-mode processing during Stroop task performance in youths with ADHD. Am J Psychiatry. 2009; 166:1286–94.
237. Fair DA, Cohen AL, Power JD, et al. Functional brain networks develop from a "local to distributed" organization. PLoS Comput Biol. 2009;5(5): e1000381.
238. Lin W, Zhu Q, Gao W, et al. Functional connectivity MR imaging reveals cortical functional connectivity in the developing brain. AJNR Am J Neuroradiol. 2008;29(10):1883–9.
239. Cao X, Cao Q, Long X, et al. Abnormal resting-state functional connectivity patterns of the putamen in medication-naive children with attention deficit hyperactivity disorder. Brain Res. 2009;1303: 195–206.
240. Kennedy DP, Redcay E, Courchesne E. Failing to deactivate: resting functional abnormalities in autism. Proc Natl Acad Sci USA. 2006;103(21):8275–80.
241. Monk CS, Peltier SJ, Wiggins JL, et al. Abnormalities of intrinsic functional connectivity in autism spectrum disorders. Neuroimage. 2009;47(2):764–72.
242. Shimony JS, Zhang D, Johnston JM, Fox MD, Roy A, Leuthardt EC. Resting-state spontaneous fluctuations in brain activity: a new paradigm for presurgical planning using fMRI. Acad Radiol. 2009; 16(5):578–83.

fMRI of the Central Auditory System

15

Deborah A. Hall

Introduction

During the last two decades, auditory neuroscience has made significant progress in understanding the functional organization of the auditory system in both normally hearing listeners and patients with sensorineural hearing impairments. Modern brain imaging techniques have made an enormous contribution to that progress by enabling the in vivo study of human central auditory function. Significant contributions have come from positron emission tomography (PET), functional magnetic resonance imaging (fMRI), electroencephalography (EEG), and magnetoencephalography (MEG). Of these four, fMRI has become the tool of choice for addressing many research questions including those of auditory neuroscience. First, fMRI is suitable for research use with children as well as adults. Second, since multiple observations can be made on the same individual, fMRI permits the investigation of longer-term dynamic processes, such as functional plasticity after disease, damage, retraining, or therapy. Third, the need for averaging data across individuals is reduced, further improving the accuracy with which activations can be mapped onto subject-specific brain structure.

To date, auditory fMRI has not been widely implemented for routine clinical purposes. However, there is a growing literature on its potential clinical application. To enhance the clinical use of auditory fMRI, standardized protocols are required that are easy and quick to use with patients and yield robust replicable results. From the auditory fMRI research with normally hearing subjects, we can now transfer the most efficient protocols to study patients with hearing impairment. For example, we know which acoustic stimuli (such as temporally varying, broadband sounds presented at a level that is clearly audible) generate robust auditory activation. In addition, it has been shown that patients are more easily able to comply with a passive listening task rather than one that requires a decision or an active response, particularly if the patient is liable to make errors. A material obstacle for efficient auditory fMRI, in general, is the intense scanner acoustic sound generated during image acquisition. The background sound reduces the sensitivity for detecting stimulus-evoked activation and can be particularly troublesome for those patients who are averse to noisy environments. Acoustic reduction methods have been developed for auditory fMRI and the availability of these methods is now facilitating clinical fMRI applications.

This chapter discusses some of the theoretical and technical challenges of auditory fMRI and

D.A. Hall, BSc, PhD (✉)
National Biomedical Research Unit in Hearing, Ropewalk House, 113 The Ropewalk, Nottingham NG1 5DU, UK

Division of Psychology, School of Social Sciences, Nottingham Trent University, Nottingham NG1 4BU, UK
e-mail: deb.hall@nottingham.ac.uk

S.H. Faro and F.B. Mohamed (eds.), *Functional BOLD MRI: Principles and Applications*, DOI 10.1007/978-1-4939-1995-6_15, © Springer Science+Business Media New York 2015

some of the major clinical applications within this field. Challenges include the intense scanner acoustic sound and the effects of the magnetic field on sound delivery equipment and on electronic hearing devices. Clinical applications of auditory fMRI embrace the preoperative or intraoperative mapping of functional areas relevant to spoken language (for example, for planning surgical intervention to relieve chronic epileptic seizures), in the study of involuntary auditory hallucinations in schizophrenia and in the investigation of reorganization of spoken language processing after temporal lobe lesions. This research often evaluates patterns of distributed brain activation, including regions responsible for sound processing and for speech perception and production. This chapter reviews only several of those major clinical applications of fMRI that investigate the processing of basic (i.e., nonlinguistic) sound features. Specifically, these include studies of the functional reorganization of the central auditory system as a consequence of adaptation to hearing loss and its remediation through amplification and the assessment of candidature for cochlear implantation.

Anatomical Organization of the Central Auditory System

Subcortical Organization

The auditory system is composed of the outer and middle ear, the cochlea, the auditory nerve, a chain of subcortical nuclei, and multiple cortical areas (Fig. 15.1). The cochlea acts as a mechanical spectrum analyzer separating the frequency components of the sound input such that the sensory hair cells at its base are excited by high frequencies, to low frequencies at its apex. The central auditory system refers to those structures and processes beyond the cochlea. The same orderly map of sound frequency is functionally represented throughout the system.

Several ascending central pathways from each cochlea support serial and parallel processing of auditory input (shown in Fig. 15.1). Reciprocal descending connections enable top-down modulatory influences. A greater density of ascending projections cross over to the contralateral side, such that at the inferior colliculus and above, activity on one side generally reflects the coding of sound input delivered to the opposite ear. This pattern is called contralateral dominance. Using fMRI, it has been possible to measure sound-related activity in cochlear nucleus, inferior colliculus, and medial geniculate nucleus. The small anatomical volumes of these nuclei pose challenges for detecting activation. Approximate sizes in humans are 0.02 cm^3 for the cochlea nucleus, 0.25 cm^3 for the inferior colliculus, and 0.08 cm^3 for the medial geniculate nucleus. Given that the spatial resolution of fMRI is typically 0.03 cm^3 (for a voxel size of 3 × 3 × 3 mm), scanning methods tend to be optimized for detecting activity in subcortical nuclei only if that is the main goal of the research question. In addition to their small size, difficulties may also be due to the characteristics of the metabolic activity or of the neurovasculature in these areas, or the fact that the brain moves with each arterial pulsation. Cardiac-related motion can be eliminated by synchronizing image acquisition with a fixed point in the cardiac cycle [1], and robust activation in the inferior colliculus has been achieved in single subjects using this gating technique [2]. Auditory activation can also be detected in the subcortical nuclei with multi-subject averaging, without the use of cardiac gating [3].

Cortical Organization

One of the goals of neuroimaging research in human listeners is to seek evidence for the anatomical and physiological systems known from studies in other mammals (particularly primates). Thus, the interpretation of imaging data often relates the patterns of brain activation to the underlying anatomy and draws links with what is known from animal neurophysiological studies. Kaas and Hackett [4, 5] present a model of auditory cortical organization in nonhuman primates in which a primary "core" region, located upon the lower bank of the lateral sulcus, is encircled by non-primary belt and parabelt regions.

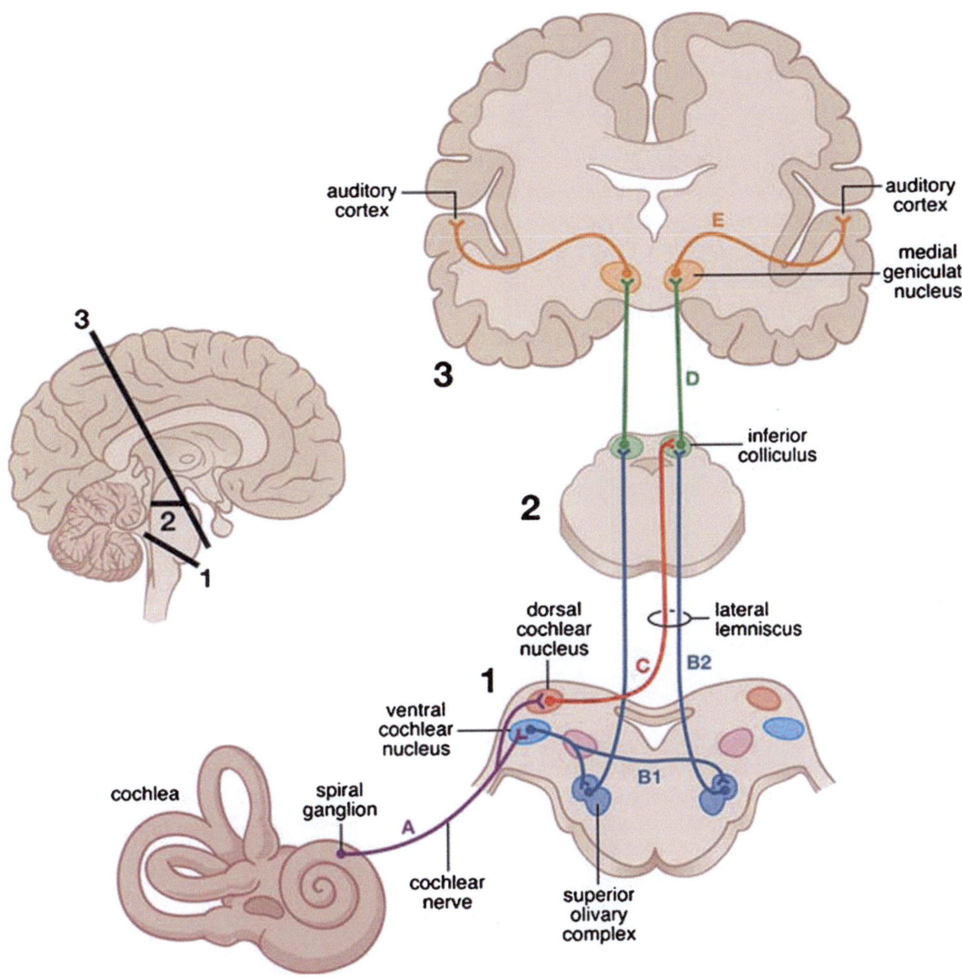

Fig. 15.1 Schematic diagram of the bilateral ascending auditory pathway from the cochlea, including auditory structures within the brainstem (1), midbrain (2), and cortex (3). Unilateral auditory pathway: cochlear nerve (A), ventral cochlear nucleus to contralateral and ipsilateral superior olivary complex (B1), superior olivary complex to inferior colliculus (B2), dorsal cochlear nucleus to contralateral inferior colliculus (C), inferior colliculus to medial geniculate nucleus (D), and medial geniculate nucleus to auditory cortex (E)

The core and belt regions are predominantly hidden from view by the overlying frontal lobe, while parabelt regions extend onto the lateral aspect of the superior temporal gyrus (STG) (Fig. 15.2). Processing is generally believed to proceed in a hierarchical manner, whereby increasingly more complex attributes of the stimulus input are coded. The organization of primate auditory cortex is generally thought to be a good model for the organization of the auditory areas of the human brain. Again, in humans, the arrangement of auditory fields is localized to the surface of the STG, along the inferior margin of the lateral sulcus (Sylvian sulcus). Although different authors have proposed a variety of classification schemes of the human auditory cortex (in terms of the number and location of areas, and nomenclature), they all identify an elongated primary area, surrounded by numerous non-primary auditory fields [6–8].

Primary Core Region

The primary core region receives inputs from the ventral medial geniculate nucleus (MGN) and

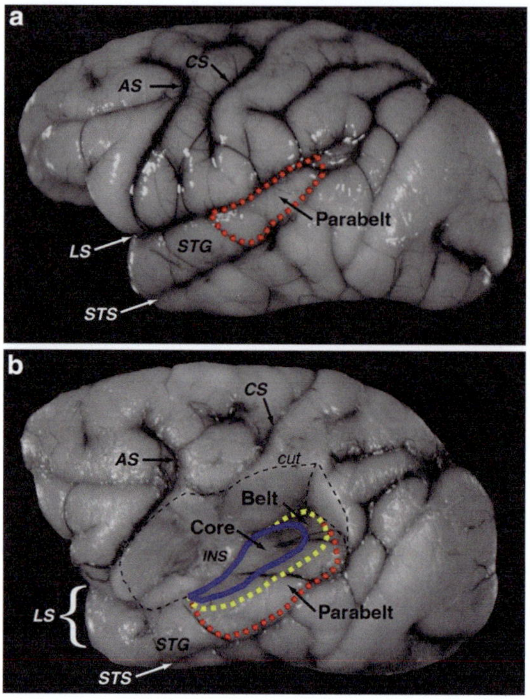

Fig. 15.2 A lateral view of the left hemisphere of the macaque brain. (**a**) The approximate location of the parabelt region on the lateral aspect of the superior temporal gyrus (*dashed red line*). (**b**) Dorsolateral view of the same brain after removal of the overlying frontal and parietal cortex, exposing the ventral bank of the lateral sulcus and insula. The *dashed black line* defines the portion of cortex cut away. The approximate location of the core region (*solid blue line*) posterior and lateral portions of the belt region (*dashed yellow line*) and the parabelt region (*dashed red line*) are shown. The medial portion of the belt region and the anterior part of the core are not visible. *AS* arcuate sulcus, *CS* central sulcus, *INS* insula, *LS* lateral sulcus, *STG* superior temporal gyrus, *STS* superior temporal sulcus. Reprinted with permission from Kaas and Hackett [5]. Copyright © 2000 National Academy of Sciences, USA

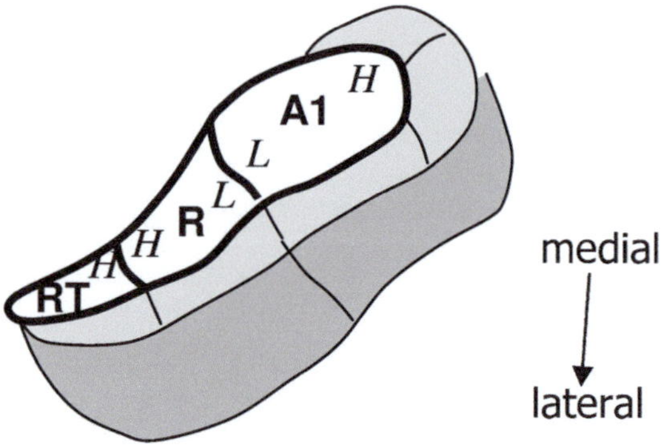

Fig. 15.3 Further subdivisions of the macaque auditory cortex illustrated in Fig. 15.2b. Auditory core fields (A1, R, and RT) are surrounded by belt (*light gray*) and parabelt (*dark gray*) fields. The core fields A1 and R are tonotopically organized. High-frequency (H) acoustic stimuli are represented posteromedially in A1, anteromedially in R. Low-frequency (L) stimuli are represented antterolaterally in A1 and posterolaterally in R. Tonotopic organization in RT is uncertain, but may mirror that found in R. Putative borders within belt and parabelt regions are depicted by the *black lines*

projects to ipsilateral and contralateral core auditory regions, as well as to adjacent non-primary regions. Neurons in the core respond well and with short latencies to pure tones, with narrow frequency tuning at their characteristic frequency [9, 10]. Neurons with a similar characteristic frequency are arranged in rows that are organized along a frequency-gradient [11]. Three distinguishable frequency gradients have been reported in the core region of the macaque monkey (Fig. 15.3). These subdivisions are referred to as fields A1, R, and RT. A1 and R share a common low-frequency border, and R and RT may share a high-frequency border [12].

In humans, the core region extends about 15 mm and is generally located on the medial two-thirds of the anterior-most long axis of Heschl's gyrus (HG). In some studies, architectonic criteria have been used to subdivide the core area. Galaburda and Sanides [6] distinguished a medial and a lateral zone in six hemispheres, while Morosan et al. [13] identified three core fields in 20 hemispheres. In both studies, boundaries were perpendicular to the long axis of HG. In terms of the functional properties of the core region, fMRI has revealed at least two frequency gradients on HG that share a low-frequency border [14, 15]. The endpoints of the two proposed gradients are illustrated in Fig. 15.4, as reported by Paltoglou et al. [16]. It has been proposed that this tonotopic arrangement is the human homologue of A1 and R reported in the macaque.

Non-Primary Belt and Parabelt Regions

In the macaque, the belt region includes seven or eight non-primary fields. Each belt field receives

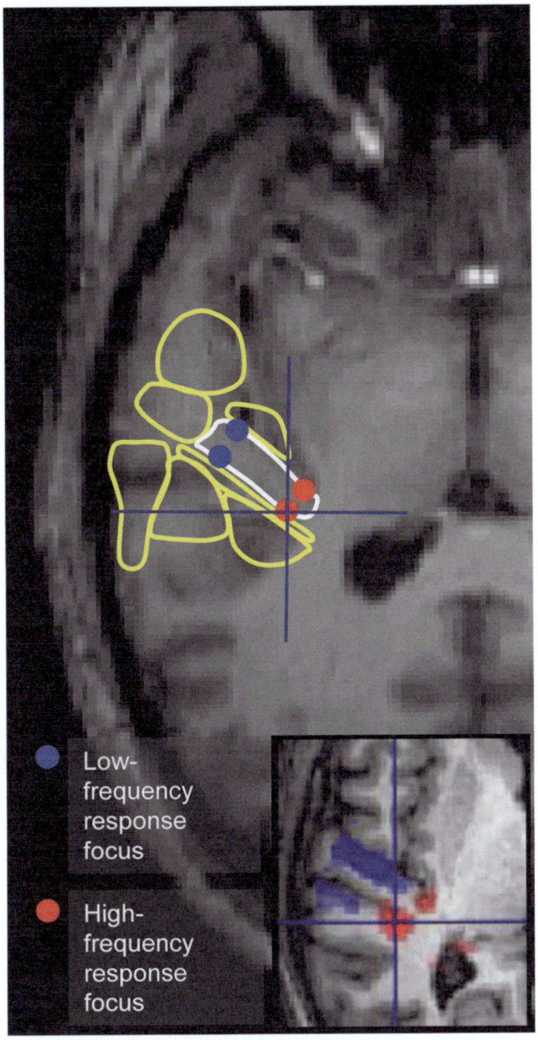

Fig. 15.4 Multiple auditory areas on the superior surface of the temporal lobe of left hemisphere in humans. The core auditory region is shown in *white* with the tonotopic gradient from low to high frequencies (as reported in Paltoglou et al. [16]). Surrounding the core region, seven non-primary regions have been identified by Wallace et al. [8] on the basis of histochemical staining. These are shown in *yellow*. The *inserted panel* presents an illustrative example of frequency-dependent activity in the vicinity of Heschl's gyrus

major inputs from the adjacent core field and from the dorsal and medial divisions of the MGN. Belt neurons respond less well to pure tones, but sufficiently to indicate tonotopicity [9, 11]. Neurons in the belt region generally have broader frequency tuning than those in the core [17]. Activation results from integration between converging inputs and so neurons have complex receptive field properties. For example, in the lateral belt region (on the STG), neurons respond vigorously to spectrally complex stimuli such as vocalizations [9, 18, 19]. The physiological characteristics of the surrounding parabelt are not well established and anatomical subdivisions are rather poorly specified [5]. The belt and parabelt connect with multiple areas in the superior temporal sulcus and anterior and posterior zones of the STG, which may have more than just an auditory function.

In the human brain, between five and six non-primary anatomical regions have been proposed on the basis of histochemical staining [7, 8] (see Fig. 15.4). As the primate, these areas surround the primary core region and extend to the convexity of the STG. The distinction between belt and parabelt non-primary regions has also been rather difficult to ascertain in humans, partly due to a lack of postmortem information [20].

Technical Challenges Involved in Auditory fMRI

The MR environment has three different types of electromagnetic fields. For 3 T MR systems, the static magnetic field is 60,000 times stronger than the earth's magnetic field. Weaker magnetic fields include the time-varying gradient magnetic fields and the pulsed radio-frequency fields. These electromagnetic fields pose three technical challenges: (1) for developing suitable equipment for the presentation of auditory signals to listeners in the scanner bore, (2) for the safe scanning of patients who wear hearing devices, and (3) for the intense scanner acoustic sound generated by the flexing of the gradient coils in the static magnetic field.

Sound Presentation in the MR Scanner

Studies of central auditory function require the presentation of low distortion acoustic signals for which the frequency spectrum and intensity at the ear can be calibrated. Some systems have utilized transducers, placed away from the high static magnetic field, from which sound is delivered through plastic tubes inserted into the subjects' ear canal through a protective ear-defender. One general disadvantage of the tube phone system is that the tubing distorts both the phase and amplitude of the acoustic signal, for example, by imposing a severe ripple on the spectra and reducing sound level, especially at higher frequencies. Nevertheless, these systems are acceptable for delivering low-frequency stimuli and they are commercially available for use in auditory fMRI.

Electronic systems for psychophysical research deliver high quality signals, but unless designed with this specific purpose in mind, these systems are unsuitable for use in the MR environment. Ordinary headphones use an electromagnet to push and pull on a diaphragm to vibrate the air and generate sound, but this does not work in the high static magnetic field. Headphone components constructed from ferromagnetic material also disrupt the magnetic fields locally and induce signal loss or spatial distortion in areas close to the ears. In addition, the electronic components can be damaged by the static magnetic field, while electromagnetic interference generated by the equipment is detected by the MR receiver coil and impairs image quality. Despite the restriction on the materials that can be used in a scanner, a number of different MR-compatible active headphone driving units have been commercially produced or built "in-house" for research (Fig. 15.5a). Electrostatic transducers ensure high-fidelity performance (Fig. 15.5b) without compromising image quality or safety. Electrostatic headphones generate sound using a conductive diaphragm placed next to a fixed conducting panel. A high voltage polarizes the fixed panel and the audio signal passing through the diaphragm rapidly switches between a positive and a negative signal, attracting or repelling it to the fixed panel and thus vibrating the air. For use in the MR scanner, the headset needs to have good passive sound-attenuating properties (Fig. 15.5c). Furthermore, to prevent radio-frequency interference, the digital audio source, electronics, and power supply that drive the system are housed outside the MR scanner room to avoid electromagnetic interference with MR scanning and all electrical signals passing into the screened room are filtered to eliminate radio-frequency interference.

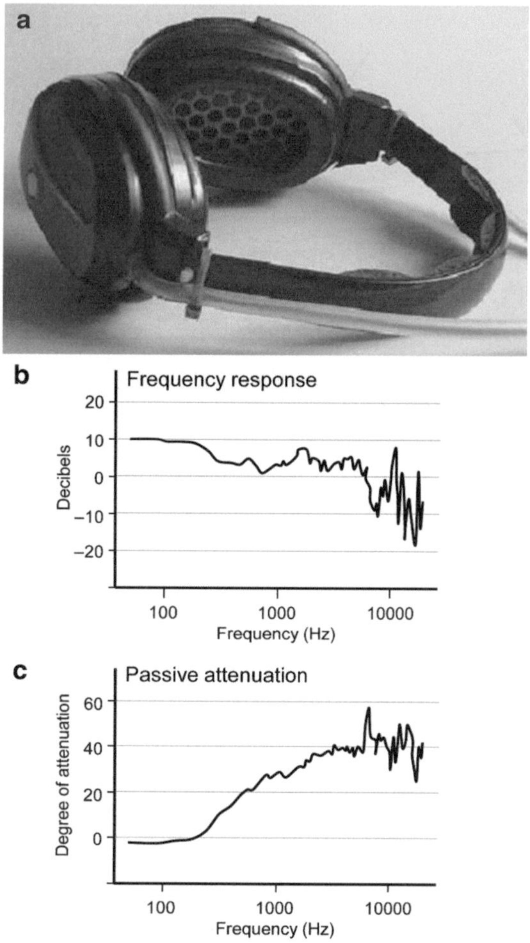

Fig. 15.5 (**a**) An example of a bespoke MR-compatible headset for auditory fMRI. A polypropylene protective grille can be seen inside the circumaural cushion to protect the front of the electrostatic capsule. Interference-free signals are delivered using carbon fiber leads with thick plastic cable protection. (**b**) This headset is capable of delivering frequencies up to 24 kHz (limited by the digital sampling rate). The frequency response is relatively flat between 50 and 10 kHz. (**c**) The headset reduces free-field noise by 30 dB between 500 and 10 kHz. Measurements were taken using a KEMAR mannikin equipped with a microphone at the ear drum to simulate real head listening. Plots have been corrected for the frequency response of the mannikin

Safe Scanning of Patients Who Are Wearing Listening Devices in the MR Scanner

There are restrictions on scanning people who are wearing electronic listening devices including hearing aids, cochlear implants, and brainstem implants. Hearing aids are battery-operated electronic devices that amplify sound for people who have moderate to profound hearing loss. External sounds are amplified and the resulting signals are passed to a receiver in the hearing aid where they are converted back into audible sounds. The aid is worn in or around the ear and can easily be removed by the patient. Other types of devices are available to people who have profound or complete hearing loss. Cochlear implants bypass damaged portions of the inner ear (the cochlea) and directly stimulate the auditory nerve, while auditory brainstem implants bypass the vestibulocochlear nerve in cases when it is damaged by tumors or surgery. Both devices directly stimulate the lower part of the auditory brain (the cochlear nucleus). In general, both types of implant consist of an external portion that sits behind the ear and a second portion that is surgically placed under the skin. The devices contain a microphone; a sound processor (which converts sounds picked up by the microphone into an electrical code); a transmitter and receiver/stimulator (which receive signals from the processor and convert them into electric impulses); and finally an electrode array (which is a set of electrodes that collect the impulses from the stimulator and stimulate groups of auditory neurons). Coded information from the sound processor is delivered across the skin via electromagnetic induction to the implanted receiver/stimulator, which is surgically placed on a bone behind the ear.

No ferromagnetic components can be placed in the MR scanner as they would experience a strong attraction by the static magnetic field, and potentially cause damage not only to the scanner and the listening device but also to the patient. Magnetizable elements induce artifacts in the brain images that are visible as areas of signal loss or spatial distortion (see Fig. 15.6). Cochlear implants contain a magnet to hold the external transmitter coil in place, and this should be removed before scanning. In modern implants, this magnet is reasonably easy to remove under local anesthetic.

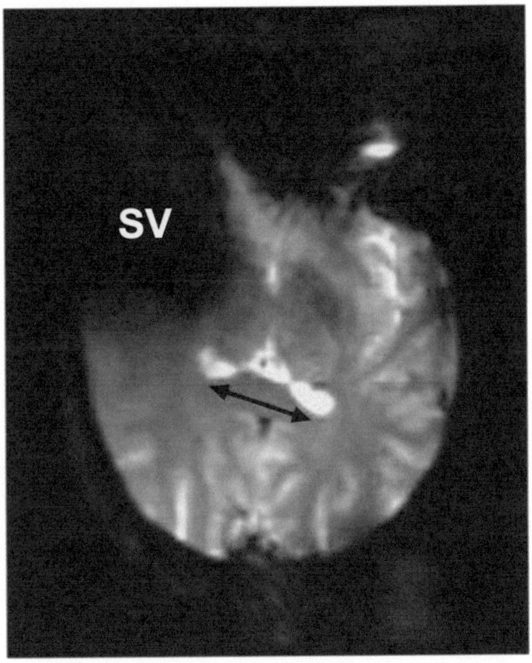

Fig. 15.6 Magnetizable elements in the electrode preparation causing a signal void (SV) can be seen in the right frontal region in this figure from Obler et al. [21]. The right ventricle is distorted (compare with the *black arrow* between the right and left ventricle). The artifact remains ipsilateral. Reprinted with permission from Obler et al. [21]; John Wiley & Sons, Inc

Induced current in the electronics, caused directly by the time-varying gradient magnetic fields or the radio-frequency pulses, presents the main hazard to electronic devices. Induced currents can damage the electronic components, while some materials can also absorb the radiofrequency energy, causing local tissue heating and even burns if in contact with soft tissue. For further discussion of the risks in using a nerve stimulating device in the MR environment, see Obler et al. [21].

The issue of MR compatibility is particularly important given the number of adults and children receiving implants who should not be excluded from MR scanning for the rest of their

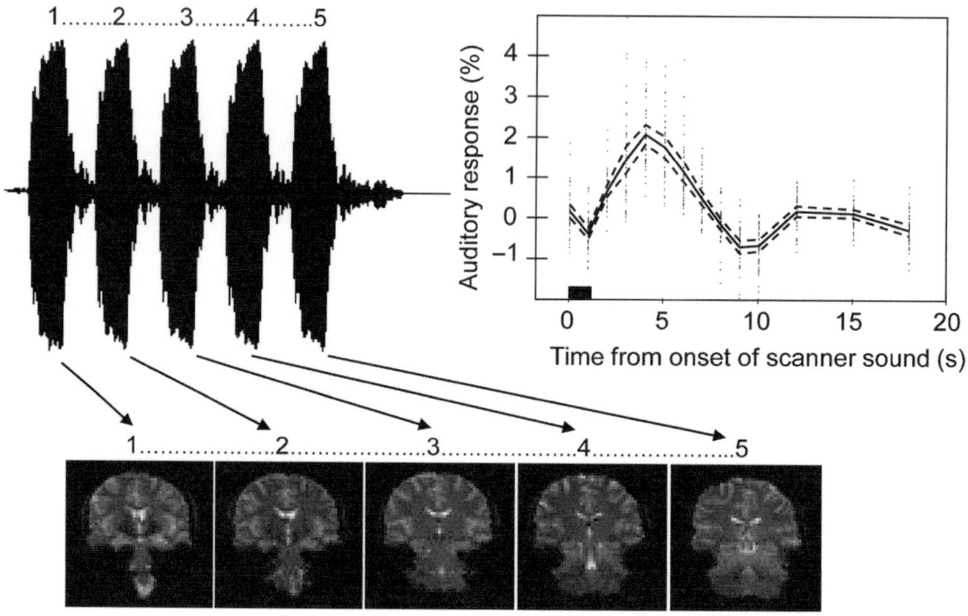

Fig. 15.7 On the *left*, a sample waveform demonstrates the pulses of acoustic energy generated during EPI acquisition of a set of five coronal brain slices. Each energy burst corresponds to the acquisition of a single slice. In the *top right-hand panel* is an example of the auditory cortical response to the pulses of scanner sound. The duration of the scanner sound is denoted by the *black square* on the time axis. Within each plot, *dots* indicate the signal change at each voxel within the region of interest. The *solid line* indicates the mean signal change and the *dashed lines* indicate the 95% confidence limits. Auditory fMRI data are taken from Hall et al. [39]

lives. Some implant designs have been proven to be MR compatible [22–25], but they have not been routinely provided in clinical practice. For these safety reasons, clinical imaging research of implantees has generally used other imaging methods, particularly PET.

Intense Scanner Acoustic Sound

The time-varying gradient magnetic fields are switched rapidly on and off during image acquisition and are central to the formation of each image slice through the brain. Currents through three sets of coiled wire induce small magnetic field gradients that are orthogonal and parallel to the long axis of the static magnetic field. The currents are rapidly switched within a large magnetic field, and interactions between the gradient coils and the static magnetic field induce pulsed Lorentz forces, which act upon the gradient coils to deform them. These abrupt flexing movements generate a compression wave in the air, which is heard as background sound during imaging (Fig. 15.7). Secondary noise can be produced if the vibration of the coils and the core on which they are wound conducts through the core supports to the rest of the structure. The background sound can reach up to 122–131 dB SPL (sound pressure level) and can be damaging without hearing protection [26].

The acoustic properties of the scanner sound (e.g., bandwidth, fundamental frequency, and spectral envelope) depend on the mechanical resonances of the coil assemblies, on the type of imaging sequence used, and on its switching frequency. The dominant components of the sound are spectral peaks at the switching frequency and its higher harmonics, mostly within the frequency range of 0–3 kHz (Fig. 15.8). In fast functional imaging sequences [e.g., echoplanar imaging (EPI)], one brain slice is acquired in one radiofrequency excitation. EPI sequences tend to have extremely fast gradient switching times and high

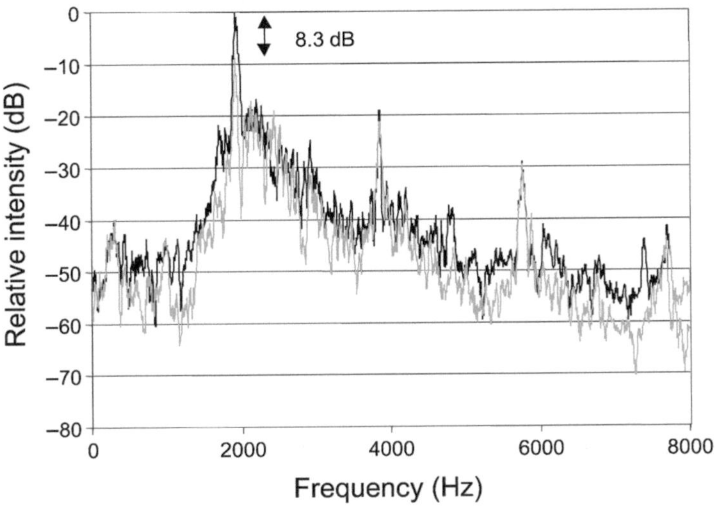

Fig. 15.8 Sample spectrum of the scanner acoustic noise computed by performing a Fourier transform on one acoustic pulse that corresponds to the acquisition of a single slice. The *black line* represents the frequency spectrum for the scanner noise measured within the center of the head coil. The *gray line* represents the frequency spectrum for the same pulse sequence after installing energy-absorbing foam on the entire inner surface of the scanner bore. Values on the *upper horizontal axis* mark the frequencies of the prominent spectral peaks at 1,921, 3,842, 5,763, and 7,684 Hz. On the *intensity axis*, 0 dB corresponds to 129 dB SPL (sound pressure level), which is the sound level of the most dominant frequency. The foam installation reduces this dominant peak by 8.3 dB. (Unpublished data from the author)

gradient amplitudes, and thus produce high levels of background sound. The aggregate noise dosage for EPI studies can be reduced by acquiring a single, or very few, brain slices [27], but at the expense of only a partial view of brain activity. During fMRI, the auditory system is, therefore, subject to continuous quasi-tonal stimulation, which materially interferes with the pattern of stimulus-related activation that the experimenter wishes to measure in the auditory cortex. Areas of stimulus-evoked activation are those that show a statistically significant difference between two experimental conditions. The simplest case is one in which one condition contains a sound stimulus and the other does not. Since the scanner sound is present throughout, the sound condition contains both stimulus and background sound and the baseline condition also contains ambient sound (i.e., it is not silent). Background sound can affect the stimulus-evoked activation pattern in two ways. First, even with hearing protection, the stimulus can be rather difficult to hear, therefore increasing the demands on attention. In particular, the frequency range of the background scanner sound is crucial for speech intelligibility. Thus, the activation pattern can include a cognitive component that reflects the attention cost of filtering out the background sound. Second, stimulus-related activations tend to be on the order of 1–3% from baseline. Thus, higher levels of baseline activation, caused by the ambient sound, are likely to make the experimentally induced auditory activation more difficult to detect statistically. Indeed several studies have reported a reduced activation signal (i.e., the difference between stimulation and baseline conditions) in the auditory cortex when the amount of prior scanner sound is increased, indicating that the sound does mask the detection of auditory activation [28–31].

Perhaps the simplest approach to reducing the airborne sound energy involves passive attenuation. Ravicz et al. [32] demonstrated that wearing ear defenders substantially reduced the ambient sound level measured at the subject's ear by 31–38 dB. However, passive treatments do not fully eliminate the airborne energy that reaches the cochlea. Active noise cancellation is a treatment method that can provide additional sound-attenuating benefits. The active noise cancellation method uses an acoustically controlled headset to deliver a cancellation signal that adds destructively with the sound at the listener's ear. Its application to auditory fMRI has recently been demonstrated [30, 33]. Cancellation is most effective at the dominant peak in the power spectrum of the background scanner sound. Specifically, Hall et al. demonstrated that, at the peak of 600 Hz, microphone measurements at the ear demonstrated 35 dB of additional acoustic attenuation in addition to that already achieved by ear defenders alone. In contrast, the benefit to perception was more modest. Masked detection thresholds improved by 20 dB. This difference can be explained by considering the relative contribution of airborne and bone-conducted transmission routes of sound energy to the cochlea. When active noise cancellation is most effective, the conduction of sound energy through the head and body perhaps becomes the more dominant mode of hearing than the airborne transmission route, thus limiting the perceptual gains that can be realized.

In this case, alternative steps can be made to reduce the scanner sound at source through either hardware or software modifications. Novel designs for the MR system hardware include the construction of "quiet" gradient coils in which the net Lorentz force is compensated between current pathways [34, 35] and encasing the gradient coils in a vacuum chamber (Pianissimo technology, http://www.medical.toshiba.com). Software modifications principally slowdown the gradient switching to reduce the intensity of the scanner sound. This approach is based on the premise that the spectrum of the acoustic signal is determined by the product of the frequency spectrum of the gradient waveforms and the frequency response function of the gradient system [36]. The frequency response function is generally substantially reduced at low frequencies (below 200 Hz) and so the acoustic energy can be reduced by using gradient pulse sequences whose spectra are band-limited to this low-frequency range using soft or sinusoidally ramped pulse shapes [37]. For example, when compared with a manufacturer-provided standard EPI sequence, Schmitter et al. [38] were able to achieve a 20-dB reduction of the background scanner sound. However, the low-sound level is achieved at the expense of slower gradient switching, extending the total imaging time. The next section discusses an experimental protocol that avoids these limitations to minimize the effect of the background scanner sound on the measured patterns of auditory cortical activation for whole brain, multi-slice EPI.

Example fMRI Paradigms

The auditory fMRI response to a single burst of sound is smoothed and delayed in time. It typically rises to a peak by 4–5 s after stimulus onset and decays by 5–8 s after stimulus offset [39] (see the top right-hand panel in Fig. 15.7). Therefore, a brief burst of sound does not generate its maximal auditory response until a few seconds after the stimulus event. Typical functional imaging paradigms measure state-related responses for a stimulus that is presented repeatedly over a period of time. These experiments generally consist of cycles of stimulation and baseline epochs, throughout which whole brain slices are acquired at regular intervals. This imaging protocol produces a burst of scanner sound that is repeated at a rate determined by the time between the acquisition of each whole brain dataset.

During a functional imaging experiment, the background sound induces an auditory response that spans two different temporal scales. First, the sound generated by the acquisition of one slice early in the brain volume may induce activation in an imaging slice, which covers the auditory cortex and is acquired later in the same volume. I shall call this "interslice noise interference." Second, scanner sound may induce auditory activation that extends across time to subsequent volumes. I shall call this second effect "inter-volume noise interference." By manipulating the timing intervals of the slice and the volume acquisitions in the scanning protocol, we can reduce the interslice and inter-volume noise interference,

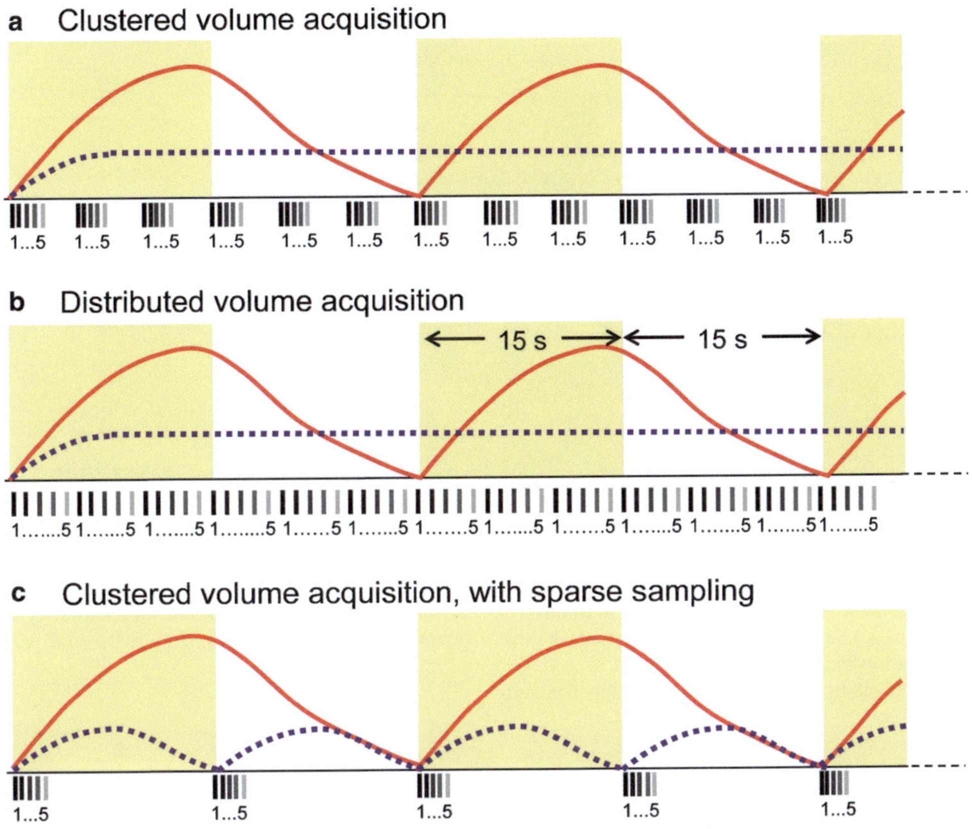

Fig. 15.9 Comparison of the temporal acquisition of sets of five brain slices for three different image acquisition protocols. Each slice acquisition is illustrated by a *line* and numbered 1–5. The experiment involves 30-s cycles of stimulus (denoted by the *yellow shaded areas*), followed by a baseline (shown in *white*). The estimated auditory response evoked by the scanner noise is shown by the *dotted lines*, while the *solid red line* shows the response to the stimulus. (**a**) The clustered volume acquisition sequence in which the five slices are acquired at a rate of 0.6 s, generating a 3-s burst of pulses, followed by a 2-s silent gap. (**b**) A distributed volume acquisition sequence in which the five slices are evenly distributed throughout the 5-s TR period. This sequence generates scanner noise that is characterized by a train of acoustic pulses at 1 Hz. Note that the same number of slices are acquired in both (**a**) and (**b**). (**c**) A combination of clustered volume acquisition with sparse sampling so that each 3-s burst of pulses is followed by 12 s of silence. Sparse sampling permits the auditory response evoked by the scanner noise to decay to baseline level before the next acquisition

respectively, and independently, of one another. The interslice interval is shortest using a clustered-volume acquisition sequence in which all slices are acquired in rapid succession, followed by a gap (Fig. 15.9a). Somewhat longer slice timing is achieved using a distributed volume acquisition sequence in which slices are acquired at slower, equally spaced intervals (Fig. 15.9b). The relative amount of interslice noise interference has been compared for clustered volume and distributed volume acquisition sequences, when the inter-volume interval is fixed. Edmister et al. [31] found that the clustered volume acquisition sequence was more sensitive to the detection of stimulus-evoked activation, over a range of inter-volume intervals. In addition, using a clustered volume acquisition sequence preceded by scanner sound, Talavage et al. [29] found that the interslice interference can be maximally reduced when the duration of each volume acquisition (and hence the burst of scanner sound) was 2 s or less. Reducing the inter-volume noise interference can be achieved by prolonging the inter-volume interval

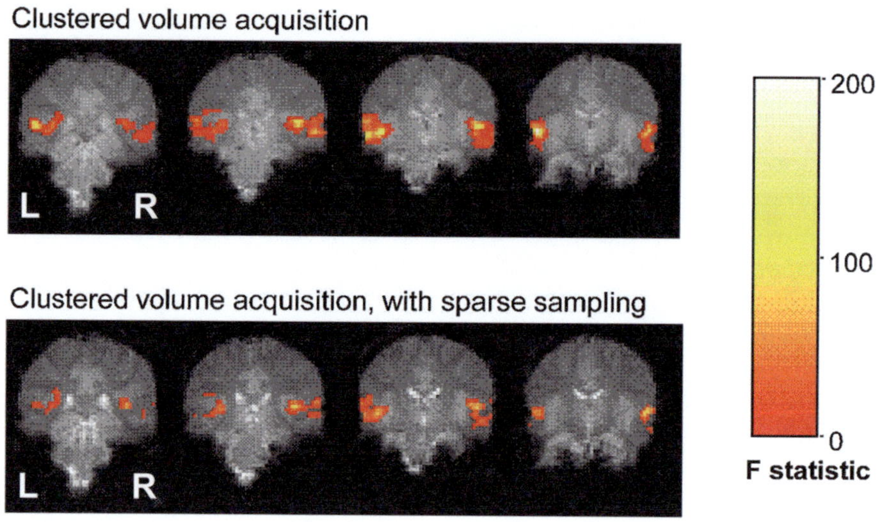

Fig. 15.10 Pattern of activation in a single subject who was scanned using the two types of temporal sampling for clustered volume acquisition. The first used an inter-volume interval of 2.33 s and the second of 14 s (sparse sampling). Activation maps were thresholded at $P < 0.001$, uncorrected for multiple comparisons, and regions of activation are shown whose size exceeds 100 voxels. Both techniques succeeded in detecting auditory activation in Heschl's gyrus, superior and middle temporal gyri. Figure adapted from Hall et al. [40]. Reprinted with permission of John Wiley & Sons, Inc

(Fig. 15.9c). Effectively, this approach acquires single sets of images using clustered volume acquisition at the end of stimulus and baseline conditions. Hall et al. [40] showed that this sparse sampling is actually more effective at detecting sound-evoked activation than the clustered volume acquisition protocol shown in Fig. 15.9b, despite the many fewer data samples (see Fig. 15.10). A sparse sampling technique has been used by many groups to identify auditory cortical evoked responses in the absence of background sound [16, 41, 42].

Major Clinical Applications of Auditory fMRI

fMRI of the auditory system has not yet been widely implemented for routine clinical purposes. However, over the past few years the number of clinical research studies has grown rapidly (Table 15.1). The mature brain can show significant changes in functional organization as a result of learning or trauma. The adult central auditory system exhibits a startling capacity for plasticity following any such changes in hearing experience. There are three ways in which central auditory plasticity might have clinical relevance for the management of adults with acquired hearing loss [43]. First, reduced auditory input from cochlear pathology may cause functional changes in the central auditory system [42–44] that affect auditory perception. Second, provision of amplification may lead to secondary plasticity because of altered input to the auditory system, and this in turn might provoke further changes in auditory perception. Third, auditory learning can cause functional changes in the auditory system [45] that might plausibly lead to alterations in perception. The next section highlights some of the more interesting developments in the field and illustrates how acquired hearing loss might affect plasticity in the central auditory system and how the treatment of those problems will in turn also affect plasticity.

Plasticity Related to Unilateral Hearing Loss as Measured by fMRI

From the normal crossover organization of the ascending auditory pathways (Fig. 15.1), it is expected that monaural stimulation will lead to

Table 15.1 Summary of key literature

Authors	Auditory fMRI	Summary
Neuman 2005 [43]	Central auditory system plasticity and aural rehabilitation of adults	This review article considers the evidence for auditory system plasticity in humans with sensorineural hearing loss, for auditory system plasticity after hearing aid use and auditory cortial reorganization after EEG training and learning. Behavioral and neuroimaging (fMRI) results are presented
Formisano et al. 2003 [14]	Mirror-symmetric tonotopic maps in human primary auditory cortex	This original research article presents high-field fMRI evidence for two adjacent frequency gradients across the human primary auditory cortex
Langers et al. 2005 [44]	Lateralization, connectivity, and plasticity in the human central auditory system	This original research article seeks evidence for plastic reorganization in the human central auditory system using fMRI following unilateral deafness. Plasticity is examined both in terms of contralateral dominance of auditory activity and in terms of the functional connectivity between subcortical and cortical centers
Neumann et al. 2008 [57]	Testing the diagnostic value of electrical ear canal stimulation in cochlear implant candidates by fMRI	This original research article explores the prognostic values of electrical ear canal stimulation and fMRI to evaluate robust predictors for cochlear implant benefit
Kaas et al. 2000 [5]	Subdivisions of auditory cortex and processing streams in primates	This landmark paper presents a summary of the anatomical organization and connectivity of the primate auditory system, with a specific focus on the cortical level
Rivier et al. 1997 [7]	Cytochrome oxidase, acetylcholinesterase, and NADPH-diaphorase staining in human supratemporal and insular cortex: evidence for multiple auditory areas	This landmark paper presents a classification scheme for the human auditory cortex. Possible cortical areas are defined using a set of anatomical and metabolic staining methods
Merzenich et al. 1973 [11]	Representation of the cochlear partition on the superior temporal plane of the macaque monkey	This seminal study reports the results of microelectrode recordings in the macaque money that clearly demonstrated several areas of the auditory cortex that were tonotopically organized
Hall et al. 1999 [40]	Sparse Temporal Sampling in auditory fMRI	This original research paper describes a method for fMRI that reduces the effect of background scanner sound. This has become the method of choice whenever auditory features are being mapped across human auditory cortex
Neuman 2005 [43]	Central auditory system plasticity and aural rehabilitation of adults	This short paper demonstrates, using a single case study, the potential of the adult human auditory cortex to undergo dynamic changes in cortical organization. The results indicate a slow, gradual increase in the ipsilateral response to monaural stimulus
Schmidt et al. 2001 [59]	fMRI of the auditory cortex as a diagnostic tool in cochlear implant candidates	This article reviews some of the uses of fMRI on cochlear implantees. It presents several illustrative cases of auditory cortical fMRI in profoundly deaf patients using the promontory testing method

bilateral cortical activity, but with greater contralateral than ipsilateral activation. For example, in ten normally hearing volunteers, Scheffler et al. [42] showed that the extent of the auditory cortical response to monaural sounds was approximately three to five times greater in the contralateral hemisphere than in the ipsilateral hemisphere. The response to binaural sounds was almost balanced between the two hemispheres, but it was approximately one-third greater than the sum of the two monaural components. This superadditive effect is known as binaural summation and probably results from some form of interaural interaction in the ascending auditory pathway.

Profound unilateral hearing loss disrupts the normal balance of interhemispheric differences in response to a monaural stimulus. The balance between ipsilateral and contralateral activation is often quantified by the "lateralization index;" i.e. (contralateral–ipsilateral activation)/(sum of contralateral and ipsilateral activation) × 100. A lateralization index of zero indicates symmetrical activity. A lateralization index of +100 indicates strong contralateral dominance and an index of −100 indicates strong ipsilateral dominance. For all five patients reported by Scheffler et al. [42], monaural stimulation of the healthy ear revealed a symmetrical pattern of bilateral activation on the STG without any effect of binaural summation. Reduced contralateral dominance after long-term profound unilateral deafness has been replicated in a cohort of 14 patients [46] and in a cohort of 7 patients [47]. These results are intriguing but require replication. One particular methodological weakness was that the ratio of ipsilateral and contralateral activation was based on a simple count of the significant ($p < 0.01$) voxels in each hemisphere. Ratio statistics based on voxel counts can be affected by volume differences between the hemispheres and by the choice of an arbitrary statistical threshold and are highly susceptible to noise (see Chap. 19). Mindful of this issue, Moore et al. [48] used a different metric based on the mean percent signal change within a predefined region of interest that encompassed Heschl's Gyrus (primary auditory cortex). Results from their cohort of 11 patients with moderate-to-profound deafness suggested that a long-standing unilateral loss did not necessarily cause a significant shift in the laterality of primary auditory cortical activation. However, this study also reported a rather atypical pattern of ipsilateral dominance for left-ear stimulation in the normally hearing controls. This particular pattern has not been reported by other groups and so it perhaps limits the generality of their interpretations.

More recently, Langers et al. [44] conducted a comprehensive analysis of contralateral dominance in five adults who had long-term complete unilateral deafness, compared with contralateral dominance in eight normally hearing controls. Within predefined auditory regions of interest, ratio statistics for stimulation of the hearing ear were based on three different metrics: a count of the significant ($p < 0.001$) voxels, the average activation level, and the mean z value of the 10% most-active voxels. The second two metrics are considered to be rather more resistant to the choice of statistical threshold than is the first. Regions were broadly defined in each hemisphere using a brain atlas and these were cochlear nucleus, superior olivary complex, inferior colliculus, medial geniculate nucleus, and auditory cortex. Activation in the cochlear nucleus and superior olivary complex was inconsistent across participants and so was not reported. Not all patients showed activity in both left and right inferior colliculi or medial geniculate nuclei, but there were sufficient data to explore general trends. Stimulation of the hearing ear led to activation patterns in the inferior colliculi and medial geniculate nuclei that were similar in the deaf and normally hearing adults; i.e. activation was largely contralateral (top and middle panels of Fig. 15.11). Meanwhile the response in left and right auditory cortices appeared to be somewhat more symmetrical in the deaf adults than in controls, especially for the two indices computed using the mean activation levels and z values (bottom panel of Fig. 15.11). However, there was a lot of variability between patients and so these differences did not reach statistical significance. The authors concluded that plastic reorganization of response lateralization takes place in the

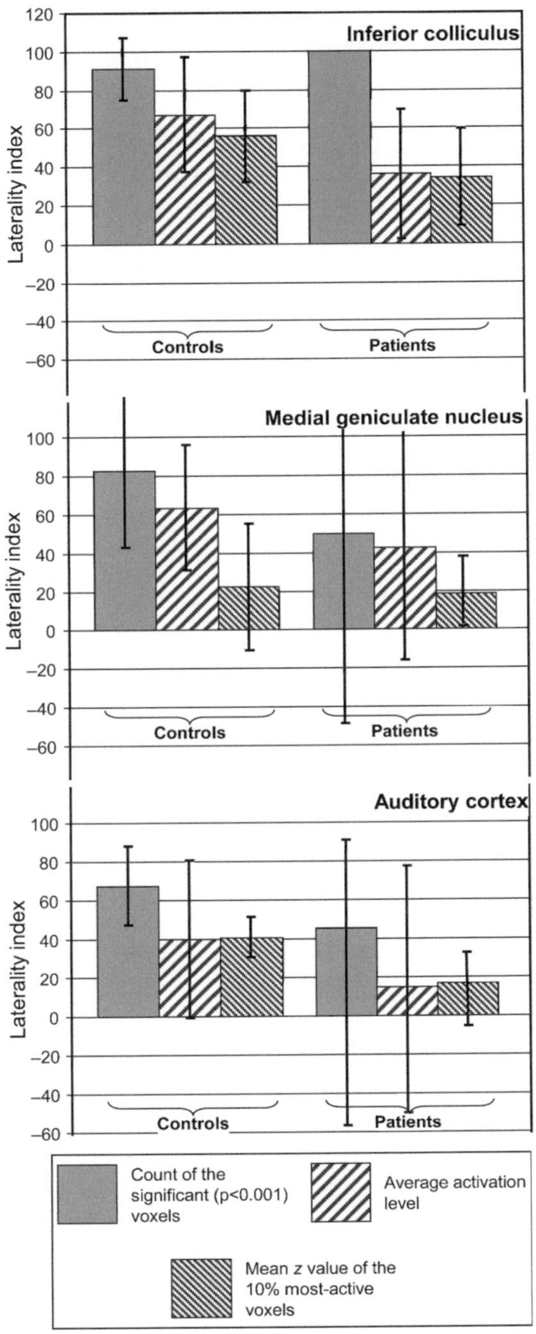

Fig. 15.11 Mean laterality indices for eight normally hearing controls and five patients with unilateral deafness. Laterality index for the controls represents the average response for the left and right ear stimulus presentations. For the patients, the laterality index has been computed for the response to the stimulus presented to the hearing ear only. *Error bars* denote ± 1 standard deviation around the mean. The graphs have been plotted by the author using data reported by Langers et al. [44]

cortex, and not in the brainstem or thalamus. This finding is perhaps surprising given the animal studies on plasticity. However, here one should not forget that fMRI is more sensitive to synaptic activity than to mean neural firing rate. A greater degree of fMRI sensitivity to cortical than to subcortical processing might be explained, if one considers the greater relative amounts of inhibitory and excitatory activity that take place within the cortical laminar. A relative increase in the ipsilateral cortical response to a monaural stimulus may reflect a general central auditory compensation process following reduced input. The precise neurophysiological mechanisms underlying functional plasticity are unknown, but one explanation is that ipsilateral connections, which are normally suppressed, become disinhibited when contralateral inhibitory inputs are removed. Langers et al. speculated that disinhibition might be mediated by interhemispheric connections through the corpus callosum.

The time dependence of such changes has been explored in a single case using a repeated measures design [49]. On initial fMRI testing, the patient had preserved bilateral hearing, but hearing was completely lost in the right ear after surgery for acoustic neuroma resection, which destroyed the auditory nerve. For sounds presented to the left ear, at 4 weeks before the surgery, the patient showed the normal pattern with greater activation in the contralateral auditory cortex. At 1 week after surgery, greater contralateral activation was still observed. However, after 1 year, the response to left ear stimulation was almost the same in both hemispheres (Fig. 15.12). Again, as for the deaf patients previously mentioned, the emergence of symmetry was largely the result of an increase in ipsilateral activity, rather than a decrease in contralateral activity.

The issues of the sites of central auditory plasticity and its time course should be addressed in future studies by collecting longitudinal data for people experiencing sudden onset unilateral hearing loss. Statistical reliability could be ascertained by exploring the data using a range of different ratio statistics applied within predefined regions of interest.

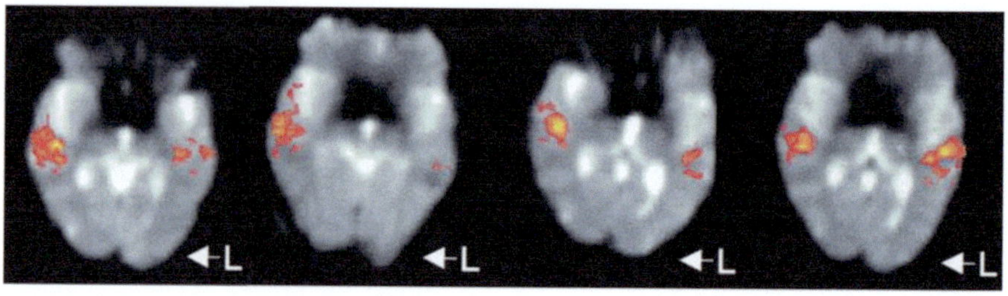

Fig. 15.12 Auditory activation pattern evoked by unilateral (*left*) presentation of a 1-kHz tone. Before surgery (at −4 weeks), a chiefly contralateral response pattern was found. After surgery, stimulation of the left healthy ear produced a progressively more balanced, bilateral a ctivation pattern. Figure adapted with permission from Bilecen et al. [49]

Plasticity Related to Amplification as Measured by fMRI

The auditory perception of hearing aid users is known to change over time and two different behavioral phenomena have been well documented in the clinical literature.

The first refers to the observation that people who have a bilateral symmetrical hearing loss and who wear one hearing aid tend to perform poorly on speech perception when tested using their unaided ear [50]. This is called "late-onset auditory deprivation." Performance has been compared with that following asymmetric hearing loss [51], suggesting that cortical plasticity might be responsible for the behavioral effects of late-onset auditory deprivation. For example, introducing an asymmetry might reduce the perceptual salience for stimuli presented to the unaided ear because of the greater ipsilateral cortical response to stimulus input presented to the aided ear. However, no research has so far combined audiological, behavioral, and neurophysiological measures, yet this convergent approach will be essential for examining direct evidence for changes in the central auditory system.

The second phenomenon refers to the observation that the benefit to speech perception from wearing a hearing aid may not manifest itself until up to about 12 weeks after fitting. This is called "hearing aid acclimatization." The question of whether or not acclimatization occurs has been controversial and the behavioral evidence is rather mixed [43]. Neuman has suggested that neuroimaging measures could be helpful for determining whether or not secondary cortical plasticity occurs in the hearing aid user. However, reliable metrics based on neuroimaging data will be needed to establish changes in the same patient over time as a result of hearing aid use. Certainly, a within-subjects design should be able to account for a number of extraneous influences on auditory activation patterns, but at present, it is unclear whether or not the within-subject test–retest reliability of auditory fMRI is adequate for this clinical application.

One such fMRI study combined speech perception scores for stimuli presented separately to the aided and the unaided ear with fMRI measures of the speech-related auditory cortical activation in the same participants [52]. Eight patients had congenital, bilateral, symmetric, moderate-to-severe hearing loss. At the start of the study, none had any experience using hearing aids, but they agreed to use an aid in their right ear for at least 8 h every day. Participants completed a speech discrimination test and fMRI at three time intervals: (1) immediately before fitting, (2) 3 months after fitting, and (3) 9 months after fitting. Behavioral performance was quantified using a percent speech discrimination score, while fMRI activity was quantified using an intensity-weighted volume, defined as the product of the size of a significant activation cluster and the averaged local maximum T statistic.

The results are summarized in Fig. 15.13. Although the mean speech discrimination score

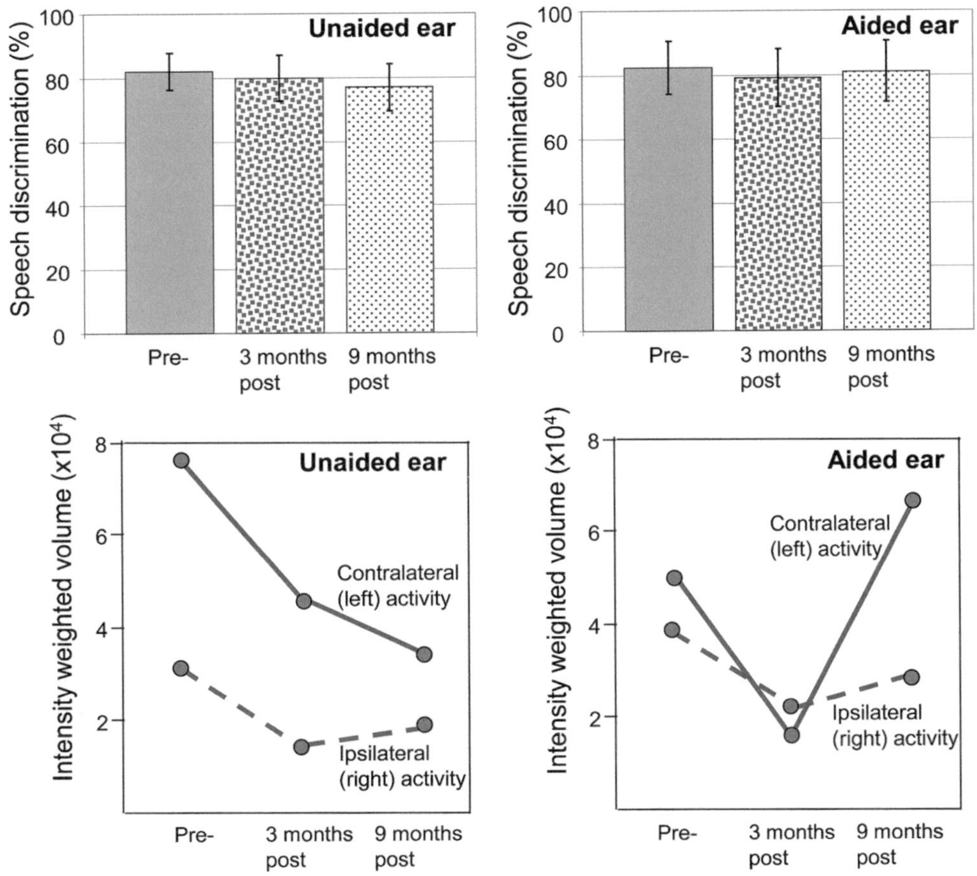

Fig. 15.13 Mean speech discrimination scores and intensity-weighted fMRI volumes for eight patients. Change scores plot the functional adaptation to wearing a hearing aid that was fitted in the right ear. The graphs have been plotted by the author using data reported by Hwang et al. [51]

in the unaided ear decreased over time (consistent with late-onset auditory deprivation), this was not statistically significant. There was no systematic change in the aided ear (no acclimatization). The fMRI results also present a challenge for interpretation. After amplification, speech-related activation decreased for stimuli presented to both unaided and aided ears, but largely recovered in the contralateral hemisphere during stimulation of the aided ear. In terms of changes in laterality, contralateral dominance decreased for the unaided ear of presentation and increased for the aided ear. This pattern of reorganization runs counter to the predictions that the ipsilateral response to the aided ear of stimulation should significantly increase over time and the response overall should become more symmetrical across the hemispheres.

In another interesting clinical application of auditory fMRI, Suzuki and colleagues [53] evaluated responses to monaural stimulation in acute and recovery phases of 11 patients with idiopathic sudden onset deafness in the right ear. Deafness was asymmetrical and hearing thresholds ranged from 32 to 105 dB in the affected ear and 0 to 40 dB in the opposite ear. Within 1 week of the deafness onset (acute phase), patients were scanned while listening to monosyllables. They were then treated in the clinic. The steroid treatment resulted in either partial (N = 5) or complete (N = 5) recovery of hearing. Patients were scanned again 3–4 weeks after the onset of deafness (recovery phase). The results are presented separately for the acute and recovery phases. Because there was no direct statistical analysis of the treatment outcome, assessing the degree of change is only possible through visual inspection of the separate sets of activation images for acute and recovery phases. Sounds presented to the affected ear produced a clear increase in contralateral auditory cortical activation, although this can be attributed to an improvement in audibility, not an effect of plasticity. Sounds presented to the unaffected ear showed a more subtle effect of treatment. Both pre- and posttreatment, there was an overall ipsilateral dominance in the patient group; not observed in the control group. According to the lateralization ratios computed from the count of significant voxels in each hemisphere, the strength of the ipsilateral dominance diminished somewhat after treatment. The authors interpreted this result as evidence for some restoration of the cross projection within the rather short time window of several weeks. However, the rather atypical pattern of ipsilateral dominance in the patient group somewhat limits the generality of the conclusion.

The use of convergent methods that include fMRI to study the effects of hearing loss and amplification should contribute to a better understanding of auditory deprivation and treatment. However, the results from the different studies that have been published to date are rather too disparate to synthesize into a coherent model that accounts for the possible role of plasticity in the central auditory system.

Cochlear Implantation: Assessment of Candidature and Evaluation of Hearing Recovery

A cochlear implant is an artificial hearing device for profoundly deaf people and is designed to produce useful auditory sensations by electrically stimulating the cochlear nerve. The system consists of an external microphone and a speech processing and battery unit, which transmits its signal to an electrode array that is inserted into the cochlea of the inner ear. As previously discussed, cochlear implants are not generally compatible with MRI, and so PET is generally the neuroimaging tool of choice in such studies. PET has been used to address two general questions (see Giraud et al. [54] for a review). First, the effects of the preceding deafness on functional brain organization have been investigated by studying the effects of cochlear implantation on prelingually and postlingually deaf patients. The duration of auditory deprivation plays an important role in determining outcome, possibly because it drives the process of brain reorganization [55]. Second, the manifestations of cortical reorganization after implant switch-on have been measured in the same patients imaged at different stages in their aural rehabilitation, so tracking the effects of aural habilitation.

fMRI has primarily been used prior to implantation to evaluate whether brain imaging can provide an additional, objective diagnostic tool for measuring the potential benefit of cochlear implantation in patients. However, several recent fMRI studies have begun to consider the application of fMRI for predicting outcomes from cochlear implantation.

The basic requirements for a positive outcome of cochlear implantation are a sufficient number of spiral ganglion cells in the medial wall of the cochlea (where the implant electrode is placed), a functional auditory nerve, and an intact central auditory pathway. To assess the integrity of the neural pathway, and hence the potential for benefit from cochlear implantation, patients are sometimes tested preoperatively using direct electrical stimulation applied to the promontory of the cochlea to elicit the perception of auditory sensations. The test has several drawbacks. First, the patient's judgment about whether or not the procedure produces auditory sensations is subjective. It is possible that the patient cannot report a subjective auditory sensation, and yet their cochlear nerve is intact. Hence, in reality, many surgeons base their decision to implant on patient history, traditional audiometry, and auditory brainstem response audiometry rather than on electrical stimulation. Second, electrical stimulation occurs some way away from the ganglion cells and pain receptors may be stimulated before auditory receptors, leading to somewhat inconsistent results. The absence of a promontory response is not, by itself, a contraindication for cochlear implantation. It has been proposed that fMRI mapping of the evoked auditory cortical response would provide an objective method of verifying the functional integrity of primary and/or non-primary auditory cortical regions. Auditory cortical activation in deaf patients has so far been identified using both ear-canal stimulation [56, 57] and transtympanic stimulation [58–61]. fMRI mapping of direct electrical stimulation is not without technical challenge as the electrodes that are routinely used in clinical practice are ferromagnetic and the electrode currents can cause ipsilateral image artifacts (see Obler et al. [21], for a discussion). These image artifacts can be eliminated by using a gold-plated tungsten electrode and carbon fiber cables, thus enabling the imaging of both hemispheres [58]. The fMRI results indicate that monaural stimulation activates the contralateral auditory cortex only. From a cohort of 35 patients, Schmidt et al. [59] estimated that fMRI could detect contralateral auditory cortical activation in approximately 85% of those patients who reported auditory sensations from promontory stimulation. Schmidt et al. concluded that fMRI may aid the decision for or against an implant as well as the decision on which side to place the implant (Fig. 15.14). However, a more recent study reported rather less optimistic results. Neumann et al. [57] studied 18 profoundly deaf adults who were candidates for cochlear implantation. All patients underwent ear canal stimulation during fMRI with either one (N = 13) or two (N = 5) ears stimulated during successive periods. Activation patterns were subjectively assessed for their statistical robustness and their localization to primary auditory cortex. In 11 of 17 ears that could be included in the fMRI analysis, stimulation led to "acceptable" or "perfect" auditory cortical activation, and in nine of these cases (82%) stimulation also produced an auditory sensation. However, to compare the results to those reported by Schmidt et al. [59], it is important to consider all of the patients who reported an auditory sensation, not just a "better" subset. Looking at the data this way yielded "acceptable" or "perfect" contralateral activation in only 56%. Lateralization indices were also calculated for the patients with "acceptable" or "perfect" activation, using a voxel counting method. It is interesting to note that despite all patients being deaf in both ears, the laterality index was more symmetrical (mean = 41) than in normally hearing controls (mean = 72). Hence it is possible that compensatory reorganization in the form of inter-hemispheric disinhibition occurs even when both ears are deprived of acoustic input.

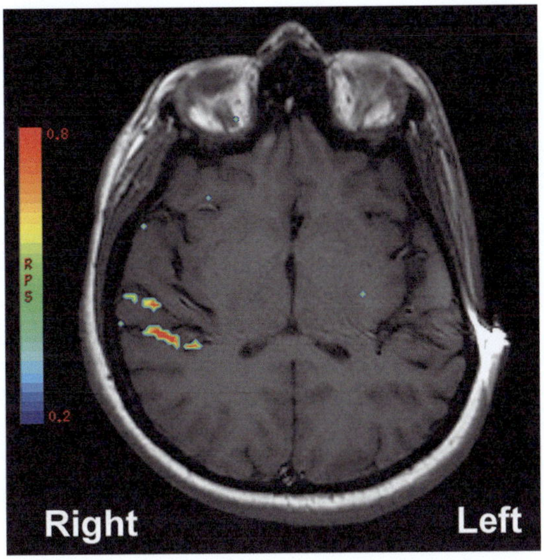

Fig. 15.14 An illustrative example of the application of fMRI to examine candidates for cochlear implantation. A 31-year-old woman with congenital blindness exhibited progressive and profound hearing loss since age 12. Promontory testing revealed weak but positive responses at 50, 100, and 200 Hz. Stimulating the left ear elicited a large activation in the vicinity of the posterior non-primary auditory cortex on the right side. Implantation was carried out on the left ear with a satisfactory outcome. Reproduced from Schmidt et al. [59]. Copyright © 2000, with permission from Elsevier

Sixteen patients from the original cohort of 18 that were tested by Neumann et al. [57] received a cochlear implant. Speech tests were conducted 6 weeks before surgery and 6 months after surgery. Outcomes were tested against a number of measures including preoperative residual hearing, result of ear canal stimulation, and fMRI activations. Rather disappointingly, neither sensations during electrical stimulation nor resulting fMRI activations correlated with the cochlear implant outcome measures. The conclusion from this study was that preoperative residual hearing still remained the most robust predictor for cochlear implant benefit.

Conclusion

While the results from a number of neuroimaging studies in humans provide some evidence of plasticity in the central auditory system, much more information is needed to understand those patterns of reorganization. It is possible to summarize our current lack of understanding as three key questions. (1) What type of hearing loss is needed to evoke auditory reorganization? (2) What is the neural basis of that reorganization? (3) What are the perceptual consequences of that reorganization and how does that affect treatment outcome? The ultimate goal is for fMRI to provide the information necessary for evidence-based clinical provision of hearing aids and implants. However, to date, auditory fMRI has not been widely implemented for routine clinical purposes in the ear, nose, throat (ENT) or audiology clinic.

The major limitation in the use of fMRI for clinical diagnosis is the large inter-subject variability. In this review, variability has been reported in terms of the presence or absence of auditory activity as well as in terms of its extent and precise localization (when activity is present). The clinician should bear in mind that a null fMRI result does not necessarily indicate the *absence* of neural activity in a particular brain region. For example, should we conclude that the seven cochlear implant candidates reported by Neumann et al. [57] who failed to show auditory cortical activity despite reporting a clear hearing sensation, all have an abnormality in the ascending auditory system and so should not receive an implant? No, such a decision would be inexcusable. Even a simple auditory task such as monaural listening can evoke a range of fMRI response patterns (from contralateral dominance on the one hand to ipsilateral dominance on the other) without any clear explanation why this should be so. Results obtained using the laterality index do not always fit the expected pattern of a shift in contralateral dominance as a consequence of long-term adaptation to hearing loss. At the moment, it would be inadvisable to rely on fMRI alone to guide important clinical decisions, although there may be cases where it can certainly supplement the decision-making process.

References

1. Guimaraes AR, Melcher JR, Talavage TM, Baker JR, Ledden P, Rosen BR, et al. Imaging subcortical auditory activity in humans. Hum Brain Mapp. 1998; 6:33–41.
2. Melcher JR, Sigalovsky IS, Guinan JJ, Levine RA. Lateralised tinnitus studied with functional magnetic resonance imaging: abnormal inferior colliculus activation. J Neurophysiol. 2000;83:1058–72.
3. Griffiths TD, Uppenkamp S, Johnsrude I, Josephs O, Patterson RD. Encoding of the temporal regularity of sound in the human brainstem. Nat Neurosci. 2001;4: 633–7.
4. Kaas JH, Hackett TA. Subdivisions of auditory cortex and levels of processing in primates. Audiol Neurootol. 1998;3:73–85.
5. Kaas JH, Hackett TA. Subdivisions of auditory cortex and processing streams in primates. Proceedings of the National Academy of Sciences. 2000;97: 11793–11799.
6. Galaburda AM, Sanides F. Cytoarchitectonic organisation of the human auditory cortex. J Comp Neurol. 1980;221:169–84.
7. Rivier F, Clarke S. Cytochrome oxidase, acetylcholinesterase, and NADPH-diaphorase staining in human supratemporal and insular cortex: evidence for multiple auditory areas. Neuroimage. 1997; 6:288–304.
8. Wallace MN, Johnston PW, Palmer AR. Histochemical identification of cortical areas in the auditory region of the human brain. Exp Brain Res. 2002;143: 499–508.
9. Rauschecker JP, Tian B, Hauser M. Processing of complex sounds in the macaque nonprimary auditory cortex. Science. 1995;268:111–4.
10. Rauschecker JP, Tian B, Pons T, Mishkin M. Serial and parallel processing in rhesus monkey auditory cortex. J Comp Neurol. 1997;382:89–103.
11. Merzenich MM, Brugge JF. Representation of the cochlear partition on the superior temporal plane of the macaque monkey. Brain Res. 1973;50:275–96.
12. Morel A, Garraghty PE, Kaas JH. Tonotopic organisation, architectonic fields, and connections of auditory cortex in macaque monkeys. J Comp Neurol. 1993; 335:437–59.

13. Morosan P, Rademacher J, Schleicher A, Amunts K, Schormann T, Zilles K. Human primary auditory cortex: cytoarchitectonic subdivisions and mapping into a spatial reference system. Neuroimage. 2001;13: 684–701.
14. Formisano E, Kim DS, Di Salle F, van de Moortele PF, Ugurbil K, Goebel R. Mirror-symmetric tonotopic maps in human primary auditory cortex. Neuron. 2003;40(4):859–69.
15. Talavage TM, Sereno MI, Melcher JR, Ledden PJ, Rosen BR, Dale AM. Tonotopic organization in human auditory cortex revealed by progressions of frequency sensitivity. J Neurophysiol. 2004;91: 1282–96.
16. Paltoglou A, Sumner CJ, Hall DA. Examining the role of frequency specificity in the enhancement and suppression of human auditory cortical activity by auditory selective attention. Hear Res. 2009;257(1–2): 106–18.
17. Recanzone GH. Spatial processing in the auditory cortex of the macaque monkey. Proceedings of the National Academy of Sciences. 2000;97: 11829–11835.
18. Rauschecker JP, Tian B. Mechanisms and streams for processing of "what" and "where" in auditory cortex. Proceedings of the National Sciences. 2000;97: 11800–11806.
19. Tian B, Reser D, Durham A, Kustov A, Rauschecker JP. Functional specialisation in rhesus monkey auditory cortex. Science. 2001;292:290–3.
20. Morosan P, Schleicher A, Amunts K, Zilles K. Multimodal architectonic mapping of human superior temporal gyrus. J Anat Embryol. 2005;210: 401–6.
21. Obler R, Köstler H, Weber B-P, Mack KF, Becker B. Safe electrical stimulation of the cochlear nerve at the promontory during functional magnetic resonance imaging. Magn Reson Med. 1999;42:371–8.
22. Heller JW, Brackmann DE, Tucci DL, Nyenhuis JA, Chou C-K. Evaluation of MRI compatibility of the modified nucleus multichannel auditory brainstem and cochlear implants. Am J Otol. 1996;17:724–9.
23. Weber BP, Neuberger J, Battmer RD, Lenarz T. Magnetless cochlear implant: relevance of adult experience for children. Am J Otol. 1997;18:S50–1.
24. Chou CK, McDougall JA, Chan KW. Absence of radiofrequency heating from auditory implants during magnetic resonance imaging. Bioelectromagnetics. 1995;16:307–16.
25. Shellock FG, Morisoli S, Kanal E. MR procedures and biomedical implants, materials and devices: 1993 update. Radiology. 1993;189:587–99.
26. Foster JR, Hall DA, Summerfield AQ, Palmer AR, Bowtell RW. Sound-level measurements and calculations of safe noise dosage during EPI at 3T. J Magn Reson Imaging. 2000;12:157–63.
27. Harms MP, Melcher JR. Sound repetition rate in the human auditory pathway: representations in the human auditory pathway – representations in the waveshape and amplitude of fMRI activation. J Neurophysiol. 2002;88(3):1433–50.
28. Bandettini PA, Jesmanowicz A, Van Kylen J, Birn RA, Hyde J. Functional MRI of brain activation induced by scanner acoustic noise. Magn Reson Med. 1998;39:410–6.
29. Talavage TM, Edmister WB, Ledden PJ, Weisskoff RM. Quantitative assessment of auditory cortex responses induced by imager acoustic noise. Hum Brain Mapp. 1999;7:79–88.
30. Hall DA, Chambers J, Akeroyd MA, Foster JR, Coxon R, Palmer AR. Acoustic, psychophysical, and neuroimaging measurements of the effectiveness of active cancellation during auditory functional magnetic resonance imaging. J Acoust Soc Am. 2009; 25:347–59.
31. Edmister WB, Talavage TM, Ledden PJ, Weisskoff RM. Improved auditory cortex imaging using clustered volume acquisitions. Hum Brain Mapp. 1999; 7:89–97.
32. Ravicz ME, Melcher JR, Kiang NYS. Acoustic noise during functional magnetic resonance imaging. J Acoust Soc Am. 2000;108:1683–96.
33. Chambers J, Akeroyd MA, Summerfield AQ, Palmer AR. Active control of the volume acquisition noise in functional magnateic resonance imaging: method and psychoacoustical investigation. J Acoust Soc Am. 2001;110:3041–54.
34. Mansfield P, Chapman BLW, Bowtell R, Glover P, Coxon R, Harvey PR. Active acoustic screening: reduction of noise in gradient coils by Lorentz force balancing. Magn Reson Med. 1995;33:276–81.
35. Bowtell R, Mansfield P. Quiet transverse gradient coils: Lorentz force balanced designs using geometric similitude. Magn Reson Med. 1995;34:494–7.
36. Hedeen RA, Edelstein WA. Characterisation and prediction of gradient acoustic noise in MR imagers. Magn Reson Med. 1997;37:7–10.
37. Hennel F, Girard F, Loenneker T. "Silent" MRI with soft gradient pulses. Magn Reson Med. 1999;42: 6–10.
38. Schmitter S, Diesch E, Amann M, Kroll A, Moayer M, Schad LR. Silent echo-planar imaging for auditory FMRI. Magma. 2008;21(5):317–25.
39. Hall DA, Summerfield AQ, Gonçalves MS, Foster JR, Palmer AR, Bowtell RW. Time-course of the auditory BOLD response to scanner noise. Magn Reson Med. 2000;43:601–6.
40. Hall DA, Haggard MP, Akeroyd MA, Palmer AR, Summerfield AQ, Elliott MR, et al. Sparse temporal sampling in auditory fMRI. Hum Brain Mapp. 1999; 7:213–23.
41. Belin P, Zatorre RJ, Hoge R, Evans AC, Pike B. Event-related fMRI of auditory cortex. Neuroimage. 1999;10:417–29.
42. Scheffler K, Bilecen D, Schmid N, Tschopp K, Seelig J. Auditory cortical responses in hearing subjects and unilateral deaf patients as detected by functional magnetic resonance imaging. Cereb Cortex. 1998;8: 156–63.
43. Neuman AC. Central auditory system plasticity and aural rehabilitation of adults. J Rehabil Res Dev. 2005;42(4):169–86.

44. Langers DR, van Dijk P, Backes WH. Lateralization, connectivity and plasticity in the human central auditory system. Neuroimage. 2005;28:490–9.
45. Jäncke L, Gaab N, Wüstenberg T, Scheich H, Heinze HJ. Short-term functional plasticity in the human auditory cortex: an fMRI study. Cogn Brain Res. 2001;12:479–85.
46. Tschopp K, Schillinger C, Schmid N, Rausch M, Bilecen D, Scheffler K. Evidence of central auditory compensation in unilateral deaf patients detected by functional MRI. Laryngol Rhinol Otol. 2000;79: 753–7.
47. Firszt J, Ulmer J, Gaggl W. Differential representation of speech sounds in the human cerebral hemispheres. Anat Rec A. 2006;288A:345–57.
48. Moore DR, Devlin JT, Raley J, Tunbridge E, Lanary K, Floyer-Lea A, et al. Effects of long term unilateral hearing loss on the lateralization of fMRI measured activation in human auditory cortex. In: Syka J, Merzenich MM, editors. Plasticity of the central auditory system and processing of complex acoustic signals. New York: Kluwer-Plenum; 2004. p. 1–11.
49. Bilecen D, Seifritz E, Radü EW, Schmid N, Wetzel S, Probst R, et al. Cortical reorganization after acute unilateral hearing loss traced by fMRI. Neurology. 2000;54:765.
50. Neuman AC. Late-onset auditory deprivation: a review of past research and an assessment of future research needs. Ear Hear. 1996;17(3 Suppl):S3–S13.
51. Silverman CA, Emmer MB. Auditory deprivation and recovery in adults with asymmetric sensorineural hearing impairment. J Am Acad Audiol. 1993;4(5): 338–46.
52. Hwang JH, Wu CW, Chen JH, Liu TC. Changes in activation of the auditory cortex following long-term amplification: an fMRI study. Acta Otolaryngol. 2006;126:1275–80.
53. Suzuki M, Kouzaki H, Nishida Y, Shiino A, Ito R, Kitano H. Cortical representation of hearing restoration in patients with sudden deafness. Neuroreport. 2002;13:1829–32.
54. Giraud AL, Truy E, Frackowiak R. Imaging plasticity in cochlear implant patients. Audiol Neurootol. 2001; 6:381–93.
55. Lee HJ, Giraud AL, Kang E, Oh SH, Kang H, Kim CS, et al. Cortical activity at rest predicts cochlear implantation outcome. Cereb Cortex. 2007;17:909–17.
56. Hofmann E, Preibisch C, Knaus C, Muller J, Kremser C, Teissl C. Noninvasive direct stimulation of the cochlear nerve for functional MR imaging of the auditory cortex. Am J Neuroradiol. 1999;20:1970–2.
57. Neumann K, Preibisch C, Spreer J, Raab P, Hamm J, Euler HA, et al. Testing the diagnostic value of electrical ear canal stimulation in cochlear implant candidates by functional magnetic resonance imaging. Audiol Neurootol. 2008;13(5):281–92.
58. Alwatban AZ, Ludman CN, Mason SM, O'Donoghue GM, Peters AM, Morris PG. A method for the direct electrical stimulation of the auditory system in deaf subjects: a functional magnetic resonance imaging study. J Magn Reson Imaging. 2002;16:6–12.
59. Schmidt AM, Weber BP, Becker H. Functional magnetic resonance imaging of the auditory cortex as a diagnostic tool in cochlear implant candidates. Neuroimaging Clin N Am. 2001;11:297–304.
60. Schmidt AM, Weber BP, Vahid M, Zacharias R, Neuburger J, Witt M, et al. Functional MR imaging of the auditory cortex with electrical stimulation of the promontory in 35 deaf patients before cochlea implantation. Am J Neuroradiol. 2003;24:201–7.
61. Berthezène Y, Truy E, Morgon A, Giard HM, Hermier M, Franconi JM, et al. Auditory cortex activation in deaf subjects during cochlear electrical stimulation. Investig Radiol. 1997;32:297–301.

fMRI of Epilepsy

16

Karsten Krakow

Introduction

Since the demonstration about 20 years ago that functional magnetic resonance imaging (fMRI) is able to provide high spatial resolution maps of brain function, considerable effort has been directed at applying this technique to study patients with epilepsy, in particular patients with intractable epilepsy considered for epilepsy surgery. Successful epilepsy surgery is vitally dependent on the accurate determination of the epileptogenic zone and of the risks of postoperative neurological deficits [1]. Functional MRI can be used to address these issues in different ways. The most established application of fMRI is the determination of eloquent cortical areas, which enables fMRI to predict deficits in cognitive (e.g., language and memory) or sensorimotor functions that might arise from surgical intervention. In many centers, fMRI studies of sensorimotor and cognitive function are already established as a routine procedure in the presurgical workup of patients with medically refractory focal epilepsy. The other more experimental application of fMRI in the field of epilepsy is the localization of focal epileptogenic regions through ictal or interictal blood-oxygen-level-dependent (BOLD) signal changes.

K. Krakow, MD, PhD (✉)
Asklepios Neurologische Klinik Falkenstein,
Asklepiosweg 15, Königstein 61462, Germany
e-mail: k.krakow@asklepios.com

Special Issues in Patients with Epilepsy

Only in the last 15 years has fMRI been increasingly applied to larger numbers of neurological patients. Working with clinical populations, in general, and patients with epilepsy, in particular, require special considerations.

The issues of task difficulty, compliance, and motivation compliance have to be carefully addressed in neurological patients. Patients may be less motivated than normal volunteers to perform well on tasks. If the epilepsy is associated with intellectual impairment, patients may be less able to perform cognitive tasks that were developed for neurologically normal subjects.

Emotional distress from MRI scanning is reported to interfere with completion of the procedure in as many as 20% of patients [2, 3]. Although these situations are often managed with tranquilizing agents in standard MRI studies, use of such drugs in fMRI complicates the interpretation of cognitive activation pattern, especially in epilepsy. The effects of medication on the BOLD signal response have not been systematically studied yet. In a study by Jokeit et al. [4], the extent of fMRI activation of the mesial temporal lobes induced by a task based on the retrieval of individually visuospatial knowledge [5] was correlated with the carbamazepine serum level in 21 patients with refractory temporal lobe epilepsy. When compared with normal controls, the activation over the

S.H. Faro and F.B. Mohamed (eds.), *Functional BOLD MRI: Principles and Applications*,
DOI 10.1007/978-1-4939-1995-6_16, © Springer Science+Business Media New York 2015

supposedly normal mesial temporal lobe (i.e., contralateral to the seizure onset) was smaller in patients. More interestingly, in the patient group, the extent of the BOLD activation over the mesial temporal lobes was inversely correlated to the carbamazepine drug level. The reduction of fMRI cluster size was most marked when the drug levels were close to toxic levels. No behavioral data concerning memory function were described for the patient group, and a potential bias of the study was the possibility that a high carbamazepine level is associated with more severe epilepsy. However, these preliminary data provide some evidence that antiepileptic drug treatment may significantly influence fMRI activation of cognitive tasks.

Another consideration with epilepsy patients relates to the effects of epileptic activity to fMRI activation. There is evidence that epileptic activity can influence the lateralization of mesiotemporal memory functions studied by memoryactivated fMRI [6]. In a case report, a patient was described in whom fMRI falsely lateralized language cortex to the right hemisphere when performed after a cluster of left temporal lobe seizures [7]. More recently, it was shown that significant BOLD signal changes can occur several minutes before the onset of a seizure (preictal BOLD signal changes) [8]. These changes can comprise both signal increases and decreases and can be localized to the site of the presumed seizure focus, as well as to distant brain regions. The complex interaction between ictal and interictal activity with fMRI activation tasks is unclear and requires further investigation. In patients with frequent seizures or epileptiform discharges, the results of fMRI activation studies should be interpreted carefully, and in some patients, electroencephalogram (EEG) monitoring before or during the fMRI study might be necessary.

fMRI Applications in the Definition of Eloquent Cortical Areas in Epilepsy

No technique used in the identification of eloquent cortical areas is without a limiting sensitivity and specificity, including the gold standard direct cortical stimulation. Whereas cortical stimulation is essentially a "lesion" study, fMRI measures endogenous function. Thus, these modalities may be expected to differ somewhat in functional localization.

fMRI has the advantage of being able to acquire functional and anatomic maps concurrently and preoperatively, it is equally sensitive to superficial and deep regions, noninvasive, cost effective, and easy to employ, even using routine clinical scanners [9].

Lateralization and Localization of Language

Just 3 years after the first reports on fMRI, a preliminary study showed that the BOLD signal contrast obtained in simple tests of language and motor function was very similar between subjects with epilepsy and normal controls, demonstrating the feasibility of the technique in studies of patients with epilepsy [10]. Since then, fMRI of language processing has become one of the most clinically relevant applications in the field of epilepsy. The main aim of localizing language functions is to predict and minimize postoperative language deficits in patients considered for epilepsy surgery, who are mainly with temporal lobe epilepsy [11]. By that, fMRI is expected to displace Wada testing as the standard of care for determining language and memory dominance in candidates for epilepsy surgery or at least to minimize the use of this invasive test with considerable methodological disadvantages [12]. In general, fMRI is predominantly used for language lateralization (i.e., determination of hemispheric dominance) and only to a lesser extent for intrahemispheric distribution of eloquent cortex.

An overview of the application of fMRI to identify language hemispheric dominance is given in Chap. 9, and a comparison of language and memory fMRI to Wada testing in Chap. 11.

Memory Function

In addition to investigation of language functions, the study of long-term memory systems is central to the presurgical evaluation of patients with temporal lobe epilepsy. The use of fMRI in the prediction of postoperative memory deficits is more challenging than for language. This is partly due to the different components involved in memory processing, such as encoding and retrieval, and the fact that the nature of the material being encoded or retrieved influences which brain areas are activated. A further difficulty is how to separate brain activity related specifically to memory from that related to other cognitive processes [5].

There is long-standing evidence from animal and clinical lesional studies that memory function depends on the functional integrity of the hippocampus and parahippocampal regions in the mesial temporal lobe [13–15]. Whereas the hippocampus proper is the brain region most commonly associated with episodic memory function [16], fMRI studies have often demonstrated activation more posteriorly in the parahippocampal formation. The explanation for this is poorly understood.

Functional imaging studies of these structures are potentially useful in two ways. First, identification of functionally hypoactive temporal lobe structures may have predictive value for lateralization of seizure foci in temporal lobe epilepsy. Second, maps of fMRI activation associated with memory tasks may help in predicting the risk of postoperative memory deficits from temporal lobe surgery and could assist in planning surgical strategies that spare functional tissue.

Tasks, which reliably activate the mesial temporal structures in normal subjects using fMRI, have been developed only relatively recently [17–19] and have rarely been used in patients with epilepsy [5, 20–27]. These studies suggest that (1) complex visual and especially spatial memory tasks are generally superior to verbal memory tasks in activating mesial temporal lobe structures, (2) nonverbal materials activate bilateral mesial temporal lobe structures, (3) encoding as well as retrieval recruit overlapping mesial temporal lobe structures, and (4) retrieval rather than encoding tends to activate bilateral mesial temporal lobe structures [5].

Two studies have compared the fMRI activation of memory tasks with the memory assessment procedures in the Wada test. In 1998, Detre et al. were the first who demonstrated that fMRI could be used to detect clinically relevant asymmetries in memory activation in patients with temporal lobe epilepsy [21]. They used an environmental scene-encoding task [19] in which subjects were asked to memorize each stimulus. In the baseline condition, subjects passively viewed a repeating nonsense stimulus (a spatially scrabbled picture). Region-of-interest analysis of the resulting bilateral activation of posterior mesial temporal lobe structures was then used to calculate a memory lateralization score. fMRI lateralization scores were compared with lateralization indices derived from Wada memory scores. While temporal lobe activation was symmetrical in a normal control group, significant asymmetries were observed in the epilepsy group. In all nine patients, the asymmetry of the activation concurred with the assessment of memory skills from the Wada test, including two patients in which memory was paradoxically located ipsilateral to the seizure focus.

In a 2002 study by Golby et al., fMRI was used to study the lateralization of memory-encoding processes (patterns, faces, scenes, and words) within the mesial temporal lobe in nine patients with temporal lobe epilepsy [24]. In eight of nine subjects, lateralization of memory encoding was concordant with that obtained from the Wada test. Group level analysis demonstrated greater activation in the mesial temporal lobe contralateral to the presumed seizure focus. Furthermore, results suggested that there is reorganization of memory encoding to the contralateral mesial temporal lobe.

Jokeit et al. [5] used a task employing mental navigation and recall of landmarks based on the retrieval of individually familiar visuospatial knowledge (Roland's Hometown Walking), which is known to be associated with symmetrical mesial temporal lobe activation. In 14 of 16 patients with left-sided temporal lobe epilepsy and 13 of 14 patients with right-sided temporal lobe epilepsy, interhemispheric differences in mesial temporal lobe activation lateralized the side of seizure onset correctly, resulting in a correct classification rate of 90%.

A study using a verbal memory encoding and retrieval paradigm compared seven patients with left temporal lobe epilepsy with a normal control group [23]. During retrieval, normal controls activated bilateral parahippocampal regions, right more than left. In the patient group, this pattern was less marked, but an additional left frontal region was also activated. The authors interpret this different activation pattern as a dysfunctional response due to the epilepsy and left hippocampal sclerosis. However, there was a vast difference in performance between patients and normal control groups, which makes a comparison between groups difficult.

The tasks in the studies previously mentioned were partly chosen because they produced bilateral and broadly symmetrical temporal lobe activations in normal controls. Other investigators have utilized memory tasks that produce rather unilateral activations. Bellgowan et al. (1998) reported that mesial temporal lobe activation during a verbal encoding task could differentiate between patients with left and right temporal lobe epilepsy [20]. The group with right temporal lobe epilepsy showed much stronger activation of the left mesial temporal lobe than did the left temporal lobe epilepsy group. Neither group showed activation in the corresponding regions of the right hemisphere. However, these findings were on the group level only and do not allow inferences to be made on an individual-subject basis.

More recently, it could be shown that fMRI of memory function can also be used to predict the individual postsurgical memory outcome in patients undergoing temporal epilepsy surgery [25–29]. In 2004, Rabin et al. used a complex visual scene-encoding task that causes symmetrical mesial-temporal-lobe activation in control, to determine a relation between mesial temporal lobe activation asymmetry ratios and postsurgical memory outcome. It was shown that increased activation ipsilateral to the seizure focus is associated with greater memory decline [25]. In an event-related linguistic encoding fMRI study in patients with temporal lobe epilepsy and left hippocampal sclerosis, greater verbal memory encoding activity in the left hippocampus compared with the right hippocampus predicted the extent of verbal memory decline after the left anterior temporal lobectomy [26]. fMRI was shown to be a stronger independent predictor of memory decline than both preoperative hippocampal volume and preoperative verbal memory function. These studies are the first examples of fMRI showing predictive value for postsurgical memory outcome at the individual subject level in a clinical setting.

Sensorimotor Systems

Among the earliest clinical applications of fMRI was the localization of motor cortices, in particular, in patients with mass lesions around the central sulcus [29–48]. Lesions in the vicinity of the central sulcus are often associated with epilepsy. However, the treatment strategies are often dependent on the nature of the underlying lesion rather than the epilepsy. In any case, it is important to avoid new, unacceptable deficits, or at least to predict a possible loss of function as a consequence of a surgical treatment. Since activation of the primary sensory and motor areas yield robust BOLD signals (near 5% signal change on a 1.5 T scanner), it is relatively easy to determine precise boundaries of functional tissue in these regions with fMRI [33, 49, 50]. Motor cortex representing tongue, hand, finger, arm, and foot areas are readily identified with tongue movement, finger tapping, and toe wiggling; analogous sensory areas are identified with brushing or an air puff. With more complex motor paradigms, the supplementary motor area and cerebellar areas are also activated [51]. Somatotopic activation has been demonstrated by many studies [52–54]. Most of the clinical studies used fMRI for identifying eloquent cortical areas in preparation for tumor or vascular malformation surgery. Several studies have compared the fMRI localization of the sensorimotor cortex with invasive electrocortical stimulation [32, 33, 35, 42, 45, 49, 55, 56]. The differences in fMRI versus cortical stimulation localization varied from 0 to 20 mm and are typically below 10 mm. The greatest differences were found in tumors surrounded by significant perilesional edema.

The most frequent causes for fMRI failure in sensorimotor mapping are stimulus-correlated head movement, inability to move adequately because of existing neurological deficit, and altered hemodynamic response, e.g., due to arteriovenous malformations or vascular tumors [40].

Malformations of Cortical Development

Malformations of cortical development (MCD) are the second most common cause for refractory epilepsy in adults and children [57]. Epileptogenesis in these disorders is not well understood and may depend on the type of MCD. The results of surgical treatment of MCD are less favorable compared with mesial temporal lobe epilepsy, with about 40% of patients rendered seizure-free over a minimum 2-year follow-up period. Space-occupying lesions of the brain primarily displace functional cortex. For this reason, resection within the boundaries of a lesion should not directly damage eloquent cortex and result in a significant deficit. In contrast, cortical stimulation studies showed functional reorganization within dysplastic cortex as well as functional overlap between dysplastic cortex and normal brain tissue. Over the last years, fMRI has shown its ability to demonstrate coactivation of MCD during physiological activation tasks [58]. Two studies on patients with subcortical laminar heterotopia [59, 60] showed fMRI activation both in the outer cortex and the subcortical band heterotopia during performance of a motor task. In another patient with epilepsy and a microgyric visual cortex, the dysplastic cortex was activated by visual stimulation [61].

In contrast, another case report found a common cortical representation of both hands on the unaffected hemisphere and no activation in the hemisphere with a complex malformation [62]. Cortical reorganization and participation of ectopic neuronal tissue in physiologic cerebral functions are of clinical importance in patients who are considered for epilepsy surgery with resection of cortical dysplasia. In addition to localize physiological activation, fMRI has the potential to identify epileptogenicity of dysplastic cortex by imaging ictal or interictal events [63–65]. In 2005, Kobayashi et al. analyzed BOLD signal changes associated with interictal epileptiform discharges (IED) in 14 patients with nodular heterotopia and band heterotopia using EEG-correlated fMRI (for technical details of this technique see the following section) [66]. BOLD signal changes in response to epileptiform discharges were observed within the heterotopia in the surrounding cortex and in distant brain regions. These results suggest that both focal and widespread epileptogenesis areas can occur in malformation of cortical development. In some patients, the heterotopia seems to be the primary epileptogenic region, while in others it appears to be of secondary importance to the epileptogenesis.

In 2008, Tyvaert et al. used EEG-correlated fMRI to study both interictal and ictal events in eight epilepsy patients with different types of MCD. In patients with focal cortical dysplasia, ictal and interictal BOLD signal changes were mainly localized within the dysplastic cortex. Heterotopic and normal appearing cortices were involved in BOLD signal changes during interictal and ictal events in patients with subcortical band heterotopia. In patients with nodular heterotopia, the maximum of the ictal activity was in the overlying cortex and not in the heterotopia [67].

Localization of the Epileptic Focus

Besides the identification of eloquent cortices and the prediction of functional deficits caused by epilepsy surgery, fMRI is also capable of providing evidence for the localization of the epileptic focus by identifying ictal or interictal epileptic activity, as described in the next sections.

Ictal fMRI

Ictal fMRI activation has the advantage that it can be expected to reflect changes within the epileptogenic region itself (and propagation sites).

Currently, only a few anecdotal reports and small studies on ictal fMRI are published.

The first attempt to use fMRI for the localization of epileptic activity was reported in 1994 by Jackson et al. [68]. This case report dealt with a 4-year-old patient with the diagnosis of Rasmussen's encephalitis. A standard MRI of the patient's brain showed widespread right hemispheric atrophy primarily over the more dorsal lateral frontal region and inferior Rolandic area. The patient was prone to frequent and prolonged focal motor seizures that involved the left arm, hand, and face. These bouts of epilepsia partialis continua were then targeted for investigation using a fast low-angle shot (FLASH) sequence to obtain susceptibility-weighted images every 8 s from a single slice only. This study demonstrated that seizure-related perfusion changes over the right inferior motor cortex corresponding to the area of maximum atrophy seen on the conventional MRI and to the region of maximum abnormality as identified with an ictal single photon emission tomography (SPECT) study [68]. Another case was reported by Warach et al. in 1994. This patient had prolonged focal status epilepticus and demonstrated a perfusion MRI abnormality over the left parietofrontal region using a susceptibility-weighted sequence and dynamic enhancement with gadolinium. This abnormal region was in keeping with the localization of the spike focus of scalp EEG and the hyperperfusion defect detected with ictal SPECT. The EEG, perfusion-based MRI abnormality, and SPECT findings normalized after more aggressive medical management [69]. Further case reports with equal findings were subsequently published [63, 70, 71]. In none of these reports was EEG recording available during MR image acquisition. Seizure detection was only possible by clinical observation of the patient in the MR scanner. The first ictal fMRI with simultaneous EEG recording was reported by Salek-Haddadi et al. in 2002. A patient with partial and generalized tonic-clonic seizures showed ictal EEG changes (rhythmic delta and theta activity maximum over F7/T3 lasting for about 40 s) in the EEG recorded inside the MR scanner. A continuous BOLD-fMRI series was simultaneously acquired and revealed a 2.5% signal increase, mainly over the left temporal lobe, peaking at around 6 s into the seizure followed later by a prolonged undershoot [72].

Further studies of ictal fMRI were performed in reflex epilepsies, in particular reading epilepsy [73]. In a study of nine patients with reading epilepsy using simultaneous EEG, EMG, and fMRI, ictal fMRI revealed patterns of BOLD activation in cortical and subcortical areas overlapping or adjacent to areas physiologically activated during language and facial motor tasks, such as left motor and premotor areas, left striatum, and mesiotemporal/limbic areas [74].

In summary, ictal fMRI studies have demonstrated that fMRI, analogous to ictal SPECT, is capable of imaging reversible perfusion or BOLD abnormalities associated with epileptic seizures, with the abnormality localized closely to the site of maximum electric abnormality. However, in contrast to ictal SPECT (which is costly but feasible in specialized epilepsy units), ictal fMRI is not routinely practicable for a number of reasons: Most ictal events are associated with head and body movement and impairment of consciousness usually to a degree that the required level of cooperation for an MRI scan cannot be achieved. Furthermore, BOLD-fMRI is not sensitive to detecting low frequency state-related changes due to large intersessional effects and scanner noise characteristics. Together with the slow hemodynamic response function (HRF), this limits detection power to a narrow frequency band and will tend to necessitate capturing both seizure onset and termination. Seizures, however, are usually short lasting and unpredictable. It is impracticable for a patient, even with frequent seizures, to lie for hours in an MR scanner awaiting the onset of one or several seizures. fMRI studies with concurrent EEG recording are complicated further by the extra time involved in attaching electrodes and equipment set up. For these practical reasons, the investigation of ictal activity will be limited to selected patients who have very frequent seizures without gross head movement, in particular seizure series, status epilepticus, or epilepsia partialis continua, or have epilepsy syndromes with seizures occurring predictably, e.g., reflex epilepsy.

Interictal fMRI

As physiological brain activity (and epileptic seizures), IED are associated with alterations of cerebral blood flow and deoxyglobin concentration in the venous bed. Hence, fMRI should be capable to identify the sources of IED in the same way that it can identify sources of functional activation from movement or cognitive processing. This is in contrast to methods such as dipole modeling, which can find only possible intracerebral sources of surface potentials and rely on assumptions that are not always easy to justify.

When compared with ictal fMRI, mapping of interictal activity has several advantages: (1) IED are a common phenomenon in patients with epilepsy, (2) IED are not associated with stimulus-correlated motion, and (3) fMRI activation associated with single discharges are less likely to be confounded with propagation effects compared with ongoing ictal activity.

On the other hand, fMRI correlated with IED localizes brain areas involved in generating these particular EEG events. The area of cortex that generates IED is labeled as the "irritative zone," which is not necessarily indicatory for the epileptogenic zone, the area of cortex that is indispensable for the generation of epileptic seizures [1].

As IED are usually a subclinical phenomenon, a second modality is necessary to identify these events. Hence, this approach was only made possible by recording EEG inside the MR scanner (EEG-correlated fMRI).

Methodological Aspects of EEG-Correlated fMRI

The MRI scanner is a hostile environment for EEG recordings. MR-compatible EEG recording equipment must ensure patient safety, sufficient quality of the EEG signals, and avoid compromising MR image quality. Since the first report on human EEG recording during MR imaging almost 20 years ago by Ives et al. [75], these issues have been addressed by several studies and technical solutions have been proposed [76–80]. Several commercial systems for intra-MR EEG recordings are now available. The main specific features implemented in these systems are a battery-powered nonmagnetic amplifier with a fiber-optic link, a high dynamic range of the amplifier, a high sampling rate, and careful choice of materials for the electrode assembly.

The most crucial practical difficulty that must be overcome before useful functional data can be acquired is EEG quality. The two most relevant artifacts obscuring the EEG recorded inside the MR scanner are (1) *pulse artifact* (or *cardioballistogram*) and (2) *image-acquisition artifact* [77, 79–82].

Cardioballistic and other movement-related artifacts are caused by movements of the body and EEG leads relative to the magnetic field of the MR scanner. It can be reduced by minimizing the area of the EEG wire loops, lead fixation, and bipolar montage of the EEG with small interelectrode distances. Remaining pulse artifacts can be removed by averaging and subtraction of the artifacts synchronized to the electrocardiogram (ECG) (Figs. 16.1a, b) [77, 81, 83]. These methods provide a degree of EEG quality sufficient for the accurate identification not only of IED [84], but also sleep stages [85], physiological EEG rhythms [86], and evoked potentials [87] in the intervals between image acquisitions.

During MR image acquisition, the EEG is obscured completely by large artifacts, mainly due to induced voltages in the EEG leads subjected to the rapidly changing gradient fields.

Several solutions to the problem of EEG-imaging artifact removal have been proposed [79, 83]. These techniques rely on amplification with sufficient dynamic range to avoid saturation of the EEG amplifier due to the artifact and a high sampling rate. The method developed by Allen et al. [77] uses a scanner-generated slice-timing pulse. For each channel, online subtraction of a running time-averaged waveform is performed, followed by adaptive noise cancelation to reduce any residual artifact. Hoffmann et al. [83] proposed a post-processing filtering method based on the fast Fourier transform (FFT): Segments of EEG without MR activity are compared with the FFT of the EEG recorded during imaging. Frequencies with amplitudes over a threshold

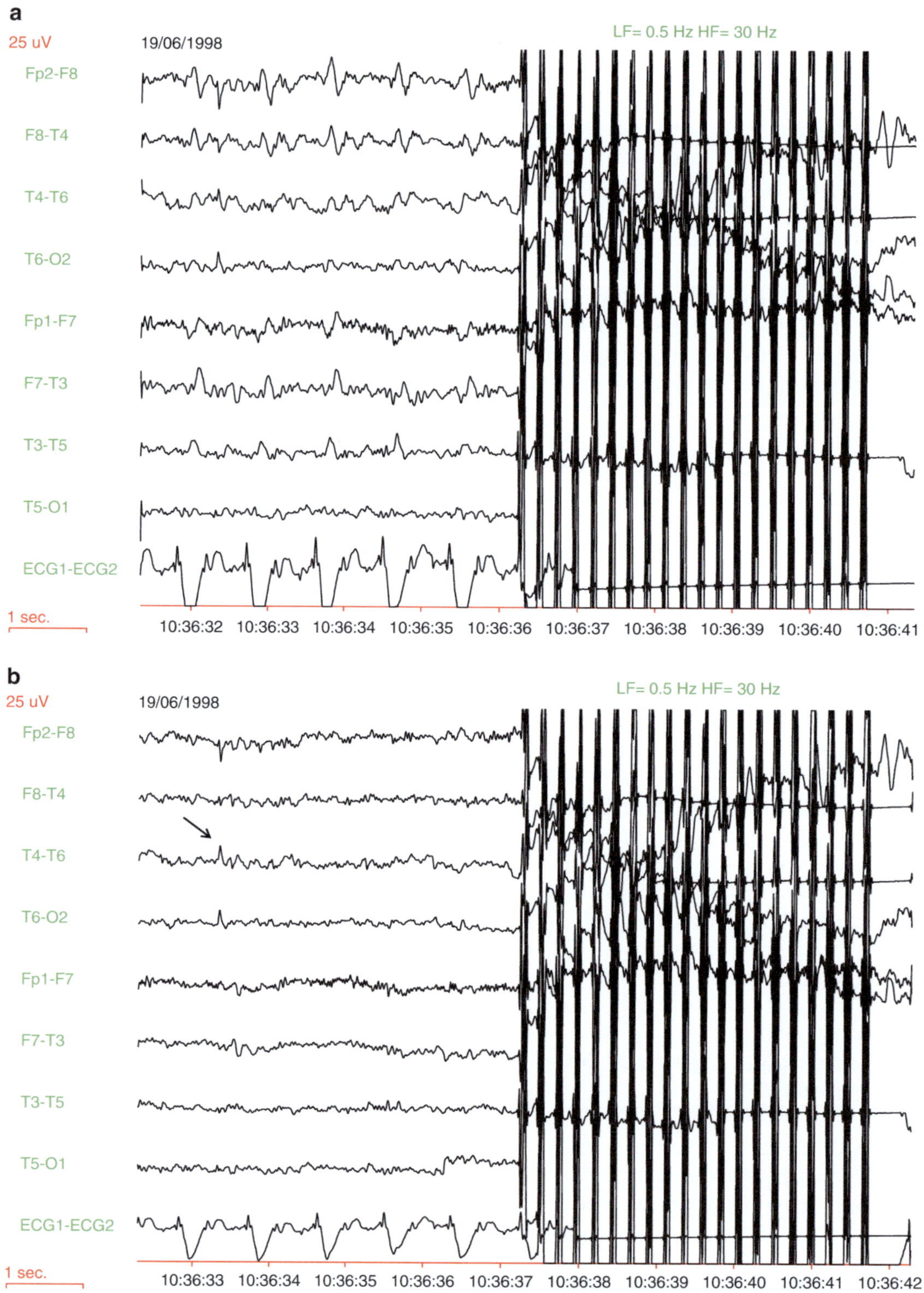

Fig. 16.1 Electroencephalogram recorded inside a 1.5 T scanner. In (**a**) an ECG-related artifact is obscuring the EEG activity (pulse artifact, cardioballistogram), making the identification of IED difficult; (**b**) shows the identical EEG sequence after on-line pulse artifact subtraction. A small amplitude spike is clearly detectable over the right hemisphere. Three-and-a-half seconds after the spike, a 20-slice EPI sequence is triggered, leading to a large EEG artifact (image acquisition artifact). The imaging result of the spike-triggered fMRI experiment is demonstrated in Fig. 16.2

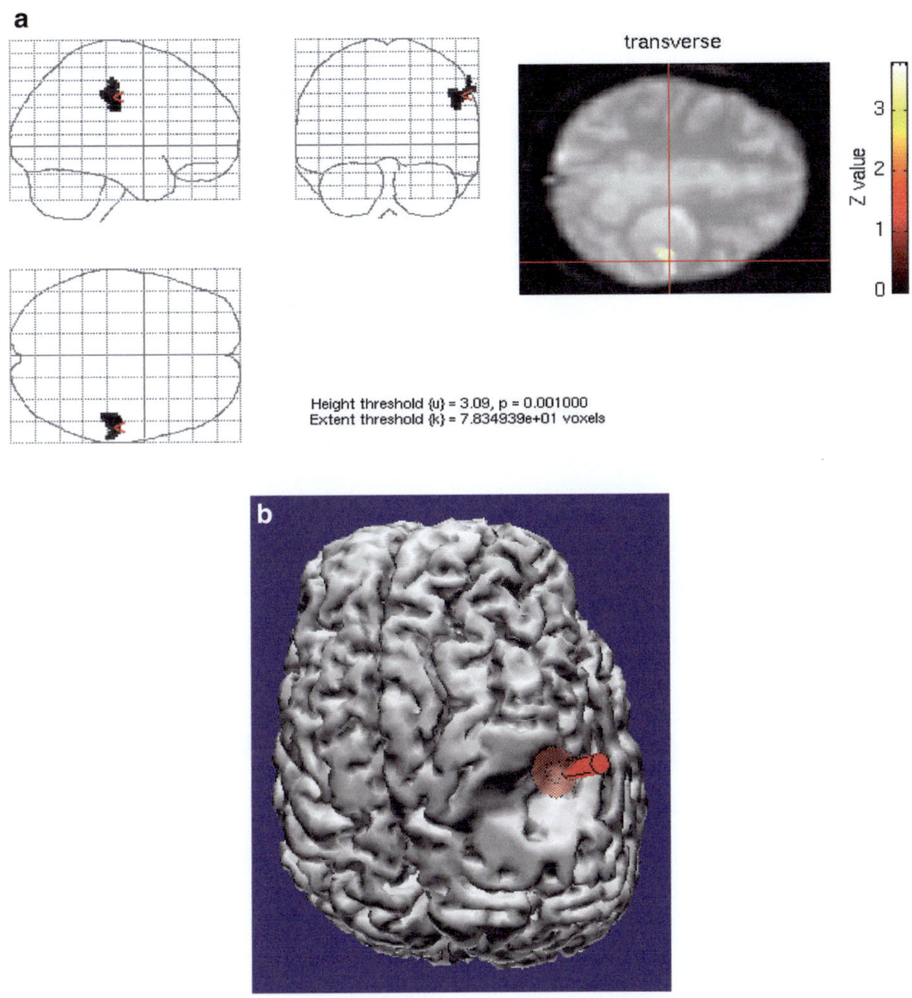

Fig. 16.2 (**a**) The statistical parametric mapping BOLD activation map of a spike-triggered fMRI experiment, which was performed on a 22-year-old patient with refractory partial and secondarily generalized seizures. Standard MRI showed subcortical nodular heterotopia of the right hemisphere with a large mass in the central region. Interictal EEG demonstrated frequent focal IED over the temporal and parasagittal region of the right hemisphere. Functional MRI result shows an axial image with crosshair through the center of the activation (overlaid in *yellow*), in the center of the nodular heterotopia of the right hemisphere. (**b**) Result of a 64-channel EEG source analysis (multiple unconstrained moving dipole model, CURRY 3.0), superimposed on a T1-weighted anatomical scan, showing colocalization with the result of the spike-triggered fMRI (Neurologic coordinates)

determined based on the FFT of the normal EEG are then discarded. The inverted FFT gives the corrected EEG. More recently, introduced methods of minimizing image acquisition artifacts comprise temporal principal component analysis (PCA), which can identify a set of basis functions that describe the temporal variations of the artifacts. These basis functions can then fitted to, and subtracted from, EEG data to reduce EEG artifacts [88]. Anami et al. [89] proposed a method that relies on synchronization between the EEG sampling and a modified fMRI sequence ("stepping stone sampling").

The ability to remove image artifacts determines the data acquisition of EEG-correlated fMRI experiments. Without image artifact removal, the EEG is obscured during imaging and interleaved data acquisition has to be applied. In epilepsy studies, this approach was introduced as spike-triggered fMRI (Figs. 16.2a, b). This

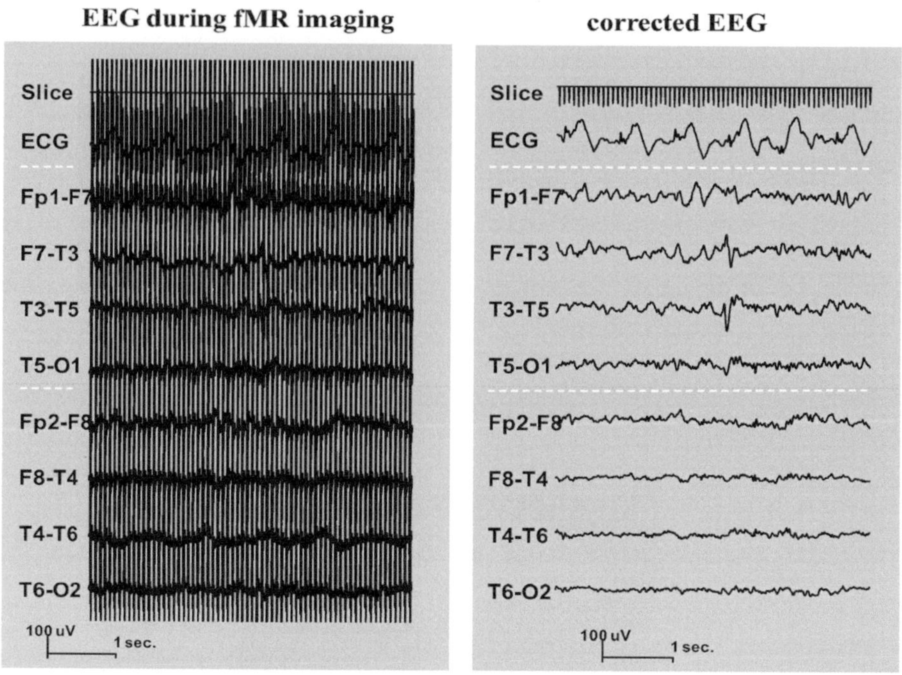

Fig. 16.3 Two segments of an EEG recording made during a continuous EEG/fMRI experiment before and after image artifact subtraction. The possibility of removing image acquisition artifact enables continuous and simultaneous EEG/fMRI in contrast to spike-triggered fMRI

method takes advantage of the delayed BOLD response after a neuronal event. This makes it possible to observe the EEG recording on-line (which requires the presence of an experienced electroencephalographer during data acquisition) and start image acquisitions manually at a fixed interval after the event of interest (usually 3 s, as the BOLD response peaks at 2–7 s after an event) or during control periods. However, spike-triggered fMRI suffers from two main limitations, both linked to the obliteration of the EEG during the image acquisition. First, there are constraints on the scanning rate and the duration of each scan. The minimum time gap between successive image acquisitions must be of the order of 15 s to avoid signal variations due to the T1-signal decay, and the maximum duration of each image acquisition must be less than the expected duration of the BOLD response to ensure proper separation of the responses from events that may occur during image acquisition, and therefore remain undetected. Second, as mentioned previously, the spike-triggered approach relies on assumptions about the BOLD response peak time and duration. However, spike-triggered fMRI is not able to reveal the HRF due to a delayed image acquisition and the lack of pre-activity baseline images.

With the possibility of image artifact subtraction, these limitations can be overcome by continuous and simulta-neous EEG-correlated fMRI (Fig. 16.3). In contrast to spike-triggered fMRI, continuous EEG/fMRI recording allows for full exploration of the temporal dynamics of activation in addition to spatial localization (Figs. 16.4 and 16.5). For each voxel, an entire time series is available for interrogation in contrast to the limited number of time points available for comparison in spike-triggered fMRI. Another advantage is that continuous EEG/fMRI allows for post hoc analysis of the EEG events of interest. Regarding image analysis, in spike-triggered fMRI there are no requirements to model the hemodynamic response. Scans can be simply grouped into spike and rest categories, and a *t*-test can be performed to judge significance. In continuous EEG/fMRI,

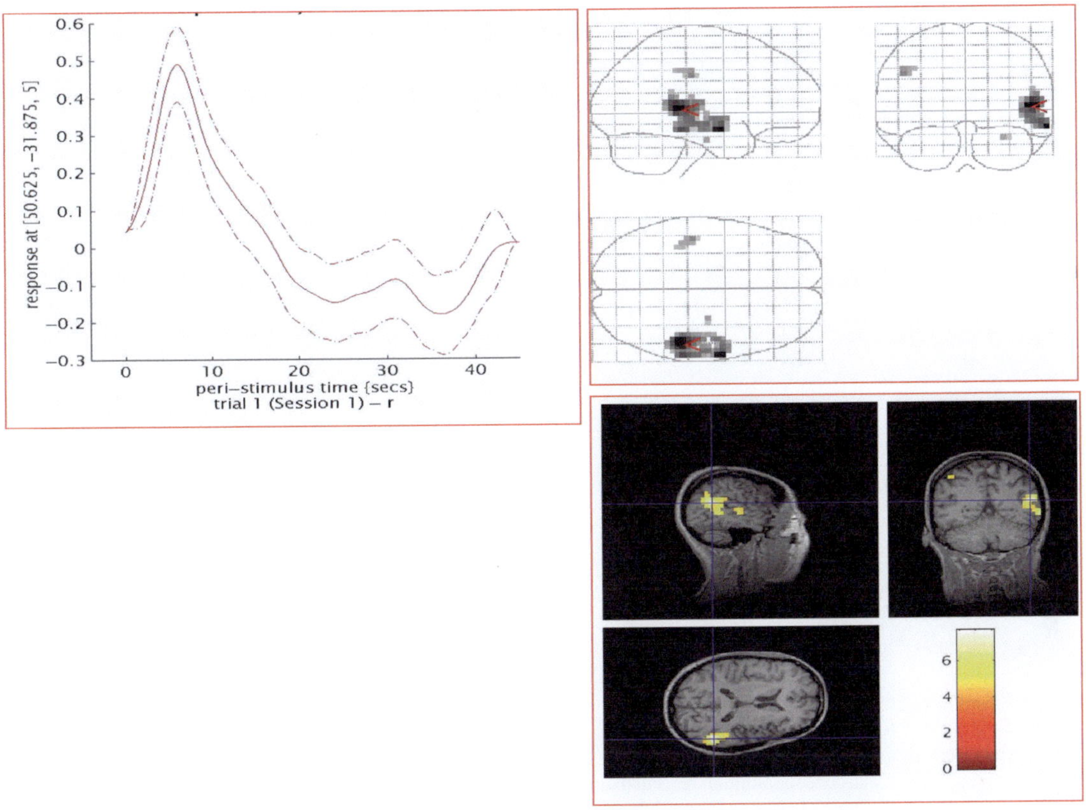

Fig. 16.4 Result of a continuous and simultaneous EEG/fMRI experiment in a patient with partial seizures due to a right temporoparietal malformation of cortical development and frequent right temporal spikes. The fMRI activation is located within the subtle cortical dysplasia. *Left*: The time course of the event-related response at location of the crosshair

the IED are treated as events of interest in an event-related analysis of the fMRI data. This involves creating a model time course for the IED and convolving this function with an appropriate HRF. This basis function is included in the analysis, and variance correlated to this model is compared with residual variance. Voxels are considered to be activated during IED when the modeled variance is significant compared with residual variance. As summarized by Salek-Haddadi et al. [84], EEG/fMRI studies in epilepsy vary considerably in their analysis approach, including acquisition method, HRF model, as well as the statistical threshold reported as significant.

In general, the continuous EEG/fMRI technique is thought to lead to a greater sensitivity to identify BOLD signal changes associated with IED compared with the spike-triggered approach [90]. Continuous EEG/fMRI has largely replaced EEG-triggered fMRI not only in the field of epilepsy, but also in EEG/fMRI studies of sleep [91], physiological EEG rhythms [92], and evoked potentials [93].

EEG-Correlated fMRI of Interictal Activity

So far, about 30 studies applying EEG-correlated fMRI to patients with epilepsy have been published. The first study using EEG-correlated fMRI in patients with epilepsy was reported by Warach et al. in 1996 [94]. In two patients with epilepsy, IED were associated with fMRI activations. In the following years, several studies followed using

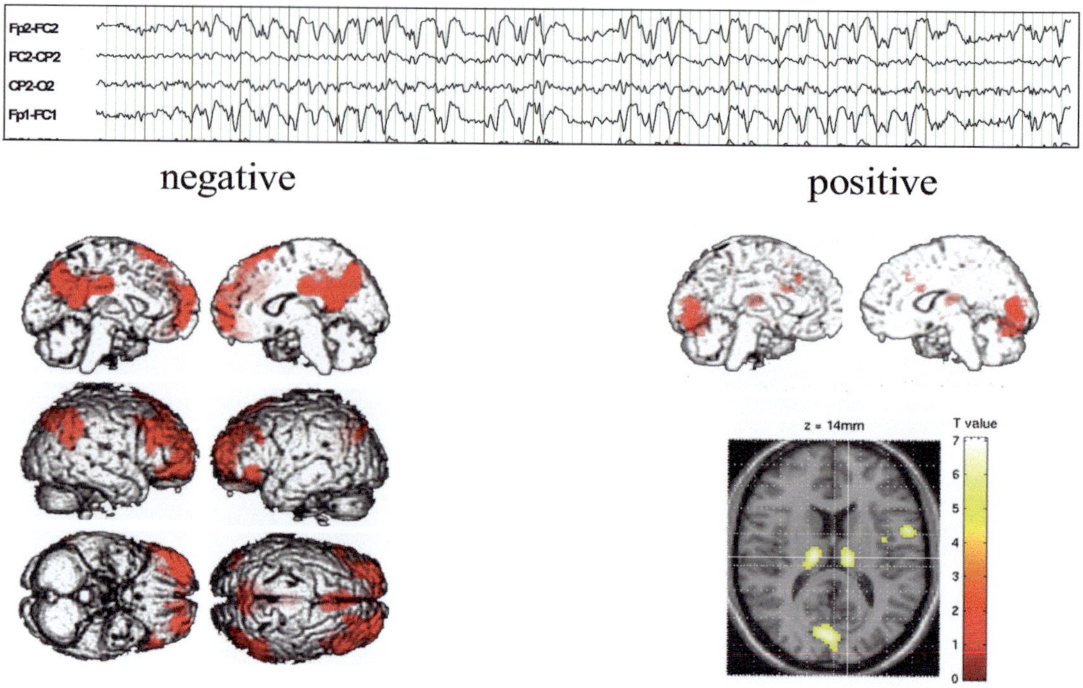

Fig. 16.5 Result of a continuous and simultaneous EEG/fMRI experiment in a patient with idiopathic epilepsy and absence seizures. The electroencephalogram recorded during functional magnetic resonance imaging shows intermittent ~2/s GSWD with frontal emphasis after image artifact reduction. Maps of fMRI signal changes during GSWD on EEG indicate brain areas where fMRI signal is significantly negatively or positively correlated with GSWD. Negative correlations ("deactivations") with GSWD are detected bilaterally in dorsal prefrontal and temporoparietal cortices and the precuneus and posterior cingulum. Regions with significant positive activations include the posterior thalamus

spike-triggered fMRI [95–100]. Since 2001, an increasing number of studies using continuous EEG/fMRI have been reported [66, 101–104]. Most of the studies were performed in patients with focal epilepsy, often medically refractory epilepsy. A few studies concentrated on defined epilepsy syndromes, such as benign epilepsy with controtemporal spikes (BECTS and rolandic epilepsy) in children [105, 106] and idiopathic generalized epilepsy [107–112].

In summary, the studies showed that EEG-correlated fMRI is a practicable method to be applied to patients with epilepsy showing frequent IED on scalp EEG (Table 16.1). The EEG quality was sufficient to detect spontaneous IED off- or on-line. Discomfort or injuries of the patients due to the EEG-recording were not reported, and the MR image quality was not significantly compromised by the EEG recording. In the patients with focal epilepsy, the activations were, in general, anatomically related to the proposed epileptic focus (as defined by interictal EEG, EEG source analysis, structural MRI, ictal video-EEG, or, in a few patients, intracranial EEG). In one of the first studies in a clinical population, Krakow et al. [99] reported 24 patients investigated with EEG-triggered fMRI. Between 12 and 50 IED were captured per session. Twelve of the 24 patients showed reproducible focal activation, which occurred in close spatial relationship to the maximum of the IED on scalp EEG. The range of pathologies included encephalitis, cortical dysgenesis, hippocampal sclerosis, low-grade astrocytoma, and dysembryoplastic neuroepithelial tumors (DNET). Nine patients had no detectable structural abnormalities. Of the

Table 16.1 Summary of EEG-correlated fMRI studies in patients with epilepsy

Authors	Subjects	EEG/fMRI technique	Results
Krakow et al., 1999 [96]	Ten consecutively recruited patients with focal epilepsy	Spike-triggered fMRI, two or more experiments in each patient, 1.5 T	Reproducible significant BOLD signal changes in six of ten patients in close relation to the presumed epileptic focus
Salek-Haddadi et al., 2006 [114]	63 consecutively recruited patients with focal epilepsy	Simultaneous EEG/ fMRI, 1.5 T	Significant BOLD signal changes in 68% of patients with epileptic spikes
Benar et al., 2006 [123]	Five patients with focal epilepsy	Simultaneous EEG/ fMRI, comparison with EEG and intracranial EEG results	Intracranial EEG largely validated the fMRI signal increases and decreases associated with epileptic spikes
Laufs et al., 2006 [111]	One patient with absence seizures	Simultaneous EEG/ fMRI, 3 T	Generalized spike-and-wave discharges were associated with signal decreases bilateral frontal, temporoparietal and in the precuneus, reflecting suspension of the "default mode" of brain function
Zijlmans et al., 2007 [115]	29 patients with focal epilepsy, no structural lesion, presurgical evaluation	Simultaneous EEG/ fMRI, 1.5 T	Positive results in 8/29 patients. EEG/fMRI can contribute to (negative) decision regarding candidacy for epilepsy surgery.

six patients with cortical dysgenesis, four showed activation in all cases located within the cortical malformation. In a patient with DNET, BOLD activation was shown adjacent to the lesion. In accordance with more recent studies using continuous EEG/fMRI [104, 113], these results support the concept of varying relationships between the epileptogenic lesion and the irritative zone. Gray matter within cortical dysgenesis may have intrinsic epileptogenic properties, while other lesions, for example tumors, may generate IED in the vicinity.

The largest group of patients studied with EEG-correlated fMRI was reported by Salek-Haddadi et al. in 2006 [114]. In 68% of 63 consecutively recruited patients with focal epilepsy, significant BOLD signal changes associated with IED were detected. The BOLD signal changes were highly concordant with the site(s) of presumed seizure generation, although deactivations provided less specific information of the localization. It could be shown that focal activations were more likely when there was good electroclinical localization, frequent stereotyped spikes, less head motion, and less background EEG abnormality.

In patients with refractory focal epilepsy, EEG/fMRI results could be compared with results of the presurgical evaluation, and in a few patients surgery was carried out after the EEG/fMRI experiment. The largest of the studies correlating invasive EEG recordings with EEG/fMRI activations was reported by Lazeyras et al. [98]. A total of 11 patients were investigated with EEG-triggered fMRI, who also underwent presurgical evaluation for their epilepsy with video-EEG, PET, and SPECT studies. In 8 of 11 patients, intracranial recordings were carried out, and in five of them, the irritative zone as determined by fMRI was affirmed.

In 2007, Zijlmans et al. assessed the potential added value of EEG/fMRI in the presurgical evaluation of patients with complex source localization (unclear focus and/or presumed multifocality on the basis of EEG) [115]. Twenty-nine patients were included; eight of these patients had a BOLD activation that was considered as significant. The main impact on the clinical decision was a corroboration of a negative decision regarding surgical candidacy and an improvement of source localization.

Despite this study investigating the value of EEG/fMRI in clinical practice, it still remains unclear whether EEG-correlated fMRI has the potential to replace invasive techniques to identify the irritative zone in a larger scale or, at least, provide additional information to guide the placement of invasive intracranial electrodes where necessary. The clinical implementation of EEG-correlated fMRI and the interpretation of the fMRI activation maps are difficult for various reasons:

1. The limitations of surface EEG affect the clinical application of EEG-correlated fMRI.

   It is well known by electroencephalographers that the majority of EEGs recorded in patients with epilepsy are entirely normal or show only unspecific slowing. Cortical spiking in epileptic patients as recorded directly from cortex is often not accessible by surface EEG. Therefore, EEG-correlated fMRI remains limited to the minority of patients with frequent IED on surface EEG.

   To overcome the limitations of surface EEG, methods have been suggested to detect IED-related BOLD signal changes without concurrent EEG recording. An example of such an exploratory, data-driven technique is temporal clustering analysis (TCA). It is based on the premise that activation would cause the number of voxels reaching their individual maximum values at any given point to rise beyond a certain threshold. It makes no assumptions with regards to the proximity of the voxels that constitute the clusters and is limited in that each voxel will reach its maximum only once in the time series. Using this approach, Morgan et al., in 2004, analyzed fMRI data in nine patients with focal epilepsy acquired during rest in an attempt to localize brain activation associated with IED [116]. By looking for a particular subset of variance, specifically changes of between 2 and 10% from the resting BOLD intensity level, focal fMRI activations with a high degree of concordance to electroclinical data could be identified in six patients. It was proposed that resting fMRI with temporal clustering analyses without EEG could contribute to localize the irritative zone. However, these findings have not been reproduced by other groups yet, and theoretical and methodological problems of this approach have been asserted, e.g., the association of the fMRI activations with head movement [117].

2. The size of the fMRI activation cluster is greatly variable between studies and also between subjects in individual studies. Some patients have a widespread, multifocal activation, others show a circumscribed activation. The extent of the activation is critically dependent on the applied statistical threshold, which partly explains differences between studies. EEG-correlated fMRI may contribute to localize the source of IED, but currently it cannot provide information about its extent. The reason for the variability between patients who were studied with identical methodology and thresholds remains unclear. No significant correlations between clinical characteristics (e.g., epilepsy syndrome and spike amplitude) and the size of the fMRI activation were found. The same applies for the number of IEDs that have been analyzed: In some patients, even individual IEDs are associated with large activations [118] in other patients as many as 50 IEDs are not associated with significant activations [99].

   In patients with widespread fMRI activation, another problem is to distinguish the primary sources from activation, which may represent areas of propagation. In such cases with equivocal information on localization, a combination of fMRI data with EEG source analysis may provide complementary information [95, 119].

3. Until now, the results of EEG-correlated fMRI have not been systematically validated with a gold standard, which are intracranial recordings and outcome after epilepsy surgery. Before EEG-triggered fMRI can be used as a decisive method to identify the irritative zone (and therewith provide information for localization of the epileptogenic zone), the relation between fMRI results, invasive EEG recordings, and surgical outcome in relation to resection of the activated area has to be established.

Furthermore, in all EEG/fMRI studies previously mentioned, only about 250 patients were reported in total. Patients for EEG/fMRI experiments were, in general, highly selected, particularly with regard to the frequency of their IEDs. It is questionable if EEG/fMRI has the potential to be applied to relevant numbers of patients in a clinical setting.

4. The high percentage of negative results even in the highly selected patients (up to 50% in the larger studies using spike-triggered fMRI) [97–100] currently hinders the wider clinical application of EEG-correlated fMRI. The physiological explanation of a negative fMRI result is that most likely a nonsignificant difference in the blood oxygenation exists between activation and control states. This might be due to there being only a modest cerebral hyperperfusion following an IED or due to an absence of a true control state, e.g., such as ongoing epileptic activity not detected on scalp EEG. In both cases, the relative signal change within the spike generator may not achieve significance.

   As previously mentioned, it is conceivable that continuous and simultaneous EEG/fMRI will increase the sensitivity of the method. However, this has to be proven by larger-scale studies using this technique and comparative studies between spike-triggered and simultaneous EEG/fMRI. Further, the use of higher strength magnets will increase the signal-to-noise ratio and hence fMRI sensitivity. Multichannel EEG has already been recorded in a 4 T MR scanner on humans and in a 7 T MR scanner in animals [120].

   An improved signal-to-noise ratio may not only increase the proportion of fMRI-positive experiments, but may also reduce the number of analyzed IEDs necessary for a significant fMRI activation, thus rendering this method applicable to patients with less frequent IEDs.

5. The significance of BOLD signal changes associated with IED is currently not well understood. In focal epilepsy, positive BOLD signal changes typically localize the generators of IED, i.e., the irritative zone. However, some patients show widespread or multifocal activations not related to the irritative zone. In addition, many patients show solely or additional negative BOLD signal changes in association with IED, especially associated with polyspike and spike-and-slow wave discharges of longer duration (bursts) [121]. These "deactivations" were observed in most EEG/fMRI studies, but yet not systematically investigated. As IEDs are a marker of the neural hyperexcitability underlying epilepsy, the observation of fMRI "deactivation" is intriguing. In some patients, negative BOLD signal changes are in good spatial agreement with the presumed irritative zone and may represent processes of focal inhibition. More frequently, negative BOLD signal changes occur widespread and bilaterally. In patients with idiopathic epilepsy, generalized spike and wave discharges (GSWD) were associated with negative BOLD signal changes in bilateral frontal, parietal cortices, and retrosplenial areas (precuneus, posterior cingulum) [110, 111]. Together with bilateral frontal and temporoparietal areas, restrosplenial areas constitute a functional network that may be active in a default mode of brain function during rest [122]. This activation pattern may indicate an aberrant suspension of this network's functionality due to the generalized IED. However, similar deactivation patterns occur also with focal IED, indicating that the BOLD signal changes associated with epileptiform activity do not only localize generators of IED within the irritative zone, but also indicate complex changes of functional connectivity.

Conclusion

Functional MRI of sensorimotor, language, and memory function can be considered as clinical tools to identify eloquent cortex and to predict postoperative deficits of specific functions. It already offers a valid alternative to invasive methods such as the Wada test for establishing language dominance, and it is likely that fMRI will also replace the Wada test for assessing presurgical memory function in the nearer future.

EEG-correlated fMRI has proved useful to provide insights into the generation of IED in patients with focal and generalized epilepsy. In selected patients with frequent IED, EEG-correlated fMRI has the potential to reproducibly identify cortical areas involved in generating IED, i.e., the irritative zone. So far, the sensitivity of the method is in the range of 50–70%. To determine the specificity of the method, further studies are necessary to compare the EEG/fMRI results with the diagnostic gold standards, which are intracranial EEG recordings and postoperative outcome after epilepsy surgery. Until these results are available, the utility of EEG-correlated fMRI in clinical epileptology cannot be definitely determined.

References

1. Rosenow F, Luders H. Presurgical evaluation of epilepsy. Brain. 2001;124:1683–700.
2. Melendez JC, McCrank E. Anxiety-related reactions associated with magnetic resonance imaging examinations. JAMA. 1993;270:745–7.
3. Thorp D, Owens RG, Whitehouse G, Dewey ME. Subjective experiences of magnetic resonance imaging. Clin Radiol. 1990;41:276–8.
4. Jokeit H, Okujava M, Woermann FG. Carbamazepine reduces memory induced activation of mesial temporal lobe structures: a pharmacological fMRI-study. BMC Neurol. 2001;1:6.
5. Jokeit H, Okujava M, Woermann FG. Memory fMRI lateralizes temporal lobe epilepsy. Neurology. 2001; 57:1786–93.
6. Janszky J, Ollech I, Jokeit H, Kontopoulou K, Mertens M, Pohlmann-Eden B, et al. Epileptic activity influences the lateralization of mesiotemporal fMRI activity. Neurology. 2004;63:1813–7.
7. Jayakar P, Bernal B, Santiago Medina L, Altman N. False lateralization of language cortex on functional MRI after a cluster of focal seizures. Neurology. 2002;58:490–2.
8. Federico P, Abbott DF, Briellmann RS, Harvey AS, Jackson GD. Functional MRI of the pre-ictal state. Brain. 2005;128:1811–7.
9. Fernandez G, de Greiff A, von Oertzen J, et al. Language mapping in less than 15 minutes: real-time functional MRI during routine clinical investigation. Neuroimage. 2001;14:585–94.
10. Morris 3rd GL, Mueller WM, Yetkin FZ, et al. Functional magnetic resonance imaging in partial epilepsy. Epilepsia. 1994;35:1194–8.
11. Hermann BP, Perrine K, Chelune GJ, et al. Visual confrontation naming following left anterior temporal lobectomy: a comparison of surgical approaches. Neuropsychology. 1999;13:3–9.
12. Haag A, Knake S, Hamer HM, Boesebeck F, Freitag H, Schulz R, et al. The Wada test in Austrian, Dutch, German, and Swiss epilepsy centers from 2000 to 2005: a review of 1421 procedures. Epilepsy Behav. 2008;13:83–9.
13. McGaugh JL. Memory–a century of consolidation. Science. 2000;287:248–51.
14. Sass KJ, Spencer DD, Kim JH, Westerveld M, Novelly RA, Lencz T. Verbal memory impairment correlates with hippocampal pyramidal cell density. Neurology. 1990;40:1694–7.
15. Scoville WB, Milner B. Loss of recent memory after bilateral hippocampal lesions. 1957. J Neuropsychiatry Clin Neurosci. 2000;12:103–13.
16. Squire LR. Memory and the hippocampus: a synthesis from findings with rats, monkeys, and humans. Psychol Rev. 1992;99:195–231.
17. Fernandez G, Weyerts H, Schrader-Bolsche M, et al. Successful verbal encoding into episodic memory engages the posterior hippocampus: a parametrically analyzed functional magnetic resonance imaging study. J Neurosci. 1998;18:1841–7.
18. Gabrieli JD, Brewer JB, Desmond JE, Glover GH. Separate neural bases of two fundamental memory processes in the human medial temporal lobe. Science. 1997;276:264–6.
19. Stern CE, Corkin S, Gonzalez RG, et al. The hippocampal formation participates in novel picture encoding: evidence from functional magnetic resonance imaging. Proc Natl Acad Sci USA. 1996;93: 8660–5.
20. Bellgowan PS, Binder JR, Swanson SJ, et al. Side of seizure focus predicts left medial temporal lobe activation during verbal encoding. Neurology. 1998;51:479–84.
21. Detre JA, Maccotta L, King D, et al. Functional MRI lateralization of memory in temporal lobe epilepsy. Neurology. 1998;50:926–32.
22. Dupont S, Samson Y, Van de Moortele PF, et al. Delayed verbal memory retrieval: a functional MRI study in epileptic patients with structural lesions of the left medial temporal lobe. Neuroimage. 2001;14:995–1003.
23. Dupont S, Van de Moortele PF, Samson S, et al. Episodic memory in left temporal lobe epilepsy: a functional MRI study. Brain. 2000;123:1722–32.
24. Golby AJ, Poldrack RA, Illes J, Chen D, Desmond JE, Gabrieli JD. Memory lateralization in medial temporal lobe epilepsy assessed by functional MRI. Epilepsia. 2002;43:855–63.
25. Rabin ML, Narayan VM, Kimberg DY, Casasanto DJ, Glosser G, Tracy JI, et al. Functional MRI predicts post-surgical memory following temporal lobectomy. Brain. 2004;127:2286–98.
26. Richardson MP, Strange BA, Thompson PJ, Baxendale SA, Duncan JS, Dolan RJ. Pre-operative verbal memory fMRI predicts post-operative memory decline after left temporal lobe resection. Brain. 2004;127:2419–26.
27. Janszky J, Jokeit H, Kontopoulou K, Mertens M, Ebner A, Pohlmann-Eden B, et al. Functional MRI predicts memory performance after right mesiotemporal epilepsy surgery. Epilepsia. 2005;46:244–50.
28. Powell HW, Richardson MP, Symms MR, Boulby PA, Thompson PJ, Duncan JS, et al. Preoperative

fMRI predicts memory decline following anterior temporal lobe resection. J Neurol Neurosurg Psychiatry. 2008;79:686–93.
29. Frings L, Wagner K, Halsband U, Schwarzwald R, Zentner J, Schulze-Bonhage A. Lateralization of hippocampal activation differs between left and right temporal lobe epilepsy patients and correlates with postsurgical verbal learning decrement. Epilepsy Res. 2008;78(2–3):161–70.
30. Yetkin FZ, Mueller WM, Morris GL, et al. Functional MR activation correlated with intraoperative cortical mapping. AJNR Am J Neuroradiol. 1997;18:1311–5.
31. Ruge MI, Victor J, Hosain S, et al. Concordance between functional magnetic resonance imaging and intraoperative language mapping. Stereotact Funct Neurosurg. 1999;72:95–102.
32. Jack Jr CR, Thompson RM, Butts RK, et al. Sensory motor cortex: correlation of presurgical mapping with functional MR imaging and invasive cortical mapping. Radiology. 1994;190:85–92.
33. Puce A, Constable RT, Luby ML, et al. Functional magnetic resonance imaging of sensory and motor cortex: comparison with electrophysiological localization. J Neurosurg. 1995;83:262–70.
34. Cosgrove GR, Buchbinder BR, Jiang H. Functional magnetic resonance imaging for intracranial navigation. Neurosurg Clin N Am. 1996;7:313–22.
35. Yousry TA, Schmid UD, Schmidt D, Hagen T, Jassoy A, Reiser MF. The central sulcal vein: a landmark for identification of the central sulcus using functional magnetic resonance imaging. J Neurosurg. 1996;85:608–17.
36. Roux FE, Ranjeva JP, Boulanouar K, et al. Motor functional MRI for presurgical evaluation of cerebral tumors. Stereotact Funct Neurosurg. 1997;68:106–11.
37. Roux FE, Boulanouar K, Ranjeva JP, et al. Cortical intraoperative stimulation in brain tumors as a tool to evaluate spatial data from motor functional MRI. Invest Radiol. 1999;34:225–9.
38. Dymarkowski S, Sunaert S, Van Oostende S, et al. Functional MRI of the brain: localisation of eloquent cortex in focal brain lesion therapy. Eur Radiol. 1998;8:1573–80.
39. Krings T, Reul J, Spetzger U, et al. Functional magnetic resonance mapping of sensory motor cortex for image-guided neurosurgical intervention. Acta Neurochir (Wien). 1998;140:215–22.
40. Krings T, Reinges MH, Erberich S, et al. Functional MRI for presurgical planning: problems, artefacts, and solution strategies. J Neurol Neurosurg Psychiatry. 2001;70:749–60.
41. Nitschke MF, Melchert UH, Hahn C, et al. Preoperative functional magnetic resonance imaging (fMRI) of the motor system in patients with tumours in the parietal lobe. Acta Neurochir (Wien). 1998;140:1223–9.
42. Pujol J, Conesa G, Deus J, Lopez-Obarrio L, Isamat F, Capdevila A. Clinical application of functional magnetic resonance imaging in presurgical identification of the central sulcus. J Neurosurg. 1998;88:863–9.
43. Schulder M, Maldjian JA, Liu WC, et al. Functional image-guided surgery of intracranial tumors located in or near the sensorimotor cortex. J Neurosurg. 1998;89:412–8.
44. Wildforster U, Falk A, Harders A. Operative approach due to results of functional magnetic resonance imaging in central brain tumors. Comput Aided Surg. 1998;3:162–5.
45. Achten E, Jackson GD, Cameron JA, Abbott DF, Stella DL, Fabinyi GC. Presurgical evaluation of the motor hand area with functional MR imaging in patients with tumors and dysplastic lesions. Radiology. 1999;210:529–38.
46. Bittar RG, Olivier A, Sadikot AF, Andermann F, Pike GB, Reutens DC. Presurgical motor and somatosensory cortex mapping with functional magnetic resonance imaging and positron emission tomography. J Neurosurg. 1999;91:915–21.
47. Fandino J, Kollias SS, Wieser HG, Valavanis A, Yonekawa Y. Intraoperative validation of functional magnetic resonance imaging and cortical reorganization patterns in patients with brain tumors involving the primary motor cortex. J Neurosurg. 1999;91:238–50.
48. Lee CC, Ward HA, Sharbrough FW, et al. Assessment of functional MR imaging in neurosurgical planning. AJNR Am J Neuroradiol. 1999;20:1511–9.
49. Mueller WM, Yetkin FZ, Hammeke TA, et al. Functional magnetic resonance imaging mapping of the motor cortex in patients with cerebral tumors. Neurosurgery. 1996;39:515–20. discussion 520–1.
50. Atlas SW, Howard 2nd RS, Maldjian J, et al. Functional magnetic resonance imaging of regional brain activity in patients with intracerebral gliomas: findings and implications for clinical management. Neurosurgery. 1996;38:329–38.
51. Rao SM, Binder JR, Bandettini PA, et al. Functional magnetic resonance imaging of complex human movements. Neurology. 1993;43:2311–8.
52. Kleinschmidt A, Nitschke MF, Frahm J. Somatotopy in the human motor cortex hand area. A high-resolution functional MRI study. Eur J Neurosci. 1997;9:2178–86.
53. Maldjian JA, Gottschalk A, Patel RS, Detre JA, Alsop DC. The sensory somatotopic map of the human hand demonstrated at 4 Tesla. Neuroimage. 1999;10:55–62.
54. Lotze M, Erb M, Flor H, Huelsmann E, Godde B, Grodd W. fMRI evaluation of somatotopic representation in human primary motor cortex. Neuroimage. 2000;11:473–81.
55. Schlosser MJ, McCarthy G, Fulbright RK, Gore JC, Awad IA. Cerebral vascular malformations adjacent to sensorimotor and visual cortex. Functional magnetic resonance imaging studies before and after therapeutic intervention. Stroke. 1997;28:1130–7.

56. Chapman PH, Buchbinder BR, Cosgrove GR, Jiang HJ. Functional magnetic resonance imaging for cortical mapping in pediatric neurosurgery. Pediatr Neurosurg. 1995;23:122–6.
57. Sisodiya SM. Surgery for malformations of cortical development causing epilepsy. Brain. 2000;123: 1075–91.
58. Salek-Haddadi A, Lemieux L, Fish DR. Role of functional magnetic resonance imaging in the evaluation of patients with malformations caused by cortical development. Neurosurg Clin N Am. 2002; 13:63–9. viii.
59. Spreer J, Martin P, Greenlee MW, et al. Functional MRI in patients with band heterotopia. Neuroimage. 2001;14:357–65.
60. Pinard J, Feydy A, Carlier R, Perez N, Pierot L, Burnod Y. Functional MRI in double cortex: functionality of heterotopia. Neurology. 2000;54:1531–3.
61. Innocenti GM, Maeder P, Knyazeva MG, Fornari E, Deonna T. Functional activation of microgyric visual cortex in a human. Ann Neurol. 2001;50:672–6.
62. Staudt M, Pieper T, Grodd W, Winkler P, Holthausen H, Krageloh-Mann I. Functional MRI in a 6-year-old boy with unilateral cortical malformation: concordant representation of both hands in the unaffected hemisphere. Neuropediatrics. 2001;32:159–61.
63. Schwartz TH, Resor Jr SR, De La Paz R, Goodman RR. Functional magnetic resonance imaging localization of ictal onset to a dysplastic cleft with simultaneous sensorimotor mapping: intraoperative electrophysiological confirmation and postoperative follow-up: technical note. Neurosurgery. 1998;43: 639–44. discussion 644–5.
64. Krakow K, Wieshmann UC, Woermann FG, et al. Multimodal MR imaging: functional, diffusion tensor, and chemical shift imaging in a patient with localization-related epilepsy. Epilepsia. 1999;40:1459–62.
65. Krakow K, Lemieux L, Messina D, et al. Spatio-temporal imaging of focal interictal epileptiform activity using EEG-triggered functional MRI. Epileptic Disord. 2001;3:67–74.
66. Kobayashi E, Bagshaw AP, Jansen A, Andermann F, Andermann E, Gotman J, et al. Intrinsic epileptogenicity in polymicrogyric cortex suggested by EEG-fMRI BOLD responses. Neurology. 2005;64:1263–6.
67. Tyvaert L, Hawco C, Kobayashi E, LeVan P, Dubeau F, Gotman J. Different structures involved during ictal and interictal epileptic activity in malformations of cortical development: an EEG-fMRI study. Brain. 2008;131:2042–60.
68. Jackson GD, Connelly A, Cross JH, Gordon I, Gadian DG. Functional magnetic resonance imaging of focal seizures. Neurology. 1994;44:850–6.
69. Warach S, Levin JM, Schomer DL, Holman BL, Edelman RR. Hyperperfusion of ictal seizure focus demonstrated by MR perfusion imaging. AJNR Am J Neuroradiol. 1994;15:965–8.
70. Detre JA, Sirven JI, Alsop DC, O'Connor MJ, French JA. Localization of subclinical ictal activity by functional magnetic resonance imaging: correlation with invasive monitoring. Ann Neurol. 1995; 38:618–24.
71. Krings T, Topper R, Reinges MH, et al. Hemodynamic changes in simple partial epilepsy: a functional MRI study. Neurology. 2000;54:524–7.
72. Salek-Haddadi A, Merschhemke M, Lemieux L, Fish DR. Simultaneous EEG-correlated ictal fMRI. Neuroimage. 2002;16:32–40.
73. Archer JS, Briellmann RS, Syngeniotis A, Abbott DF, Jackson GD. Spike-triggered fMRI in reading epilepsy: Involvement of left frontal cortex working memory area. Neurology. 2003;60:415–21.
74. Salek-Haddadi A, Mayer T, Hamandi K, Symms M, Josephs O, Fluegel D, et al. Imaging seizure activity: a combined EEG/EMG-fMRI study in reading epilepsy. Epilepsia. 2009;50(2):256–64.
75. Ives JR, Warach S, Schmitt F, Edelman RR, Schomer DL. Monitoring the patient's EEG during echo planar MRI. Electroencephalogr Clin Neurophysiol. 1993;87:417–20.
76. Lemieux L, Allen PJ, Franconi F, Symms MR, Fish DR. Recording of EEG during fMRI experiments: patient safety. Magn Reson Med. 1997;38:943–52.
77. Allen PJ, Polizzi G, Krakow K, Fish DR, Lemieux L. Identification of EEG events in the MR scanner: the problem of pulse artifact and a method for its subtraction. Neuroimage. 1998;8:229–39.
78. Krakow K, Allen PJ, Symms MR, Lemieux L, Josephs O, Fish DR. EEG recording during fMRI experiments: image quality. Hum Brain Mapp. 2000; 10:10–5.
79. Allen PJ, Josephs O, Turner R. A method for removing imaging artifact from continuous EEG recorded during functional MRI. Neuroimage. 2000;12:230–9.
80. Krakow K, Allen PJ, Lemieux L, Symms MR, Fish DR. Methodology: EEG-correlated fMRI. Adv Neurol. 2000;83:187–201.
81. Bonmassar G, Purdon P, Jaaskelainen I, et al. Motion and Ballistocardiogram Artifact Removal for Interleaved Recording of EEG and EPs during MRI. Neuroimage. 2002;16:1127.
82. Salek-Haddadi A, Lemieux L, Merschhemke M, Diehl B, Allen PJ, Fish DR. EEG quality during simultaneous functional MRI of interictal epileptiform discharges. Magn Reson Imaging. 2003;21: 1159–66.
83. Hoffmann A, Jager L, Werhahn KJ, Jaschke M, Noachtar S, Reiser M. Electroencephalography during functional echo-planar imaging: detection of epileptic spikes using post-processing methods. Magn Reson Med. 2000;44:791–8.
84. Salek-Haddadi A, Friston KJ, Lemieux L, Fish DR. Studying spontaneous EEG activity with fMRI. Brain Res Brain Res Rev. 2003;43:110–33.
85. Portas CM, Krakow K, Allen P, Josephs O, Armony JL, Frith CD. Auditory processing across the sleep-wake cycle: simultaneous EEG and fMRI monitoring in humans. Neuron. 2000;28:991–9.

86. Goldman RI, Stern JM, Engel Jr J, Cohen MS. Simultaneous EEG and fMRI of the alpha rhythm. Neuroreport. 2002;13:2487–92.
87. Bonmassar G, Anami K, Ives J, Belliveau JW. Visual evoked potential (VEP) measured by simultaneous 64-channel EEG and 3 T fMRI. Neuroreport. 1999;10:1893–7.
88. Niazy RK, Beckmann CF, Iannetti GD, Brady JM, Smith SM. Removal of FMRI environment artifacts from EEG data using optimal basis sets. Neuroimage. 2005;28:720–37.
89. Anami K, Mori T, Tanaka F, Kawagoe Y, Okamoto J, Yarita M, et al. Stepping stone sampling for retrieving artifact-free electroencephalogram during functional magnetic resonance imaging. Neuroimage. 2003;19:281–95.
90. Al-Asmi A, Benar CG, Gross DW, Khani YA, Andermann F, Pike B, et al. fMRI activation in continuous and spike-triggered EEG-fMRI studies of epileptic spikes. Epilepsia. 2003;44:1328–39.
91. Kaufmann C, Wehrle R, Wetter TC, Holsboer F, Auer DP, Pollmacher T, et al. Brain activation and hypothalamic functional connectivity during human non-rapid eye movement sleep: an EEG/fMRI study. Brain. 2006;129:655–67.
92. Laufs H, Kleinschmidt A, Beyerle A, Eger E, Salek-Haddadi A, Preibisch C, et al. EEG-correlated fMRI of human alpha activity. Neuroimage. 2003;19:1463–76.
93. Becker R, Ritter P, Moosmann M, Villringer A. Visual evoked potentials recovered from fMRI scan periods. Hum Brain Mapp. 2005;26:221–30.
94. Warach S, Ives JR, Schlaug G, Patel MR, Darby DG, Thangaraj V, et al. EG-triggered echo-planar functional MRI in epilepsy. Neurology. 1996;47:89–93.
95. Seeck M, Lazeyras F, Michel CM, Blanke O, Gericke CA, Ives J, et al. Non-invasive epileptic focus localization using EEG-triggered functional MRI and electromagnetic tomography. Electroencephalogr Clin Neurophysiol. 1998;106:508–12.
96. Krakow K, Woermann FG, Symms MR, Allen PJ, Lemieux L, Barker GJ, et al. EEG-triggered functional MRI of interictal epileptiform activity in patients with partial seizures. Brain. 1999;122: 1679–88.
97. Patel MR, Blum A, Pearlman JD, Yousuf N, Ives JR, Saeteng S, et al. Echo-planar functional MR imaging of epilepsy with concurrent EEG monitoring. AJNR Am J Neuroradiol. 1999;20:1916–9.
98. Lazeyras F, Blanke O, Perrig S, Zimine I, Golay X, Delavelle J, et al. EEG-triggered functional MRI in patients with pharmacoresistant epilepsy. J Magn Reson Imaging. 2000;12:177–85.
99. Krakow K, Lemieux L, Messina D, Scott CA, Symms MR, Duncan JS, et al. Spatio-temporal imaging of focal interictal epileptiform activity using EEG-triggered functional MRI. Epileptic Disord. 2001;3:67–74.
100. Jager L, Werhahn KJ, Hoffmann A, Berthold S, Scholz V, Weber J, et al. Focal epileptiform activity in the brain: detection with spike-related functional MR imaging – preliminary results. Radiology. 2002;223:860–9.
101. Lemieux L, Salek-Haddadi A, Josephs O, Allen P, Toms N, Scott C, et al. Event-related fMRI with simultaneous and continuous EEG: description of the method and initial case report. Neuroimage. 2001;14:780–7.
102. Baudewig J, Bittermann HJ, Paulus W, Frahm J. Simultaneous EEG and functional MRI of epileptic activity: a case report. Clin Neurophysiol. 2001; 112:1196–200.
103. Iannetti GD, Di Bonaventura C, Pantano P, Giallonardo AT, Romanelli PL, Bozzao L, et al. fMRI/EEG in paroxysmal activity elicited by elimination of central vision and fixation. Neurology. 2002;58:976–9.
104. Kobayashi E, Bagshaw AP, Grova C, Gotman J, Dubeau F. Grey matter heterotopia: what EEG-fMRI can tell us about epileptogenicity of neuronal migration disorders. Brain. 2006;129:366–74.
105. Archer JS, Briellman RS, Abbott DF, Syngeniotis A, Wellard RM, Jackson GD. Benign epilepsy with centro-temporal spikes: Spike triggered fMRI shows somato-sensory cortex activity. Epilepsia. 2003;44:200–4.
106. Boor S, Vucurevic G, Pfleiderer C, Stoeter P, Kutschke G, Boor R. EEG-related functional MRI in benign childhood epilepsy with centrotemporal spikes. Epilepsia. 2003;44:688–92.
107. Archer JS, Abbott DF, Waites AB, Jackson GD. fMRI "deactivation" of the posterior cingulate during generalized spike and wave. Neuroimage. 2003;20:1915–22.
108. Salek-Haddadi A, Lemieux L, Merschhemke M, Friston K, Duncan JS, Fish DR. Functional MRI of human absence seizures. Ann Neurol. 2003;53:663–7.
109. Aghakhani Y, Bagshaw AP, Benar CG, Hawco C, Andermann F, Dubeau F, et al. fMRI activation during spike and wave discharges in idiopathic generalized epilepsy. Brain. 2004;127:1127–44.
110. Gotman J, Grova C, Bagshaw A, Kobayashi E, Aghakhani Y, Dubeau F. Generalized epileptic discharges show thalamocortical activation and suspension of the default state of the brain. Proc Natl Acad Sci USA. 2005;102:15236–40.
111. Laufs H, Lengler U, Khalid H, Kleinschmidt A, Krakow K. Linking generalized spike-and-wave dischrges and resting brain activity by using EEG/fMRI in a patient with absence seizures. Epilepsia. 2006; 47:444–8.
112. Vaudano AE, Laufs H, Kiebel SJ, Carmichael DW, Hamadi K, Guye M, et al. Causal hierarchy within the thalamo-cortical network in spike and wave discharges. PLoS ONE. 2009;49:6475.
113. Federico P, Archer JS, Abbott DF, Jackson GD. Cortical/subcortical BOLD changes associated with epileptic discharges: an EEG-fMRI study at 3 T. Neurology. 2005;64:1125–30.
114. Salek-Haddadi A, Diehl B, Hamadi K, Merschhemke M, Liston A, Friston K, et al. Hemodynamic correlates

of epileptiform discharges: an EEG-fMRI study of 63 patients with focal epilepsy. Brain Res. 2006;1088: 148–66.

115. Zijlmans J, Evans A, Fontes F, Katzenschlager R, Gacinovic S, Lees AJ, et al. EEG-fMRI in the preoperative work-up for epilepsy surgery. Brain. 2007; 130:2343–53.

116. Morgan VL, Price RR, Arain A, Modur P, Abou-Khalil B. Resting functional MRI with temporal clustering analysis for localization of epileptic activity without EEG. Neuroimage. 2004;21:473–81.

117. Hamandi K, Salek Haddadi A, Liston A, Laufs H, Fish DR, Lemieux L. fMRI temporal clustering analysis in patients with frequent interictal epileptiform discharges: comparison with EEG-driven analysis. Neuroimage. 2005;26:309–16.

118. Krakow K, Messina D, Lemieux L, Duncan JS, Fish DR. Functional MRI activation of individual interictal epileptiform spikes. Neuroimage. 2001;13:502–5.

119. Lemieux L, Krakow K, Fish DR. Comparison of spike-triggered functional MRI BOLD activation and EEG dipole model localization. Neuroimage. 2001;14:1097–104.

120. Sijbers J, Michiels I, Verhoye M, Van Audekerke J, Van der Linden A, Van Dyck D. Restoration of MR-induced artifacts in simultaneously recorded MR/EEG data. Magn Reson Imaging. 1999;17:1383–91.

121. Kobayashi E, Bagshaw AP, Grova C, Dubeau F, Gotman J. Negative BOLD responses to epileptic spikes. Hum Brain Mapp. 2006;27:488–97.

122. Raichle ME, MacLeod AM, Snyder AZ, Powers WJ, Gusnard DA, Shulman GL. A default mode of brain function. Proc Natl Acad Sci USA. 2001;98:676–82.

123. Benar CG, Grova C, Kobayashi E, Bagshaw AP, Aghakhani Y, Dubeau F, et al. EEG-fMRI of epileptic spikes: concordance with EEG source localization and intracranial EEG. Neuroimage. 2006;30: 1161–70.

Applications of fMRI to Psychiatry 17

Melissa Lopez-Larson
and Deborah A. Yurgelun-Todd

Introduction

The application of functional neuroimaging to characterize cortical dysfunction in patients with psychiatric disorders provides one of the most exciting in vivo techniques for the identification of both pathophysiologic factors and treatment effects. Functional magnetic resonance imaging (fMRI) refers to a noninvasive method to assess cortical activation by measuring changes in oxidation and regional blood flow. The most frequently used fMRI paradigms involve primary sensory stimulation, including visual stimulation and motor sequencing, and affective and cognitive paradigms. Functional brain imaging studies have historically been limited both by the need to use radioactive tracers and by poor temporal resolution. Developments in the area of magnetic resonance imaging (MRI) may largely surmount these limitations. First, the development of high-speed, echo-planar imaging devices has greatly enhanced the temporal resolution of MRI. With echo-planar imaging, single image planes can be acquired in 50–100 ms or multiple image planes can be acquired each second. Studies, which may be performed with or without a high-speed MR scanner, selectively detect image parameters that are proportional to cerebral blood flow (CBF) or blood volume (CBV). This strategy capitalizes on the fact that in general, focal changes in neuronal activity are coupled closely to changes in CBF and CBV.

Functional MRI studies generally are divided into two separate classes. The first includes studies that make use of endogenous physiologic factors to detect changes in cerebral activation, often referred to as the non-contrast techniques [1]. The second group of studies requires the intravenous administration of a paramagnetic agent and comprises the contrast techniques [2]. Non-contrast techniques make use of either T1-weighted pulse sequences to detect changes in blood flow or, more commonly, T2-weighted pulse sequences to detect changes in the local concentration of paramagnetic deoxyhemoglobin. The latter method has been referred to as blood oxygen level-dependent (BOLD) imaging.

In a BOLD experiment, regional brain activation is associated with changes in both blood flow and blood volume, generally leading to a washout of paramagnetic deoxyhemoglobin, which results in an increase in local signal intensity. BOLD studies have several limitations from the perspective of performing clinical research studies. At 1.5 Tesla (T), the magnitude of the observed signal intensity changes is relatively small. For instance, photic stimulation, which induces a substantial increase in occipital cortical blood flow, produces only a 2–4% MR signal

M. Lopez-Larson, MD (✉) • D.A. Yurgelun-Todd, PhD
Department of Psychiatry, The Brain Institute,
University of Utah, 383 Colorow Drive,
Salt Lake City, UT 84108, USA
e-mail: melissa.lopez-larson@hsc.utah.edu;
deborah.yurgelun-todd@hsc.utah.edu

S.H. Faro and F.B. Mohamed (eds.), *Functional BOLD MRI: Principles and Applications*,
DOI 10.1007/978-1-4939-1995-6_17,

intensity increase. The application of functional imaging techniques during complex cognitive functions may result in even smaller changes in signal intensity. One reason is that higher order functions, such as attentional processing, are subserved by widely distributed networks. Furthermore, studies of more medial cortical regions, such as the cingulate cortex, have been difficult to carry out because of the limited signal available in functional activation and MRI experiments completed with standard imaging hardware [3]. These factors reduce the likelihood of finding unique anatomical correlates for higher cognitive functions and may contribute to the relatively small cortical activation observed during cognitive tasks compared with primary sensory activation.

Previous investigations also have suggested that the magnitude of BOLD signal intensity changes may vary with subject age and gender. To investigate the effects of age and sex on cortical activation, Ross and colleagues [4] measured signal intensity changes during photic stimulation in a group of young adults and in a group of elderly subjects. The older study subjects produced significantly less signal change in response to photic stimulation compared with younger subjects. An examination of the younger group revealed that women demonstrated significantly less signal change in response to photic stimulation compared with men, and men produced greater activation in the right occipital lobe. This study suggests that both age and sex are important covariates in analyzing fMRI data.

Furthermore, a number of medications directly alter vascular tone and modify BOLD signal changes, presenting an important confound for studies of subjects with psychiatric illness. Finally, the uncoupling of CBF and CBV, which occurs acutely after cerebral activation and produces the BOLD effect, appears to resolve with prolonged stimulation. In response to these problems, many research groups are developing noncontrast fMRI methods, which have a greater sensitivity to changes in cerebral flow.

The contrast method is a tracer kinetic technique using a bolus injection of a paramagnetic contrast agent to produce changes in tissue magnetic susceptibility and MR image intensity. During the first pass of the contrast agent, MR signal intensity may decrease by as much as 20–40%. This method may be used to map the distribution of CBV at rest or to measure changes in response to cerebral activation. Resting CBV maps have been shown to correlate well with positron emission tomography (PET) images of fluorodeoxyglucose uptake and with hexamethyl propyleneamine oxime (HMPAO) single-photon emission computed tomography (SPECT) images of CBF. Additionally, the development of a multiple bolus method for performing dynamic susceptibility contrast (DSC-MRI) studies may facilitate the measurement of drug effects on cerebral hemodynamics.

Magnetic resonance brain imaging technologies offer exceptional promise for greater clarification and understanding of psychopathology. Neuroimaging techniques may one day make or confirm psychiatric diagnoses, and neuroimaging profiles may even be incorporated into the diagnostic criteria for certain psychiatric disorders. Moreover, the potential clinical applications extend beyond diagnosis. Ultimately, neuroimaging data may be valuable for predicting natural course of illness and for monitoring treatment response. Currently, the clinical utility of fMRI to patients has thus far been limited, as no findings have been shown to be diagnostically specific for any psychiatric illness or treatment. Although many hospitals and research facilities MRI on psychiatric patients, this information cannot as yet be used reliably to generate a psychiatric diagnosis; however, scans are often used to rule out the presence of a neurologic illness. This chapter highlights the promise that fMRI studies hold for the evaluation of patients with mental illness by briefly reviewing applications of fMRI to the study of developmental disorders, schizophrenia, major depression, bipolar disorder, substance abuse, and anxiety disorders.

Developmental Disorders

Autism spectrum disorders (ASD) are classified in the Diagnostic and Statistical Manual of Mental Disorders, Fourth Edition (DSM-IV), as developmental disabilities with behavioral deficits existing in each of the three main domains of functioning: social interactions, communication, and interests or activities [5]. Research related to the clinical application of neuroimaging techniques to the study of autistic disorder and Asperger's disorder, both found under the ASD umbrella, has increased tremendously over the last decade. Currently, the application of modern medical technology to clinical populations is used to rule out more general medical conditions. The clinical diagnosis of ASD continues to rely solely on behavior-oriented diagnostic tools designed to identify deficits in children through observation, clinical testing, and parental reports [6]. While these diagnostic tools have shown better reliability and validity in identifying an overall population of children with ASD, overall scores have been inadequate in distinguishing between the vast combination and degrees of symptomology [7, 8]. The importance of distinguishing subsets of autism sharing common symptoms and symptom degrees may play an essential role in clinical diagnosis, etiology, and treatment planning.

ASD is a developmental disorder of dysconnectivity, dyschrony, and atypical recruitment of brain circuits resulting in deficits in language, auditory processing, social cognition, face processing, and executive functioning (see Table 17.1). For example, brain regions involved in social communication and interaction, such as the amygdala, inferior frontal gyrus, fusiform, and superior temporal gyrus, are thought to be responsible for impairments in both perceiving and expressing social information [9]. Furthermore, the "theory of mind" hypothesis, originated by Premack and Woodruff, suggests that a special class of motor neurons, the mirror neurons, may also be involved in ASD. This theory is based on the concept of one's ability to attribute mental states such as beliefs, desires, emotions, perceptions, and intentions to self and to others in order to understand and predict behaviors [10]. The mirror neurons involved in the "theory of mind" hypothesis reside in regions of the inferior frontal gyrus, inferior parietal lobule, and superior temporal sulcus, and disruptions of these regions may also result in social and communicative abnormalities [11]. Based on neuroanatomic reports of significant differences in amygdalar volume in ASD individuals compared to normal control subjects [12–15], researchers have begun to explore the functional role of the amygdala and other regions associated with affect processing during facial affect tasks in ASD. Overall, fMRI studies have demonstrated atypical face or emotional processing in ASD patients when compared to healthy controls (HC), particularly when viewing emotion-laden faces or gestures, or when viewing self versus other tasks [16–22]. The most consistently reported abnormality in facial/affect studies include reduced activation of the amygdala in ASD patients, and abnormal recruitment of alternative brain regions compared to that in HC.

Language delay and impairment, particularly semantic and pragmatic difficulties, have also been studied in ASD utilizing fMRI techniques. Converging evidence suggests that abnormal and dyschronous brain activation between the left inferior frontal gyrus (Broca's area) and left superior and middle temporal gyrus (Wernicke's area) play a central role in the language impairment seen in ASD [23]. For example, an fMRI study in ASD patients during a semantic sentence comprehension task found reduced activation in Broca's area and greater activation in Wernicke's area [23]. Abnormal activation patterns in these language centers and atypical brain recruitment in other brain regions such as the visual cortex have been replicated in other studies of ASD [24–27]. Studies of cognition have also found impaired connectivity between frontal and parietal areas in ASD individuals performing a Tower of London Task [28] and an imagery task [27]. In addition, a study of verbal working memory found that compared to HC, ASD patients had more activation in posterior brain regions such as the posterior inferior temporal and the occipital lobe rather than expected frontal regions typically activated during working memory tasks [29]. These findings suggest that individuals with ASD process information at a more basic sensory level and do not utilize higher level integrative cortical brain processing. Furthermore, the evidence supports a reduction in regional functional specialization in

Table 17.1 Summary of fMRI research in autistic spectrum disorders population by paradigm category

Author-Year	Subjects	fMRI paradigm	Results
Affect/social			
Grezes et al. 2009 [18]	12 medication-free, ASD[a]; 12 HC[b]	Static or dynamic emotional body postures	Similar but greater activation in HC compared to ASD patients. ASD patients had decreased activation of amygdala, inferior frontal gyrus, and dorsal premotor cortex relative to HC
Hadjikhani et al. 2009 [19]	10 adult high-functioning ASD; 7 HC	Neutral or fearful body pictures	ASD group was more accurate in identifying neutral conditions than emotional conditions. Relative to HC, activation differences between the two stimuli in ASD patients were found in the striate and the extrastriate visual cortex
Bookheimer et al. 2008 [9]	12 male ASD children; 12 age-matched HC	Facial perception task using upright/inverted faces	Similar activation patterns between groups were seen specifically in fusiform and lingual gyrus bilaterally. PFC and amygdalar activation was found in HC only, while ASD patients exhibited only demonstrated precuneus activation
Silani et al. 2008 [21]	15 high-functioning adult ASD; 15 gender-, age-, and IQ-matched HC	Two experiments presenting identical sets of pictures subject indicates un/pleasantness of image by button press	ASD patients showed increased activity of the parietal and occipital cortex and decreased activity in the left temporal pole, cerebellum, precuneus, ACC,[c] and medial PFC[d] relative to HC
Uddin et al. 2008 [22]	18 medication-free, high-functioning male ASD children; 12 age- and IQ- matched male HC	Images of self and morphed self and asked to make "self/other" judgments	In HC, activation of the right premotor/prefrontal system was evident for "self/other" stimuli. ASD group showed this system activation only when presented with "self" stimuli
Pierce et al. 2001 [20]	7 male, medication-free, ASD adults; 8 sex- and age-matched HC	Facial perception task	ASD patients had decreased activation in the fusiform gyrus and left amygdala compared to HC
Critchley et al. 2001 [17]	9 high-functioning male ASD adults; 8 HC	Facial emotional/neutral stimuli	
Baron-Cohen et al. 1999 [16]	6 adult autistic or Asperger's disorder patients; 12 matched controls	Two tasks using visual viewing of photographs eyes	ASD patients showed increased activations in superior temporal gyrus bilaterally, whereas controls showed an increase in left inferior frontal gyrus, right insula, and left amygdala
Cognition/language			
Groen et al. 2010 [25]	16 high-functioning, medication-free, adolescent ASD; 26 HC	Word/semantic-knowledge task	The word-knowledge task revealed greater activation of the language association areas in HC versus ASD patients. The semantic-knowledge condition showed activation in the language areas and contralateral cerebellum in HC. ASD patients showed activation in language centers, but not in temporal areas

(continued)

Table 17.1 (continued)

Author-Year	Subjects	fMRI paradigm	Results
Solomon et al. 2009 [33]	22 ASD adolescents; 23 gender-, age-, and IQ-matched HC	Slow event-related design using a prepotency task	ASD patients displayed less network integration and lower levels of functional connectivity between frontal, parietal, and occipital regions
Tesink et al. 2009 [198]	24 adult high-functioning ASD; 2 HC	Speaker-inference sentences and sentences with lexical semantic or word knowledge anomalies	Compared to HC, ASD patients showed increased activation of the right inferior frontal gyrus in speaker-incongruent sentences compared to speaker-congruent sentences. In contrast, the HC exhibited decreased activation in the right ventral medial PFC during the same task
Shafritz et al. 2008 [32]	18 high-functioning, medication-free ASD; 15 neurotypical HC	Target detection task using presentation of geometric shapes	ASD patients demonstrated diminished activation in parietal, striatal, and frontal areas relative to HC. Activation of the ACC and posterior parietal regions was also negatively correlated with severity of restricted repetitive behaviors in ASD patients
Gaffrey et al. 2007 [24]	10 high-functioning ASD; 10 HC	Target/nontarget sequences with a semantic decision-making condition and a perceptual control task	During the control condition, results show significant activation of the left inferior frontal gyrus in HC relative to ASD patients, while the semantic condition showed significantly greater activation of the extrastriate visual cortex bilaterally in the ASD subjects compared to HC
Schmitz et al. 2006 [31]	10 high-functioning ASD males; 12 HC males	Go/No-Go, Stroop, & SWITCH tasks	Compared to HC, ASD patients showed increased activation of the left inferior and orbitofrontal cortex, left insula, and left inferior and right mesial parietal cortex (respectively)
Just et al. 2004 [23]	17 high-functioning ASD; 17 HC	Sentence comprehension task	ASD patients showed increased activation in the left latero-superior temporal area and decreased activation in the left inferior frontal gyrus relative to controls

[a]Autism spectrum disorder
[b]Healthy controls
[c]Anterior cingulate cortex
[d] Prefrontal cortex

ASD patients [30–33]. The use of alternative functional and dysfunctional pathways for social interactions, communication, and cognitive functions in ASD may be related to altered early neuronal migration [11]. The identification of various alternative activation patterns during similar tasks for ASD patients illustrates a physiologic variation within the broader diagnosis of autism, which may or may not be identified behaviorally. This variation further supports the importance of identifying additional markers in understanding and treatment of these disorders (Fig. 17.1).

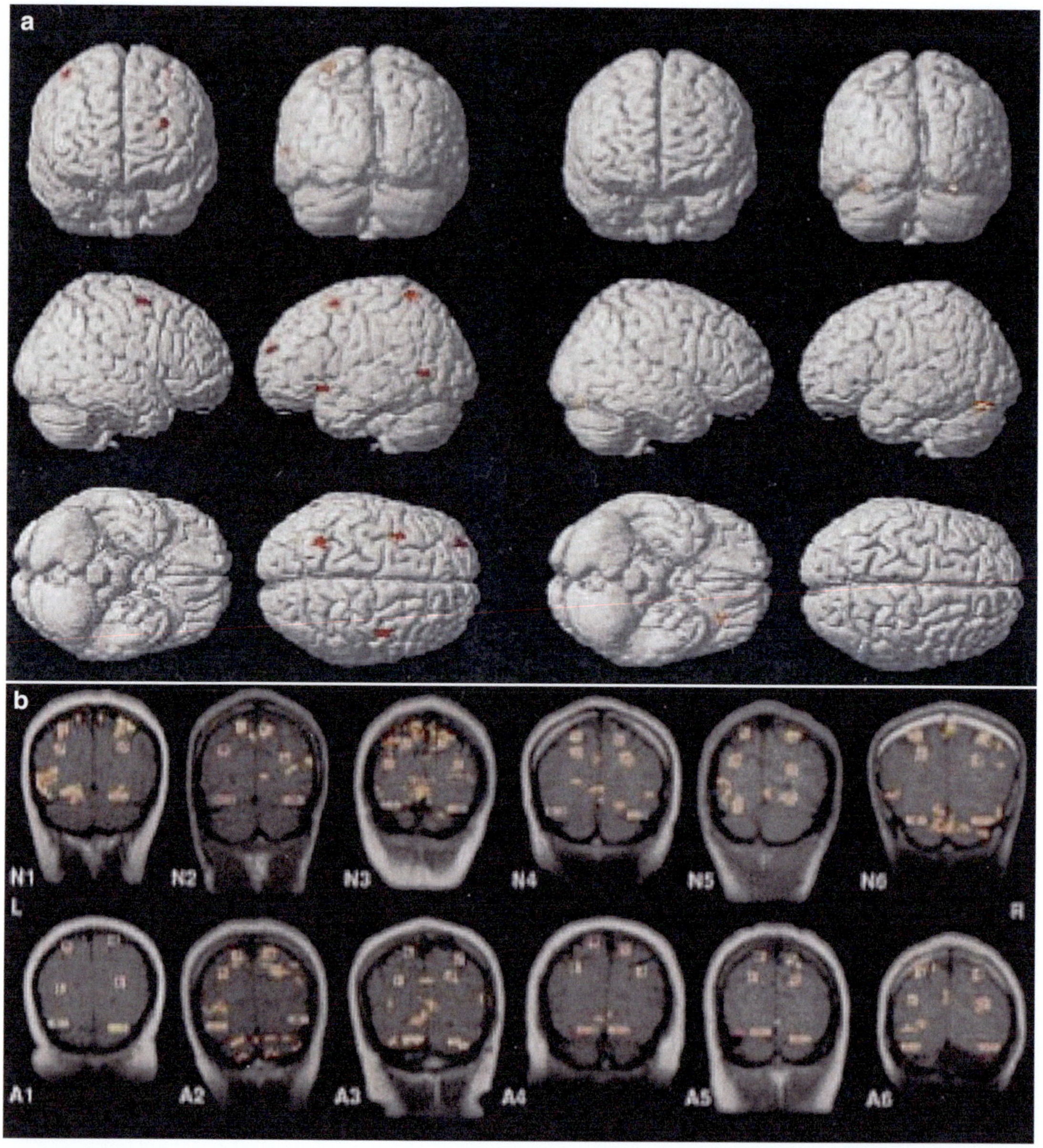

Fig. 17.1 (**a**) Surface views for normal (*left*) and autistic (*right*) subjects [199]. (**b**) Single slice projections of functional regions of interest during task versus fixation in normal (*top*) and autistic (*bottom*) subjects [199]

Substance Use

Drug abuse and addiction remain critical public health problems in the USA, associated with serious adverse behavioral, health, and social consequences for individuals, their families, and society. Recent data indicate that 20.1 million Americans aged 12 years and older were current users of illegal drugs in 2008 [34]. The American Psychiatric Association considers the abuse of alcohol, amphetamines, caffeine, cannabis, cocaine, hallucinogens, inhalants, nicotine, opioids, phencyclidine, and sedatives to be diagnosable disorders. Despite aggressive intervention efforts during the last decade, the overall

Table 17.2 Summary of fMRI research in marijuana users

Author-Year	Subjects	fMRI paradigm	Results
Jager et al. 2006 [41]	20 MJ[a]; 20 HC[b]	Associative learning task	MJ users showed lower activation in parahippocampal regions with more distinct hypoactivation visible in left hippocampus and parahippocampal gyrus than in the right side, versus HC
Chang et al. 2006 [39]	12 MJ abstinent & 12 MJ users; 19 HC	Visual-attention task	Compared with MJ users showed greater activation in the middle frontal gyrus bilaterally, the right medial cerebellum, and dorsal medial and right precuneus. Both MJ groups showed increased activation in the left occipital lingual area versus HC, while HC showed increased activation in the right cerebellum relative to both MJ groups
Gruber and Yurgelun-Todd 2005 [40]	9 MJ users; 9 HC	Modified Stroop task	MJ users showed lower AC[c] activity and higher midcingulate activity versus HC. MJ users also showed a more diffuse, bilateral pattern of DLPFC[d] activation versus HC, who showed increased activity within the right DLPFC
Kanayama et al. 2004 [38]	12 MJ users; 10 HC	Spatial working memory task	Compared with HC, MJ users showed greater activation of the superior, middle, and inferior frontal gyrus; right superior temporal gyrus; AC gyrus bilaterally; right precentral gyrus; and regions of the caudate and putamen
Pillay 2004 [36]	9 MJ users; 16 HC	Finger-sequencing task	MJ users showed decreased activation in supplementary motor cortex and AC regions versus controls

[a]Marijuana
[b]Healthy controls
[c]Anterior cingulate
[d]Dorsolateral prefrontal cortex

prevalence of drug use has remained relatively constant. Ominously, drug use among youths has increased significantly over this same time period. Medically, drug-induced deaths have increased over the last decade, reaching a total of 15,973 in 1997, and the Drug Abuse Warning Network has noted consistent increases in hospital emergency room mentions of marijuana-, heroin-, and cocaine-related episodes. Economically, illegal drug use accounted for an estimated 110 billion dollars in expenses and lost revenue in the USA in 1995 [35].

It has been reported that the reinforcing effects of abused drugs may be related to their effects on specific neural circuits, and neuroimaging methods provide an important set of techniques for the identification of pathways that mediate the cognitive changes and reinforcing effects of drugs. Magnetic resonance techniques are particularly well suited for identifying withdrawal and treatment effects. While fMRI has yet to be applied clinically to drug abuse, research has begun to exemplify the importance of functional brain activity on understanding both the phenomenon of craving and the neurophysiologic effects of addiction (see Table 17.2).

Marijuana

Functional MRI techniques have been applied in an effort to better understand the psychomotor, memory, attention, and other cognitive differences seen between marijuana (MJ) users and healthy controls (HC) (see Table 17.2). In a simple motor task, chronic heavy MJ users demonstrated significantly less activation than HC in supplementary motor cortex and anterior cingulate regions [36]. In a longitudinal study, Yurgelun-Todd et al. [37] administered a visual working memory task to chronic marijuana users and healthy controls and found that marijuana smokers demonstrated diminished activation in the dorsolateral prefrontal cortex (DLPFC) after 24 h and 28 days of abstinence. In addition, MJ smokers produced increased activation in the cingulate cortex at both time points, while control subjects did not. In a spatial working memory task, chronic MJ users also showed significantly greater activation than HC in prefrontal brain regions [38]. Furthermore, compared to HC, both active and abstinent MJ subjects were found to have abnormal activation patterns in the right prefrontal and medial cerebellar regions, which normalized with duration of abstinence during a visual-attention task [39]. In a pilot investigation of inhibitory processing in MJ users, Gruber and Yurgelun-Todd [40] administered a modified Stroop task to MJ users and HC. While the groups performed the task equally well, MJ smokers demonstrated significantly lower anterior cingulate activity and higher midcingulate activity relative to controls. Controls also demonstrated increased activity within the right DLPFC during the interference condition, while MJ smokers demonstrated a more diffuse, bilateral pattern of DLPFC activation. These findings suggest that despite similar task performance as HC, marijuana smokers exhibit different patterns of BOLD response. In addition to activation abnormalities and atypical recruitment of brain regions seen in motor and cognitive tasks, recent studies also have reported that MJ use impacts learning and affective processing. For example, during an associative learning task, MJ users displayed overall lower activation in hippocampal/parahippocampal regions [41]. Furthermore, on an affective task, MJ users had decreased activity in the anterior cingulate and amygdala compared to HC while viewing masked faces, suggesting differences in processing affective stimuli compared to healthy controls (Fig. 17.2).

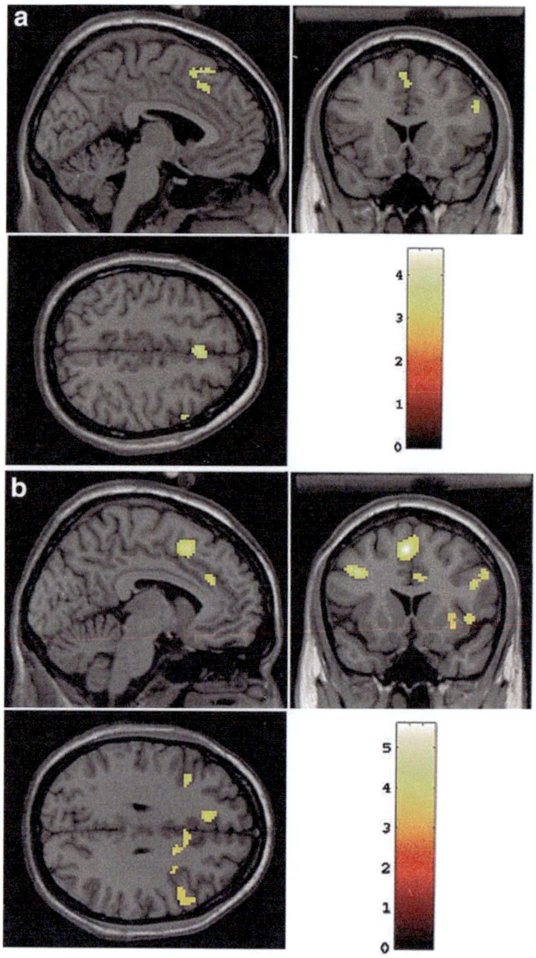

Fig. 17.2 Illustration of brain activation during a working memory task in heavy cannabis users after 1–24 h discontinuation and in control subjects. (**a**) Control subjects. (**b**) Heavy cannabis users

Methamphetamine

Functional imaging studies of methamphetamine users have also provided evidence for affective and executive system dysfunction after drug exposure (see Table 17.3). Executive functions and decision making may remain compromised during abstinence and lead to relapse, particularly under conditions in which negative mood states are present [42–45]. Cross-sectional fMRI studies of abstinent chronic methamphetamine users during decision-making tasks have reported that compared to controls, abstinent methamphetamine-dependent subjects have

Table 17.3 Summary of fMRI research in methamphetamine

Author-Year	Subjects	fMRI paradigm	Results
Kim et al. 2010 [53]	19 MA[a] (20.5 ± 8.3 days abstinent); 19 HC[b]	Visual activation task	HC showed more activation in the orbitofrontal cortex on an empathy task. HC also showed greater activation in the DLPFC,[c] temporal poles, and hippocampus versus MA
Salo et al. 2009 [48]	12 MA (4.1 ± 2.8 months abstinent); 16 age-matched HC	Modified Stroop task	MA showed lower activation in the right PFC.[d] No difference between HC and MA was evident in the ACC[e]
Payer et al. 2010 [52]	12 MA (dependent); 12 HC	Affective task	HC showed higher activation in the right hemisphere ventrolateral PFC, temporoparietal junction, anterior and posterior temporal cortex, fusiform gyrus, and left hemisphere cuneus; MA showed increased activity in the dorsal ACC
Hoffman et al. 2008 [50]	19 MA (48 ± 17 days abstinent); 17 HC	Delay discounting task	HC showed increased activation in the precuneus, right caudate nucleus, ACC, and DLPFC
Paulus et al. 2003 [46]	14 MA (25 ± 2.7 days abstinent); 14 HC	Decision-making/choice prediction task	MA showed less activation in the bilateral inferior PFC, DLPFC, bilateral parietal cortex, left postcentral gyrus, and left superior temporal gyrus. MA also showed increased activation in the left insula, inferior frontal gyrus, middle frontal gyrus, precuneus, and inferior parietal lobule versus HC
Paulus et al. 2002 [47]	10 MA (22.4 ± 3.5 days abstinent); 10 HC	Decision-making/choice prediction tasks	MA showed less activation in the DLOFC. MA did not show activation of the ventromedial cortex, left PFC, and right orbitofrontal cortex during tasks

[a]Methamphetamine abusers
[b]Healthy controls
[c]Dorsolateral prefrontal cortex
[d]Prefrontal cortex
[e]Anterior cingulate cortex

shown decreased task-related activity in prefrontal brain regions [46, 47]. Decreased activity has also been shown in the prefrontal cortex (PFC) in abstinent methamphetamine abusers in a modified Stroop task [48]. Abstinent and current methamphetamine abusers show deficits in their ability to wait for larger rewards in delay discounting tasks and they show decreased activity in the anterior cingulate cortex (ACC) and dorsolateral PFC [49–51]. Differences in affective processing in methamphetamine users compared to that in healthy controls have also been described. For instance, one study demonstrated that active methamphetamine users had increased activation in the dorsal ACC, while healthy controls (HC) showed more activation in the ventrolateral PFC, temporoparietal junction, anterior and posterior temporal cortex, and right hemisphere fusiform gyrus, on a facial affect-matching task [52]. Furthermore, in an empathy processing study, abstinent methamphetamine users showed lower activation in the dorsolateral and orbitofrontal cortex, temporal poles, and hippocampus compared to HC [53]. Activity within the cingulate cortex, insula, and temporal cortex has also been shown to be predictive of relapse [54]. Together these studies suggest impairments in task performance with a particular emphasis on abnormal task-related activity in frontal regions that persist during abstinence and may be predictive of increased risk of relapse.

Cocaine Use

Cocaine dependence has become a significant public health problem, with one of the highest rates of use in the USA (World Health Organization [55]). Medical and social issues such as the spread of infectious disease, crime, and violence are major concerns linked to chronic cocaine use. fMRI methods may provide a means to characterize more fully brain regions that produce the euphoria associated with cocaine [56]. Additionally, recent functional neuroimaging studies have explored the effects of cocaine use on reward processing, the role of craving, and predictions for relapse (see Table 17.4). These investigators have noted increased signal activity in notable regions of interest such as the anterior cingulate [57–59], the orbitofrontal cortex (OFC) [60, 61], and the amygdala [58, 60]. Altered reward processing after repeated cocaine use was observed in a study in which cocaine users displayed decreased sensitivity to monetary values during a monetary reward task. This was charac-

Table 17.4 Summary of fMRI research in cocaine users

Author-Year	Subjects	fMRI paradigm	Results
Hanlon et al. 2010 [57]	14 CD,[a] 15 HC[b]	Finger-tapping task	CD patients showed increased bilateral activation and increased activity in the primary motor cortex, ACC[c], and putamen
Goldstein et al. 2009 [63]	15 CD, 15 HC	Viewing and matching the color of the drug-related or neutral words and a word fluency task	In response to drug words, CD patients displayed bilateral mesencephalon activation, suggesting drug cue reactivity
Kufahl et al. 2008 [58]	13 CD	Expected and unexpected cocaine and saline infusions	For expected and unexpected cocaine infusions, activation occurred in the medial orbitofrontal gyrus and the ACC. During unexpected cocaine infusions (but not expected), activation was observed in the amygdala and lateral orbitofrontal cortex
Li et al. 2008 [200]	15 abstinent CD males, 15 HC	Stop signal task	The CD group showed less activation than HC in the rostral ACC, indicating altered impulse control
Tomasi et al. 2007 [201]	16 CD, 16 HC	0-, 1-, 2-back working memory task	Decreased activation occurred in the thalamus, mesencephalon, ACC, amygdala, parahippocampal gyrus and putamen in CD patients compared to HC. Increased activation in the prefrontal and parietal cortices was detected in CD patients compared to HC
Goldstein et al. 2007 [60]	16 CD, 13 HC	Monetary reward task	Decreased sensitivity to monetary values was found only in CD patients, which correlated with increased activation in the left orbitofrontal cortex and amygdala, and decreased activation in the right middle frontal gyrus

(continued)

Table 17.4 (continued)

Author-Year	Subjects	fMRI paradigm	Results
Kosten et al. 2006 [61]	17 abstinent CD with relapse history, 8 abstinent CD.	Viewing of cocaine cue and neutral videos	Activation was observed in the left precentral and the right superior cortices during the viewing of cocaine-related versus neutral videos for CD patients. Relapsers had increased activation in the right precentral cortex and right posterior cingulate from cue to baseline compared to nonrelapsers
Kufahl et al. 2005 [62]	15 CD	Cocaine or saline infusions, while providing ratings describing affective state	The cocaine infusion, compared to saline infusion, correlated with activation in the mesolimbic region, the anterior prefrontal cortex, and the orbitofrontal cortex
Sinha et al. 2005 [202]	20 CD, 8 HC	Stress imagery/neutral-relaxing scripts played on an audiotape during scanning	Relative to HC, during the stress cue, CD patients displayed decreased activation in the ACC, left hippocampal region, right fusiform gyrus, and the right postcentral gyrus, and increased activation in the caudate and dorsal striatum
Kubler et al. 2005 [203]	14 CD, 14 HC	Attention switching within verbal or visuospatial working memory and an additional verbal only task	CD patients displayed decreased activation in the cingulate gyrus during all switching demands compared to HC

[a]Cocaine dependent
[b]Healthy controls
[c]Anterior cingulate cortex

terized by increased activation in the left OFC and amygdala and decreased activation in the right middle frontal gyrus [60]. Investigations involving the role of craving and predictions for relapses have also utilized functional neuroimaging. For example, subjects in cocaine abuse treatment participated in a study that involved a cocaine cue videotape that elicited prior relapsers in the group (compared to nonrelapsers) to have increased activation in the precentral cortex and posterior cingulate [61]. Drug cue activity was also observed in an investigation with a task that involved viewing of drug-related and neutral words. In response to the drug words, the cocaine-dependent subjects displayed mesencephalon activation, a region associated with dopaminergic mechanisms, the neurotransmitter that suffers from signaling dysfunction with cocaine use [62]. Investigations involving cocaine exposure have demonstrated an association with cognitive and affective neurocircuitry dysfunction.

Alcohol

A growing body of evidence in alcohol use disorders (AUD) has identified abnormal neural response patterns in association with a host of affective, working memory, and reward perception tasks in fMRI. Studies assessing BOLD changes and ratings of alcohol craving in response to alcohol-associated cue images, non-alcoholic beverage, and visual control images found that activity in limbic regions such as the left nucleus accumbens, anterior cingulate, and left orbitofrontal cortex (OFC) significantly correlated with subjective craving ratings in alcohol subjects but not in control subjects [63, 64]. The notion that limbic activation is one component of cue-induced craving for addictive drugs such as alcohol is consistent with more recent work that identified the nucleus accumbens, OFC, fusiform gyri, temporal gyri, parahippocampal gyrus, uncus, frontal gyri, and precuneus as areas directly associated with craving in individuals with AUD [65, 66]. Furthermore, affect-based fMRI studies have found distinct activation patterns in alcoholic and social drinkers in response to positive, neutral, or alcohol-related images, including an attenuated response to fearful stimuli in visual and limbic regions and increased activation of a "limbic" fronto-striato-thalamic loop, including the anterior cingulate cortex (ACC), ventral striatum, and thalamus in response to pleasant pictures [67, 68]. A recent finding of decreased amygdala activation during risk taking in moderate/heavy alcohol drinkers compared to non/light drinkers suggests that altered amygdala activation during risk taking may also be a key neural process underlying early habitual alcohol use and a potential marker for the transition to alcohol dependence [69]. Furthermore, there is evidence to suggest that alcohol use directly affects reward centers in the brain, sensitizing areas in the limbic system and associated regions to the rewarding effects of alcohol, which is reflected in a devaluation of nonalcohol rewards [70, 71]. Working memory and memory encoding deficits have also been reported in AUD and in non-AUD subjects during alcohol use, with fMRI activation abnormalities detected in dorsal ACC, cerebellum, and parahippocampal gyrus [64, 72–74]. Taken together, these findings indicate widespread affective, rewards, and cognitive neurocircuitry deficits in both acute and chronic alcohol use, and the potential use of fMRI for their assessment (see Table 17.5).

Table 17.5 Summary of fMRI research in alcohol use disorders

Author-Year	Subjects	fMRI paradigm	Results
Yan and Li 2009 [70]	12 non- or light drinkers; 9 moderate or heavy drinkers	Simple reaction time task in a stop signal paradigm	While the two groups did not significantly differ in prefrontal activation during inhibitory control, nondependent heavy drinkers, compared to non- or light drinkers, showed decreased amygdala activation during risk-taking decisions in the stop signal task
Beck et al. 2009 [71]	19 detoxified males w/ AUD[a]; 19 age-matched HC[b]	MID[c] task	AUD patients showed significant reduced activation in the right ventral striatum during gain anticipation and a trend-wise decrease in right ventral striatum during loss anticipation
Gundersen et al. 2008 [73]	25 HC randomly assigned to a control group (N = 13) or an alcohol group (N = 12)	Working memory n-back task presented at a BAC[d] of 0.02% and a BAC of 0.08%	AUD patients exhibited a decrease in neuronal activation in the dorsal ACC[e] and cerebellum at the BAC of 0.08%
Bragulat et al. 2008 [66]	10 hazardous drinkers (average drinks per drinking day = 5.9)	IV[f] of 6% alcohol coupled with administration of appetitive alcohol odors (AO), non-appetitive odors (NApO), and appetitive control odors	Alcohol infusion enhanced the contrast between AO and NApO in the NAcc, and in the orbitofrontal, medial frontal, and precuneus/posterior cingulate regions. The most robust finding was a potentiated response in the posterior cingulate/retrosplenial area
Gilman et al. 2008 [68]	12 HC	IV administration of placebo or 6% alcohol solution during the presentation of 45 neutral and 45 fearful faces	Alcohol robustly activated striatal reward circuits including left NAcc and left caudate while attenuating response to fearful stimuli in visual and limbic regions including right amygdala and right parahippocampal gyrus. Self-report ratings of intoxication were found to correlate with striatal activation

(continued)

Table 17.5 (continued)

Author-Year	Subjects	fMRI paradigm	Results
Heinz et al. 2007 [69]	12 detoxified AUD patients; 12 gender-matched HC	Visual affect paradigm consisting of 18 alcohol-associated stimuli and neutral, positive, and negative pictures	Alcohol-associated cues elicited increased activation in the prefrontal and dorsal cingulate cortex and precuneus in AUD patients, while pleasant pictures activated a "limbic" fronto-striato-thalamic loop, which includes the ACC, ventral striatum, and thalamus
Park et al. 2007 [67]	9 AUD subjects; 9 HC	Presentation of images associated with alcohol, nonalcoholic beverages, and visual control images	Brain areas associated with the level of craving in the AUD subjects included the fusiform gyri, temporal gyri, parahippocampal gyrus, uncus, frontal gyri, and precuneus
Soderlund et al. 2007 [74]	24 HC divided into a placebo and alcohol condition.	Memory encoding battery consisting of four conditions: words, object pairs, face-name pairs, and phrase-word pairs	Alcohol impaired memory for object pairs and face-name pairs, but not for words and phrase-word pairs. Impaired performance was associated with reduced bilateral prefrontal activation and nonspecific activation of the parahippocampal gyrus
Wrase et al. 2007 [72]	16 male AUD patients; 16 male age-matched HC	MID task and presentation of a series of alcohol-associated and affectively neutral pictures	Abstinent AUD showed reduced activation of the ventral striatum including the NAcc[g] during anticipation of conventional (i.e., monetary) rewards. Reduction was correlated with increased alcohol craving. AUD patients also displayed increased activation in the ventral striatum when confronted with alcohol cues, which was also associated with increased alcohol craving
Myrick et al. 2004 [64]	10 nontreatment-seeking AUD patients; 10 HC	A cue-induced paradigm consisting of alcohol and nonalcohol beverage pictures as well as visual control pictures	AUD patients reported higher craving ratings and had increased activity in the PFC[h] and anterior limbic regions. Brain activity in the left NAcc, ACC, and left orbitofrontal cortex significantly correlated with subjective craving rating in AUD patients but not in HC

[a]Alcohol use disorder
[b]Healthy controls
[c]Monetary incentive delay
[d]Blood alcohol content
[e]Anterior cingulate cortex
[f]Intravenous
[g]Nucleus accumbens
[h]Prefrontal cortex

Psychotic Disorders

Schizophrenia

Schizophrenia (SCZ) is often considered the most serious psychiatric disorder, with classic symptoms of auditory hallucinations and bizarre delusions. Affecting approximately 1% of the population in late adolescence or early adulthood, the illness is lifelong, with significant morbidity and disability. Because of its severity, fMRI research directed at psychiatric illnesses has dedicated more time to schizophrenia than any other illness. Despite these exhaustive efforts, the clinical applications of fMRI in SCZ are still preliminary (see Table 17.6). Investigations of altered functional brain activation in schizophrenic

Table 17.6 Summary of fMRI research in schizophrenia by paradigm category

Author-Year	Subjects	fMRI paradigm	Results
Sensory/motor			
Chen et al. 2008 [76]	10 SCZ[a] or SCZA[b]; 8 HC[c]	Three visual discrimination tasks were used: direction, speed, and contrast	For direction and speed discrimination tasks, patients showed decreased BOLD response in the middle temporal area and increased activation in the prefrontal cortex. The groups did not differ in the contrast discrimination tasks
Keedy et al. 2009 [77]	9 SCZ (scanned before and after antipsychotic treatment)	Processing visually guided saccades to unpredictable targets	Before treatment, patients had less activation in frontal and parietal eye fields, cerebellum, and sensory and ventromedial prefrontal cortex
Morey et al. 2008 [80]	26 SCZ; 17 HC	Automatic auditory detection task and controlled auditory processing task	Patients showed reduced activation in inferior frontal gyrus, middle frontal gyrus, anterior cingulate gyrus, basal ganglia, thalamus, and insula during the controlled auditory task and reduced activation in the right middle frontal gyrus, thalamus, and superior temporal gyrus during automatic auditory processing
Szycik et al. 2009 [204]	15 SCZ; 15 HC	Audiovisual stimuli presented as congruent and incongruent	Patients showed lower activation than controls during the incongruent tasks in the right medial frontal gyrus, the middle temporal gyrus, the fusiform gyrus, the left head of the caudate nucleus, and the left precuneus
Attention, executive function, and memory			
Benetti et al. 2009 [205]	10 SCZ, 16 ARMS[d]; 14 HC	Modified version of DMTS[e] test from the Cambridge Neuropsychological Test Automated Battery	Decreased connectivity from the hippocampus to the inferior frontal gyrus, lateralized on the right. Patients also showed greater activation in the bilateral inferior frontal gyrus, bilateral superior temporal gyrus, and the right insula and middle temporal gyrus during recognition
Elsabagh et al. 2009 [86]	25 SCZ; 25 HC	0-back, 1-back, and 2-back tasks	"Duration of illness correlated with reduced dorsolateral prefrontal cortex activity in males and reduced cerebellum activity in females, regardless of performance and age"

(continued)

Table 17.6 (continued)

Author-Year	Subjects	fMRI paradigm	Results
Hamilton et al. 2009 [87]	20 SCZ, 21 BPD,[f] and 38 HC	Shown four stimuli and then decided if fifth stimulus was in the previous four.	Patients with schizophrenia showed less activation than controls in the left inferior frontal gyrus and the left dorsolateral prefrontal cortex
Kaladjian et al. 2007 [83]	36 SCZ; 30 HC	Go/No-go task	During motor response inhibition, patients showed a decrease in activation in the right ventrolateral prefrontal cortex
Karch et al. 2009 [91]	61 SCZ; 61 HC	0-, 1-, 2-, and 3-back tasks	Patients showed increased activation in frontal, temporal, and subcortical regions of the brain. Compensatory strategies were seen in both groups
Karlsgodt et al. 2009 [88]	14 SCZ; 18 HC	A Sternberg-style item recognition task	In patients as performance increased, activation in the dorsolateral prefrontal cortex also increased, but the opposite was true for controls
Kim et al. 2009 [79]	66 SCZ; 71 HC	Auditory oddball task	Areas implicated included bilateral temporal network containing the superior and middle temporal gyrus, the default-mode network (posterior cingulate, precuneus, and middle frontal gyrus), and multiple dorsolateral prefrontal cortex networks
Meda et al. 2009 [90]	37 SCZ; 54 HC	Modified Sternberg Item Recognition Paradigm	Patients showed reduced activation in the bilateral posterior parietal, bilateral dorsolateral prefrontal cortex, cingulate, basal ganglia, and the default mode network during encoding. MORE
Rametti et al. 2009 [206]	22 SC; 24 HC	Word and face recognition tasks	Patients displayed reduced activation in the amygdala, basal ganglia, thalamus, and posterior cingulate during word recognition and reduced activation in the inferior frontal gyrus, cerebellum, insula, postcentral and precentral gyrus, cuneus and precuneus, superior frontal gyrus, and posterior cingulate gyrus during face recognition

(continued)

Table 17.6 (continued)

Author-Year	Subjects	fMRI paradigm	Results
Vink et al. 2006 [85]	21 SCZ; 15 unaffected siblings; 36 HC	Motor inhibition GO/STOP tasks	In general, patients showed slightly increased motor activation in the thalamus. Patients also showed reduced striatal activation when an inhibiting stimuli was more likely
Weiss et al. 2009 [207]	18 SCZ; 18 HC	Old–new recognition item task	Patients showed lateralization to the left hemisphere, where controls showed bilateral activation, in the prefrontal and posterior parietal regions
Emotional processing			
Benedetti et al. 2009 [208]	24 SCZ; 20 HC	Participant had to select correct story ending related to theory of mind, affective empathy, and two controls based on physical causality	In the theory of mind task, patients showed greater activation in the right superior-transverse temporal gyrus. In the affective empathy task, patients showed greater activation in an area near the right superior temporal gyrus
Gur et al. 2007 [92]	16 SCZ; 17 HC	Participants responded to five different facial expressions: fear, anger, sad, happy, and neutral	Patients showed less activation in the amygdala, hippocampus, thalamus, fusiform gyrus, and frontal and visual association cortex during the task
Park et al. 2008 [209]	14 SCZ; 14 HC	Modified emotional Stroop task	During emotional incongruence, patients did not display the deactivation in the subgenual cingulate gyrus and then ventrolmedial prefrontal cortex that was seen in the healthy controls
Reske et al. 2009 [210]	18 First-episode SCZ; 18 HC	View happy, sad, and neutral faces and null-events and determine the emotion	Patients showed reduced activation in the inferior parietal and orbitofrontal areas and the hippocampus during emotion decision compared to controls
Reske et al. 2007 [93]	10 first-episode SCZ; 10 HC	Induced sad and happy moods through facial expressions	Patients showed reduced activation in the anterior cingulate, orbitofrontal and temporal areas, the hippocampus, and other regions of emotional processing
Whalley et al. 2009 [211]	15 SCZ; 14 BPD; 14 HC	Recognition of positive and neutral emotional stimuli	Schizophrenic patients showed reduced activation in the bilateral amygdala in viewing emotional scenes

(continued)

Table 17.6 (continued)

Author-Year	Subjects	fMRI paradigm	Results
Hallucinatory correlations			
Kang et al. 2009 [212]	14 hallucinating SCZ, 14 non-hallucinating SCZ; 28 HC	Processing laughing, crying, and neutral sounds	When processing crying sounds, the hallucinating patients showed reduced activation in the left amygdala and bilaterally in the hippocampus
Plaze et al. 2006 [213]	15 hallucinating SCZ	Listening to sentence in spoken French	A negative correlation was found between the severity of chronic auditory hallucinations and activation in the left superior temporal gyrus
Raij et al. 2009 [95]	11 SCZ	Press button at beginning and end of auditory verbal hallucination	Auditory hallucinations elicited activation in the inferior frontal gyri, the ventral striatum, the auditory cortex, the right posterior temporal lobe, and the cingulate cortex
Sommer et al. 2008 [96]	24 SCZ-SD[g]	Squeeze ball at beginning and release ball at end of auditory verbal hallucination	Extended activation found in the right inferior frontal area. Other regions included the bilateral supramarginal gyri and the right superior temporal gyrus
Wible et al. 2009 [98]	74 SCZ	Sternberg Item Recognition Paradigm	Hallucinating patients had decreased activation in the superior temporal and inferior parietal areas
Zhang et al. 2008 [99]	13 hallucinating SCZ, 13 non-hallucinating SCZ; 13 HC	Listen to sentences and determine if it was presented in the left or right ear	In the hallucinating group, the supramarginal gyrus, angular gyurs, and superior temporal gyurs showed increased activation in both right- and left-sided auditory stimulation

[a]Schizophrenia
[b]Schizoaffective
[c]Healthy control
[d]At-risk mental state
[e]Delayed matching to sample
[f] Bipolar disorder
[g]Schizophrenia-spectrum disorder

patients utilizing fMRI originally began with sensory and motor paradigms. For example, it has been demonstrated that the mean signal intensity change in the primary visual cortex was significantly greater in patients with SCZ than in comparison subjects when presented with alternating blocks of flash photic stimulation and darkness [75]. More recent studies of visual processing in SCZ have implicated other areas of dysfunction, including regions of the prefrontal cortex (PFC) [76, 77].

Furthermore, primary sensory paradigms have shown dysfunction in frontal, striatal, and temporal areas during auditory tasks [77–80] and in

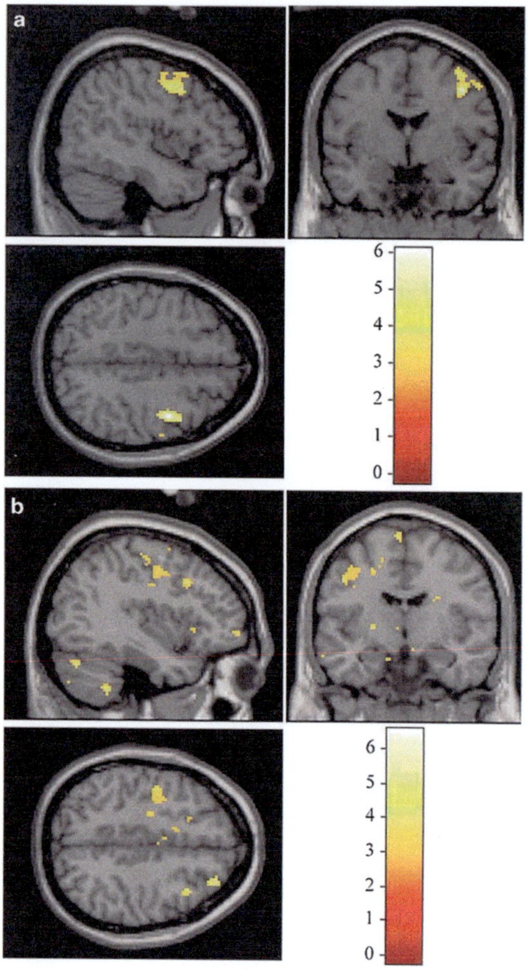

Fig. 17.3 Illustrating activation from a schizophrenic patient during (**a**) left and (**b**) right finger tapping. Images are based on SPM analysis of data

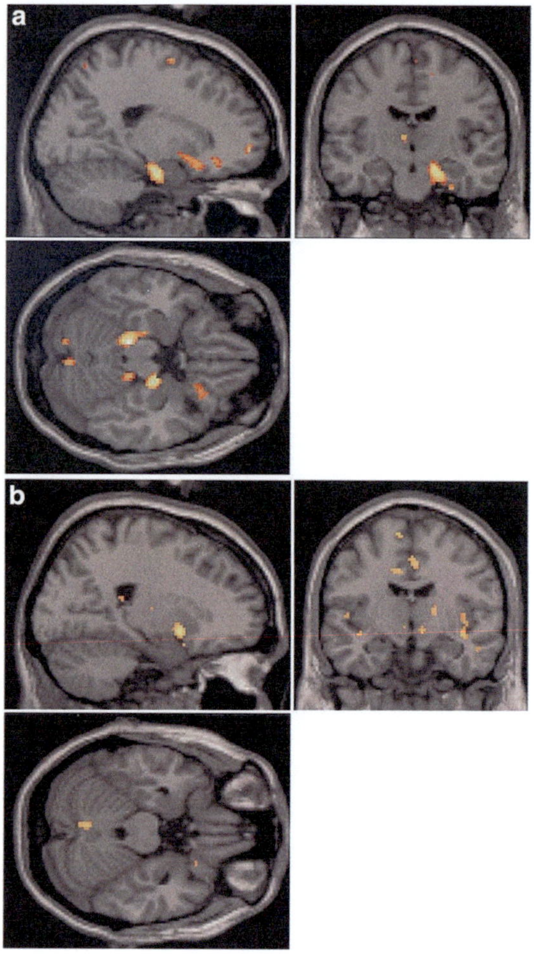

Fig. 17.4 Illustration of contrast of activation between schizophrenic and control subjects during a semantic priming task. (**a**) Shows increased activation in patients with schizophrenia during an indirect priming task with an ISI of 50 ms. (**b**) shows increased activation in schizophrenics during an indirect priming task with an ISI of 750 ms

sensorimotor cortices and the supplementary motor area during a finger-to-thumb opposition task [81] (Fig. 17.3).

A number of investigations also assessed brain activation during language, memory, and executive function tasks as a method of determining altered neural processing between schizophrenic patients and healthy control (HC) subjects. For example, in a verbal cognitive challenge paradigm [82], HC subjects produced higher frontal lobe activation and lower temporal lobe activation compared to schizophrenic patients. On motor response inhibition tasks, schizophrenic patients have generally shown decreased activation in PFC and striatal areas [83–85] (Fig. 17.4). Decreased performance and altered activation in the dorsolateral PFC during working memory tasks have also been reported in SCZ [86–90], with compensatory activations seen in other frontal, temporal, and subcortical areas of the brain [91].

Functional MRI paradigms utilizing affective-inducing tasks such as viewing facial expressions of fear, anger, disgust, and happiness have been used to examine the altered emotional processing in SCZ (Fig. 17.5). Overall, schizophrenic

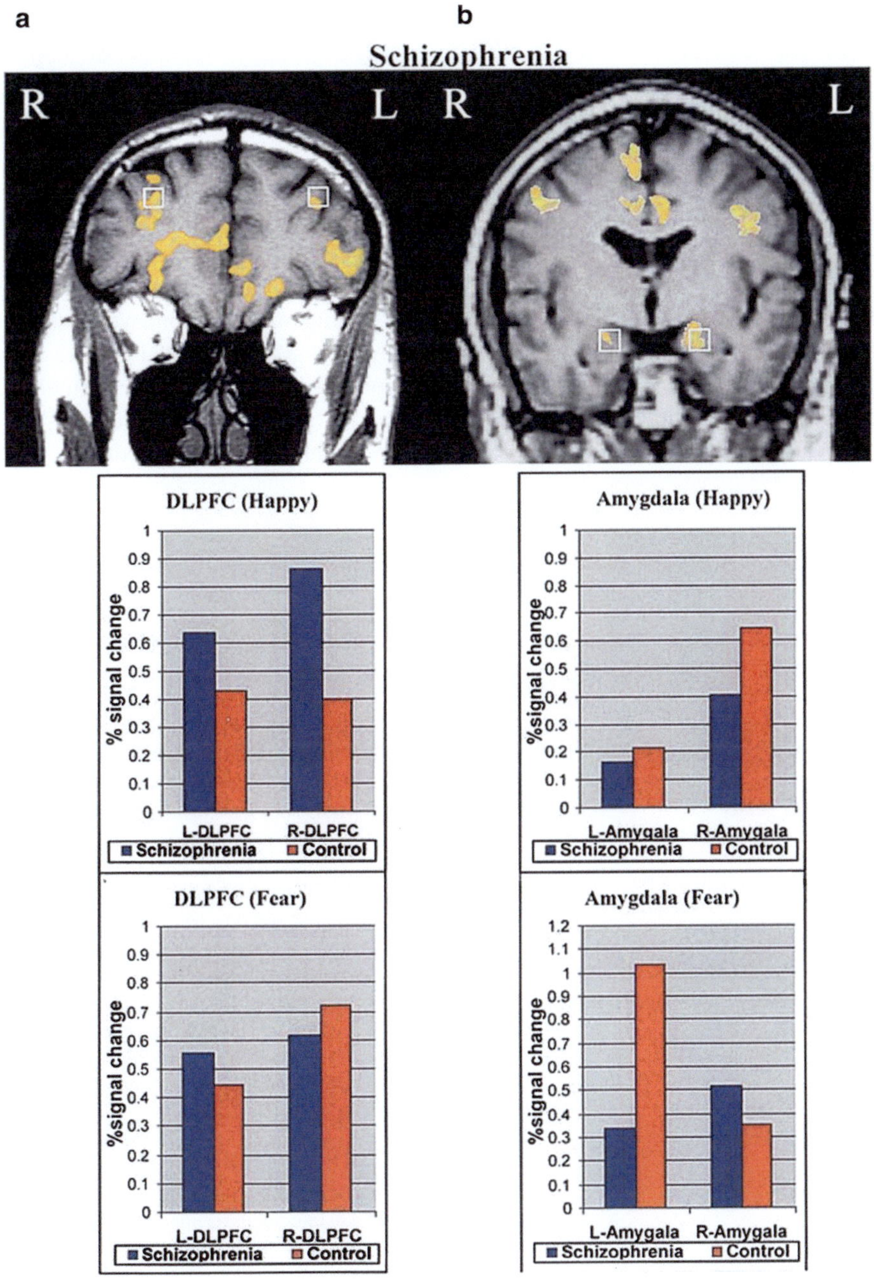

Fig. 17.5 Location of regions of interest (ROIs) selected for study, shown on a coronal section of a control subject as an example. Image A was obtained while the subject was viewing a happy face; image B was obtained while the subject was viewing a fearful face. (**a**) Squares indicate right and left dorsolateral prefrontal cortex. (**b**) Squares indicate right and left amygdala. Average overall percent signal change in the left and right amygdala, and dorsolateral prefrontal cortex (DLPFC) in response to happy affect ("Happy") and fearful affect ("Fear") in schizophrenic and control subjects

patients showed reduced activation in amygdala, hippocampus, fusiform gyrus, inferior parietal, and prefrontal (OFC and ACC) brain regions [92, 93] compared to HC subjects on affective tasks involving viewing emotional faces. Studies have also begun to look at the functional neuroanatomic correlates of hallucinations. Studies evaluating the activation patterns during auditory hallucinations in SCZ have found increased activation in the auditory cortex (including Heschl's gyrus), the cingulate cortex, and the inferior frontal gyri, superior temporal lobe, and ventral striatum [94–99].

Mood Disorders

Major Depression Disorder

Major depression disorder (MDD) is characterized by persistent feelings of deep despair accompanied by at least four of the following symptoms: sleep disturbances, disruption of appetite, apathy, lethargy, feelings of hopelessness or worthlessness, difficulty concentrating, or suicidal thoughts. The World Health Organization (WHO) [55] has concluded that by the year 2020, major depression will be the second most debilitating disease to affect mankind, followed only by ischemic heart disease. While fMRI research investigating major depression and bipolar disorder compared to nonpsychiatric populations shows consistent regional activation differences, empirical studies remain limited, causing a restraint on its ability to be used as a clinical tool (see Table 17.7). Functional neuroimaging

Table 17.7 Summary of fMRI research in major depression disorder

Author-Year	Subjects	fMRI paradigm	Results
Affect			
Chen et al. 2008 [76]	19 MDD[a] on fluoxetine; 19 HC[b]	Implicit facial affect task. Pre- and post-fluoxetine therapy	In MDD subjects, greater activity in the right fronto-striato-thalamic system was associated with a unit change in amygdala activity. A significant time-related increase in functional coupling was also observed between the right prefrontal, anterior cingulate cortex, and the amygdala
Fales et al. 2008 [104]	27 MDD unmedicated; 24 HC	Attentional interference task w/pictures of houses and faces	MDD subjects displayed increased amygdala response in fear-related versus neutral stimuli. HC exhibited increased activity in the right dorsolateral prefrontal cortex that depressed patients did not, while ignoring fear stimuli
Siegle et al. 2007 [109]	27 MDD unmedicated; 25 never-depressed HC	Digit-sorting and emotional information processing tasks	MDD subjects exhibited decreased dorsolateral prefrontal cortex (DLPFC) activity on the digit-sorting task and increased and sustained bilateral amygdalar activation on the emotion task, relative to HC. Decreased DLPFC and amygdala relationships were also prevalent in MDD subjects
Chen et al. 2007 [112]	17 MDD unmedicated	Facial affect processing task	Subjects demonstrated a negative correlation between baseline symptom severity and activation in the anterior cingulate cortex, right rectus gyrus, left medial frontal and orbitofrontal cortices, and caudate nucleus. Functional activation and gray matter volume were significantly correlated. MDD subjects also demonstrated an anatomical overlap between structural and functional MRI correlates in the anterior cingulate cortex relative to symptom severity (possibly to multimodal)
Anand et al. 2005 [101]	15 MDD unmedicated; 15 HC	Block design activation during exposure to negative versus neutral stimuli	MDD subjects demonstrated decreased low-frequency BOLD fluctuation (LFBF) correlations between the anterior cingulate cortex, pallidostriatum, and thalamic regions. In the negative versus neutral task, greater activation was also evident in the amygdala, pallidostriatum, insula, anteriomedial prefrontal cortex, and anterior cingulate cortex in MDD

(continued)

Table 17.7 (continued)

Author-Year	Subjects	fMRI paradigm	Results
Anand et al. 2005 [101]	12 MDD on sertraline; 11 HC	Visual picture sequence	MDD subjects exhibited decreased cortico-limbic LFBF correlations compared to controls during baseline resting state. Following sertraline treatment, MDD subjects displayed a significant increase in LFBF correlation between anterior cingulate cortex and limbic regions. Cortico-limbic LFBF correlations remained decreased in MDD subjects when exposed to negative pictures (possibly to multimodal)
Canli et al. 2004 [214]	15 MDD; 15 HC	Lexical decision task composed of happy, sad, threat-related, and neutral words	MDD patients demonstrated increased activation in the inferior parietal lobule and decreased activation in the superior temporal gyrus and cerebellum relative to HC
Sheline et al. 2001 [115]	27 MDD unmedicated; 25 never-depressed HC	Personal relevance rating and digit-sorting tasks	MDD patients exhibited decreased activity in the dorsolateral prefrontal cortex on the digit-sorting task and sustained amygdala reactivity relative to HC
Cognitive/executive functioning			
Matthews et al. 2009 [125]	16 MDD; 16 HC	Stop-signal task	MDD patients showed decreased activation in the bilateral IFG/IC and left supragenual ACC relative to controls, on an easy error trial. Inhibition-related subgenual activation was correlated with symptom severity in MDD patients
Schoning et al. 2009 [124]	28 MDD; 28 HC	*n*-back continuous performance task	Between-group activation differences were found in terms of hyperactivation of the cingulate cortex in HC relative to MDD patients, whereas lateral prefrontal activation was observed more so in MDD patients versus HC
Smoski et al. 2009 [127]	14 MDD unmedicated; 15 HC	Wheel of fortune task	HC showed increased activation in the paracingulate gyrus and middle frontal gyrus versus MDD patients, whereas MDD patients showed increased activation in left orbitofrontal cortex and other occipital areas relative to controls
Fitzgerald et al. 2008 [120]	13 MDD; 13 HC	TOL[c] and *n*-back tasks	Relative to HC, MDD patients showed increased activation of the inferior and middle frontal gyrus as well as the right angular gyrus on the TOL task and increased activation in the middle, medial, and inferior frontal gyri bilaterally; thalamus; anterior cingulate gyrus; cuneus/precuneus; and precentral gyrus
Matsuo et al. 2007 [122]	15 MDD unmedicated; 15 HC	*n*-back task	MDD patients showed increased activation in the ACC and the left dorsolateral cortex relative to HC
Harvey et al. 2005 [121]	10 MDD; 10 HC	*n*-back task	MDD patients showed increased activation in the ACC, bilateral inferior frontal gyri, superior parietal lobule, and the left middle frontal gyrus, relative to HC

[a]Major depressive disorder
[b]Healthy controls
[c] Tower of London

studies of depression have primarily focused on probing brain regions involved in emotion regulation, including regions of the PFC, amygdala, hippocampus, striatum, and hypothalamus [100]. Emotional dysregulation has been hypothesized to be secondary to a loss of top (PFC)-down (limbic structures) control or, alternatively, the result of a disinhibited limbic drive overriding cortical executive control. Emotional paradigms attempting to induce feelings of sadness, happiness, or fear have shown significant differences in regions of the prefrontal, cingulate gyrus, and amygdala between depressed and normal control subjects (Fig. 17.6). For example, increased amygdala and dysfunctional PFC activity, including the anterior cingulate cortex (ACC), is a commonly reported finding during tasks of negatively valenced stimuli [101–110]. Furthermore, authors have reported a "decoupling" of the dorsolateral PFC and amygdala, which may be secondary to impaired integration of cognitive and emotional processing within the ACC [109, 111]. Interestingly, faster and more robust response to antidepressant treatment has been associated with greater functional activation in the ACC on affective tasks [112, 113]. In addition, exaggerated amygdala activation to faces has been reported to be normalized following treatment with antidepressants [113–115]. Furthermore, the functional coupling/connectivity between cortico-limbic brain regions has also been shown to increase following antidepressant treatment [112, 116]. In addition to the amygdala, the hippocampus/parahippocampal gyrus has also been associated with increased activity in MDD [101, 117], with normalization of activation with recovery from depression [118]. Lastly, several studies have reported abnormal activity of the striatum and basal ganglia in MDD [101, 118], providing further support for a limbic cortico-striato-pallido-thalamic circuit abnormality in the pathophysiology of depression [119].

Cognitive deficits have been described both during a depressive episode and during euthymia. Studies utilizing tasks of working memory in medicated and unmedicated depressed individuals have found increased activation in limbic and lateral PFC and ACC regions, presumably in an attempt to recruit additional cognitive resources to accomplish the task [120–123]. Interestingly, a study of working memory in recently remitted individuals with MDD found persistent hyperactivation of the cingulate cortex but not lateral PFC regions, suggesting that the ACC hyperactivity may be a trait or endophenotypic marker for depression [124]. Abnormal activation patterns of the ACC in MDD have also been reported in tasks of inhibitory control such as the stop-signal task [125] and Stroop [126], and in reward

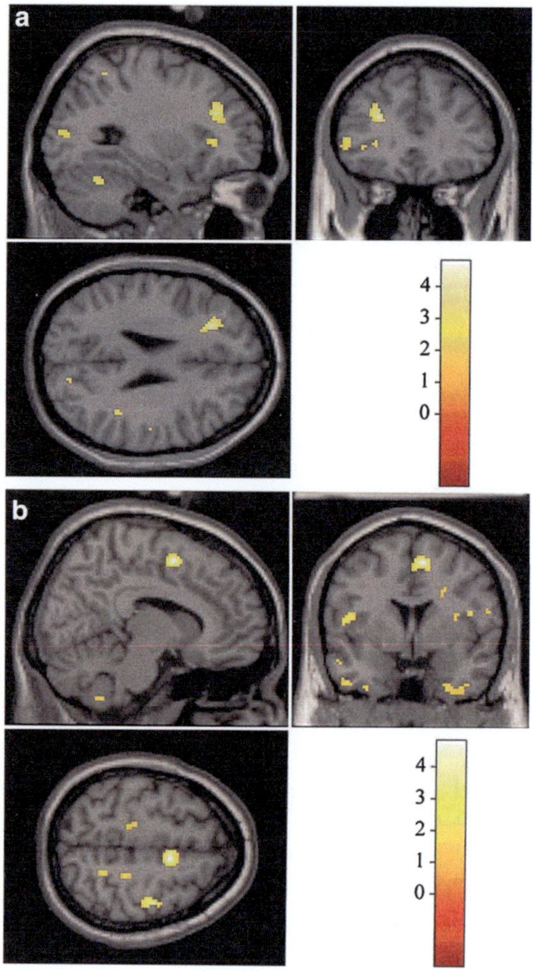

Fig. 17.6 (**a**) Illustrating increased frontal activation in control subjects compared with depressed subjects during the viewing of fearful faces. (**b**) Comparison of activation in depressed adolescents and healthy comparison adolescents during the viewing of happy facial affect. Nonpsychiatric subjects produced significantly greater cingulate activation than depressed subjects during this task

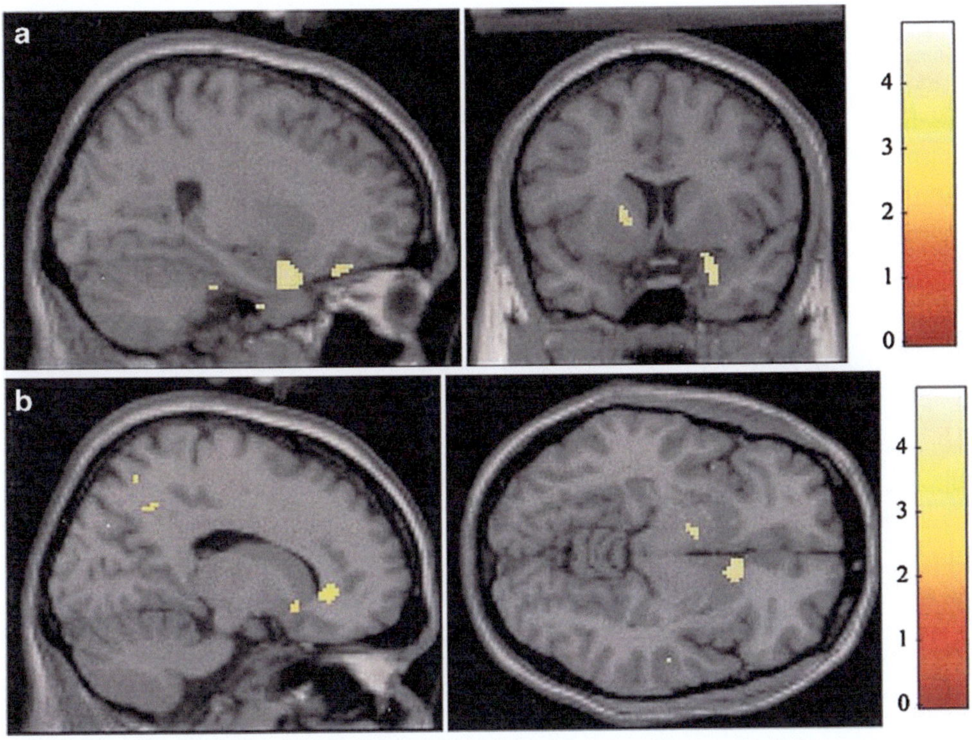

Fig. 17.7 (**a**) Illustration of increased parahippocampal activation in patients with bipolar disorder compared with controls during the viewing of fearful faces. (**b**) Illustration of increased cingulate activation in patients with bipolar disorder compared with controls during the viewing of fearful faces

selection and anticipation [127], providing further evidence for its role in the pathophysiology of MDD.

Bipolar Disorder

Abnormalities in brain activation recorded using fMRI during cognitive and emotional tasks in bipolar disorder (BD) patients report similar frontal-subcortico-limbic activation patterns as seen in major depression disorder. In order to be diagnosed with BD, an individual has to have at least one hypomanic or manic episode, which is characterized by elevated, expansive, or irritable mood, and is usually accompanied by altered cognitive processing, heightened energy levels, pressured thought and speech, and distractibility. Unlike depressed individuals, manic patients show an increased interest in pleasurable activities and a resultant increase in reward-directed behavior. Thus, depressive and manic episodes involve a complex mix and interplay of mood, motivational, cognitive, and behavioral symptoms [128, 129]. The euthymic state (in the absence of depressive or manic symptoms) is also associated with residual cognitive and emotional deficits [130, 131]. These varied clinical presentations point to aberrant functioning of discrete and interacting brain regions and networks including the ACC, DLPFC, and the amygdala (Fig. 17.7). Furthermore, current models of BD converge in suggesting that two major groups of brain regions – a "dorsal" and "ventral" network – account for the formation and modulation of the varied symptoms of affective illness. The ventromedial system includes regions of the parahippocampal gyrus, hippocampus, subgenual ACC, and ventromedial and dorsomedial PFC, while the dorsal system is comprised of dorsal and lateral prefrontal cortical regions [132, 133]. These two systems in concert with the subcortico-limbic regions including the amygdala, ventral striatum, and thalamus appear to regulate mood [132, 133], and dysfunction of regions within these circuits is state dependent.

Compared to healthy controls (HC), increased subcortico-limbic activation and abnormal dorsolateral and ventromedial activity during emotional processing tasks have been reported in individuals with BD during remission [134–139], depression [137, 140], and mania [141–144] (see Table 17.8). Increased limbic activity has been reported to be greater in unmedicated BD, but

Table 17.8 Summary of fMRI research in bipolar disorder

Author-Year	Subjects	fMRI paradigm	Results
Affect			
Almeida et al. 2009 [151]	21 BD, euthymic; 25 HC	Facial affect-processing task of mild, intense happy, and neutral faces	No between-group effective connectivity differences were evident in the sgCG[a]-DLPFC[b]; however, BD patients showed increased right parahippocampal gyrus-sgCG effective connectivity relative to HC
Hassel et al. 2008 [136]	19 BD, euthymic BD; 24 HC	Facial affect-processing task of mild and intense happy, fearful, and neutral faces	BD patients had increased left striatal activity in response to mild happy faces, decreased DLPFC activity in response to neutral, mild, and intense happy faces and fearful faces, relative to HC
Wang et al. 2009 [147] May move to multimodal section	33 BD (16 euthymic, 10 manic/mixed or hypomanic, 7 depressed); 31 HC	Facial affect-processing task. Functional magnetic resonance imaging (fMRI) during processing of face stimuli and diffusion tensor imaging (DTI) were performed	Functional connectivity was decreased between the perigenual ACC and amygdala in BD patients compared with HC, during the processing of fearful and happy faces. A significant positive association between perigenual ACC-amygdala functional coupling and FA in ventrofrontal white matter, including the region of the uncinate fasciculus, was identified
Hassel et al. 2009 [135]	14 BD, euthymic; 16 HC	Facial affect-processing task of neutral, mild, and intense happy and fearful faces	Relative to HC, BD patients scored higher on all spectrum measures as determined by activity in subcortical-striatal and prefrontal regions. Reduced dorsal prefrontal-cortical activity was seen in BD patients in response to all faces, and BD only demonstrated greater subcortical-striatal activity in response to happy/neutral faces
Bermpohl et al. 2008 [215]	10 BD mania or hypomania; 10 HC	Facial affect-processing task during which subjects rated the emotional valence and intensity of each picture	In response to positive versus neutral pictures in BD, higher valence ratings were associated with larger BOLD responses in the left amygdala
Killgore et al. 2008 [216]	14 BD, mixed; 13 HC	Two-block fearful face perception task	During the late stage of task, HC had increased orbitofrontal, ACC,[c] and striatum activity, whereas BD patients did not show normal task-related activity in these regions
Jogia et al. 2008 [145]	12 BD; 12 HC	Sad facial affect recognition task pre- and post-12 weeks of lamotrigine monotherapy	At baseline and compared to HC, BD patients showed underactivity in the dorsal medial and right ventrolateral PFC,[d] and the dorsal cingulate gyrus and overactivity in temporal regions. Lamotrigine therapy for BD patients resulted in reduced temporal and increased prefrontal activation compared with study baseline

(continued)

Table 17.8 (continued)

Author-Year	Subjects	fMRI paradigm	Results
Foland et al. 2008 [146]	10 BD, manic; 10 HC	Emotion labeling and perception tasks	During the emotion-labeling task, BD patients showed decreased ventrolateral PFC regulation of amygdala response relative to HC
Blumberg et al. 2005 [134]	33 BD (16 euthymic, 10 manic/mixed or hypomanic, 7 depressed); 31 HC	Facial affect-processing task of mild and intense happy and neutral faces	Compared to HC, unmedicated BD patients showed decreased rostral ACC activation, while medicated BD patients showed activation in the same area similar to HC. Amygdala increases were greater in unmedicated BD, but lower in medicated BD patients
Executive functioning tasks			
Kaladjian et al. 2009 [152]	10 BD, manic; 10 HC Longitudinal study with fMRI obtained while manic and again when remitted	Inhibitory Go/No-Go task	BD demonstrated amygdalar hyperactivity during mania with normalization of activity with remission. Group differences were found for the left amygdala between HC and BD patients, with the BD group exhibiting hyperactivity in the amygdala during mania with normalization of activity with remission
Kaladjian et al. 2009 [153]	20 BD, euthymic; 20 HC	Inhibitory Go/No-Go task	BD patients exhibited decreased activation in the left fronto-polar cortex and bilateral dorsal amygdala compared with HC during response inhibition
Mazzola-Pomietto et al. 2009 [154]	16 BD, manic; 16 HC	Inhibitory Go/No-Go task	In BD patients, decreased ventrolateral PFC activation was evident when compared to HC
Altshuler et al. 2005 [141]	11 patients with manic BPD; 13 healthy controls	Inhibitory Go-No-Go task	Increased activation in right orbitofrontal cortex in HC compared to BD patients
Gruber et al. 2010 [159]	18 BD, euthymic; 18 HC	Working memory task (articulatory rehearsal)	Compared to HC, BD patients had increased activation of the right amygdala, right frontal and intraparietal cortex, and in the right cerebellum
Deckersbach et al. 2008 [165]	9 BD, depressed; 17 HC	2-back working memory task under no mood induction, neutral state, or acute sadness	BD individuals exhibited sadness-specific activation increases in the left DLPFC and left dorsal ACC
Thermenos et al. 2010 [164]	19 BD, euthymic; 18 unmedicated, first-degree relatives of persons with BD (AR), and 19 HC	Working memory task; fMRI signal was measured during 2-back and 0-back working memory tasks	During the working memory task, HC suppressed left anterior insular activation while BD patients and AR failed to do the same. Compared to HC, AR also failed to suppress activation in the orbitofrontal cortex and superior parietal cortex. HC and AR exhibited greater activation in the left fronto-polar cortex compared to BD patients
Haldane et al. 2008 [163]	12 BD; lamotrigine therapy	Verbal working memory (*n*-back sequential letter task) and an angry facial affect recognition task; scanned pre- and post-12-week lamotrigine (LTG) therapy	Compared to baseline, both tasks demonstrated increased activation in the medial and superior frontal regions as well as the ACC. This increase was associated with lamotrigine monotherapy

[a]Subgenual cingulate gyrus
[b]Dorsolateral prefrontal cortex
[c]Anterior cingulate gyrus
[d]Prefrontal cortex

lower in medicated BD [134, 145]. Furthermore, underactivity of PFC in unmedicated BD appears to normalize with treatment [134, 145]. Studies of functional connectivity have found reduced coherence between ventrolateral PFC (VLPFC), the pregenual ACC, and amygdala in patients with BD versus HC during an emotion-labeling task [146, 147]. Furthermore, there are reports of reduced activity in patients with remitted and manic BD versus HC in ventromedial PFC (vmPFC) during emotional Stroop and risk-taking tasks [148–150]. Right parahippocampal-subgenual cingulate (sgCG) effective connectivity was significantly greater in patients with remitted BD than HC, but no difference was observed in sgCG-DLPFC effective connectivity between groups [151].

Deficits in inhibitory control and increased impulsivity have been reported in bipolar patients. A Go/No Go task, which measures inhibitory control, showed that in a longitudinal study, the left amygdala was hyperactive during a manic state and normalized with remission [152]. Cross-sectional studies of response inhibition have also found abnormal activation patterns in the orbito frontal cortex (OFC) VLPFC, fronto-polar cortices BD HC [141, 153–155]. When performing the Stroop task, an attentional and behavioral inhibition task, euthymic bipolar patients demonstrated significantly decreased activation within the ACC and increased activation in the DLPFC compared with HC [156]. In studies of working memory, BD patients displayed atypical activation in the PFC (frontopolar, VLPFC/OFC), the temporal cortex/limbic regions, regions of the parietal cortex/precuneus, the basal ganglia, cerebellum, and the thalamus compared with HC, suggesting that these regions could make up an alternate working memory network for BD [157–162]. Activation abnormalities during euthymia in the amygdala, insula, and PFC in working memory tasks may serve as an endophenotypic marker of BD [158–160, 163, 164]. In a study of depressed BD individuals using a working memory task, sadness-specific abnormalities were found in the left DLPFC and the left dACC, suggesting difficulties in the integration of emotion and cognition [165].

Brain activation patterns that have emerged for BD patients include a pattern of subcortical/limbic hyperactivity with either increased or decreased activation in cortical regions compared with HC. The interpretation of this imaging data is complicated since the neural circuits involved are composed of both inhibitory and excitatory connections, which may be differentially affected. One common interpretation is that BD is characterized by a reduction in the inhibitory input from subcortical regions, resulting in increased cortical activation, particularly in the manic state. The use of different activation paradigms of varying complexity also makes it difficult to compare study results directly. Nevertheless, the data suggest that there are abnormalities in a number of regions that are structurally linked via neural networks that are known to underlie cognition and emotional processing [166–168].

Anxiety Disorders

Posttraumatic Stress Disorder

Posttraumatic stress disorder (PTSD) is a psychiatric disorder characterized by exposure to trauma followed by significant functional and emotional impairment. Symptoms related to impairment include re-experiencing the trauma (flashbacks or dreams); avoidance and numbing; and hyperarousal (hypervigilance, sleep difficulties, poor concentration, etc.). Functional neuroimaging studies with PTSD participants have focused primarily on regions involved in emotional-regulation and memory – primarily the amygdala, hippocampus, insula, and frontal cortex. Tasks used to probe these brain regions in PTSD include affective tasks such as participants viewing faces with positive (e.g., happy) and negative (e.g., angry) expressions, cognitive tasks such as the Stroop, and combined tasks such as the Emotional Stroop task (see Table 17.9).

The amygdala is a primary structure of the limbic system, involved in emotional learning and memory. It has been identified as being involved in PTSD due to its importance in

Table 17.9 Summary of fMRI Research in PTSD

Author-Year	Subjects	fMRI paradigm	Results
Thomaes et al. 2009 [175]	9 PTSD[a]; 9 HC[b]	Verbal declarative memory task with neutral/negative words	PTSD patients exhibited enhanced BOLD response in left hippocampus during deep encoding of negative words and during correct recognition of negative words compared with HC
Werner et al. 2009 [176]	12 PTSD; 12 HC	Associative learning paradigm (encoding/retrieval)	Relative to HC, PTSD patients showed increased hippocampal and decreased prefrontal activation during encoding and reduced left parahippocampal gyrus activation during retrieval
Shin et al. 2005 [173]	26 males (veterans or firefighters); 13 PTSD; 13 HC	Affective task: picture presentation of fearful, happy, and neutral facial expressions	Compared to HC, PTSD patients showed exaggerated amygdala response and decreased mPFC[c] response to fearful faces compared to happy faces. Amygdala activity was negatively correlated with BOLD changes in mPFC
Protopopescu et al. 2005 [171]	9 PTSD; 14 HC	Participants presented with 48 negative/anxiety words, 48 positive safety words, and 48 neutral words	Increased amygdala response to trauma-related negative words but not to non-trauma negative words in PTSD patients compared to HC
Lanius et al. 2004 [178]	11 PTSD; 13 HC	Autobiographical script of neutral/traumatic event read to subject during scan	Both groups exhibited activation in the middle frontal gyrus and parts of cingulate gyrus. Functional connectivity maps showed that PTSD patients had greater correlations in right posterior cingulate gyrus, right caudate, right parietal lobe, and right occipital lobe. HC showed greater correlations in left superior frontal gyrus, left anterior cingulate gyrus, left striatum (caudate), left parietal lobe, and left insula
Shin et al. 2001 [174]	8 PTSD (Vietnam veterans); 8 HC (Vietnam veterans)	Emotional counting Stroop: words were neutral (e.g., mirror), generally negative (e.g., combat), and combat related (e.g., firefight)	HC showed increased activity in rostral ACC[d] with combat words and in medial frontal cortex, left hippocampus, left parahippocampal gyrus, and right midcingulate cortex in response to generally negative words. PTSD patients showed increased BOLD signal in dorsal ACC but no signal increase in rostral ACC with combat words
Rauch et al. 2000 [172]	8 PTSD (Vietnam veterans); 8 HC (Vietnam veterans)	Masked faces: Pictures of faces (fearful, happy, and neutral) masked by neutral faces	PTSD patients exhibited greater amygdala response than HC; PTSD patients showed exaggerated amygdala response to masked-fear faces compared to masked-happy faces

[a]Posttraumatic stress disorder
[b]Healthy controls
[c]Medial prefrontal cortex
[d]Anterior cingulate cortex

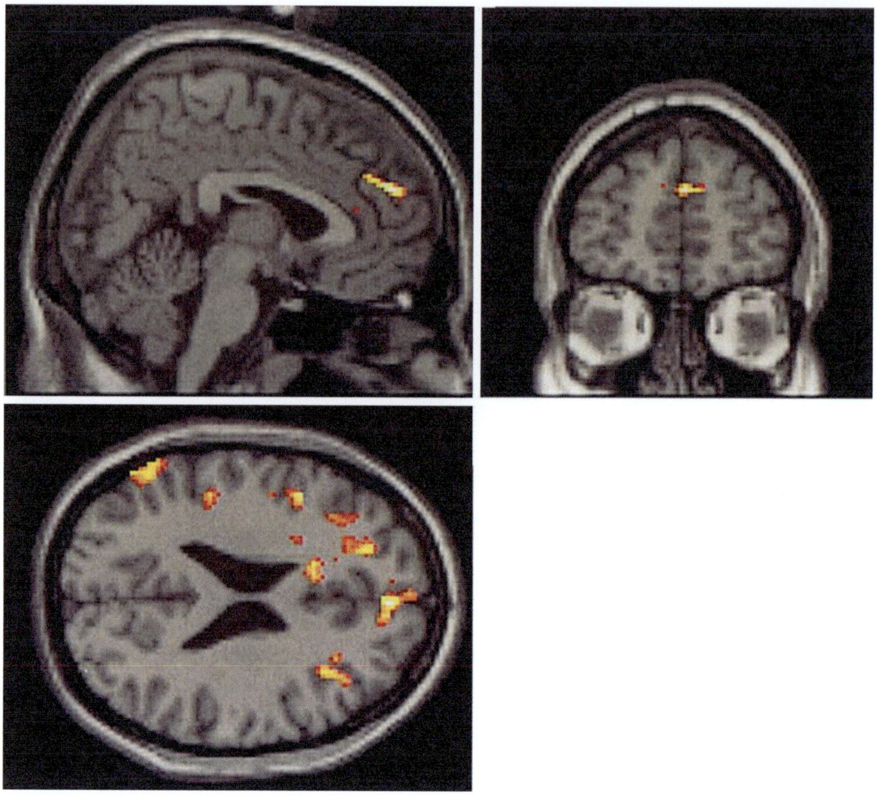

Fig. 17.8 Illustrating increased activation in subjects with panic disorder compared with activation in healthy controls. All subjects were completing interference subtest of the Stroop test

behavior regulation and emotional response [169]. Using affective and cognitive tasks, researchers have found increased amygdala response (Fig. 17.8) in individuals with PTSD, including combat- and noncombat-related PTSD [170–173]. The hippocampus is another structure important in the limbic system; it is implicated in stress-inhibition, working memory, declarative memory, and memory for episodic events. The hippocampus has been identified as a primary structure with differential activation in individuals with PTSD. Increases in activation in the left hippocampus, left parahippocampal gyrus, and right midcingulate cortex have been shown in non-PTSD Vietnam veterans exposed to combat-related words during an Emotional Stroop task [174]. Participants with comorbid Borderline Personality Disorder (BPD) and PTSD have shown increased right parahippocampal activity compared to patients with BPD without PTSD [170]. Enhanced BOLD activation in the hippocampus has been shown during both encoding and recognition tasks [175, 176].

The PFC including the anterior ACC is involved in fear response and in the extinction of fear responses [177]. In individuals with PTSD, sensitization and habituation to negative stimuli (e.g., triggers) do not occur as they do in healthy controls [171]. Several studies suggest that the lack of habituation/sensitization may be due to dysfunctional activity of PFC regions [173, 174, 178]. For example, Vietnam veterans without PTSD have exhibited increased activity in the rostral ACC, while Vietnam veterans with PTSD showed greater BOLD signal activity in the dorsal ACC [174]. Furthermore, another study reported that PTSD participants had decreased medial PFC activation to overt fearful faces compared to overt happy faces (Shin et al. [173]). Researchers have also found associations between the vmPFC and the amygdala, suggesting that the vmPFC aids in inhibiting the amygdala, which is differentially activated in PTSD [173, 177, 179, 180].

Obsessive–Compulsive Disorder

Obsessive–compulsive disorder (OCD) is an anxiety disorder in which patients experience recurrent obsessions and compulsions that cause significant distress and occupy a significant portion of the affected person's life. Lifetime prevalence of this disorder is 2–3%. Blood oxygenation level-dependent fMRI studies have afforded much insight into the brain–behavior relationships in patients with OCD (see Table 17.10). Medicated patients with OCD have exhibited increased activation in the medial orbitofrontal, lateral frontal, anterior temporal, anterior cingulate, and insular cortex, as well as caudate, lenticulate, and amygdalar regions in association

Table 17.10 Summary of fMRI research in obsessive–compulsive disorder

Author-Year	Subjects	fMRI paradigm	Results
Nakao et al. 2009 [186]	40 OCD[a]; 25 HC[b]	*n*-back task, 2-back task	OCD patients had increased activation in right DLPFC,[c] left superior temporal gyrus, left insula, and cuneus during 2-back task. OCD patients with primary obsessions/checking showed less activation of the postcentral gyrus and more memory deficits than OCD patients with primary washing
Ursu and Carter 2009 [194]	15 OCD; 15 HC (age and handedness matched)	Modified continuous performance task	OCD patients showed increased activation of lateral OFC[d] in response to conflict probes. OFC activation was correlated with anxiety symptoms
An et al. 2009 [217]	29 OCD (13 with primary hoarding, 16 without); 21 HC	Subjects shown pictures of common hoarding items, disgusting/anxiety provoking stimuli, and pictures of neutral/pleasant scenes	OCD patients with hoarding had increased activation in the bilateral anterior vmPFC.[e] For both OCD groups, anxiety was related to increased activation in the anterior vmPFC, bilateral medial temporal structures, left thalamus, bilateral precentral gyri and postcentral gyri, right vlPFC,[f] and bilateral cerebellum
den Braber et al. 2008 [190]	12 monozygotic twin pairs discordant for OCD	Tower of London task	OCD twin showed decreased activation in the DLPFC, thalamus, and inferior parietal cortex during planning compared to non-OCD twin
Rauch et al. 2007 [192]	12 OCD; 12 HC (gender, age, and education matched)	Serial reaction time task (implicit learning versus random contrast)	During implicit learning, OCD patients showed increased activation in the right hippocampus and right OFC (near significant in left OFC)
Roth et al. 2007 [189]	12 OCD (6 medicated and 6 unmedicated); 14 HC	Go/no-go task	Activation for HC was concentrated in the right hemisphere, whereas OCD patients showed bilateral activation during response inhibition. HC showed greater activation of the right inferior and medial frontal gyrus, fusiform gyrus, right superior frontal gyrus, middle temporal gyrus, and thalamus, whereas OCD patients showed increased activation in the left supramarginal gyrus, right cuneus, and postcentral gyrus

(continued)

Table 17.10 (continued)

Author-Year	Subjects	fMRI paradigm	Results
Fitzgerald et al. 2005 [196]	8 OCD; 7 HC	Flanker interference task	OCD patients showed dorsal ACC activation during error commission and greater activation in rostral ACC compared to HC
Nakao et al. 2005 [191]	24 OCD unmedicated; 14 HC	Chinese character Stroop task	OCD patients showed decreased activation in the ACC and right caudate nucleus compared to HC
Schienle et al. 2005 [218]	10 OCD (5 medicated and 5 unmedicated), 10 HC (age, gender, handedness, education, and SES matched)	Visual task with disgust-evoking, fear-inducing, and neutral pictures; personally relevant OCD pictures	For personally relevant pictures, OCD patients had greater activation of prefrontal cortex (especially bilateral OFC and left dorsolateral prefrontal cortex), left insula, right supramarginal gyrus, left caudate nucleus, and right thalamus. In disgust- and fear-evoking pictures, OCD patients had greater activation of the insula compared to HC

[a]Obsessive–compulsive disorder
[b]Healthy controls
[c]Dorsolateral prefrontal cortex
[d]Orbitofrontal cortex
[e]Ventromedial prefrontal cortex
[f] Ventrolateral prefrontal cortex

with OCD symptoms. In contrast, healthy controls (HC) did not exhibit activation of any of these regions after provocation. These same findings have been replicated using unmedicated patients with OCD [181].

Functional MRI techniques have been used to examine the neuroanatomic correlates of OCD in patients and control subjects using symptom provocation [182]. In one symptom provocation study, OCD participants with hoarding symptoms showed increased activation in bilateral anterior vmPFC compared to non-hoarding OCD participants and HC [183]. Anxiety was related to activation in the vmPFC, medial temporal, thalamus, and sensorimotor cortex for OCD participants with and without hoarding [184]. Schienle et al. [185] examined neural response differences in OCD participants exposed to personally relevant OCD trigger pictures and OCD-irrelevant disgust-inducing, fear-inducing, and neutral pictures. OCD participants exhibited increased activation in the bilateral prefrontal cortex, left insula, right supramarginal gyrus, left caudate nucleus, and right thalamus when shown personally relevant OCD trigger stimuli. OCD participants exhibited increased insula activation in response to disgust-inducing and fear-inducing stimuli when compared to HC. Differential neural response has also been observed between two more specific OCD symptoms: washing and checking. OCD subjects predominately concerned with washing were shown to have similar neural activations during the viewing of disgusting pictures and washer-relevant pictures. Patients predominately concerned with checking instead showed decreased activity in the postcentral gyrus [186] and increased activations in the fronto-striatal regions, seen to be associated with the urge to ritualize in OCD [187]. Checking behavior has also been hypothesized as related to deficits in working memory, and data have shown that OCD participants (especially those focused on checking more than washing) perform more poorly on immediate and delayed recall measures compared to HC [186]. While OCD participants and HC exhibit neural activation in similar brain regions during working memory tasks (frontal and parietal), OCD patients have exhibited higher levels of activation in these regions [188] when compared to HC.

It has been hypothesized that OCD may be related to inhibitory dysfunction and disruption in the fronto-striatal-thalamic-cortical (FSTC) circuitry. Based on this hypothesis, researchers have examined inhibitory control in participants with OCD. Researchers have found that while HC show mainly right hemisphere activation during inhibitory tasks, participants with OCD show more bilateral activation. OCD participants have also shown less right hemisphere activation in the inferior and medial frontal gyri compared to HC [189]. In a monozygotic twin study, twins with obsessive–compulsive symptoms showed less activity in DLPFC, thalamus pulvinar, and inferior parietal cortex compared to the healthy control twins during an executive function task [190]. Decreased activation of the ACC and right caudate nucleus has also been observed in OCD participants compared to healthy controls during an inhibition/executive function task [191]. Researchers have also documented differential activity in the orbitofrontal cortex in participants with OCD compared to healthy controls [183, 191–194]. The importance of identifying differential neural responses associated with varying symptomatology and symptom degrees in OCD has great implications for the future use of fMRI as a tool for treatment development and evaluation. Several studies have found associations between clinical severity and neural activation. Specifically, Levine and colleagues [195] identified a negative correlation between clinical ratings of OCD symptomatology and the activation of the DLPFC during verbal fluency, and Fitzgerald and colleagues [196] found an association between activation of the rostral ACC and severity of OCD symptoms.

Functional MRI and Treatment Response

Recently, fMRI techniques have increasingly been applied to evaluate medication effects on both brain function and predictors of treatment response. For instance, in a study by Chen and colleagues, a group of adults with MDD, who received 8 weeks of fluoxetine, found that faster rates of improvement in depressive symptoms were found in individuals with greater gray matter in the ACC, insula, and right temporoparietal cortex and in individuals with greater functional activation in the ACC on an affective facial task [112]. A similar study of depressed individuals who received venlafaxine treatment also noted that greater ACC activation to negative stimuli at baseline was associated with more robust treatment response [113]. Studies attempting to address the impact of medication on brain functioning utilizing fMRI have been performed in other psychiatric illnesses as well, including BD and SCZ [77, 163]. In general, studies that have investigated medication effects on activation signal have observed a more "normalized" brain activation response after treatment [77, 163, 166, 167], suggesting that altered activation is indeed related to the pathophysiology of illness. Future fMRI studies should continue to evaluate brain activation patterns that predict treatment response in order to one day allow clinicians to provide timely and effective treatment for patients and reduce the risk of medication complications.

Multimodal Neuroimaging

It is evident that additional analytical techniques are needed to characterize neural network function, as measured by fMRI, so that it can be used to examine cognitive and affective processing deficits in psychiatric disorders. A key challenge is how researchers can best model these neurophysiologic changes. More recent studies of patients with psychiatric disorders have attempted to address these issues using multimodal neuroimaging techniques in combination, including fMRI data with structural MR results, diffusion tensor imaging, and magnetic resonance spectroscopy. For example, to further examine the relationship between D2 receptor dysfunction in the ventral striatum, central processing of alcohol-associated cues, and alcohol craving, Heinz et al. [197] used fMRI together with PET to study detoxified male alcoholics. A multimodal study of MDD, utilizing both structural data and fMRI, demonstrated an anatomical overlap between structural and functional MRI correlates in the anterior cingulate cortex relative to symptom severity [112]. In another study, authors combined fMRI and DTI data to assess structural and functional connectivity of fronto-limbic circuits in BD [147]. The authors found a significant positive association between perigenual ACC–amygdala functional coupling and fractional anisotropy (a measure of white matter integrity) in ventrofrontal white matter, including the region of the uncinate fasciculus [147]. Together, these studies imply that multi-modal neuroimaging data may provide complimentary and convergent evidence for brain dysfunction in psychiatric disorder on a gross, network, and cellular level.

Conclusion: Future Implications

There is little question that fMRI methods are considered to play a critical role in psychiatric research. The ability to monitor brain function noninvasively using fMRI techniques in individuals with brain disorders is compelling, especially considering that the months of work often can be summarized in a single image on the cover of a scientific journal. These tools are even more important in psychiatry, as opposed to other medical disciplines, in the context of limited existing knowledge with respect to the pathophysiology of mental illnesses and an absence of valid or compelling animal models of disease. However, research studies conducted to date have not yet identified a role for fMRI as a diagnostic imaging method in psychiatric practice. While it is likely that future fMRI research will provide new insights into psychiatric brain dysfunction, there are obstacles that stand in the way of clinical method development.

The majority of ongoing psychiatric neuroimaging research is focused on studies of brain activity occurring in groups of subjects with specific disorders. Indeed, National Institutes of Health-funded investigations increasingly involve the use of methods such as single-event fMRI, where averaging across subjects is essential for statistically significant results to be obtained. In a parallel vein, cognitive neuroscience studies often make use of complex paradigms that may not be performed well in persons with psychotic or affective illness. Deconvolving the effects of changes in brain activity with differences in task performance remains a challenging problem. Moreover, there exists a relatively limited understanding of the effects of psychotropic agents – many of which have vasoactive properties – on fMRI parameters.

At the present time, the future use of fMRI in psychiatry is uncertain and progress toward this end has been limited; for example, little effort is being devoted to the identification of relatively simple challenges that can be presented in a block design and that provide distinct patterns of brain activation in single subjects with a specific psychiatric illness. The elucidation of fMRI methods that provide task-independent assessments of cerebral activity, such as DSCI, may help to clarify this area of study. Research along these lines would be facilitated greatly if it were to be driven by the vendors of MRI devices. Given the substantial prevalence of psychiatric disorders, these vendors would benefit greatly from the development of psychiatrically relevant fMRI strategies as a means to address a substantial new market.

References

1. Kwong KK, Belliveau JW, Chesler DA, Goldberg IE, Weisskoff RM, Poncelet BP, et al. Dynamic magnetic resonance imaging of human brain activity during primary sensory stimulation. Proc Natl Acad Sci USA. 1992;89(12):5675–9.
2. Belliveau JW, Rosen BR, Kantor HL, Rzedzian RR, Kennedy DN, McKinstry RC, et al. Functional cerebral imaging by susceptibility-contrast NMR. Magn Reson Med. 1990;14(3):538–46.
3. Yurgelun-Todd DA, Renshaw PF. Applications of functional MR imaging to research in psychiatry. Neuroimaging Clin N Am. 1999;9(2):295–308.
4. Ross MH, Yurgelun-Todd DA, Renshaw PF, Maas LC, Mendelson JH, Mello NK, et al. Age-related reduction in functional MRI response to photic stimulation. Neurology. 1997;48(1):173–6.
5. American Psychiatric Association, Task Force on DSM-IV. Diagnostic and statistical manual of mental disorders: DSM-IV. 4th ed. Washington, DC: American Psychiatric Association; 1994.
6. Filipek PA, Accardo PJ, Ashwal S, Baranek GT, Cook Jr EH, Dawson G, et al. Practice parameter: screening and diagnosis of autism: report of the Quality Standards Subcommittee of the American Academy of Neurology and the Child Neurology Society. Neurology. 2000;55(4):468–79.

7. Hill A, Bolte S, Petrova G, Beltcheva D, Tacheva S, Poustka F. Stability and interpersonal agreement of the interview-based diagnosis of autism. Psychopathology. 2001;34(4):187–91.
8. Lord C, Risi S, Lambrecht L, Cook Jr EH, Leventhal BL, DiLavore PC, et al. The autism diagnostic observation schedule-generic: a standard measure of social and communication deficits associated with the spectrum of autism. J Autism Dev Disord. 2000;30(3):205–23.
9. Bookheimer SY, Wang AT, Scott A, Sigman M, Dapretto M. Frontal contributions to face processing differences in autism: evidence from fMRI of inverted face processing. J Int Neuropsychol Soc. 2008;14(6):922–32.
10. Premack D, Woodruff G. Does the chimpanzee have a theory of mind? Behav Brain Sci. 1978;1:515–26.
11. Verhoeven JS, De Cock P, Lagae L, Sunaert S. Neuroimaging of autism. Neuroradiology. 2010; 52(1):3–14.
12. Abell F, Krams M, Ashburner J, Passingham R, Friston K, Frackowiak R, et al. The neuroanatomy of autism: a voxel-based whole brain analysis of structural scans. Neuroreport. 1999;10(8):1647–51.
13. Aylward EH, Minshew NJ, Goldstein G, Honeycutt NA, Augustine AM, Yates KO, et al. MRI volumes of amygdala and hippocampus in non-mentally retarded autistic adolescents and adults. Neurology. 1999;53(9):2145–50.
14. Howard MA, Cowell PE, Boucher J, Broks P, Mayes A, Farrant A, et al. Convergent neuroanatomical and behavioural evidence of an amygdala hypothesis of autism. Neuroreport. 2000;11(13):2931–5.
15. Sparks BF, Friedman SD, Shaw DW, Aylward EH, Echelard D, Artru AA, et al. Brain structural abnormalities in young children with autism spectrum disorder. Neurology. 2002;59(2):184–92.
16. Baron-Cohen S, Ring HA, Wheelwright S, Bullmore ET, Brammer MJ, Simmons A, et al. Social intelligence in the normal and autistic brain: an fMRI study. Eur J Neurosci. 1999;11(6):1891–8.
17. Critchley HD, Daly EM, Bullmore ET, Williams SC, Van Amelsvoort T, Robertson DM, et al. The functional neuroanatomy of social behaviour: changes in cerebral blood flow when people with autistic disorder process facial expressions. Brain. 2000;123(Pt 11):2203–12.
18. Grezes J, Wicker B, Berthoz S, de Gelder B. A failure to grasp the affective meaning of actions in autism spectrum disorder subjects. Neuropsychologia. 2009;47(8–9):1816–25.
19. Hadjikhani N, Joseph RM, Manoach DS, Naik P, Snyder J, Dominick K, et al. Body expressions of emotion do not trigger fear contagion in autism spectrum disorder. Soc Cogn Affect Neurosci. 2009; 4(1):70–8.
20. Pierce K, Muller RA, Ambrose J, Allen G, Courchesne E. Face processing occurs outside the fusiform 'face area' in autism: evidence from functional MRI. Brain. 2001;124(Pt 10):2059–73.
21. Silani G, Bird G, Brindley R, Singer T, Frith C, Frith U. Levels of emotional awareness and autism: an fMRI study. Soc Neurosci. 2008;3(2):97–112.
22. Uddin LQ, Davies MS, Scott AA, Zaidel E, Bookheimer SY, Iacoboni M, et al. Neural basis of self and other representation in autism: an FMRI study of self-face recognition. PLoS ONE. 2008; 3(10):e3526.
23. Just MA, Cherkassky VL, Keller TA, Minshew NJ. Cortical activation and synchronization during sentence comprehension in high-functioning autism: evidence of underconnectivity. Brain. 2004;127(Pt 8):1811–21.
24. Gaffrey MS, Kleinhans NM, Haist F, Akshoomoff N, Campbell A, Courchesne E, et al. Atypical [corrected] participation of visual cortex during word processing in autism: an fMRI study of semantic decision. Neuropsychologia. 2007;45(8):1672–84.
25. Groen WB, Tesink C, Petersson KM, van Berkum J, van der Gaag RJ, Hagoort P, et al. Semantic, factual, and social language comprehension in adolescents with autism: an FMRI study. Cereb Cortex. 2010;20(8):1937–45.
26. Harris GJ, Chabris CF, Clark J, Urban T, Aharon I, Steele S, et al. Brain activation during semantic processing in autism spectrum disorders via functional magnetic resonance imaging. Brain Cogn. 2006; 61(1):54–68.
27. Kana RK, Keller TA, Cherkassky VL, Minshew NJ, Just MA. Sentence comprehension in autism: thinking in pictures with decreased functional connectivity. Brain. 2006;129(Pt 9):2484–93.
28. Just MA, Cherkassky VL, Keller TA, Kana RK, Minshew NJ. Functional and anatomical cortical underconnectivity in autism: evidence from an FMRI study of an executive function task and corpus callosum morphometry. Cereb Cortex. 2007;17(4): 951–61.
29. Koshino H, Carpenter PA, Minshew NJ, Cherkassky VL, Keller TA, Just MA. Functional connectivity in an fMRI working memory task in high-functioning autism. Neuroimage. 2005;24(3):810–21.
30. Muller JL, Roder CH, Schuierer G, Klein H. Motor-induced brain activation in cortical, subcortical and cerebellar regions in schizophrenic inpatients. A whole brain fMRI fingertapping study. Prog Neuropsychopharmacol Biol Psychiatry. 2002;26(3): 421–6.
31. Schmitz N, Rubia K, Daly E, Smith A, Williams S, Murphy DG. Neural correlates of executive function in autistic spectrum disorders. Biol Psychiatry. 2006;59(1):7–16.
32. Shafritz KM, Dichter GS, Baranek GT, Belger A. The neural circuitry mediating shifts in behavioral response and cognitive set in autism. Biol Psychiatry. 2008;63(10):974–80.
33. Solomon M, Ozonoff SJ, Ursu S, Ravizza S, Cummings N, Ly S, et al. The neural substrates of cognitive control deficits in autism spectrum disorders. Neuropsychologia. 2009;47(12):2515–26.

34. Office of Applied Studies. Results from the 2008 National Survey on Drug Use and Health: National Findings. MD: Rockville; 2009.
35. www.ncjrs.gov/ondcppubs/publications/policy/ndcs00/chap2_10.html, last accessed Oct. 1, 2010
36. Pillay SS, Rogowska J, Kanayama G, Jon DI, Gruber S, Simpson N, et al. Neurophysiology of motor function following cannabis discontinuation in chronic cannabis smokers: an fMRI study. Drug Alcohol Depend. 2004;76(3):261–71.
37. Yurgelun-Todd DA, Gruber SA, Hanson RA et al. (1998). Residual effects of marijuana use: an fMRI study. Paper presented at the College on Problems of Drug Dependence, Sixtieth Annual Scientific Meeting.
38. Kanayama G, Rogowska J, Pope HG, Gruber SA, Yurgelun-Todd DA. Spatial working memory in heavy cannabis users: a functional magnetic resonance imaging study. Psychopharmacol (Berl). 2004;176(3–4):239–47.
39. Chang L, Yakupov R, Cloak C, Ernst T. Marijuana use is associated with a reorganized visual-attention network and cerebellar hypoactivation. Brain. 2006;129(Pt 5):1096–112.
40. Gruber SA, Yurgelun-Todd DA. Neuroimaging of marijuana smokers during inhibitory processing: a pilot investigation. Brain Res Cogn Brain Res. 2005;23(1):107–18.
41. Jager G, Kahn RS, Van Den Brink W, Van Ree JM, Ramsey NF. Long-term effects of frequent cannabis use on working memory and attention: an fMRI study. Psychopharmacol (Berl). 2006;185(3):358–68.
42. Bechara A. Decision making, impulse control and loss of willpower to resist drugs: a neurocognitive perspective. Nat Neurosci. 2005;8(11):1458–63.
43. Hartz DT, Frederick-Osborne SL, Galloway GP. Craving predicts use during treatment for methamphetamine dependence: a prospective, repeated-measures, within-subject analysis. Drug Alcohol Depend. 2001;63(3):269–76.
44. Nakama H, Chang L, Cloak C, Jiang C, Alicata D, Haning W. Association between psychiatric symptoms and craving in methamphetamine users. Am J Addict. 2008;17(5):441–6.
45. Schonfeld L, Rohrer GE, Dupree LW, Thomas M. Antecedents of relapse and recent substance use. Community Ment Health J. 1989;25(3):245–9.
46. Paulus MP, Hozack N, Frank L, Brown GG, Schuckit MA. Decision making by methamphetamine-dependent subjects is associated with error-rate-independent decrease in prefrontal and parietal activation. Biol Psychiatry. 2003;53(1):65–74.
47. Paulus MP, Hozack NE, Zauscher BE, Frank L, Brown GG, Braff DL, et al. Behavioral and functional neuroimaging evidence for prefrontal dysfunction in methamphetamine-dependent subjects. Neuropsychopharmacology. 2002;26(1):53–63.
48. Salo R, Ursu S, Buonocore MH, Leamon MH, Carter C. Impaired prefrontal cortical function and disrupted adaptive cognitive control in methamphetamine abusers: a functional magnetic resonance imaging study. Biol Psychiatry. 2009; 65(8):706–9.
49. Hoffman WF, Moore M, Templin R, McFarland B, Hitzemann RJ, Mitchell SH. Neuropsychological function and delay discounting in methamphetamine-dependent individuals. Psychopharmacol (Berl). 2006;188(2):162–70.
50. Hoffman WF, Schwartz DL, Huckans MS, McFarland BH, Meiri G, Stevens AA, et al. Cortical activation during delay discounting in abstinent methamphetamine dependent individuals. Psychopharmacol (Berl). 2008;201(2):183–93.
51. Monterosso JR, Ainslie G, Xu J, Cordova X, Domier CP, London ED. Frontoparietal cortical activity of methamphetamine-dependent and comparison subjects performing a delay discounting task. Hum Brain Mapp. 2007;28(5):383–93.
52. Payer DE, Lieberman MD, Monterosso JR, Xu J, Fong TW, London ED. Differences in cortical activity between methamphetamine-dependent and healthy individuals performing a facial affect matching task. Drug Alcohol Depend. 2008;93(1–2):93–102.
53. Kim YT, Lee JJ, Song HJ, Kim JH, Kwon DH, Kim MN, et al. Alterations in cortical activity of male methamphetamine abusers performing an empathy task: fMRI study. Hum Psychopharmacol. 2010; 25(1):63–70.
54. Paulus MP, Tapert SF, Schuckit MA. Neural activation patterns of methamphetamine-dependent subjects during decision making predict relapse. Arch Gen Psychiatry. 2005;62(7):761–8.
55. World Health Organization, www.who.int, last accessed October 1, 2010.
56. Breiter HC, Gollub RL, Weisskoff RM, Kennedy DN, Makris N, Berke JD, et al. Acute effects of cocaine on human brain activity and emotion. Neuron. 1997;19(3):591–611.
57. Hanlon CA, Wesley MJ, Roth AJ, Miller MD, Porrino LJ. Loss of laterality in chronic cocaine users: An fMRI investigation of sensorimotor control. Psychiatry Res. 2010;181(1):15–23.
58. Kufahl P, Li Z, Risinger R, Rainey C, Piacentine L, Wu G, et al. Expectation modulates human brain responses to acute cocaine: a functional magnetic resonance imaging study. Biol Psychiatry. 2008; 63(2):222–30.
59. Wexler BE, Gottschalk CH, Fulbright RK, Prohovnik I, Lacadie CM, Rounsaville BJ, et al. Functional magnetic resonance imaging of cocaine craving. Am J Psychiatry. 2001;158(1):86–95.
60. Goldstein RZ, Tomasi D, Alia-Klein N, Cottone LA, Zhang L, Telang F, et al. Subjective sensitivity to monetary gradients is associated with frontolimbic activation to reward in cocaine abusers. Drug Alcohol Depend. 2007;87(2–3):233–40.
61. Kosten TR, Scanley BE, Tucker KA, Oliveto A, Prince C, Sinha R, et al. Cue-induced brain activity changes and relapse in cocaine-dependent patients. Neuropsychopharmacology. 2006;31(3):644–50.

62. Kufahl PR, Li Z, Risinger RC, Rainey CJ, Wu G, Bloom AS, et al. Neural responses to acute cocaine administration in the human brain detected by fMRI. Neuroimage. 2005;28(4):904–14.
63. Goldstein RZ, Tomasi D, Alia-Klein N, Honorio Carrillo J, Maloney T, Woicik PA, et al. Dopaminergic response to drug words in cocaine addiction. J Neurosci. 2009;29(18):6001–6.
64. Myrick H, Anton RF, Li X, Henderson S, Drobes D, Voronin K, et al. Differential brain activity in alcoholics and social drinkers to alcohol cues: relationship to craving. Neuropsychopharmacology. 2004; 29(2):393–402.
65. Yoon HW, Chung JY, Oh JH, Min HK, Kim DJ, Cheon Y, et al. Differential activation of face memory encoding tasks in alcohol-dependent patients compared to healthy subjects: an fMRI study. Neurosci Lett. 2009;450(3):311–6.
66. Bragulat V, Dzemidzic M, Talavage T, Davidson D, O'Connor SJ, Kareken DA. Alcohol sensitizes cerebral responses to the odors of alcoholic drinks: an fMRI study. Alcohol Clin Exp Res. 2008;32(7): 1124–34.
67. Park MS, Sohn JH, Suk JA, Kim SH, Sohn S, Sparacio R. Brain substrates of craving to alcohol cues in subjects with alcohol use disorder. Alcohol Alcohol. 2007;42(5):417–22.
68. Gilman JM, Ramchandani VA, Davis MB, Bjork JM, Hommer DW. Why we like to drink: a functional magnetic resonance imaging study of the rewarding and anxiolytic effects of alcohol. J Neurosci. 2008;28(18):4583–91.
69. Heinz A, Wrase J, Kahnt T, Beck A, Bromand Z, Grusser SM, et al. Brain activation elicited by affectively positive stimuli is associated with a lower risk of relapse in detoxified alcoholic subjects. Alcohol Clin Exp Res. 2007;31(7):1138–47.
70. Yan P, Li CS. Decreased Amygdala activation during risk taking in non-dependent habitual alcohol users: a preliminary fMRI study of the stop signal task. Am J Drug Alcohol Abuse. 2009;35(5):284–9.
71. Beck A, Schlagenhauf F, Wustenberg T, Hein J, Kienast T, Kahnt T, et al. Ventral striatal activation during reward anticipation correlates with impulsivity in alcoholics. Biol Psychiatry. 2009;66(8): 734–42.
72. Wrase J, Schlagenhauf F, Kienast T, Wustenberg T, Bermpohl F, Kahnt T, et al. Dysfunction of reward processing correlates with alcohol craving in detoxified alcoholics. Neuroimage. 2007;35(2):787–94.
73. Gundersen H, Gruner R, Specht K, Hugdahl K. The effects of alcohol intoxication on neuronal activation at different levels of cognitive load. Open Neuroimag J. 2008;2:65–72.
74. Soderlund H, Grady CL, Easdon C, Tulving E. Acute effects of alcohol on neural correlates of episodic memory encoding. Neuroimage. 2007;35(2): 928–39.
75. Renshaw PF, Yurgelun-Todd DA, Cohen BM. Greater hemodynamic response to photic stimulation in schizophrenic patients: an echo planar MRI study. Am J Psychiatry. 1994;151(10):1493–5.
76. Chen Y, Grossman ED, Bidwell LC, Yurgelun-Todd D, Gruber SA, Levy DL, et al. Differential activation patterns of occipital and prefrontal cortices during motion processing: evidence from normal and schizophrenic brains. Cogn Affect Behav Neurosci. 2008;8(3):293–303.
77. Keedy SK, Rosen C, Khine T, Rajarethinam R, Janicak PG, Sweeney JA. An fMRI study of visual attention and sensorimotor function before and after antipsychotic treatment in first-episode schizophrenia. Psychiatry Res. 2009;172(1):16–23.
78. Hazlett EA, Buchsbaum MS, Zhang J, Newmark RE, Glanton CF, Zelmanova Y, et al. Frontal-striatal-thalamic mediodorsal nucleus dysfunction in schizophrenia-spectrum patients during sensorimotor gating. Neuroimage. 2008;42(3):1164–77.
79. Kim DI, Mathalon DH, Ford JM, Mannell M, Turner JA, Brown GG, et al. Auditory oddball deficits in schizophrenia: an independent component analysis of the fMRI multisite function BIRN study. Schizophr Bull. 2009;35(1):67–81.
80. Morey RA, Mitchell TV, Inan S, Lieberman JA, Belger A. Neural correlates of automatic and controlled auditory processing in schizophrenia. J Neuropsychiatry Clin Neurosci. 2008;20(4): 419–30.
81. Schroder J, Wenz F, Schad LR, Baudendistel K, Knopp MV. Sensorimotor cortex and supplementary motor area changes in schizophrenia. A study with functional magnetic resonance imaging. Br J Psychiatry. 1995;167(2):197–201.
82. Yurgelun-Todd DA, Waternaux CM, Cohen BM, Gruber SA, English CD, Renshaw PF. Functional magnetic resonance imaging of schizophrenic patients and comparison subjects during word production. Am J Psychiatry. 1996;153(2):200–5.
83. Kaladjian A, Jeanningros R, Azorin JM, Grimault S, Anton JL, Mazzola-Pomietto P. Blunted activation in right ventrolateral prefrontal cortex during motor response inhibition in schizophrenia. Schizophr Res. 2007;97(1–3):184–93.
84. Snitz BE, MacDonald 3rd A, Cohen JD, Cho RY, Becker T, Carter CS. Lateral and medial hypofrontality in first-episode schizophrenia: functional activity in a medication-naive state and effects of short-term atypical antipsychotic treatment. Am J Psychiatry. 2005;162(12):2322–9.
85. Vink M, Ramsey NF, Raemaekers M, Kahn RS. Striatal dysfunction in schizophrenia and unaffected relatives. Biol Psychiatry. 2006;60(1):32–9.
86. Elsabagh S, Premkumar P, Anilkumar AP, Kumari V. A longer duration of schizophrenic illness has sex-specific associations within the working memory neural network in schizophrenia. Behav Brain Res. 2009;201(1):41–7.
87. Hamilton LS, Altshuler LL, Townsend J, Bookheimer SY, Phillips OR, Fischer J, et al. Alterations in functional activation in euthymicbipolar disorder and

schizophrenia during a working memory task. Hum Brain Mapp. 2009;30(12):3958–69.

88. Karlsgodt KH, Sanz J, van Erp TG, Bearden CE, Nuechterlein KH, Cannon TD. Re-evaluating dorsolateral prefrontal cortex activation during working memory in schizophrenia. Schizophr Res. 2009; 108(1–3):143–50.
89. Manoach DS, Press DZ, Thangaraj V, Searl MM, Goff DC, Halpern E, et al. Schizophrenic subjects activate dorsolateral prefrontal cortex during a working memory task, as measured by fMRI. Biol Psychiatry. 1999;45(9):1128–37.
90. Meda SA, Stevens MC, Folley BS, Calhoun VD, Pearlson GD. Evidence for anomalous network connectivity during working memory encoding in schizophrenia: an ICA based analysis. PLoS ONE. 2009;4(11):e7911.
91. Karch S, Leicht G, Giegling I, Lutz J, Kunz J, Buselmeier M, et al. Inefficient neural activity in patients with schizophrenia and nonpsychotic relatives of schizophrenic patients: evidence from a working memory task. J Psychiatr Res. 2009; 43(15):1185–94.
92. Gur RE, Turetsky BI, Loughead J, Snyder W, Kohler C, Elliott M, et al. Visual attention circuitry in schizophrenia investigated with oddball event-related functional magnetic resonance imaging. Am J Psychiatry. 2007;164(3):442–9.
93. Reske M, Kellermann T, Habel U, Jon Shah N, Backes V, von Wilmsdorff M, et al. Stability of emotional dysfunctions? A long-term fMRI study in first-episode schizophrenia. J Psychiatr Res. 2007; 41(11):918–27.
94. Jardri R, Pins D, Bubrovszky M, Lucas B, Lethuc V, Delmaire C, et al. Neural functional organization of hallucinations in schizophrenia: multisensory dissolution of pathological emergence in consciousness. Conscious Cogn. 2009;18(2):449–57.
95. Raij TT, Valkonen-Korhonen M, Holi M, Therman S, Lehtonen J, Hari R. Reality of auditory verbal hallucinations. Brain. 2009;132(Pt 11):2994–3001.
96. Sommer IE, Diederen KM, Blom JD, Willems A, Kushan L, Slotema K, et al. Auditory verbal hallucinations predominantly activate the right inferior frontal area. Brain. 2008;131(Pt 12):3169–77.
97. van de Ven VG, Formisano E, Roder CH, Prvulovic D, Bittner RA, Dietz MG, et al. The spatiotemporal pattern of auditory cortical responses during verbal hallucinations. Neuroimage. 2005;27(3):644–55.
98. Wible CG, Lee K, Molina I, Hashimoto R, Preus AP, Roach BJ, et al. fMRI activity correlated with auditory hallucinations during performance of a working memory task: data from the FBIRN consortium study. Schizophr Bull. 2009;35(1):47–57.
99. Zhang Z, Shi J, Yuan Y, Hao G, Yao Z, Chen N. Relationship of auditory verbal hallucinations with cerebral asymmetry in patients with schizophrenia: an event-related fMRI study. J Psychiatr Res. 2008;42(6):477–86.
100. Ongur D, Price JL. The organization of networks within the orbital and medial prefrontal cortex of rats, monkeys and humans. Cereb Cortex. 2000; 10(3):206–19.
101. Anand A, Li Y, Wang Y, Wu J, Gao S, Bukhari L, et al. Activity and connectivity of brain mood regulating circuit in depression: a functional magnetic resonance study. Biol Psychiatry. 2005;57(10): 1079–88.
102. Beauregard M, Leroux JM, Bergman S, Arzoumanian Y, Beaudoin G, Bourgouin P, et al. The functional neuroanatomy of major depression: an fMRI study using an emotional activation paradigm. Neuroreport. 1998;9(14):3253–8.
103. Dichter GS, Felder JN, Smoski MJ. Affective context interferes with cognitive control in unipolar depression: an fMRI investigation. J Affect Disord. 2009;114(1–3):131–42.
104. Fales CL, Barch DM, Rundle MM, Mintun MA, Snyder AZ, Cohen JD, et al. Altered emotional interference processing in affective and cognitive-control brain circuitry in major depression. Biol Psychiatry. 2008;63(4):377–84.
105. Frodl T, Scheuerecker J, Albrecht J, Kleemann AM, Muller-Schunk S, Koutsouleris N, et al. Neuronal correlates of emotional processing in patients with major depression. World J Biol Psychiatry. 2009; 10(3):202–8.
106. Johnstone T, van Reekum CM, Urry HL, Kalin NH, Davidson RJ. Failure to regulate: counterproductive recruitment of top-down prefrontal-subcortical circuitry in major depression. J Neurosci. 2007; 27(33):8877–84.
107. Mayberg HS, Liotti M, Brannan SK, McGinnis S, Mahurin RK, Jerabek PA, et al. Reciprocal limbic-cortical function and negative mood: converging PET findings in depression and normal sadness. Am J Psychiatry. 1999;156(5):675–82.
108. Peluso MA, Glahn DC, Matsuo K, Monkul ES, Najt P, Zamarripa F, et al. Amygdala hyperactivation in untreated depressed individuals. Psychiatry Res. 2009;173(2):158–61.
109. Siegle GJ, Thompson W, Carter CS, Steinhauer SR, Thase ME. Increased amygdala and decreased dorsolateral prefrontal BOLD responses in unipolar depression: related and independent features. Biol Psychiatry. 2007;61(2):198–209.
110. Surguladze S, Brammer MJ, Keedwell P, Giampietro V, Young AW, Travis MJ, et al. A differential pattern of neural response toward sad versus happy facial expressions in major depressive disorder. Biol Psychiatry. 2005;57(3):201–9.
111. Chen CH, Suckling J, Ooi C, Fu CH, Williams SC, Walsh ND, et al. Functional coupling of the amygdala in depressed patients treated with antidepressant medication. Neuropsychopharmacology. 2008; 33(8):1909–18.
112. Chen CH, Ridler K, Suckling J, Williams S, Fu CH, Merlo-Pich E, et al. Brain imaging correlates of

depressive symptom severity and predictors of symptom improvement after antidepressant treatment. Biol Psychiatry. 2007;62(5):407–14.
113. Davidson RJ, Irwin W, Anderle MJ, Kalin NH. The neural substrates of affective processing in depressed patients treated with venlafaxine. Am J Psychiatry. 2003;160(1):64–75.
114. Fu CH, Williams SC, Cleare AJ, Brammer MJ, Walsh ND, Kim J, et al. Attenuation of the neural response to sad faces in major depression by antidepressant treatment: a prospective, event-related functional magnetic resonance imaging study. Arch Gen Psychiatry. 2004;61(9):877–89.
115. Sheline YI, Barch DM, Donnelly JM, Ollinger JM, Snyder AZ, Mintun MA. Increased amygdala response to masked emotional faces in depressed subjects resolves with antidepressant treatment: an fMRI study. Biol Psychiatry. 2001;50(9):651–8.
116. Anand A, Li Y, Wang Y, Gardner K, Lowe MJ. Reciprocal effects of antidepressant treatment on activity and connectivity of the mood regulating circuit: an FMRI study. J Neuropsychiatry Clin Neurosci. 2007;19(3):274–82.
117. Videbech P, Petersen TH. Depression, stress and brain function. Ugeskr Laeger. 2001;163(47): 6568–72.
118. Kennedy SH, Evans KR, Kruger S, Mayberg HS, Meyer JH, McCann S, et al. Changes in regional brain glucose metabolism measured with positron emission tomography after paroxetine treatment of major depression. Am J Psychiatry. 2001;158(6): 899–905.
119. Drevets WC. Neuroimaging and neuropathological studies of depression: implications for the cognitive-emotional features of mood disorders. Curr Opin Neurobiol. 2001;11(2):240–9.
120. Fitzgerald PB, Srithiran A, Benitez J, Daskalakis ZZ, Oxley TJ, Kulkarni J, et al. An fMRI study of prefrontal brain activation during multiple tasks in patients with major depressive disorder. Hum Brain Mapp. 2008;29(4):490–501.
121. Harvey PO, Fossati P, Pochon JB, Levy R, Lebastard G, Lehericy S, et al. Cognitive control and brain resources in major depression: an fMRI study using the n-back task. Neuroimage. 2005;26(3):860–9.
122. Matsuo K, Glahn DC, Peluso MAM, Hatch JP, Monkul ES, Najt P, et al. Prefrontal hyperactivation during working memory task in untreated individuals with major depressive disorder. Mol Psychiatry. 2007;12(2):158–66.
123. Rose EJ, Simonotto E, Ebmeier KP. Limbic overactivity in depression during preserved performance on the n-back task. Neuroimage. 2006;29(1): 203–15.
124. Schoning S, Zwitserlood P, Engelien A, Behnken A, Kugel H, Schiffbauer H, et al. Working-memory fMRI reveals cingulate hyperactivation in euthymic major depression. Hum Brain Mapp. 2009;30(9): 2746–56.
125. Matthews S, Simmons A, Strigo I, Gianaros P, Yang T, Paulus M. Inhibition-related activity in subgenual cingulate is associated with symptom severity in major depression. Psychiatry Res. 2009; 172(1):1–6.
126. Wagner G, Sinsel E, Sobanski T, Kohler S, Marinou V, Mentzel HJ, et al. Cortical inefficiency in patients with unipolar depression: an event-related FMRI study with the Stroop task. Biol Psychiatry. 2006; 59(10):958–65.
127. Smoski MJ, Felder J, Bizzell J, Green SR, Ernst M, Lynch TR, et al. fMRI of alterations in reward selection, anticipation, and feedback in major depressive disorder. J Affect Disord. 2009;118(1–3):69–78.
128. Coffman JA, Bornstein RA, Olson SC, Schwarzkopf SB, Nasrallah HA. Cognitive impairment and cerebral structure by MRI in bipolar disorder. Biol Psychiatry. 1990;27(11):1188–96.
129. Joseph R. Frontal lobe psychopathology: mania, depression, confabulation, catatonia, perseveration, obsessive compulsions, and schizophrenia. Psychiatry. 1999;62(2):138–72.
130. Murphy FC, Sahakian BJ. Neuropsychology of bipolar disorder. Br J Psychiatry Suppl. 2001;41:s120–7.
131. Murphy FC, Sahakian BJ. Neuropsychology of bipolar disorder. Br J Psychiatry. 2001;178 Suppl 41: S120–7.
132. Phillips ML, Drevets WC, Rauch SL, Lane R. Neurobiology of emotion perception I: the neural basis of normal emotion perception. Biol Psychiatry. 2003;54(5):504–14.
133. Phillips ML, Ladouceur CD, Drevets WC. A neural model of voluntary and automatic emotion regulation: implications for understanding the pathophysiology and neurodevelopment of bipolar disorder. Mol Psychiatry. 2008;13(9):829, 833–57.
134. Blumberg HP, Donegan NH, Sanislow CA, Collins S, Lacadie C, Skudlarski P, et al. Preliminary evidence for medication effects on functional abnormalities in the amygdala and anterior cingulate in bipolar disorder. Psychopharmacol (Berl). 2005;183(3):308–13.
135. Hassel S, Almeida JR, Frank E, Versace A, Nau SA, Klein CR, et al. Prefrontal cortical and striatal activity to happy and fear faces in bipolar disorder is associated with comorbid substance abuse and eating disorder. J Affect Disord. 2009;118(1–3):19–27.
136. Hassel S, Almeida JR, Kerr N, Nau S, Ladouceur CD, Fissell K, et al. Elevated striatal and decreased dorsolateral prefrontal cortical activity in response to emotional stimuli in euthymic bipolar disorder: no associations with psychotropic medication load. Bipolar Disord. 2008;10(8):916–27.
137. Lawrence NS, Williams AM, Surguladze S, Giampietro V, Brammer MJ, Andrew C, et al. Subcortical and ventral prefrontal cortical neural responses to facial expressions distinguish patients with bipolar disorder and major depression. Biol Psychiatry. 2004;55(6):578–87.

138. Robinson JL, Monkul ES, Tordesillas-Gutierrez D, Franklin C, Bearden CE, Fox PT, et al. Fronto-limbic circuitry in euthymic bipolar disorder: evidence for prefrontal hyperactivation. Psychiatry Res. 2008; 164(2):106–13.
139. Yurgelun-Todd DA, Gruber SA, Kanayama G, Killgore WD, Baird AA, Young AD. fMRI during affect discrimination in bipolar affective disorder. Bipolar Disord. 2000;2(3 Pt 2):237–48.
140. Malhi GS, Lagopoulos J, Ward PB, Kumari V, Mitchell PB, Parker GB, et al. Cognitive generation of affect in bipolar depression: an fMRI study. Eur J Neurosci. 2004;19(3):741–54.
141. Altshuler L, Bookheimer S, Proenza MA, Townsend J, Sabb F, Firestine A, et al. Increased amygdala activation during mania: a functional magnetic resonance imaging study. Am J Psychiatry. 2005; 162(6):1211–3.
142. Chen CH, Lennox B, Jacob R, Calder A, Lupson V, Bisbrown-Chippendale R, et al. Explicit and implicit facial affect recognition in manic and depressed States of bipolar disorder: a functional magnetic resonance imaging study. Biol Psychiatry. 2006; 59(1):31–9.
143. Elliott R, Ogilvie A, Rubinsztein JS, Calderon G, Dolan RJ, Sahakian BJ. Abnormal ventral frontal response during performance of an affective go/no go task in patients with mania. Biol Psychiatry. 2004;55(12):1163–70.
144. Malhi GS, Lagopoulos J, Sachdev P, Mitchell PB, Ivanovski B, Parker GB. Cognitive generation of affect in hypomania: an fMRI study. Bipolar Disord. 2004;6(4):271–85.
145. Jogia J, Haldane M, Cobb A, Kumari V, Frangou S. Pilot investigation of the changes in cortical activation during facial affect recognition with lamotrigine monotherapy in bipolar disorder. Br J Psychiatry. 2008;192(3):197–201.
146. Foland LC, Altshuler LL, Bookheimer SY, Eisenberger N, Townsend J, Thompson PM. Evidence for deficient modulation of amygdala response by prefrontal cortex in bipolar mania. Psychiatry Res. 2008;162(1):27–37.
147. Wang F, Kalmar JH, He Y, Jackowski M, Chepenik LG, Edmiston EE, et al. Functional and structural connectivity between the perigenual anterior cingulate and amygdala in bipolar disorder. Biol Psychiatry. 2009;66(5):516–21.
148. Malhi GS, Lagopoulos J, Sachdev PS, Ivanovski B, Shnier R. An emotional Stroop functional MRI study of euthymic bipolar disorder. Bipolar Disord. 2005;7 Suppl 5:58–69.
149. Malhi GS, Lagopoulos J, Sachdev PS, Ivanovski B, Shnier R, Ketter T. Is a lack of disgust something to fear? A functional magnetic resonance imaging facial emotion recognition study in euthymic bipolar disorder patients. Bipolar Disord. 2007;9(4): 345–57.
150. Rubinsztein JS, Fletcher PC, Rogers RD, Ho LW, Aigbirhio FI, Paykel ES, et al. Decision-making in mania: a PET study. Brain J Neurol. 2001; 124(12):2550–63.
151. Almeida JR, Mechelli A, Hassel S, Versace A, Kupfer DJ, Phillips ML. Abnormally increased effective connectivity between parahippocampal gyrus and ventromedial prefrontal regions during emotion labeling in bipolar disorder. Psychiatry Res. 2009;174(3):195–201.
152. Kaladjian A, Jeanningros R, Azorin JM, Nazarian B, Roth M, Anton JL, et al. Remission from mania is associated with a decrease in amygdala activation during motor response inhibition. Bipolar Disord. 2009;11(5):530–8.
153. Kaladjian A, Jeanningros R, Azorin JM, Nazarian B, Roth M, Mazzola-Pomietto P. Reduced brain activation in euthymic bipolar patients during response inhibition: an event-related fMRI study. Psychiatry Res. 2009;173(1):45–51.
154. Mazzola-Pomietto P, Kaladjian A, Azorin J-M, Anton J-L, Jeanningros R. Bilateral decrease in ventrolateral prefrontal cortex activation during motor response inhibition in mania. J Psychiatr Res. 2009;43(4):432–41.
155. Wessa M, Houenou J, Paillere-Martinot ML, Berthoz S, Artiges E, Leboyer M, et al. Fronto-striatal overactivation in euthymic bipolar patients during an emotional go/nogo task. Am J Psychiatry. 2007; 164(4):638–46.
156. Gruber SA, Rogowska J, Yurgelun-Todd DA. Decreased activation of the anterior cingulate in bipolar patients: an fMRI study. J Affect Disord. 2004;82(2):191–201.
157. Adler CM, Holland SK, Schmithorst V, Tuchfarber MJ, Strakowski SM. Changes in neuronal activation in patients with bipolar disorder during performance of a working memory task. Bipolar Disord. 2004; 6(6):540–9.
158. Frangou S, Kington J, Raymont V, Shergill SS. Examining ventral and dorsal prefrontal function in bipolar disorder: a functional magnetic resonance imaging study. Eur Psychiatry. 2008;23(4):300–8.
159. Gruber O, Tost H, Henseler I, Schmael C, Scherk H, Ende G, et al. Pathological amygdala activation during working memory performance: Evidence for a pathophysiological trait marker in bipolar affective disorder. Hum Brain Mapp. 2010;31(1):115–25.
160. Lagopoulos J, Ivanovski B, Malhi GS. An event-related functional MRI study of working memory in euthymic bipolar disorder. J Psychiatry Neurosci. 2007;32(3):174–84.
161. Monks PJ, Thompson JM, Bullmore ET, Suckling J, Brammer MJ, Williams SC, et al. A functional MRI study of working memory task in euthymic bipolar disorder: evidence for task-specific dysfunction. Bipolar Disord. 2004;6(6):550–64.
162. Strakowski SM, Adler CM, Holland SK, Mills N, DelBello MP. A preliminary FMRI study of sustained attention in euthymic, unmedicated bipolar disorder. Neuropsychopharmacology. 2004;29(9): 1734–40.

163. Haldane M, Jogia J, Cobb A, Kozuch E, Kumari V, Frangou S. Changes in brain activation during working memory and facial recognition tasks in patients with bipolar disorder with Lamotrigine monotherapy. Eur Neuropsychopharmacol. 2008;18(1):48–54.
164. Thermenos HW, Goldstein JM, Milanovic SM, Whitfield-Gabrieli S, Makris N, Laviolette P, et al. An fMRI study of working memory in persons with bipolar disorder or at genetic risk for bipolar disorder. Am J Med Genet B Neuropsychiatr Genet. 2010;153B(1):120–31.
165. Deckersbach T, Rauch SL, Buhlmann U, Ostacher MJ, Beucke JC, Nierenberg AA, et al. An fMRI investigation of working memory and sadness in females with bipolar disorder: a brief report. Bipolar Disord. 2008;10(8):928–42.
166. Caligiuri MP, Brown GG, Meloy MJ, Eberson SC, Kindermann SS, Frank LR, et al. An fMRI study of affective state and medication on cortical and subcortical brain regions during motor performance in bipolar disorder. Psychiatry Res. 2003;123(3):171–82.
167. Caligiuri MP, Brown GG, Meloy MJ, Eyler LT, Kindermann SS, Eberson S, et al. A functional magnetic resonance imaging study of cortical asymmetry in bipolar disorder. Bipolar Disord. 2004;6(3):183–96.
168. Cummings JL. Frontal-subcortical circuits and human behavior. Arch Neurol. 1993;50(8):873–80.
169. Woon FL, Hedges DW. Hippocampal and amygdala volumes in children and adults with childhood maltreatment-related posttraumatic stress disorder: a meta-analysis. Hippocampus. 2008;18(8):729–36.
170. Driessen M, Beblo T, Mertens M, Piefke M, Rullkoetter N, Silva-Saavedra A, et al. Posttraumatic stress disorder and fMRI activation patterns of traumatic memory in patients with borderline personality disorder. Biol Psychiatry. 2004;55(6):603–11.
171. Protopopescu X, Pan H, Tuescher O, Cloitre M, Goldstein M, Engelien W, et al. Differential time courses and specificity of amygdala activity in posttraumatic stress disorder subjects and normal control subjects. Biol Psychiatry. 2005;57(5):464–73.
172. Rauch SL, Whalen PJ, Shin LM, McInerney SC, Macklin ML, Lasko NB, et al. Exaggerated amygdala response to masked facial stimuli in posttraumatic stress disorder: a functional MRI study. Biol Psychiatry. 2000;47(9):769–76.
173. Shin LM, Wright CI, Cannistraro PA, Wedig MM, McMullin K, Martis B, et al. A functional magnetic resonance imaging study of amygdala and medial prefrontal cortex responses to overtly presented fearful faces in posttraumatic stress disorder. Arch Gen Psychiatry. 2005;62(3):273–81.
174. Shin LM, Whalen PJ, Pitman RK, Bush G, Macklin ML, Lasko NB, et al. An fMRI study of anterior cingulate function in posttraumatic stress disorder. Biol Psychiatry. 2001;50(12):932–42.
175. Thomaes K, Dorrepaal E, Draijer NP, de Ruiter MB, Elzinga BM, van Balkom AJ, et al. Increased activation of the left hippocampus region in Complex PTSD during encoding and recognition of emotional words: a pilot study. Psychiatry Res. 2009;171(1):44–53.
176. Werner NS, Meindl T, Engel RR, Rosner R, Riedel M, Reiser M, et al. Hippocampal function during associative learning in patients with posttraumatic stress disorder. J Psychiatr Res. 2009;43(3):309–18.
177. Shin LM, Rauch SL, Pitman RK. Amygdala, medial prefrontal cortex, and hippocampal function in PTSD. Ann N Y Acad Sci. 2006;1071:67–79.
178. Lanius RA, Williamson PC, Densmore M, Boksman K, Neufeld RW, Gati JS, et al. The nature of traumatic memories: a 4-T FMRI functional connectivity analysis. Am J Psychiatry. 2004;161(1): 36–44.
179. Koenigs M, Grafman J. Posttraumatic stress disorder: the role of medial prefrontal cortex and amygdala. Neuroscientist. 2009;15(5):540–8.
180. Rauch SL, Shin LM, Phelps EA. Neurocircuitry models of posttraumatic stress disorder and extinction: human neuroimaging research–past, present, and future. Biol Psychiatry. 2006;60(4):376–82.
181. Adler CM, McDonough-Ryan P, Sax KW, Holland SK, Arndt S, Strakowski SM. fMRI of neuronal activation with symptom provocation in unmedicated patients with obsessive compulsive disorder. J Psychiatr Res. 2000;34(4–5):317–24.
182. Breiter HC, Rauch SL, Kwong KK, Baker JR, Weisskoff RM, Kennedy DN, et al. Functional magnetic resonance imaging of symptom provocation in obsessive-compulsive disorder. Arch Gen Psychiatry. 1996;53(7):595–606.
183. Rotge JY, Guehl D, Dilharreguy B, Cuny E, Tignol J, Bioulac B, et al. Provocation of obsessive-compulsive symptoms: a quantitative voxel-based meta-analysis of functional neuroimaging studies. J Psychiatry Neurosci. 2008;33(5):405–12.
184. An SK, Mataix-Cols D, Lawrence NS, Wooderson S, Giampietro V, Speckens A, et al. To discard or not to discard: the neural basis of hoarding symptoms in obsessive-compulsive disorder. Mol Psychiatry. 2009;14(3):318–31.
185. Schienle A, Schafer A, Stark R, Walter B, Vaitl D. Neural responses of OCD patients towards disorder-relevant, generally disgust-inducing and fear-inducing pictures. Int J Psychophysiol. 2005;57(1):69–77.
186. Nakao T, Nakagawa A, Nakatani E, Nabeyama M, Sanematsu H, Yoshiura T, et al. Working memory dysfunction in obsessive-compulsive disorder: a neuropsychological and functional MRI study. J Psychiatr Res. 2009;43(8):784–91.
187. Phillips ML, Marks IM, Senior C, Lythgoe D, O'Dwyer AM, Meehan O, et al. A differential neural response in obsessive-compulsive disorder patients with washing compared with checking symptoms to disgust. Psychol Med. 2000;30(5):1037–50.

188. Henseler I, Gruber O, Kraft S, Krick C, Reith W, Falkai P. Compensatory hyperactivations as markers of latent working memory dysfunctions in patients with obsessive-compulsive disorder: an fMRI study. J Psychiatry Neurosci. 2008;33(3):209–15.
189. Roth RM, Saykin AJ, Flashman LA, Pixley HS, West JD, Mamourian AC. Event-related functional magnetic resonance imaging of response inhibition in obsessive-compulsive disorder. Biol Psychiatry. 2007;62(8):901–9.
190. den Braber A, Ent D, Blokland GA, van Grootheest DS, Cath DC, Veltman DJ, et al. An fMRI study in monozygotic twins discordant for obsessive-compulsive symptoms. Biol Psychol. 2008;79(1):91–102.
191. Nakao T, Nakagawa A, Yoshiura T, Nakatani E, Nabeyama M, Yoshizato C, et al. A functional MRI comparison of patients with obsessive-compulsive disorder and normal controls during a Chinese character Stroop task. Psychiatry Res. 2005;139(2):101–14.
192. Rauch SL, Wedig MM, Wright CI, Martis B, McMullin KG, Shin LM, et al. Functional magnetic resonance imaging study of regional brain activation during implicit sequence learning in obsessive-compulsive disorder. Biol Psychiatry. 2007;61(3):330–6.
193. Remijnse PL, Nielen MM, van Balkom AJ, Hendriks GJ, Hoogendijk WJ, Uylings HB, et al. Differential frontal-striatal and paralimbic activity during reversal learning in major depressive disorder and obsessive-compulsive disorder. Psychol Med. 2009;39(9):1503–18.
194. Ursu S, Carter CS. An initial investigation of the orbitofrontal cortex hyperactivity in obsessive-compulsive disorder: exaggerated representations of anticipated aversive events? Neuropsychologia. 2009;47(10):2145–8.
195. Levine JB, Gruber SA, Baird AA, Yurgelun-Todd D. Obsessive-compulsive disorder among schizophrenic patients: an exploratory study using functional magnetic resonance imaging data. Compr Psychiatry. 1998;39(5):308–11.
196. Fitzgerald KD, Welsh RC, Gehring WJ, Abelson JL, Himle JA, Liberzon I, et al. Error-Related Hyperactivity of the Anterior Cingulate Cortex in Obsessive-Compulsive Disorder. Biol Psychiatry. 2005;57(3):287–94.
197. Heinz A, Siessmeier T, Wrase J, Hermann D, Klein S, Grusser SM, et al. Correlation between dopamine D(2) receptors in the ventral striatum and central processing of alcohol cues and craving. Am J Psychiatry. 2004;161(10):1783–9.
198. Tesink CM, Buitelaar JK, Petersson KM, van der Gaag RJ, Kan CC, Tendolkar I, et al. Neural correlates of pragmatic language comprehension in autism spectrum disorders. Brain. 2009;132(Pt 7):1941–52.
199. Belmonte MK, Yurgelun-Todd DA. Functional anatomy of impaired selective attention and compensatory processing in autism. Brain Res Cogn Brain Res. 2003;17(3):651–64.
200. Li CS, Huang C, Yan P, Bhagwagar Z, Milivojevic V, Sinha R. Neural correlates of impulse control during stop signal inhibition in cocaine-dependent men. Neuropsychopharmacology. 2008;33(8):1798–806.
201. Tomasi D, Goldstein RZ, Telang F, Maloney T, Alia-Klein N, Caparelli EC, et al. Widespread disruption in brain activation patterns to a working memory task during cocaine abstinence. Brain Res. 2007;1171:83–92.
202. Sinha R, Lacadie C, Skudlarski P, Fulbright RK, Rounsaville BJ, Kosten TR, et al. Neural activity associated with stress-induced cocaine craving: a functional magnetic resonance imaging study. Psychopharmacology (Berl). 2005;183(2):171–80.
203. Kubler A, Murphy K, Garavan H. Cocaine dependence and attention switching within and between verbal and visuospatial working memory. Eur J Neurosci. 2005;21(7):1984–92.
204. Szycik GR, Munte TF, Dillo W, Mohammadi B, Samii A, Emrich HM, et al. Audiovisual integration of speech is disturbed in schizophrenia: an fMRI study. Schizophr Res. 2009;110(1–3):111–18.
205. Benetti S, Mechelli A, Picchioni M, Broome M, Williams S, McGuire P. Functional integration between the posterior hippocampus and prefrontal cortex is impaired in both first episode schizophrenia and the at risk mental state. Brain. 2009;132(Pt 9):2426–36.
206. Rametti G, Junque C, Vendrell P, Catalan R, Penades R, Bargallo N, et al. Hippocampal underactivation in an fMRI study of word and face memory recognition in schizophrenia. Eur Arch Psychiatry Clin Neurosci. 2009;259(4):203–11.
207. Weiss AP, Ellis CB, Roffman JL, Stufflebeam S, Hamalainen MS, Duff M, et al. Aberrant frontoparietal function during recognition memory in schizophrenia: a multimodal neuroimaging investigation. J Neurosci. 2009;29(36):11347–59.
208. Benedetti F, Bernasconi A, Bosia M, Cavallaro R, Dallaspezia S, Falini A, et al. Functional and structural brain correlates of theory of mind and empathy deficits in schizophrenia. Schizophr Res. 2009;114(1–3):154–60.
209. Park IH, Park HJ, Chun JW, Kim EY, Kim JJ. Dysfunctional modulation of emotional interference in the medial prefrontal cortex in patients with schizophrenia. Neurosci Lett. 2008;440(2):119–24.
210. Reske M, Habel U, Kellermann T, Backes V, Jon Shah N, von Wilmsdorff M, et al. Differential brain activation during facial emotion discrimination in first-episode schizophrenia. J Psychiatr Res. 2009;43(6):592–9.
211. Whalley HC, McKirdy J, Romaniuk L, Sussmann J, Johnstone EC, Wan HI, et al. Functional imaging of emotional memory in bipolar disorder and schizophrenia. Bipolar Disord. 2009;11(8):840–56.
212. Kang JI, Kim JJ, Seok JH, Chun JW, Lee SK, Park HJ. Abnormal brain response during the auditory

emotional processing in schizophrenic patients with chronic auditory hallucinations. Schizophr Res. 2009;107(1):83–91.
213. Plaze M, Bartres-Faz D, Martinot JL, Januel D, Bellivier F, De Beaurepaire R, et al. Left superior temporal gyrus activation during sentence perception negatively correlates with auditory hallucination severity in schizophrenia patients. Schizophr Res. 2006;87(1–3):109–15.
214. Canli T, Sivers H, Thomason ME, Whitfield-Gabrieli S, Gabrieli JD, Gotlib IH. Brain activation to emotional words in depressed vs healthy subjects. Neuroreport. 2004;15(17):2585–8.
215. Bermpohl F, Dalanay U, Kahnt T, Sajonz B, Heimann H, Ricken R, et al. A preliminary study of increased amygdala activation to positive affective stimuli in mania. Bipolar Disord. 2009;11(1): 70–75.
216. Killgore WD, Gruber SA, Yurgelun-Todd DA. Abnormal corticostriatal activity during fear perception in bipolar disorder. Neuroreport. 2008;19(15): 1523–7.
217. An SK, Mataix-Cols D, Lawrence NS, Wooderson S, Giampietro V, Speckens A, et al. To discard or not to discard: the neural basis of hoarding symptoms in obsessive-compulsive disorder. Mol Psychiatry. 2009;14(3):318–31.
218. Schienle A, Schafer A, Stark R, Walter B, Vaitl D. Neural responses of OCD patients towards disorder-relevant, generally disgust-inducing and fear-inducing pictures. Int J Psychophysiol. 2005;57(1): 69–77.

Applications of fMRI to Neurodegenerative Disease

18

Shamseldeen Y. Mahmoud, Stephen E. Jones, and Michael D. Phillips

Introduction

The age distribution in developed countries is shifting, with more seniors living to age 80 and 90 years, and beyond. This shift has created a challenge for medical professionals caring for geriatric patients, as an aging population means an increased prevalence of age-related neurodegenerative brain diseases with signs and symptoms such as memory impairment, frank dementia, and motor deterioration.

Neurodegenerative diseases progress through stages of synaptic dysfunction, synaptic loss, neuronal degeneration, and neuronal loss [1, 2]. The earlier stages may be asymptomatic and may occur over a period of months or even years. Because the early stages may be more responsive to treatment than the later stages, early diagnosis is essential; however, because the disease is often clinically silent in the earliest stages, clinicians may not diagnose the condition at this stage. There is great interest, therefore, in the development of cutting-edge techniques such as functional magnetic resonance imaging (fMRI), which may allow for earlier diagnosis and thereby permit earlier treatment [3].

Alzheimer's disease (AD) can serve as an example of this process. In the earliest stage of AD, before cell loss and independent of amyloid plaque and neurofibrillary tangle formation, synaptic loss affecting the basal functional properties of neurons is found. In theory, synaptic loss can be detected by measuring AD-induced changes in basal function or by measuring stimulus-evoked responses on top of basal changes [4]. Functional MRI is sensitive to both basal changes and evoked responses, and therefore offers two approaches to pinpoint the location and timing of synaptic loss in AD [4].

S.Y. Mahmoud, MD (✉)
Department of Radiology, Cleveland Clinic,
9500 Euclid Avenue, MC U-15, Cleveland,
OH 44195, USA

Assiut University, Asyut, Egypt
e-mail: mahmous@ccf.org

S.E. Jones, MD, PhD
Department of Neuroradiology, Cleveland Clinic,
9500 Euclid Avenue, MC U-15, Cleveland,
OH 44195, USA
e-mail: Joness19@ccf.org

M.D. Phillips, MD
Research and Academic Affairs, Imaging Institute,
Department of Radiology, Cleveland Clinic,
9500 Euclid Avenue, MC U-15, Cleveland,
OH 44195, USA
e-mail: phillim@ccf.org

Aging Brain

Although the effects of aging on the brain may share some features with the effects of degenerative disease (such as diminished function), it is important to distinguish between these states. This distinction can be most difficult during the earliest stages of disease, as many of the "normal"

S.H. Faro and F.B. Mohamed (eds.), *Functional BOLD MRI: Principles and Applications*,
DOI 10.1007/978-1-4939-1995-6_18, © Springer Science+Business Media New York 2015

physiologic changes are similar to the changes seen in early pathologic degeneration. In addition, chronic diseases such as diabetes and hypertension can lead to superimposed variability of white matter content and cortical volume. Thus, a thorough understanding of normal aging and its variations is essential for clinicians to differentiate between normal aging and disease.

Neurodegenerative Diseases

Neurodegenerative disease can be defined as the gradual loss of neurons and replacement by gliosis, with functional impairment occurring in affected regions. Affected territories may be diffuse or regional, cortical or subcortical, and may include any neuron type or only certain subsets. Clinical manifestations are often determined by the location of degeneration, which may not respect functional boundaries; pathologically, different diseases may have very similar signs and symptoms if they affect comparable brain regions. For the purposes of this chapter, it is useful to divide neurodegenerative diseases into two broad categories based on the major neurologic system affected: cognition and movement. These disease categories manifest as dementia or movement disorders, with dementia being the most common symptom (Table 18.1). The precise definition of dementia is elusive, but the condition can be defined generally as the deterioration of intellectual and cognitive function, including the modalities of memory, learning, language, numerical skills, visual-spatial perception, and deductive reasoning [5].

fMRI in Neurodegenerative Diseases

Over the past 15 years, the number of fMRI studies performed for research and clinical purposes has increased substantially. The role of fMRI in mapping motor, visual, and some higher functions (such as language) is relatively well established, and researchers are now studying the ability of fMRI to assess more complex facets of cognition, such as memory and emotions.

Briefly, fMRI studies compare the blood oxygen level-dependent (BOLD) signals obtained during two cognitive conditions: an "active" phase and a "control" phase. Because the BOLD signal-to-noise ratio of primary cortex activation can be robust, it is possible to obtain reliable mapping of the sensorimotor, visual, and auditory cortex during a single fMRI acquisition. However, because these cognitive systems are very robust, involve primary cortex, and are well localized, they are often the last to be affected by degenerative diseases. Conversely, higher cognitive functions that are affected earlier in the degenerative disease process often have lower signal-to-noise ratios and are more difficult to visualize reliably in a single patient. Therefore, current research is focused on extending the techniques of fMRI for the assessment of higher cognitive function such as memory and emotions, thus allowing clinicians to look for earlier manifestations of a degenerative disease. The paradigms used for higher cognitive function are more complex; event-related paradigms are often needed rather than the block paradigms that are used for primary cortical activation.

Table 18.1 Neurodegenerative disease categories [5]

Neurodegenerative disease with dementia as the major symptom	Neurodegenerative disease with combined movement disorders and dementia	Neurodegenerative disease with movement disorders as the major symptom
AD	Multiple system atrophy	Leigh's disease
Creutzfeldt–Jakob disease	Parkinson's disease (PD)	Wilson's disease
Frontotemporal dementia	Huntington's disease (HD)	
Multi-infarct dementia	Hallervorden–Spatz disease	
Vascular dementia	Amyotrophic lateral sclerosis (ALS)	
	Normal pressure hydrocephalus	

A variation of fMRI is another functional technique conducted on patients inside the MRI who are in a resting state, revealing low-frequency BOLD fluctuations, and is known as resting-state fMRI (rsfMRI). When compared throughout the brain, these fluctuations have surprisingly long-range correlations that form networks suggestive of underlying functional connections. Many of these independent resting-state networks appear highly correlated with functional modalities, including the "default mode" of human brain activity [6, 7].

Because the hallmark of many degenerative diseases is dementia, which includes memory loss, much early fMRI research has focused on normal memory systems, including complex memory formation [8, 9]. These studies have confirmed the central physiologic role of the hippocampus and neighboring parahippocampal cortices in encoding new events into long-term memory [10, 11]. fMRI can, therefore, be used as an in vivo tool to investigate the dysfunction of the medial temporal lobes and related memory networks during memory encoding and retrieval. The specific application of clinical fMRI is best established in the setting of AD [12, 13], with the goal of improving early diagnostic and therapeutic options. In addition, fMRI offers great potential for monitoring disease progression, in effect becoming an objective noninvasive biomarker.

This chapter will focus on the application of fMRI to degenerative diseases. The diseases will be divided into two groups: those with dementia as the main symptom and those with movement disorders as the main symptom.

Dementias

Mild Cognitive Impairment

There is a spectrum of cognitive change as dementias progress; mild cognitive impairment (MCI) is considered an early and transitional stage between normal brain aging and frank dementia. MCI can affect an array of cognitive or motor functions [14] while the patient is still largely independent in daily life [15], and this condition may last for a number of years [16, 17]. Some individuals with MCI do not have AD neuropathology and will never progress to clinical AD [18]. Most studies suggest that approximately 12–15% of patients with MCI will progress to dementia within 1 year; in these individuals, the early symptoms of MCI actually represent the first manifestations of frank dementia [19]. Because MCI has twice the prevalence of dementia [20] and is associated with an increased risk of death in addition to incipient dementia [21], the public health implications are vast.

When MCI is predominately associated with episodic memory loss, it is commonly referred to as amnestic MCI (a-MCI). Within a-MCI, a subjective memory complaint is corroborated with an objective memory impairment, as revealed by clinical testing. Amnestic MCI is diagnosed if the clinician determines that the patient has otherwise normal general cognitive functions, intact activities of daily living, and no frank dementia [22]. Because a-MCI has been associated with an increased risk of incident AD [20, 22], early detection of the a-MCI subtype has become an area of interest. Within a-MCI, there is occasional reference to a subcategory of patients whose deficit encompasses only a single domain; these cases are referred to as sd-a-MCI.

Because this early stage of disease may be more responsive to treatments that slow decline and delay the onset of clinically diagnosed AD, early diagnosis is important [21, 23–25]. In general, the accurate identification of early AD phenotype [26] may involve assessing early memory impairment, performing imaging studies, and evaluating cerebrospinal fluid biomarkers. In particular, fMRI may be especially useful for detecting alterations in brain function present in patients with MCI.

Alzheimer's Disease

The prevalence of dementia is approximately 5% in individuals aged less than 75 years and approximately 10% in those who are in their early 80s. After age 85 years, the incidence is approximately 20%; after age 90 years, approximately

40% [5]. AD is the most common cause of dementia among the elderly people, comprising about two-thirds of all neurodegenerative illnesses. According to recent estimates, as many as 2.4–4.5 million Americans and approximately 20 million people worldwide are living with AD.

In 1906, Dr. Alois Alzheimer first noticed changes in the brain tissue of a woman who had died of a mental illness that included symptoms of memory loss, language problems, and unpredictable behavior. The postmortem examination revealed brain tissue with many extracellular abnormalities (now called amyloid plaques) and intracellular abnormalities (now called neurofibrillary tangles), which are now considered pathologic hallmarks of AD. A third hallmark is the loss of synaptic connections between neurons. Much progress has been made in understanding the molecular biology of amyloid plaques and neurofibrillary tangles, yet the exact cause of AD remains unknown.

Although there is no cure for AD, four therapies (donepezil, rivastigmine, galantamine, and memantine) are in wide use for the treatment of symptoms, and more than 100 drugs are in clinical trials for treating or preventing AD. Today, a clinical diagnosis of probable AD can be made with high accuracy using clinical, neuropsychological, and imaging assessments. A definitive diagnosis, by convention, can be made only pathologically. Newer developments may expand the use of imaging to monitor preclinical AD changes in patients at risk, serve as outcomes in trials of neuroprotective agents, and eventually become tools for definitive diagnosis [27].

fMRI Studies of Memory

A clinical hallmark of early AD, as well as MCI, is the inability to form new and enduring episodic memories. Because the medial temporal lobe and hippocampus are central to memory formation, it is not surprising that early pathologic changes in AD and MCI occur in the medial temporal lobe, including synaptic alterations, selective neuronal loss, and neurofibrillary tangles [28–30]. These changes also lead to regional atrophy, for which detailed structural MRI studies show macroscopic volume loss of the medial temporal lobe. Although medial temporal lobe volume loss is a common finding in AD, it is not specific and can also be found in diseases such as cerebrovascular disease or hippocampal sclerosis [31].

Given the wealth of evidence of neuropathology and structural atrophy in the medial temporal lobe in early AD, pioneering fMRI studies in AD patients used memory tasks to investigate alterations in the medial temporal lobe activation pattern [13, 32–35]. There are two major aspects to memory – encoding and retrieval – and fMRI tasks have been designed to assess both. Although both block- and event-related paradigms have been used, event-related paradigms are often more useful for memory tasks. Functional MRI studies have consistently reported decreased hippocampal and/or parahippocampal activity in patients with AD compared with that in healthy elderly individuals during the encoding of novel information [12, 13, 32–41]. These studies used a wide variety of visually presented stimulus material for memorization, including faces [36], face-name pairs [12, 13], line-drawings [32, 41], scenes [38], words [39], and geometric shapes [34].

These studies and others [42, 43] highlight the importance of carefully recording and incorporating behavioral data when interpreting fMRI results in patients with cognitive difficulty. Particularly with episodic memory tasks, the performance of patients with AD may not be comparable to the performance of cognitively intact elderly individuals; therefore, any fMRI data analyses should take into account task performance. New event-related fMRI techniques are likely to allow for trials based on behavioral results (i.e., successfully memorized versus forgotten stimuli) in patients with mild memory problems relative to healthy elderly individuals. When imaging older and cognitively impaired individuals, it is particularly important to familiarize the patients with the scanner environment and to ensure adequate practice of the cognitive task before image acquisition.

Despite the relative infancy of the field, there have already been a number of promising fMRI studies in both AD and MCI, highlighting the potential use of fMRI in both the cognitive neuroscience and the clinical spheres of investigation.

These studies, which will be discussed in the following sections, found that early manifestations of network dysfunction in the early phases of AD and MCI may paradoxically be associated with increased neural activity, whereas the later phases of AD are associated with decreased neural activity. The underlying mechanisms remain unclear, but may involve reactive compensation in early disease and nonengagement of the hippocampus in later disease. A recent article by Sperling et al. [44] provides a thorough review of the recent advances in fMRI in AD.

fMRI in Patients with MCI

The term MCI, and a-MCI in particular, is used to refer to a presumed transitional state between the cognitive changes of healthy aging and fully developed clinical dementia [45, 46]. The MCI patient population is very heterogeneous, and not all patients with MCI show continued progressive decline. Results from fMRI studies are likewise variable in this patient population. For example, given the strong symptomology involving memory systems, most fMRI studies focus on the medial temporal lobe. In these studies, the medial temporal lobe demonstrates wide-ranging activation patterns from hyperactivation [37, 40, 41, 47, 48] to hypoactivation [35, 49, 50]. In general, however, patients with more advanced MCI who have more severely impaired memory typically demonstrate decreased activity in the medial temporal lobe compared with healthy elderly individuals [35, 40, 50] – a pattern similar to that observed in patients with AD.

Most studies demonstrate increased activation in the medial temporal lobe in both older patients with very mild cognitive impairment and patients with MCI. Dickerson et al. [37] used an associative face-name-encoding paradigm to compare medial temporal lobe activation in patients with very mild MCI, patients with AD, and control individuals (see Fig. 10.3 in Chap. 10). Compared with controls, patients with MCI showed a greater extent of hippocampal activation and a trend toward greater entorhinal activation. Furthermore, there was minimal atrophy of the hippocampal formation or entorhinal cortex in this group. Lenzi et al. [51] investigated brain activation in 16 patients with a-MCI who had only a memory deficit (single domain) (sd-a-MCI) and in 14 controls during four different tasks assessing language, memory, attention, and empathy functions. The investigators found greater activation in patients with sd-a-MCI than in controls in the left inferior temporal gyrus (language), the right superior temporal gyrus (memory), and the right dorsal precentral gyrus (attention). Moreover, the activation correlated significantly with neuropsychological scores on tests exploring the corresponding functions. Other investigators have reported a similar phenomenon of hyperactivation in patients with MCI when visual object-encoding paradigms [41] and event-related verbal memory paradigms [48, 52] were used. Another recent study, which combined structural MRI and fMRI analysis, reported increased posterior medial temporal lobe activity during novel associative encoding in patients with incipient atrophy in the anterior parts of the medial temporal lobe [41].

A common aspect among these studies is that the patients with MCI were able to perform the fMRI tasks reasonably well. In particular, the event-related fMRI studies found that the hyperactivity was observed specifically during successful memory trials, suggesting that the increased activity may serve as a compensatory mechanism in the setting of early AD pathology [53]. Again, these patients typically have minimal medial temporal lobe atrophy [37, 47].

A handful of fMRI studies have demonstrated decreased medial temporal lobe activation in patients with MCI versus controls [33, 35, 54]. Mandzia et al. [55] found that patients with MCI had decreased activation in the bilateral medial temporal lobe and in the inferior frontal lobes during deep (left only) and superficial (bilateral) encoding. However, when performance was added as a covariate, medial temporal lobe activation was similar to that in control patients. In a region of interest analysis, the extent of activation during deep encoding in the bilateral parahippocampi and left hippocampus correlated with subsequent recognition accuracy in control individuals but not in patients with MCI. This may reflect the heterogeneity of activation responses resulting from varying degrees of pathology burden and progression status in the MCI group [55]. Petrella et al. [50] found no differences between patients with MCI and controls in medial temporal lobe activation during encoding, but the researchers observed hippocampal hypoactivation in patients with MCI versus controls during retrieval. Hippocampal hypoactivation in MCI was no longer observed when memory performance was included as a covariate. Johnson et al. [56] used a paradigm involving the repetitive presentation of faces to demonstrate that patients with MCI do not show the same habituation of hippocampal activation with face repetition as is seen in older control individuals, suggesting disruption of this "adaptive" response in the medial temporal lobe.

Several fMRI studies have assessed mechanisms and regions other than the medial temporal lobe. For example, one recent fMRI study of memory retrieval reported reduced posterior cingulate activity during recognition of previously learned items in patients with MCI compared with older controls [49]. One event-related fMRI study used a verbal recognition memory paradigm requiring discrimination of studied versus new words and showed more prefrontal activity in patients with MCI than in controls during correct behavioral responses [52]. In two other recent studies, a combination of visual episodic recognition and autobiographical self-appraisal tasks was used to investigate potential dysfunction of the posteromedial cortical regions in patients with MCI [57, 58]. Interestingly, impaired activity of the posteromedial cortices was observed during the episodic retrieval but not during the self-appraisal task, suggesting disruption of memory-related processing in the posteromedial cortices in patients with MCI [57].

The detailed mechanisms of medial temporal lobe hypoactivation or hyperactivation remain unclear. In particular, it is unclear whether the phenomenon of hyperactivity is related to compensatory mechanisms, excitotoxicity, and impending neural failure [44], or to cholinergic or other neurotransmitter upregulation [59]. Alternatively, increased regional brain activation may be a marker of the pathophysiologic process of AD itself, such as aberrant sprouting of cholinergic fibers [60] or inefficiency in synaptic transmission [61]. Multiple non-neural factors may confound the BOLD response, including resting hypoperfusion and reduced metabolism in MCI and AD, which may significantly alter the fMRI signal during activation [62, 63].

In summary, these findings suggest that fMRI is sensitive to changes in MCI and possibly early AD. Most studies have shown hyperactivation of the medial temporal lobe, with some studies showing the opposite effect. Most changes have been noted within the medial temporal lobe, although changes may also be seen in the remaining neocortex. These functional changes of increased activation may reflect growing early compensatory mechanisms that reduce cognitive deficits associated with the progressive accumulation of brain damage [51]. Additional studies employing event-related fMRI paradigms will be helpful to further investigate the mechanisms of increased activation and to exclude possible confounders such as increased effort and altered baseline perfusion and metabolism.

fMRI in Patients with AD

The pathophysiologic process of frank AD is associated with mature alterations in large-scale functional brain networks, in particular the distributed networks supporting memory function. As with MCI, fMRI primarily demonstrates changes in the activation patterns of the medial temporal lobe. Some of these changes are similar in mature and early AD (e.g., using face-name associative memory encoding tasks) [13, 64, 65]. Contrary to fMRI studies of MCI, however, most fMRI studies of AD have shown decreased medial temporal lobe activation, with a few studies reporting the opposite effect.

Over the past decade, a number of fMRI studies have reported decreased activation in medial temporal lobe regions in patients with clinically diagnosed AD compared to that in older controls during episodic encoding tasks [32–35, 38, 41, 66–68]. These studies have employed a variety of unfamiliar visual stimuli, including faces [12, 33, 69], face-name pairs [66], scenes [38], line-drawings [32, 41], geometric shapes [34], and verbal stimuli [39]. These studies have consistently reported decreased hippocampal and/or parahippocampal activity in patients with AD compared to that in healthy older controls during the encoding of novel stimuli.

Three recent studies demonstrated increased medial temporal lobe activity in patients with AD and in patients with MCI during processing of repeatedly presented stimuli, which became highly familiar during the fMRI protocol to healthy elderly controls but not to patients with AD [38, 56, 70]. There have also been reports of increased neural activity in prefrontal regions in patients with AD performing memory tasks [66, 71]. Altogether, there is growing evidence that increased activation may reflect impaired inhibition, rather than intrinsic hyperactivity. Pihlajamaki et al. [70] demonstrated that normal suppression of medial temporal lobe activity with repeated face-name stimuli is significantly impaired in patients with AD. This suggests that intact medial temporal lobe repetition suppression may be part of normal memory encoding and consolidation processes, and that failure of medial temporal lobe repetition suppression is a potential indicator of impaired medial temporal lobe and memory function early in the course of AD [72]. Several studies have investigated the notion of compensatory increased cortical brain responses in patients with AD in relation to their ability to perform the fMRI task [31, 42]. No significant differences in fMRI activity were found between patients with AD who performed an easy version of the visuospatial paired-associates learning task and controls who performed a difficult version of the task [43]. In contrast, when task performance was not equated between groups, greater recruitment of cortical brain regions was found in the patients with AD, perhaps representing a compensatory response related to their compromised cognitive abilities [42].

AD affects not only the medial temporal lobe memory structures but also the interconnected large-scale networks outside of the medial temporal lobe [10, 28, 29, 73]. In contrast to the consistent finding of decreased medial temporal lobe activity during novel encoding, several studies have found increased activity in other widespread neocortical regions, such as prefrontal and parietal cortices, in patients with mild AD [12, 13, 40, 71]; for a review, see Buckner [74]. A recent meta-analysis [75] reported that patients with AD had increased encoding-related activation in the ventrolateral prefrontal, orbitofrontal, dorsolateral prefrontal, superior temporal, and fusiform regions. Regions involved in the so-called cognitive control network (dorsolateral prefrontal, posterolateral parietal, anterior cingulate, and anterior insula) were less engaged in patients with AD, indicating the contribution of dysfunction in other cortical networks to impaired memory function in AD. Often the patterns are mixed, including opposite changes within both the medial temporal lobe and distal cortices [76], and may represent a compensatory process in the setting of neuropathological changes within and outside of the medial temporal lobe. On the whole, many studies show consistent, if complex, patterns of brain activation differences between patients and controls.

Several fMRI studies of language systems have investigated the neural basis of semantic memory difficulties in patients with clinical AD [77, 78]. For example, Grossman et al. [78] investigated processing of words versus pseudowords and showed degraded word-category knowledge with preserved semantic memory networks in patients with AD compared with that in controls. Reduced fMRI activity during an associative semantic memory task has also been reported in the lateral temporal neocortex in patients with MCI [79]. Naming deficits are common in dementia, and assessment can be obtained through either visual confrontation naming or auditory response naming, methods that exemplify different aspects of the language networks. Recently, Miller et al. [80] used fMRI to compare these two naming networks in a group of 50 patients with dementia of mixed etiologies. Patients performed significantly worse on auditory responsive naming than on visual confrontation naming, suggesting a more widespread topographical distribution of auditory naming sites within the temporal lobe. These findings may also be influenced by demands on working memory and cognitive flexibility.

Attention, working memory, and long-term memory are closely related higher-order cognitive functions. Often, studies exploring these domains are difficult to accomplish with AD patients, due to the cognitive nature of their impairment. Thus, many studies focus on early AD or advanced MCI. One recent study investigated divided attention and reported reduced prefrontal activity in patients with a-MCI compared with that in age-matched controls, but no differences between the groups during passive sensory processing [81]. Two fMRI studies used a face-matching task in patients with MCI and found that alterations in functional connectivity of the inferotemporal regions (such as the fusiform gyrus) might be a sensitive indicator of emerging AD pathology [82, 83].

Thiyagesh et al. [84] investigated the neural basis of visuospatial perception in patients with AD compared with healthy elderly individuals. The control group had activated V5, superior parietal lobe, parieto-occipital cortex, and premotor cortices, whereas the AD group demonstrated hypoactivation in these regions and hyperactivation in the inferior parietal lobule. There was no associated confounding structural atrophy. These functional deficits may help to form a pathophysiologic explanation for the clinically important symptom of visuospatial disorientation in patients with AD.

Most applications of fMRI for AD have been presented at the research stage, but there is growing movement toward routine clinical usage. For example, Tripoliti et al. [85] presented an automated fMRI method that assists in the diagnosis of AD and helps clinicians to monitor disease progression. This method consists of six stages: (1) preprocessing of fMRI data, (2) modeling of fMRI voxel time series using a generalized linear model, (3) feature extraction from the fMRI data, (4) feature selection, (5) classification using classical and improved variations of the random forests algorithm and support vector machines, and (6) calculation of rules that have physical meaning. The method was applied to a dataset of 41 patients and demonstrated accuracies of 94 and 97% for AD diagnosis and disease progression monitoring, respectively.

Overall, these fMRI memory studies provide accumulating evidence that the characteristic inability to memorize new events observed in patients with AD is related to significant medial temporal lobe dysfunction, most commonly reported during memory encoding and manifested as decreased activation in the medial temporal lobe during fMRI memory tasks.

BOLD Resting-State Connectivity in MCI and AD

The significance of multiple "resting-state networks" (discovered in the 1990s) is gaining acceptance. These MRI acquisitions are known as resting-state fMRI, during which the patient performs no task and the images present as regions or maps of coherent low-frequency BOLD fluctuations. These maps tend to form networks that conform to known underlying functional networks. One network in particular is most active when the mind is at rest: the default-mode network, which involves the posteromedial and anterior cingulate and medial prefrontal cortices. It is important to note, however, that the concepts of the default-mode network and the resting state are not always interpreted similarly throughout the neuroscience and neuroimaging communities, and these concepts are being actively researched [6, 7, 86].

A major advantage of rsfMRI over fMRI is that imaging of the resting state requires no patient task or active participation, therefore eliminating the performance-related variability seen with fMRI. Furthermore, rsfMRI is easier to acquire and standardize and may be more effective in identifying functional pathology associated with AD than fMRI [87].

Recent work applying these observations to degenerative disease has shown that the resting-state networks are significantly affected in patients with MCI, even when accounting for atrophy [40, 50, 88–90]. In particular, studies have found that the default-mode network demonstrates markedly abnormal responses during memory tasks in patients with clinical AD and in those at risk for AD [40, 70, 72, 89, 91]. Interestingly, the same default-mode network regions that typically demonstrate beneficial deactivations in healthy young individuals [92], especially the posterior cingulate/precuneus cortex, tend to demonstrate a paradoxical increase in fMRI activity above baseline in patients with AD. It is unclear whether this aberrant default-mode network activity is the result of alterations in baseline synaptic activity, as these regions typically demonstrate hypoactivation at rest in patients with AD [93–95] and in those at risk for AD [96–98]. These regions demonstrating aberrant default-mode network activity overlap with regions that show a high amyloid burden in early AD [99]. Qi et al. [100] investigated default-mode network activity in 14 patients with a-MCI and in 14 healthy elderly individuals and found that patients with a-MCI had decreased default-mode network activity. In addition, patients with a-MCI had increased activity in the left prefrontal cortex, inferior parietal lobule, and middle temporal gyrus, which may indicate a compensatory process.

Recently, several studies using a combination of fMRI and rsfMRI have found reduced resting-state connectivity and decreased fMRI task-induced deactivation responses in patients with MCI or AD compared with that in healthy controls [40, 88, 90, 101–106]. Interestingly, the posteromedial cortical areas (e.g., the posterior cingulum and precuneus), which have demonstrated altered fMRI activity and connectivity in MCI and AD, are largely the same brain regions that have demonstrated abnormal uptake in Pittsburgh compound B (PiB)-positron emission tomography (PET) studies [99, 107–109] and hypometabolism [110, 111]. Studies have consistently found progressively disrupted fMRI deactivation responses and altered resting-state connectivity along the continuum of patients, from healthy elderly individuals to those with clinical AD. In one study only, patients with AD showed no difference versus controls in task-induced deactivation during successful encoding and retrieval of visuospatial paired associates [112].

The ability of the default-mode network to coordinate its activity with other cognitive networks may be important for healthy brain function, as indicated by recent studies in young adults and older adults [65, 113, 114]. More specifically, the ability of the default-mode network to suspend its activity may be quite important, as this ability may, for example, allow for reallocation of neurocognitive resources to other networks, thereby optimizing task performance. A disruption in this ability may be one of the earliest signs of memory impairment in aging [65]. Furthermore, it is possible that the brain of a patient with AD is no longer capable of flexibly modulating the balance of activity among large-scale neural networks. These ideas are supported by a recent study that used both structural MRI and rsfMRI and found reduced functional connectivity between the medial temporal lobe and posteromedial cortices in patients with MCI and with concordant bilateral medial temporal lobe atrophy [90].

fMRI Studies in Individuals at Genetic Risk for AD

The *APOE* ε4 allele is the main known genetic susceptibility factor for late-onset AD [115, 116]. Posteromedial association cortices have consistently demonstrated glucose hypometabolism in cognitively normal carriers of *APOE* ε4 [117, 118], similar to [^{18}F]fluorodeoxyglucose (FDG) PET findings in patients with MCI and AD [110, 111]. Suthana et al. [119] used high-resolution fMRI in *APOE* ε4 carriers and noncarriers to measure activity in the hippocampus and medial temporal lobe. The investigators found reduced left CA2, CA3, and dentate gyrus activity in cognitively intact *APOE* ε4 carriers. These results suggest that reduced neural activity in hippocampal subregions may underlie the compensatory increase in extrahippocampal activity before the onset of cognitive deficits in individuals with a genetic risk for AD.

A study by Dennis et al. [120] found that the *APOE* ε4 allele may influence both functional activations within the medial temporal lobe and functional connectivity of the medial temporal lobe to other regions involved in memory encoding. The study demonstrated enhanced functional connectivity of the medial temporal lobe to the posterior cingulate in young adult *APOE* ε4 carriers – a result suggesting that *APOE* may be expressed early in brain regions known to be involved in AD.

Similar to fMRI studies in patients with MCI, results of fMRI studies comparing activation in *APOE* ε4 carriers versus noncarriers have been variable, despite careful matching of carriers and noncarriers. Increased medial temporal lobe and cortical activity has been observed in several studies in carriers; this increased activity is generally believed to be compensatory in nature [37, 121–127]. In contrast, several studies have demonstrated reduced functional brain activity in the medial temporal lobe and other brain areas in carriers [128–131]. Therefore, it is currently difficult to draw firm conclusions regarding the effects of *APOE* ε4 on the BOLD fMRI activation pattern. It is possible that the discrepant findings in studies of patients at genetic risk for AD may be related to factors such as how challenging the memory task is and how close the individuals are to symptom onset. Interestingly, the most recent large-scale fMRI studies have suggested more complex patterns of alterations in fMRI activity affected by *APOE* ε4 and family history of AD [54, 132].

Fleisher et al. [133] compared the fMRI response with the arterial spin labeling perfusion response during an associative encoding in patients at high risk or low risk for AD. Within the medial temporal lobe, the high-risk group demonstrated elevated resting perfusion, with relatively decreased perfusion and functional activity during the encoding task. However, there was no difference between the groups in absolute cerebral blood flow during the task, suggesting that individuals with increased risk for AD have elevated medial temporal lobe resting cerebral blood flow, which significantly influences apparent differences in BOLD activations. Thus, BOLD activations should be interpreted with caution, as they may not necessarily reflect differences in neuronal activation.

fMRI to Assess Pharmacologic Therapy for AD

There is considerable need for objective biomarkers to evaluate the efficacy of pharmacologic interventions for AD, and noninvasive techniques for measuring these biomarkers are particularly attractive options. There are a number of disease-modifying therapies entering clinical trials for AD, despite the recent failures of several large phase 3 trials. Such phase 3 trials typically require hundreds of patients, run for a minimum of 18 months, and are costly. Structural imaging techniques are increasingly included as outcome measures in these clinical trials, but structural imaging is unlikely to show any acute drug effects or evidence of improvement during short follow-up periods. Therefore, additional techniques such as rsfMRI or fMRI might be useful in early-stage clinical trials to detect a signal of efficacy and perhaps even to predict subsequent clinical response. Functional imaging of pharmacologically induced neurochemical changes may also enhance our understanding of the mechanisms by which these medications exert their effects [134, 135].

Currently available treatments for AD include the cholinesterase inhibitors donepezil, galantamine, and rivastigmine, and the *N*-methyl-D-ASPARTATE antagonist memantine [136, 137]. Several fMRI studies have demonstrated improved fMRI activation with improved task performance in patients with AD after acute or prolonged treatment with the cholinesterase inhibitors donepezil [138, 139], galantamine [140–143], or rivastigmine [144]. Some of these studies included patients with MCI; their results were generally similar to the results in patients with AD [138, 140–142]. However, Goekoop et al. [141] noted that acute exposure to galantamine in patients with MCI increased activation in the posterior cingulate, parietal, and anterior temporal cortices, whereas in patients with AD, activation was most increased in the hippocampal regions. The authors speculated that these differences may reflect varying levels of dysfunction of the cholinergic system in patients with MCI or AD [145].

An important requirement for incorporation of fMRI tests in clinical trials is sufficiently high test–retest reliability. It has been demonstrated in young individuals that fMRI can detect pharmacologic effects and that the test–retest reliability of fMRI during memory encoding is reasonably good in terms of both the extent and magnitude of regional brain activation [134, 146]. However, there have not yet been adequate validation studies of fMRI reliability in healthy older individuals and patients with AD. Efforts have been made to correlate fMRI activation in AD with clinical dementia assessment scales obtained from standardized tests, such as the Alzheimer's Disease Assessment Scale, the Free and Cued Selective Reminding Test [147], and the California Verbal Learning Test [148]. These early validation studies demonstrated potential reproducibility in tracking clinical changes in cognitive function, suggesting that fMRI may be useful for monitoring therapeutic response.

Overall Picture

Based on the data presented previously, it can be hypothesized that there is an initial phase of medial temporal lobe hyperactivation in the early stages of AD, followed by hypoactivation with progression of pathology and memory impairment. The neural basis of this fMRI hyperactivation is not fully understood but may involve aberrant sprouting of cholinergic fibers [60], inefficiency of synaptic transmission [61], upregulated hippocampal choline acetyltransferase activity in MCI [59], or compensatory efforts to overcome presymptomatic neural dysfunction [149]. See Table 18.2 for a summary of the key literature that reviews MCI and AD.

Frontotemporal Dementia

Frontotemporal dementia (FTD) is a clinically and pathologically heterogeneous group of neurodegenerative disorders that predominantly affects the frontal and temporal lobes. The syndrome was earlier known as Pick's disease, but Pick's disease is now recognized as a subset of this disorder. Other terms include "frontotemporal lobar degeneration," "frontal dementia," "frontal lobe dementia," and "Pick complex." Although there can be some clinical overlap of symptoms of FTD with that of AD, the histopathology of FTD lacks the plaques and tangles seen in AD. On gross pathology, there is circumscribed and often asymmetric lobar atrophy of the frontal lobes, adjacent anterior temporal regions, or both. On microscopic examination, there are microvacuoles and gliosis with or without inclusion bodies [151–153]. Patients with Pick's disease have frontotemporal lobar degeneration with argentophilic, tau-positive intranuclear inclusions (Pick bodies) [154]; however, most patients with FTD lack tau-positive inclusions and may have tau-negative, ubiquitin-positive inclusions with TDP-43 protein [155, 156].

Behavioral symptoms in patients with FTD result from disproportionate degeneration of the frontal and temporal lobes; FTD, therefore, presents as a focal clinical syndrome characterized by profound changes in personality and social conduct. As with AD, neuropsychiatric symptoms develop in later stages [157]. These behavioral changes most commonly emerge when patients are in their 50s [158–160], although the age of onset for FTD can range from the third to the ninth decade [158]. FTD is one of the most common dementias of early onset; the syndrome accounts for 20–50% of all cases of dementia, with an age of onset younger than 65 years [160–163]. The median survival is approximately 8 years.

Heterogeneity of FTD syndromes is likely related to variability of the pathology within the frontal and temporal lobes. Patients with left hemisphere FTD have early speech and language difficulty, whereas those with right hemisphere FTD have socially undesirable behavior and a flattened affect [164–166]. Patients with frontal FTD demonstrate apathy, decreased social dominance, and personality change [166–168], and those with temporal FTD have impairments in language and emotional processing, interpersonal coldness, and hypomania-like behavior [167–169].

fMRI in Patients with FTD

Berthoz et al [170] used event-related fMRI in healthy volunteers to investigate abnormal social behavior using stories describing normal behavior, embarrassing situations, or violations of social norms. Consistent with *a priori* hypotheses, the investigators found that the neural response to intentional and unintentional violations of social

Table 18.2 Key mild cognitive impairment (MCI) and Alzheimer's disease (AD) imaging studies

Study	Patients	fMRI paradigm	Results
Kato et al. 2001 [34]	7 Patients with mild AD; 8 control individuals	Geometric designs for 45 s	Patients with AD showed activation only in visual association areas, with very poor recall of the geometric designs; the control individuals showed activations of the right entorhinal cortex, right supramarginal gyrus, right prefrontal regions, and left anterior–inferior temporal lobe; the control individuals had good recall of the designs
Sperling et al. 2003 [13]	7 Patients with mild AD; 10 young control individuals; 10 elderly control individuals	Face-name association encoding task (block design with three conditions: novel face-name pairs, repeated face-name pairs, and visual fixation)	Patients with AD showed significantly less activation in the hippocampal formation but greater activation in the medial parietal and posterior cingulate; the young and elderly control individuals differed in prefrontal and parietal cortices: the elderly controls showed significantly less activation in both superior and inferior prefrontal cortices but greater activation in parietal regions
Remy et al. 2005 [39]	8 Patients with probable AD; 11 healthy elderly control individuals	Verbal episodic encoding and recognition tasks	Patients with AD showed reduced activations during encoding and recognition in the medial temporal lobes and inferior parietal/superior temporal associative areas; fMRI activity during the recognition task positively correlated with hippocampal gray matter volume; patients with AD also showed increased left prefrontal activity that was correlated with memory performance
Rombouts et al. 2005 [69]	28 Patients with MCI; 18 patients with AD; 41 healthy elderly control individuals	Face-encoding task	Patients with AD showed diminished early-phase BOLD activation in widespread regions throughout the brain, with no differences in the late (slow) phase; in the occipital lobe, the early-phase response was also significantly diminished in patients with MCI (although still distinguishable from the very decreased activation in patients with AD)
Vandenbulcke et al. 2007 [79]	13 Patients with a-MCI; 13 control individuals	Word reading and picture naming	In control individuals, the lower bank of the posterior third of the left superior temporal sulcus was activated during an associative-semantic condition with words compared with the visuoperceptual control condition; in patients with a-MCI, this word-specific activation was significantly reduced
Braskie et al. 2009 [150]	32 Cognitively intact older individuals (mean age, 60 years)	Verbal word-pair encoding and recall	Patients showed increased activation during both encoding and retrieval in most regions throughout the brain
Lenzi et al. 2009 [51]	16 Patients with sd-a-MCI; 14 control individuals	Four paradigms assessing language, memory, attention, and empathy	Patients with sd-a-MCI showed greater activation in the left inferior temporal gyrus (language), right superior temporal gyrus (memory), and right dorsal precentral gyrus (attention)
Mandzia et al. 2009 [55]	14 Patients with MCI; 14 control individuals	Encoding and recognition tasks and behaviors	Patients with MCI showed reduced inferior frontal activation during deep (left only) and superficial (bilateral) encoding and in both medial temporal lobes; there was no difference with covariance of performance; during recognition testing of deeply encoded items, the control individuals showed increased activation in both prefrontal and left medial temporal lobe regions

(continued)

Table 18.2 (continued)

Study	Patients	fMRI paradigm	Results
Fleisher et al. 2009 [133]	13 Patients with a family history of AD and at least one copy of *APOE* ε4; 10 control individuals	Associative encoding task and resting perfusion signal	The high-risk group showed increased resting perfusion, with decreased task-related BOLD and perfusion activation in the medial temporal lobes; there was no difference in absolute cerebral blood flow during the task
Thiyagesh et al. 2009 [84]	12 Patients with AD; 13 elderly control individuals	Visuospatial stimuli	Patients with AD showed hypoactivation in V5, superior parietal lobe, parieto-occipital cortex, and premotor cortices, with greater activation in inferior parietal lobule
Fleisher et al. 2009 [87]	17 Cognitively normal individuals with a family history of AD and at least one copy of *APOE* ε4; 12 controls individuals	Memory encoding and resting-state default mode network	There were no significant differences in encoding-associated activations; encoding-associated deactivations were greater in the low-risk group in the medial and right lateral parietal cortex; resting-state analysis demonstrated nine regions in the prefrontal, orbital frontal, temporal, and parietal lobes that distinguished the risk groups
Peters et al. 2009 [76]	16 Patients with mild AD; 16 elderly control individuals	Short-term memory task (lists of four words followed by a probe word)	Patients with AD showed reduced activation in the bilateral middle frontal, left inferior frontal gyri, and transverse temporal gyri
Miller et al. 2010 [80]	50 Patients with dementia of various etiologies	Visual confrontation naming task and auditory responsive naming	Patients performed significantly worse on auditory responsive naming than on visual confrontation naming; patients with mixed AD/vascular dementia performed worse on auditory responsive naming than did patients with probable AD; there were no group differences for visual confrontation naming
Qi et al. 2010 [100]	14 Patients with a-MCI; 14 healthy elderly individuals	Resting-state fMRI	Patients with a-MCI showed increased activity in the left prefrontal cortex, inferior parietal lobule, and middle temporal gyrus; healthy elderly individuals exhibited increased activity in the default-mode network regions, and in right medial temporal lobe

norms involved systems previously found to be implicated in the representation of the mental states of others; namely, medial prefrontal and temporal areas. This neural response involved systems that respond to the aversive emotional reactions of others, particularly others' anger; which include the lateral orbitofrontal (BA 47) and medial prefrontal cortices. Although not yet applied to patients with FTD, these results may provide insight into the mechanisms of FTD behavior.

Rombouts et al. [171] used a working memory task to compare frontal lobe activation in patients with early FTD to activation in patients with early AD. Although both groups activated the working memory network of the frontal lobes, parietal lobes, and thalamus, patients with FTD had decreased activation in the frontal and parietal lobes (Fig. 18.1). In addition, the frontal regions in patients with FTD showed less activation correlated with working memory load. The investigators concluded that regional functional loss within the frontal lobes can help identify early FTD even when results on structural MRI are normal.

Werner et al. [172] investigated higher cognitive function using two aspects of emotional processing: emotional reactivity and emotion recognition. The researchers found that patients with FTD had emotional reactivity similar to that of control individuals when viewing film clips with fearful, happy, and sad valences. In addition, patients with FTD had emotional recognition similar to that of control individuals when viewing film clips with a happy valence. However, patients with FTD were significantly impaired in emotion recognition for film clips with fearful and sad valences. Volumetric analyses revealed that deficits in emotion recognition were associated with decreased lobar volumes in the frontal and temporal lobes. The investigators concluded that the socio-emotional decline typically seen in patients with frontotemporal lobar degeneration may result more from an inability to process certain emotions in other people than from deficits in emotional reactivity. For a summary of the key literature that reviews this topic, see Table 18.3.

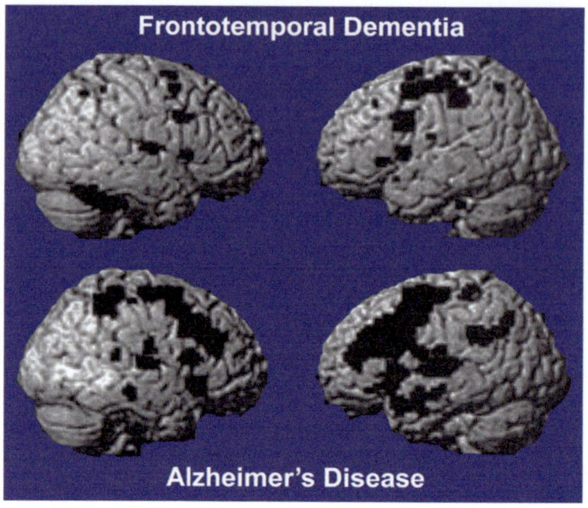

Fig. 18.1 Cortical surface projection of the right and left hemispheres, with overlaid regions (*black*) showing significant activation ($p > 0.05$) during an n-back working memory task, compared to fixation. The *top images* show averaged data from FTD patients, whereas the *bottom images* show averaged data from AD patients. The extent of activation in the frontal cortex in AD resembles frontal activation in healthy controls more than FTD. Most activation is found in both groups in the frontal cortex. The predominant effect is a reduction of activation in patients with FTD compared with that in controls and those with AD. These results suggest that fMRI could be used to discriminate between FTD and AD. Adapted from [171]

Vascular Dementia

Vascular dementia (VaD) is the second most common dementia after AD [173]. VaD risk is known to be correlated with AD risk, but the nature of this relationship remains unclear. Braskie et al. [174] investigated the early stages of VaD, studying the association between vascular health risks and fMRI activity during a memory task. The researchers found that VaD risk factors such as increased systolic blood pressure and body mass index were significantly correlated with increased activation in the posterior cingulate cortex and frontal, temporal, and parietal regions. This pattern of increased activation is similar to the pattern in those at risk for AD, and raises questions about the relationship between vascular risk and cognition.

Table 18.3 Key frontotemporal dementia (FTD) imaging studies

Study	Patients	fMRI paradigm	Results
Rombouts et al. 2003 [171]	7 Patients with FTD; 7 patients with AD	Parametric working memory task to assess frontal activation as a function of working memory load	Patients with FTD showed significantly reduced activation in the frontal and parietal lobes compared to patients with AD; frontal regions in patients with FTD showed less linear activation increase with working memory load
Werner et al. 2007 [172]	28 Patients with FTD; 16 control individuals	Emotional reactivity (self-reported emotional experience, emotional facial behavior, and autonomic nervous system response to film stimuli) and emotion recognition (ability to identify a target emotion of fear, happiness, or sadness experienced by film characters)	Patients with FTD were comparable to control individuals in emotional reactivity to fearful, happy, and sad film clips and were comparable to control individuals in emotional recognition for the happy film clip; patients with FTD showed significant emotion recognition for fearful and sad film clips

Table 18.4 Key imaging studies of vascular dementia

Study	Patients	fMRI paradigm	Results
Braskie et al. 2008 [174]	30 Cognitively intact, primarily normotensive older adults; vascular risk measures included systolic blood pressure, body mass index, and total cholesterol	Memory task	Higher systolic blood pressure and body mass index (but not total cholesterol) were significantly correlated with increased fMRI activation in posterior cingulate cortex and frontal, temporal, and parietal regions
Haley et al. 2007 [175]	13 Patients with cardiovascular disease	Working memory task and carotid ultrasound	Increased carotid disease was associated with lower working memory activation in the right middle frontal gyrus

fMRI in Patients with VaD

Intimal-medial thickening of the carotid wall is an accepted peripheral marker of atherosclerosis, correlating with increased risk for myocardial infarction, stroke, and lower attention-executive-psychomotor functioning. Haley et al. [175] examined the relationship between intimal-media thickening and brain activity during an fMRI verbal working memory task in patients with cardiovascular disease. The investigators found that higher intimal-medial thickening was associated with decreased fMRI activation of working memory regions in the right middle frontal gyrus. This correlation was independent of age and nonspecific white matter change. The authors suggested that fMRI may be useful as an additional sensitive marker of peripheral vascular health. For a summary of the key literature that reviews vascular dementia, see Table 18.4.

Normal Pressure Hydrocephalus

Idiopathic normal pressure hydrocephalus (NPH) is a syndrome that includes hypokinetic-rigid gait, incontinence, and cognitive decline, together constituting the classical "Adams triad" [176, 177]. Radiologic features include dilated ventricles out of proportion to the extra-axial cerebrospinal fluid spaces without corresponding volume loss [178, 179]. Symptoms can sometimes be relieved by insertion of a shunt catheter [180], but the exact mechanism of improved brain function remains unknown. These results are also confounded by uncertainty about patient selection criteria, which is an active field of research.

fMRI in Patients with Normal Pressure Hydrocephalus

One study used fMRI to investigate changes in cortical activity after placement of a shunt catheter. In 11 patients, there was behavioral improvement in both finger-tapping rates and reaction times. Similarly, there was improved fMRI activation in the bilateral supplementary motor area (SMA), but there was no improvement in cognitive functioning. These findings suggest that treatment-related recovery of motor function centers in the motor areas of the medial frontal cortex, in regions considered crucial for motor planning. Furthermore, NPH likely represents a reversible suppression of frontal periventricular cortico-basal ganglia-thalamo-cortical pathways [181].

Movement Disorders

Parkinson's Disease

Parkinson's disease (PD) is a chronic, progressive, neurodegenerative disorder of unknown etiology characterized by bradykinesia, rigidity, tremor, and postural instability. It is the second most common neurodegenerative disorder next to AD [182–184]. Despite being generally thought of as a movement disorder, PD is also associated with significant cognitive deficits. Patients with PD have significant morbidity and disability, with an overall higher mortality rate [185–187]. This disease also results in a considerable societal burden in terms of lost wages, medical resources, and human suffering [185, 188, 189].

The primary risk factor for PD is age: the prevalence is 0.3% in the general US population and increases to 1–2% in patients aged at least 65 years. Some data indicate a prevalence of 4–5% in patients aged at least 85 years [182, 184, 190]. Although the typical age of onset is approximately 60 years, about 10% of patients begin displaying symptoms before they turn 45 years of age; these patients have what is known as "young-onset" PD [190, 191].

Pathologically, the hallmark of PD is degeneration of the dopaminergic neurons in the substantia nigra pars compacta, which results in depletion of the striatal dopamine. This neurotransmitter controls excitatory and inhibitory outflow of the basal ganglia [182, 192].

The architecture of systems involving the basal ganglia centers on a series of parallel cortico-striatal loops [193]. The specific function of each loop is determined by the characteristics of the associated cortical area. For example, the sensorimotor, cognitive, and limbic regions of the striatum are differentiated by the locations and character of the associated cortex, which provides the dominant axonal input [194, 195]. Respectively, these regions are the posterior putamen (sensorimotor), caudate plus anterior putamen (cognitive), and ventral striatum or nucleus accumbens (limbic) [196]. Differential dysfunction of individual pathways produces the variety of symptoms associated with PD. Task-dependent fMRI and rsMRI measures are particularly well suited to assess individual dopamine pathways affected by PD; individual motor, cognitive, and affective components will be discussed in the following sections.

Motor fMRI in Patients with PD

PD symptoms typically begin when at least 70% of dopamine cells are lost from the substantia nigra [197]. Corresponding alterations in fMRI activation have been demonstrated throughout the motor system, principally affecting the SMA, primary motor cortex, and lateral premotor cortex regions. These changes are widely thought to reflect neural deafferentation (inhibition) from the loss of dopaminergic neurons within the substantia nigra. Other factors affecting fMRI activation include disease-related bradykinesia and the degree of attention. In addition to functional connectivity changes, there are structural connectivity changes in patients with PD. Changes in fMRI activation while patients are on and off levodopa have been correlated to clinical response, providing additional insights into the mechanisms of the disease.

To date, many fMRI motor paradigms in patients with PD show hypoactivation within the rostral SMA; overall, this is the most consistent abnormality associated with the motor system [198–200]. However, there can be variation throughout the entire SMA. For example, Sabatini et al. [199] found decreased activation in the rostral SMA and increased activation in the caudal SMA. This finding may argue against SMA deafferentiation being the direct cause of bradykinesia in patients with PD.

An important confounder for fMRI activation in the SMA is attention: the degree of activation may depend on the degree of attention paid by the patient during task performance. For example, Rowe et al. [201] found that when patients with PD performed simple paced finger movements, they had greater SMA activation than controls, consistent with the results obtained by Sabatini et al. However, when patients were asked to attend to their movements, the investigators observed greater SMA activation in the control group than in the PD group. The authors suggested that the SMA hypoactivation commonly seen on images is mostly the result of deficient attention to movements. Another study showed similar SMA hypoactivation in patients with PD during the generation of random numbers [202]. These findings suggest that cortical hypoactivation in the SMA in patients with PD may not be the cause or substrate of observed bradykinesia. Rather, it may reflect a more general deficit in attention [196].

Functional MRI has demonstrated mixed activation results within the primary motor, premotor, and prefrontal cortex in patients with PD. Sabatini et al. [199] used fMRI to assess activation during a complex, well-rehearsed sequential motor task and found greater activation in patients with PD than in controls in the primary motor cortex, caudal SMA, cingulate cortex, and lateral premotor cortex – regions that are involved in direct motor control. Interestingly, controls showed greater activation in the rostral SMA and dorsolateral prefrontal cortex – areas that are more involved in planning, monitoring, and sequencing of movements. The primary motor cortex and lateral premotor cortex areas have direct projections from the cortico-striatal loops involving the globus pallidus internal (GPI) segment [203], which is known to be affected in PD. Similarly, Haslinger et al. [198] showed increased premotor cortex activity in patients with PD who were evaluated with event-related fMRI during self-selected joystick movements. Not all investigators have found increased activation in direct motor control regions. Buhmann et al. [200], using simple self-chosen paced finger movements, demonstrated a reduced extent of BOLD activation in patients with hemiparkinsonian disease versus controls in contralateral primary motor cortex, primarily on the side of the affected hand. This result was not observed with the unaffected hand. The inconsistency of findings across these studies may reflect differences in the tasks assessed, particularly in the degree of motor planning and complexity.

Functional MRI changes in the motor system have been correlated with genetic mutations in familial PD. Mutations in the *parkin* (PARK2) and *PINK1* genes (PARK6) can cause recessively inherited PD. The specific mutations are associated with dopaminergic nigrostriatal dysfunction [204]. Motor fMRI performed in asymptomatic *parkin* mutation carriers demonstrated stronger activation of rostral SMA and right dorsal premotor cortex during a simple motor sequence task, and stronger activation of anterior cingulate motor area and left rostral premotor cortex during internal movement selection versus externally cued movements [204]. The additional recruitment of the rostral SMA and right rostral premotor cortex during the finger sequence task was also observed in a group of asymptomatic heterozygous *PINK1* mutation carriers. It is possible that the increased activation in motor areas may reflect compensation, with recruitment of additional brain regions to maintain function in the face of developing nigrostriatal loss/dysfunction. Interestingly, these brain regions demonstrate decreased activation in patients with PD and, as will be discussed later, demonstrate normalized or increased activation after levodopa therapy. The results of these studies suggest a more generalized pattern for cortical involvement in compensation and restoration of function in PD [204].

Studies of patients with hemiparkinsonian disease [205] have also shown activation in the ipsilateral primary motor cortex when the patients perform joystick movements with their most affected hand. Palmer et al. [206] demonstrated increased recruitment of brain regions in PD patients within the cerebellum and premotor cortex during a visually guided force sinusoidal task, which partially normalized with levodopa therapy. These findings may represent cortical compensation to maintain function, as is seen in other neurodegenerative diseases, rather than a direct manifestation of pathology. Peters et al. [207] assessed hemiparkinsonian disease cases through the use of a simple finger opposition task when patients were off and on apomorphine therapy. Finger movements with both the affected and unaffected hand, while patients were off medication, were associated with activation in the contralateral primary motor cortex and lateral premotor cortex, posterior parietal cortex, and cerebellum. Apomorphine significantly reduced the patients' bradykinesia and resulted in focused activation confined to the contralateral primary motor cortex.

Functional connectivity rsfMRI is a relatively new method that uses a variety of BOLD techniques to study the function of brain networks. Wu et al. [208] assessed automatic movements that are difficult for PD patients to perform. The investigators found differences between patients with PD and control cases in the degree of network activity involving the prefrontal cortex during the learning process. There was also diminished functional connectivity within the rostral SMA, cerebellum, and cingulate motor area in patients with PD; this decreased connectivity was negatively correlated with the Unified Parkinson's Disease Rating Scale (UPDRS), suggesting worsening

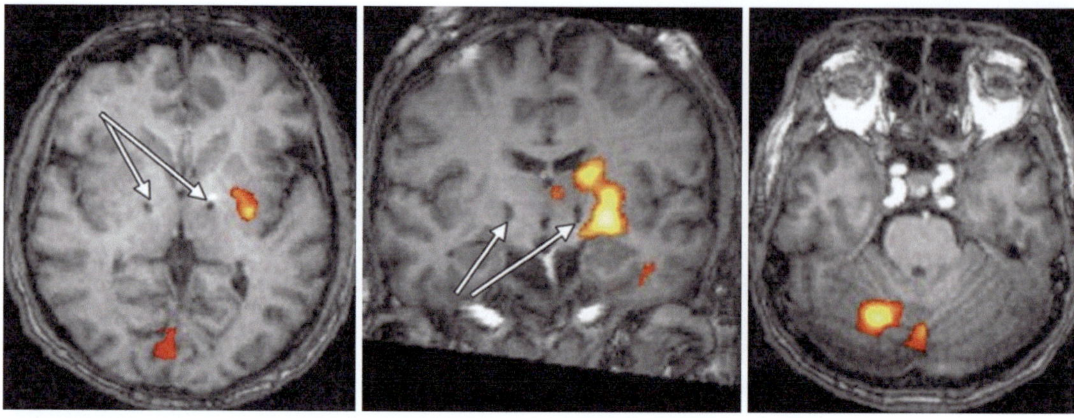

Fig. 18.2 Colorized fMRI activation data displayed in *yellow*, *orange*, and *red* on anatomic magnetization-prepared rapid acquisition gradient-echo images displayed in transverse, coronal, and transverse planes from *left* to *right*. Only left-sided deep brain stimulation was performed. *Arrows* point to bilateral deep brain stimulation electrodes. Areas of activation were identified within left posterior globus pallidus external (*left and middle images*), posterior putamen (*left and middle images*), left thalamus (*middle image*), and right cerebellum (*right image*). Adapted from [213]

connectivity with disease progression. In another study, patients with PD were found to have diminished resting-state functional connectivity in the SMA, left dorsolateral prefrontal cortex, and left putamen, and increased connectivity in the left cerebellum, left premotor cortex, and left parietal cortex. These changes were correlated with the UPDRS and normalized with levodopa therapy, suggesting that changes in connectivity contribute fractures to the motor dysfunction in PD [209].

Functional MRI has been used in multiple studies to study the effect of therapy on PD, most commonly levodopa. In general, levodopa therapy causes a normalization of abnormal fMRI activation and functional connectivity [198, 206, 209, 210]. Interpretation of these findings is difficult, however, as levodopa therapy typically produces a marked improvement in motor function. Results may reflect improved task performance, which could be reasonably expected to produce a pattern of activation in connectivity closely approximating the normal state. Interestingly, levodopa therapy in patients with hemiparkinsonian disease appears to affect the activation pattern only during movements of the affected hand [200]. Kaft et al. [211] have suggested that the putamen and thalamus may be preferentially affected by levodopa therapy, demonstrating more prominent changes in fMRI activation than cortical structures. This theory may provide some insight into the mechanism of action for effective therapy.

Deep brain stimulation is an effective therapy for the treatment of late-stage PD, and several investigators have used fMRI to evaluate this therapy. Deep brain stimulation placed in the subthalamic nucleus appears to produce a consistent pattern of activation in the ipsilateral basal ganglia and thalamus. These brain regions have been implicated in the pathways involved in the abnormal motor functioning seen in patients with PD. fMRI may provide confirmation of appropriate deep brain stimulation placement and function in the future, particularly for placement within the MRI environment (Fig. 18.2) [212–214].

Cognitive fMRI in Patients with PD

Cognitive dysfunction is common in PD and contributes significantly to reduced quality of life [215, 216]. Patients with PD frequently have cognitive deficits that meet the criteria for dementia [196, 217]; the incidence of dementia is increased sixfold in these patients compared to that in the general population [218]. Frontal lobe abnormalities are the most common cognitive changes seen early in PD [196]. The abnormalities may include deficits in attention, planning, habit and skill learning, and cognitive flexibility. Functional imaging studies involving frontal lobe tasks, such as the Wisconsin Card-Sorting [219] and Tower of London tasks [220], appear to involve a network of regions including the caudate nucleus, anterior cingulate cortex, prefrontal cortex, and posterior parietal cortex. These regions make up the cognitive cortico-striatal loop described by Alexander et al. [193], which is affected during disease progression in PD. These pathways have been studied by multiple investigators using fMRI to gain insight into PD-related cognitive dysfunction.

Cognitive function can vary among patients with PD even at the same stage of disease. Lewis et al. [221] compared two groups of patients with PD with and without executive dysfunction who were matched by disease duration, motor dysfunction, and mini-mental state examination; these patients were also compared to age-matched controls. Functional MRI was performed using a working memory task. The patients with PD and with executive dysfunction had diminished activation in the prefrontal cortex and caudate bilaterally compared with the PD group without executive dysfunction. The degree of activation correlated with task performance. PD patients without executive dysfunction had an activation pattern no different than that of age-matched controls. These findings may reflect a dopamine deficiency in either the caudate or the prefrontal cortex (or both). The results also suggest that the cognitive cortico-striatal loop (prefrontal cortex-caudate) may be affected in PD independently of the motor cortico-striatal loops (cortical motor areas – posterior putamen), thus producing different degrees of disease progression in the cognitive and motor domains in individual patients [196].

The relative independence of motor and cognitive systems can also be seen by assessing the effects of levodopa therapy. Mattay et al. [222] performed fMRI using both a motor and a working memory task. The investigators found greater BOLD activation in numerous cortical areas (including dorsolateral prefrontal cortex, anterior cingulate cortex, and posterior parietal cortex) when patients with PD were off levodopa therapy than when they were on therapy. Interestingly, the degree of cortical activation was positively correlated with increasing errors in task performance. These results suggest improved performance with decreased activation when patients are on medication, which may reflect a focusing of activity and/or reduction of unwanted neuronal activity by effects on the caudate nucleus and a larger cortico-striatal system [223, 224]. In contrast, levodopa therapy produced increased activation in motor and premotor regions during performance of the motor task. Increased activation was accompanied by improved task performance. Jubault et al. [225] observed a similar differential effect, with increased activation in motor pathways and decreased activation in cognitive pathways, in response to levodopa therapy when patients were given the Wisconsin Card-Sorting Task. In addition to confirming the relative independence of the cognitive and motor systems, these results also refute the concept that levodopa therapy may be having a direct effect on cerebral blood flow, which may be affecting fMRI results.

Not all studies have demonstrated improved performance on cognitive tasks with levodopa therapy. Cools et al. [226] used a probabilistic reversal learning task to test the effect of levodopa in patients with PD. Previous studies have suggested that this task involves the ventral striatum and ventrolateral prefrontal cortex in normal individuals and that the ventral striatum has relatively preserved dopamine innervation compared to the dorsal striatum in patients with PD [227]. In the study by Cools et al., patients performed better on this task when they were off medication than when they were on medication, and fMRI demonstrated that levodopa modulated reversal-related activity within the nucleus accumbens but not in the dorsal striatum or prefrontal cortex. These results are consistent with the so-called overmedication hypothesis of PD, originally proposed by Gotham et al. [228]. This hypothesis suggests that some parts of the dopamine system are more preserved than others [227] and that while some cognitive functions may improve with levodopa treatment, others may worsen. Similarly, this hypothesis may help explain the differential effect of dopamine on motor and cognitive functions.

Cognitive performance and activation patterns in patients with PD appear to be dependent on whether or not the striatum is used for task performance. In one study, patients with PD who were given the Wisconsin Card-Sorting Task displayed diminished ventrolateral prefrontal cortex activation but increased dorsolateral prefrontal cortex activation [229]. The ventrolateral prefrontal cortex may be activated as part of the cortical loop involving the striatum, thus explaining the diminished activation. The increased activation of the dorsolateral prefrontal cortex likely reflects task activity in a portion of the network that does not involve the striatum. This hypothesis was supported by a more recent study using a modified card-sorting task, which demonstrated that prefrontal cortex hypoactivation in patients with PD is seen only during the phases of the task that also recruit the caudate [230]. Task phases that did not normally involve the caudate showed cortical hyperactivation in patients with PD compared with the control group.

The striatum is extensively connected to the entire cortex and is involved in numerous cognitive functions that rely on large-scale neural networks. Grossman et al. [231] used fMRI to study the processing of complex sentences in patients with PD. Processing of long sentences requires working memory and grammatical processing and involves the striatum, lateral temporal cortex, anterior cingulate cortex, and left inferior frontal cortex. Patients with PD showed decreased activation in these areas but displayed recruitment of other cortical areas (posterior parietal and ventrolateral prefrontal cortex). Recruitment of prefrontal cortex areas may represent compensation, recruitment of latent pathways, or manifestation of the disease process. Regardless of etiology, these findings suggest that the striatal dysfunction in PD has manifestations in multiple cognitive domains, including linguistic processing.

Visual fMRI in Patients with PD

Visual hallucinations occur in 8–40% of patients with PD undergoing long-term therapy [232]. fMRI has been suggested as a potential tool to better understand changes in visual circuitry and processing in PD.

Meppelink et al. [233] studied activation patterns both before and during recognition of objects appearing gradually out of random visual noise in patients with PD and visual hallucinations, patients with PD but without visual hallucinations, and healthy controls. Bilateral activation of the fusiform and lingual gyri was seen during image recognition in all groups. Several seconds before image recognition, patients with PD and visual hallucinations showed reduced activation of the lateral occipital cortex and extrastriate temporal visual cortices, suggesting an association between increased vulnerability for visual hallucinations in PD and impaired visual object processing in the occipital and temporal extrastriate visual cortices. Ramirez-Ruiz et al. [234] showed that patients with PD and visual hallucinations had significant reductions in activation in the right prefrontal regions, including the superior, anterior, and middle frontal gyri, and in the anterior cingulate during a face-detection task. These results suggest that there may be attentional components associated with abnormal processing of visual stimuli. Combined attention and visual processing abnormalities may play a role in visual hallucinations in PD.

Olfaction fMRI in Patients with PD

Loss of olfaction (hyposmia) is common in patients with idiopathic PD. Event-related potentials (ERPs) in patients with idiopathic PD who have hyposmia are typically found to be delayed or absent, suggesting the presence of neuronal damage. Welge-Lussen et al. [235] analyzed ERPs and fMRI scans of hyposmic patients with idiopathic PD. Patients were divided into groups based on the presence or absence of ERPs. The group with intact ERPs (suggesting relatively intact function) demonstrated greater activation in the amygdale, parahippocampal cortex, inferior frontal gyrus insula, cingulate gyrus, striatum, and inferior temporal gyrus. Patients with PD and without detectable ERPs had decreased activation of primary olfactory areas, suggesting a severe disruption of olfactory processing in these patients [235].

Westermann et al. [236] found that patients with PD and control individuals had activated brain regions relevant to olfactory processing (i.e., the amygdaloid complex, lateral orbitofrontal cortex, striatum, thalamus, midbrain, and hippocampal formation). Controls, however, demonstrated bilateral activation of the amygdala and hippocampus, whereas patients with PD showed activation of these areas in the left hemisphere only. Patients with PD had increased activation bilaterally in the inferior frontal gyrus (BA 44/45), anterior cingulate gyrus (BA 24/32), and left dorsal and right ventral striatum. The results of this study suggest that patients with PD have reduced neuronal activity in the amygdala and hippocampus when they perform olfactory tasks, whereas neuronal activity in the cortico-striatal loops may be upregulated, possibly reflecting compensation.

Overall Picture

Parkinson's disease is a global neurodegenerative process involving motor, cognitive, and visual olfactory systems, which has been extensively studied using fMRI. The most consistent motor effect is diminished activation within an SMA during past performance. Other portions of the motor pathway demonstrate less consistent results and patterns of fMRI activation are dependent on many factors such as subject attention and task complexity. In general, medical therapy for PD produces normalization of activation patterns. Findings in cognitive fMRI of Parkinson's disease are variable and task dependent, with tasks involving the stratum being preferentially affected demonstrating decreased activation. The response to levodopa therapy is complex, task dependent, and differs from that of the motor system. The nonuniform response to levodopa therapy may reflect differential loss of dopamine in pathways responsible for individual functions, producing appropriate therapeutic effect in some pathways and possible overdosing in others. For a summary of the key Parkinson's disease imaging studies, see Table 18.5.

Huntington's Disease

Huntington's disease (HD) is an autosomal dominant neurodegenerative disease characterized by progressive loss of movement control, cognition, and emotional regulation over a relatively prolonged period [243]. HD is caused by an expansion of a trinucleotide cytosine–adenine–guanine (CAG) sequence in the short arm of chromosome 4 [244]; the length of CAG expansion is inversely correlated with age at diagnosis [245]. The characteristic pathologic finding in HD is the loss of small to medium spiny neurons, beginning in the dorsal medial head of the caudate and progressing to the ventrolateral striatum [246, 247], with less pronounced neuronal loss in other subcortical and cortical structures [248].

Imaging evaluations of HD over the last 20 years have largely focused on structural changes with loss of size in the basal ganglia, particularly the caudate head. These changes correlate with disease duration, severity, and time of diagnosis and may be present decades before HD is diagnosed [249–252]. These changes also depend on the CAG repeat length [253–256]. Functional imaging has become more prevalent in recent years; a recently published comprehensive review of functional imaging in HD is recommended for readers interested in more details regarding these techniques [257]. fMRI may provide new insights regarding the underlying neuronal dysfunction that may precede neuronal loss in HD.

fMRI in Patients with HD

Multiple investigators have used fMRI and various cognitive paradigms, including maze learning [258], clock reading [259], the response conflict Simon task [260, 261] (Fig. 18.3), serial reaction time [262], and working memory [263, 264], to assess HD. In most cases, patients with HD had impaired task performance with significantly lower task-related activations in several subcortical and cortical regions [262–264]. Interestingly, many patients demonstrated increased activation in various cortical areas [258–260], which is typically interpreted as cortical recruitment and/or compensation. Only one

Table 18.5 Key imaging studies of Parkinson's disease

Study	Patients	fMRI paradigm	Results
Motor studies			
Peran et al. 2009 [238]	14 Patients with PD and without dementia	Event-related fMRI during 2 overt oral language tasks (object naming and generation of action verbs in using object drawings). Objects used were either man-made or manipulable biological objects	Positive correlations between the severity of the motor deficit and language activity suggest a relationship between motor system dysfunction in PD and the extent of activation in verb generation
Wu et al. 2009 [209]	22 Patients with PD before and after levodopa administration; age- and sex-matched control individuals	Total connectivity degree of each region within the motor network was calculated and compared between patients and controls	Before levodopa administration, patients with PD had decreased functional connectivity in the supplementary motor area, left dorsal lateral prefrontal cortex, and left putamen and had increased functional connectivity in the left cerebellum, left primary motor cortex, and left parietal cortex; administration of levodopa produced a relatively normal pattern of functional connectivity
Palmer et al. 2009 [206]	10 Patients with PD off and on medication; 10 age-matched control individuals	Visually guided sinusoidal force task at 0.25, 0.5, and 0.75 Hz	Controls monotonically increased activity within striato-thalamo-cortical and cerebello-thalamo-cortical regions with increasing speed; PD patients at low speeds were similar to controls at higher speeds; PD patients off medication demonstrated novel areas of recruitment of the bilateral cerebellum and primary motor cortex, which were incompletely normalized by levodopa
Palmer et al. 2009 [210]	8 Patients with PD off and on levodopa; 10 age-matched control individuals	Simultaneous and unimanual motor tasks in an fMRI scanner	Patients with PD demonstrated alterations in both effective connectivity and temporal dynamics compared with control individuals during the performance of a simultaneous task; levodopa treatment was able to normalize effective connectivity and temporal patterns of activity partially in patients with PD
Kraft et al. 2009 [211]	12 Right-handed patients with PD (Hoehn–Yahr stages I–II) after at least 12 h without medication (OFF state) and 1 h after oral administration of single levodopa dose (sdLD) (ON state);12 age-matched control individuals	2 unilateral and 2 bimanual grip force movements with a defined movement amplitude and force (10 N) in a block design	Bimanual grip force tasks activated a specific pattern of cortical and subcortical structures in all patients during the OFF and ON states, with statistically significant differences between these states in the putamen and thalamus; no significant changes were observed in cortical structures; between-group analysis revealed higher putaminal activity in controls than in patients in the OFF state when they were performing bimanual tasks, but these differences disappeared after levodopa administration
Wu et al. 2010 [208]	12 Patients with PD; 12 age- and sex-matched control individuals	Patients were asked to perform 2 sequences of right-hand finger tapping. All sequential movements were self-initiated, self-paced, and executed at 0.5 Hz. Automaticity was evaluated by having patients perform a visual letter-counting task simultaneously with movements	During automaticity, the rostral supplementary motor area, cerebellum, and cingulate motor area had increased effective connectivity with brain networks in patients with PD

(continued)

Table 18.5 (continued)

Study	Patients	fMRI paradigm	Results
Sen et al. 2009 [237]	5 Patients with PD; 5 control individuals	Patients performed either externally or internally guided sequential finger movements performed at baseline and follow-up	Controls showed changes from baseline to follow-up in cerebello-thalamo-cortical circuits. PD subjects had increased recruitment of both cortical motor-associated and cerebellar areas and demonstrated augmented recruitment of cerebello-thalamo-cortical circuits over time
Genetic studies			
Van Nuenen et al. 2009 [204]	12 Patients with nonmanifesting *Parkin* mutations, and 12 healthy age-matched noncarriers	2 Separate experiments: a simple motor sequence task and internal movement selection as opposed to externally cued movements	*Parkin* carriers displayed stronger activation of rostral supplementary motor area and right dorsal premotor cortex during a simple motor sequence task, and stronger activation of anterior cingulate motor area and left rostral premotor cortex during internal movement selection than during externally cued movements; the additional recruitment of the rostral supplementary motor area and right rostral premotor cortex during the finger sequence task was also observed in a separate group of nonmanifesting mutation carriers with a single heterozygous *PINK1* mutation
Cognitive studies			
Williams-Gray et al. 2008 [240]	29 Patients with early-stage PD	Cognitive task designed to fractionate components of attentional control. Investigated impact of the COMT Val158Met genotype and dopaminergic medication	Attentional control in PD is critically determined by genetic and pharmacologic influences on dopaminergic activity in frontoparietal networks
Tinaz et al. 2008 [241]	13 Patients with early-stage PD and without dementia; and 13 matched control individuals	Semantic event-sequencing task that required patients to examine 4 pictures of meaningful events, determine the correct temporal relationship among pictures, and reorder the pictures into a coherent sequence	Abnormal activation within the prefrontal cortex and the "default" network in patients with PD; distinct areas of the prefrontal cortex showed both hypoactivation and hyperactivation, whereas the "default" network showed reduced levels of resting activation in PD; left caudate hyperactivation was observed in patients with PD
Rowe et al. 2008 [242]	19 Patients with PD in OFF and ON states induced by dopaminergic medication withdrawal	Two competing performance tasks coupled with a reward mechanism to examine how patients with PD evaluate rewards and switch tasks	Lateral prefrontal cortex and caudate nucleus showed a nonlinear, U-shaped relationship between motor disease severity and regional brain activation; dopaminergic treatment led to a shift in this function, supporting the hypothesis of differential neurodegeneration in separate motor and cognitive cortico-striato-thalamo-cortical circuits
Jubault et al. 2009 [225]	11 Patients with PD	Wisconsin Card-Sorting Task was administered using customized software	Levodopa helped restore a normal pattern of activity when matching was required but not planning by increasing cortical activity in the premotor cortex; this effect was even stronger in the motor loop; medication did not change the pattern of activity in conditions relying primarily on a cognitive loop

(continued)

Table 18.5 (continued)

Study	Patients	fMRI paradigm	Results
Cardoso et al. 2009 [239]	36 Patients with idiopathic PD (20 diagnosed with major depression disorder)	Event-related parametric emotional perception paradigm with test–retest design	Decreased activation in the left mediodorsal thalamus and in medial prefrontal cortex in patients with PD with depression compared to those without depression
Visual studies			
Ramirez-Ruiz et al. 2009 [234]	10 Patients with PD and visual hallucinations; 10 patients with PD and without visual hallucinations; 10 control individuals matched for age and education	The fMRI task consisted of 3 blocks of 21-face stimuli (activation condition) and 3 blocks of 21-colored mosaics (control condition). Patients were asked to press a key when 2 identical stimuli were presented consecutively	During the face condition, PD patients with visual hallucinations showed significant reductions in the activation of several right prefrontal areas, such as the inferior (BA 10, 47), superior (BA 6/8), middle frontal (BA 8), and anterior cingulate gyrus (BA 31/32), versus PD patients without visual hallucinations; in the control condition, patients with PD and visual hallucinations showed hyperactivation in the right inferior frontal gyrus versus patients with PD and without visual hallucinations
Meppelink et al. 2008 [233]	9 Patients with PD and visual hallucinations; 14 patients with PD and without visual hallucinations; 13 control individuals	Static images of animals and objects appearing gradually out of random visual noise were used in an event-related design paradigm.	Bilateral activation of the fusiform and lingual gyri was seen during image recognition in all groups; several seconds before image recognition, PD subjects with visual hallucinations showed reduced activation of the lateral occipital cortex versus PD patients without visual hallucinations and control individuals; reduced activation of extrastriate temporal visual cortices was seen just before image recognition in patients with PD and visual hallucinations
Olfactory studies			
Westermann et al. 2008 [236]	12 Hyposmic patients with PD; 16 age-matched control individuals	fMRI was used to investigate brain activity related to olfactory processing in hyposmic patients with mild-to-moderate PD	In PD and control individuals, olfactory stimulation activated brain regions relevant for olfactory processing; in control individuals, a bilateral activation of the amygdala and hippocampus was observed, whereas in PD patients, these structures were involved in the left hemisphere only; group comparison showed that regions of higher activation in PD were located bilaterally in the inferior frontal gyrus (BA 44/45), anterior cingulate gyrus (BA 24/32), and left dorsal and right ventral striatum
Welge-Lussen et al. 2009 [235]	18 Hyposmic patients with idiopathic PD (9 with ERPs, 9 without ERPs)	ERPs and fMRI central activation were analyzed during olfactory stimulation in hyposmic patients with IPD	Both ERP+ and ERP– patients showed activity in brain areas relevant to olfactory processing, such as the amygdala, parahippocampal regions, and temporal regions (BA 37, 21/22); comparison of groups revealed higher activation in ERP+ patients, especially in the amygdala, parahippocampal cortex, inferior frontal gyrus (BA 47), insula, cingulate gyrus, striatum, and inferior temporal gyrus

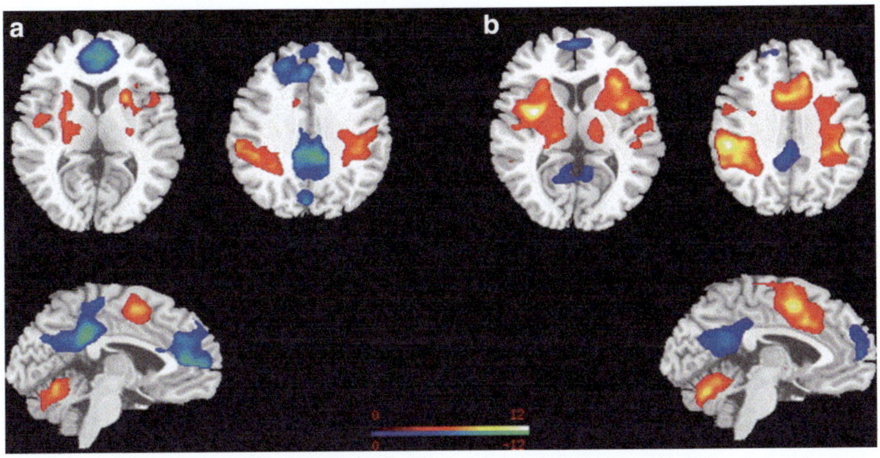

Fig. 18.3 Significant activation and deactivation during the Simon task, compared to baseline, in control individuals (A) and in patients with HD (B). Activation is shown in *red–yellow* and deactivation is shown in *blue–green*. Images are in radiological format. Adapted with permission from Georgiou-Karistianis N, Sritharan A, Farrow M, et al. Increased cortical recruitment in Huntington's disease using a Simon task. Neuropsychologia. 2007;45(8):1791–800. For interpretation of the references to color in this figure legend, the reader is referred to the online version of the article

study has examined functional connectivity in patients with HD [261]. This study showed that patients with HD had impaired functional connectivity between the anterior cingulate and lateral prefrontal regions, which correlated with reduced task performance.

fMRI in Patients with Pre-HD

Several studies have evaluated patients with the gene for HD in pre-HD time periods using a variety of paradigms, including time discrimination, global local interference [265, 266], time production [267], and working memory [268]. Studies have consistently shown that participants with pre-HD, but with normal performance and no evidence of brain atrophy, have increased activation in cortical brain regions during task performance [265, 266, 268], which has been interpreted as recruitment of cortical brain regions for maintenance of normal cognitive performance. Results varied in participants with pre-HD and with either striatal atrophy on structural MRI analyses or cognitive deficits. These patients had reduced striatal, cingulate, and frontal activation [265–267], as well as increased activation in the frontoparietal cortex [268]. The variability among these results may be caused by differences in study populations, with some populations having larger numbers of CAG repeats and earlier onset of disease.

Wolf et al [264, 268] evaluated functional connectivity in patients with pre-HD. The investigators used a working memory task to assess memory-related patterns of functional connectivity in healthy control individuals and patients with pre-HD. The patients with pre-HD exhibited lower functional connectivity in the left lateral prefrontal, parietal, and bilateral putamen. The identified functional networks were not confined to frontostriatal pathways but included frontoparietal networks with sparing of the striatum. This finding suggests that cortical structures may play a primary role in the underlying mechanisms of HD. For a summary of the key literature that reviews Huntington's disease, see Table 18.6.

Amyotrophic Lateral Sclerosis

Amyotrophic Lateral Sclerosis (ALS) is a progressive, usually fatal, neurodegenerative disease caused by degeneration involving the upper motor neurons, including the large corticospinal pyramidal neurons of the motor cortex (Betz cells), and the lower motor neurons, including the large pyramid-like neurons of the ventral spinal

Table 18.6 Key Huntington's disease imaging studies

Study	Patients	fMRI paradigm	Results
Dierks et al. 1999 [259]	1 Patient with HD with dementia and pronounced parieto-frontal atrophy and 6 healthy control subjects	fMRI and FDG-PET	Parietal area in HD showed extensive atrophy and reduced resting glucose metabolism; HD patient performed with similar accuracy but with longer response time in a visuospatial task compared with healthy control subjects; the BOLD fMRI signal in these areas which are involved in visuospatial processing, showed a similar task-dependent modulation in patient and control individuals; the signal amplitude of the task-dependent activation was even higher for the patient with HD than for the control group
Clark et al. 2002 [258]	3 Patients with HD; 3 control individuals	Porteus Maze task	Reduced fMRI signal was observed in patients with HD relative to controls in occipital, parietal, and somato-motor cortex and in the caudate; increased signal was found in patients with HD in the left post-central and right middle frontal gyri
Reading et al. 2004 [266]	7 Patients with HD with genetic mutation who were presymptomatic for movement symptoms; 6 matched controls	fMRI "interference" protocol, a task known to be mediated in part by cortico-striatal circuitry	Despite normal cognitive performance, presymptomatic patients with HD had significantly and specifically less activation in the left anterior cingulate cortex (BA 24, 32) compared with matched controls
Georgiou-Karistianis et al. 2007 [260]	20 Patients with mild to moderate HD; 17 healthy control individuals	Simon task that required a button press response to congruent or incongruent arrow stimuli	HD patients recruited frontal and parietal cortical regions to perform the task and showed significantly greater activation, versus controls, in the caudal anterior cingulate, insula, inferior parietal lobules, superior temporal gyrus bilaterally, right inferior frontal gyrus, right precuneus/superior parietal lobule, left precentral gyrus, and left dorsal premotor cortex
Wolf et al. 2007 [268]	16 Patients with pre-HD; 16 healthy control individuals	Parametric verbal working memory paradigm comprising 3 different WM load levels. Voxel-based morphometry was used to control potentially confounding brain atrophy	Working memory performance did not differ significantly between patients with pre-HD and healthy controls. Pre-HD showed a significantly decreased activation of the left dorsolateral prefrontal cortex at intermediate and high working memory load levels only; this region was not affected by early cortical atrophy, as revealed by voxel-based morphometry; patients with pre-HD who were nearing the onset of motor symptoms showed an increased activation of the left inferior parietal lobule and the right superior frontal gyrus compared with both healthy controls and patients with pre-HD who were far from symptom onset; the activation level in the left dorsolateral prefrontal cortex was positively correlated with the UHDRS cognitive subscore in patients with pre-HD
Zimbelman et al. 2007 [267]	26 Patients with pre-HD (13 "far" [>12 years to estimated onset of manifest HD] and 13 "close" [<12 years to estimated onset of manifest HD]); 13 demographically matched healthy control individuals	Time reproduction task	Close patients demonstrated behavioral deficits, striatal atrophy, and reduced neural activation in the left putamen, supplementary motor area, left anterior insula, and right inferior frontal gyrus; far patients showed reduced neural activation in the right anterior cingulate and right anterior insula; far patients also demonstrated increased neural activation in the left sensorimotor, left medial frontal gyrus, left precentral gyrus, bilateral superior temporal gyri, and right cerebellum; the fMRI changes in the far group occurred in the relative absence of striatal atrophy and behavioral performance deficits

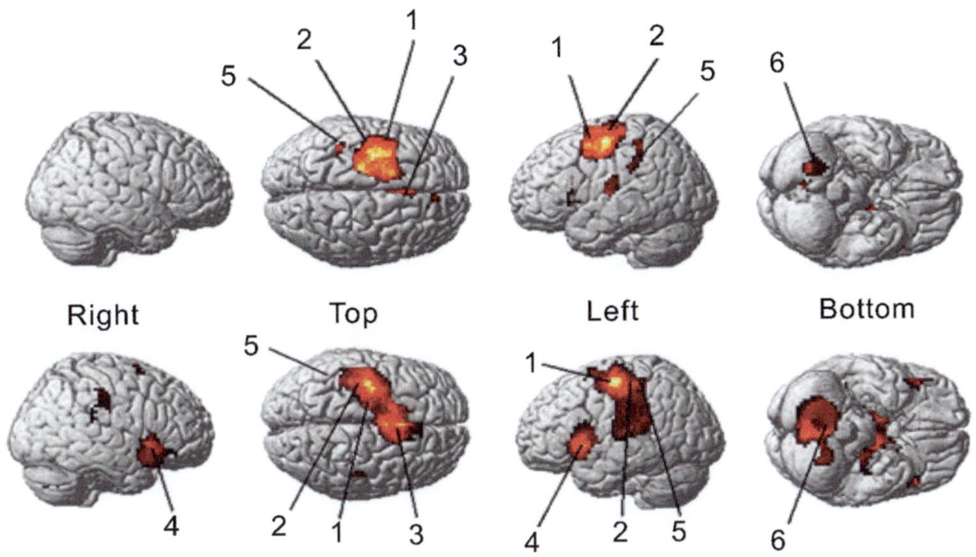

Fig. 18.4 Relative increases in neural activity associated with the right-hand finger flexion task relative to rest (random-effect analysis, $P < .001$, uncorrected) for the control group (*top*) and for patients with ALS (*bottom*). Only clusters with a size of at least five activated voxels are displayed. Activated brain areas: *1*, left primary motor and premotor area (BA 4, 6); *2*, left somatosensory area (BA 1,2,3); *3*, supplementary motor area and cingulate motor areas (BA 6, 24, 32); *4*, inferior lateral premotor area (BA 6); *5*, left parietal motor area (BA 40); *6*, cerebellum. Adapted with permission from Konrad C, Jansen A, Henningsen H, et al. Subcortical reorganization in amyotrophic lateral sclerosis. Exp Brain Res. 2006;172(3):361–9

cord (anterior horn cells) [269]. Typically, patients with ALS have normal MRIs until the occurrence of advanced disease; imaging may then show subtle abnormal increases in T2 and fluid-attenuated inversion recovery (FLAIR) signal along the corticospinal motor tracts, specifically along the intracranial portion of the tracts down to the pons. Within the spinal cord, only atrophic changes are observed [5].

fMRI of Motor Paradigms in Patients with ALS

A recent review of the role of functional neuroimaging in ALS is available from Lule et al. [270]. The most common fMRI finding in ALS is an increase in the volume and of hyperactivation in regions associated with motor tasks [269, 271–274]. It has been suggested that these changes represent potential cortical plasticity and/or adaptation to maintain function. Studies have shown that activation tends to shift to more anterior border regions, including the SMA and premotor cortex (i.e., Brodmann area [BA] 6) [271, 272, 275] (Fig. 18.4). These results are similar to those from previous functional imaging studies with PET [276, 277]. Longitudinal fMRI studies have suggested that there is progressive involvement of the premotor area in upper limb motor tasks over the course of the disease [278].

Patients with ALS performing upper limb motor tasks have demonstrated enlarging regions of activation in multiple additional brain regions, including the anterior insular cortex, anterior cingulate cortex, sensorimotor cortices, bilateral inferior parietal lobe (BA 40), and bilateral superior temporal gyrus (BA 22) [269, 271–273, 275–277, 279–281]. fMRI changes in ALS have also been demonstrated on the subcortical level, with motor execution tasks resulting in increased activation in the basal ganglia, cerebellum, and brain stem [272, 279, 281]. Whether the changed pattern of activity in motor and nonmotor regions, including higher cognitive areas, during motor tasks represents the recruitment of redundant parallel motor system pathways or true functional reorganization remains unclear.

Motor fMRI also demonstrates increased ipsilateral cortical activity within the motor regions during unilateral task performance in patients with ALS [272, 274, 280]. Healthy control individuals often recruit ipsilateral areas as tasks increase in complexity, suggesting that ipsilateral involvement may reflect difficulty-dependent compensation and not necessarily cortical reorganization in ALS. Instead, these results may reflect recruitment of existing neuronal pathways to compensate for functional loss in the primary motor cortex [274].

The use of motor imagery tasks has several potential benefits in studies of ALS. Importantly, it allows for the inclusion of some patients with diminished motor function and may provide unique information regarding motor planning during disease progression. Lule et al. [278] demonstrated that motor imagery led to increased activation in the SMA and primary motor regions. Interestingly, motor imagery tasks did not lead to increased activation in all brain regions evaluated. Decreased activation has been demonstrated in the left anterior parietal lobe, the anterior cingulate, and medial prefrontal cortex regions [280]. This reduction in cortical activation during motor imagery may reflect disruption of normal motor imagery networks by ALS pathology outside the primary motor cortex [278, 280].

fMRI of Extra-Motor Paradigms in Patients with ALS

Data from electrophysiologic, histopathologic, and PET studies clearly demonstrate that ALS affects multiple systems outside of the motor pathway. Changes in sensory, auditory, language, and cognitive function have been demonstrated in patients with ALS [282–291]. Cognitive impairment has been found to be more pronounced in patients with ALS with a bulbar onset than in those with spinal onset [292–295], and is also evident in patients with primary lateral sclerosis [296]. Longitudinal investigation of ALS cases has shown that cognitive changes may progress more slowly than motor decline [295]. PET functional imaging studies have demonstrated hypoperfusion in the frontal cortex when patients with ALS are in the resting state; these studies have also found evidence of decreased activity in different cortical areas during the performance of varying tasks [289–291, 297, 298].

Abrahams et al. [299] evaluated cognitive function using a letter fluency and confrontation naming task in 28 patients with ALS but without dementia, compared to 18 healthy control individuals. Patients with ALS had significantly impaired activation in the middle and inferior frontal gyri, anterior cingulate gyrus, and regions of the parietal and temporal lobes versus control individuals. The confrontation naming fMRI task in ALS demonstrated decreased activation less extensively in prefrontal regions, including the inferior frontal gyrus and regions of the temporal, parietal, and occipital lobes. Control individuals and patients with ALS had matched task performance despite the differences in activation. The researchers found that activation patterns corresponded to the presence of cognitive deficits for both letter fluency and confrontation naming in the ALS group. This study provides evidence of cerebral abnormalities in patients with ALS in the network of regions involved in language and executive functions [299].

Emotional responses in ALS have also been studied using fMRI. Lule et al. [300] studied social-emotional information processing in ALS using pictures of social interactions and facial expressions. Patients with ALS showed increased activation in the right supramarginal area and reduced activation in extrastriate visual areas compared with control individuals. In patients with ALS, there was a reduced response in the anterior insula. The authors suggested that the reduced response in the anterior insula in extrastriate visual areas indicated reduced arousal, whereas increased brain response in the right supramarginal area of patients with ALS might represent an altered sensitivity to social-emotional cues. For a summary of key ALS imaging literature, see Table 18.7.

Multiple System Atrophy

Several systems are involved in this collection of diseases. The associated cell degeneration causes

Table 18.7 Key amyotrophic lateral sclerosis (ALS) imaging studies

Author	Patients	fMRI paradigm	Results
Brooks et al. 2000 [269]	5 Patients with ALS; 5 control individuals	Standard hand motor test (index–thumb opposition or pinch)	ALS patients had higher volumes of activated brain areas during motor tasks compared with controls
Konrad et al. 2002 [271]	11 Patients with ALS; 13 healthy control individuals	Patients performed a multiple finger flexion task by squeezing the plastic handle of a specially developed handgrip force transducer	In ALS, motor cortex activation was located more anteriorly, encompassing the premotor gyrus; the cluster volume within the supplementary motor area was higher and shifted toward the pre-supplementary motor area; contralateral inferior area 6 and bilateral parietal area 40 revealed higher cluster volumes
Abrahams et al. 2004 [299]	28 Patients with ALS and without dementia; 18 healthy control individuals	Letter fluency and confrontation naming	In ALS subjects relative to controls, the letter fluency task showed impaired activation in the middle and inferior frontal gyri, anterior cingulate gyrus, and regions of the parietal and temporal lobes; the confrontation naming task also revealed impaired activation in less extensive prefrontal regions, including the inferior frontal gyrus and regions of the temporal, parietal, and occipital lobes; these changes were present despite matched performance
Han et al. 2006 [272]	15 Patients with definite or probable ALS; 15 age- and sex-matched control individuals	Sequential finger tapping movement at the frequency of 1–2 Hz during a block-design motor task	Bilateral primary sensorimotor cortex, bilateral premotor area, bilateral supplementary motor area, bilateral parietal region, contralateral inferior lateral premotor area, and ipsilateral cerebellum showed activation in patients with ALS and control individuals when they were executing the same motor task; the activation areas in bilateral primary sensorimotor cortex, bilateral premotor area, bilateral supplementary motor area, and ipsilateral cerebellum were larger in patients with ALS than in controls; extra activation areas, including ipsilateral inferior lateral premotor area, bilateral posterior limb of internal capsule, and contralateral cerebellum, were detected only in patients with ALS
Konrad et al. 2006 [279]	10 Patients with ALS; 10 healthy control individuals	Simple finger flexion task. Cued by an acoustic trigger, participants squeezed a handgrip force transducer with their right hand at 10% of their maximum voluntary contraction force. Movement frequency, amplitude, and force were controlled	Increased activation in ALS versus healthy controls; the main activation increases were found in the supplementary motor area, basal ganglia, brain stem, and cerebellum
Lule et al. 2007 [278]	14 Patients with ALS; 15 healthy control individuals; a subgroup of 11 patients and 14 controls.	Grip force paradigm comprising imagery and execution tasks	Motor imagery activated similar neural networks as motor execution in patients with ALS and healthy controls in the primary motor (BA 4), premotor, and supplementary motor (BA 6) cortex. ALS patients presented a stronger response within premotor and primary motor areas for imagery and execution than controls. After 6 months, these differences persisted, with patients with ALS demonstrating additional activity in the precentral gyrus and in a frontoparietal network for motor imagery, in which activity increased with impairment

problems with movement, balance, and automatic functions of the body, such as bladder control. There are no specific imaging findings for this group of diseases [5].

Wilson's Disease (Hepatolenticular Degeneration)

This is one of the few movement disorders in which there is a specific imaging finding. On T2-weighted MRI, prominent hyperintensities in the putamen, thalami, brain stem, and dentate nuclei have been reported. Within the putamen, irregular hypointensities may be present, secondary to focal iron depositions causing susceptibility artifact. The deposition of copper may also cause a similar finding [5].

Conclusion

Because neurodegenerative diseases progress through stages that may occur over a period of months or even years, early diagnosis and treatment are essential. Early signs of disease, however, can be hard to detect and may often go undiagnosed. New developments in fMRI detection techniques may allow for earlier diagnosis and as a result lead to earlier treatments.

References

1. Selkoe DJ. Alzheimer's disease is a synaptic failure. Science. 2002;298(5594):789–91.
2. Coleman P, Federoff Kurlan R. A focus on the synapse for neuroprotection in Alzheimer disease and other dementias. Neurology. 2004;63(7):1155–62.
3. DeKosky ST, Marek K. Looking backward to move forward: early detection of neurodegenerative disorders. Science. 2003;302(5646):830–4.
4. Brickman AM, Small SA, Fleisher A. Pinpointing synaptic loss caused by Alzheimer's disease with fMRI. Behav Neurol. 2009;21(1):93–100.
5. Essig M. Degenerative brain disease. In: Diseases of the brain, head & neck, spine. Milan: Springer; 2008.
6. Raichle ME, Mintun MA. Brain work and brain imaging. Annu Rev Neurosci. 2006;29:449–76.
7. Buckner RL, Andrews-Hanna JR, Schacter DL. The brain's default network: anatomy, function, and relevance to disease. Ann N Y Acad Sci. 2008; 1124:1–38.
8. Pihlajamäki M, Tanila H, Hänninen T, et al. Encoding of novel picture pairs activates the perirhinal cortex: an fMRI study. Hippocampus. 2003;13(1):67–80.
9. Sperling RA, Bates JF, Cocchiarella AJ, Schacter DL, Rosen BR, Albert MS. Encoding novel face-name associations: a functional MRI study. Hum Brain Mapp. 2001;14(3):129–39.
10. Eichenbaum H. A cortical-hippocampal system for declarative memory. Nat Rev Neurosci. 2000;1(1): 41–50.
11. Scoville WB, Milner B. Loss of recent memory after bilateral hippocampal lesions. J Neurol Neurosurg Psychiatry. 1957;20(1):11–21.
12. Pariente J, Cole S, Henson R, et al. Alzheimer's patients engage an alternative network during a memory task. Ann Neurol. 2005;58(6):870–9.
13. Sperling RA, Bates JF, Chua EF, et al. fMRI studies of associative encoding in young and elderly controls and mild Alzheimer's disease. J Neurol Neurosurg Psychiatry. 2003;74(1):44–50.
14. Yan JH, Dick MB. Practice effects on motor control in healthy seniors and patients with mild cognitive impairment and Alzheimer's disease. Neuropsychol Dev Cogn B Aging Neuropsychol Cogn. 2006; 13(3–4):385–410.
15. Dickerson BC, Sperling RA. Neuroimaging biomarkers for clinical trials of disease-modifying therapies in Alzheimer's disease. NeuroRx. 2005; 2(2):348–60.
16. Dickerson BC, Miller SL, Greve DN, et al. Prefrontal-hippocampal-fusiform activity during encoding predicts intraindividual differences in free recall ability: an event-related functional-anatomic MRI study. Hippocampus. 2007;17(11):1060–70.
17. Amieva H, Le Goff M, Millet X, et al. Prodromal Alzheimer's disease: successive emergence of the clinical symptoms. Ann Neurol. 2008;64(5):492–8.
18. Petersen RC, Parisi JE, Dickson DW, et al. Neuropathologic features of amnestic mild cognitive impairment. Arch Neurol. 2006;63(5):665–72.
19. Morris JC, Cummings J. Mild cognitive impairment (MCI) represents early-stage Alzheimer's disease. J Alzheimers Dis. 2005;7(3):235–9. discussion 255–62.
20. Morris JC, Storandt M, Miller JP, et al. Mild cognitive impairment represents early-stage Alzheimer disease. Arch Neurol. 2001;58(3):397–405.
21. Bennett DA, Wilson RS, Schneider JA, et al. Natural history of mild cognitive impairment in older persons. Neurology. 2002;59(2):198–205.
22. Petersen RC, Smith GE, Waring SC, Ivnik RJ, Tangalos EG, Kokmen E. Mild cognitive impairment: clinical characterization and outcome. Arch Neurol. 1999;56(3):303–8.
23. Bowen J, Teri L, Kukull W, McCormick W, McCurry SM, Larson EB. Progression to dementia in patients with isolated memory loss. Lancet. 1997;349(9054): 763–5.

24. Lyketsos CG, Lopez O, Jones B, Fitzpatrick AL, Breitner J, DeKosky S. Prevalence of neuropsychiatric symptoms in dementia and mild cognitive impairment: results from the cardiovascular health study. JAMA. 2002;288(12):1475–83.
25. Vogel A, Stokholm J, Gade A, Andersen BB, Hejl AM, Waldemar G. Awareness of deficits in mild cognitive impairment and Alzheimer's disease: do MCI patients have impaired insight? Dement Geriatr Cogn Disord. 2004;17(3):181–7.
26. Dubois B, Feldman HH, Jacova C, et al. Research criteria for the diagnosis of Alzheimer's disease: revising the NINCDS-ADRDA criteria. Lancet Neurol. 2007;6(8):734–46.
27. National Institute on Aging. Alzheimer's disease fact sheet. Bethesda, MD: US National Institute of Health National Institute on Aging; 2008.
28. Braak H, Braak E. Neuropathological stageing of Alzheimer-related changes. Acta Neuropathol. 1991;82(4):239–59.
29. Hyman BT, Van Hoesen GW, Damasio AR, Barnes CL. Alzheimer's disease: cell-specific pathology isolates the hippocampal formation. Science. 1984; 225(4667):1168–70.
30. Scheff SW, Price DA, Schmitt FA, Mufson EJ. Hippocampal synaptic loss in early Alzheimer's disease and mild cognitive impairment. Neurobiol Aging. 2006;27(10):1372–84.
31. Jagust WJ, Zheng L, Harvey DJ, et al. Neuropathological basis of magnetic resonance images in aging and dementia. Ann Neurol. 2008; 63(1):72–80.
32. Rombouts SA, Barkhof F, Veltman DJ, et al. Functional MR imaging in Alzheimer's disease during memory encoding. AJNR Am J Neuroradiol. 2000;21(10):1869–75.
33. Small SA, Perera GM, DeLaPaz R, Mayeux R, Stern Y. Differential regional dysfunction of the hippocampal formation among elderly with memory decline and Alzheimer's disease. Ann Neurol. 1999; 45(4):466–72.
34. Kato T, Knopman D, Liu H. Dissociation of regional activation in mild AD during visual encoding: a functional MRI study. Neurology. 2001;57(5): 812–6.
35. Machulda MM, Ward HA, Borowski B, et al. Comparison of memory fMRI response among normal, MCI, and Alzheimer's patients. Neurology. 2003;61(4):500–6.
36. Gron G, Riepe MW. Neural basis for the cognitive continuum in episodic memory from health to Alzheimer disease. Am J Geriatr Psychiatry. 2004; 12(6):648–52.
37. Dickerson BC, Salat DH, Greve DN, et al. Increased hippocampal activation in mild cognitive impairment compared to normal aging and AD. Neurology. 2005;65(3):404–11.
38. Golby A, Silverberg G, Race E, et al. Memory encoding in Alzheimer's disease: an fMRI study of explicit and implicit memory. Brain. 2005;128(Pt 4):773–87.
39. Rémy F, Mirrashed F, Campbell B, Richter W. Verbal episodic memory impairment in Alzheimer's disease: a combined structural and functional MRI study. Neuroimage. 2005;25(1):253–66.
40. Celone KA, Calhoun VD, Dickerson BC, et al. Alterations in memory networks in mild cognitive impairment and Alzheimer's disease: an independent component analysis. J Neurosci. 2006;26(40): 10222–31.
41. Hämäläinen A, Pihlajamäki M, Tanila H, et al. Increased fMRI responses during encoding in mild cognitive impairment. Neurobiol Aging. 2007;28(12):1889–903.
42. Gould RL, Arroyo B, Brown RG, Owen AM, Bullmore ET, Howard RJ. Brain mechanisms of successful compensation during learning in Alzheimer disease. Neurology. 2006;67(6):1011–7.
43. Gould RL, Brown RG, Owen AM, Bullmore ET, Williams SC, Howard RJ. Functional neuroanatomy of successful paired associate learning in Alzheimer's disease. Am J Psychiatry. 2005;162(11):2049–60.
44. Sperling RA, Dickerson BC, Pihlajamaki M, et al. Functional alterations in memory networks in early Alzheimer's disease. Neuromolecular Med. 2010; 12(1):27–43.
45. Petersen RC, Doody R, Kurz A, et al. Current concepts in mild cognitive impairment. Arch Neurol. 2001;58(12):1985–92.
46. Petersen RC. Mild cognitive impairment: current research and clinical implications. Semin Neurol. 2007;27(1):22–31.
47. Dickerson BC, Salat DH, Bates JF, et al. Medial temporal lobe function and structure in mild cognitive impairment. Ann Neurol. 2004;56(1):27–35.
48. Kircher TT, Weis S, Freymann K, et al. Hippocampal activation in patients with mild cognitive impairment is necessary for successful memory encoding. J Neurol Neurosurg Psychiatry. 2007;78(8):812–8.
49. Johnson SC, Schmitz TW, Moritz CH, et al. Activation of brain regions vulnerable to Alzheimer's disease: the effect of mild cognitive impairment. Neurobiol Aging. 2006;27(11):1604–12.
50. Petrella JR, Krishnan S, Slavin MJ, Tran TT, Murty L, Doraiswamy PM. Mild cognitive impairment: evaluation with 4-T functional MR imaging. Radiology. 2006;240(1):177–86.
51. Lenzi D, Serra L, Perri R, et al. Single domain amnestic MCI: A multiple cognitive domains fMRI investigation. Neurobiol Aging. 2009. Article in Press, Corrected Proof.
52. Heun R, Freymann K, Erb M, et al. Mild cognitive impairment (MCI) and actual retrieval performance affect cerebral activation in the elderly. Neurobiol Aging. 2007;28(3):404–13.
53. Dickerson BC, Sperling RA. Functional abnormalities of the medial temporal lobe memory system in mild cognitive impairment and Alzheimer's disease:

insights from functional MRI studies. Neuropsychologia. 2008;46(6):1624–35.
54. Johnson SC, Schmitz TW, Trivedi MA, et al. The influence of Alzheimer disease family history and apolipoprotein E epsilon4 on mesial temporal lobe activation. J Neurosci. 2006;26(22):6069–76.
55. Mandzia JL, McAndrews MP, Grady CL, Graham SJ, Black SE. Neural correlates of incidental memory in mild cognitive impairment: an fMRI study. Neurobiol Aging. 2009;30(5):717–30.
56. Johnson SC, Baxter LC, Susskind-Wilder L, Connor DJ, Sabbagh MN, Caselli RJ. Hippocampal adaptation to face repetition in healthy elderly and mild cognitive impairment. Neuropsychologia. 2004;42(7):980–9.
57. Ries ML, Schmitz TW, Kawahara TN, Torgerson BM, Trivedi MA, Johnson SC. Task-dependent posterior cingulate activation in mild cognitive impairment. Neuroimage. 2006;29(2):485–92.
58. Ries ML, Jabbar BM, Schmitz TW, et al. Anosognosia in mild cognitive impairment: relationship to activation of cortical midline structures involved in self-appraisal. J Int Neuropsychol Soc. 2007;13(3):450–61.
59. DeKosky ST, Ikonomovic MD, Styren SD, et al. Upregulation of choline acetyltransferase activity in hippocampus and frontal cortex of elderly subjects with mild cognitive impairment. Ann Neurol. 2002;51(2):145–55.
60. Hashimoto M, Masliah E. Cycles of aberrant synaptic sprouting and neurodegeneration in Alzheimer's and dementia with Lewy bodies. Neurochem Res. 2003;28(11):1743–56.
61. Stern EA, Bacskai BJ, Hickey GA, Attenello FJ, Lombardo JA, Hyman BT. Cortical synaptic integration in vivo is disrupted by amyloid-beta plaques. J Neurosci. 2004;24(19):4535–40.
62. Davis TL, Kwong KK, Weisskoff RM, Rosen BR. Calibrated functional MRI: mapping the dynamics of oxidative metabolism. Proc Natl Acad Sci U S A. 1998;95(4):1834–9.
63. Cohen ER, Ugurbil K, Kim SG. Effect of basal conditions on the magnitude and dynamics of the blood oxygenation level-dependent fMRI response. J Cereb Blood Flow Metab. 2002;22(9):1042–53.
64. Rand-Giovannetti E, Chua EF, Driscoll AE, Schacter DL, Albert MS, Sperling RA. Hippocampal and neocortical activation during repetitive encoding in older persons. Neurobiol Aging. 2006; 27(1):173–82.
65. Miller SL, Celone K, DePeau K, et al. Age-related memory impairment associated with loss of parietal deactivation but preserved hippocampal activation. Proc Natl Acad Sci U S A. 2008;105(6):2181–6.
66. Sperling R, Chua E, Cocchiarella A, et al. Putting names to faces: successful encoding of associative memories activates the anterior hippocampal formation. Neuroimage. 2003;20(2):1400–10.
67. Grön G, Bittner D, Schmitz B, Wunderlich AP, Riepe MW. Subjective memory complaints: objective neural markers in patients with Alzheimer's disease and major depressive disorder. Ann Neurol. 2002;51(4):491–8.
68. Rémy F, Mirrashed F, Campbell B, Richter W. Mental calculation impairment in Alzheimer's disease: a functional magnetic resonance imaging study. Neurosci Lett. 2004;358(1):25–8.
69. Rombouts SA, Goekoop R, Stam CJ, Barkhof F, Scheltens P. Delayed rather than decreased BOLD response as a marker for early Alzheimer's disease. Neuroimage. 2005;26(4):1078–85.
70. Pihlajamäki M, DePeau KM, Blacker D, Sperling RA. Impaired medial temporal repetition suppression is related to failure of parietal deactivation in Alzheimer disease. Am J Geriatr Psychiatry. 2008; 16(4):283–92.
71. Grady CL, McIntosh AR, Beig S, Keightley ML, Burian H, Black SE. Evidence from functional neuroimaging of a compensatory prefrontal network in Alzheimer's disease. J Neurosci. 2003;23(3):986–93.
72. Pihlajamäki M, O' Keefe K, Bertram L, et al. Evidence of altered posteromedial cortical fMRI activity in subjects at risk for Alzheimer disease. Alzheimer Dis Assoc Disord. 2010;24(1):28–36.
73. Mesulam MM. From sensation to cognition. Brain. 1998;121(Pt 6):1013–52.
74. Buckner RL. Memory and executive function in aging and AD: multiple factors that cause decline and reserve factors that compensate. Neuron. 2004; 44(1):195–208.
75. Schwindt GC, Black SE. Functional imaging studies of episodic memory in Alzheimer's disease: a quantitative meta-analysis. Neuroimage. 2009;45(1):181–90.
76. Peters F, Collette F, Degueldre C, Sterpenich V, Majerus S, Salmon E. The neural correlates of verbal short-term memory in Alzheimer's disease: an fMRI study. Brain. 2009;132(Pt 7):1833–46.
77. Saykin AJ, Flashman LA, Frutiger SA, et al. Neuroanatomic substrates of semantic memory impairment in Alzheimer's disease: patterns of functional MRI activation. J Int Neuropsychol Soc. 1999;5(5):377–92.
78. Grossman M, Koenig P, Glosser G, et al. Neural basis for semantic memory difficulty in Alzheimer's disease: an fMRI study. Brain. 2003;126(Pt 2):292–311.
79. Vandenbulcke M, Peeters R, Dupont P, Van Hecke P, Vandenberghe R. Word reading and posterior temporal dysfunction in amnestic mild cognitive impairment. Cereb Cortex. 2007;17(3):542–51.
80. Miller KM, Finney GR, Meador KJ, Loring DW. Auditory responsive naming versus visual confrontation naming in dementia. Clin Neuropsychol. 2010;24(1):103–18.
81. Dannhauser TM, Walker Z, Stevens T, Lee L, Seal M, Shergill SS. The functional anatomy of divided attention in amnestic mild cognitive impairment. Brain. 2005;128(Pt 6):1418–27.
82. Bokde AL, Lopez-Bayo P, Meindl T, et al. Functional connectivity of the fusiform gyrus during a face-matching task in subjects with mild cognitive impairment. Brain. 2006;129(Pt 5):1113–24.

83. Teipel SJ, Bokde AL, Born C, et al. Morphological substrate of face matching in healthy ageing and mild cognitive impairment: a combined MRI-fMRI study. Brain. 2007;130(Pt 7):1745–58.
84. Thiyagesh SN, Farrow TF, Parks RW, et al. The neural basis of visuospatial perception in Alzheimer's disease and healthy elderly comparison subjects: an fMRI study. Psychiatry Res. 2009;172(2):109–16.
85. Tripoliti EE, Fotiadis DI, Argyropoulou M, Manis G. A six stage approach for the diagnosis of the Alzheimer's disease based on fMRI data. J Biomed Inform. 2010;43(2):307–20.
86. Morcom AM, Fletcher PC. Does the brain have a baseline? Why we should be resisting a rest. Neuroimage. 2007;37(4):1073–82.
87. Fleisher AS, Sherzai A, Taylor C, Langbaum JB, Chen K, Buxton RB. Resting-state BOLD networks versus task-associated functional MRI for distinguishing Alzheimer's disease risk groups. Neuroimage. 2009;47(4):1678–90.
88. Rombouts SA, Barkhof F, Goekoop R, Stam CJ, Scheltens P. Altered resting state networks in mild cognitive impairment and mild Alzheimer's disease: an fMRI study. Hum Brain Mapp. 2005; 26(4):231–9.
89. Petrella JR, Prince SE, Wang L, Hellegers C, Doraiswamy PM. Prognostic value of posteromedial cortex deactivation in mild cognitive impairment. PLoS One. 2007;2(10):e1104.
90. Sorg C, Riedl V, Mühlau M, et al. Selective changes of resting-state networks in individuals at risk for Alzheimer's disease. Proc Natl Acad Sci U S A. 2007;104(47):18760–5.
91. Lustig C, Buckner RL. Preserved neural correlates of priming in old age and dementia. Neuron. 2004; 42(5):865–75.
92. Daselaar SM, Fleck MS, Dobbins IG, Madden DJ, Cabeza R. Effects of healthy aging on hippocampal and rhinal memory functions: an event-related fMRI study. Cereb Cortex. 2006;16(12):1771–82.
93. Meltzer CC, Zubieta JK, Brandt J, Tune LE, Mayberg HS, Frost JJ. Regional hypometabolism in Alzheimer's disease as measured by positron emission tomography after correction for effects of partial volume averaging. Neurology. 1996;47(2):454–61.
94. Silverman DH, Small GW, Chang CY, et al. Positron emission tomography in evaluation of dementia: regional brain metabolism and long-term outcome. JAMA. 2001;286(17):2120–7.
95. Alexander GE, Chen K, Pietrini P, Rapoport SI, Reiman EM. Longitudinal PET evaluation of cerebral metabolic decline in dementia: a potential outcome measure in Alzheimer's disease treatment studies. Am J Psychiatry. 2002;159(5):738–45.
96. Small GW, Ercoli LM, Silverman DH, et al. Cerebral metabolic and cognitive decline in persons at genetic risk for Alzheimer's disease. Proc Natl Acad Sci U S A. 2000;97(11):6037–42.
97. Reiman EM, Chen K, Alexander GE, et al. Functional brain abnormalities in young adults at genetic risk for late-onset alzheimer's dementia. Proc Natl Acad Sci U S A. 2004;101(1):284–9.
98. Jagust W, Gitcho A, Sun F, Kuczynski B, Mungas D, Haan M. Brain imaging evidence of preclinical Alzheimer's disease in normal aging. Ann Neurol. 2006;59(4):673–81.
99. Klunk WE, Engler H, Nordberg A, et al. Imaging brain amyloid in Alzheimer's disease with Pittsburgh Compound-B. Ann Neurol. 2004;55(3):306–19.
100. Qi Z, Wu X, Wang Z, et al. Impairment and compensation coexist in amnestic MCI default mode network. Neuroimage. 2010;50(1):48–55.
101. Lustig C, Snyder AZ, Bhakta M, et al. Functional deactivations: change with age and dementia of the Alzheimer type. Proc Natl Acad Sci U S A. 2003;100(24):14504–9.
102. Greicius MD, Srivastava G, Reiss AL, Menon V. Default-mode network activity distinguishes Alzheimer's disease from healthy aging: evidence from functional MRI. Proc Natl Acad Sci U S A. 2004;101(13):4637–42.
103. Wang L, Zang Y, He Y, et al. Changes in hippocampal connectivity in the early stages of Alzheimer's disease: evidence from resting state fMRI. Neuroimage. 2006;31(2):496–504.
104. Wang K, Liang M, Wang L, et al. Altered functional connectivity in early Alzheimer's disease: a resting-state fMRI study. Hum Brain Mapp. 2007;28(10):967–78.
105. He Y, Wang L, Zang Y, et al. Regional coherence changes in the early stages of Alzheimer's disease: a combined structural and resting-state functional MRI study. Neuroimage. 2007;35(2):488–500.
106. Petrella JR, Wang L, Krishnan S, et al. Cortical deactivation in mild cognitive impairment: high-field-strength functional MR imaging. Radiology. 2007; 245(1):224–35.
107. Buckner RL, Snyder AZ, Shannon BJ, et al. Molecular, structural, and functional characterization of Alzheimer's disease: evidence for a relationship between default activity, amyloid, and memory. J Neurosci. 2005;25(34):7709–17.
108. Mintun MA, Larossa GN, Sheline YI, et al. [11C] PIB in a nondemented population: potential antecedent marker of Alzheimer disease. Neurology. 2006; 67(3):446–52.
109. Forsberg A, Engler H, Almkvist O, et al. PET imaging of amyloid deposition in patients with mild cognitive impairment. Neurobiol Aging. 2008;29(10): 1456–65.
110. Minoshima S, Giordani B, Berent S, Frey KA, Foster NL, Kuhl DE. Metabolic reduction in the posterior cingulate cortex in very early Alzheimer's disease. Ann Neurol. 1997;42(1):85–94.
111. Nestor PJ, Fryer TD, Smielewski P, Hodges JR. Limbic hypometabolism in Alzheimer's disease and mild cognitive impairment. Ann Neurol. 2003; 54(3):343–51.
112. Gould RL, Brown RG, Owen AM, Bullmore ET, Howard RJ. Task-induced deactivations during suc-

cessful paired associates learning: an effect of age but not Alzheimer's disease. Neuroimage. 2006; 31(2):818–31.
113. Grady CL, Springer MV, Hongwanishkul D, McIntosh AR, Winocur G. Age-related changes in brain activity across the adult lifespan. J Cogn Neurosci. 2006;18(2):227–41.
114. Daselaar SM, Prince SE, Cabeza R. When less means more: deactivations during encoding that predict subsequent memory. Neuroimage. 2004;23(3): 921–7.
115. Bertram L, McQueen MB, Mullin K, Blacker D, Tanzi RE. Systematic meta-analyses of Alzheimer disease genetic association studies: the AlzGene database. Nat Genet. 2007;39(1):17–23.
116. Saunders AM, Strittmatter WJ, Schmechel D, et al. Association of apolipoprotein E allele epsilon 4 with late-onset familial and sporadic Alzheimer's disease. Neurology. 1993;43(8):1467–72.
117. Small GW, Mazziotta JC, Collins MT, et al. Apolipoprotein E type 4 allele and cerebral glucose metabolism in relatives at risk for familial Alzheimer disease. JAMA. 1995;273(12):942–7.
118. Reiman EM, Caselli RJ, Yun LS, et al. Preclinical evidence of Alzheimer's disease in persons homozygous for the epsilon 4 allele for apolipoprotein E. N Engl J Med. 1996;334(12):752–8.
119. Suthana NA, Krupa A, Donix M, et al. Reduced hippocampal CA2, CA3, and dentate gyrus activity in asymptomatic people at genetic risk for Alzheimer's disease. Neuroimage. 2010;53(3):1077–84.
120. Dennis NA, Browndyke JN, Stokes J, et al. Temporal lobe functional activity and connectivity in young adult APOE varepsilon4 carriers. Alzheimers Dement. 2010;6:303–11.
121. Bookheimer SY, Strojwas MH, Cohen MS, et al. Patterns of brain activation in people at risk for Alzheimer's disease. N Engl J Med. 2000;343(7): 450–6.
122. Burggren AC, Small GW, Sabb FW, Bookheimer SY. Specificity of brain activation patterns in people at genetic risk for Alzheimer disease. Am J Geriatr Psychiatry. 2002;10(1):44–51.
123. Smith CD, Andersen AH, Kryscio RJ, et al. Women at risk for AD show increased parietal activation during a fluency task. Neurology. 2002;58(8):1197–202.
124. Bondi MW, Houston WS, Eyler LT, Brown GG. fMRI evidence of compensatory mechanisms in older adults at genetic risk for Alzheimer disease. Neurology. 2005;64(3):501–8.
125. Fleisher AS, Houston WS, Eyler LT, et al. Identification of Alzheimer disease risk by functional magnetic resonance imaging. Arch Neurol. 2005;62(12):1881–8.
126. Wishart HA, Saykin AJ, Rabin LA, et al. Increased brain activation during working memory in cognitively intact adults with the APOE epsilon4 allele. Am J Psychiatry. 2006;163(9):1603–10.
127. Han SD, Houston WS, Jak AJ, et al. Verbal paired-associate learning by APOE genotype in non-demented older adults: fMRI evidence of a right hemispheric compensatory response. Neurobiol Aging. 2007;28(2):238–47.
128. Smith CD, Andersen AH, Kryscio RJ, et al. Altered brain activation in cognitively intact individuals at high risk for Alzheimer's disease. Neurology. 1999;53(7):1391–6.
129. Lind J, Persson J, Ingvar M, et al. Reduced functional brain activity response in cognitively intact apolipoprotein E epsilon4 carriers. Brain. 2006; 129(Pt 5):1240–8.
130. Trivedi MA, Schmitz TW, Ries ML, et al. Reduced hippocampal activation during episodic encoding in middle-aged individuals at genetic risk of Alzheimer's disease: a cross-sectional study. BMC Med. 2006;4:1.
131. Borghesani PR, Johnson LC, Shelton AL, et al. Altered medial temporal lobe responses during visuospatial encoding in healthy APOE*4 carriers. Neurobiol Aging. 2008;29(7):981–91.
132. Bassett SS, Yousem DM, Cristinzio C, et al. Familial risk for Alzheimer's disease alters fMRI activation patterns. Brain. 2006;129(Pt 5):1229–39.
133. Fleisher AS, Podraza KM, Bangen KJ, et al. Cerebral perfusion and oxygenation differences in Alzheimer's disease risk. Neurobiol Aging. 2009; 30(11):1737–48.
134. Sperling R, Greve D, Dale A, et al. Functional MRI detection of pharmacologically induced memory impairment. Proc Natl Acad Sci U S A. 2002; 99(1):455–60.
135. Bentley P, Driver J, Dolan RJ. Cholinesterase inhibition modulates visual and attentional brain responses in Alzheimer's disease and health. Brain. 2008;131(Pt 2):409–24.
136. Kaduszkiewicz H, Zimmermann T, Beck-Bornholdt HP, van den Bussche H. Cholinesterase inhibitors for patients with Alzheimer's disease: systematic review of randomised clinical trials. BMJ. 2005;331(7512):321–7.
137. McShane R, Areosa Sastre A, Minakaran N. Memantine for dementia. Cochrane Database Syst Rev 2006;(2):CD003154.
138. Saykin AJ, Wishart HA, Rabin LA, et al. Cholinergic enhancement of frontal lobe activity in mild cognitive impairment. Brain. 2004;127(Pt 7):1574–83.
139. Kircher TT, Erb M, Grodd W, Leube DT. Cortical activation during cholinesterase-inhibitor treatment in Alzheimer disease: preliminary findings from a pharmaco-fMRI study. Am J Geriatr Psychiatry. 2005;13(11):1006–13.
140. Goekoop R, Rombouts SA, Jonker C, et al. Challenging the cholinergic system in mild cognitive impairment: a pharmacological fMRI study. Neuroimage. 2004;23(4):1450–9.
141. Goekoop R, Scheltens P, Barkhof F, Rombouts SA. Cholinergic challenge in Alzheimer patients and mild cognitive impairment differentially affects hippocampal activation – a pharmacological fMRI study. Brain. 2006;129(Pt 1):141–57.

142. Grön G, Brandenburg I, Wunderlich AP, Riepe MW. Inhibition of hippocampal function in mild cognitive impairment: targeting the cholinergic hypothesis. Neurobiol Aging. 2006;27(1):78–87.
143. Shanks MF, McGeown WJ, Forbes-McKay KE, Waiter GD, Ries M, Venneri A. Regional brain activity after prolonged cholinergic enhancement in early Alzheimer's disease. Magn Reson Imaging. 2007; 25(6):848–59.
144. Rombouts SA, Barkhof F, Van Meel CS, Scheltens P. Alterations in brain activation during cholinergic enhancement with rivastigmine in Alzheimer's disease. J Neurol Neurosurg Psychiatry. 2002;73(6): 665–71.
145. Pihlajamäki M, Sperling RA. fMRI: use in early Alzheimer's disease and in clinical trials. Future Neurol. 2008;3(4):409–21.
146. Machielsen WC, Rombouts SA, Barkhof F, Scheltens P, Witter MP. FMRI of visual encoding: reproducibility of activation. Hum Brain Mapp. 2000;9(3):156–64.
147. Diamond EL, Miller S, Dickerson BC, et al. Relationship of fMRI activation to clinical trial memory measures in Alzheimer disease. Neurology. 2007;69(13):1331–41.
148. Johnson SC, Saykin AJ, Flashman LA, McAllister TW, Sparling MB. Brain activation on fMRI and verbal memory ability: functional neuroanatomic correlates of CVLT performance. J Int Neuropsychol Soc. 2001;7(1):55–62.
149. Mondadori CR, Buchmann A, Mustovic H, et al. Enhanced brain activity may precede the diagnosis of Alzheimer's disease by 30 years. Brain. 2006;129(Pt 11):2908–22.
150. Braskie MN, Small GW, Bookheimer SY. Entorhinal cortex structure and functional MRI response during an associative verbal memory task. Hum Brain Mapp. 2009;30(12):3981–92.
151. Hodges JR, Davies RR, Xuereb JH, et al. Clinicopathological correlates in frontotemporal dementia. Ann Neurol. 2004;56(3):399–406.
152. McKhann GM, Albert MS, Grossman M, et al. Clinical and pathological diagnosis of frontotemporal dementia: report of the Work Group on Frontotemporal Dementia and Pick's Disease. Arch Neurol. 2001;58(11):1803–9.
153. Mott RT, Dickson DW, Trojanowski JQ, et al. Neuropathologic, biochemical, and molecular characterization of the frontotemporal dementias. J Neuropathol Exp Neurol. 2005;64(5):420–8.
154. Kertesz A, Munoz DG. Frontotemporal dementia. Med Clin North Am. 2002;86(3):501–18. vi.
155. Forman MS, Farmer J, Johnson JK, et al. Frontotemporal dementia: clinicopathological correlations. Ann Neurol. 2006;59(6):952–62.
156. Josephs KA, Petersen RC, Knopman DS, et al. Clinicopathologic analysis of frontotemporal and corticobasal degenerations and PSP. Neurology. 2006;66(1):41–8.
157. Mendez MF, Lauterbach EC, Sampson SM. An evidence-based review of the psychopathology of frontotemporal dementia: a report of the ANPA Committee on Research. J Neuropsychiatry Clin Neurosci. 2008;20(2):130–49.
158. Johnson JK, Diehl J, Mendez MF, et al. Frontotemporal lobar degeneration: demographic characteristics of 353 patients. Arch Neurol. 2005; 62(6):925–30.
159. Mendez MF, Selwood A, Mastri AR, Frey 2nd WH. Pick's disease versus Alzheimer's disease: a comparison of clinical characteristics. Neurology. 1993;43(2):289–92.
160. Pasquier F, Delacourte A. Non-Alzheimer degenerative dementias. Curr Opin Neurol. 1998;11(5): 417–27.
161. The Lund and Manchester Groups. Clinical and neuropathological criteria for frontotemporal dementia. J Neurol Neurosurg Psychiatry. 1994;57(4):416–8.
162. Ratnavalli E, Brayne C, Dawson K, Hodges JR. The prevalence of frontotemporal dementia. Neurology. 2002;58(11):1615–21.
163. Robert PH, Lafont V, Snowden JS, Lebert F. Diagnostic criteria for fronto-temporal lobe degeneration. Encephale. 1999;25(6):612–21.
164. Mychack P, Kramer JH, Boone KB, Miller BL. The influence of right frontotemporal dysfunction on social behavior in frontotemporal dementia. Neurology. 2001;56(11 Suppl 4):S11–5.
165. Edwards-Lee T, Miller BL, Benson DF, et al. The temporal variant of frontotemporal dementia. Brain. 1997;120(Pt 6):1027–40.
166. Liu W, Miller BL, Kramer JH, et al. Behavioral disorders in the frontal and temporal variants of frontotemporal dementia. Neurology. 2004;62(5):742–8.
167. Miller BL, Cummings J, Mishkin F, et al. Emergence of artistic talent in frontotemporal dementia. Neurology. 1998;51(4):978–82.
168. Rankin KP, Kramer JH, Mychack P, Miller BL. Double dissociation of social functioning in frontotemporal dementia. Neurology. 2003;60(2):266–71.
169. Rosen HJ, Hartikainen KM, Jagust W, et al. Utility of clinical criteria in differentiating frontotemporal lobar degeneration (FTLD) from AD. Neurology. 2002;58(11):1608–15.
170. Berthoz S, Armony JL, Blair RJ, Dolan RJ. An fMRI study of intentional and unintentional (embarrassing) violations of social norms. Brain. 2002;125(Pt 8):1696–708.
171. Rombouts SA, van Swieten JC, Pijnenburg YA, Goekoop R, Barkhof F, Scheltens P. Loss of frontal fMRI activation in early frontotemporal dementia compared to early AD. Neurology. 2003;60(12): 1904–8.
172. Werner KH, Roberts NA, Rosen HJ, et al. Emotional reactivity and emotion recognition in frontotemporal lobar degeneration. Neurology. 2007;69(2):148–55.
173. Whitehouse PJ, Sciulli CG, Mason RM. Dementia drug development: use of information systems to

harmonize global drug development. Psychopharmacol Bull. 1997;33(1):129–33.

174. Braskie MN, Small GW, Bookheimer SY. Vascular health risks and fMRI activation during a memory task in older adults. Neurobiol Aging. 2010;31(9):1532–42. Epub 2008 Oct 1.

175. Haley AP, Sweet LH, Gunstad J, et al. Verbal working memory and atherosclerosis in patients with cardiovascular disease: an fMRI study. J Neuroimaging. 2007;17(3):227–33.

176. Snijders AH, van de Warrenburg BP, Giladi N, Bloem BR. Neurological gait disorders in elderly people: clinical approach and classification. Lancet Neurol. 2007;6(1):63–74.

177. Adams RD, Fisher CM, Hakim S, Ojemann RG, Sweet WH. Symptomatic occult hydrocephalus with "normal" cerebrospinal-fluid pressure. A treatable syndrome. N Engl J Med. 1965;273:117–26.

178. Tullberg M, Hultin L, Ekholm S, Månsson JE, Fredman P, Wikkelsø C. White matter changes in normal pressure hydrocephalus and Binswanger disease: specificity, predictive value and correlations to axonal degeneration and demyelination. Acta Neurol Scand. 2002;105(6):417–26.

179. Malm J, Eklund A. Idiopathic normal pressure hydrocephalus. Pract Neurol. 2006;6(1):14–27.

180. Malm J, Kristensen B, Stegmayr B, Fagerlund M, Koskinen LO. Three-year survival and functional outcome of patients with idiopathic adult hydrocephalus syndrome. Neurology. 2000;55(4):576–8.

181. Lenfeldt N, Larsson A, Nyberg L, et al. Idiopathic normal pressure hydrocephalus: increased supplementary motor activity accounts for improvement after CSF drainage. Brain. 2008;131(Pt 11):2904–12.

182. McNaught KS, Olanow CW. Protein aggregation in the pathogenesis of familial and sporadic Parkinson's disease. Neurobiol Aging. 2006;27(4):530–45.

183. Miyasaki JM, Shannon K, Voon V, et al. Practice Parameter: evaluation and treatment of depression, psychosis, and dementia in Parkinson disease (an evidence-based review): report of the Quality Standards Subcommittee of the American Academy of Neurology. Neurology. 2006;66(7):996–1002.

184. Rao SS, Hofmann LA, Shakil A. Parkinson's disease: diagnosis and treatment. Am Fam Physician. 2006;74(12):2046–54.

185. Leibson CL, Long KH, Maraganore DM, et al. Direct medical costs associated with Parkinson's disease: a population-based study. Mov Disord. 2006;21(11):1864–71.

186. Chaudhuri KR, Healy DG, Schapira AH. Non-motor symptoms of Parkinson's disease: diagnosis and management. Lancet Neurol. 2006;5(3):235–45.

187. Poewe W. The natural history of Parkinson's disease. J Neurol. 2006;253 Suppl 7:VII2–6.

188. Dowding CH, Shenton CL, Salek SS. A review of the health-related quality of life and economic impact of Parkinson's disease. Drugs Aging. 2006; 23(9):693–721.

189. Huse DM, Schulman K, Orsini L, Castelli-Haley J, Kennedy S, Lenhart G. Burden of illness in Parkinson's disease. Mov Disord. 2005;20(11): 1449–54.

190. Weintraub D, Comella CL, Horn S. Parkinson's disease – Part 1: pathophysiology, symptoms, burden, diagnosis, and assessment. Am J Manag Care. 2008;14(2 Suppl):S40–8.

191. Pallone JA. Introduction to Parkinson's disease. Dis Mon. 2007;53(4):195–9.

192. Jenner P, Olanow CW. The pathogenesis of cell death in Parkinson's disease. Neurology. 2006;66(10 Suppl 4):S24–36.

193. Alexander GE, DeLong MR, Strick PL. Parallel organization of functionally segregated circuits linking basal ganglia and cortex. Annu Rev Neurosci. 1986;9:357–81.

194. Haber SN, Fudge JL, McFarland NR. Striatonigrostriatal pathways in primates form an ascending spiral from the shell to the dorsolateral striatum. J Neurosci. 2000;20(6):2369–82.

195. Parent A. Extrinsic connections of the basal ganglia. Trends Neurosci. 1990;13(7):254–8.

196. Dagher A, Nagano-Saito A. Functional and anatomical magnetic resonance imaging in Parkinson's disease. Mol Imaging Biol. 2007;9(4):234–42.

197. Fearnley JM, Lees AJ. Ageing and Parkinson's disease: substantia nigra regional selectivity. Brain. 1991;114(Pt 5):2283–301.

198. Haslinger B, Erhard P, Kämpfe N, et al. Event-related functional magnetic resonance imaging in Parkinson's disease before and after levodopa. Brain. 2001;124(Pt 3):558–70.

199. Sabatini U, Boulanouar K, Fabre N, et al. Cortical motor reorganization in akinetic patients with Parkinson's disease: a functional MRI study. Brain. 2000;123(Pt 2):394–403.

200. Buhmann C, Glauche V, Stürenburg HJ, Oechsner M, Weiller C, Büchel C. Pharmacologically modulated fMRI – cortical responsiveness to levodopa in drug-naive hemiparkinsonian patients. Brain. 2003; 126(Pt 2):451–61.

201. Rowe J, Stephan KE, Friston K, Frackowiak R, Lees A, Passingham R. Attention to action in Parkinson's disease: impaired effective connectivity among frontal cortical regions. Brain. 2002;125(Pt 2):276–89.

202. Dirnberger G, Frith CD, Jahanshahi M. Executive dysfunction in Parkinson's disease is associated with altered pallidal-frontal processing. Neuroimage. 2005;25(2):588–99.

203. Middleton FA, Strick PL. Basal ganglia and cerebellar loops: motor and cognitive circuits. Brain Res Brain Res Rev. 2000;31(2–3):236–50.

204. van Nuenen BF, van Eimeren T, van der Vegt JP, et al. Mapping preclinical compensation in Parkinson's disease: an imaging genomics approach. Mov Disord. 2009;24 Suppl 2:S703–10.

205. Thobois S, Dominey P, Decety J, Pollak P, Gregoire MC, Broussolle E. Overactivation of primary motor cortex is asymmetrical in hemiparkinsonian patients. Neuroreport. 2000;11(4):785–9.

206. Palmer SJ, Ng B, Abugharbieh R, Eigenraam L, McKeown MJ. Motor reserve and novel area

recruitment: amplitude and spatial characteristics of compensation in Parkinson's disease. Eur J Neurosci. 2009;29(11):2187–96.

207. Peters S, Suchan B, Rusin J, et al. Apomorphine reduces BOLD signal in fMRI during voluntary movement in Parkinsonian patients. Neuroreport. 2003;14(6):809–12.
208. Wu T, Chan P, Hallett M. Effective connectivity of neural networks in automatic movements in Parkinson's disease. Neuroimage. 2010;49(3):2581–7. Epub 2009 Oct 22.
209 Wu T, Wang L, Chen Y, Zhao C, Li K, Chan P. Changes of functional connectivity of the motor network in the resting state in Parkinson's disease. Neurosci Lett. 2009;460(1):6–10.
210. Palmer SJ, Eigenraam L, Hoque T, McCaig RG, Troiano A, McKeown MJ. Levodopa-sensitive, dynamic changes in effective connectivity during simultaneous movements in Parkinson's disease. Neuroscience. 2009;158(2):693–704.
211. Kraft E, Loichinger W, Diepers M, et al. Levodopa-induced striatal activation in Parkinson's disease: a functional MRI study. Parkinsonism Relat Disord. 2009;15(8):558–63.
212. Hesselmann V, Sorger B, Girnus R, et al. Intraoperative functional MRI as a new approach to monitor deep brain stimulation in Parkinson's disease. Eur Radiol. 2004;14(4):686–90.
213. Phillips MD, Baker KB, Lowe MJ, et al. Parkinson disease: pattern of functional MR imaging activation during deep brain stimulation of subthalamic nucleus – initial experience. Radiology. 2006;239(1): 209–16.
214. Stefurak T, Mikulis D, Mayberg H, et al. Deep brain stimulation for Parkinson's disease dissociates mood and motor circuits: a functional MRI case study. Mov Disord. 2003;18(12):1508–16.
215. Schrag A, Jahanshahi M, Quinn N. What contributes to quality of life in patients with Parkinson's disease? J Neurol Neurosurg Psychiatry. 2000;69(3): 308–12.
216. Weintraub D, Moberg PJ, Duda JE, Katz IR, Stern MB. Effect of psychiatric and other nonmotor symptoms on disability in Parkinson's disease. J Am Geriatr Soc. 2004;52(5):784–8.
217. Owen AM, James M, Leigh PN, et al. Fronto-striatal cognitive deficits at different stages of Parkinson's disease. Brain. 1992;115(Pt 6):1727–51.
218. Aarsland D, Andersen K, Larsen JP, Lolk A, Nielsen H, Kragh-Sørensen P. Risk of dementia in Parkinson's disease: a community-based, prospective study. Neurology. 2001;56(6):730–6.
219. Monchi O, Petrides M, Petre V, Worsley K, Dagher A. Wisconsin Card Sorting revisited: distinct neural circuits participating in different stages of the task identified by event-related functional magnetic resonance imaging. J Neurosci. 2001;21(19):7733–41.
220. Dagher A, Owen AM, Boecker H, Brooks DJ. Mapping the network for planning: a correlational PET activation study with the Tower of London task. Brain. 1999;122(Pt 10):1973–87.
221. Lewis SJ, Dove A, Robbins TW, Barker RA, Owen AM. Cognitive impairments in early Parkinson's disease are accompanied by reductions in activity in frontostriatal neural circuitry. J Neurosci. 2003; 23(15):6351–6.
222. Mattay VS, Tessitore A, Callicott JH, et al. Dopaminergic modulation of cortical function in patients with Parkinson's disease. Ann Neurol. 2002;51(2):156–64.
223. Sawaguchi T, Matsumura M, Kubota K. Catecholaminergic effects on neuronal activity related to a delayed response task in monkey prefrontal cortex. J Neurophysiol. 1990;63(6):1385–400.
224. Mink JW. The basal ganglia: focused selection and inhibition of competing motor programs. Prog Neurobiol. 1996;50(4):381–425.
225. Jubault T, Monetta L, Strafella AP, Lafontaine AL, Monchi O. L-dopa medication in Parkinson's disease restores activity in the motor cortico-striatal loop but does not modify the cognitive network. PLoS One. 2009;4(7):e6154.
226. Cools R, Lewis SJ, Clark L, Barker RA, Robbins TW. L-DOPA disrupts activity in the nucleus accumbens during reversal learning in Parkinson's disease. Neuropsychopharmacology. 2007;32(1):180–9.
227. Kish SJ, Shannak K, Hornykiewicz O. Uneven pattern of dopamine loss in the striatum of patients with idiopathic Parkinson's disease. Pathophysiologic and clinical implications. N Engl J Med. 1988; 318(14):876–80.
228. Gotham AM, Brown RG, Marsden CD. 'Frontal' cognitive function in patients with Parkinson's disease 'on' and 'off' levodopa. Brain. 1988;111(Pt 2):299–321.
229. Monchi O, Petrides M, Doyon J, Postuma RB, Worsley K, Dagher A. Neural bases of set-shifting deficits in Parkinson's disease. J Neurosci. 2004; 24(3):702–10.
230. Monchi O, Petrides M, Mejia-Constain B, Strafella AP. Cortical activity in Parkinson's disease during executive processing depends on striatal involvement. Brain. 2007;130(Pt 1):233–44.
231. Grossman M, Cooke A, DeVita C, et al. Grammatical and resource components of sentence processing in Parkinson's disease: an fMRI study. Neurology. 2003;60(5):775–81.
232. Barnes J, David AS. Visual hallucinations in Parkinson's disease: a review and phenomenological survey. J Neurol Neurosurg Psychiatry. 2001;70(6): 727–33.
233. Meppelink AM, de Jong BM, Renken R, Leenders KL, Cornelissen FW, van Laar T. Impaired visual processing preceding image recognition in Parkinson's disease patients with visual hallucinations. Brain. 2008;132(Pt 11):2980–93.
234. Ramírez-Ruiz B, Martí MJ, Tolosa E, et al. Brain response to complex visual stimuli in Parkinson's patients with hallucinations: a functional magnetic resonance imaging study. Mov Disord. 2009;23(16): 2335–43.
235. Welge-Lüssen A, Wattendorf E, Schwerdtfeger U, et al. Olfactory-induced brain activity in Parkinson's

disease relates to the expression of event-related potentials: a functional magnetic resonance imaging study. Neuroscience. 2009;162(2):537–43.

236. Westermann B, Wattendorf E, Schwerdtfeger U, et al. Functional imaging of the cerebral olfactory system in patients with Parkinson's disease. J Neurol Neurosurg Psychiatry. 2008;79(1):19–24.
237. Sen S, Kawaguchi A, Truong Y, Lewis MM, Huang X. Dynamic changes in cerebello-thalamo-cortical motor circuitry during progression of Parkinson's disease. Neuroscience. 2010;166(2):712–9. Epub 2009 Dec 24.
238. Péran P, Cardebat D, Cherubini A, et al. Object naming and action-verb generation in Parkinson's disease: a fMRI study. Cortex. 2009;45(8):960–71.
239. Cardoso EF, Maia FM, Fregni F, et al. Depression in Parkinson's disease: convergence from voxel-based morphometry and functional magnetic resonance imaging in the limbic thalamus. Neuroimage. 2009;47(2):467–72.
240. Williams-Gray CH, Hampshire A, Barker RA, Owen AM. Attentional control in Parkinson's disease is dependent on COMT val 158 met genotype. Brain. 2008;131(Pt 2):397–408.
241. Tinaz S, Schendan HE, Stern CE. Fronto-striatal deficit in Parkinson's disease during semantic event sequencing. Neurobiol Aging. 2008;29(3):397–407.
242. Rowe JB, Hughes L, Ghosh BC, et al. Parkinson's disease and dopaminergic therapy – differential effects on movement, reward and cognition. Brain. 2008;131(Pt 8):2094–105.
243. Gusella JF, McNeil S, Persichetti F, et al. Huntington's disease. Cold Spring Harb Symp Quant Biol. 1996;61:615–26.
244. The Huntington's Disease Collaborative Research Group. A novel gene containing a trinucleotide repeat that is expanded and unstable on Huntington's disease chromosomes. Cell. 1993;72(6):971–83.
245. Duyao M, Ambrose C, Myers R, et al. Trinucleotide repeat length instability and age of onset in Huntington's disease. Nat Genet. 1993;4(4):387–92.
246. Gutekunst CA, Li SH, Yi H, et al. Nuclear and neuropil aggregates in Huntington's disease: relationship to neuropathology. J Neurosci. 1999;19(7):2522–34.
247. Vonsattel JP, DiFiglia M. Huntington disease. J Neuropathol Exp Neurol. 1998;57(5):369–84.
248. Myers RH, Sax DS, Koroshetz WJ, et al. Factors associated with slow progression in Huntington's disease. Arch Neurol. 1991;48(8):800–4.
249. Rosas HD, Salat DH, Lee SY, et al. Cerebral cortex and the clinical expression of Huntington's disease: complexity and heterogeneity. Brain. 2008;131(Pt 4):1057–68.
250. Sax DS, O'Donnell B, Butters N, Menzer L, Montgomery K, Kayne HL. Computed tomographic, neurologic, and neuropsychological correlates of Huntington's disease. Int J Neurosci. 1983;18(1–2):21–36.
251. Starkstein SE, Brandt J, Folstein S, et al. Neuropsychological and neuroradiological correlates in Huntington's disease. J Neurol Neurosurg Psychiatry. 1988;51(10):1259–63.
252. Starkstein SE, Brandt J, Bylsma F, Peyser C, Folstein M, Folstein SE. Neuropsychological correlates of brain atrophy in Huntington's disease: a magnetic resonance imaging study. Neuroradiology. 1992;34(6):487–9.
253. Aylward EH, Li Q, Stine OC, Ranen N, et al. Longitudinal change in basal ganglia volume in patients with Huntington's disease. Neurology. 1997;48(2):394–9.
254. Rosas HD, Goodman J, Chen YI, et al. Striatal volume loss in HD as measured by MRI and the influence of CAG repeat. Neurology. 2001;57(6):1025–8.
255. Aylward EH, Codori AM, Barta PE, Pearlson GD, Harris GJ, Brandt J. Basal ganglia volume and proximity to onset in presymptomatic Huntington disease. Arch Neurol. 1996;53(12):1293–6.
256. Paulsen JS, Langbehn DR, Stout JC, et al. Detection of Huntington's disease decades before diagnosis: the Predict-HD study. J Neurol Neurosurg Psychiatry. 2008;79(8):874–80.
257. Paulsen JS. Functional imaging in Huntington's disease. Exp Neurol. 2009;216(2):272–7.
258. Clark VP, Lai S, Deckel AW. Altered functional MRI responses in Huntington's disease. Neuroreport. 2002;13(5):703–6.
259. Dierks T, Linden DE, Hertel A, et al. Multimodal imaging of residual function and compensatory resource allocation in cortical atrophy: a case study of parietal lobe function in a patient with Huntington's disease. Psychiatry Res. 1999;90(1):67–75.
260. Georgiou-Karistianis N, Sritharan A, Farrow M, et al. Increased cortical recruitment in Huntington's disease using a Simon task. Neuropsychologia. 2007;45(8):1791–800.
261. Thiruvady DR, Georgiou-Karistianis N, Egan GF, et al. Functional connectivity of the prefrontal cortex in Huntington's disease. J Neurol Neurosurg Psychiatry. 2007;78(2):127–33.
262. Kim JS, Reading SA, Brashers-Krug T, Calhoun VD, Ross CA, Pearlson GD. Functional MRI study of a serial reaction time task in Huntington's disease. Psychiatry Res. 2004;131(1):23–30.
263. Wolf RC, Sambataro F, Vasic N, Schönfeldt-Lecuona C, Ecker D, Landwehrmeyer B. Aberrant connectivity of lateral prefrontal networks in presymptomatic Huntington's disease. Exp Neurol. 2008;213(1):137–44.
264. Wolf RC, Vasic N, Schönfeldt-Lecuona C, Ecker D, Landwehrmeyer GB. Functional imaging of cognitive processes in Huntington's disease and its presymptomatic mutation carriers. Nervenarzt. 2008;79(4):408–20.
265. Paulsen JS, Zimbelman JL, Hinton SC, et al. fMRI biomarker of early neuronal dysfunction in presymptomatic Huntington's disease. AJNR Am J Neuroradiol. 2004;25(10):1715–21.
266. Reading SA, Dziorny AC, Peroutka LA, et al. Functional brain changes in presymptomatic

Huntington's disease. Ann Neurol. 2004;55(6):879–83.
267. Zimbelman JL, Paulsen JS, Mikos A, Reynolds NC, Hoffmann RG, Rao SM. fMRI detection of early neural dysfunction in preclinical Huntington's disease. J Int Neuropsychol Soc. 2007;13(5):758–69.
268. Wolf RC, Vasic N, Schönfeldt-Lecuona C, Landwehrmeyer GB, Ecker D. Dorsolateral prefrontal cortex dysfunction in presymptomatic Huntington's disease: evidence from event-related fMRI. Brain. 2007;130(Pt 11):2845–57.
269. Brooks BR, Bushara K, Khan A, et al. Functional magnetic resonance imaging (fMRI) clinical studies in ALS – paradigms, problems and promises. Amyotroph Lateral Scler Other Motor Neuron Disord. 2000;1 Suppl 2:S23–32.
270. Lule D, Ludolph AC, Kassubek J. MRI-based functional neuroimaging in ALS: an update. Amyotroph Lateral Scler. 2009;10(5–6):258–68.
271. Konrad C, Henningsen H, Bremer J, et al. Pattern of cortical reorganization in amyotrophic lateral sclerosis: a functional magnetic resonance imaging study. Exp Brain Res. 2002;143(1):51–6.
272. Han J, Ma L. Functional magnetic resonance imaging study of the brain in patients with amyotrophic lateral sclerosis. Chin Med Sci J. 2006;21(4):228–33.
273. Stanton BR, Williams VC, Leigh PN, et al. Altered cortical activation during a motor task in ALS. Evidence for involvement of central pathways. J Neurol. 2007;254(9):1260–7.
274. Schoenfeld MA, Tempelmann C, Gaul C, et al. Functional motor compensation in amyotrophic lateral sclerosis. J Neurol. 2005;252(8):944–52.
275. Weiller C, May A, Sach M, Buhmann C, Rijntjes M. Role of functional imaging in neurological disorders. J Magn Reson Imaging. 2006;23(6):840–50.
276. Kew JJ, Leigh PN, Playford ED, et al. Cortical function in amyotrophic lateral sclerosis. A positron emission tomography study. Brain. 1993;116(Pt 3):655–80.
277. Kew JJ, Brooks DJ, Passingham RE, Rothwell JC, Frackowiak RS, Leigh PN. Cortical function in progressive lower motor neuron disorders and amyotrophic lateral sclerosis: a comparative PET study. Neurology. 1994;44(6):1101–10.
278. Lulé D, Diekmann V, Kassubek J, et al. Cortical plasticity in amyotrophic lateral sclerosis: motor imagery and function. Neurorehabil Neural Repair. 2007;21(6):518–26.
279. Konrad C, Jansen A, Henningsen H, et al. Subcortical reorganization in amyotrophic lateral sclerosis. Exp Brain Res. 2006;172(3):361–9.
280. Stanton BR, Williams VC, Leigh PN, et al. Cortical activation during motor imagery is reduced in Amyotrophic Lateral Sclerosis. Brain Res. 2007;1172:145–51.
281. Tessitore A, Esposito F, Monsurrò MR, et al. Subcortical motor plasticity in patients with sporadic ALS: an fMRI study. Brain Res Bull. 2006;69(5):489–94.
282. Isaacs JD, Dean AF, Shaw CE, Al-Chalabi A, Mills KR, Leigh PN. Amyotrophic lateral sclerosis with sensory neuropathy: part of a multisystem disorder? J Neurol Neurosurg Psychiatry. 2007;78(7):750–3.
283. Mai R, Facchetti D, Micheli A, Poloni M. Quantitative electroencephalography in amyotrophic lateral sclerosis. Electroencephalogr Clin Neurophysiol. 1998;106(4):383–6.
284. Pugdahl K, Fuglsang-Frederiksen A, de Carvalho M, et al. Generalised sensory system abnormalities in amyotrophic lateral sclerosis: a European multicentre study. J Neurol Neurosurg Psychiatry. 2007;78(7):746–9.
285. Pekkonen E, Osipova D, Laaksovirta H. Magnetoencephalographic evidence of abnormal auditory processing in amyotrophic lateral sclerosis with bulbar signs. Clin Neurophysiol. 2004;115(2):309–15.
286. Münte TF, Tröger MC, Nusser I, et al. Alteration of early components of the visual evoked potential in amyotrophic lateral sclerosis. J Neurol. 1998;245(4):206–10.
287. Vieregge P, Wauschkuhn B, Heberlein I, Hagenah J, Verleger R. Selective attention is impaired in amyotrophic lateral sclerosis–a study of event-related EEG potentials. Brain Res Cogn Brain Res. 1999;8(1):27–35.
288. Pinkhardt EH, Jürgens R, Becker W, et al. Signs of impaired selective attention in patients with amyotrophic lateral sclerosis. J Neurol. 2008;255(4):532–8.
289. Ludolph AC, Langen KJ, Regard M, et al. Frontal lobe function in amyotrophic lateral sclerosis: a neuropsychologic and positron emission tomography study. Acta Neurol Scand. 1992;85(2):81–9.
290. Kew JJ, Goldstein LH, Leigh PN, et al. The relationship between abnormalities of cognitive function and cerebral activation in amyotrophic lateral sclerosis. A neuropsychological and positron emission tomography study. Brain. 1993;116(Pt 6):1399–423.
291. Abrahams S, Goldstein LH, Kew JJ, et al. Frontal lobe dysfunction in amyotrophic lateral sclerosis. A PET study. Brain. 1996;119(Pt 6):2105–20.
292. Abrahams S, Goldstein LH, Al-Chalabi A, et al. Relation between cognitive dysfunction and pseudobulbar palsy in amyotrophic lateral sclerosis. J Neurol Neurosurg Psychiatry. 1997;62(5):464–72.
293. Strong MJ, Grace GM, Orange JB, Leeper HA, Menon RS, Aere C. A prospective study of cognitive impairment in ALS. Neurology. 1999;53(8):1665–70.
294. Lomen-Hoerth C, Anderson T, Miller B. The overlap of amyotrophic lateral sclerosis and frontotemporal dementia. Neurology. 2002;59(7):1077–9.
295. Schreiber H, Gaigalat T, Wiedemuth-Catrinescu U, et al. Cognitive function in bulbar- and spinal-onset amyotrophic lateral sclerosis. A longitudinal study in 52 patients. J Neurol. 2005;252(7):772–81.

296. Piquard A, Le Forestier N, Baudoin-Madec V, et al. Neuropsychological changes in patients with primary lateral sclerosis. Amyotroph Lateral Scler. 2006;7(3):150–60.
297. Anzai E, Shiozawa Z, Shindo K, Tsunoda S, Koizumi K, Uchiyama G. 123I-iodoamphetamine single photon emission computed tomography in three patients with amyotrophic lateral sclerosis. Kaku Igaku. 1990;27(8):863–7.
298. Tanaka M, Kondo S, Hirai S, Sun X, Yamagishi T, Okamoto K. Cerebral blood flow and oxygen metabolism in progressive dementia associated with amyotrophic lateral sclerosis. J Neurol Sci. 1993;120(1): 22–8.
299. Abrahams S, Goldstein LH, Simmons A, et al. Word retrieval in amyotrophic lateral sclerosis: a functional magnetic resonance imaging study. Brain. 2004;127(Pt 7):1507–17.
300. Lulé D, Diekmann V, Anders S, et al. Brain responses to emotional stimuli in patients with amyotrophic lateral sclerosis (ALS). J Neurol. 2007;254(4): 519–27.

Applications of MRI to Psychopharmacology

19

Dan J. Stein, Yihong Yang, and Betty Jo Salmeron

Introduction

Pharmacological functional magnetic resonance (pharmacoMRI or phMRI) refers to the use of functional magnetic resonance imaging (fMRI) after administration of a psychotropic agent [1], but can be defined more broadly as the application of MRI methods to basic and clinical psychopharmacology questions. There has been significant growth in this field over the past decade, with a steady increase in published papers, perhaps attesting to the significant potential of phMRI for advancing psychopharmacological knowledge in important ways [2–9]. In this chapter, we begin by outlining some general issues in phMRI, outlining some of its advantages and limitations. We then go on to illustrate the potential value of phMRI by discussing both animal and clinical work.

D.J. Stein, MD, PhD
Department of Psychiatry and Mental Health, University of Cape Town, Groote Schuur Hospital (J-2), Anzio Road, Observatory, 7925 Cape Town, South Africa
e-mail: dan.stein@uct.ac.za

Y. Yang, PhD
FMRI Section, Neuroimaging Research Branch, National Institute on Drug Abuse, NIH, 251 Bayview Boulevard, Suite 200, Room 07A709, Baltimore, MD, 21224, USA
e-mail: yihongyang@mail.nih.gov

B.J. Salmeron, MD (✉)
Neuroimaging Research Branch, National Institute on Drug Abuse, NIH, 251 Bayview Boulevard, Suite 200, Room 07A717, Baltimore, MD, 21224, USA
e-mail: bsalmeron@mail.nih.gov

Background

Perhaps the earliest and best known application of functional brain imaging to psychopharmacological research is so-called molecular imaging [10], where positron emission tomography (PET) and single photon emission computed tomography (SPECT) radioligands allow the direct assessment of neuroreceptors, transporters, or enzymes. Although enormously valuable, molecular imaging has a number of important limitations, including exposure to radioactivity, dosimetry limitations, and relatively poor spatial and temporal resolution. The newer magnetic resonance imaging technologies provide a complementary set of tools for psychopharmacological investigation – they are not yet linked to investigation of single molecules, but they are noninvasive, can be used to study acute and chronic medication dosing, and have relatively high spatial and temporal resolution.

Typically, phMRI relies on blood-oxygen-level-dependent (BOLD) fMRI, with neuronal activation leading to a local increase in blood flow [11] and an uncoupled increase in oxidative metabolism [12], with subsequent decrease in deoxyhemoglobin concentration, greater local magnetic field homogeneity, and an increase in

S.H. Faro and F.B. Mohamed (eds.), *Functional BOLD MRI: Principles and Applications*, DOI 10.1007/978-1-4939-1995-6_19, © Springer Science+Business Media New York 2015

Table 19.1 Selected clinical studies using pharmacological MRI: acute drug effects (challenge phMRI)

Authors	Subjects	FMRI paradigm	Results
Breiter et al. 1997 [22]	17 cocaine-dependent subjects	Double-blind placebo-controlled cocaine injection (single dose, two sessions)	ʿsignal in multiple areas including VTA, NAcc, cingulate, frontal areas, hippocampus, and insula
Stein et al. 1998 [23]	16 healthy smokers	Saline and three doses of nicotine given 20 min apart in ascending order in cumulative dosing paradigm	Dose-related activation in NAcc, cingulate, amygdala, and frontal lobes
Risinger et al. 2005 [24]	Eight male cocaine-dependent subjects	IV cocaine self-administration with ratings of subjective effects	"High" correlated negatively with activity in limbic, paralimbic, and mesocortical regions while "Craving" correlated positively in same regions
Mckie et al. 2005 [25]	12 healthy adult males, 19–36 years old	Single-blind, placebo-controlled crossover study with 7.5 min IV injection of 7.5 mg citalopram in the middle of 22.5 min BOLD scan	Signal increases in caudate, amygdala, hippocampus, striatum, and thalamus
Rose et al. 2006 [26]	18 healthy adult males, 19–33 years old	Double-blind, placebo-controlled crossover DSC perfusion imaging 2 h after 20 mg oral d-amphetamine at 1.5 and 4 T	Widespread CBF increases, which were more significant at 4 T in amygdala and striatal structures
Kofke et al. 2007 [15]	27 healthy male and female adults, 20–30 years old, genotyped for ApoE4	CBF using pulsed ASL, global and in cortical and subcortical ROIs	Widespread dose-related CBF increases before $PaCO_2$ correction With $PaCO_2$ correction, ↑CBF in cingulate ↓CBF in hippocampus and amygdala; corrected changes absent with ApoE4
Addicott et al. 2009 [27]	45 low, moderate, and high caffeine users (25 female)	Gray matter CBF following placebo or 250 mg caffeine in abstinent or satiated state	In abstinence, high and moderate users had increased CBF. Acute caffeine reduced CBF

the MR signal [13]. However, other MRI methods are also possible. For example, perfusion imaging based on arterial spin labeling (ASL) may also be used to measure cerebral blood flow after administration of psychotropic agents [14–18], and superparamagnetic contrast agents may be used, particularly in animals, to detect cerebral blood volume changes accompanying changes in neuronal activity [1, 19, 20]. It may also be useful to draw a distinction between "challenge phMRI" – in which the focus is on direct alteration of the fMRI signal in response to a psychotropic or combination of psychotropics – and "modulatory phMRI" – where the emphasis is on investigating changes in fMRI during cognitive/affective paradigms after acute or chronic administration of such an agent [21] (see Table 19.1 for a summary of selected challenge phMRI studies [15, 22–27] and Table 19.2 for a summary of selected modulatory phMRI studies [28–40]). Both approaches can be used in healthy animals or humans, as well as in lesioned or diseased subjects.

A good deal has been written on the precise nature of the relationship of the BOLD signal to neuronal activity. Along these lines, a number of issues are particularly relevant for phMRI. First, although psychotropics can have a broad range of neuronal effects (e.g., both excitatory and inhibitory effects), the precise relationship of such effects to the BOLD signal remains a matter of some dispute [21, 41]. Nevertheless, it has been argued that the local field potential (LFP) reflecting neuronal input to a region is a better predictor of the BOLD signal than multiunit activity (MUA), which reflects the activity of the local neurons [42]. Indeed, phMRI has been used to contribute to the debate on the precise relationship between BOLD and neuronal activation. Rauch et al. [43] found that infusion into the visual cortex of a $5HT_{1A}$ agonist acting on efferent

Table 19.2 Selected clinical studies using pharmacological MRI: drug on task effects (modulatory phMRI)

Authors	Subjects	FMRI paradigm	Results
Levin et al. 1998 [30]	15 healthy adults	Photic stimulation before and after oral ETOH (n = 10) or placebo (n = 5)	33% ↓ in visual cortex activation after ETOH
Loubinoux et al. 1999 [35]	12 healthy right-handed adults (six male)	Auditorily paced sequential opposition of thumb and fingers before and after fenozolone or fluoxetine	Both drugs produced more focused activation in sensorimotor areas, greater involvement of posterior supplemental motor area and ↓ cerebellar activation
Furey et al. 2000 [28]	Seven healthy adults	Delayed face match-to-sample paradigm on tow occasions: i.v. bolus + drip physostigmine or saline prior to and during experiment	Physostigmine ↓ selectivity of extrastriate response, esp. during encoding; ↓ ventral extrastriate, ↓ prefrontal cortex during maintenance
Mattay et al. 2000 [31]	Ten healthy adults	no-back, 2-back, and 3-back WM task 2° after D-amph. or placebo	D-amph. ↓ activation in no-back, ↑ activation in 3-back, especially in those whose performance worsened
Seifritz et al. 2000 [32]	11 healthy adults	Two sessions: tone presented three times before and after oral ETOH or placebo	ETOH ↓ response to acoustic stimulation
Kimberg et al. 2001 [29]	11 healthy adults	Verbal 2-back WM, WCST, motor response task on and off bromocriptine	Bromocriptine generally reduced task-related activity in all three tasks
Sperling et al. 2002 [36]	Ten right-handed healthy male adults	Face-name associative encoding paradigm after scopolamine, lorazepam, or placebo (x2) (four sessions, total)	↓ extent and magnitude of activation in hippocampal, fusiform, and prefrontal regions after scopolamine or lorazepam
Thiel et al. 2002 [33]	47 healthy adults	Scopolamine, lorazepam, or placebo given prior to showing faces to subjects. Scanning in a face recognition paradigm followed	Scopolamine impaired priming and showed none of the repetition effects seen after placebo and lorazepam
Paulus et al. 2005 [37]	15 (6 female) healthy subjects, 18–39 years old	Double-blind, placebo-controlled crossover study of oral lorazepam (0.25 or 1.0 mg) 1 h before face recognition task	Dose-dependent attenuation of BOLD response in amygdala and insula but not medial prefrontal cortex
Vollm et al. 2006 [38]	45 healthy males, 18–45 years old	Double-blind, parallel groups design, 30 mg oral mirtazepine 3 h before fMRI study including go/no-go, reward/no-reward and loss/no-loss tasks	Mirtazepine-enhanced BOLD in R OFC during response inhibition and in bilateral parietal cortex during reward task
Norbury et al. 2007 [39]	24 healthy adults	Gender identification of covertly and overtly presented happy, fearful and neutral faces after 7 days of reboxetine or placebo	↓ R amygdala activation to covert fearful faces and ↓ R fusiform activation to covert happy faces under reboxetine
Wise et al. 2007 [34]	8 healthy male adults	Double-blind, placebo-controlled crossover study of 30 μg/kg IV midazolam before thermal pain conditioning experiment	Midazolam ↓ BOLD response to pain cue especially in insula with no effect on pain-related responses
Simmons et al. 2009 [40]	15 healthy subjects	Double-blind, placebo-controlled crossover study of effect of 21 days of 10 mg escitalopram on anticipation of aversive or pleasant images	Escitalopram ↓ mid-, post-insula activation to all anticipation and ↓ ACC and medial prefrontal activation during aversive anticipation

i.v. intravenous, *THC* tetrahydrocannabinol, *NAcc* nucleus accumbens, *VTA* ventral tegmental area, *ACC* anterior cingulate, *L* left, *R* right, *Post. Cing.* posterior cingulate, *WCST* Wisconsin card sorting task, *ETOH* ethanol, *WM* working memory, D-*amph.* dextro-amphetamine

neurons reduced MUA without affecting either LFP or BOLD activity. They concluded that the efferents of a neuronal network pose relatively little metabolic burden compared with the overall presynaptic and postsynaptic processing of incoming afferents.

Second, whatever the precise mechanisms are linking neuronal activation with regional cerebral

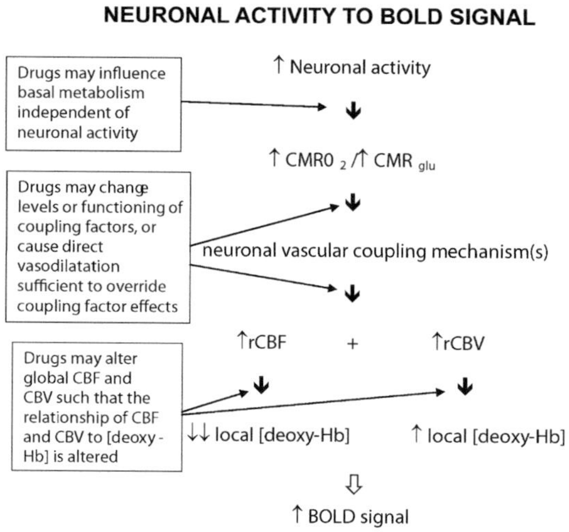

Fig. 19.1 Pharmacologic agents might alter the relationship of BOLD signal to neuronal activity independent of direct changes in neural activity at any point indicated by a *closed arrow*

blood flow (rCBF), it is possible that certain psychotropics or disorders may alter the nature of this neurovascular coupling (Fig. 19.1). Proposed mechanisms underlying such coupling include direct innervation of blood vessels by neurons or glial cells (the "neurogenic hypotheses") and/or the release of diffusible coupling factors by activated neurons or glial cells (the "metabolic hypotheses") [44]. Diffusible coupling factors may include metabolic byproducts and/or small molecules directly or indirectly involved in cell-signaling (whether ions or neurotransmitters). Psychotropics affecting these factors may alter the BOLD signal independent of changing neuronal activity [45]. Nevertheless, in many cases, psychotropic administration does not lead to a change in BOLD during performance of well-characterized tasks. Rao and colleagues, for example, found no change in BOLD response to a finger-tapping task after methylphenidate administration, suggesting that coupling mechanisms were not affected by this agent, and emphasizing the value of including a sensorimotor procedural control in phMRI studies [46].

Similarly, it is possible that certain psychotropic agents may alter global cerebral blood flow and blood volume, so affecting the BOLD signal [47–51]. This may be of particular concern with centrally acting agents that are also vasoactive such as cocaine. Gollub et al. [52], for example, demonstrated the possibility of using BOLD to examine activation under drug effect even when the drug alters central nervous system (CNS) perfusion. They found no significant difference in percentage BOLD signal change to visual stimulation after acute cocaine administration despite a modest decrease in global cerebral blood flow. An alternative approach to this issue was taken by Seifritz et al., modeling the change in BOLD due to alcohol-induced vasodilation and attributing the excess BOLD reduction to a direct neuronal effect of alcohol [32].

A special note about caffeine is warranted. Caffeine has cerebral vasoconstrictive actions, resulting in changes in the BOLD signal to other stimuli. Indeed, it has been suggested as a "contrast booster" in fMRI studies [53]. As caffeine is readily available and widely used, with varying effects depending on the baseline level of use [54], it is important to keep caffeine use in mind when conducting clinical studies. Some subject populations may use more caffeine than controls, thus skewing results. When comparing effects of a drug over time periods of days or more, subjects may use more caffeine while on drug to counter sedative side effects, thus introducing a systematic confound into the data. Careful attention to caffeine use in clinical studies is important.

In animal phMRI, with some exceptions [55–60], the bulk of research uses anesthetics, often $GABA_A$ receptor potentiators, again leading to questions about the precise nature of the BOLD signal, which is often altered in such paradigms [61–64]. In clinical phMRI, on the other hand, the use of particular tasks raises a range of methodological questions, with neuronal activation critically dependent on task parameters [5]. Since BOLD data is acquired in arbitrary units, analysis of task-induced activation relies on comparison with a control condition, making it difficult to determine if a change in activation following a drug manipulation is due to a change in the active task activation or in the control condition or both. ASL can provide a quantitative measure of blood flow changes to resolve such issues, but produces a less sensitive signal than BOLD, sometimes

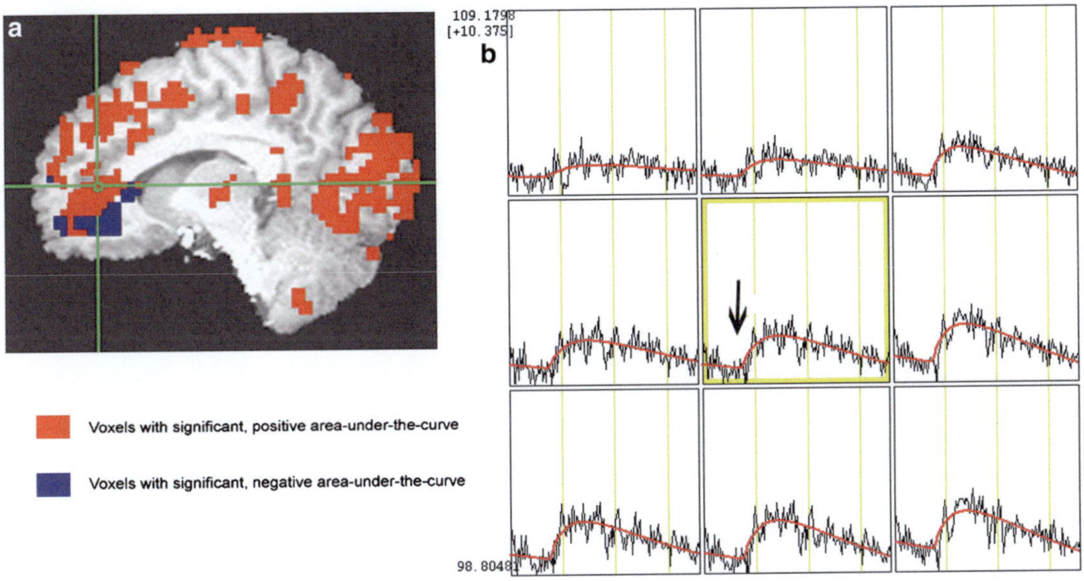

Fig. 19.2 Example of nonlinear regression model fitting of data gathered after an injection of nicotine. Data were fit using $Y_i = k[e^{-\alpha 1(ti-t0)} - e^{-\alpha 2(ti-t0)}]$, where Y_i = signal response at time t_i, $\alpha 1$ = elimination rate constant, $\alpha 2$ = absorption rate constant, $t0$ = time delay, and k = multiplicative constant. (**a**) Sagittal view showing voxels with a significant model fit. (**b**) Time series data from nine voxels centered on the crosshairs in (**a**) with the best model fit in each voxel overlaid on the data. *Arrow* indicates start of 30 s injection (unpublished data)

limiting interpretability. Careful cross-validation of fMRI measures of psychotropic action with direct measures of neuronal activity and histological changes in animals [19, 65, 66], and with electrophysiological and behavioral measures in humans [5, 67], is needed to understand how best to interpret the BOLD signal in a range of phMRI applications and is fortunately ongoing.

An additional set of methodological issues emerges from the question of how best to analyze phMRI data [21, 68]. At least three approaches are commonly used. First, given the pharmacokinetics of the administered drug, a model of the expected time course and pattern of BOLD signal increase can be applied to the data [69] (Fig. 19.2 illustrates an application of this method). However, in some cases, especially with oral administration, this time course may be too long and/or too variable to model in this way. Second, peripheral physiological or subjective psychological response to the drug can be used as regressors to model the effects of the drug in the brain. This is particularly useful in studying drugs of abuse, when the acute, subjective effect (i.e., the "high" or "rush") is of particular interest (Fig. 19.3). However, not all drugs have such effects (and indeed, the BOLD response is arguably more informative than behavioral effects as an indicator of psychobiological function [70]). Third, methods that analyze changes in BOLD signal over time can be used. This may involve comparison of averaged post- versus preinfusion scans, or more complex time series approaches [21, 22]. A similar post- versus pre-approach or drug versus placebo comparison can also be useful in evaluating the effects of drugs that emerge only after extended exposure, such as antidepressants and antipsychotics [71–73]. Finally, data-driven methods such as independent components analysis (ICA) (e.g., [74–77]) offer unique advantages in analyzing phMRI. ICA attempts to decompose data into spatially independent maps with associated time courses. While it can sometimes be difficult to identify which components are physiologically relevant, the method allows for identification of components with different time courses, whereas regression-based methods are more limited in this respect.

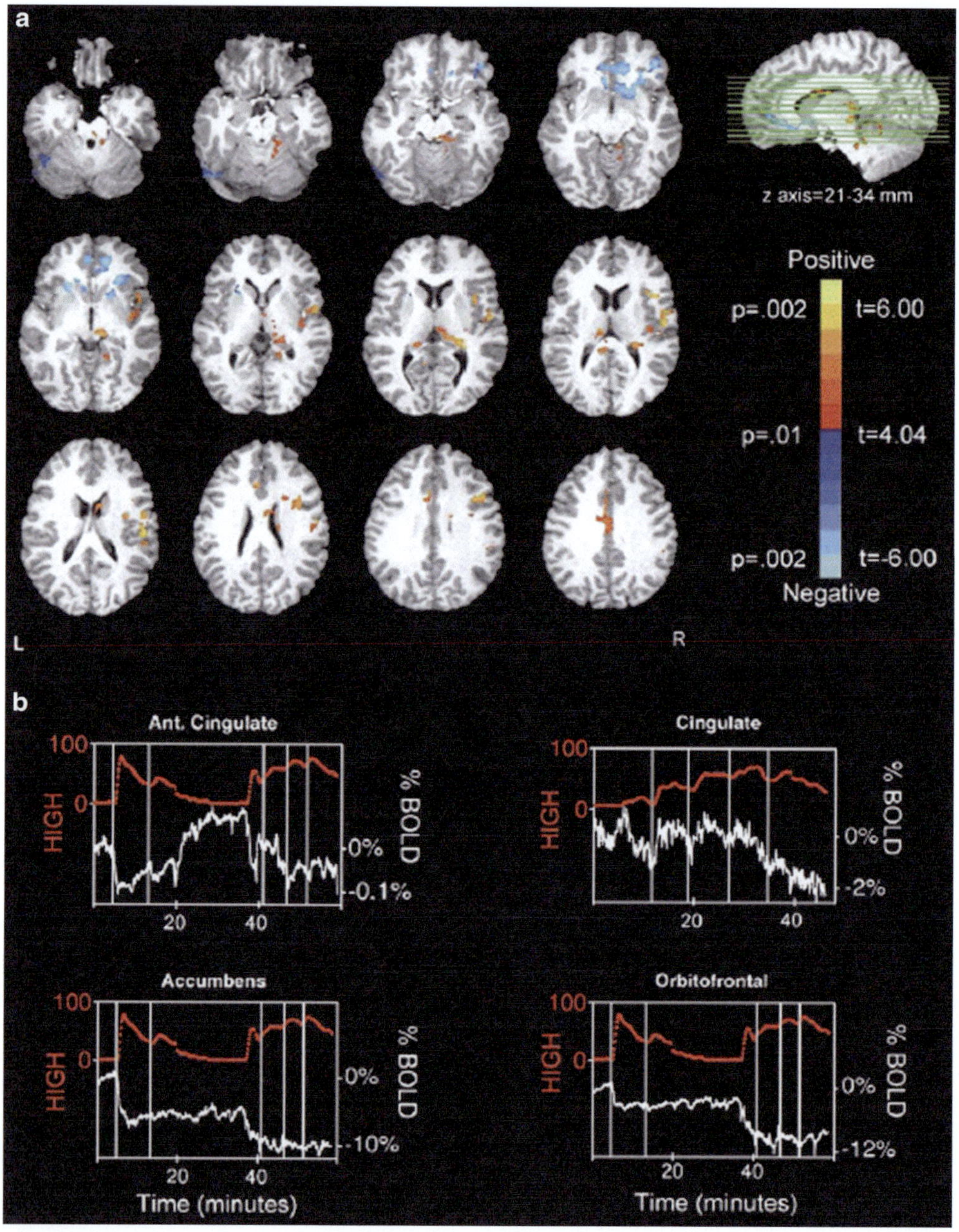

Fig. 19.3 Neural correlates of self-reported "high" during cocaine self-administration. (**a**) Regions of significant group correlation with VAS ratings of "high" (positive in *yellow*, negative in *blue*). (**b**) Plots of VAS ratings (*red tracing*) and % BOLD change averaged across the indicated ROI (*white tracing*) in selected subjects. *Vertical white lines* indicate injection events. Reprinted with permission from Risinger R C, Salmeron BJ, Ross TJ, et al. Neural correlates of high and craving during cocaine self-administration using BOLD fMRI. NeuroImage, 2005;26:1097–1108

In 2008, Dieler et al. illustrated the advantage of this approach for phMRI [78]. Applying tensorial probabilistic ICA to a placebo-controlled study of cholecystokinine-4-induced panic attacks, they identified increases in activity in 12 networks. These reproduced results obtained from a regression analysis, but also identified additional components with time courses related to the injection but not captured by the original regressors. Such approaches may allow for more complete exploration of the data and are not affected by erroneous assumptions about the neural response to the drug or the shape of the hemodynamic response function. Whichever approach is used, it is clearly important to emphasize that the signal from BOLD-fMRI measures relative rather than quantitative change and to consider whether changes after drug administration are due to observed neural changes and/or to the psychological effects of the drug or to cerebrovascular effects or both, employing experimental designs that include appropriate controls relevant to the psychopharmacological questions at hand [6]. As in other MRI analyses, it is also important to define regions of interest judiciously [79].

Animal Research

Much of our knowledge of psychopharmacology is based on preclinical or animal studies. Similarly, with the advent of small-bore magnetic resonance imaging machines, there is now the opportunity to undertake phMRI in animal investigations. An early set of rodent studies focused on the dopamine system, and was important in demonstrating that the BOLD-fMRI response to pharmacological stimulation with amphetamine, which increases synaptic dopamine, showed a tight coupling to regional distribution of dopamine transporters using PET, to the release of dopamine as studied using microdialysis, and to behavioral measures [1, 80, 81].

Although linear dose-dependent changes in BOLD-fMRI in rodents can be demonstrated with some psychostimulants, or opposite BOLD-fMRI effects with certain dopaminergic agonists and antagonists, more complex patterns are seen with other psychotropics [64]. Similarly, mismatches between the distribution of particular receptors and the apparent downstream functional sites of drug action have been described and are again apparent in the phMRI literature [64].

Studies combining dopaminergic drugs with different mechanisms of action may allow the contribution of particular receptor subtypes, such as D_1 versus D_2 to the overall response to increased synaptic dopamine to be investigated [82, 83]. A range of rodent studies have gone on to explore not only the dopamine system and receptor subtypes [57, 84–89], but also the serotonin system and receptor subtypes [66, 90–93], as well as an expanding range of other neurochemical systems [16, 60, 91, 94–114]. For example, in a series of studies utilizing an *N*-methyl-D-aspartate (NMDA) receptor antagonist (PCP) model of schizophrenia, Gozzi and colleagues demonstrated differential ability of dopamine receptor D2 antagonism and various manipulations of glutamate and related receptors to block the widespread effects of PCP thought to relate to psychotic symptoms [105, 106] (Fig. 19.4).

Pharmacological functional MRI work has been undertaken not only in rodents but also in nonhuman primates. Another early set of studies used fMRI to study response to levodopa in hemiparkinsonian rhesus monkeys [115, 116]. Sites of increased activity in the lesioned hemisphere following levodopa included the lateral putamen, the ventral region of the caudate head, septal areas, and midlateral amygdala. Furthermore, the increases in neuronal activity following levodopa treatment were temporally correlated with increases in striatal dopamine levels. Finally, chronic levodopa treatment reduced behavioral responsiveness to levodopa and abolished the fMRI response. Taken together, this work indicated that fMRI provides a useful tool for studying neuronal changes in response to dopaminergic agents in primates. It may also ultimately allow for the monitoring of neurorestorative therapies in Parkinson's disease [117].

Pharmacological functional MRI work in rodent and nonhuman primate models seems particularly promising insofar as it provides a solid foundation for translational studies. For example, administration of addictive substances to animals activates reward neurocircuitry [1, 20, 50, 56, 58, 94, 104, 118–120], allowing more detailed subsequent studies of tolerance to and withdrawal from such agents [59, 121–125] and encouraging analogous work in humans. Pharmacological functional MRI

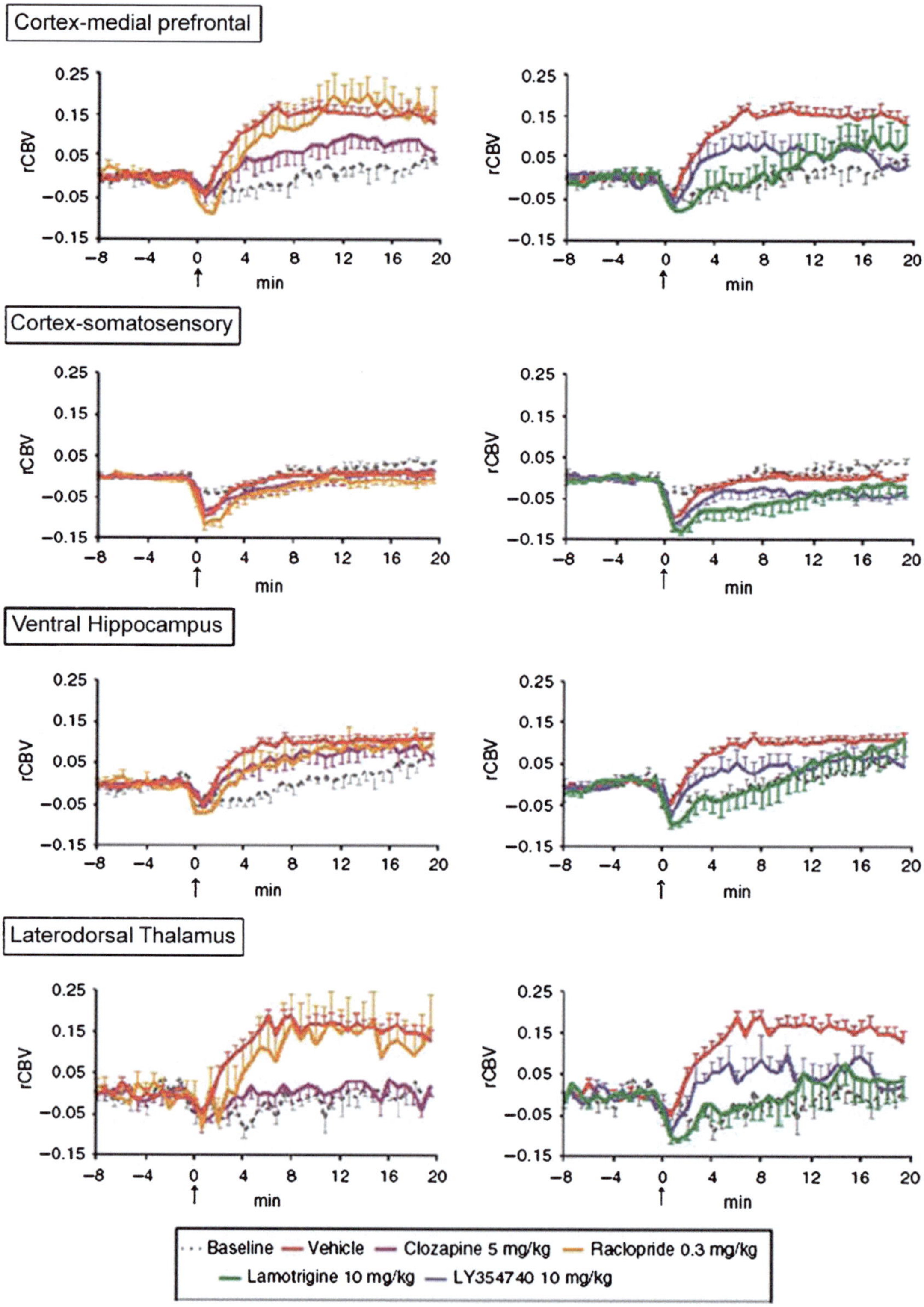

Fig. 19.4 rCBV time course in anesthetized rat following phencyclidine injection (*arrows*) as a function of pretreatment in four representative brain structures. Baseline data were obtained in animals

studies of animal models of depression and anxiety may also demonstrate parallels with clinical research [126]. Studies of the effects of pharmacological treatment on functional connectivity (the correlation of low frequency fluctuations in the BOLD time series between various brain regions) [127–129] may elucidate network level effects of drugs and, again, provide an important foundation for human work. The range of available animal models in psychopharmacology, including knockout models [130], remains to be exploited fully by phMRI. At the same time, consistent with the limitations of translational paradigms, phMRI does not always reveal parallel changes in response to the administration of pharmacological agents in animals and man [64].

Advances in experimental and analytic aspects of phMRI, including anesthesia, physiological monitoring, scanning protocol, and statistical analysis methods are important for advancing this kind of research [64, 131]. For example, Lu and colleagues [132] have developed a standard procedure for registering rat fMRI data into common space in which further analysis can be performed at a group level. A standard rat brain atlas is used to facilitate the identification of activated areas in common space. Lu and colleagues have also developed software for real-time fMRI studies in rodents, allowing for online monitoring and manipulation of psychopharmacological experiments [133]. See Table 19.3 for a summary of selected preclinical studies [60, 89, 105, 106, 110].

Table 19.3 Selected preclinical studies using pharmacological MRI

Authors	Subjects	FMRI paradigm	Results
Chen et al. 2005 [89]	Halothane-anesthetized male Sprague–Dawley rats	MION-enhanced rCBV in response to amphetamine challenge combined with D2 agonist and antagonist compared with DA microdialysis results	D2 antag → ↑ amph-induced rCBV changes in striatum and paralleled DA release in NAcc. D2 agonist → ↓ amph-induced rCBV changes in striatum
Chin et al. 2008 [60]	Awake and α-chloralose anesthetized male Sprague–Dawley rats	Contrast-enhanced rCBV pre- and post-α4β2 nicotinic receptor agonists compared with autoradiography of α4β2 receptor distribution	Awake: increased rCBV matching distribution of receptors Anesthetized: rCBV changes limited to cortex
Chin et al. 2008 [110]	Awake male Sprague–Dawley rats	Contrast-enhanced rCBV pre- and post-CB1 and CB2 agonists	CB1 agonist → ↑ rCBV in distribution of CB1 receptor, blocked by CB1 antag CB2 agonist no rCBV changes
Gozzi et al. 2008 [106]	Halothane-anesthetized male Sprague–Dawley rats	rCBV pre- and post-PCP with and without pretreatment with D2 antag, clozapine, lamotrigine and mGluR2/3 agonist	D2 antag: no change in rCBV response to PCP Clozapine: regional ↓ in rCBV response Lamotrigine and mGluR2/3 agonist: complete suppression of rCBV response to PCP
Gozzi et al. 2008 [105]	Male Sprague–Dawley rats with variable concentrations of halothane and doses of PCP	rCBV pre- and post-PCP under variable halothane concentrations	Qualitatively different patterns of activation with varying concentrations of halothane and doses of PCP

pretreated and challenged with saline. Differential blockade of PCP effects by a D2 antagonist (raclopride), an atypical antipsychotic (clozapine), an anticonvulsant (lamotrigine), and an mGluR2/3 agonist (LY363740). Reprinted by permission from Macmillan Publishers Ltd: Neuropsychopharmacology, Gozzi A, Large CH, Schwarz A, Bertani S, Crestan V, Bifone A. Differential effects of antipsychotic and glutamatergic agents on the phMRI response to phencyclidine. Neuropsychopharmacology, 2008;33: 1690–1703

Clinical Research

Although animal research is key for understanding basic mechanisms, human work is ultimately needed, given the unique nature of the human brain-mind and given the need to address clinical questions. Once again, although a good deal of work has focused on the dopamine and serotonin systems, several other neurochemical systems have also been explored with phMRI. In addition, phMRI has been used to explore the psychobiology of fundamental cognitive/affective phenomena (such as emotion), as well as of a number of major psychiatric disorders (including substance use disorders). Here we briefly review some key exemplars of this work.

One important set of phMRI findings has emerged from work on the dopamine system in general [26, 29, 46, 67, 134–139], and the role of the catechol-*O*-methyltransferase (COMT) gene in particular [140]. Prefrontal activation during a working memory task was studied after administration of D-amphetamine, which increases synaptic dopamine; subjects who had high performance at baseline tended to deteriorate, while subjects with a low performance at baseline had improved performance and increased prefrontal activation [31]. Methylphenidate, which also increases synaptic dopamine, and sulpiride, a D2 receptor antagonist, both attenuate adaptive response of a fronto-striatal network to cognitive load in an object-location learning task [141]. These kind of results can be modeled by suggesting an "inverted-U" relationship between dopamine tone and cognitive performance. Furthermore, responses to D-amphetamine are influenced strongly by a single functional variant in COMT; those with valine (Val^{158}) alleles (increased COMT activity and lower prefrontal synaptic dopamine) showed improved performance and reduced BOLD activation on amphetamine, while those with the methionine (Met^{158}) substitution showed impaired performance and increased activation on amphetamine. Both results were interpreted as changes in efficiency of prefrontal cortex (PFC) processing and illustrate how the "inverted-U" relationship between dopamine tone and cognitive performance is manifest in PFC activity (Fig. 19.5) [140]. Val^{158} alleles

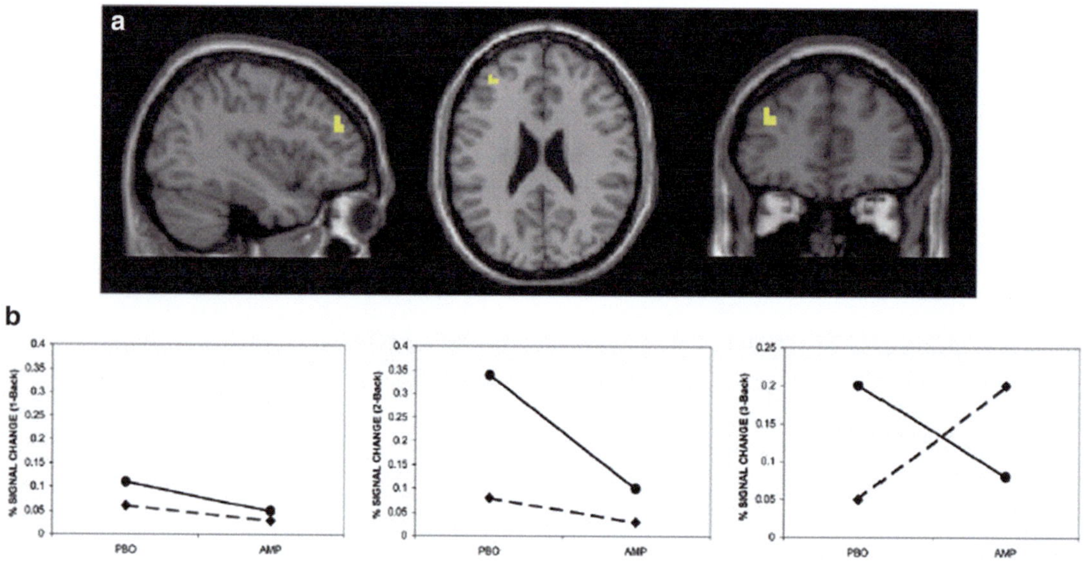

Fig. 19.5 (**a**) Representative sagittal, axial, and coronal slices from a group analysis showing locales of a drug [amphetamine(AMP)/placebo(PBO)] X COMT genotype interaction in the left PFC during a working memory task. (**b**) Percent change in BOLD signal in the left PFC during the *N*-back relative to the control task on AMP and PBO conditions. There is a main effect of genotype at baseline (PBO), as *val_val* (•) individuals are less efficient than *met/met* individuals (♦) at all levels of task difficulty. Reprinted with permission from Mattay VS, Goldberg TE, Fera F, et al. Catechol *O*-methyltransferase val(158)-met genotype and individual variation in the brain response to amphetamine. Proceedings of the National Academy of Sciences of the United States of America, 2003; 100, 6186–6191

may be associated with an advantage in the processing of aversive stimuli (warrior strategy), while Met^{158} alleles may be associated with an advantage in memory and attention tasks (worrier strategy) [142].

A range of phMRI investigations have shed light on the serotonin system; studies have, for example, assessed cognitive/affective tasks after serotonin depletion, after selective serotonin reuptake inhibitor (SSRI) administration in healthy volunteers, and after SSRI treatment of patients [21]. Taken together, this work provides significant evidence that serotonin does influence emotional processing occurring in the amygdala. Once again, key functional gene variants may play an important role; in particular, variants in the serotonin transporter gene (5-HTTLPR) may account for a significant proportion of variance in cognitive/affective and functional imaging data [143]. Pharmacological functional MRI has demonstrated considerable promise as a new tool to delineate both the complexity of the genetic influences on emotional processing (many other genes undoubtedly play a role) and the complexity of the underlying neurotransmitter systems (indeed, phMRI also reveals that the dopamine system contributes to emotional processing by the amygdala [134]).

Another valuable set of findings has emerged from work on the acetylcholine system in general, and the "cholinergic model" of Alzheimer's disorder in particular [36, 141]. Furey et al. [28] reported that administration of physostigmine, a cholinesterase inhibitor, led to increased visual working memory performance, increased selectivity of neural responses in extrastriate cortices particularly during encoding, as well as increased participation of ventral extrastriate cortex and decreased participation of anterior PFC during memory maintenance. They argued that this pattern of findings indicates that cholinergic enhancement improves memory performance by augmenting the selectivity of perceptual processing during encoding, so simplifying processing demands during memory. Administration of the selective muscarinic acetylcholine receptor antagonist scopolamine, on the other hand, disrupts repetition priming [33, 144]. Cholinergic stimulation does not, however, have uniformly positive effects [145–147], and it may interfere with retrieval at a neural level [148].

A range of other neurotransmitter systems has been studied with phMRI, including the noradrenaline, glutamate, GABA, opioid, and cannabinoid systems [34, 37, 47, 103, 144, 149–161], and there is also a growing area of psychoneuroendocrine imaging [162]. This work may be particularly useful in generating and testing system-level hypotheses, such as an inverted-U model of the relationship between GABA tone and adaptivity to repeated tasks [149].

An immediate question, however, is the potential utility of phMRI for testing neurotransmitter models of disorders, predicting treatment response, and supporting the development of novel compounds in neuropsychiatry. An early phMRI study, for example, focused on the hypodopaminergic hypothesis of schizophrenia, and suggested that in comparison with typical antipsychotics, an atypical agent was associated with increased activation of PFC during performance of a working memory task [73]. A more recent review of several additional studies came to a similar conclusion [163].

Similarly, a series of promising studies has explored the way in which serotonergic and noradrenergic drugs or depleting agents affect fMRI during various cognitive/affective paradigms in healthy controls [25, 38–40, 71, 164–174], as well as in mood and anxiety disorders [72, 175–179]. Studies have also begun to characterize the effects of pharmacological treatment on connectivity; a dopamine blocker increases caudate connectivity in healthy volunteers [136] and in patients with schizophrenia. Functional connectivity is also altered by the antipsychotic olanzapine [180], the cholinesterase inhibitor donepezil [181], and nicotine administration [182].

In addition to work on schizophrenia and mood and anxiety disorders, phMRI studies have been undertaken on various addictive substances (including cocaine, heroin, nicotine, alcohol, and caffeine) and in substance use disorders [22–24, 27, 30, 32, 52–54, 183–199], attention deficit hyperactivity disorder [200–203], in Parkinson's disorder and in a range of other neurological disorders [2]. Such work is consistent with, and has helped extend, prior neurobiological knowledge;

for example, phMRI of addictive substances implicates reward circuitry. Ultimately, such work may have an important role in delineating "brain signatures" of particular psychotropics and in the development of novel agents for a range of psychiatric disorders [5, 7, 9].

Although most clinical work in the area of phMRI has focused on BOLD-fMRI, a range of other MRI technologies may be of value for psychopharmacology. Dynamic susceptibility contrast MRI, utilizing a bolus injection of a contrast agent to enhance MR signal, has been used in humans [204, 205], and such so-called molecular MRI, using agents such as certain nanoparticles with particular biological and magnetic properties as targeted contrast agents to study particular biological processes, [206] may ultimately have an important role in psychopharmacology research. There is growing interest, also, in the use of magnetic resonance spectroscopy to investigate the relationship between drug dose and plasma and brain levels of several medications [6], as well as the effects of psychotropic agents on specific metabolites. At present, given the ability of MRS to measure glutamate and GABA, this method may have a particularly important role to play in the study of these amino acid neurotransmitter systems [207]. By combining BOLD phMRI, MRS, and even PET [208], it may be possible to integrate functional and metabolic consequences of drug administration.

Conclusion

The field of phMRI is at a relatively early stage; its basic assumptions (e.g., relationship of BOLD activity to neuronal activity) are still under investigation, and its methods (e.g., registration of anatomical brain images and analysis of data) are still under development. Nevertheless, during the last decade, the field has developed from only a few studies (see Table 19.1) to many dozens, with investigations ranging from animal to clinical work, and from work on cognitive/affective processing in healthy individuals to work on subjects with psychiatric and substance use disorders. While such work has not yet led to paradigm-shifting insights in psychopharmacology, phMRI has certainly contributed significantly to psychopharmacology, including understanding the pharmacodynamics and pharmacokinetics of various psychotropics, the implications of gene variants on psychotropic effects, neurotransmitter mechanisms underlying different cognitive/affective paradigms, and the psychopharmacology of psychiatric disorders. Perhaps more importantly, it has laid a foundation for future translational research and development, in which phMRI could potentially be productively integrated and into a range of other methodologies including longitudinal endophenotype assessment, genetic and proteomic research, and randomized clinical trials.

Acknowledgments This work was supported in part by NIH/NIDA.

References

1. Chen YCI, Galpern WR, Brownell AL, Matthews RT, Bogdanov M, Isacson O, et al. Detection of dopaminergic neurotransmitter activity using pharmacologic MRI: correlation with PET, microdialysis, and behavioral data. Magn Reson Med. 1997;38:389–98.
2. Honey G, Bullmore E. Human pharmacological MRI. Trends Pharmacol Sci. 2004;25:366–74.
3. Shah YB, Marsden CA. The application of functional magnetic resonance imaging to neuropharmacology. Curr Opin Pharmacol. 2004;4:517–21.
4. Leslie RA, James MF. Pharmacological magnetic resonance imaging: a new application for functional MRI. Trends Pharmacol Sci. 2000;21:314–8.
5. Paulus MP, Stein MB. Role of functional magnetic resonance imaging in drug discovery. Neuropsychol Rev. 2007;17:179–88.
6. Salmeron BJ, Stein EA. Pharmacological applications of magnetic resonance imaging. Psychopharm Bull. 2002;36:179–88.
7. Wise RG, Tracey I. The role of fMRI in drug discovery. J Magn Reson Imaging. 2006;23:862–76.
8. Rudin M, Beckmann N, Porszasz R, Reese T, Bochelen D, Sauter A. In vivo magnetic resonance methods in pharmaceutical research: current status and perspectives. NMR Biomed. 1999;12:69–97.
9. Borsook D, Bleakman D, Hargreaves R, Upadhyay J, Schmidt KF, Becerra L. A "BOLD" experiment in defining the utility of fMRI in drug development. Neuroimage. 2008;42:461–6.
10. Cropley VL, Fujita M, Innis RB, Nathan PJ. Molecular imaging of the dopaminergic system and

its association with human cognitive function. Biol Psychiatry. 2006;59:898–907.

11. Roy CS, Sherrington CS. On the regulation the blood supply of the brain. J Physiol. 1896;11:85–108.
12. Fox PT, Raichle ME. Focal physiological uncoupling of cerebral blood flow and oxidative metabolism during somatosensory stimulation in human subjects. Proc Natl Acad Sci USA. 1986;83(4):1140–4.
13. Ogawa S, Lee TM, Kay AR, Tank DW. Brain magnetic-resonance-imaging with contrast dependent on blood oxygenation. Proc Natl Acad Sci US Am. 1990;87:9868–72.
14. MacIntosh BJ, Pattinson KTS, Gallichan D, Ahmad I, Miller KL, Feinberg DA, et al. Measuring the effects of remifentanil on cerebral blood flow and arterial arrival time using 3D GRASE MRI with pulsed arterial spin labelling. J Cereb Blood Flow Metab. 2008;28:1514–22.
15. Kofke WA, Blissitt PA, Rao H, Wang JJ, Addya K, Detre J. Remifentanil-induced cerebral blood flow effects in normal humans: dose and ApoE genotype. Anesth Analg. 2007;105:167–75.
16. Kochanek PM, Hendrich KS, Robertson CL, Williams DS, Melick JA, Ho C, et al. Assessment of the effect of 2-chloroadenosine in normal rat brain using spin-labeled MRI measurement of perfusion. Magn Reson Med. 2001;45:924–9.
17. Silva AC, Zhang WG, Williams DS, Koretsky AP. Multislice Mri of rat-brain perfusion during amphetamine stimulation using arterial spin-labeling. Magn Reson Med. 1995;33:209–14.
18. Bruns A, Kunnecke B, Risterucci C, Moreau JL, von Kienlin M. Validation of cerebral blood perfusion imaging as a modality for quantitative pharmacological MRI in rats. Magn Reson Med. 2009;61:1451–8.
19. Lu HB, Xi ZX, Gitajn L, Rea W, Yang YH, Stein EA. Cocaine-induced brain activation detected by dynamic manganese-enhanced magnetic resonance imaging (MEMRI). Proc Natl Acad Sci US Am. 2007;104:2489–94.
20. Marota JJA, Mandeville JB, Weisskoff RM, Moskowitz MA, Rosen BR, Kosofsky BE. Cocaine activation discriminates dopaminergic projections by temporal response: an fMRI study in rat. Neuroimage. 2000;11:13–23.
21. Anderson IM, Mckie S, Elliott R, Williams SR, Deakin JFW. Assessing human 5-HT function in vivo with pharmacoMRI. Neuropharmacology. 2008;55:1029–37.
22. Breiter HC, Gollub RL, Weisskoff RM, Kennedy DN, Makris N, Berke JD, et al. Acute effects of cocaine on human brain activity and emotion. Neuron. 1997;19:591–611.
23. Stein EA, Pankiewicz J, Harsch HH, Cho JK, Fuller SA, Hoffmann RG, et al. Nicotine-induced limbic cortical activation in the human brain: a functional MRI study. Am J Psychiatry. 1998;155:1009–15.
24. Risinger RC, Salmeron BJ, Ross TJ, Amen SL, Sanfilipo M, Hoffmann RG, et al. Neural correlates of high and craving during cocaine self-administration using BOLD fMRI. Neuroimage. 2005;26:1097–108.
25. Mckie S, Del Ben C, Elliott R, Williams S, del Vai N, Anderson I, et al. Neuronal effects of acute citalopram detected by pharmacoMRI. Psychopharmacology. 2005;180:680–6.
26. Rose SE, Janke AL, Strudwick MW, McMahon KL, Chalk JB, Snyder P, et al. Assessment of dynamic susceptibility contrast cerebral blood flow response to amphetamine challenge: a human pharmacological magnetic resonance imaging study at 1.5 and 4 T. Magn Reson Med. 2006;55:9–15.
27. Addicott MA, Yang LL, Peiffer AM, Burnett LR, Burdette JH, Chen MY, et al. The effect of daily caffeine use on cerebral blood flow: how much caffeine can we tolerate? Hum Brain Mapp. 2009;30:3102–14.
28. Furey ML, Pietrini P, Haxby JV. Cholinergic enhancement and increased selectivity of perceptual processing during working memory. Science. 2000;290:2315-+
29. Kimberg DY, Aguirre GK, Lease J, D'Esposito M. Cortical effects of bromocriptine, a D-2 dopamine receptor agonist, in human subjects, revealed by fMRI. Hum Brain Mapp. 2001;12:246–57.
30. Levin JM, Ross MH, Mendelson JH, Kaufman MJ, Lange N, Maas LC, et al. Reduction in BOLD fMRI response to primary visual stimulation following alcohol ingestion. Psychiatry Res Neuroimaging. 1998;82:135–46.
31. Mattay VS, Callicott JH, Bertolino A, Heaton I, Frank JA, Coppola R, et al. Effects of dextroamphetamine on cognitive performance and cortical activation. Neuroimage. 2000;12:268–75.
32. Seifritz E, Bilecen D, Hanggi D, Haselhorst R, Radu EW, Wetzel S, et al. Effect of ethanol on BOLD response to acoustic stimulation: implications for neuropharmacological fMRI. Psychiatry Res Neuroimaging. 2000;99:1–13.
33. Thiel CM, Henson RNA, Dolan RJ. Scopolamine but not lorazepam modulates face repetition priming: a psychopharmacological fMR1 study. Neuropsychopharmacology. 2002;27:282–92.
34. Wise RG, Lujan BJ, Schweinhardt P, Peskett GD, Rogers R, Tracey I. The anxiolytic effects of midazolam during anticipation to pain revealed using fMRI. Magn Reson Imaging. 2007;25:801–10.
35. Loubinoux I, Boulanouar K, Ranjeva JP, Carel C, Berry I, Rascol O, et al. Cerebral functional magnetic resonance imaging activation modulated by a single dose of the monoamine neurotransmission enhancers fluoxetine and fenozolone during hand sensorimotor tasks. J Cereb Blood Flow Metab. 1999;19(12):1365–75.
36. Sperling R, Greve D, Dale A, Killiany R, Holmes J, Rosas HD, et al. Functional MRI detection of pharmacologically induced memory impairment. Proc Natl Acad Sci US Am. 2002;99:455–60.
37. Paulus MP, Feinstein JS, Castillo G, Simmons AN, Stein MB. Dose-dependent decrease of activation in

bilateral amygdala and insula by lorazepam during emotion processing. Arch Gen Psychiatry. 2005; 62:282–8.

38. Vollm B, Richardson P, Mckie S, Elliott R, Deakin JFW, Anderson IM. Serotonergic modulation of neuronal responses to behavioural inhibition and reinforcing stimuli: an fMRI study in healthy volunteers. Eur J Neurosci. 2006;23:552–60.
39. Norbury R, Mackay CE, Cowen PJ, Goodwin GM, Harmer CJ. Short-term antidepressant treatment and facial processing – functional magnetic resonance imaging study. Br J Psychiatry. 2007;190:531–2.
40. Simmons AN, Arce E, Lovero KL, Stein MB, Paulus MP. Subchronic SSRI administration reduces insula response during affective anticipation in healthy volunteers. Int J Neuropsychopharmacol. 2009;12: 1009–20.
41. Rother J, Knab R, Hamzei F, Fiehler J, Reichenbach JR, Buchel C, et al. Negative dip in BOLD fMRI is caused by blood flow – Oxygen consumption uncoupling in humans. Neuroimage. 2002;15:98–102.
42. Logothetis NK, Pauls J, Augath M, Trinath T, Oeltermann A. Neurophysiological investigation of the basis of the fMRI signal. Nature. 2001; 412(6843):150–7.
43. Rauch A, Rainer G, Logothetis NK. The effect of a serotonin-induced dissociation between spiking and perisynaptic activity on BOLD functional MRI. Proc Natl Acad Sci US Am. 2008;105:6759–64.
44. Schmidt KF, Febo M, Shen Q, Luo F, Sicard KM, Ferris CF, et al. Hemodynamic and metabolic changes induced by cocaine in anesthetized rat observed with multimodal functional MRI. Psychopharmacology. 2006;185:479–86.
45. Choi JK, Chen YI, Hamel E, Jenkins BG. Brain hemodynamic changes mediated by dopamine receptors: role of the cerebral microvasculature in dopamine-mediated neurovascular coupling. Neuroimage. 2006;30:700–12.
46. Rao SM, Salmeron BJ, Durgerian S, Janowiak JA, Fischer M, Risinger RC, et al. Effects of methylphenidate on functional MRI blood-oxygen-level-dependent contrast. Am J Psychiatry. 2000;157:1697–9.
47. Pattinson KTS, Rogers R, Mayhew SD, Tracey I, Wise RG. Pharmacological FMRI: measuring opioid effects on the BOLD response to hypercapnia. J Cereb Blood Flow Metab. 2007;27:414–23.
48. Luo F, Wu GH, Li Z, Li SJ. Characterization of effects of mean arterial blood pressure induced by cocaine and cocaine methiodide on BOLD signals in rat brain. Magn Reson Med. 2003;49:264–70.
49. Luo F, Schmidt KF, Fox GB, Ferris CF. Differential responses in CBF and CBV to cocaine as measured by fMRI: implications for pharmacological MRI signals derived oxygen metabolism assessment. J Psychiatr Res. 2009;43:1018–24.
50. Schwarz A, Gozzi A, Reese T, Bertani S, Crestan V, Hagan J, et al. Selective dopamine D-3 receptor antagonist SB-277011-A potentiates phMRI response to acute amphetamine challenge in the rat brain. Synapse. 2004;54:1–10.
51. Gozzi A, Ceolin L, Schwarz A, Reese T, Bertani S, Crestan V, et al. A multimodality investigation of cerebral hemodynamics and autoregulation in pharmacological MRI. Magn Reson Imaging. 2007;25:826–33.
52. Gollub RL, Breiter HC, Kantor H, Kennedy G, Gastfriend D, Mathew RT, et al. Cocaine decreases cortical cerebral blood flow but does not obscure regional activation in functional magnetic resonance imaging in human subjects. J Cereb Blood Flow Metab. 1998;18:724–34.
53. Mulderink TA, Gitelman DR, Mesulam MM, Parrish TB. On the use of caffeine as a contrast booster for BOLD fMRI studies. Neuroimage. 2002;15:37–44.
54. Laurienti PJ, Field AS, Burdette JH, Maldjian JA, Yen YF, Moody DM. Dietary caffeine consumption modulates fMRI measures. Neuroimage. 2002; 17:751–7.
55. Zhang ZM, Andersen AH, Avison MJ, Gerhardt GA, Gash DM. Functional MRI of apomorphine activation of the basal ganglia in awake rhesus monkeys. Brain Res. 2000;852:290–6.
56. Zhang ZM, Andersen A, Grondin R, Barber T, Avison R, Gerhardt G, et al. Pharmacological MRI mapping of age-associated changes in basal ganglia circuitry of awake rhesus monkeys. Neuroimage. 2001;14:1159–67.
57. Hagino H, Tabuchi E, Kurachi M, Saitoh O, Sun YJ, Kondoh T, et al. Effects of D-2 dopamine receptor agonist and antagonist on brain activity in the rat assessed by functional magnetic resonance imaging. Brain Res. 1998;813:367–73.
58. Febo M, Segarra AC, Tenney JR, Brevard ME, Duong TQ, Ferris CF. Imaging cocaine-induced changes in the mesocorticolimbic dopaminergic system of conscious rats. J Neurosci Meth. 2004;139:167–76.
59. Febo M, Segarra AC, Nair G, Schmidt K, Duong TQ, Ferris CF. The neural consequences of repeated cocaine exposure revealed by functional MRI in awake rats. Neuropsychopharmacology. 2005;30: 936–43.
60. Chin CL, Pauly JR, Surber BW, Skoubis PD, Mcgaraughty S, Hradil VP, et al. Pharmacological MRI in awake rats predicts selective binding of alpha(4)beta(2) nicotinic receptors. Synapse. 2008;62:159–68.
61. Peeters RR, Tindemans I, De Schutter E, Van der Linden A. Comparing BOLD fMRI signal changes in the awake and anesthetized rat during electrical forepaw stimulation. Magn Reson Imaging. 2001;19: 821–6.
62. Lahti KM, Ferris CF, Li FH, Sotak CH, King JA. Comparison of evoked cortical activity in conscious and propofol-anesthetized rats using functional MRI. Magn Reson Med. 1999;41:412–6.
63. Gozzi A, Schwarz A, Crestan V, Bifone A. Drug-anaesthetic interaction in phMRI: the case of the psychotomimetic agent phencyclidine. Magn Reson Imaging. 2008;26:999–1006.
64. Steward CA, Marsden CA, Prior MJW, Morris PG, Shah YB. Methodological considerations in rat

brain BOLD contrast pharmacological MRI. Psychopharmacology. 2005;180:687–704.

65. Rauch A, Rainer G, Augath M, Elterinann A, Logothetis NK. Pharmacological MRI combined with electrophysiology in non-human primates: effects of Lidocaine on primary visual cortex. Neuroimage. 2008;40:590–600.
66. Stark JA, Davies KE, Williams SR, Luckman SM. Functional magnetic resonance imaging and c-Fos mapping in rats following an anorectic dose of m-chlorophenylpiperazine. Neuroimage. 2006;31:1228–37.
67. Arthurs OJ, Stephenson CME, Rice K, Lupson V, Spiegelhalter DJ, Boniface SJ, et al. Dopaminergic effects on electrophysiological and functional MRI measures of human cortical stimulus-response power laws. Neuroimage. 2004;21:540–6.
68. Pohlmann A, Barjat H, Tilling LC. James MF. Pharmacological fMRI – Challenges in analysing drug-induced single-event BOLD responses. Conf Proc IEEE Eng Med Biol Soc. 2007;2007:3411–6.
69. Bloom AS, Hoffmann RG, Fuller SA, Pankiewicz J, Harsch HH, Stein EA. Determination of drug-induced changes in functional MRI signal using a pharmacokinetic model. Hum Brain Mapp. 1999;8:235–44.
70. Wilkinson D, Halligan P. Opinion – the relevance of behavioural measures for functional-imaging studies of cognition. Nat Rev Neurosci. 2004;5:67–73.
71. Norbury R, Mackay CE, Cowen PJ, Goodwin GM, Harmer CJ. The effects of reboxetine on emotional processing in healthy volunteers: an fMRI study. Mol Psychiatry. 2008;13:1011–20.
72. Sheline YI, Barch DM, Donnelly JM, Ollinger JM, Snyder AZ, Mintun MA. Increased amygdala response to masked emotional faces in depressed subjects resolves with antidepressant treatment: an fMRI study. Biol Psychiatry. 2001;50:651–8.
73. Honey GD, Bullmore ET, Soni W, Varatheesan M, Williams SCR, Sharma T. Differences in frontal cortical activation by a working memory task after substitution of risperidone for typical antipsychotic drugs in patients with schizophrenia. Proc Natl Acad Sci US Am. 1999;96:13432–7.
74. Smith SM, Jenkinson M, Woolrich MW, Beckmann CF, Behrens TEJ, Johansen-Berg H, et al. Advances in functional and structural MR image analysis and implementation as FSL. Neuroimage. 2004;23:S208–19.
75. McKeown MJ, Hansen LK, Sejnowski TJ. Independent component analysis of functional MRI: what is signal and what is noise? Curr Opin Neurobiol. 2003;13:620–9.
76. Whitcher B, Schwarz AJ, Barjat H, Smart SC, Grundy RI, James MF. Wavelet-based cluster analysis: data-driven grouping of voxel time courses with application to perfusion-weighted and pharmacological MRI of the rat brain. Neuroimage. 2005;24:281–95.
77. Schwarz AJ, Whitcher B, Gozzi A, Reese T, Bifone A. Study-level wavelet cluster analysis and data-driven signal models in pharmacological MRI. J Neurosci Meth. 2007;159:346–60.
78. Dieler AC, Sämann PG, Leicht G, Eser D, Kirsch V, Baghai TC, et al. Independent component analysis applied to pharmacological magnetic resonance imaging (phMRI): new insights into the functional networks underlying panic attacks as induced by CCK-4. Curr Pharm Des. 2008;14:3492–507.
79. Mitsis GD, Iannetti GD, Smart TS, Tracey I, Wise RG. Regions of interest analysis in pharmacological fMRI: how do the definition criteria influence the inferred result? Neuroimage. 2008;40:121–32.
80. Chen YI, Brownell AL, Galpern W, Isacson O, Bogdanov M, Beal MF, et al. Detection of dopaminergic cell loss and neural transplantation using pharmacological MRI, PET and behavioral assessment. Neuroreport. 1999;10:2881–6.
81. Nguyen TV, Brownell AL, Chen YCI, Livni E, Coyle JT, Rosen BR, et al. Detection of the effects of dopamine receptor supersensitivity using pharmacological MRI and correlations with PET. Synapse. 2000;36:57–65.
82. Dixon AL, Prior M, Morris PM, Shah YB, Joseph MH, Young AMJ. Dopamine antagonist modulation of amphetamine response as detected using pharmacological MRI. Neuropharmacology. 2005;48:236–45.
83. Schwarz AJ, Zocchi A, Reese T, Gozzi A, Garzotti M, Varnier G, et al. Concurrent pharmacological MRI and in situ microdialysis of cocaine reveal a complex relationship between the central hemodynamic response and local dopamine concentration. Neuroimage. 2004;23:296–304.
84. Preece M, Mukherjee B, Huang CLH, Hall LD, Leslie RA, James MF. Detection of pharmacologically mediated changes in cerebral activity by functional magnetic resonance imaging: the effects of sulpiride in the brain of the anaesthetised rat. Brain Res. 2001;916:107–14.
85. Ireland MD, Lowe AS, Reavill C, James MF, Leslie RA, Williams SCR. Mapping the effects of the selective dopamine D-2/D-3 receptor agonist quinelorane using pharmacological magnetic resonance imaging. Neuroscience. 2005;133:315–26.
86. Nordquist RE, Risterucci C, Moreau JL, von Kienlin M, Kunnecke B, Maco M, et al. Effects of aripiprazole/OPC-14597 on motor activity, pharmacological models of psychosis, and brain activity in rats. Neuropharmacology. 2008;54:405–16.
87. Easton N, Marshall FH, Marsden CA, Fone KCF. Mapping the central effects of methylphenidate in the rat using pharmacological MRI BOLD contrast. Neuropharmacology. 2009;57:653–64.
88. Canese R, Adriani W, Marco EM, De Pasquale F, Lorenzini P, De Luca N, et al. Peculiar response to methylphenidate in adolescent compared to adult rats: a phMRI study. Psychopharmacol Berl. 2009;203:143–53.
89. Chen YC, Choi JK, Andersen SL, Rosen BR, Jenkins BG. Mapping dopamine D2/D3 receptor function using pharmacological magnetic resonance imaging. Psychopharmacol Berl. 2005;180:705–15.

90. Martin C, Sibson NR. Pharmacological MRI in animal models: a useful tool for 5-HT research? Neuropharmacology. 2008;55:1038–47.
91. Houston GC, Papadakis NG, Carpenter TA, Hall LD, Mukherjee B, James MF, et al. Mapping of brain activation in response to pharmacological agents using fMRI in the rat. Magn Reson Imaging. 2001; 19:905–19.
92. Stark JA, Mckie S, Davies KE, Williams SR, Luckman SM. 5-HT2C antagonism blocks blood oxygen level-dependent pharmacological-challenge magnetic resonance imaging signal in rat brain areas related to feeding. Eur J Neurosci. 2008;27:457–65.
93. Scanley BE, Kennan RP, Gore JC. Changes in rat cerebral blood volume due to modulation of the 5-HT1A receptor measured with susceptibility enhanced contrast MRI. Brain Res. 2001;913: 149–55.
94. Shah YB, Prior MJW, Dixon AL, Morris PG, Marsden CA. Detection of cannabinoid agonist evoked increase in BOLD contrast in rats using functional magnetic resonance imaging. Neuropharmacology. 2004; 46:379–87.
95. Shah YB, Haynes L, Prior MJ, Marsden CA, Morris PG, Chapman V. Functional magnetic resonance imaging studies of opioid receptor-mediated modulation of noxious-evoked BOLD contrast in rats. Psychopharmacology. 2005;180:761–73.
96. Malisza KL, Docherty JC. Capsaicin as a source for painful stimulation in functional MRI. J Magn Reson Imaging. 2001;14:341–7.
97. Kochanek PM, Hendrich KS, Jackson EK, Wisniewski SR, Melick JA, Shore PM, et al. Characterization of the effects of adenosine receptor agonists on cerebral blood flow in uninjured and traumatically injured rat brain using continuous arterial spin-labeled magnetic resonance imaging. J Cereb Blood Flow Metab. 2005;25:1596–612.
98. Fabene PF, Marzola P, Sbarbati A, Bentivoglio M. Magnetic resonance imaging of changes elicited by status epilepticus in the rat brain: diffusion-weighted and T2-weighted images, regional blood volume maps, and direct correlation with tissue and cell damage. Neuroimage. 2003;18:375–89.
99. Van Camp N, D'Hooge R, Verhoye M, Peeters RR, De Deyn PP, Van der Linden A. Simultaneous electroencephalographic recording and functional magnetic resonance imaging during pentylenetetrazol-induced seizures in rat. Neuroimage. 2003;19:627–36.
100. Reese T, Bjelke B, Porszasz R, Baumann D, Bochelen D, Sauter A, et al. Regional brain activation by bicuculline visualized by functional magnetic resonance imaging. Time-resolved assessment of bicuculline-induced changes in local cerebral blood volume using an intravascular contrast agent. NMR Biomed. 2000;13:43–9.
101. Gozzi A, Schwarz AJ, Reese T, Crestan V, Bertani S, Turrini G, et al. Functional magnetic resonance mapping of intracerebroventricular infusion of a neuroactive peptide in the anaesthetised rat. J Neurosci Meth. 2005;142:115–24.
102. Burdett NG, Menon DK, Carpenter TA, Jones JG, Hall LD. Visualization of changes in regional cerebral blood-flow (Rcbf) produced by ketamine using long Te gradient-Echo sequences – preliminary-results. Magn Reson Imaging. 1995;13:549–53.
103. Dodd GT, Stark JA, Mckie S, Williams SR, Luckman SM. Central cannabinoid signaling mediating food intake: a pharmacological-challenge magnetic resonance imaging and functional histology study in rat. Neuroscience. 2009;163:1192–200.
104. Gozzi A, Schwarz A, Reese T, Bertani S, Crestan V, Bifone A. Region-specific effects of nicotine on brain activity: a pharmacological MRI study in the drug-naive rat. Neuropsychopharmacology. 2006;31: 1690–703.
105. Gozzi A, Herdon H, Schwarz A, Bertani S, Crestan V, Turrini G, et al. Pharmacological stimulation of NMDA receptors via co-agonist site suppresses fMRI response to phencyclidine in the rat. Psychopharmacology. 2008;201:273–84.
106. Gozzi A, Large CH, Schwarz A, Bertani S, Crestan V, Bifone A. Differential effects of antipsychotic and glutamatergic agents on the phMRI response to phencyclidine. Neuropsychopharmacology. 2008; 33:1690–703.
107 Chen Z, Silva AC, Yang J, Shen J. Elevated endogenous GABA level correlates with decreased fMRI signals in the rat brain during acute inhibition of GABA transaminase. J Neurosci Res. 2005; 79:383–91.
108. Yao BB, Hsieh G, Daza AV, Fan Y, Grayson GK, Garrison TR, et al. Characterization of a cannabinoid CB2 receptor-selective agonist, A-836339 [2,2,3,3-tetramethyl-cyclopropanecarboxylic acid [3-(2-methoxy-ethyl)-4,5-dimethyl-3H-thiazol-(2Z)-ylidene]-amide], using in vitro pharmacological assays, in vivo pain models, and pharmacological magnetic resonance imaging. J Pharmacol Exp Ther. 2009;328:141–51.
109. Roberts TJ, Williams SCR, Modo M. A pharmacological MRI assessment of dizocilpine (MK-801) in the 3-nitroproprionic acid-lesioned rat. Neurosci Lett. 2008;444:42–7.
110. Chin CL, Tovcimak AE, Hradil VP, Seifert TR, Hollingsworth PR, Chandran P, et al. Differential effects of cannabinoid receptor agonists on regional brain activity using pharmacological MRI. Br J Pharmacol. 2008;153:367–79.
111. Easton N, Shah YB, Marshall FH, Fone KC, Marsden CA. Guanfacine produces differential effects in frontal cortex compared with striatum: assessed by phMRI BOLD contrast. Psychopharmacology. 2006;189:369–85.
112. Easton N, Marshall F, Fone K, Marsden C. Atomoxetine produces changes in cortico-basal thalamic loop circuits: assessed by phMRI BOLD contrast. Neuropharmacology. 2007;52:812–26.

113. Littlewood CL, Jones N, O'Neill MJ, Mitchell SN, Tricklebank M, Williams SCR. Mapping the central effects of ketamine in the rat using pharmacological MRI. Psychopharmacology. 2006;186:64–81.
114. Jones N, O'Neill MJ, Tricklebank M, Libri V, Williams SC. Examining the neural targets of the AMPA receptor potentiator LY404187 in the rat brain using pharmacological magnetic resonance imaging. Psychopharmacol Berl. 2005;180:743–51.
115. Chen Q, Andersen AH, Zhang Z, Ovadia A, Gash DM, Avison MJ. Mapping drug-induced changes in cerebral R(2)* by Multiple Gradient Recalled Echo functional MRI. Magn Reson Imaging. 1996; 14:469–76.
116. Chen Q, Andersen AH, Zhang ZM, Ovadia A, Cass WA, Gash DM, et al. Functional MRI of basal ganglia responsiveness to levodopa in parkinsonian rhesus monkeys. Exp Neurol. 1999;158:63–75.
117. Luan LM, Ding F, Ai Y, Andersen A, Hardy P, Forman E, et al. Pharmacological MRI (phMRI) monitoring of treatment in hemiparkinsonian rhesus monkeys. Cell Transplant. 2008;17:417–25.
118. Xu HY, Li SJ, Bodurka J, Zhao XL, Xi ZX, Stein EA. Heroin-induced neuronal activation in rat brain assessed by functional MRI. Neuroreport. 2000;11:1085–92.
119. Calderan L, Chiamulera C, Marzola P, Fabene PF, Fumagalli GF, Sbarbati A. Sub-chronic nicotine-induced changes in regional cerebral blood volume and transversal relaxation time patterns in the rat: a magnetic resonance study. Neurosci Lett. 2005; 377:195–9.
120. Easton N, Marshall F, Fone KCF, Marsden CA. Differential effects of the D- and L-isomers of amphetamine on pharmacological MRI BOLD contrast in the rat. Psychopharmacology. 2007;193: 11–30.
121. Xi ZX, Wu GH, Stein EA, Li SJ. GABAergic mechanisms of heroin-induced brain activation assessed with functional MRI. Magn Reson Med. 2002; 48:838–43.
122. Xi ZX, Wu GH, Stein EA, Li SJ. Opiate tolerance by heroin self-administration: an MRI study in rat. Magn Reson Med. 2004;52:108–14.
123. Luo F, Xi ZX, Wu GH, Liu C, Gardner EL, Li SJ. Attenuation of brain response to heroin correlates with the reinstatement of heroin-seeking in rats by fMRI. Neuroimage. 2004;22:1328–35.
124. Lowe AS, Williams SCR, Symms MR, Stolerman IP, Shoaib M. Functional magnetic resonance neuroimaging of drug dependence: naloxone-precipitated morphine withdrawal. Neuroimage. 2002;17:902–10.
125. Shoaib M, Lowe AS, Williams SCR. Imaging localised dynamic changes in the nucleus accumbens following nicotine withdrawal in rats. Neuroimage. 2004;22:847–54.
126. Kalisch R, Salome N, Platzer S, Wigger A, Czisch M, Sommer W, et al. High trait anxiety and hyporeactivity to stress of the dorsomedial prefrontal cortex: a combined phMRI and Fos study in rats. Neuroimage. 2004;23:382–91.
127. Schwarz AJ, Gozzi A, Reese T, Heidbreder CA, Bifone A. Pharmacological. modulation of functional connectivity: the correlation structure underlying the phMRI response to d-amphetamine modified by selective dopamine D-3 receptor antagonist SB277011A. Magn Reson Imaging. 2007;25:811–20.
128. Schwarz AJ, Gozzi A, Reese T, Bifone A. In vivo mapping of functional connectivity in neurotransmitter systems using pharmacological MRI. Neuroimage. 2007;34:1627–36.
129. Schwarz AJ, Gozzi A, Bifone A. Community structure in networks of functional connectivity: resolving functional organization in the rat brain with pharmacological MRI. Neuroimage. 2009;47:302–11.
130. Kuriwaki J, Nishijo H, Kondoh T, Uwano T, Torii K, Katsuki M, et al. Comparison of brain activity between dopamine D2 receptor-knockout and wild mice in response to dopamine agonist and antagonist assessed by fMRI. Neurosignals. 2004;13:227–40.
131. Schwarz AJ, Danckaert A, Reese T, Gozzi A, Paxinos G, Watson C, et al. A stereotaxic MRI template set for the rat brain with tissue class distribution maps and co-registered anatomical atlas: application to pharmacological MRI. Neuroimage. 2006;32:538–50.
132. Lu H, Scholl CA, Zuo Y, Demny S, Rea W, Stein EA, et al. Registering and analyzing rat fMRI data in the stereotaxic framework by exploiting intrinsic anatomical features. Magn Reson Imaging. 2010;28: 146–52.
133. Lu HB, Yang SL, Zuo YT, Demny S, Stein EA, Yang YH. Real-time animal functional magnetic resonance imaging and its application to neurophamacological studies. Magn Reson Imaging. 2008;26: 1266–72.
134. Hariri AR, Mattay VS, Tessitore A, Fera F, Smith WG, Weinberger DR. Dextroamphetamine modulates the response of the human amygdala. Neuropsychopharmacology. 2002;27:1036–40.
135. Brassen S, Tost H, Hoehn F, Weber-Fahr W, Klein S, Braus DF. Haloperidol challenge in healthy male humans: a functional magnetic resonance imaging study. Neurosci Lett. 2003;340:193–6.
136. Honey GD, Suckling J, Zelaya F, Long C, Routledge C, Jackson S, et al. Dopaminergic drug effects on physiological connectivity in a human cortico-striato-thalamic system. Brain. 2003;126:1767–81.
137. Murphy A, Mckie S, Deakin JFW. Aripiprazole and risperidone improve working memory in healthy volunteers; an fMRI study. Eur Neuropsychopharmacol. 2009;19:S188–9.
138. Vollm BA, de Araujo IE, Cowen PJ, Rolls ET, Kringelbach ML, Smith KA, et al. Methamphetamine activates reward circuitry in drug naive human subjects. Neuropsychopharmacology. 2004;29:1715–22.
139. Fischer H, Nyberg L, Karlsson S, Karlsson P, Brehmer Y, Rieckmann A, et al. Simulating neurocognitive aging: effects of a dopaminergic antagonist

on brain activity during working memory. Biol Psychiatry. 2010;67:575–80.
140. Mattay VS, Goldberg TE, Fera F, Hariri AR, Tessitore A, Egan MF, et al. Catechol O-methyltransferase val(158)-met genotype and individual variation in the brain response to amphetamine. Proc Natl Acad Sci US Am. 2003;100:6186–91.
141. Bullmore E, Suckling J, Zelaya F, Long C, Honey G, Reed L, et al. Practice and difficulty evoke anatomically and pharmacologically dissociable brain activation dynamics. Cereb Cortex. 2003;13:144–54.
142. Stein DJ, Newman TK, Savitz J, Ramesar R. Warriors vs worriers: the role of COMT gene variants. CNS Spectr. 2006;11:745–8.
143. Munafo MR, Brown SM, Hariri AR. Serotonin transporter (5-HTTLPR) genotype and amygdala activation: a meta-analysis. Biol Psychiatry. 2008;63: 852–7.
144. Thiel CM, Henson RNA, Morris JS, Friston KJ, Dolan RJ. Pharmacological modulation of behavioral and neuronal correlates of repetition priming. J Neurosci. 2001;21:6846–52.
145. Bentley P, Vuilleumier P, Thiel CM, Driver J, Dolan RJ. Cholinergic enhancement modulates neural correlates of selective attention and emotional processing. Neuroimage. 2003;20:58–70.
146. Bentley P, Vuilleumier P, Thiel CM, Driver J, Dolan RJ. Effects of attention and emotion on repetition priming and their modulation by cholinergic enhancement. J Neurophysiol. 2003;90:1171–81.
147. Bentley P, Husain M, Dolan RJ. Effects of cholinergic enhancement on visual stimulation, spatial attention, and spatial working memory. Neuron. 2004; 41:969–82.
148. Kukolja J, Thiel CM, Fink GR. Cholinergic stimulation enhances neural activity associated with encoding but reduces neural activity associated with retrieval in humans. J Neurosci. 2009;29:8119–28.
149. Stephenson CME, Suckling J, Dirckx SG, Ooi C, McKenna PJ, Bisbrown-Chippendale R, et al. GABAergic inhibitory mechanisms for repetition-adaptivity in large-scale brain systems. Neuroimage. 2003;19:1578–88.
150. Coull JT, Nobre AC, Frith CD. The noradrenergic alpha 2 agonist clonidine modulates behavioural and neuroanatomical correlates of human attentional orienting and alerting. Cereb Cortex. 2001;11:73–84.
151. Northoff G, Witzel T, Richter A, Gessner M, Schlagenhauf F, Fell J, et al. GABA-ergic modulation of prefrontal spatio-temporal activation pattern during emotional processing: a combined fMRI/MEG study with placebo and lorazepam. J Cogn Neurosci. 2002;14:348–70.
152. Fu CHY, Abel KM, Allin MPG, Gasston D, Costafreda SG, Suckling J, et al. Effects of ketamine on prefrontal and striatal regions in an overt verbal fluency task: a functional magnetic resonance imaging study. Psychopharmacology. 2005;183:92–102.
153. Abel KM, Allin MPG, Kucharska-Pietura K, David A, Andrew C, Williams S, et al. Ketamine alters neural processing of facial emotion recognition in healthy men: an fMRI study. Neuroreport. 2003; 14:387–91.
154. Wise RG, Rogers R, Painter D, Bantick S, Ploghaus A, Williams P, et al. Combining fMRI with a pharmacokinetic model to determine which brain areas activated by painful stimulation are specifically modulated by remifentanil. Neuroimage. 2002;16: 999–1014.
155. Wise RG, Williams P, Tracey I. Using fMRI to quantify the time dependence of remifentanil an algesia in the human brain. Neuropsychopharmacology. 2004;29:626–35.
156. Pattinson KTS, Governo RJ, MacIntosh BJ, Russell EC, Corfield DR, Tracey I, et al. Opioids depress cortical centers responsible for the volitional control of respiration. J Neurosci. 2009;29: 8177–86.
157. Arce E, Miller DA, Feinstein JS, Stein MB, Paulus MP. Lorazepam dose-dependently decreases risk-taking related activation in limbic areas. Psychopharmacology. 2006;189:105–16.
158. Deakin JFW, Lees J, Mckie S, Hallak JEC, Williams SR, Dursun SM. Glutamate and the neural basis of the subjective effects of ketamine. Arch Gen Psychiatry. 2008;65:154–64.
159. Borras MC, Becerra L, Ploghaus A, Gostic JM, DaSilva A, Gonzalez RG, et al. fMRI measurement of CNS responses to naloxone infusion and subsequent mild noxious thermal stimuli in healthy volunteers. J Neurophysiol. 2004;91:2723–33.
160. Kukolja J, Schlapfer TE, Keysers C, Klingmuller D, Maier W, Fink GR, et al. Modeling a negative response bias in the human amygdala by noradrenergic-glucocorticoid interactions. J Neurosci. 2008;28:12868–76.
161. Hurlemann R, Walter H, Rehme AK, Kukolja J, Santoro SC, Schmidt C, Schnell K, Musshoff F, Keysers C, Maier W, Kendrick KM, Onur OA. Human amygdala reactivity is diminished by the beta-noradrenergic antagonist propranolol. Psychol Med. 2010;40:1–10
162. van Honk J, Pruessner JC. Psychoneuroendocrine Imaging: a special issue of psychoneuroendocrinology. Psychoneuroendocrinology. 2010;35:1–4.
163. Alves FS, Figee M, Vamelsvoort T, Veltman D, de Haan L. The revised dopamine hypothesis of schizophrenia: evidence from pharmacological MRI studies with atypical antipsychotic medication. Psychopharmacol Bull. 2008;41:121–32.
164. Harmer CJ, Mackay CE, Reid CB, Cowen PJ, Goodwin GM. Antidepressant drug treatment modifies the neural processing of nonconscious threat cues. Biol Psychiatry. 2006;59:816–20.
165. Arce E, Simmons AN, Lovero KL, Stein MB, Paulus MP. Escitalopram effects on insula and amygdala BOLD activation during emotional processing. Psychopharmacology. 2008;196:661–72.
166. Harmer CJ, Shelley NC, Cowen PJ, Goodwin GM. Increased positive versus negative affective perception and memory in healthy volunteers following

selective serotonin and norepinephrine reuptake inhibition. Am J Psychiatry. 2004;161:1256–63.
167. Norbury R, Taylor MJ, Selvaraj S, Murphy SE, Harmer CJ, Cowen PJ. Short-term antidepressant treatment modulates amygdala response to happy faces. Psychopharmacology. 2009;206:197–204.
168. Murphy SE, Norbury R, O'Sullivan U, Cowen PJ, Harmer CJ. Effect of a single dose of citalopram on amygdala response to emotional faces. Br J Psychiatry. 2009;194:535–40.
169. Harmer CJ, Bhagwagar Z, Perrett DI, Vollm BA, Cowen PJ, Goodwin GM. Acute SSRI administration affects the processing of social cues in healthy volunteers. Neuropsychopharmacology. 2003;28:148–52.
170. Cools R, Calder AJ, Lawrence AD, Clark L, Bullmore E, Robbins TW. Individual differences in threat sensitivity predict serotonergic modulation of amygdala response to fearful faces. Psychopharmacology. 2005;180:670–9.
171. Evers EAT, Cools R, Clark L, van der Veen FM, Jolles J, Sahakian BJ, et al. Serotonergic modulation of prefrontal cortex during negative feedback in probabilistic reversal learning. Neuropsychopharmacology. 2005;30:1138–47.
172. Del Ben CM, Deakin JFW, Mckie S, Delvai NA, Williams SR, Elliott R, et al. The effect of citalopram pretreatment on neuronal responses to neuropsychological tasks in normal volunteers: an fMRI study. Neuropsychopharmacology. 2005;30:1724–34.
173. Anderson IM, Del Ben CM, Mckie S, Richardson P, Williams SR, Elliott R, et al. Citalopram modulation of neuronal responses to aversive face emotions: a functional MRI study. Neuroreport. 2007; 18:1351–5.
174. Vollm B, Richardson P, McKie S, Reniers R, Elliott R, Anderson IM, et al. Neuronal correlates and serotonergic modulation of behavioural inhibition and reward in healthy and antisocial individuals. J Psychiatr Res. 2010;44:123–31.
175. Kalin NH, Davidson RJ, Irwin W, Warner G, Orendi JL, Sutton SK, et al. Functional magnetic resonance imaging studies of emotional processing in normal and depressed patients: effects of venlafaxine. J Clin Psychiatry. 1997;58:32–9.
176. Kalin NH, Irwin W, Anderle M, Davidson RJ. Venlafaxine induces early and later changes in the neural circuitry of emotion that correlate with treatment response. Biol Psychiatry. 2001;49:321.
177. Davidson RJ, Irwin W, Anderle MJ, Kalin NH. The neural substrates of affective processing in depressed patients treated with venlafaxine. Am J Psychiatry. 2003;160:64–75.
178. Whalen PJ, Johnstone T, Somerville LH, Nitschke JB, Polis S, Alexander AL, et al. A functional magnetic resonance imaging predictor of treatment response to venlafaxine in generalized anxiety disorder. Biol Psychiatry. 2008;63:858–63.
179. Bhagwagar Z, Cowen PJ, Goodwin GM, Harmer CJ. Normalization of enhanced fear recognition by acute SSRI treatment in subjects with a previous history of depression. Am J Psychiatry. 2004; 161:166–8.
180. Stephan KE, Magnotta VA, White T, Arndt S, Flaum M, O'Leary DS, et al. Effects of olanzapine on cerebellar functional connectivity in schizophrenia measured by fMRI during a simple motor task. Psychol Med. 2001;31:1065–78.
181. Nahas Z, George MS, Horner MD, Markowitz JS, Li XB, Lorberbaum JP, et al. Augmenting atypical Antipsychotics with a cognitive enhancer (donepezil) improves regional brain activity in schizophrenia patients: a pilot double-blind placebo controlled BOLD fMRI study. Neurocase. 2003;9:274–82.
182. Jacobsen LK, D'Souza DC, Mencl WE, Pugh KR, Skudlarski P, Krystal JH. Nicotine effects on brain function and functional connectivity in schizophrenia. Biol Psychiatry. 2004;55:850–8.
183. Sell LA, Simmons A, Lemmens GM, Williams SCR, Brammer M, Strang J. Functional magnetic resonance imaging of the acute effect of intravenous heroin administration on visual activation in long-term heroin addicts: results from a feasibility study. Drug Alcohol Depend. 1997;49:55–60.
184. Lowen SB, Nickerson LD, Levin JM. Differential effects of acute cocaine and placebo administration on visual cortical activation in healthy subjects measured using BOLD fMRI. Pharmacol Biochem Behav. 2009;92:277–82.
185. Li SJ, Biswal B, Li Z, Risinger R, Rainey C, Cho JK, et al. Cocaine administration decreases functional connectivity in human primary visual and motor cortex as detected by functional MRI. Magn Reson Med. 2000;43:45–51.
186. Hong LE, Gu H, Yang Y, Ross TJ, Salmeron BJ, Buchholz B, et al. Association of nicotine addiction and nicotine's actions with separate cingulate cortex functional circuits. Arch Gen Psychiatry. 2009;66:431–41.
187. Lawrence NS, Ross TJ, Stein EA. Cognitive mechanisms of nicotine on visual attention. Neuron. 2002;36:539–48.
188. Hahn B, Ross TJ, Yang YH, Kim I, Huestis MA, Stein EA. Nicotine enhances visuospatial attention by deactivating areas of the resting brain default network. J Neurosci. 2007;27:3477–89.
189. Hahn B, Ross TJ, Wolkenberg FA, Shakleya DM, Huestis MA, Stein EA. Performance effects of nicotine during selective attention, divided attention, and simple stimulus detection: an fMRI study. Cereb Cortex. 2009;19:1990–2000.
190. Jacobsen LK, Gore JC, Skudlarski P, Lacadie CM, Jatlow P, Krystal JH. Impact of intravenous nicotine on BOLD signal response to photic stimulation. Magn Reson Imaging. 2002;20:141–5.
191. Jacobsen LK, Pugh KR, Mencl WE, Gelernter J. C957T polymorphism of the dopamine D2 receptor gene modulates the effect of nicotine on working memory performance and cortical processing efficiency. Psychopharmacology. 2006;188:530–40.
192. Wrase J, Grusser SM, Klein S, Diener C, Hermann D, Flor H, et al. Development of alcohol-associated

cues and cue-induced brain activation in alcoholics. Eur Psychiatry. 2002;17:287–91.
193. Hermann D, Smolka MN, Wrase J, Klein S, Nikitopoulos J, Georgi A, et al. Blockade of cue-induced brain activation of abstinent alcoholics by a single administration of amisulpride as measured with fMRI. Alcohol Clin Exp Res. 2006;30:1349–54.
194. Schneider F, Habel U, Wagner M, Franke P, Salloum JB, Shah NJ, et al. Subcortical correlates of craving in recently abstinent alcoholic patients. Am J Psychiatry. 2001;158:1075–83.
195. Thiel CM, Fink GR. Effects of the cholinergic agonist nicotine on reorienting of visual spatial attention and top-down attentional control. Neuroscience. 2008;152:381–90.
196. Kano M, Gyoba J, Kamachi M, Mochizuki H, Hongo M, Yanai K. Low doses of alcohol have a selective effect on the recognition of happy facial expressions. Hum Psychopharmacol Clin Exp. 2003;18:131–9.
197. Koppelstaetter F, Poeppel TD, Siedentopf CM, Ischebeck A, Verius M, Haala I, et al. Does caffeine modulate verbal working memory processes? An fMRI study. Neuroimage. 2008;39:492–9.
198. Koppelstaetter F, Poeppel TD, Siedentopf CM, Ischebeck A, Kolbitsch C, Mottaghy FM, et al. Caffeine and Cognition in Functional Magnetic Resonance Imaging. Dis: J Alzheimers; 2010.
199. Langleben DD, Ruparel K, Elman I, Busch-Winokur S, Pratiwadi R, Loughead J, et al. Acute effect of methadone maintenance dose on brain FMRI response to heroin-related cues. Am J Psychiatry. 2008;165:390–4.
200. Vaidya CJ, Austin G, Kirkorian G, Ridlehuber HW, Desmond JE, Glover GH, et al. Selective effects of methylphenidate in attention-deficit/hyperactivity disorder: a functional magnetic resonance study. Proc Natl Acad Sci USA. 1998;95:14494–9.
201. Anderson CM, Polcari A, Lowen SB, Renshaw PF, Teicher MH. Effects of methylphenidate on functional magnetic resonance relaxometry of the cerebellar vermis in boys with ADHD. Am J Psychiatry. 2002;159:1322–8.
202. Silveri MM, Anderson CM, Mcneil JF, Diaz CI, Lukas SE, Mendelson JH, et al. Oral methylphenidate challenge selectively decreases putaminal T2 in healthy subjects. Drug Alcohol Depend. 2004;76:173–80.
203. Anderson CM, Lowen SB, Renshaw PF. Emotional task-dependent low-frequency fluctuations and methylphenidate: Wavelet scaling analysis of 1/f-type fluctuations in fMRI of the cerebellar vermis. J Neurosci Meth. 2006;151:52–61.
204. Kaufman MJ, Levin JM, Maas LC, Kukes TJ, Villafuerte RA, Dostal K, et al. Cocaine-induced cerebral vasoconstriction differs as a function of sea and menstrual cycle phase. Biol Psychiatry. 2001;49:774–81.
205. Streeter CC, Ciraulo DA, Harris GJ, Kaufman MJ, Lewis RF, Knapp CM, et al. Functional magnetic resonance imaging of alprazolam-induced changes in humans with familial alcoholism. Psychiatry Res Neuroimaging. 1998;82:69–82.
206. Sosnovik DE, Weissleder R. Emerging concepts in molecular MRI. Curr Opin Biotechnol. 2007;18:4–10.
207. Soares DP, Law M. Magnetic resonance spectroscopy of the brain: review of metabolites and clinical applications. Clin Radiol. 2009;64:12–21.
208. Judenhofer MS, Wehrl HF, Newport DF, Catana C, Siegel SB, Becker M, et al. Simultaneous PET-MRI: a new approach for functional and morphological imaging. Nat Med. 2008;14:459–65.

Functional MRI: Cognitive Neuroscience Applications

20

Mark D'Esposito, Andrew S. Kayser, and Anthony J.W. Chen

Introduction

Cognitive neuroscience is a discipline that attempts to determine the neural mechanisms underlying cognitive processes. Specifically, cognitive neuroscientists test hypotheses about brain–behavior relationships that can be organized along two conceptual domains: (1) *functional specialization* – the idea that functional modules exist within the brain, i.e., areas of the cerebral cortex that are specialized for a specific cognitive process; and (2) *functional integration* – the idea that a cognitive process can be an emergent property of interactions among a network of brain regions, which suggests that a brain region can play a different role across many functions.

Early investigations of brain–behavior relationships consisted of careful observation of individuals with neurological injury resulting in focal brain damage. The idea of functional specialization evolved from the hypotheses that damage to a particular brain region was responsible for a given behavioral syndrome that was characterized by a precise neurological examination. For instance, the association of nonfluent aphasia with right-sided limb weakness implicated the left hemisphere as the site of language abilities. Moreover, upon death of a patient with a neurological disorder, clinicopathological correlations provided confirmatory information about the site of damage causing a specific neurobehavioral syndrome, such as aphasia. For example, in 1861, Paul Broca's observations of nonfluent aphasia in the setting of a damaged left inferior frontal gyrus cemented the belief that this brain region was critical for speech output [1]. The introduction of structural brain imaging more than 100 years after Broca's observations, first with computerized tomography (CT) and later with magnetic resonance imaging (MRI), paved the way for more precise anatomical localization in the living patient of the cognitive deficits that develop after brain injury. The superb spatial resolution of structural neuroimaging has reduced the reliance on the infrequently obtained autopsy for making brain–behavior correlations.

M. D'Esposito, MD (✉)
Brain Imaging Center, Helen Wills Neuroscience Institute, University of California, Berkeley, 132 Barker Hall, Berkeley, CA 94720-3190, USA
e-mail: despo@berkley.edu

A.S. Kayser, MD, PhD
Department of Neurology, Ernest Gallo Clinic & Research Center, University of California at San Francisco, 5858 Horton Street, Suite 200, Emeryville, CA 94608, USA
e-mail: akayser@gallo.ucsf.edu

A.J.W. Chen, MA, MD
Department of Neurology, VA Medical Center – San Francisco, Helen Wills Neuroscience Institute, University of California, San Francisco, 132 Barker Hall, Berkeley, CA 94720, USA
e-mail: Anthony.chen@va.gov

S.H. Faro and F.B. Mohamed (eds.), *Functional BOLD MRI: Principles and Applications*, DOI 10.1007/978-1-4939-1995-6_20, © Springer Science+Business Media New York 2015

Functional neuroimaging, broadly defined as techniques that measure brain activity, has expanded our ability to study the neural basis of cognitive processes. One such method, functional magnetic resonance imaging (fMRI), has emerged as an extremely powerful technique that affords excellent spatial and temporal resolution. Measuring regional brain activity in healthy subjects while they perform cognitive tasks links localized brain activity with specific behaviors. For example, functional neuroimaging studies have demonstrated that the left inferior frontal gyrus is consistently activated during the performance of speech production tasks in healthy individuals [2]. Such findings from functional neuroimaging are complementary to findings derived from observations of patients with focal brain damage. This chapter focuses on the principles underlying fMRI as a cognitive neuroscience tool for exploring brain–behavior relationships.

Inference in Functional Neuroimaging Studies of Cognitive Processes

Insight regarding the link between brain and behavior can be gained through a variety of approaches. It is unlikely that any single neuroscience method is sufficient to investigate any particular question regarding the mechanisms underlying cognitive function fully. From a methodological point of view, each method will offer different temporal and spatial resolution. From a conceptual point of view, each method will provide data that will support different types of inferences that can be drawn from it. Thus, data obtained by addressing a single question but derived from multiple methods can provide more comprehensive and inferentially sound conclusions.

Functional neuroimaging studies support inferences about the association of a particular brain system with a cognitive process. However, it is difficult to prove in such a study that the observed activity is necessary for an isolated cognitive process because perfect control over a subject's cognitive processes during a functional neuroimaging experiment is never possible. Even if the task a subject performs is well designed, it is difficult to demonstrate conclusively that he or she is differentially engaging a single, identified cognitive process. The subject may engage in unwanted cognitive processes that either have no overt, measurable effects or are perfectly confounded with the process of interest. Consequently, the neural activity measured by the functional neuroimaging technique may result from some confounding neural computation that is itself not necessary for executing the cognitive process seemingly under study. In other words, functional neuroimaging is an observational, correlative method [3]. It is important to note that the inferences that can be drawn from functional neuroimaging studies such as fMRI apply to all methods of physiological measurement, e.g., electroencephalography (EEG) or magnetoencephalography (MEG).

The inference of necessity cannot be made without showing that inactivating a brain region disrupts the cognitive process in question. However, lesions in patients are often extensive, damaging local neurons and "fibers of passage." For example, damage to prominent white matter tracts can cause cognitive deficits similar to those produced by cortical lesions, such as the amnesia resulting from lesions of the fornix, the main white matter pathway projecting from the hippocampus [4]. In addition, connections from region "A" may support the continued metabolic function of region "B," but region A may not be computationally involved in certain processes undertaken by region B. Thus, damage to region A could impair the function of region B via two possible mechanisms: (1) diaschisis [5] and (2) retrograde transsynaptic degeneration. Consequently, studies of patients with focal lesions cannot conclusively demonstrate that the neurons within a specific region are themselves critical to the computational support of an impaired cognitive process.

Empirical studies using lesion and electrophysiological methods demonstrate these issues regarding the types of inferences that can be logically drawn from them. For example, in monkeys, single-unit recording reveals neurons in the lateral prefrontal cortex (PFC) that increase their firing during the delay between the presentation of information to be remembered and a few seconds later when that information must be recalled [6, 7]. These studies are taken as evidence that persistent neural activity in the PFC is involved in temporary storage of information, a cognitive process known as working memory. The necessity of PFC for working memory was demonstrated in other monkey studies showing that prefrontal lesions impair performance on working memory tasks, but not on tasks that do not require temporarily holding information in memory [8]. Persistent neural activity during working memory tasks is also found in the hippocampus [9, 10]. Hippocampal lesions, however, do not impair performance on most working memory tasks [11], which suggests that the hippocampus is *involved* in maintaining information over short periods of time, but is not *necessary* for this cognitive operation. Observations in humans support this notion. For example, the well-studied patient H.M., with complete bilateral hippocampal damage and severe inability to learn new information, could nevertheless perform normally on working memory tasks such as digit span [12]. The hippocampus is implicated in long-term memory, especially when relations between multiple items or multiple features of a complex novel item must be retained. Thus, the hippocampus may only be engaged during working memory tasks that require someone to remember novel information subsequently [13].

When the results from lesion and functional neuroimaging studies are combined, a stronger level of inference emerges. As in the examples of Broca's aphasia or working memory, a lesion of a specific brain region causes impairment of a given cognitive process, and when engaged by an intact individual, that cognitive process evokes neural activity in the same brain region. Given these findings, the inference that this brain region is computationally necessary for the cognitive process is stronger than data derived from each study performed in isolation. Thus, lesion and functional neuroimaging studies are complementary, each providing inferential support that the other lacks.

Other types of inferential failure can occur in the interpretation of functional neuroimaging studies when other common assumptions do not hold true. First, it is assumed that if a cognitive process activates a particular brain region (evoked by a particular task), the neural activity in that brain region must depend on engaging that particular cognitive process. For example, a brain region showing greater activation during the presentation of faces than to other types of stimuli, such as photographs of cars or buildings, is considered to engage face perception processes. However, this region may also support other higher level cognitive processes, such as memory processes, in addition to lower level perceptual processes [14]. See Henson [15] for a further discussion of this issue.

The opposite type of inference is made when it is assumed that if a particular brain region is activated during the performance of a cognitive task, the subject must have engaged the cognitive process supported by that region during the task (referred to as a "reverse inference"). For example, observing activation of the frontal lobes during a mental rotation task, it was proposed that subjects engaged working memory processes to recall the identity of the rotated target [16]. (They derived this assumption from other imaging studies showing activation of the frontal lobes during working memory tasks.) However, in this example, because some other cognitive processes supported by the frontal lobes could have activated this region [17], one cannot be sure that working memory was engaged, leading to the activation of the frontal lobes. Unfortunately, this potentially faulty logic is a fairly common practice in fMRI studies. See Poldrack [18] for a further discussion of this issue.

In summary, interpretation of the results of functional neuroimaging studies attempting to link brain and behavior rests on numerous assumptions. Familiarity with the types of inferences that can and cannot be drawn from these studies is helpful for assessing the validity of the findings reported by such studies.

Functional MRI as a Cognitive Neuroscience Tool

Functional MRI has become the predominant functional neuroimaging method for studying the neural basis of cognitive processes in humans. Compared to its predecessor, positron emission tomography (PET) scanning, fMRI offers many advantages. For example, MRI scanners are much more widely available, and imaging costs are less expensive since MRI does not require a cyclotron to produce radioisotopes. MRI is also a noninvasive procedure since there is no requirement for injection of a radioisotope into the bloodstream. Also, given the half-life of available radioisotopes, PET scanning is unable to provide temporal resolution comparable to that of fMRI, which can provide images of behavioral events occurring on the order of seconds rather than the summation of many behavioral events occurring over tens of seconds.

In selected circumstances, however, PET can provide an advantage over fMRI for studying certain questions concerning the neural basis of cognition. For example, at present, fMRI does not adequately image the regions within the orbitofrontal cortex and the anterior or inferior temporal lobe because of the susceptibility artifact near the interface of the brain and sinuses. These artifacts worsen at higher magnetic fields (i.e., 3 or 4 T) and such scanners are becoming commonly available and increasingly utilized by cognitive neuroscientists. Improvements in pulse sequences for acquiring fMRI data and development of algorithms for limiting susceptibility loss of signal and distortion correction of images should eventually eliminate or reduce these artifacts [19–21]. Currently, however, such sequences and methods are not widely available and implemented.

PET scanning may remain desirable or necessary when studying certain populations of individuals. For example, amnesic patients resulting from cerebral anoxia often have implanted cardiac pacemakers, precluding them from having MRI scans due to the magnetic field. However, PET scanning is unacceptable for studies of children due to the radiation exposure. A particular advantage of PET scanning in the study of cognition that can nicely complement fMRI studies is its ability to assess neurochemical (neurotransmitter and neuromodulator) systems. Radioactively labeled ligands may be used to measure directly the density and distribution of particular receptors and even receptor subtypes, distribution of presynaptic terminals, or enzymes involved in the production or breakdown of particular neurochemicals [22].

The MRI scanner, compared to a behavioral testing room, is less than ideal for performing most cognitive neuroscience experiments. Experiments are performed in the awkward position of lying on one's back, often requiring subjects to visualize the presentation of stimuli through a mirror, in an acoustically noisy environment. Moreover, most individuals develop some degree of claustrophobia due to the small bore of the MRI scanner and find it difficult to remain completely motionless for the long duration of time that is required for most experiments, e.g., usually 60–90 min. These constraints of the MRI scanner make it especially difficult to scan children or certain patient populations (e.g., Parkinson's disease patients), which has resulted in many fewer fMRI studies involving children than adults and neurological patients in general. However, mock scanners have been built in many imaging centers, with motion devices, which acclimate children to the scanner environment before they participate in an fMRI study. This approach has led to an increasing number of fMRI studies of children being reported in the literature, which are providing tremendous insight regarding the mechanisms underlying the developing brain [23, 24].

All sensory systems have been investigated with fMRI including the visual, auditory, somatosensory, olfactory, and gustatory systems. Each system requires different technologies for successful presentation of relevant stimuli within an MRI environment. At the time of this writing, very few off-the-shelf commercial products exist that are MRI compatible, and most in use today have been engineered locally by individual laboratories. Most published fMRI studies have utilized visual stimuli, although great strides have been made to allow the presentation of other types of stimuli. Details regarding the issues related to presenting visual and auditory stimuli in the MRI environment are further reviewed in a comprehensive chapter by Savoy and colleagues in ref. [25]. In brief, the most common means of presenting visual stimuli is via a liquid crystal display (LCD) projector system, with the sophistication of the system depending on the quality of image resolution required for the experiment. Several options exist for auditory stimuli such as piezoelectric or electrostatic headphones. However, the biggest challenge is the acoustically noisy scanner environment. The pulsing of the fMRI gradient coils is the source of such noise, making the study of auditory processes challenging [26, 27]. For example, during echo-planar imaging within a 4-T magnet using a high-performance head gradient set, sound levels can reach 130 dB. As a reference point, Food and Drug Administration (FDA) safety regulations require no greater than an average of 105 dB for one hour. With placement of absorbing materials within the scanner and on the walls of the room, as well as a fiberglass bore liner surrounding the gradient set, we have been able to reduce sound levels by about 25 dB. One of the biggest technical challenges within an MRI scanner has been the ability to present olfactory stimuli. However, sophisticated MR-compatible olfactometers have been designed and utilized successfully. Such methods use a nasal mask in which the change from odorant to no-odorant conditions occurs within a few milliseconds [28, 29].

Acquiring ancillary electrophysiological data, such as electromyographic recordings to measure muscle contraction or electrodermal responses to measure autonomic activity, enhances many cognitive neuroscience experiments. Devices have been developed that are MR compatible for these types of measurements and other physiological measures such as heart rate, electrocardiography, oxygen saturation, and respiratory rate. The recording of eye movements is becoming commonplace in MRI scanners, predominantly with the use of infrared video camera equipped with long-range optics [30, 31]. Video images of the pupil–corneal reflection can be sampled at 60/120/240 Hz, allowing for the accurate (<1°) localization of gaze within 50 horizontal and 40 vertical degrees of visual angle. Although most behavioral tasks used in cognitive neuroscience experiments rely on collecting manual responses, the ability to collect verbal responses reliably without significant artifact introduced into the data has been demonstrated by several laboratories [32–34].

EEG recordings have also been successfully performed during MRI scanning (e.g., [35, 36]). However, the recording of event-related potentials (ERP), a signal that is much smaller in amplitude than the signal in EEG, can be more difficult in a magnetic field due to artifacts induced by gradient pulsing and head movement from cardiac pulsation. New monitoring devices and algorithms to remove artifacts are being developed, allowing for reliable measurements of ERPs during MRI scanning [37, 38]. In summary, most initial challenges facing performing cognitive experiments within the MRI environment have been overcome, creating an environment that is comparable to standard psychophysical testing laboratories outside of a scanner. Although individual laboratories have achieved most of these advancements, MRI scanners originally designed for clinical use by manufacturers are now being designed with consideration of many of these research-related issues.

Temporal Resolution

Two types of temporal resolution need to be considered for cognitive neuroscience experiments. First, what is the briefest neural event that can be detected as an fMRI signal? Second, how close apart can two neural events occur and be resolved as separable fMRI signals?

The timescale on which neural changes occur are quite rapid. For example, neural activity in the lateral intraparietal area of monkeys increases within 100 ms of the visual presentation of a saccade target [39]. In contrast, the fMRI signal gradually increases to its peak magnitude within 4–6 s after an experimentally induced brief (<1 s) change in neural activity, and then decays back to baseline after several more seconds [40–42]. This slow time course of fMRI signal change in

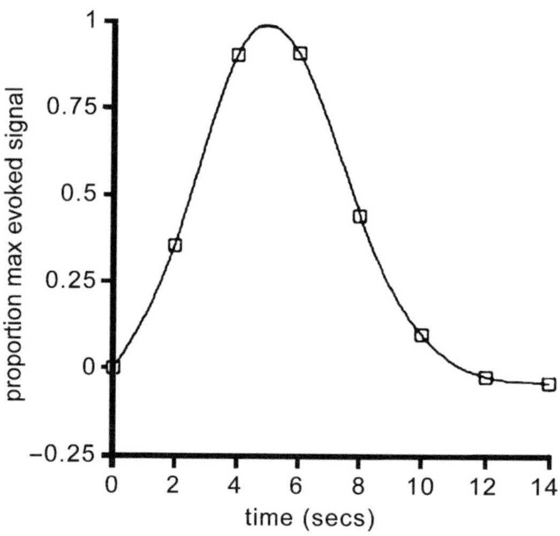

Fig. 20.1 A typical hemodynamic response (i.e., fMRI signal change in response to a brief increase in neural activity) from the primary sensorimotor cortex. The fMRI signal peaked approximately 5 s after the onset of the motor response (at time zero)

response to such a brief increase in neural activity is informally referred to as the blood-oxygen level-dependent (BOLD) fMRI hemodynamic response or simply, the hemodynamic response (Fig. 20.1). Thus, neural dynamics and neurally evoked hemodynamics, as measured with fMRI, are on quite different timescales.

The sluggishness of the hemodynamic response limits the temporal resolution of the fMRI signal to hundreds of milliseconds to seconds, as opposed to the millisecond temporal resolution of electrophysiological recordings of neural activity. However, it has been clearly demonstrated that brief changes in neural activity can be detected with reasonable statistical power using fMRI. For example, appreciable fMRI signal can be observed in sensorimotor cortex in association with single finger movements [43] and in visual cortex during very briefly presented (34 ms) visual stimuli [44]. In contrast, the temporal resolution of fMRI limits the detection of sequential changes in neural activity that occurs rapidly with respect to the hemodynamic response. That is, the ability to resolve the changes in the fMRI signal associated with two neural events often requires the separation of the events by a relatively long period of time compared with the width of the hemodynamic response. This is because two neural events closely spaced in time will produce a hemodynamic response that reflects the accumulation from both neural events, making it difficult to estimate the contribution of each individual neural event. In general, evoked fMRI responses to discrete neural events separated by at least 4 s appear to be within the range of resolution [45]. However, provided that the stimuli are presented randomly, studies have shown significant differential functional responses between two events (e.g., flashing visual stimuli) spaced as closely as 500 ms apart [46–48]. The effect of fixed and randomized intertrial intervals on the BOLD signal is illustrated in Fig. 20.2.

In some tasks, the order of individual trial events cannot be randomized. For example, in certain types of working memory tasks, the presentation of the information to be remembered during the delay period, and the period when the subject must recall the information are individual trial events whose order cannot be randomized. In these types of tasks, short timescales (<4 s) cannot be temporally resolved. These temporal resolution issues in fMRI have been extensively considered regarding their impact on experimental design [49, 50].

Spatial Resolution

It is yet to be determined how precisely the measured BOLD fMRI signal, which arises from the vasculature, reflects adjacent neural activity. Thus, the ultimate spatial resolution of BOLD fMRI is unknown. Functional MRI studies in both monkey and man at high field (4–4.7 T) have demonstrated that BOLD signal can be obtained with high spatial resolution – approximately $0.75 \times 0.75\ \text{mm}^2$ in-plane resolution [51, 52]. In monkeys, with novel approaches such as using a small, tissue-compatible, intraosteally implanted radiofrequency coil, ultra high spatial resolution of $125 \times 125\ \mu\text{m}^2$ has been obtained [53]. Using this method, Logothetis and colleagues demonstrated cortical lamina-specific activation in a task that compared responses to moving stimuli with those elicited by flickering

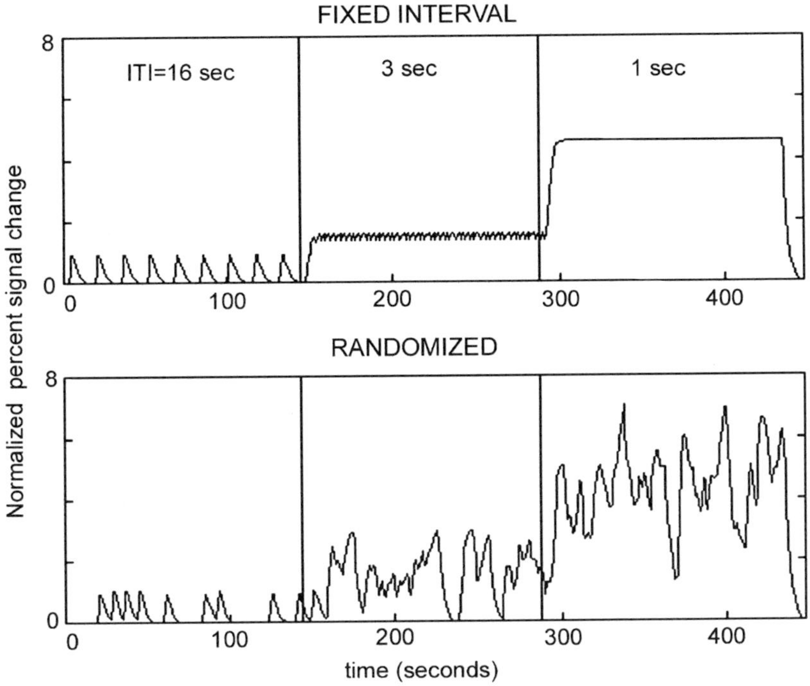

Fig. 20.2 Effect of fixed versus randomized intertrial intervals on the BOLD fMRI signal [46]

stimuli. This contrast elicited BOLD signal mostly in the granular layers of the striate cortex of the monkey, which is known to have a high concentration of directionally selective cells. Advances in such methods would allow for imaging of hundreds of neurons per voxel as opposed to hundreds of thousands of neurons per voxel, which is more typical for a human cognitive neuroscience fMRI experiment.

Virtually all fMRI studies model the large BOLD signal increase, which is due to a local low-deoxyhemoglobin state, in order to detect changes correlating with a behavioral task. However, optical imaging studies have demonstrated that preceding this large positive response, there is an initial negative response reflecting a localized increase in oxygen consumption causing a high-deoxyhemoglobin state [54]. This early hemodynamic response is called the "initial dip" and is thought to be more tightly coupled to the actual site of neural activity evoking the BOLD signal compared to the later positive portion of the BOLD response. For example, Kim and colleagues, scanning cats in a high field scanner, demonstrated that the early-negative BOLD response (e.g., initial dip) produced activation maps that were consistent with orientation columns within visual cortex. This finding is quite remarkable given that the average spacing between two adjacent orientation columns in cortex is approximately 1 mm. In contrast, the activation maps produced by the delayed positive BOLD response appeared more diffuse, and cortical columnar organization could not be identified [55]. Thus, empirical evidence suggests that deriving activation maps by correlating behavioral responses with the initial dip may markedly improve spatial resolution. However, it is important to note that the initial dip of the BOLD signal has been inconsistently observed in humans across laboratories for reasons that are still unclear. Several groups, however, were able to detect columnar architecture (in this case, ocular dominance columns) by modeling the positive BOLD response in humans scanned at 4 T [52, 56]. These investigators attributed their success to optimized radiofrequency coils, limiting head motion, optimizing slice orientation, and the enhanced signal-to-noise ratio provided by a high magnetic field.

Another unique method for improving spatial resolution has been called functional magnetic resonance adaptation (fMR-A), which could provide a means for identifying and assessing the functional attributes of sharply defined neuronal populations within a given region of the brain [57]. Even if the spatial resolution of fMRI evolves to the point of being able to resolve a population of a few hundred neurons within a voxel, it is still likely that this small population will contain neurons with very different functional properties that will be averaged together. The adaptation method is based on several basic principles. First, repeated presentation of the same type of stimuli (i.e., a picture of an object) causes neurons to adapt to those stimuli (i.e., neuronal firing is reduced). Second, if these neurons are then exposed to a different type of stimulus (i.e., a picture of another object) or a change in some property of the stimulus (i.e., the same object in a different orientation), recovery from adaptation can be assessed (i.e., whether or not the BOLD signal returns to its original state). If the signal remains adapted, it implies that the neurons are invariant to the attribute that was changed, or if the signal recovers from the adapted state, it would imply that the neurons are sensitive to that attribute. For example, Grill-Spector and colleagues demonstrated that an area of lateral occipital cortex thought to be important for object recognition was less sensitive to changes in object size and position compared to changes in illumination and viewpoint [58]. Thus, with this method, it is possible to investigate the functional properties of neuronal populations with a level of spatial resolution that is beyond that obtained using conventional fMRI data analysis methods.

Considering all the neuroscientific methods available today for studying human brain–behavior relationships, fMRI provides an excellent balance of temporal and spatial resolution. Improvements on both fronts will clearly add to the increasing popularity of this method.

Issues in Functional MRI Experimental Design

Numerous options exist for designing experiments using fMRI. The prototypical fMRI experimental design consists of two behavioral tasks presented in blocks of trials alternating over the course of a scanning session, and the fMRI signal between the two tasks is compared. This is known as a block design. For example, a given block might present a series of faces to be viewed passively, which evokes a particular cognitive process, such as face perception. The "experimental" block alternates with a "control" block, which is designed to evoke all of the cognitive processes present in the experimental block, except for the cognitive process of interest. In this experiment, the control block may comprise a series of objects. In this way, the stimuli used in experimental and control tasks have similar visual attributes, but differ in the attribute of interest (i.e., faces). The inferential framework of "cognitive subtraction" [59] attributes differences in neural activity between the two tasks to the specific cognitive process (i.e., face perception). Cognitive subtraction was originally conceived by Donders in the late 1800s for studying the chronometric substrates of cognitive processes (see Sternberg [60]) and was a major innovation in imaging [59, 61].

The assumptions required for cognitive subtraction may not always hold and could produce erroneous interpretation of functional neuroimaging data [45]. Cognitive subtraction relies on two assumptions: "pure insertion" and linearity. Pure insertion implies that a cognitive process can be added to a preexisting set of cognitive processes without affecting them. This assumption is difficult to prove because one needs an independent measure of the preexisting processes in the absence and presence of the new process [60]. If pure insertion fails as an assumption, a difference in the neuroimaging signal between the two tasks might be observed, not because a specific cognitive process was engaged in one task and not the other, but because the added cognitive process and the preexisting cognitive processes interact.

An example of this point is illustrated in working memory studies using delayed response tasks [62]. These tasks (for an example, see Jonides et al. [63]) typically present information that the subject must remember (engaging an *encoding* process), followed by a delay period during which the subject must hold the information in memory over a short period of time (engaging a *memory* process), followed by a probe that requires the subject to make a decision based on the stored information (engaging a *retrieval* process). The brain regions engaged by evoking the *memory* process theoretically are revealed by subtracting the BOLD signal measured by fMRI during a block of trials that the subject performs that do not have a delay period (only engaging the *encoding* and *retrieval* processes) from a block of trials with a delay period (engaging the *encoding*, *memory*, and *retrieval* processes). In this example, if the addition or "insertion" of a delay period between the *encoding* and *retrieval* processes affects these other behavioral processes in the task, the result is failure to meet the assumptions of cognitive subtraction. That is, these "non-memory" processes may differ in delay trials and no-delay trials, resulting in a failure to cancel each other out in the two types of trials that are being compared.

Empirical evidence of such failure exists [64]. For example, Fig. 20.3 demonstrates BOLD signal derived from the PFC of a subject performing a delayed response task similar to the tasks described previously. The left side of the figure illustrates BOLD signal consistent with delay period activity, whereas the right side of the figure illustrates BOLD signal from another region of PFC that did not display sustained activity during the delay, yet showed greater activity in the delay trials compared to the trials without a delay. In any block functional neuroimaging study that compares delay versus no-delay trials with subtraction, such a region would be detected and likely assumed to be a "memory" region. Thus, this result provides empirical grounds for adopting a

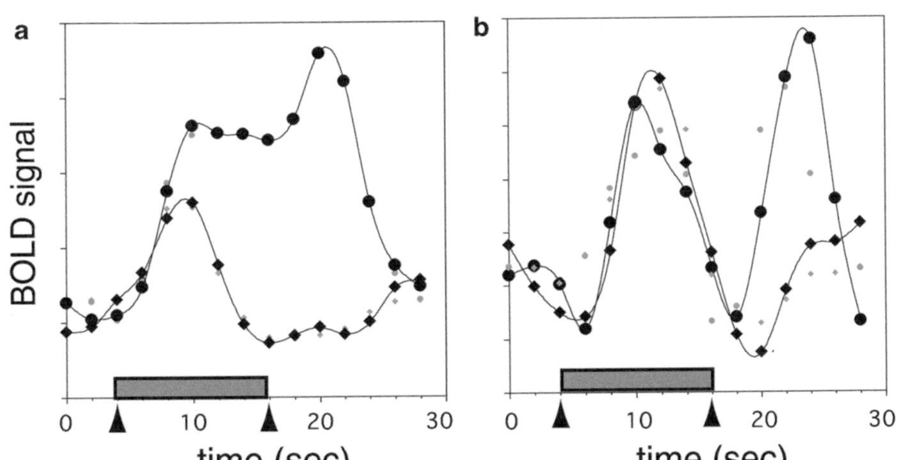

Fig. 20.3 Data derived from the performance of a normal subject on a spatial delayed-response task [64]. This task comprised both delay trials (circles) and trials without a delay period (no-delay trials; diamonds). (**a**) Trial-averaged fMRI signal from prefrontal cortex that displayed delay-correlated activity. The gray bar along the *X*-axis denotes the 12-s delay period during delay trials. The delay trials display a level of fMRI signal greater than baseline throughout the period of time corresponding to the retention delay (taking into account the delay and dispersion of the fMRI signal). The peaks seen in the signal correspond to the encoding and retrieval periods. (**b**) Trial-averaged fMRI signal from a region in prefrontal cortex that did not display the characteristics of delay-correlated activity. This region displays a significant functional change associated with the no-delay trials, and significant functional changes associated with the encoding and retrieval periods of the delay trials, but not one associated with the retention delay of delay trials

healthy doubt regarding the inferences drawn from imaging studies that rely exclusively on cognitive subtraction.

In functional neuroimaging, the transform between the neural signal and the hemodynamic response (measured by fMRI) must also be linear for the cognitive subtractive method to yield valid results. In other words, it is assumed that the BOLD signal being measured is approximately proportional to the local neural activity that evokes it. Surprisingly, although thousands of empirical studies using fMRI to study brain–behavior relationships have been published, only a handful exist that have explored the neurophysiological basis of the BOLD signal (for reviews, see Attwell et al. [65] and Heeger et al. [66]). In several studies, linearity did not strictly hold for the BOLD fMRI system, but the linear transform model was reasonably consistent with the data. For example, Boynton and colleagues tested whether BOLD signal in response to long duration stimuli can be predicted by summing the responses to shorter duration stimuli [42]. Using pulses of flickering checkerboard patterns and measuring within human primary visual cortex, these investigators found that the BOLD signal response to various durations of stimulus presentation (6, 12, or 24 s) could be predicted from the responses they obtained from shorter stimulus presentations. For example, the BOLD signal response to a 6-s pulse could be predicted from the summation of the BOLD signal response to the 3-s pulse with a copy of the same response delayed by 3 s. However, temporal summation did not always hold, and there are clearly nonlinear effects in the transform of neural activity to a hemodynamic response that must be considered [67–70]. If these nonlinearities lead to saturation of the BOLD effect at a certain stimulus intensity, erroneous interpretation of particular results of fMRI experiments may occur.

Another class of experimental designs, called event-related fMRI, attempts to detect changes associated with individual trials, as opposed to the larger unit of time comprising a block of trials [71, 72]. Each individual trial may be composed of one behavioral "event," such as the presentation of a single stimulus (e.g., a face or object to be perceived), or several behavioral events, such as in the delayed response task described previously (e.g., an item to be remembered, a delay period, and a motor response in a delayed response task). For example, with an event-related design, activity within the PFC has consistently been shown to correlate with the delay period [64], supporting the role of the PFC in temporarily maintaining information. Event-related designs offer numerous advantages. For example, it allows for stimulus or trial randomization, avoiding the behavioral confounds of block trials. It also permits the separate analysis of functional responses, which are identified only in retrospect (i.e., trials on which the subject made a correct or incorrect response). Of course, an experiment does not have to be limited to either a block or an event-related design – a mixed type (both event-related and block) design where particular trial types are randomized within a block is perfectly feasible. In this type of design, both item-related processes (e.g., transient responses to stimuli) and state-related processes (processes sustained throughout a block of trials or a task [73, 74]) are perfectly feasible.

Overall, much flexibility exists in the type of experimental design that can be utilized in fMRI experiments, and continued innovation in this area will greatly expand the types of neuroscientific questions that can be addressed.

Issues in Interpretation of FMRI Data

Statistics

Many statistical techniques are used for analyzing fMRI data, but no single method has emerged as the ideal or "gold standard." The analysis of any fMRI experiment designed to contradict the null hypothesis (i.e., there is no difference between experimental conditions) requires inferential statistics. If the difference between two experimental conditions is too large to be reasonably due to chance, then the null hypothesis is rejected in favor of the alternative hypothesis, which typically is the experimenter's hypothesis (e.g., the fusiform gyrus is activated to a greater extent by viewing faces than objects). Unfortunately, since errors can occur in any statistical test, experimenters will never know when an error is committed and can only try to minimize them [75]. Knowledge of several basic statistical issues provides a solid foundation for the correct interpretation of the data derived from fMRI studies.

Two types of statistical errors can occur. A type I error is committed when the null hypothesis is falsely rejected when it is true, that is, a difference between experimental conditions is found but a difference does not truly exist. This type of error is also called a false-positive error. In an fMRI study, a false-positive error would be finding a brain region activated during a cognitive task, when actually it is not. A type II error is committed when the null hypothesis is accepted when it is false, that is, no difference between experimental conditions exists when a difference does exist. This type of error is also called a false-negative error. A false-negative error in an fMRI study would be failure to find a brain region activated during the performance of a cognitive task when actually it is. The concept of type II error is closely related to the idea of statistical power. If the false-negative rate for a given study design is 20%, for instance, then the *power* of that design to detect an activation is "100–20%", or 80%.

In cognitive neuroscience studies, much emphasis has been placed on avoiding type I errors. The negative effects of incorrectly identifying a brain region as task active include the expenditures of time, money, and effort spent in replicating and/or expanding upon a false-positive result. Type II error, on the contrary, is seen as less damning; failure to detect brain activity in a research study has fewer implications for future research, provided that one is careful to interpret the so-called null results correctly. For example, cognitive neuroscience studies (due to factors such as the expense and the difficulty of finding research participants, for example) tend to employ a small number of subjects – 15 would not be atypical – and, therefore, frequently lack the power to detect significant brain activations. One must consequently be careful to avoid interpreting a lack of activation in one part of the brain as true inactivity during the task.

In a clinical research study, on the contrary, the emphasis may be different, especially when fMRI studies are being used diagnostically in single patients. A type II error – failing to detect active brain regions related to movement or language in the vicinity of a brain tumor, for example – may lead to a larger surgical resection that leaves the patient with avoidable residual deficits. On the contrary, a type I error – for example, identifying motor activity adjacent to a tumor when in fact none exists – may erroneously lead to a more cautious surgical resection, or to use of a different treatment modality. Which error is deemed more tolerable may depend on the clinical situation.

In fMRI experiments, as in all experiments, a tolerable probability for type I error, typically less than 5%, is chosen for adequate control of specificity, that is, control of false-positive rates. Two features of fMRI data can cause unacceptable false-positive rates, even with traditional parametric statistical tests. First, there is the problem of multiple comparisons. For the typical resolution of images acquired during fMRI scans, the full extent of the human brain could comprise as many as 15,000 voxels. Thus, with any given statistical comparison of two experimental conditions, there are actually 15,000 statistical comparisons being performed. With such a large number of statistical tests, the probability of finding a false-positive activation, that is, committing a type I error, somewhere in the brain increases. Several methods exist to deal with this problem. One method, Bonferroni correction, assumes that each statistical test is independent and calculates the probability of type I error by dividing the chosen probability ($p = 0.05$) by the number of statistical tests performed. Another method is based on Gaussian field theory [76], and calculates the probability of type I error when imaging data are spatially smoothed. Many other methods for determining thresholds of statistical maps are proposed and utilized [77, 78], but unfortunately no single method has been universally accepted. Nevertheless, all fMRI studies must apply some type of correction for multiple comparisons to control for the false-positive rate.

The second feature that might increase the false-positive rate is the "noise" in fMRI data. Data from BOLD fMRI are temporally autocorrelated with more noise at some frequencies than at others. The shape of this noise distribution is characterized by a 1/frequency function, with increasing noise at lower frequencies [79]. Traditional parametric and nonparametric statistical tests assume that the noise is not temporally autocorrelated, that is, each observation is independent. Therefore, any statistical test used in fMRI studies must account for the noise structure of fMRI data. If not, the false-positive rates will inflate [79, 80].

Type II error is rarely considered in functional neuroimaging studies. When a brain map from an fMRI experiment is presented, several areas of activation are typically attributed to some experimental manipulation. The focus of most fMRI studies is on brain activation, whereas it is often implicitly assumed that all of the other areas (typically most of the brain) are not activated during the experiment. Power as a statistical concept refers to the probability of correctly rejecting the null hypothesis [75]. As the power of an fMRI study to detect changes in brain activity increases, the false-negative rate decreases. Unfortunately, power calculations for particular fMRI experiments are rarely performed, although this methodology is evolving [81–83]. Reports that specific brain areas were not active during an experimental manipulation should provide an estimate of the power required for detection of a change in the region. All experiments should be designed to maximize power. Relatively simple strategies can increase power in an fMRI experiment in certain circumstances, such as increasing the amount of imaging data collected or increasing the number of subjects studied. It is also important to note that task designs can affect sensitivity [84]. For example, since BOLD fMRI data are temporally autocorrelated, experiments with fundamental frequencies in the lower range (e.g., a boxcar design with 60-s epochs) will have reduced sensitivity, due to the presence of greater noise at these lower frequencies. Finally, in a study that simultaneously measured neural signal via intracortical recording and BOLD signal in a monkey, it was observed that the signal-to-noise ratio of the neural signal was on average at least one order of magnitude higher than that of the BOLD signal. The investigators of this study concluded that "the statistical and thresholding methods applied to the hemodynamic responses probably underestimate a great deal of actual neural activity related to a stimulus or task" [85]. Thus, the magnitude of type II error in BOLD fMRI may currently be underestimated and warrants further consideration in the interpretation of almost any cognitive neuroscience experiment.

Altered Hemodynamic Response

When comparing changes in fMRI BOLD signal levels within the brain of an individual subject across different cognitive tasks and making conclusions regarding changes in neural activity and the pattern of activity, numerous assumptions are made regarding the steps comprising neurovascular coupling (stimulus → neural activity → hemodynamic response → BOLD signal) and the regional variability of the metabolic and vascular parameters influencing the BOLD signal. It should be obvious that fMRI studies of cognition of individuals with local vascular compromise or diffuse vascular disease (e.g., patients with strokes or normal elderly people) are potentially problematic. For example, many fMRI studies have sought to identify age-related changes in the neural substrates of cognitive processes. These studies that directly compare changes in fMRI BOLD signal intensity across age groups rely upon the assumption of age-equivalent coupling of neural activity to BOLD signal. However, there is empirical evidence that suggests that this general assumption may not hold true. Extensive research on the aging neurovascular system has revealed that it undergoes significant changes in multiple domains in a continuum throughout the human lifespan, probably as early as the fourth decade (for review, see reference [86]). These changes affect the vascular ultrastructure [87], the resting cerebral blood flow [88, 89], the vascular responsiveness of the vessels [90], and the cerebral metabolic rate of oxygen consumption [91, 92]. Aging is also frequently associated with comorbidities such as diabetes, hypertension, and hyperlipidemia, all of which may affect the fMRI BOLD signal by influencing cerebral blood flow and neurovascular coupling [93]. Any one of these age-related differences in the vascular system could conceivably produce age-related differences in BOLD fMRI signal responsiveness, greatly affecting the interpretation of results from such studies.

Our laboratory compared the hemodynamic response function (HRF) characteristics in the sensorimotor cortex of young and older subjects in response to a simple motor reaction time task [71]. The provisional assumption was made that there was identical neural activity between the two populations based on physiological findings of equivalent movement-related electrical potentials in subjects under similar conditions [94]. Thus, we presumed that any changes that we observed in BOLD fMRI signal between young and older individuals in the motor cortex would be due to vascular, and not neural, activity changes in normal aging. Several important similarities and differences were observed between age groups. Although there was no significant difference in the shape of the hemodynamic response curve or peak amplitude of the signal, we found a significantly decreased signal-to-noise ratio in the fMRI BOLD signal in older individuals compared to that in young individuals. This was attributed to a greater level of noise in the older individuals. We also observed a decrease in the spatial extent of the BOLD signal in older individuals compared to that in younger individuals in the sensorimotor cortex (i.e., the median number of suprathreshold voxels). Similar results have been replicated by two other laboratories [95, 96]. These findings suggest that there is some property of the coupling between neural activity and fMRI BOLD signal that changes with age.

The notion that vascular differences among individuals may affect BOLD signal is especially a concern when considering studies of patient populations with known vascular changes such as stroke. A recent fMRI study addressed the issue of the influence of vascular factors on the BOLD signal in a symptomatic stroke population [97]. They analyzed the time course of the BOLD HRF in the sensorimotor cortex of patients with an isolated subcortical lacunar stroke compared to that in a group of age-matched controls. They found a decrease in the rate of rise and the maximal fMRI BOLD HRF to a finger- or hand-tapping task in the sensorimotor cortex of both the hemisphere affected by the stroke and the unaffected hemisphere. These investigators proposed that given the widespread changes of these fMRI BOLD signal differences, the change was unlikely a direct consequence of the subcortical lacunar stroke, but rather a manifestation of preexisting diffuse vascular pathology.

In summary, comparing BOLD signal in two different groups of individuals who may differ in their vascular system should be done with caution. For example, in one scenario, a comparison of activation of young and elderly individuals during a cognitive task may show less activation by elderly people (compared to young subjects) in some brain regions, but greater activation in other regions (e.g., Rypma et al. [98]). In this scenario, it is unlikely that regional variations in the hemodynamic coupling of neural activity to fMRI signal would account for such age-related differences in patterns of activation. In another scenario, a comparison of young and elderly subjects may show less activation by elderly subjects (compared to young subjects) in some brain regions, but no evidence of greater activation in any other region. In this case, it is possible that the observed age-related differences are not due to differences in intensity of neural activity, but rather to other nonneuronal contributions to the imaging signal, i.e., neurovascular coupling.

Consequently, BOLD contrast methods yield signal changes that result from a complex mix of vascular effects and provide only relative, rather than absolute, measures. One approach to account for the influence of purely vascular effects is to measure regional and individual variability directly in vascular reactivity via a breathholding task, which increases carbon dioxide concentration in the blood and leads to vascular dilatation [99]. The task-related BOLD signal in each subject can then be corrected for particular region- and subject-specific vascular effects.

An alternative functional neuroimaging approach, based on more direct measurements of cerebral blood flow to active brain areas, is known as arterial spin labeling (ASL). In the various ASL techniques, the MRI scanner selectively magnetizes flowing blood with a particular range of locations and/or velocities, and then waits for the appearance of the magnetic "tag" in downstream vessels. It thus becomes possible to obtain absolute measures of cerebral perfusion [99], thereby opening up the possibility of a more quantitative distinguishing between the differential influence of a disease on blood flow, and its effect on brain activity [100]. Additionally, relative to BOLD contrast, these absolute measurements appear to be more stable over long experiments [101], to show less between-subject and between-session variability [102], and to produce decreased susceptibility artifact in areas such as medial temporal lobe [103]. The current major limitation is temporal resolution: one must both wait for the generation of sufficient magnetic label, and also acquire two scans, a reference scan and a post-labeling scan, to produce a single data point. However, efforts are underway to improve this resolution. Research into the so-called turbo ASL, for example, is attempting to reduce the time required to apply the magnetic tag, and to optimize image acquisition with respect to the arrival time of the tag in downstream areas [104]. A final potential disadvantage somewhat related to the temporal issues is the lower signal-to-noise ratio of ASL relative to BOLD, but this decline may be compensated by the observation that ASL methods appear to be less variable across subjects [100].

Types of Hypotheses Tested Using FMRI

Functional neuroimaging experiments test hypotheses regarding the anatomical specificity for cognitive processes (functional specialization), or direct or indirect interactions among brain regions (functional integration). The experimental design and statistical analyses chosen will determine the types of questions that can be addressed. Ultimately, the most powerful approach for the testing of theories on brain–behavior relationships is the analysis of converging data from multiple methods.

Functional Specialization

The major focus of fMRI studies of cognition is testing theories on functional specialization. The concept of functional specialization is based on the premise that functional modules exist within the brain, that is, areas of the cerebral cortex are specialized for a specific cognitive process. For example, facial recognition is a critical primary function likely served by a functional module. Prosopagnosia is the selective inability to recognize faces. Patients with prosopagnosia, however, can recognize familiar faces, such as those of relatives, by other means, such as the voice, dress, or body shape. Other types of visual recognition, such as identifying common objects, are normal. Prosopagnosia arises from lesions of the inferomedial temporo-occipital lobe, which are usually due to a stroke within the posterior cerebral artery circulation. No lesion studies have precisely localized the area crucial for facial perception. However, they provide strong evidence that a brain area is specialized for processing faces. Functional imaging studies have provided anatomical specificity for such a module. For example, Kanwisher and colleagues [105] used fMRI to test a group of healthy individuals and found that the fusiform gyrus was significantly more active when the subjects viewed faces than when they viewed assorted common objects. The specificity of a "fusiform face area" was further demonstrated by the finding that this area also responded significantly more strongly to passive viewing of faces than to scrambled two-tone faces, front-view photographs of houses, and photographs of human hands. These elegant experiments allowed the investigators to reject alternative functions of the face area, such as visual attention, subordinate level classification, or general processing of any animate or human forms, demonstrating that this region selectively perceives faces.

Of course, the existence of brain areas specialized for certain functions does not exclude the strong possibility that those areas are part of larger networks. Recent neuroimaging work has focused on pattern classification methods, i.e., on techniques to explore whether a distributed spatial pattern of brain activity corresponds to object (or more abstract) representations. This area of research, still in its infancy, draws on results from physics, computer science, and statistics, among other disciplines, to search for more broadly distributed structure in neuroimaging data. As such, the techniques themselves differ. For example, to distinguish between voxel activity patterns across experimental conditions, various reports have used correlations between the set of activations in visual responses to faces and other objects [106]; neural network classifiers to identify particular patterns correlated with particular memories [107]; and variants of a matrix algebra transformation known as singular value decomposition to look for distributed spatial correlates of memory storage and search [108]. A large number of other techniques – too large to be reviewed here – are also being tested. As such research continues, this type of pattern classification will need to be validated via comparison with behavioral responses, in order to ensure that these patterns are not epiphenomenal [109].

Functional Integration

Functional neuroimaging experiments can also test hypotheses about interactions between brain regions by focusing on covariances of activation levels between regions [110, 111]. These covariances reflect "functional connectivity," a concept that was originally developed in reference to temporal interactions among individual neurons [112].

In addition to providing information about the specialization of various brain regions, functional neuroimaging can also address the interactions between brain regions that underlie cognitive processing. Understanding the various techniques that permit these types of analyses comprises a very active area of current research [113]. However, most, if not all, of the techniques used to test for regional interactions are ultimately based on the covariance of activation levels in different brain regions across time – in other words, on the way in which activity levels in different areas of the brain rise or fall with relation to each other. Such statistical techniques are commonly known as "multivariate," both because they rely on interactions between two or more brain areas, and to distinguish them from the "univariate" methods applied in most tests of functional specialization.

The universe of multivariate techniques is further subdivided into two types, determined by whether the method in question is designed to assess connectivity in a model-free ("functional connectivity") or model-based ("effective connectivity") fashion. The former refers simply to methods that measure the temporal covariance in activity between brain areas without a priori notions about which brain areas are relevant or how they should interact. Examples of model-free techniques would include *correlation* and its frequency-based analog, *coherence*, which can be applied irrespective of hypotheses about the neural events that produced them. On the contrary, model-based, or effective connectivity, approaches begin with hypotheses about the interactions between different brain regions, and attempt to support/refute them by evaluating the presence/absence of specific activity covariance patterns. Examples of these techniques would include structural equation modeling and dynamic causal modeling, both of which start by postulating the existence of influences (potentially complex and potentially time-varying) between specific brain regions. Both types of statistical techniques have value, of course; their use is determined by the problem at hand. Model-free approaches are more general, and more easily deployed in exploratory analyses. However, they are not as powerful as model-based methods, which address specific hypotheses about how regions interact, but which fail if the model is mis-specified. Model-free methods, for example, may be more useful when attempting to determine which networks of brain areas might be involved in a task, whereas model-based methods may be most appropriate when the nodes of the network are

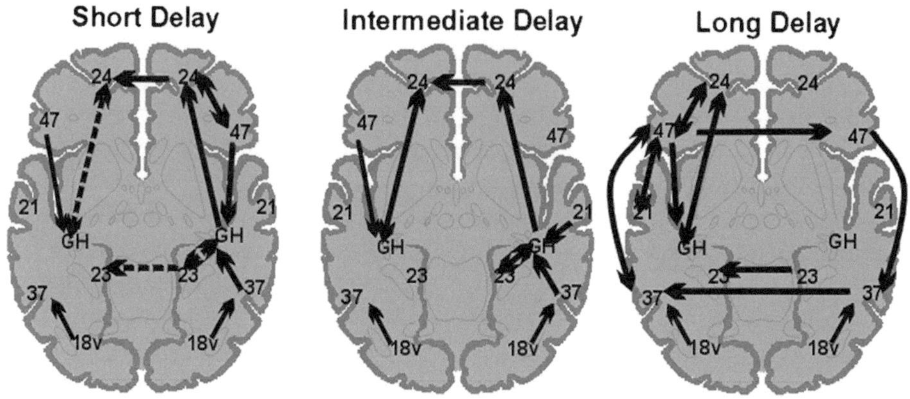

Fig. 20.4 Network analysis of fMRI data using structural equation modeling during performance of a working memory task cross three different delay periods [111]. Areas of correlated increases in activation (*solid lines*) and areas of correlated decreases in activation (*dotted lines*) are shown. Note the different pattern of interactions among brain regions at short and long delays

known, and specific notions about how they interact need to be tested.

In our own laboratory, we have developed and used functional connectivity techniques to understand how brain interactions change under different task conditions, and over time [114, 115]. For example, we have shown that functional connectivity changes as subjects learn a complex finger-tapping task [116]. In the early phases of learning, the data show that subjects not only activate wide areas of primary sensorimotor cortex, premotor cortex, and the supplementary motor area, but also that the coherence between these areas is increased relative to that of later stages. Such changes were not observed when subjects performed an already learned motor skill; and more importantly, they were not found in the univariate responses, whose means were unchanged despite the changes in the subjects' facility at the task. Similarly, in a working memory task for faces [117], we have found an interesting dissociation between their univariate and multivariate analyses in the networks that support the so-called delay period activity. In their protocol, subjects encoded a cue face, maintained the image across a delay of several seconds, and then decided whether a subsequently presented probe face matched the initial one. Interestingly, they found that despite a general decrease in the univariate activity from the cue to the delay period, there was a robust increase in the correlation between activity in the right fusiform face area and a diffuse set of brain regions including the frontal and parietal cortices, as well as the basal ganglia (Fig. 20.4).

In such known networks, effective connectivity techniques can be employed to evaluate the influence of the nodes of the network on each other more specifically. McIntosh and colleagues, for example, were able to exploit their own functional neuroimaging research on working memory networks to formulate a hypothesis about the interactions of the PFC, cingulate cortex, and other brain regions during task performance [111]. Using structural equation modeling, the authors found shifting prefrontal and limbic interactions in a working memory task for faces as the retention delay increased (Fig. 20.5). The different interactions between brain regions at short and long delays were interpreted as a functional change. For example, strong corticolimbic interactions were found at short delays, but at longer delays, when the image of the face was more difficult to maintain, strong fronto-cingulate-occipital interactions were found. The investigators postulated that the former finding was due to maintaining an iconic facial representation, and the latter due to an expanded encoding strategy, resulting in a more resilient memory. As in our own previous studies, information that was not seen in the univariate analysis was captured by an approach sensitive to regional interactions. In addition to

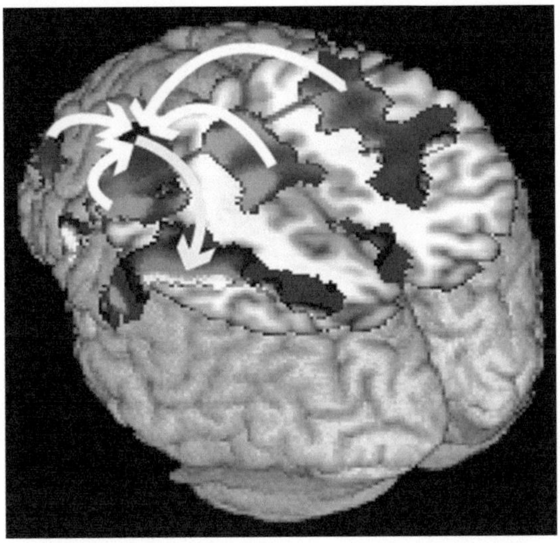

Fig. 20.5 Network analysis of fMRI data using coherence during the performance of a motor learning task. Activity of some brain regions precede activity in the region of interest, whereas activity in other areas follow in time after activation of the region of interest

structural equation modeling, other approaches have been applied to fMRI datasets to capture information regarding the relative timing of activation across brain regions such as Granger causality, information analysis, and coherence (Fig. 20.5 and [114, 115, 118]).

Cognitive Theory

An exciting new direction for studies using functional neuroimaging is those that test theories of the underlying mechanisms of cognition. For example, an fMRI study [119] attempted to answer the question, "To what extent does perception depend on attention?" One hypothesis is that unattended stimuli in the environment receive very little processing [120], but another hypothesis is that the processing load in a relevant task determines the extent to which irrelevant stimuli are processed [121]. These alternative hypotheses were tested by asking normal individuals to perform linguistic tasks of low or high load, while ignoring irrelevant visual motion in the periphery of a display. Visual motion was used as the distracting stimulus, because it activates a distinct region of the brain (cortical area MT or V5, another functional module in the visual system). Activation of area MT would indicate that irrelevant visual motion was processed. Although task and irrelevant stimuli were unrelated, fMRI of motion-related activity in MT showed a reduction in motion processing during the high-processing load condition in the linguistic task. These findings supported the hypothesis that perception of irrelevant environmental information depends on the information processing load that is currently relevant and being attended to. Thus, by the finding that perception depends on attention, this fMRI experiment provides insight regarding the underlying cognitive mechanism.

Integration of Multiple Methods

The most powerful approach toward understanding brain–behavior relationships comes from analyzing converging data from multiple methods. There are several ways in which different methods can provide complementary data. For example, one method can provide superior spatial resolution (e.g., fMRI), whereas the other can provide superior temporal resolution (e.g., ERP). Also, the data from one method may allow for different conclusions to be drawn from it, such as whether a particular brain region is necessary to implement a cognitive process (i.e., lesion methods) or whether it is only involved during its implementation (i.e., physiological methods). The following sections describe examples of such approaches.

Combined fMRI/Lesion Studies

The combined use of functional neuroimaging and lesion studies can be illustrated with studies of the neural basis of semantic memory, the cognitive system that represents our knowledge of the world. Early studies of patients with focal lesions supported the notion that the temporal lobes mediate the retrieval of semantic knowledge [122]. For example, patients with temporal lobe lesions may show a disproportionate impairment in the knowledge of living things (e.g., animals) compared with nonliving things. Other patients have a disproportionate deficit in knowledge of nonliving things [123]. These observations led to the notion that the semantic memory system is subdivided into different sensorimotor modalities: that is, living things, compared with nonliving things, are represented by their visual and other sensory attributes (e.g., a banana is yellow), while nonliving things are represented by their function (e.g., a hammer is a tool but comes in many different visual forms). The small number of patients with these deficits, and often large lesions, limits precise anatomical–behavioral relationships. However, functional neuroimaging studies in normal subjects can provide spatial resolution that the lesion method lacks [124].

These original observations regarding the neural basis of semantic memory conflicted with functional neuroimaging studies consistently showing activation of the left inferior frontal gyrus (IFG) during the retrieval of semantic knowledge. For example, an early cognitive activation PET study revealed IFG activation during a verb generation task compared with a simple word repetition task [61]. A subsequent fMRI study [125] offered a fundamentally different interpretation of the apparent conflict between lesion and functional neuroimaging studies of semantic knowledge: Left IFG activity is associated with the need to select some relevant feature of semantic knowledge from competing alternatives, not retrieval of semantic knowledge per se. This interpretation was supported by an fMRI experiment in normal individuals in which selection, but not retrieval, demands were varied across three semantic tasks. In a verb generation task, in a high selection condition, subjects generated verbs to nouns with many appropriate associated responses without any clearly dominant response (e.g., "wheel"), but in a low selection condition, nouns with few associated responses or with a clear dominant response (e.g., "scissors") were used. In this way, all tasks required semantic retrieval, and differed only in the amount of selection required. The fMRI signal within the left IFG increased as the selection demands increased (Fig. 20.6). When the degree of semantic processing varied independently of selection demands, there was no difference in left IFG activity, suggesting that selection, not

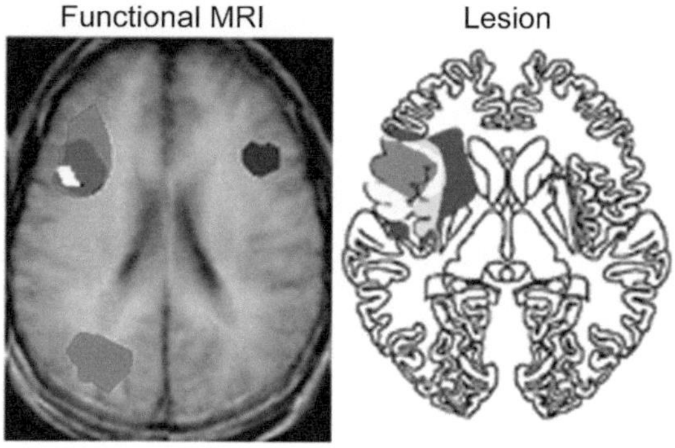

Fig. 20.6 Regions of overlap of fMRI activity in healthy human subjects (*left side of figure*) during the performance of three semantic memory tasks, with the convergence of activity within the left inferior frontal gyrus (*white region*) [125]. Regions of overlap of lesion location in patients with selection-related deficits on a verb generation task (*right side of figure*) with maximal overlap within the left inferior frontal gyrus [126]

retrieval, of semantic knowledge drives activity in the left IFG.

To determine if left IFG activity was correlated with, but not necessary for, selecting information from semantic memory, the same task used during the fMRI study was used to examine the ability of patients with focal frontal lesions to generate verbs [126]. Supporting the earlier claim regarding left IFG function derived from an fMRI study [125], the overlap of the lesions in patients with deficits on this task corresponded to the site of maximum fMRI activation in healthy young subjects during the verb generation task (Fig. 20.6). In this example, the approach of using converging evidence from lesion and fMRI studies differs in a subtle but important way from the study described earlier that isolated the face processing module. Patients with left IFG lesions do not present with an identifiable neurobehavioral syndrome reflecting the nature of the processing in this region. Guided by the fMRI results from healthy young subjects, the investigators studied patients with left IFG lesions to test a hypothesis regarding the necessity of this region in a specific cognitive process. Coupled with the well-established finding that lesions of the left temporal lobe impair semantic knowledge, these studies further our understanding of the neural network mediating semantic memory.

Combined fMRI/Transcranial Magnetic Stimulation Studies

Transcranial magnetic stimulation (TMS) is a noninvasive method that can induce a reversible "virtual" lesion of the cerebral cortex in a normal human subject [127]. Using both fMRI and TMS provides another means of combining brain activation data with data derived from the lesion method. There are several advantages for using TMS as a lesion method. First, brain injury likely results in brain reorganization after the injury and studies of patients with lesions assume that the non-lesioned brain areas have not been affected, whereas TMS is performed on the normal brain. Another advantage of using TMS is that it has excellent spatial resolution and can target specific locations in the brain, whereas lesions in patients with brain injury are markedly variable in location and size across individuals. Such an approach can be illustrated in a recent investigation of the role of the medial frontal cortex in task switching [128]. In this study, subjects first performed an fMRI study that identified the regions that were active when they stayed on the current task versus when they switched to a new task. It was found that medial frontal cortex is activated when switching between tasks. In order to determine if the medial frontal cortex was necessary for the processes involved in task switching, the same paradigm was utilized during inactivation of the medial frontal cortex with TMS. Guided by the locations of activation observed in the fMRI study, and using an MRI guided frameless stereotaxic procedure, it was found that applying a TMS pulse over the medial frontal cortex disrupted performance only during trials where the subject was required to switch between tasks. TMS over adjacent brain regions did not show this effect. Also, the excellent temporal resolution of TMS allowed the investigators to stimulate during precise periods of the task, determining that the observed effect was during the time when the subjects were presented a cue indicating they must switch tasks prior to the actual performance of the new task. Thus, combining the results from both fMRI and TMS, it was concluded that medial prefrontal cortex was essential for allowing individuals to switch to a new task intentionally.

Recently, some groups have begun to perform TMS studies not only as an adjunct to, but also concurrently with, fMRI. The advantage of this approach is clear: Applying TMS at various times during (rather than after) fMRI scans permits it to be causally linked with functional changes in the brain, even independently of behavior. In a recent study employing this technique, Ruff and colleagues [129, 130] examined the influence on early visual cortex of a parietal region (the anterior intraparietal sulcus, or aIPS) implicated in the generation of both covert spatial attention and eye movements. They chose a range of TMS stimulus intensities, all of which were thought to be in an effectively stimulatory rather than inhibitory range, and applied them to the aIPS while subjects fixated the center of a viewing screen. On some trials, a randomly moving visual stimulus was present; subjects had no other task than to maintain fixation. Using this approach, the authors were able to demonstrate a parametric, so-called top–down effect from aIPS following TMS – an increase in the BOLD response in early visual cortex with increasing TMS intensity – that could be found only when visual stimuli were absent, and that did not vary with retinotopic eccentricity. In distinction, their previous work (extended here) had shown that TMS of the frontal eye field (FEF) led to a decrease in BOLD response in the central visual field, but to an increase in BOLD response in the peripheral visual field, irrespective of the presence or absence of a visual stimulus. The authors were consequently able to conclude that the aIPS and FEF have distinct top–down effects on visual cortex, a finding that would not have been possible without concurrent TMS.

Combined fMRI/Event-Related Potential Studies

The strength of combining these two methods is coupling the superb spatial resolution of fMRI with the superb temporal resolution of ERP recording. An example of such a study was reported by Dehaene and colleagues who asked the question, "Does the human capacity for mathematical intuition depend on linguistic competence or on visuospatial representations?" [131]

In this study, subjects performed two addition tasks – one in which they were instructed to select the correct sum from two numerically close numbers (exact condition) and one in which they were instructed to estimate the result and select the closest number (approximate condition). During fMRI scanning, greater bilateral parietal lobe activation was observed in the approximation condition compared to that in the exact condition. Since this activation was outside the perisylvian language zone, it was taken as support that visuospatial processes were engaged during the cognitive operations involved in approximate calculation. Left lateralized frontal lobe activation was observed to be greater in the exact condition compared to that in the approximate condition, which was taken as evidence for language-dependent coding of exact addition facts. In order to consider an alternative explanation of the fMRI findings, the investigators also performed an ERP study. The alternative explanation was that in both the exact and approximate tasks, subjects would compute the exact result using the same representation for numbers but later processing; when they had to make a decision as to the correct choice was what led to the differences in brain activation. Since fMRI does not offer adequate temporal resolution to resolve these two behavioral events that occur on a brief time scale, ERP was the appropriate method to test this hypothesis. In the ERP study, it was demonstrated that the evoked neural response during exact and approximate trials already differed significantly during the first 400 ms of a trial before subjects had to make a decision.

Combined fMRI/Pharmacological Studies

Combining pharmacological challenges during the performance of cognitive tasks during fMRI scanning may yield significantly different information than either method alone. In isolation, fMRI cognitive task paradigms provide little information with respect to the underlying pharmacologic systems involved in cognition. On the contrary, drug administration without a brain measure cannot determine underlying neural mechanisms of the effects of neuromodulatory systems on cognition. Combining the two approaches allows the potential of probing the pharmacologic bases of behavior. One may measure the interactive effects of drug (compared to placebo, or a range of doses) with cognitive task-related modulation of brain activity. It is fair to infer that drug × task interactions reflect modulation of the underlying anatomical and chemical brain systems, and do not simply reflect nonspecific vascular effects. For example, dopaminergic agonists have been shown to have task-specific effects [132–134]: Different component processes of working memory are differentially affected by a dopaminergic drug, with effects that may differ between individuals depending on their baseline state [135]. This study demonstrated that a dopamine agonist improved the flexible updating (switching) of relevant information in working memory. However, the effect only occurred in individuals with low working memory capacity, but not in individuals with higher working memory capacity. This behavioral effect was accompanied by dissociable effects of the dopaminergic agonist on frontostriatal activity. The dopamine agonist modulated the striatum during switching but not during distraction from relevant information in working memory, while the lateral frontal cortex was modulated by the drug during distraction but not during switching.

Application of a Cognitive Neuroscience Approach Toward Clinical Studies

Use of Biomarkers Derived from Cognitive Neuroscience Studies

Cognitive neuroscience studies using fMRI may provide an important foundation for clinical studies. A biomarker is an indicator that reflects a process, event, or condition in a biological system. Biomarkers may be useful for providing a measure of exposure, effect, or susceptibility. Reliable biomarkers of a neural system could reliably quantify how such a neural system is affected by almost any input. The input may be the effects of a drug, the effects of cognitive therapy, or the effects of a disease process. For a measurement to be useful as a *biomarker* in clinical studies, it needs to have well-defined significance based on preclinical studies. That is, a change in an fMRI measurement would ideally reflect a change in a well-understood process, thus providing a clear a priori hypothesis and interpretation of the findings. Once the processes are established, fMRI biomarkers may then be useful for addressing a number of clinical questions. For any neurophysiological measurement to be a *surrogate* marker, a stable, reliable relationship between the fMRI measurement and a defined clinical outcome needs to be defined. Only in that scenario would an fMRI measurement provide a suitable surrogate for other clinical outcomes. Cognitive neuroscience studies provide the foundation for fMRI biomarkers, but the studies necessary for defining fMRI surrogate markers have not been done.

Questions regarding the mechanisms of brain function disrupted by pathologic states, processes affected by treatment interventions, or the nature of post-injury reorganization of function are examples of clinical questions that can be tested with fMRI. For example, attentional modulation of information processing-related activity in visual cortex is a well-established phenomenon, with effects measurable using fMRI. It has been shown that activity in category-selective regions of inferior temporal cortex is modulated based on the target of attention, relatively up-modulated if the target is relevant to the region and down-modulated if not relevant [136, 137]. This finding provides a biomarker of attentional control over visual processing, and has been used to test how such control is altered by aging [138]. Using this biomarker, it was shown that a mechanism of cognitive aging might be a selective deficit in goal-directed down-modulation of nonrelevant activity.

Functional MRI for Measuring the Effect of Clinical Interventions

Functional MRI may not only be useful in defining "static" brain–behavioral relationships, but may also be applied to defining changes that occur due to learning, experience, or injury. In order to assess changes, longitudinal or repeated measurements are required. Because fMRI involves no exposure-limiting factors such as radiation, it is suitable for repeated measurements. However, multi-session studies are also significantly more complicated to design, analyze, and interpret due to a number of issues that will be discussed.

There are at least two distinct approaches relevant to assessing changes within an individual. First, fMRI may be used for determining the aftereffects of a learning intervention. Functional MRI measures pre- and post-intervention may be used to address this question. For example, after two pieces of information have been strongly associated over repetitive exposures, one may find reduced activation in response to presentation of that information, but increased functional connectivity between regions of the brain that process the two types of information [110]. Second, fMRI may be used for determining the processes that occur during an intervention, such as cognitive training. To do this, one would need to acquire fMRI data *during* the process of training. An alternative approach is to use a cross-sectional approach to examine differences across individuals rather than within individuals [139]. For example, brain activation differences between long-term meditation practitioners and novices may be used to infer the neural effects of meditation training. However, other confounding effects of differences between cohorts are difficult to exclude.

The use of fMRI to define changes over time requires consideration of certain additional methodological issues. Test–retest reliability needs to be considered. Estimates of reliability depend on what is being measured. For example, in statistical parametric mapping, the question may be whether particular brain regions are stably labeled as "active" or not in serial sessions. A handful of studies have addressed this question. For example, one group showed that with a classification learning task, scans 1 year apart resulted in highly concordant results with defined regions of interest [140]. Another group showed that maps obtained from a working memory task were similar across time [141], but with a motor task, there appeared to be significant variation over time in volume and spatial location of activations [142]. The reliability of inter-regional functional connectivity fMRI measurements has not yet been systematically tested.

In longitudinal studies, sources of variability may be both physiologic and non-physiologic (e.g., MRI hardware). In some cases, the magnitudes of activation in specific brain regions of interest are themselves an outcome of interest. In these instances, the stability of BOLD signal measurements becomes an even more salient issue. It may be worthwhile to utilize within-session indices that effectively normalize parameters of interest. For example, rather than comparing estimates of the magnitudes of activation, it may be worthwhile to utilize an index of activity for one condition compared to a second controlled condition with each session. An additional statistical approach that could account for potential variability in signal-to-noise ratio is to combine data sets across sessions and then "whiten" the noise, effectively normalizing noise contribution across sessions. Other analytic approaches may be taken that are less sensitive to non-physiologic instabilities. For example, one could test for changes in the spatial *pattern* of activation that is not necessarily affected by signal magnitude changes. That is, one could test whether the patterns of activity are identical to that within a scaling factor [108]. Finally, other factors that concurrently change over time can produce confounds to the interpretation of longitudinal studies. For example, performance may change, resulting in changes in reaction time or accuracy. All of these may alter measured responses, making determination of the neural bases of the process of interest, such as a treatment intervention, more difficult. These and a number of other issues are discussed in greater depth by Poldrack in consideration of learning-related changes [139].

Conclusion

Functional MRI is an extremely valuable tool for studying brain–behavior relationships, as it is widely available, noninvasive, and has superb temporal and spatial resolution. New approaches in fMRI experimental design and data analysis are appearing in the literature at an almost exponential rate, leading to numerous options for testing hypotheses on brain–behavior relationships (Table 20.1). Combined with information from other complimentary methods, such as the study of patients with focal lesions and healthy individuals with TMS, pharmacological intervention, or event-related potentials, data from fMRI studies provide new insights regarding the organization of the cerebral cortex, and the neural mechanisms underlying cognition. Moreover, cognitive neuroscience approaches that have been developed for fMRI provide an excellent foundation for its use as clinical tool.

Table 20.1 Summary of key literature of cognitive neuroscience imaging applications

Authors	Article title	Summary
Boynton et al. 1996 [42]	Linear systems analysis of functional magnetic resonance imaging in human V1. The Journal of Neuroscience, 1996. 16: p. 4207–4221	The linear transform model of fMRI was used to estimate the temporal fMRI impulse–response function and the underlying contrast–response function of human V1
Sarter et al. 1996 [3]	Brain imaging and cognitive neuroscience: toward strong inference in attributing function to structure. American Psychologist, 1996. 51: p. 13–21	The article provides a conceptual framework to advance the interpretation of data describing the relationships between cognitive phenomena and brain structure
Dale et al. 1997 [48]	Selective averaging of rapidly presented individual trials using fMRI. Human Brain Mapping, 1997. 5: p. 1–12	Selective averaging techniques could be used to demonstrate fMRI responses to rapidly intermixed trials. The ability to analyze closely spaced single-trial, or event-related, signals provides for a class of experiments that cannot be conducted using blocked designs

(continued)

Table 20.1 (continued)

Authors	Article title	Summary
Zarahn et al. 1997 [79]	A trial-based experimental design for functional MRI. NeuroImage, 1997. 6: p. 122–138	Trial-based fMRI design is presented whose conceptual units of analysis are behavioral trials rather than blocks of trials
Aguirre et al. 1998 [40]	The variability of human, BOLD hemodynamic responses. Neuroimage, 1998. 8(4): p. 360–9	FMRI is used to determine the contribution of subject, day, and scanning session (within a day) to variability in the shape of evoked hemodynamic response. While there is significant and substantial variability in the shape of responses collected across subjects, responses collected during multiple scans within a single subject are less variable
D'Esposito et al. 1999 [50]	The effect of normal aging on the coupling of neural activity to the bold hemodynamic response. Neuroimage, 1999. 10(1): p. 6–14	Some aspects of the hemodynamic coupling between neural activity and BOLD fMRI signal change with age, cautioning against simple interpretations of the results of imaging studies that compare young and elderly subjects
Logothetis et al. 2001 [85]	Neurophysiological investigation of the basis of the fMRI signal. Nature, 2001. 412(6843): p. 150–7	A trial-by-trial linear systems analysis of the visual cortex of monkeys showed that the impulse response of the neurovascular system is both animal and site specific, and that local field potentials yield a better estimate of BOLD responses than the multi-unit responses. These findings suggest that the BOLD contrast mechanism reflects the input and intracortical processing of a given area rather than its spiking output
Heeger et al. 2002 [66]	What does fMRI tell us about neuronal activity? Nat Rev Neurosci, 2002. 3(2): p. 142–51	A clearer understanding of how neuronal activity influences the fMRI signal is needed if in order to interpret functional imaging data correctly
Sun et al. 2004 [114]	Measuring interregional functional connectivity using coherence and partial coherence analyses of fMRI data. Neuroimage, 2004. 21(2): p. 647–58	The authors measured task-related functional interactions between neural regions by applying coherence and partial coherence analyses to fMRI data. Significant increases in interhemispheric coherence were found between the primary motor (M1) and premotor (PM) regions for the task requiring more bimanual coordination
Poldrack 2006 [18]	Can cognitive processes be inferred from neuroimaging data? Trends Cogn Sci, 2006. 10(2): p. 59–63	The author explores the validity of "reverse inference," by which the engagement of a particular cognitive process is inferred from the activation of a particular brain region

References

1. Broca P. Remarques sur le siege de la faculte du langage articule suivies d'une observation d'amphemie (perte de al parole). Bulletin et Memoires de la Societe Anatomique de Paris, 1861;36: 330–357
2. Buckner RL, Raichle ME, Petersen SE. Dissociation of human prefrontal cortical areas across different speech production tasks and gender groups. J Neurophysiol. 1995;74(5):2163–73.
3. Sarter M, Bernston G, Cacioppo J. Brain imaging and cognitive neuroscience: toward strong inference in attributing function to structure. Am Psychol. 1996;51:13–21.
4. Gaffan D, Gaffan EA. Amnesia in man following transection of the fornix: a review. Brain. 1991;114: 2611–8.
5. Feeney DM, Baron JC. Diaschisis. Stroke. 1986; 17(5):817–30.
6. Fuster JM, Alexander GE. Neuron activity related to short-term memory. Science. 1971;173:652–4.
7. Funahashi S, Bruce CJ, Goldman-Rakic PS. Mnemonic coding of visual space in the monkey's dorsolateral prefrontal cortex. J Neurophysiol. 1989; 61:331–49.
8. Funahashi S, Bruce CJ, Goldman-Rakic PS. Dorsolateral prefrontal lesions and oculomotor delayed-response performance: Evidence for mnemonic "scotomas". J Neurosci. 1993;13:1479–97.
9. Watanabe T, Niki H. Hippocampal unit activity and delayed response in the monkey. Brain Res. 1985;325(1–2):241–54.
10. Cahusac PM, Miyashita Y, Rolls ET. Responses of hippocampal formation neurons in the monkey related to delayed spatial response and object-place memory tasks. Behav Brain Res. 1989;33(3): 229–40.
11. Alvarez P, Zola-Morgan S, Squire LR. The animal model of human amnesia: long-term memory

impaired and short-term memory intact. Proc Natl Acad Sci USA. 1994;91(12):5637–41.
12. Corkin S. Lasting consequences of bilateral medial temporal lobectomy: clinical course and experimental findings in H.M. Semin Neurol. 1984;4:249–59.
13. Ranganath C, D'Esposito M. Medial temporal lobe activity associated with active maintenance of novel information. Neuron. 2001;31(5):865–73.
14. Druzgal TJ, D'Esposito M. Activity in fusiform face area modulated as a function of working memory load. Brain Res Cogn Brain Res. 2001;10(3): 355–64.
15. Henson R. Forward inference using functional neuroimaging: dissociations versus associations. Trends Cogn Sci. 2006;10(2):64–9.
16. Cohen MS, Kosslyn SM, Breiter HC, et al. Changes in cortical activity during mental rotation: a mapping study using functional MRI. Brain. 1996;119:89–100.
17. D'Esposito M, Ballard D, Aguirre GK, Zarahn E. Human prefrontal cortex is not specific for working memory: a functional MRI study. Neuroimage. 1998;8(3):274–82.
18. Poldrack RA. Can cognitive processes be inferred from neuroimaging data? Trends Cogn Sci. 2006; 10(2):59–63.
19. Hutton C, Bork A, Josephs O, Deichmann R, Ashburner J, Turner R. Image distortion correction in fMRI: A quantitative evaluation. Neuroimage. 2002;16(1):217–40.
20. Jezzard P, Clare S. Sources of distortion in functional MRI data. Hum Brain Mapp. 1999;8(2–3):80–5.
21. Zeng H, Constable RT. Image distortion correction in EPI: comparison of field mapping with point spread function mapping. Magn Reson Med. 2002;48(1):137–46.
22. Grasby PM. Imaging the neurochemical brain in health and disease. Clin Med. 2002;2(1):67–73.
23. Bunge SA, Dudukovic NM, Thomason ME, Vaidya CJ, Gabrieli JD. Immature frontal lobe contributions to cognitive control in children: evidence from fMRI. Neuron. 2002;33(2):301–11.
24. Casey BJ, Cohen JD, Jezzard P, et al. Activation of prefrontal cortex in children during a nonspatial working memory task with functional MRI. Neuroimage. 1995;2(3):221–9.
25. Savoy RL, Ravicz ME, Gollub R. The psychophysiological laboratory in the magnet: stimulus delivery, response recording, and safety. In: Moonen CTW, Bandettini PA, editors, Functional MRI. Berlin: Springer; 1999. p. 347–365
26. Edmister WB, Talavage TM, Ledden PJ, Weisskoff RM. Improved auditory cortex imaging using clustered volume acquisitions. Hum Brain Mapp. 1999;7:88–97.
27. Belin P, Zatorre RJ, Hoge R, Evans AC, Pike B. Event-related fMRI of the auditory cortex. Neuroimage. 1999;10(4):417–29.
28 Sobel N, Prabhakaran V, Hartley CA, et al. Blind smell: brain activation induced by an undetected air-borne chemical. Brain. 1999;122(Pt 2):209–17.
29. Sobel N, Prabhakaran V, Desmond JE, Glover GH, Sullivan EV, Gabrieli JD. A method for functional magnetic resonance imaging of olfaction. J Neurosci Meth. 1997;78(1–2):115–23.
30. Gitelman DR, Parrish TB, LaBar KS, Mesulam MM. Real-time monitoring of eye movements using infrared video-oculography during functional magnetic resonance imaging of the frontal eye fields. Neuroimage. 2000;11(1):58–65.
31. Kimmig H, Greenlee MW, Gondan M, Schira M, Kassubek J, Mergner T. Relationship between saccadic eye movements and cortical activity as measured by fMRI: quantitative and qualitative aspects. Exp Brain Res. 2001;141(2):184–94.
32. Palmer ED, Rosen HJ, Ojemann JG, Buckner RL, Kelley WM, Petersen SE. An event-related fMRI study of overt and covert word stem completion. Neuroimage. 2001;14(1 Pt 1):182–93.
33. Fu CH, Morgan K, Suckling J, et al. A functional magnetic resonance imaging study of overt letter verbal fluency using a clustered acquisition sequence: greater anterior cingulate activation with increased task demand. Neuroimage. 2002;17(2):871–9.
34. Barch DM, Sabb FW, Carter CS, Braver TS, Noll DC, Cohen JD. Overt verbal responding during fMRI scanning: empirical investigations of problems and potential solutions. Neuroimage. 1999;10(6): 642–57.
35. Goldman RI, Stern JM, Engel Jr J, Cohen MS. Acquiring simultaneous EEG and functional MRI. Clin Neurophysiol. 2000;111(11): 1974–80.
36. Lazeyras F, Zimine I, Blanke O, Perrig SH, Seeck M. Functional MRI with simultaneous EEG recording: feasibility and application to motor and visual activation. J Magn Reson Imaging. 2001;13(6): 943–8.
37. Mantini D, Perrucci MG, Cugini S, Ferretti A, Romani GL, Del Gratta C. Complete artifact removal for EEG recorded during continuous fMRI using independent component analysis. Neuroimage. 2007;34(2):598–607.
38. Otzenberger H, Gounot D, Foucher JR. Optimisation of a post-processing method to remove the pulse artifact from EEG data recorded during fMRI: an application to P300 recordings during e-fMRI. Neurosci Res. 2007;57(2):230–9.
39. Gnadt JW, Andersen RA. Memory related motor planning activity in posterior parietal cortex of macaque. Exp Brain Res. 1988;70: 216–20.
40. Aguirre GK, Zarahn E, D'Esposito M. The variability of human, BOLD hemodynamic responses. Neuroimage. 1998;8(4):360–9.
41. Bandettini PA, Wong EC, Hinks RS, Tikofsky RS, Hyde JS. Time course of EPI of human brain function during task activation. Magn Reson Med. 1992; 25:390–7.
42. Boynton GM, Engel SA, Glover GH, Heeger DJ. Linear systems analysis of functional magnetic resonance imaging in human V1. J Neurosci. 1996; 16:4207–21.

43. Kim SG, Richter W, Ugurbil K. Limitations of temporal resolution in fMRI. Magn Reson Med. 1997;37:631–6.
44. Savoy RL, Bandettini PA, Weisskoff R, et al. Pushing the temporal resolution of fMRI: studies of very brief stimuli, onset of variability and asynchrony, and stimulu-correlated changes in noise. Proceedings of the 3rd Annual Meeting of the SMR, 1995. 3: p. 450
45. Zarahn E, Aguirre GK, D'Esposito M. A trial-based experimental design for functional MRI. Neuroimage. 1997;6:122–38.
46. Burock MA, Buckner RL, Woldorff MG, Rosen BR, Dale AM. Randomized event-related experimental designs allow for extremely rapid presentation rates using functional MRI. Neuroreport. 1998;9(16): 3735–9.
47. Clark VP, Maisog JM, Haxby JV. fMRI studies of visual perception and recognition using a random stimulus design. Soc Neurosci Abstr. 1997;23:301.
48. Dale AM, Buckner RL. Selective averaging of rapidly presented individual trials using fMRI. Hum Brain Mapp. 1997;5:1–12.
49. Miezin FM, Maccotta L, Ollinger JM, Petersen SE, Buckner RL. Characterizing the hemodynamic response: effects of presentation rate, sampling procedure, and the possibility of ordering brain activity based on relative timing. Neuroimage. 2000;11(6 Pt 1):735–59.
50. D'Esposito M, Zarahn E, Aguirre GK. Event-related functional MRI: implications for cognitive psychology. Psychol Bull. 1999;125:155–64.
51. Logothetis NK, Guggenberger H, Peled S, Pauls J. Functional imaging of the monkey brain. Nat Neurosci. 1999;2(6):555–62.
52. Cheng K, Waggoner RA, Tanaka K. Human ocular dominance columns as revealed by high-field functional magnetic resonance imaging. Neuron. 2001; 32(2):359–74.
53. Logothetis N, Merkle H, Augath M, Trinath T, Ugurbil K. Ultra high-resolution fMRI in monkeys with implanted RF coils. Neuron. 2002;35(2): 227–42.
54. Malonek D, Grinvald A. Interactions between electrical activity and cortical microcirculation revealed by imaging spectroscopy: implications for functional brain mapping. Science. 1996;272:551–4.
55. Kim SG, Duong TQ. Mapping cortical columnar structures using fMRI. Physiol Behav. 2002; 77(4–5):641–4.
56. Menon RS, Ogawa S, Strupp JP, Uğurbil K. Ocular dominance in human V1 demonstrated by functional magnetic resonance imaging. J Neurophysiol. 1997; 77(5):2780–7.
57. Grill-Spector K, Malach R. fMR-adaptation: a tool for studying the functional properties of human cortical neurons. Acta Psychol (Amst). 2001;107(1–3): 293–321.
58. Grill-Spector K, Kushnir T, Edelman S, Avidan G, Itzchak Y, Malach R. Differential processing of objects under various viewing conditions in the human lateral occipital complex. Neuron. 1999; 24(1):187–203.
59. Posner MI, Petersen SE, Fox PT, Raichle ME. Localization of cognitive operations in the human brain. Science. 1988;240:1627–31.
60. Sternberg S. The discovery of processing stages: extensions of Donders' method. Acta Psychol. 1969;30:276–315.
61. Petersen SE, Fox PT, Posner MI, Mintun M, Raichle ME. Positron emission tomographic studies of the cortical anatomy of single word processing. Nature. 1988;331:585–9.
62. Fuster J. The prefrontal cortex: anatomy, physiology, and neuropsychology of the frontal lobes. 3rd ed. Raven Press: New York; 1997.
63. Jonides J, Smith EE, Koeppe RA, Awh E, Minoshima S, Mintun MA. Spatial working memory in humans as revealed by PET. Nature. 1993;363:623–5.
64. Zarahn E, Aguirre GK, D'Esposito M. Temporal isolation of the neural correlates of spatial mnemonic processing with fMRI. Cogn Brain Res. 1999;7(3): 255–68.
65. Attwell D, Iadecola C. The neural basis of functional brain imaging signals. Trends Neurosci. 2002; 25(12):621–5.
66. Heeger DJ, Ress D. What does fMRI tell us about neuronal activity? Nat Rev Neurosci. 2002; 3(2):142–51.
67. Friston KJ, Josephs O, Rees G, Turner R. Nonlinear event-related responses in fMRI. Magn Reson Med. 1998;39(1):41–52.
68. Glover GH. Deconvolution of impulse response in event-related BOLD fMRI. Neuroimage. 1999; 9(4):416–29.
69. Miller KL, Luh WM, Liu TT, et al. Nonlinear temporal dynamics of the cerebral blood flow response. Hum Brain Mapp. 2001;13(1):1–12.
70. Vazquez AL, Noll DC. Nonlinear aspects of the BOLD response in functional MRI. Neuroimage. 1998;7(2):108–18.
71. D'Esposito M, Zarahn E, Aguirre GK, Rypma B. The effect of normal aging on the coupling of neural activity to the bold hemodynamic response. Neuroimage. 1999;10(1):6–14.
72. Rosen BR, Buckner RL, Dale AM. Event-related functional MRI: past, present, and future. Proc Natl Acad Sci USA. 1998;95(3):773–80.
73. Donaldson DI, Petersen SE, Ollinger JM, Buckner RL. Dissociating state and item components of recognition memory using fMRI. Neuroimage. 2001;13(1):129–42.
74. Mitchell KJ, Johnson MK, Raye CL, D'Esposito M. fMRI evidence of age-related hippocampal dysfunction in feature binding in working memory. Brain Res Cogn Brain Res. 2000;10(1–2):197–206.
75. Keppel G, Zedeck S. Data analysis for research design. 1989, New York: W.H. Freeman & Company
76. Worsley KJ, Friston KJ. Analysis of fMRI time-series revisited - again. Neuroimage. 1995;2: 173–82.

77. Everitt BS, Bullmore ET. Mixture model mapping of the brain activation in functional magnetic resonance images. Hum Brain Mapp. 1999;7(1):1–14.
78. Genovese CR, Lazar NA, Nichols T. Thresholding of statistical maps in functional neuroimaging using the false discovery rate. Neuroimage. 2002;15(4): 870–8.
79. Zarahn E, Aguirre GK, D'Esposito M. Empirical analyses of BOLD fMRI statistics. I. Spatially unsmoothed data collected under null-hypothesis conditions. Neuroimage. 1997;5:179–97.
80. Aguirre GK, Zarahn E, D'Esposito M. Empirical analyses of BOLD fMRI statistics. II. Spatially smoothed data collected under null-hypothesis and experimental conditions. Neuroimage. 1997;5: 199–212.
81. D'Esposito M, Ballard D, Zarahn E, Aguirre GK. The role of prefrontal cortex in sensory memory and motor preparation: an event-related fMRI study. Neuroimage. 2000;11(5 Pt 1):400–8.
82. Zarahn E, Slifstein M. A reference effect approach for power analysis in fMRI. Neuroimage. 2001; 14(3):768–79.
83. Van Horn JD, Ellmore TM, Esposito G, Berman KF. Mapping voxel-based statistical power on parametric images. Neuroimage. 1998;7(2):97–107.
84. Aguirre GK, D'Esposito M. Experimental design for brain fMRI. In: Moonen CTW, Bandettini PA, editors. Functional MRI, Berlin: Springer; 1999, p. 369–380
85. Logothetis NK, Pauls J, Augath M, Trinath T, Oeltermann A. Neurophysiological investigation of the basis of the fMRI signal. Nature. 2001; 412(6843):150–7.
86. Farkas E, Luiten PG. Cerebral microvascular pathology in aging and Alzheimer's disease. Prog Neurobiol. 2001;64(6):575–611.
87. Fang HCH. Observations on aging characteristics of cerebral blood vessels, macroscopic and microscopic features. In: Gerson S, Terry RD, editors. Neurobiology of aging, New York: Raven Press; 1976
88. Bentourkia M, Bol A, Ivanoiu A, et al. Comparison of regional cerebral blood flow and glucose metabolism in the normal brain: effect of aging. J Neurol Sci. 2000;181(1–2):19–28.
89. Schultz SK, O'Leary DS, Boles Ponto LL, Watkins GL, Hichwa RD, Andreasen NC. Age-related changes in regional cerebral blood flow among young to midlife adults. Neuroreport. 1999;10(12): 2493–6.
90. Yamamoto M, Meyer JS, Sakai F, Yamaguchi F. Aging and cerebral vasodilator responses to hypercarbia: responses in normal aging and in persons with risk factors for stroke. Arch Neurol. 1980;37(8):489–96.
91. Yamaguchi T, Kanno I, Uemura K, et al. Reduction in regional cerebral rate of oxygen during human aging. Stroke. 1986;17: 1220–8.
92. Takada H, Nagata K, Hirata Y, et al. Age-related decline of cerebral oxygen metabolism in normal population detected with positron emission tomography. Neurol Res. 1992;14(2 Suppl):128–31.
93. Claus JJ, Breteler MM, Hasan D, et al. Regional cerebral blood flow and cerebrovascular risk factors in the elderly population. Neurobiol Aging. 1998; 19(1):57–64.
94. Cunnington R, Iansek R, Bradshaw JL, Phillips JG. Movement-related potentials in Parkinson's disease. Presence and predictability of temporal and spatial cues. Brain. 1995;118(Pt 4):935–50.
95. Buckner RL, Snyder AZ, Sanders AL, Raichle ME, Morris JC. Functional brain imaging of young, nondemented, and demented older adults. J Cogn Neurosci. 2000;12 Suppl 2:24–34.
96. Huettel SA, Singerman JD, McCarthy G. The effects of aging upon the hemodynamic response measured by functional MRI. Neuroimage. 2001;13(1):161–75.
97. Pineiro R, Pendlebury S, Johansen-Berg H, Matthews PM. Altered hemodynamic responses in patients after subcortical stroke measured by functional MRI. Stroke. 2002;33(1):103–9.
98. Rypma B, Prabhakaran V, Desmond JE, Gabrieli JD. Age differences in prefrontal cortical activity in working memory. Psychol Aging. 2001;16(3):371–84.
99. Wolf RL, Detre JA. Clinical neuroimaging using arterial spin-labeled perfusion magnetic resonance imaging. Neurotherapeutics. 2007;4(3):346–59.
100. Brown GG, Clark C, Liu TT. Measurement of cerebral perfusion with arterial spin labeling: part 2 applications. J Int Neuropsychol Soc. 2007;13(3):526–38.
101. Aguirre GK, Detre JA, Zarahn E, Alsop DC. Experimental design and the relative sensitivity of BOLD and perfusion fMRI. Neuroimage. 2002; 15(3):488–500.
102. Liu TT, Brown GG. Measurement of cerebral perfusion with arterial spin labeling: part 1 methods. J Int Neuropsychol Soc. 2007;13(3):517–25.
103. Fernández-Seara MA, Wang J, Wang Z, et al. Imaging mesial temporal lobe activation during scene encoding: comparison of fMRI using BOLD and arterial spin labeling. Hum Brain Mapp. 2007;28(12):1391–400.
104. Lee GR, Hernandez-Garcia L, Noll DC. Functional imaging with Turbo-CASL: transit time and multislice imaging considerations. Magn Reson Med. 2007;57(4):661–9.
105. Kanwisher N, McDermott J, Chun MM. The fusiform face area: a module in huma extrastriate cortex specialized for face perception. J Neurosci. 1997; 17:4302–11.
106. Haxby JV, Gobbini MI, Furey ML, Ishai A, Schouten JL, Pietrini P. Distributed and overlapping representations of faces and objects in ventral temporal cortex. Science. 2001;293(5539):2425–30.
107. Polyn SM, Natu VS, Cohen JD, Norman KA. Category-specific cortical activity precedes retrieval during memory search. Science. 2005;310(5756): 1963–6.
108. Zarahn E, Rakitin BC, Abela D, Flynn J, Stern Y. Distinct spatial patterns of brain activity associated with memory storage and search. Neuroimage. 2006;33(2):794–804.
109. Williams MA, Dang S, Kanwisher NG. Only some spatial patterns of fMRI response are read out in task performance. Nat Neurosci. 2007;10(6):685–6.

110. Buchel C, Coull JT, Friston KJ. The predictive value of changes in effective connectivity for human learning. Science. 1999;283(5407): 1538–41.
111. McIntosh AR, Grady CL, Haxby JV, Ungerleider LG, Horwitz B. Changes in limbic and prefrontal functional interactions in a working memory task for faces. Cereb Cortex. 1996;6(4):571–84.
112. Gerstein GL, Perkel DH, Subramanian KN. Identification of functionally related neural assemblies. Brain Res. 1978;140(1):43–62.
113. Penny WD, Stephan KE, Mechelli A, Friston KJ. Modelling functional integration: a comparison of structural equation and dynamic causal models. Neuroimage. 2004;23 Suppl 1:S264–74.
114. Sun FT, Miller LM, D'Esposito M. Measuring interregional functional connectivity using coherence and partial coherence analyses of fMRI data. Neuroimage. 2004;21(2):647–58.
115. Sun FT, Miller LM, D'Esposito M. Measuring temporal dynamics of functional networks using phase spectrum of fMRI data. Neuroimage. 2005;28(1): 227–37.
116. Sun FT, Miller LM, Rao AA. D'Esposito M. Cereb Cortex: Functional Connectivity of Cortical Networks Involved in Bimanual Motor Sequence Learning; 2006.
117. Gazzaley A, Rissman J, Desposito M. Functional connectivity during working memory maintenance. Cogn Affect Behav Neurosci. 2004;4(4):580–99.
118. Fuhrmann Alpert G, Sun FT, Handwerker D, D'Esposito M, Knight RT. Spatio-temporal information analysis of event-related BOLD responses. Neuroimage. 2007;34(4):1545–61.
119. Rees G, Frith CD, Lavie N. Modulating irrelevant motion perception by varying attentional load in an unrelated task. Science. 1997;278(5343):1616–9.
120. Treisman AM. Strategies and models of selective attention. Psychol Rev. 1969;76(3):282–99.
121. Lavie N, Tsal Y. Perceptual load as a major determinant of the locus of selection in visual attention. Percept Psychophys. 1994;56(2):183–97.
122. McCarthy RA, Warrington EK. Disorders of semantic memory. Philos Trans R Soc Lond B Biol Sci. 1994;346(1315):89–96.
123. Warrington EST. Category specific semantic impairments. Brain. 1984;107:829–54.
124. Thompson-Schill SL. Neuroimaging studies of semantic memory: inferring "how" from "where". Neuropsychologia. 2003;41(3): 280–92.
125. Thompson-Schill SL, D'Esposito M, Aguirre GK, Farah MJ. Role of left inferior prefrontal cortex in retrieval of semantic knowledge: a reevaluation. Proc Natl Acad Sci USA. 1997;94(26): 14792–7.
126. Thompson-Schill SL, Swick D, Farah MJ, D'Esposito M, Kan IP, Knight RT. Verb generation in patients with focal frontal lesions: a neuropsychological test of neuroimaging findings. Proc Natl Acad Sci USA. 1998;95(26):15855–60.
127. Pascual-Leone A, Tarazona F, Keenan J, Tormos JM, Hamilton R, Catala MD. Transcranial magnetic stimulation and neuroplasticity. Neuropsychologia. 1999;37(2):207–17.
128. Rushworth MF, Hadland KA, Paus T, Sipila PK. Role of the human medial frontal cortex in task switching: a combined fMRI and TMS study. J Neurophysiol. 2002;87(5):2577–92.
129. Ruff CC, Bestmann S, Blankenburg F, et al. Distinct causal influences of parietal versus frontal areas on human visual cortex: evidence from concurrent TMS fMRI. Cereb Cortex. 2008;18(4):817–27.
130. Ruff CC, Blankenburg F, Bjoertomt O, et al. Concurrent TMS-fMRI and psychophysics reveal frontal influences on human retinotopic visual cortex. Curr Biol. 2006;16(15):1479–88.
131. Dehaene S, Spelke E, Pinel P, Stanescu R, Tsivkin S. Sources of mathematical thinking: behavioral and brain-imaging evidence. Science. 1999;284(5416): 970–4.
132. Gibbs SE, D'Esposito M. Individual capacity differences predict working memory performance and prefrontal activity following dopamine receptor stimulation. Cogn Affect Behav Neurosci. 2005;5(2):212–21.
133. Gibbs SE, D'Esposito M. A functional MRI study of the effects of bromocriptine, a dopamine receptor agonist, on component processes of working memory. Psychopharmacol (Berl). 2005;180(4): 644–53.
134. Gibbs SE, D'Esposito M. A functional magnetic resonance imaging study of the effects of pergolide, a dopamine receptor agonist, on component processes of working memory. Neuroscience. 2006;28;139(1):359–71.
135. Cools R, Sheridan M, Jacobs E, D'Esposito M. Impulsive personality predicts dopamine-dependent changes in frontostriatal activity during component processes of working memory. J Neurosci. 2007; 27(20):5506–14.
136. Kastner S, Pinsk MA. Visual attention as a multilevel selection process. Cogn Affect Behav Neurosci. 2004;4(4):483–500.
137. Gazzaley A, Cooney JW, McEvoy K, Knight RT, D'Esposito M. Top-down enhancement and suppression of the magnitude and speed of neural activity. J Cogn Neurosci. 2005;17(3):507–17.
138. Gazzaley A, Cooney JW, Rissman J, D'Esposito M. Top-down suppression deficit underlies working memory impairment in normal aging. Nat Neurosci. 2005;8(10):1298–300.
139. Poldrack RA. Imaging brain plasticity: conceptual and methodological issues–a theoretical review. Neuroimage. 2000;12(1): 1–13.
140. Aron AR, Gluck MA, Poldrack RA. Long-term test-retest reliability of functional MRI in a classification learning task. Neuroimage. 2006;1;29(3):1000–6.
141. Wei X, Yoo SS, Dickey CC, Zou KH, Guttmann CR, Panych LP. Functional MRI of auditory verbal working memory: long-term reproducibility analysis. Neuroimage. 2004;21(3):1000–8.
142. Yoo SS, Wei X, Dickey CC, Guttmann CR, Panych LP. Long-term reproducibility analysis of fMRI using hand motor task. Int J Neurosci. 2005;115(1):55–77.

Part IV

BOLD fMRI Paradigms

BOLD fMRI Paradigms

21

Feroze B. Mohamed and Scott H. Faro

Introduction

In this chapter, we have provided a few paradigms that are commonly used for preneurosurgical mapping of the language and motor functions. The activation tasks used in one of the most widely used language paradigms in the functional magnetic resonance imaging (fMRI) community, the sentence completion, are shown in several languages (English, Russian, Spanish, and Vietnamese). In addition, other commonly used language paradigms, including rhyming and word generations, are also provided in this chapter. We have also provided a commonly used motor paradigm and a visual paradigm as well.

The list of paradigms provided here does not represent a full list that might be used in institutions across the globe. Care should be taken while implementing these paradigms since they can influence the outcome of the results. It will be of utmost importance to gain some experience with these paradigms before testing in patient populations. Currently, the standardization of fMRI paradigms is an ongoing process. Therefore, the contents presented here do not represent an official recommendation or endorsement by the authors of this book.

Sentence Completion Paradigm

Paradigm Description

Intended to show language regions involved in comprehension and expression.

Paradigm Parameters

The paradigm consists of (30 s duration, six conditions) rest state (viewing of gibberish nonsense words), followed by activation states of sentences with blank words (30 s duration, six conditions).

F.B. Mohamed, PhD (✉) • S.H. Faro, MD
Department of Radiology, Functional Brain Imaging Center, Temple University School of Medicine, 3401 North Broad Street, Philadelphia, PA, 19140-5103, USA
e-mail: feroze@temple.edu; faros@tuhs.temple.edu

S.H. Faro and F.B. Mohamed (eds.), *Functional BOLD MRI: Principles and Applications*, DOI 10.1007/978-1-4939-1995-6_21, © Springer Science+Business Media New York 2015

Paradigm Instructions

During the control phase the subject is requested to just view the sentence with the nonsense words and try not to make any meaning of the sentence.

During the activation phase the subject is asked to covertly read the sentence and complete the blank with an appropriate word. The block diagram of the paradigm used is shown below (Fig. 21.1). The total imaging time is 6 min (Table 21.1).

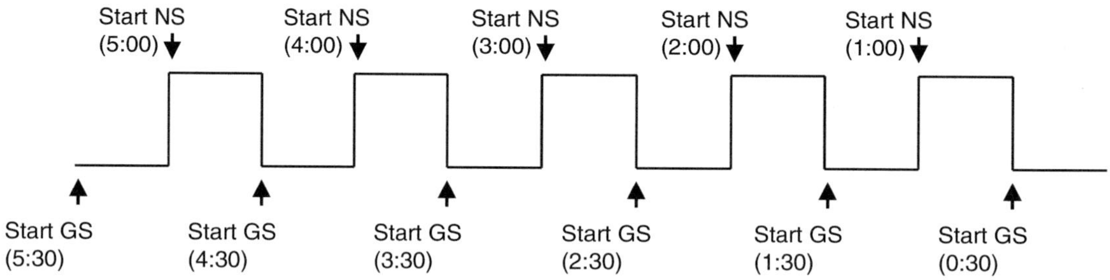

Fig. 21.1 Block diagram of sentence completion paradigm. (GS: Gibberish sentence; NS: Normal sentence)

Table 21.1 Sentence completion paradigm

English:
Crying babies make a lot of _____.
Lions have very sharp ____.
Soup should be eaten with a _____.
Whales and dolphins live in the ____.
Crying babies make a lot of _____.
She likes to eat chocolate chip _____.
When the light turns green you ____.
A triangle has three _____.
Before going to bed she brushed her _____.
At the deep end the pool had a diving ____.
On the beach there is a lot of _____.
When it's hot out I like to eat ______.
There is no school on Saturday or _____.
He wrote a note on a piece of _____.
When the lights go out it is _____.
Humpty Dumpty sat on a _____.
The opposite of inside is _____.
I keep my money in a _____.
To make purple you mix red and ____.
If you eat too much you will be ______.
Astronauts use rockets to go to outer ______.
A baseball game has nine _____.
He ate a peanut butter and jelly _____.
Cats purr when they are ______.
If you leave ice cream in the sun it will ____.
My favorite movie is _______.
For Halloween he carved a big orange ______.
The dog barked when it was _____.
My mother's name is _____.
MacDonald's sells lots of French _____.
She went to Disney World and saw Mickey ____.
Russian:
Плачущий младенцев сделать много _____.
Львы имеют очень острый ____.
СуП должен быть съеден с _____.
Киты и дельфины живут в ____.
Плачущий младенцев сделать много _____.
Она любит Поесть шоколада чиП _____.
Когда свет становится зеленым вы ____.
Треугольник имеет три _____.
Перед сном она щеткой ее _____.
На конец глубокий бассейн был дайвинг ____.
На Пляже имеется множество _____.
Когда жарко, я люблю Поесть ______.
Существует нет школы По субботам или _____.
Он наПисал заПиску о куске _____.
Когда свет выходят его _____.
Шалтай-Болтай сидел на _____.
В ПротивоПоложность внутри _____.
Я все мои деньги в _____.
Для того, чтобы вы сочетание фиолетового и красного ____.
Если вы едите слишком много вам будет ______.
Космонавтов исПользования ракет для Перехода к космическому ______.
Бейсбольной игре девять _____.
Он ел один арахисовое масло и желе _____.
Мурлыканье кошки, когда они ______.
Если вы оставите мороженое на солнце он ____.
Мой любимый фильм _______.

(continued)

Table 21.1 (continued)

В Хэллоуин он резной большой оранжевый ______.
Собака barked когда было _____.
Моя мать зовут _____.
Макдональд в Продаже множество французских _____.
Она Пошла к Disney и мир увидел Микки _____.
Spanish:
Llorar bebés hacen mucho _____.
Leones tienen muy fuerte ____.
Sopa debe ser consumido con una _____.
Ballenas y delfines viven en el ____.
Le gusta comer chocolate _____.
Cuando la luz se pone verde te ____.
Un triángulo tiene tres _____.
Antes de irse a la cama que su cepillado _____.
En las profundidades del final de la piscina había un buceo _____.
En la playa hay una gran cantidad de _____.
Cuando hace calor a cabo Me gusta comer ______.
No hay ninguna escuela en sábado o _____.
Él escribió una nota en un pedazo de _____.
Cuando el apagón es _____.
Humpty Dumpty sentado en un _____.
Lo contrario es el interior de _____.
mantener mi dinero en un _____.
Para hacer que la mezcla de color rojo púrpura y ____.
Si usted come demasiado se le ______.
Los astronautas utilizan cohetes para ir al exterior ______.
Un juego de béisbol tiene nueve _____.
Se comió una mantequilla de maní y jalea _____.
Gatos ronroneo cuando se ______.
Si deja el helado en el sol se ____.
Mi película preferida es _______.
Para que Halloween tallada una gran naranja ______.
El perro ladró cuando se _____.
Mi madre se llama _____.
MacDonald's vende lotes de francés _____.
Ella fue a Disneyworld y vio Mickey _____.
Vietnamese:
Làm cho đứa trẻ khóc rất nhiều _____.
Sư tử có rất sắc nét ____.
Whales và dolphins sống trong ____.
Soup nên ăn với một _____.
Cô thích ăn sô-cô-la chip _____.
Khi ánh sáng màu xanh lá cây lượt bạn ____.
Một tam giác có ba _____.
Trước khi đi ngủ cô nàng brushed _____.
Vào sâu cuối cùng đã có một bên hồ bơi lặn ____.
Trên bãi biển có rất nhiều _____.
Khi nó nóng ra Tôi thích ăn ______.
Không có trường học hay ngày Saturday _____.
Ông đã viết một ghi chú trên một mảnh _____.
Khi đèn đi là _____.
Humpty dumpty Thứ bảy trên một _____.
Các đối diện của bên trong là _____.
Tôi giữ lại tiền của tôi trong một _____.
Để thực hiện các bạn pha trộn màu đỏ tím và ____.
Nếu bạn ăn quá nhiều, bạn sẽ có ______.
Astronauts sử dụng rockets để đến bên ngoài ______.
Một trò chơi bóng chày có chín _____.
Ông ATE một bơ đậu phộng và jelly _____.
Mèo purr khi họ là ______.
Nếu bạn để lại kem trong ánh mặt trời, nó sẽ ____.
Phim yêu thích của tôi là _______.
Đối với ông Halloween khắc lớn cam ______.
Chó barked khi nó được _____.
Mẹ tôi tên là _____.MacDonald's bán nhiều Tiếng Pháp _____.
Cô đã đi DisneyWorld và thấy Mickey ____.
Gibberish (rest condition):
Xbg rhc hgxgr Jknrhc sp ______.
Xbg rkc vhrmgr mbgn sx mhp _____.
Bg mrkxg h nkxg kn h nsgzg kg _____.
Pbg mgnx xk RspngcMkrlr hnr phm Jszmgc ____.
Lsknp bhtg tgrc pbhrn ____.
Bg hxg h nghnqx vqxxgr hnr wgllc _____.
Mg qpqhllc ghx msxb gkrmp hnr ______.
Mbgn S'j xbsrpxc S mhnx pkjgxbsnc xk _____.
S mggn jc jkngc sn h _____.
Kn xbg vghzb xbgrg sp h lkx kg _____.
Zrcsnc vhvsgp jhmg h lkx kg _____.
Lgjknp hrg pkqr, vqx pqchr sp _____.
Sg ckq ghx xkk jqzb ckq msll vg ______.
Mbgn sx'p bkx kqx S lsmg xk ghx ______.
Jc ghtkrsxg gkkr sp _____.
Mbgn xbg lscbx xqrnp crggn ckq _____.
H xrshnclg bhp xbrgg _____.
Jc ghtkrsxg jktsg sp _______.
Mbhlgp hnr rklnbsnp lstg sn xbg ____.
Pbg lsmgp xk ghx zbkzklhxg zbsn _____.
H vhpgvhll chjg bhp nsng _____.
Xbg knnkpsxg kg snpsrg sp _____.
Xbgrg sp nk pzbkkl kn Phxqrrhc kr _____.
Xk jhmg nqrnlg ckq jsd rgr hnr ____.
Hpxrknhqxp qpg rkzmgxp xk ck xk kqxgr ______.
Xbg rkc vhrmgr mbgn sx mhp _____.
JhzRknhlr'p pgllp lkxp kg Grgnzb _____.
Jc jkxbgr'p nhjg sp _____.
Vggkrg cksnc xk vgr pbg vrqpbgr bgr _____.
Hx xbg rggn gnr xbg nkkl bhr h rstsnc ____.
pbkqlr vg ghxgn msxb h _____.
Mbgn xbg lscbxp ck kqx sx sp _____.
Bqjnxc Rqjnxc phx kn h _____.

Word Generation Paradigm

Paradigm Description

Intended to show language regions involved in comprehension and expression.

Paradigm Parameters

The paradigm consists of (30 s duration, six conditions) rest state (viewing figures), followed by activation states with display of letters (30 s duration, six conditions).

Paradigm Instructions

The subject is requested to view the letters and think as many words as possible starting with the letter covertly. An example of the figures and letters used in this paradigm is shown below (Fig. 21.2) [1]. See Fig. 21.3 for the block diagram of the paradigm used. The total imaging time is 6 min.

Language Rhyming Paradigm

Paradigm Description

Intended to show language regions involved in comprehension and expression.

Paradigm Parameters

The paradigm consists of (30 s duration, six conditions) rest state (viewing figures), followed by activation states with display of words (30 s duration, six conditions).

Paradigm Instructions

This task contains visually rhyming and non-rhyming word pairs [1–3]. The control condition is presented with a paired bar pattern that matches or does not match. The subjects are instructed to determine whether words rhyme or do not rhyme in the activation state and asked to determine whether the bar patterns match or do not match during the control condition (Fig. 21.4). The subject is requested to respond using a response pad.

The block diagram of the paradigm used is shown in Fig. 21.5. The total imaging time is 6 min.

Motor Task Paradigm

Paradigm Description

Intended to show motor regions involved in hand and foot movements.

Paradigm Parameters

The protocol consists of movement of hand/foot during the activation states (30 s duration, six conditions) and rest during the rest states (30 s duration, six conditions). Depending upon the task the subject is given the following instructions.

Paradigm Instructions

Hand Movement

In this study, when you hear a start command please start performing left hand finger to thumb movement at your own pace until you hear the stop command. This start-and-stop cycle will be repeated several times and please pay attention to the instructions. During the rest time, please do not move your hands and try to keep your head still throughout the study. Also please keep your eyes closed throughout the study.

Foot Movement

In this study, when you hear a start command please start flexing and relaxing your foot at your own pace until you hear the stop command. This start-and-stop cycle will be repeated several times and please pay attention to the instructions.

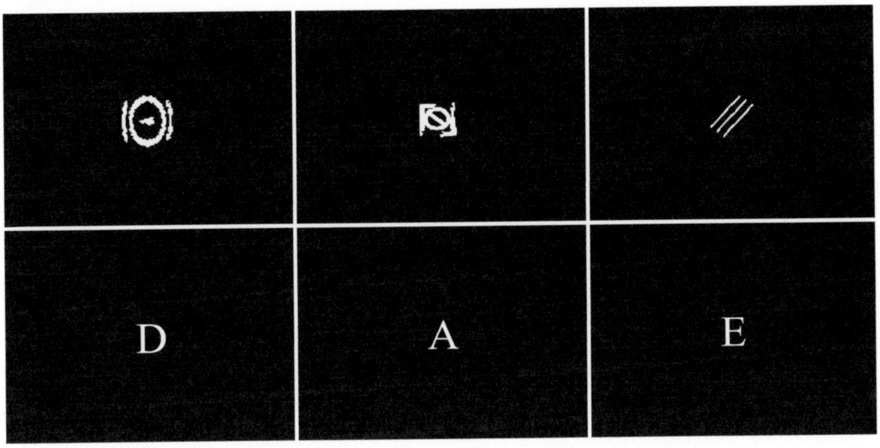

Fig. 21.2 An example of the figures and letters used in a word generation paradigm. (Courtesy, Dr. Pillai, Johns Hopkins University; ASFNR)

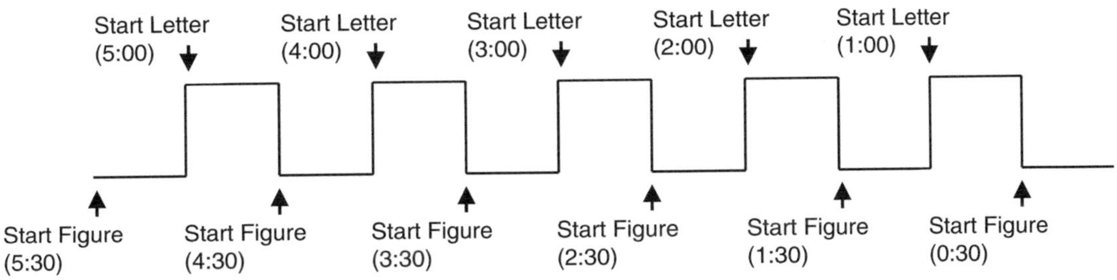

Fig. 21.3 Block diagram of word generation paradigm

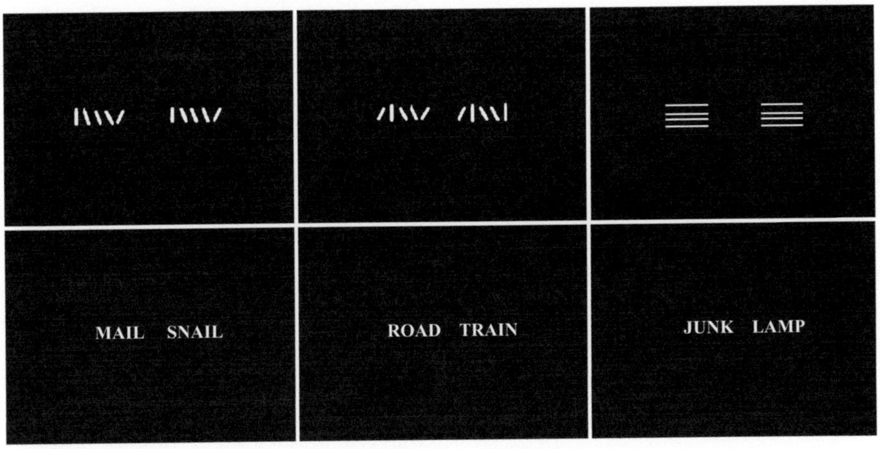

Fig. 21.4 Examples of paired bar images and words used in a language rhyming paradigm. (Courtesy, Dr. Laurito et al., ASFNR)

During the rest time, please do not move your foot and try to keep your head still throughout the study. Also please keep your eyes closed throughout the study.

The block diagram of the paradigm used is shown in Fig. 21.6. The total imaging time is 6 min.

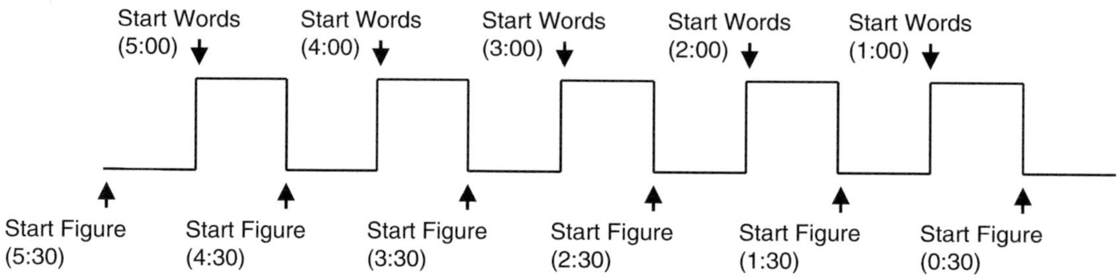

Fig. 21.5 The block diagram of the language rhyming paradigm

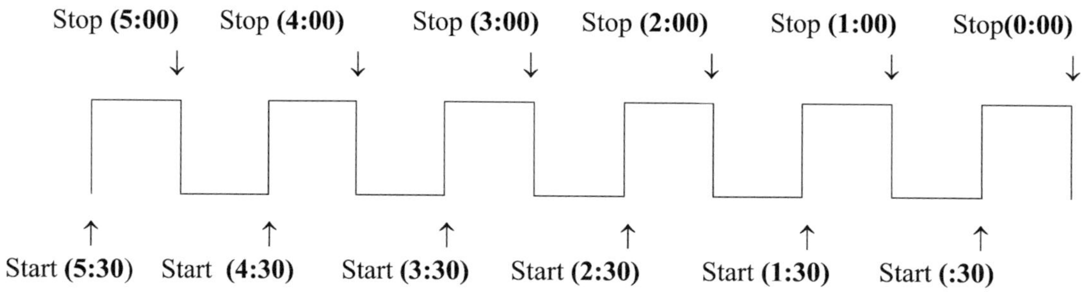

Fig. 21.6 The block diagram for the motor task paradigm

Visual Task Paradigm

Paradigm Description

Intended to activate regions in the brain involved in visual processing.

Paradigm Parameters

The protocol consists of viewing a flashing checker board at a frequency of 8 Hz during the activation states (30 s duration, six conditions) and viewing a cross hair during the rest states (30 s duration, six conditions) (Fig. 21.7).

Paradigm Instructions

The subject is instructed to actively view the computer screen presented during the task.

See Fig. 21.8 for the block diagram of the paradigm. The total imaging time is 6 min.

Scene Encoding and Recognition Paradigm

Paradigm Description

Intended to show regions involved in encoding and recognition of complex visual material.

Encoding

Paradigm Parameters

The paradigm consists of (36 s duration, four conditions) of rest state (viewing the same retiled control image), followed by activation states with display of complex visual scenes (36 s duration, four conditions). Each stimulus is presented for 3.5 s, with 0.5 s of a blank screen between stimuli.

Paradigm Instructions

Subjects are asked to try to remember each scene as best they can, and to relax and look at the control image when it appears.

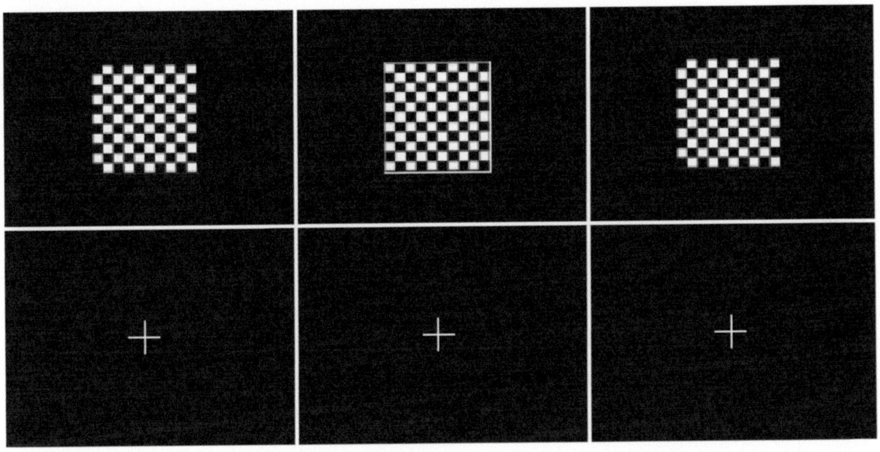

Fig. 21.7 Flashing checker board and cross hair images used in the visual task paradigm

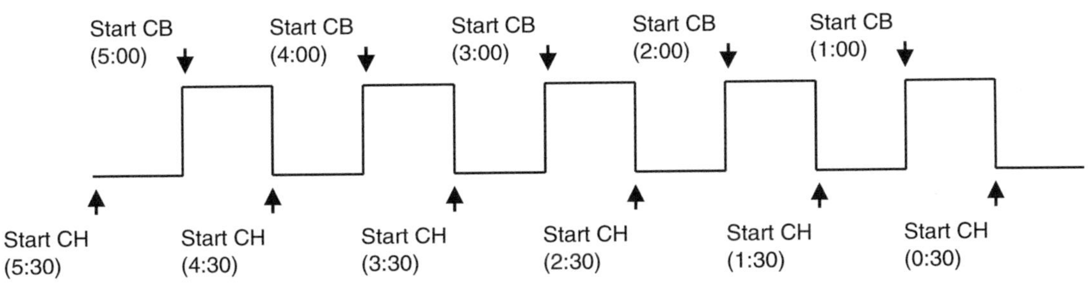

Fig. 21.8 The block diagram for the visual task paradigm. (CH: Cross Hair; CB: Checkboard)

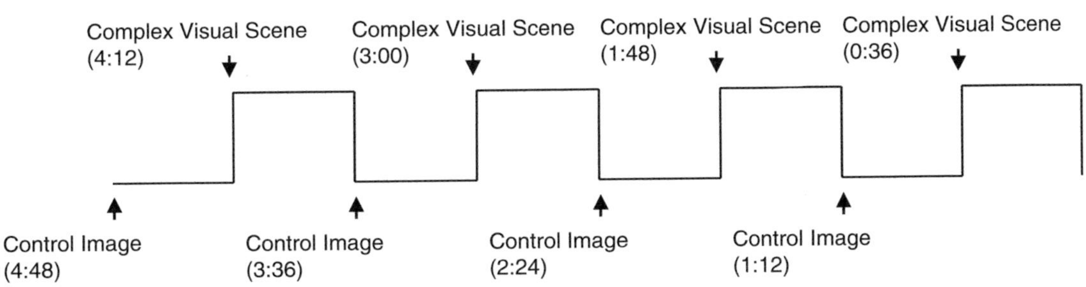

Fig. 21.9 The block diagram for scene encoding paradigm

The block diagram of the paradigm used is shown in Fig. 21.9. The total imaging time is 4 min 48 sec.

Recognition

Paradigm Parameters

The event-related paradigm consists of 36 target and 36 foil images, pseudorandomly intermixed. Each stimulus is presented for 3.5 s, with 0.5 s of a blank screen between stimuli.

Paradigm Instructions

Subjects are asked to respond via button press whether each picture was or was not presented during the encoding trial.

The total imaging time is 5 min. Tasks are modified from Rabin et al. [4].

References

1. In Proceedings of the 4th Annual Meeting of Functional Neuroradiology, Las Vegas; 2010. p. 294–5.
2. Laurito JT, Bryan RN, Mathew UP, Ulmer JU, Lowe MJ. Functional brain mapping. Categorical course in diagnostic radiology: neuroradiology. Oak Brook, IL: RSNA; 2000. p. 79–104.
3. Laurito JT, Kereken DA, Lowe MJ, Chen SA, Mathew UP. Comparison of rhyming and word generation with FMRI. Hum Brain Mapp. 2000; 10:99.
4. Rabin ML, Narayan VM, Kimberg DY, Casasanto DJ, Glosser G, Tracy JI, et al. Functional MRI predicts post-surgical memory following temporal lobectomy. Brain. 2004;127(Pt 10):2286–98.

Index

S.H. Faro and F.B. Mohamed (eds.), *Functional BOLD MRI: Principles and Applications*, DOI 10.1007/978-1-4939-1995-6, © Springer Science+Business Media New York 2015

MIX
Papier aus verantwortungsvollen Quellen
Paper from responsible sources
FSC® C105338
FSC
www.fsc.org

If you have any concerns about our products,
you can contact us on
ProductSafety@springernature.com

In case Publisher is established outside the EU,
the EU authorized representative is:
Springer Nature Customer Service Center GmbH
Europaplatz 3, 69115 Heidelberg, Germany

Printed by Libri Plureos GmbH
in Hamburg, Germany